Surgery of the Liver

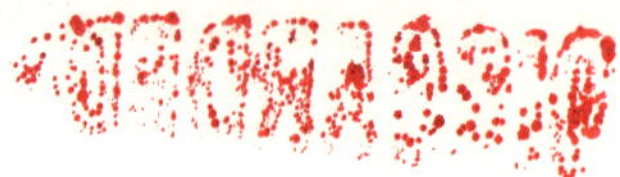

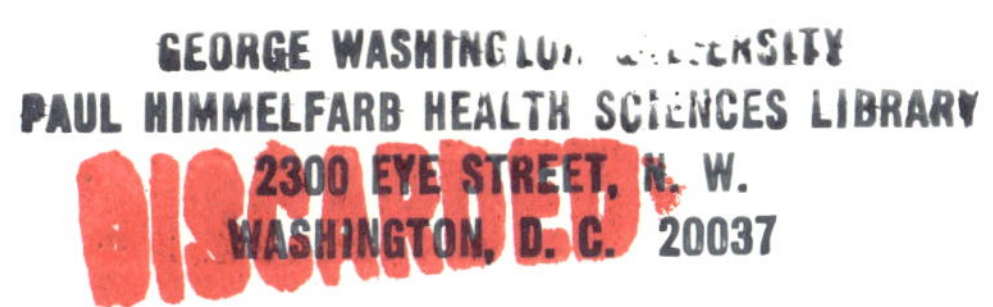

Surgery of the Liver

EDITED BY

WILLIAM V. McDERMOTT, JR., A.B., M.D., F.A.C.S.

*David W. and David Professor of Surgery Emeritus Harvard Medical School;
Chairman (Retired), Department of Surgery New England Deaconess Hospital,
Boston, Massachusetts*

Blackwell Scientific Publications

BOSTON OXFORD LONDON EDINBURGH MELBOURNE

Blackwell Scientific Publications
Editorial Offices:
Three Cambridge Center, Suite 208, Cambridge,
Massachusetts 02142, USA
Osney Mead, Oxford OX2 0EL, England
8 John Street, London, WC1N 2 ES, England
23 Ainslie Place, Edinburgh, EH3 6AJ, Scotland
107 Barry Street, Carlton, Victoria 3053, Australia

Distributors:
USA and Canada
Year Book Medical Publishers
200 North LaSalle Street
Chicago, Illinois 60601
(Orders: Telephone: 1 800 621-9262)

Australia
Blackwell Scientific Publications
(Australia) Pty Ltd
107 Barry Street
Carlton, Victoria 3053
(Orders: Telephone: 03 347-0300)

Outside North America and Australia
Blackwell Scientific Publications, Ltd.
Osney Mead
Oxford OX2 0EL
England
(Orders: Telephone: 011 44 865 240201)

Typeset by The William Byrd Press
Printed and bound by Hamilton Printing Company

Blackwell Scientific Publications, Inc.
©1989 by Blackwell Scientific Publications, Inc.
Printed in the United States of America
89 90 91 92 5 4 3 2 1

Library of Congress Cataloging-in-Publication Data

Surgery of the liver / [edited by] William V.
McDermott, p. cm.
Includes bibliographies and index.
ISBN 0-86542-039-4 : $125.00
1. Liver—Surgery. I. McDermott, William V.,
1917–
[DNLM: 1. Liver—surgery. WI 770 S9615]
RD546.S948 1988
617'.556—dc19
DNLM/DLC
for Library of Congress   88-30018
                                                 CIP

To Blanche and to Mary
and to my children —
Gwen, Shaw and Jane

Contents

Contributors

HARRY ANASTOPOULOUS, M.D. *Fellow, Gastroenterology, New England Deaconess Hospital, Boston, Massachusetts*

SANJEEV ARORA, M.D. *Staff Physician, New England Medical Center, Gastroenterology Division, Assistant Professor of Medicine, Tufts University, Boston, Massachusetts*

STACEY J. BELL, M.S., R.D. *Research Nutritionist for Nutritional Support Service, New England Deaconess Hospital, Boston, Massachusetts*

GEORGE L. BLACKBURN, M.D., Ph.D. *Associate Professor of Surgery, Harvard Medical School, Chief of Nutrition/ Metabolism Laboratory, New England Deaconess Hospital, Boston, Massachusetts*

BLAKE CADY, M.D. *Associate Professor of Surgery, Harvard Medical School, Chief of Surgical Oncology, New England Deaconess Hospital, Boston, Massachusetts*

ROY YORKE CALNE, F.R.S. *Professor and Chairman, Department of Surgery, University of Cambridge, Addenbrooke's Hospital, Cambridge, United Kingdom*

GEORGE H.S. CLOWES, Jr., M.D., F.A.C.S. *Professor of Surgery Emeritus, Harvard Medical School, Department of Surgery, New England Deaconess Hospital, Boston, Massachusetts*

ARTHUR J. DONOVAN, M.D. *Professor and Chairman, Department of Surgery, University of Southern California, School of Medicine, Director of Surgery, Los Angeles County– University of Southern California Medical Center*

WALTER H. DZIK, M.D. *Department of Medicine, Harvard Medical School, Director, Blood Bank and Tissue Typing Laboratory, New England Deaconess Hospital, Boston, Massachusetts*

Z. MYRON FALCHUCK, M.D. *Associate Professor of Medicine, Harvard Medical School, New England Deaconess Hospital, Boston, Massachusetts*

JOSEF E. FISCHER, M.D. *Christian R. Holmes Professor and Chairman, Department of Surgery, University of Cincinnati Medical Center, Cincinnati, Ohio*

BENJAMIN GERSON, M.D. *Veterans Administration Hospital, Boston, Massachusetts*

JAMES S. GESSNER, M.D. *Clinical Instructor in Anesthesia, Harvard Medical School, Staff Anesthesiologist, New England Deaconess Hospital, Staff Anesthesiologist, The Faulkner Hospital, Boston, Massachusetts*

NORMAN D. GRACE, M.D. *Associate Professor of Medicine, Tufts University Medical School, Chief Gastroenterology, Faulkner & LeMuel Shattuck Hospitals, Boston, Massachusetts*

W. HARDY HENDREN, M.D. *Robert E. Gross Professor of Surgery, Harvard Medical School, Chief of Surgery, The Children's Hospital, Visiting Surgeon, Massachusetts General Hospital, Boston, Massachusetts*

KURT J. ISSELBACHER, M.D. *Mallinckrodt Professor of Medicine, Harvard Medical School, Director, Cancer Center and Chief, Gastrointestinal Unit, Massachusetts General Hospital, Boston, Massachusetts*

ROGER L. JENKINS, M.D. *Division of Liver Transplantation, Department of Surgery, New England Deaconess Hospital, Harvard Medical School, Boston, Massachusetts*

ROBERT KANE, M.D. *Associate Professor of Radiology, Harvard Medical School, Director of Ultrasound, New England Deaconess Hospital, Boston, Massachusetts*

MARSHALL M. KAPLAN, M.D. *Chief, Gastroenterology Division, New England Medical Center Hospitals, Professor of Medicine, Tufts University School of Medicine, New England Medical Center Hospitals, Boston, Massachusetts*

ADOLF W. KARCHMER, M.D. *Associate Professor of Medicine, Harvard Medical School, Chief, Infectious Disease Section, New England Deaconess Hospital, Boston, Massachusetts*

URMILA KHETTRY, M.D. *Clinical Instructor in Pathology, Harvard Medical School, Pathologists, New England Deaconess Hospital, Boston, Massachusetts*

ISTRATI A. KUPELI, M.D. *Clinical Instructor in Anesthesiology, Harvard Medical School, Anesthesiologist, New England Deaconess Hospital, Boston, Massachusetts*

RONALD A. MALT, M.D. *Professor of Surgery, Harvard Medical School, Massachusetts General Hospital, Boston, Massachusetts*

WILLIAM V. McDERMOTT, Jr., A.B., M.D., F.A.C.S. *David W. and David Professor of Surgery Emeritus, Harvard Medical School, Chairman (Retired) Department of Surgery, New England Deaconess Hospital, Boston, Massachusetts*

DOMINIC NOMPLEGGI, M.D., Ph.D. *Hyperalimentation Fellow, New England Deaconess Hospital, Boston, Massachusetts*

MARSHALL J. ORLOFF, M.D. *Professor of Surgery, School of Medicine, University of California, San Diego, California*

ELLISON C. PIERCE, Jr., M.D.   *Assistant Professor of Anesthesia, Harvard Medical School, Chairman–Department of Anesthesia, New England Deaconess Hospital, The Faulkner Hospital, Boston, Massachusetts*

C. WRIGHT PINSON, M.D.   *Harvard Medical School, Division of Liver Transplantation, Department of Surgery, New England Deaconess Hospital, Boston, Massachusetts*

DANIEL K. PODOLSKY, M.D.   *Associate Professor of Medicine, Harvard Medical School, Gastrointestinal Unit, Massachusetts General Hospital, Boston, Massachusetts*

LOUIS B. RICE, M.D.   *Research Fellow, Harvard Medical School, Infectious Disease Research Fellow, New England Deaconess Hospital, Boston, Massachusetts*

RICARDO L. ROSSI, M.D.   *Assistant Professor of Surgery, Harvard Medical School, Chairman–Department of Surgery, Lahey Clinic, Boston, Massachusetts*

SEYMOUR I. SCHWARTZ, M.D., F.A.C.S.   *Professor and Chairman, Department of Surgery, University of Rochester, School of Medicine and Dentistry, Rochester, New York*

L.K.R. SHABHOGUE, M.B.B.S., F.R.C.S.   *Surgical Registrar, Department of Paediatric Surgery, Royal Manchester Children's Hospital, Pendlebury, Near Manchester M27 1HA, United Kingdom*

SHEILA SHERLOCK, D.B.E., M.D.   *Professor of Medicine, University of London at the Royal Free Hospital, School of Medicine, Hampstead, London, NW3 2QG, United Kingdom*

THOMAS E. STARZL, M.D., Ph.D.   *Professor of Surgery, Director of Organ Transplantation Services, University of Pittsburgh, Pittsburgh, Pennsylvania*

GLENN STEELE, Jr., M.D.   *Chairman, Department of Surgery, New England Deaconess Hospital, William V. McDermott Professor of Surgery, Harvard Medical School, Boston, Massachusetts*

MICHAEL D. STONE, M.D.   *Harvard Medical School, Division of Liver Transplantation, Department of Surgery, New England Deaconess Hospital, Boston, Massachusetts*

PROFESSOR JOHN TERBLANCHE, Ch.M., F.C.S.(S.A.), F.R.C.S.(Eng), F.R.S.P.S.(Glasg), F.A.C.S. (HON)   *Professor and Chairman, Department of Surgery, University of Cape Town and Groote Schuur Hospital Cape Town, Co-Director Medical Research Council Liver Research Center, University of Cape Town, Cape Town, South Africa*

JAMES L. TULLIS, M.D.   *Professor of Medicine Emeritus, Harvard Medical School, New England Deaconess Hospital, Boston, Massachusetts*

W. DEAN WARREN, M.D.   *Department of Surgery, Emory University School of Medicine, Atlanta, Georgia*

ALEXANDER J. WALT, M.B., Ch.B., M.S.(Minn), F.R.C.S., F.A.C.S.   *Professor of Surgery, Wayne State University, Detroit, Michigan*

CLAYTON L. WOOD, M.D.   *Clinical Instructor in Medicine, Harvard University, Department of Gastroenterology, Lahey Clinic, Boston, Massachusetts*

JOSEPH P. VACANTI, M.D.   *Assistant Professor of Surgery, Harvard Medical School, Assistant in Surgery and Director of Liver Transplantation, The Children's Hospital, Boston, Massachusetts*

Preface

Before attempting to construct a preface for this text on "Surgery of the Liver," I reviewed the preface for a book that I had undertaken to write in 1974 on "Surgery of the Liver and Portal Hypertension."

That particular book was one of single authorship, and in the preface I made a number of comments comparing the inadequacies of single authorship and the problems of books with multiple authors. I think the differences are obvious. In one, the reader has the advantage of a single, consistent viewpoint on the intricacies of surgical disorders of the liver and its circulation, but the disadvantages were also emphasized.

In persuading a number of leading authorities on the liver to write sections in this particular text, one has the advantage of a high degree of special knowledge in each subdivision of the text and one also has the opportunity to encounter the spirited environment of controversy that always exists in medicine and science and is certainly a source of stimulation to the reader.

A majority of the authors will certainly be familiar to readers, and the book provides an opportunity to savor tremendous knowledge brought to bear on a relatively small area of scientific study. The reader can enjoy the areas where sparkling controversy exist and focus attention on the future as well as the past

I have taken the liberty of writing some chapters myself and of introducing editorial comments in a number of sections that were of considerable interest to me. I would like to thank in particular Mrs. Joan Long, Mrs. Jayne McGuire Kennedy, Mrs. Marguerite Norton-Perisie and Mrs. Suzanne Jackson for their continued help with the typescript, with the endless details concerned with the final text, and with the various suggestions and criticisms that have been extremely helpful throughout. Colleagues on the medical and surgical staff of the New England Deaconess Hospital and on the faculty of the Harvard Medical School have been generous with their time in discussing various aspects of the text as well as providing individual contributions to this effort of multiple authorship.

I am grateful to the authors who provided the superb manuscripts that together make up the total text and whose lifetime of work in the area of the liver has been the real reason for the excellence of the presentations.

It is hoped that the readers will enjoy the full compilation as much as I have enjoyed absorbing the various segments as they arrived over the past two years.

William V. McDermott Jr., M.D.
Boston, Massachusetts

NOTICE

The indications and dosages of all drugs in this book have been recommended in the medical literature and conform to the practices of the general medical community. The medications described do not necessarily have specific approval by the Food and Drug Administration for use in the diseases and dosages for which they are recommended. The package insert for each drug should be consulted for use and dosage as approved by the FDA. Because standards for usage change, it is advisable to keep abreast of revised recommendations, particularly those concerning new drugs.

PART I
Historical Aspects of Liver Surgery

Chapter 1
Historical Background

SEYMOUR I. SCHWARTZ

Throughout history the liver has been regarded as a central organ, and the oldest extant representations of the liver, which are models of the sheep liver from the Assyro-Babylonian era (3000–2000 B.C.) (Fig. 1.1), present evidence that the organ was one destined to be divided. At that time, the models were used by the portenders of the future in the art of divination and prognostication. "Reading" the liver of sacrificial animals for prophetic signs, known as hepatoscopy, reached its pinnacle among the Babylonians and was also a part of haruspicy, which was "reading" the entrails of animals. The liver was regarded as the seat of the soul, and, as such, was considered a reflection of the divine being. The very origin of the word "liver" is identical to the origin of the word "life."

A history of surgery of the liver includes consideration of the management of hepatic abscesses, the treatment of hepatic trauma, hepatic resection, transplantation, biliary reconstruction, and operative procedures directed at ameliorating the manifestations of portal hypertension.

Hepatic Abscesses

The earliest surgical interventions related to the liver centered on the management of hepatic abscesses. Evacuation of a hepatic abscess with a knife or with cautery was recommended by Hippocrates about the fifth century B.C., and later by Celsus in the first century A.D. Hippocrates wrote: "When abscess of the liver is treated by cautery or incision, if the pus which is discharged be pure and white, the patients recover . . . but if it resembles the lees of oil as it flows, they die" (1). Hippocrates and the early Greeks practiced open drainage of amoebic abscesses of the liver.

In 1828, Annesly advised opening only those liver abscesses that pointed posteriorly and therefore had formed adhesions (2). Of the two types of drainage procedures currently used, the transpleural approach was actually suggested first. This approach was advocated for subphrenic abscess by Trendelenberg in 1883 (3). The more frequently used anterior drainage technique of Clairmont and Meyer was also first proposed as an extraserous approach for subphrenic abscess (4).

Hepatic Trauma

Ambrose Pare wrote that, "When the liver is wounded, much blood cometh out the wound, and pricking pain disperth it selfe even unto sword-like gristle, which hath its situation at the Lower end of the brest bone called Sternon; the blood that falleth from thence down into the intestine does often times interfere with most maligne accidents, yea and sometimes death" (5). Although sporadic cases of spontaneous recovery from serious hepatic injuries had been recorded in early medical literature, the wounds of the liver were not considered amenable to surgical therapy until the latter half of the nineteenth century. The turning point occurred in 1870 when von Bruns successfully resected the lacerated portion of a liver that had been traumatized by a gunshot wound (6).

In 1879, Tillmann demonstrated experimentally that hepatic wounds were significant only when larger vessels were involved (7). In 1887, Burckhardt reported control of a hemorrhaging liver injury (8), and in the following year, Willett performed the first successful laparotomy for traumatic rupture of the liver (9).

The major problem in the management of liver trauma both in the past and currently has been control of hemorrhage. In 1896, Kousnetzoff and

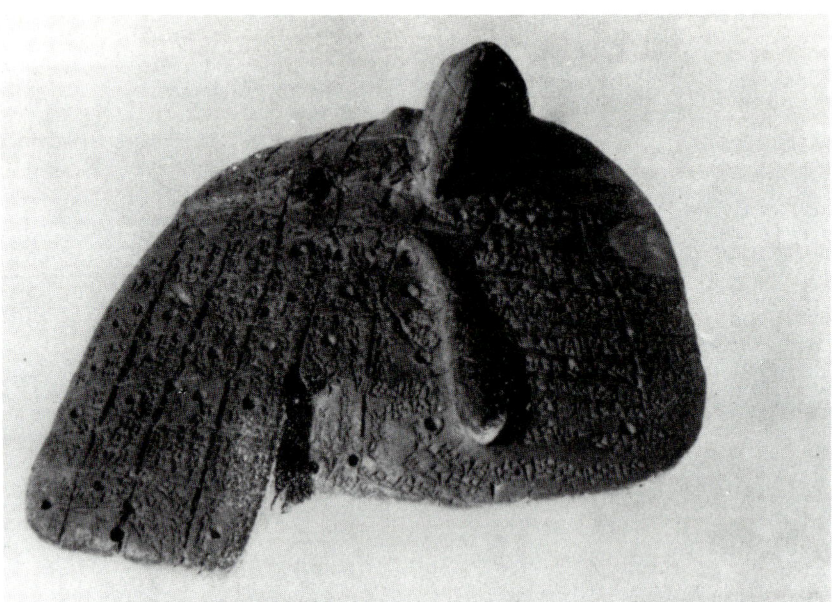

Figure 1.1 Sheep's liver from the Assyro-Babylonian era (around 2000 B.C.). (Reproduced by permission from Schwartz SI. *Surgical Diseases of the Liver*. New York: McGraw-Hill, 1964, p. viii.)

Pensky published the results of their experiments in the *St. Petersburg Surgical Review* (10). They performed experiments on dogs and rabbits and concluded that in order to secure hemorrhage, the ligature of the liver should be tied very snugly, the stump of the liver should be left in the peritoneal cavity, and it should not be experitonealized, because blunt needles prevent pricking of the wall of intrahepatic blood vessels, only blunt needles should be used, and the application of ligatures to isolated blood vessels is possible. This was a particularly significant statement because it had been felt that a blood vessel of the liver was more friable than that of any other organ. A year later, the Parisian surgeon Auvray of the Terrier Clinic described a series of mattress sutures that resembled the Kousnetzoff and Pensky suture, and first applied this technique to humans (11). Just one decade later, in the United States, Hough (12) described a new method of suturing the liver that was, in essence, a series of mattress sutures with a crossover to permit closure of Glisson's capsule.

Chronologically, the next approach to managing bleeding from the hepatic parenchyma was that of temporary inflow occlusion, which still bears the eponym, Pringle maneuver. In 1908, the Glaswegian surgeon J. Hogarth Pringle published an article in the *Annals of Surgery* on the arrest of hepatic hemorrhage due to trauma (13). It is surprising that this article should have had the impact that it did, since the author reported eight patients with hepatic trauma, only four of whom had been operated upon, while two had died on the operating table, and two died shortly thereafter. As a consequence of that experience, he experimented on rabbits and showed that inflow occlusion could be effective. He applied this technique to two patients using finger occlusion of the porta hepatis; one patient died on the table and the other died on the fourth postoperative day.

The technique of inflow occlusion was extended in 1966 by Heaney et al. (14), who recommended cross-clamping the aorta below the diaphragm and occluding the inferior vena cava above and below the liver. A more recent modification was that of Schrock et al. (15) in 1968, which achieved vascular isolation of the liver to arrest hemorrhage from the avulsed hepatic veins by inserting a large catheter into the inferior vena cava through the right atrial appendage and securing tapes about the cava within the pericardium and at the suprarenal level.

Hepatic Resection

The history of hepatic resection falls chronologically into four periods. The first period witnessed removal of portions of the liver without regard for intrahepatic planes. In the second period, hepatic resection was based on an appreciation of interlobar and major segmental planes. During the third period, technical refinements were incorporated, and the fourth period saw the introduction of segmental resection based on newer concepts of anatomy.

The first surgical removal of a portion of the human liver was recorded in 1716 by Berta (16); on the day following injury, he amputated the protruding portion of the liver from a patient with a self-inflicted knife wound to the right upper quadrant. The liver was regarded as a "noli me tangere" (do not touch me) organ, until 1870 when von Bruns resected a lacerated portion of the liver from a surgeon wounded during the Franco-Prussian War. In 1886, Luis (17) reported for the first time the removal of a solid tumor (an adenoma) from the liver; the patient died. The first successful elective hepatic resection is credited to Langenbuch (18), who excised a portion of the left lobe of the liver in 1888. He ascribed the "tumor" to the constriction caused by corsets. The abdomen was reopened for internal hemorrhage a few hours after the operation; vessels were ligated and the stump returned. The patient survived. Tiffany (19), in 1890, was the first American surgeon to report a case of hepatic resection for tumor. In 1891, Lücke (20) reported the first successful removal of a cancer from the left lobe of the liver. In 1892, W. W. Keen (21) reported the excision of a cystic adenoma of the bile ducts, using a technique of ligature through the base of the tumor, a paquelin cautery, and stripping the liver from the tumor with his thumbnail, thus preceding the so-called "finger fracture technique." His article included a collective review of 20 cases recorded from the literature, the first such review on the subject. In 1899, the same author (22) performed the first successful left hepatic lobectomy for cancer of the liver; this was actually a left lateral segmentectomy. In this procedure, five vessels were tied individually with catgut and cautery was applied. Wendel (23), in 1911, reported the first case of near-total right lobectomy. The operation was performed for a primary tumor and the patient survived 9 years.

In 1940, Cattell (24) reported the successful removal of a liver metastasis from a primary lesion in the colon and rectum. Wangensteen in 1943 (25) reported coincidental partial hepatectomy for gastric carcinoma involving the liver by direct extension. The parenchyma was cauterized and vessels were tied as they were encountered. Four patients underwent left lateral segmentectomy and two were alive 1 year after the operation.

The second period, in which hepatic resection was based on an appreciation of interlobar and major segmental planes, grew out of the demonstration of the refinement of anatomy of the liver.

The old concept that the liver is divided into right and left lobes by the falciform ligaments was disproved in 1898 by Cantlie (26), who used casts of the liver to determine that the main lobar fissure is oblique, and extends from right to left and from the visceral to the parietal surface at about a 70 degree angle. Thus, the main division between the right and left lobe extends from approximately the bed of the gallbladder anteroinferiorly to the right side of the inferior vena cava posterosuperiorly. This work was further extended by Hjorstjö (27) and by Healey and Schroy (28), who also demonstrated by using casts that the right lobe was further divided into an anterior and posterior segment, and the left lobe was divided into a medial and lateral segment by the line of the falciform ligament. These anatomic divisions were based on the topography of the intrahepatic biliary duct system. An appreciation of this refined anatomy led to the development of surgical planes of the liver, and to recommended planes for performing a right lobectomy (right hepatectomy), a left lobectomy (left hepatectomy), and a left lateral segmental resection (29).

In 1948, Raven (30) reported a left lateral segmentectomy for metastatic colon carcinoma in which the triangular and coronary ligaments were transected and the left portal vein, left hepatic artery, and left hepatic duct were ligated within the hepatoduodenal ligament. The left hepatic vein was then isolated extrahepatically and divided, following which the parenchyma was transected. This patient survived. In 1952, Lortat-Jacob and Robert (31) advanced the procedure by performing a right hepatic lobectomy, using a technique designed to control hemorrhage with ligation of the blood vessels and bile ducts to the right lobe in the hepatoduodenal ligament followed by extrahepatic ligation of the right hepatic vein prior to transection of the hepatic parenchyma. In 1953, Quattlebaum (32) reported three cases of massive hepatic resection, one of which represents the first recorded right hepatic lobectomy for primary carcinoma. In that procedure, performed in February 1952, the three structures in the hepatoduodenal

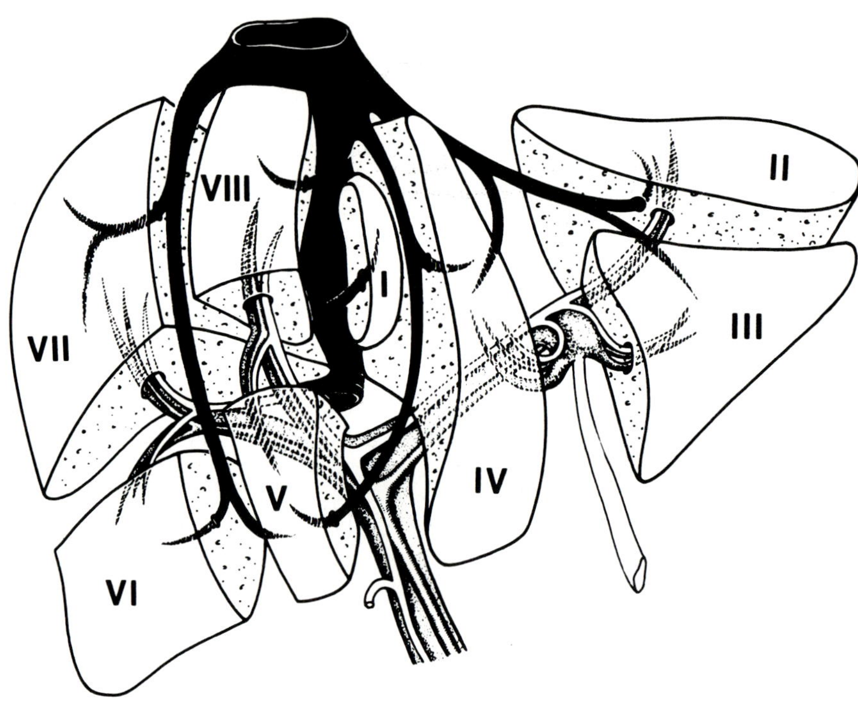

Figure 1.2 The functional division of the liver and the segments according to Couinaud's nomenclature. (Reproduced by permission from Bismuth H. Surgical anatomy and anatomical surgery of the liver. *World J Surg* 1982;6:3–9.)

ligament were ligated first and the parenchyma was transected with the handle of the scalpel. Also in 1953, Mersheimer (33) published a similar experience and Pack and Baker (34) described resection of the right lobe of the liver for a primary granulomatous process. In 1955, Pack et al. (35) reported the first hepatic lobectomy for cancer of the gallbladder.

The third period witnessed the incorporation of technical refinements of liver resection and the facilitation of the procedure by the application of finger fracture of the hepatic parenchyma. As Couinaud has insisted: "finger fracture (digitoclasia) should be a gentle technique and must be respectful of anatomy: it should be carried exactly along the fissures and lead toward well determined pedicles. It affords a quick opening of the fissures and the control of the secondary vessels which usually bleed in the plane of section" (36). In 1903, Anshutz (37) first pointed out that the liver tissue broke easily under the finger; the only structures that resisted were the portal pedicles and the hepatic veins. In 1953, Quattlebaum (32) reported deliberately breaking the liver tissue with the handle of the knife, and indicated that this permitted exposure of the vessels as they traversed the plane of transection. In 1956, Fineburg et al. (38) reported cutting the capsule of the liver by

sharp dissection and then dividing the parenchyma by means of a finger or by the back of the scalpel during a right hepatic lobectomy for primary carcinoma. At that time, a careful search of the surgical literature revealed 20 recorded cases of right hepatic lobectomy of which only 3 were for primary carcinoma of the liver. In 1958, Tien-Yu Lin et al. (39) reported "fracturing and crushing the tissue between the fingers" and indicated that when resistant ducts or vessels were encountered, they were tied or divided. This technique was then modified in 1963, by Ton That Tung (40), who occluded the portal pedicle and then transected the liver by digital laceration.

The most recent advance in hepatic resection is the consequence of an appreciation of functional anatomy based on the distribution of the portal pedicles and the location of the hepatic veins. This anatomic concept evolved from Couinaud's study of vasculobiliary casts made by plastic injection followed by corrosion of the surrounding parenchyma (41). The two lobes (hemilivers) actually consist of eight segments (Fig. 1.2). Theoretically each of the eight segments could be resected separately, and the amount of functional hepatic impairment minimized.

Segmentectomy I usually requires a preliminary left lobectomy because of its location; this was first described by Ton That Tung (42). Usually only the anterior aspect of segment IV is removed. This procedure was first performed by Caprio (43). Segmentectomy VI is performed only when total right lobectomy would precipitate hepatic failure. This was first described by Bismuth et al. (44). Segmentectomy VIII was first reported by Ton That Tung (42), who advocated this resection for chronic liver abscess in this region. Bisegmentectomy VI and VII has been reported by Ton That Tung (42) and Bismuth (44). Bisegmentectomy IV and V, which has been used for carcinoma of the gallbladder, was also reported by Bismuth et al. (44). Bisegmentectomy V and VI was proposed by Mancuso (45) and is rarely performed. Two cases have been reported by Bismuth et al. (44). Trisegmentectomy IV, VI, and VI, also known as medial hepatectomy, was proposed by Couinaud for carcinoma of the gallbladder (41).

Transplantation

The liver was the second visceral organ to be allotransplanted in humans. It was the first of the unpaired organs to be transplanted, and therefore the first dependent on a cadaver donor. Welch (46) is credited with initiating liver transplantation in the experimental animal in 1955. Moore and associates (47) and Starzl et al. (48) extended the field experimentally. On March 1, 1963, Starzl performed the first human liver transplant in a patient with biliary atresia. This patient died, as did four other patients operated on by Starzl, and one who was operated on by Moore et al. that year. After an interval of 4 years, Starzl's efforts were reinstituted, and in 1968 he performed the first hepatic transplant resulting in a long-term survival in a patient who had biliary atresia (49). Three of 12 patients operated on that year lived over a year. No other surgeon had achieved long-term survival up to that point. The first auxiliary liver transplantation was performed by Absolon et al. (50) in 1964. The patient died 2 weeks after the operation, and no success had been reported prior to 1970 (49).

Biliary Atresia

Although it is felt that the entity was described by Aristotle, the first collective review of the subject did not appear until 1891 (51). In 1916, Holmes suggested that operative relief was possible and advised an aggressive approach (52). He credited Giese and Witzel with the first operation, performed in 1896, and Treves with the first success in 1899; this was a cholecystoenterostomy using a Murphy button. In 1928, Ladd (53) reported that six of eight patients amenable to proximal decompression recovered; most of these patients had localized atresia of the common duct. In 1958, Schnug (54) reviewed the cases reported since 1951 and noted the dismal picture of a 22% incidence of correctibility and that only one-third of these potentially curable cases remained cured at the time of followup 1 year later. Kasai and Suzuki introduced hepatic portoenterostomy in 1959; this procedure revolutionized the field (55). Orthotopic liver transplantation has been applied with increasing success; the longest survival following hepatic transplantation is a patient with biliary atresia who received an orthotopic transplantation in 1968 (49).

Portal Hypertension

The surgery of portal hypertension has undergone an interesting evolution. Beginning with a focus on the treatment of ascites and the suggestion of the applicability of a total shunt to decompress the portal circulation, it has come to a point that the manifestation of concern is bleeding esophagogastric varices and the newer operative procedures are directed at partially shunting portal flow with an emphasis on maintaining hepatic perfusion.

In 1887, Nicolai Eck published his seminal work in a Russian military medical journal (56) He wrote

I am conducting these experiments with the purpose of clarifying some physiological problems as well as to determine whether it would be possible to treat some cases of mechanical ascites by means of forming such a fistula.

I consider the main reason to doubt that such an operation can be carried out on human beings has been removed because it was established that the blood of the portal vein, without any danger to the body, could be diverted directly into the general circulation and this by means of a perfectly safe operation.

In reviewing this experimental work that led to a new clinical application, it is revealing to note that only one of the eight animals survived longer than a week, and that the "unaffected" dog "which lived two and one-half months after the operation ran away so that it was impossible to determine the success of the operation by postmortem examination'' (57). That statement comes from the work of Pavlov and associates, published in 1893, who created an Eck's fistula in animals and recorded for the first time the syndrome of meat intoxication.

A year later, Banti (58) suggested splenectomy for the splenomegaly and anemia associated with cirrhosis. He maintained that the hepatosplenopathy caused by a toxic agent that first produced the splenic enlargement and was later responsible for the cirrhosis.

Attention reverted to the treatment of ascites by suturing the omentum to the peritoneum (omentopexy). This operation was first suggested by Talma in 1887, and was performed by Van der Muelen in 1889 and by Schlekly in 1891, in both cases at Talma's suggestion. An account of the operation was published by Lens in 1892 (59). Drummond and Morison (60) published their experience with omentopexy in 1896. In 1902, Tansini advocated clinical application of Eck's fistula; he based his ideas on the results of his animal experiments (61). In 1903, Vidal (62) reported the first Eck's fistula in humans. The patient was operated on for ascites, lived 14 weeks, and died of ascites. In 1907, a peritoneovenous shunt was introduced as a new approach to the management of ascites; it was reported by Ruotte (63), who implanted the proximal end of the transected saphenous vein into the peritoneal cavity.

Sporadic reports of shunts between the splanchnic and systemic venous circulations as a treatment for ascites continued to appear. In 1910, DeMartel (64) reported on an Eck fistula in a woman who died of anuria shortly after the operation. In 1912, Rosenstein (65) reported the first successful Eck's fistula in a woman who had been tapped repeatedly, and 5 months after the operation required only an occasional paracentesis and had decreased ascites.

Several attempts were made to anastomose by suture technique a branch of the splanchnic venous circulation and the ovarian or spermatic vein. In 1910, Villard and Tavernier (66) recorded an ovarian superior mesenteric venous shunt. In 1911, Gunn (67) reported an ovarian portal-venous shunt. In 1912, Meursing (68) performed a spermatic-splenic venous shunt. The following year, the Russian surgeon Bogoras reported implantation of the superior mesenteric vein into the infe-

rior vena cava (69). The superior mesenteric vein was transected at the lower end of the mesoileum, and its distal (aboral) end was implanted into the inferior vena cava. One month later the spleen had decreased in size and the ascites had disappeared.

During the hiatus between the early anecdotal reports and the monumental work of Allen O. Whipple, attention turned away from ascites and portal hypertension per se and was directed at local control of bleeding varices. In 1930, Westphal (70) introduced the concept of compression of the esophageal varices. The technique of tamponade underwent a series of modifications until the presently most popular Sengstaken-Blakemore tube evolved in 1950 (71). Esophagoscopic injection of bleeding varices with a sclerosing solution was first described by Crafoord and Freckner in 1939 (72). In 1950, Boerema (73) and Crile (74) independently reported direct surgical control of the bleeding site by transesophageal ligation.

The year 1945 marked the beginning of the modern era of surgical intervention for portal hypertension, with the publication of back-to-back reports from the Columbia-Presbyterian Medical Center. The first report by Whipple (75) offered an in-depth consideration of the portal and splenic circulation, the collateral circulation in portal obstruction, and the clinical consequences of portal hypertension. Whipple then recounted past experiences with the Eck fistula in experimental animals and in humans, and concluded with a statement that Blakemore and he had performed five end-to-end splenorenal anastomoses and five end-to-side portacaval anastomoses, using a sutureless technique. The operations were carried out in patients with repeated severe hemorrhages, all patients survived the postoperative period, and five showed a marked improvement in liver function tests and disappearance of the ascites. In that report, reference was made to personal communication with Alfred Blalock, who had performed four splenorenal shunts for portal hypertension. Two patients experienced generalized improvement and diminished ascites while the other two died of bleeding varices ascribed to occlusion of the anastomosis. The second paper, by Blakemore and Lord (76), detailed the technique of using vitallium tubes in establishing portacaval shunts.

In the 1947 publication of the first Churchill lecture, Blalock (77) incorporated a consideration of shunt operations for portal hypertension with his experience managing pulmonic stenosis. He expressed the opinion

(1) Anastomosis of the portal vein and the inferior vena cava is preferable when indicated to a splenorenal union in that it will conduct more blood and is more apt to remain patent; (2) if a splenorenal anastomosis is performed, suture of the proximal end of the splenic vein to the side of the renal vein is preferable to an end-to-end anastomosis; (3) suture of the divided distal end of the portal vein to the side of the inferior vena cava is preferable to a side-to-side anastomosis since the opening is more apt to remain patent; and (4) it is not necessary to occlude the inferior vena cava completely while performing a portacaval shunt.

He concluded that "it does appear that the principle of portacaval shunts in the treatment of ascites and gastro-intestinal bleeding is a much sounder one than those previously advocated." The same year, Linton et al. (78) reported the technique of splenectomy and splenorenal shunt with preservation of the kidney.

In 1953, Marion, (79) and Clatworthy et al. (80) in 1955 independently described a shunt between the proximal transected end of the inferior vena cava and side of the superior mesenteric vein. The next step was the facilitation of the mesenteric caval shunt by an interposition graft. This was preceded by the 1951 report by Reynolds and Southwick (81) of two patients in whom a portacaval shunt was performed using autogenous azygous vein graft as a conduit. The first mesocaval interposition graft using Teflon was reported in 1963 by de Resene-Alves (82). The first Dacron interposition mesocaval shunt was performed by Gliedman in 1967 (83).

The most recent innovation in the procedures directed at decompression of portal hypertension is the selective (distal) splenorenal shunt, introduced clinically in 1967 by Warren and colleagues as a method of preserving portal flow to the liver while reducing the hypertension in the bleeding varices (84). One month later Davidson et al. (85) published their independent animal experiment with reverse splenorenal anastomosis as a means of preventing postshunt ammonia intoxication.

The advocacy of the selective splenorenal shunt was in response to a growing lack of enthusiasm for portal-systemic shunts that demonstrated no improvements in long-term survival, and showed an acceleration of hepatic failure and the adverse consequence of encephalopathy. Another re-

sponse was the introduction of nonshunting procedures to control variceal bleeding.

In 1929, ligation of the coronary vein had been described as a method of interrupting flow to esophagogastric varices (86). In 1947, Phemister and Humphreys (87) reported their results following gastroesophageal resection with total gastrectomy for bleeding varices. In 1950, Tanner (88) suggested gastric transection and reanastomosis to interrupt channels carrying blood to the region that had the varices. These concepts were extended by Merendino and Dillard (89) in 1955 when they performed jejunal interposition, and by Koop and Roddy (90), in 1958, who interposed colon for bleeding varices.

Another approach was directed at interrupting afferent arterial flow in an effort to effect a reduction of portal flow and pressure. In 1950, Berman et al. (91) reported on the effects of ligation of the hepatic and splenic arteries and the following year Rienhoff presented his experience (92). Womack and associates, in 1953, designed an ablative procedure consisting of splenectomy, resection of the superior two-thirds of the greater curvature of the stomach, ligation of the left gastric artery and its ascending branch, transesophageal ligation of varices, and in some cases, vagotomy and pyloroplasty. The results obtained were equivalent to shunting procedures (93). The most recent variation on this theme is the procedure introduced by Sugiura and Futagawa in 1973 (94).

In 1962, 50 years after Ruotte's (63) use of a saphenoperitoneal shunt, Smith et al. (95) reported on the drainage of resistant ascites using a modification of the Spitz-Holter valve technique. A technical breakthrough was achieved in 1974 by LeVeen et al. (96) with the development of a new device with an absolutely competent valve, activated by a pressure gradient of 2 to 4 centimeters of water. New devices have incorporated a pumping mechanism. The history of procedures to shunt ascitic fluid directly into the systemic circulation extends over half a century.

References

1. *Genuine Works of Hippocrates.* Adams F, tr. Baltimore: William Wood, vol. 2, aphorism 45, p. 267
2. Cited in: Rogers Sir L. Lettsonian lectures on amoebic liver abscess; its pathology, prevention and cure: Lecture II. The varieties and treatment of amoebic liver abscess. *Lancet* 1922;I:569–571.

3. Melnikoff A. Die Chirurgischen zugänge durch den unteren rand des brustkarbes zur den organen des subdiaphragmaten raunes. *Dtsch Z Chir* 1923;182:83–151.

4. Clairmont P, Meyer M. Erfahrungen uber die behandlung der appendicitis. *Acta Chir Scand* 1926;60:55–134.

5. Keynes G, ed. *The Apologie and Treatise of Ambroise Pare.* London: Falcon Educational Books, 1951, p. 205–206.

6. von Bruns. *Beitr Klin Chir* 1870;II(1).

7. Tillmann H. Experimentelle und anatomische untersuchungen uber wunden der leber und niere: Ein beitrag zur lehre von der antiseptischen wundheilung. *Arch Pathol Anat* 1879;78:437.

8. Burckhardt. *Zentralbl Chir* 1887;14:88.

9. DaCosta JC. *Modern Surgery.* Philadelphia: WB Saunders, 1917.

10. Kousnetzoff M, Pensky J. Sur la resection partielle du foie. *Rev Chir* 1896;16:501–521, 954–992.

11. Auvray M. Etude experimentale sur la resection du foie chez l'homme et chez les animaux. *Rev Chir* 1897;17:319–331.

12. Hough FS. "Communications" (description of a new method of suturing the liver). *Iowa Med J* 1907–1908;14:238–241.

13. Pringle JH. Notes on the arrest of hepatic hemorrhage due to trauma. *Ann Surg* 1908;48:541–549.

14. Heaney JP, Stanton WR, Halbert DS, Seidel J, Vice T. An improved technic for vascular isolation of the liver. *Ann Surg* 1966;163:237–244.

15. Schrock T, Blaisdell TW, Mathewson C. Management of blunt trauma to the liver and hepatic veins. *Arch Surg* 1968;96:698–704.

16. Cited in: Paolucci Di Valmaggiore P. L'epatectomie. Proceedings of the 16th Congress of the International Society of Surgery (Copenhagen). Brussels: Imprimerie Medicale et Scientifique. 1955, p. 1009.

17. Luis. *Gazz Chir* 1896.

18. Langenbuch C. Ein fall von resection eines linksseitigen schurlappens der leber. *Berl Klin Wochenschr* 1888;25:37.

19. Tiffany L. The removal of a solid tumor from the liver by laparotomy. *Maryland Med J* 1890;23:531.

20. Lücke. *Centralbl Chir* 1891;6:115.

21. Keen WW. On resection of the liver, especially for hepatic tumors. *Bost Med Surg J* 1892;126:405–409.

22. Keen WW. Report of a case of resection of the liver for the removal of a neoplasm with a table of seventy-six cases of resection of the liver for hepatic tumor. *Ann Surg* 1899;30:267–283.

23. Wendel W. Beiträge zur Chirurgie der Leber. *Arch Klin Chir Berl* 1911;95:887–894.

24. Cattell RB. Successful removal of liver metastasis from carcinoma of the rectum. *Lahey Clin Bull* 1940;2:7–11.

25. Wangensteen OH. The surgical problem of gastric cancer. With special reference to: (1) the closed method of gastric resection, (2) coincidental hepatic resection and (3) preoperative and postoperative management. *Arch Surg* 1943;46:879–906.

26. Cantlie J. On a new arrangement of the right and left lobes of the liver. *J Anat and Physiol Lond* 1898;32:4.

27. Hjortsjö C-H. The topography of the intrahepatic duct system. *Acta Anat* 1951;11:599–615.

28. Healey JE Jr, Schroy PC. Anatomy of the biliary ducts within the human liver. *Arch Surg* 1953;66:599–616.

29. Goldsmith NA, Woodburne RT. The surgical anatomy pertaining to liver resection. *Surg Gynecol Obstet* 1957;105:310–318.

30. Raven RW. Partial hepatectomy. *Br J Surg* 1948;36:397–401.

31. Lortat-Jacob JL, Robert HG. Hepatectomie droite reglé. *Presse Med* 1952;60:549–550.

32. Quattlebaum JK. Massive resection of the liver. *Ann Surg* 1953;137:787–796.

33. Mersheimer WL. Successful right hepatolobectomy for primary neoplasm:—preliminary observations. *Bull NY Med Coll* 1953;16:121–125.

34. Pack GT, Baker HW. Total right hepatic lobectomy. *Ann Surg* 1953;138:253–258.

35. Pack GT, Miller TR, Brasfield RD. Total right hepatic lobectomy for cancer of the gallbladder. Report of three cases. *Ann Surg* 1955;142:6–16.

36. Couinaud C. Plaidoyer pour une segmentation hepatique exacte et une technique anatomique de resection reglie du foie le clampage du pedicule hepatique. *Presse Med* 1966;74:2849–2852.

37. Anschutz W. Uber die resektion der leber. *Samt K Vort* 1903;356–357.

38. Fineberg C, Goldburgh WP, Templeton JY. Right hepatic lobectomy for primary carcinoma of the liver. *Ann Surg* 1956;144:882–892.

39. Lin T-Y, Tsu KY, Mien C, Chen CS. Study on lobectomy of the liver. *J Formosa Med Assoc* 1958;57(11):742–759.

40. Tung TT. A new technic for operation on the liver. *Lancet* 1963;1:192–193.

41. Couinaud C. Le foie. *Études anatomiques et chirurgicales.* Paris: Masson, 1957.

42. Tung TT. *Les resections majeures et mineures du foie.* Paris: Masson, 1979.

43. Caprio G. Un caso de extirpacion die lobulo izquierdo die hegado. *Bull Soc Cir Urug Montevideo* 1931;2:159.

44. Bismuth H, Houssin D, Castaing D. Major and minor segmentectomies "reglées" in liver surgery. *World J Surg* 1982;6:10–24.

45. Mancuso M, Nataline E, DelGrande G. Contributo alla conoscenza della struttura segmentaria del fegato in rapporto al problema della resezione epatica. *Policlinico, Sez Chir* 1955;62(5):259–293.

46. Welch CS. A note on transplantation of the whole liver in dogs. *Transplant Bull* 1955;2:54–55.

47. Moore FD, Smith LL, Burnap TK, et al. One-stage homotransplantation of the liver following total hepatectomy in dogs. *Transplant Bull* 1959;6:103–107.

48. Starzl TE, Kaupp HA Jr, Brock DR, Lazarus RE, Johnson RV. Reconstructive problems in canine liver homotransplantation with special reference to the postoperative role of hepatic venous flow. *Surg Gynecol Obstet* 1960;111:733–743.

49. Starzl TE. *Experience in Hepatic Transplantation.* Philadelphia: WB Saunders, 1969.

50. Absolon KB, Hagihara PF, Griffen WO Jr, Lillehei RC. Experimental and clinical heterotopic liver homotransplantation. *Rev Int Hepat* 1965;15:1481.

51. Thomson J. On congenital obliteration of bile-ducts. *Edinb Med J* 1891;37:523–724.

52. Holmes JB. Congenital obliteration of the bile ducts; diagnosis and suggestions for treatment. *Am J Dis Child* 1916;11:405–431.

53. Ladd WE. Congenital atresia and stenosis of the bile ducts. *JAMA* 1928;91:1082–1085.

54. Schnug GE. Importance of early operation in congenital atresia of the extrahepatic bile ducts. Report of ten proved cases. *Ann Surg* 1958;148:931–936.

55. Kasai M, Suzuki S. A new operation for "non-correctable" biliary atresia—hepatic portoenterostomy. *Shuzutsu* 1959;13:733.

56. Child CG III. Eck's fistula. *Surg Gynecol Obstet* 1953;96:375–376.
57. Hahn M, Massen O, Nencki M, Pawlow S. Die Eck'sche Fistel zwischen der unteren hohlvene und der Pfortader und ihre Folgen für den Organismus. *Arch f exper Path u Pharmakol* 1893;32:161–210.
58. Banti G. La splenomegalia con cirrosi hepatica. *Lo Sperimentale, Sez, biol Fasc*, 1894, V–VI.
59. Lens T. Hechting von het omentum majus aan den buikwand bij cirrhosis hepatis atrophica. *Nederlansch Tijdschrift Geneeskunde* 1892;28(1):645–450.
60. Drummond D, Morison R. A case of ascites due to cirrhosis of the liver cured by operation. *Br Med J* 1986;2:728–729.
61. Tansini, Mentioned by Enderten, Hotz, and Magnus-Alsleben. Die Pathologie und Therapie des Pfortaderverschlusses. Experimentelle untersuchungen über die Ecksche Fistel. *Ztschr f d ges exper Med Berl* 1914;3:223–308.
62. Vidal M. Traitement chirurgicale des ascites. *Presse Med* 1903;2:747.
63. Ruotte M. Abouchement de la veine saphene externe au peritoines pour resorber des epanchements sciatiques. *Lyon Med* 1907;109:574–577.
64. DeMartel MF. Report of an Eck fistula in a woman. *Rev Chir (Paris)* 1910;42:1181.
65. Rosenstein P. Ueber die behandlung der Lebercirrhose durch Anlegung einer Eck'schen Fistel. *Arch f klin Chir* 1912;98:1082–1092.
66. Villard E, Tavernier L. Suture ovario-mésentérique dans un cas de cirrhose du foie. *Lyon Méd* 1910;114:1113–1119.
67. Gunn, KELG. *R Acad Ire* 1911;8:12.
68. Meursing F. *Dtsch Med Wochenschr* 1912;49.
69. Bogoras NA. The transplantation of the superior mesenteric vein into the inferior vena cava in cirrhosis of the liver. *Russki Vratch* 1913;12:48–50.
70. Westphal K. Ueber eine Kompressionsbehandlung der Blutungen aus Oesophagusvarizen. *Deutsche med Wchnschr* 56:1135–1136.
71. Sengstaken RW, Blakemore AH. Balloon tamponade for the control of hemorrhage from esophageal varices. *Ann Surg* 1950;131:781–789.
72. Crafoord C, Freckner P. Nonsurgical treatment of varicose veins of the esophagus. *Acta Otolaryngol* 1939;27:422.
73. Boerema I. Bleeding varices of the esophagus in cirrhosis of the liver and Banti's syndrome. *Arch Chir Neirc* 1949;1(3).
74. Crile G Jr. Transesophageal ligation of bleeding esophageal varices. A preliminary report of seven cases. *Arch Surg* 1950;61:654–660.
75. Whipple AO. The problem of portal hypertension in relation to the hepatosplenopathies. *Ann Surg* 1945;122:449–475.
76. Blakemore AH, Lord JW Jr. The technic of using vitallium tubes in establishing portacaval shunts for portal hypertension. *Ann Surg* 1945;122:476–489.
77. Blalock AH. The use of shunt or by-pass operations in the treatment of certain circulatory disorders including portal hypertension and pulmonic stenosis. *Ann Surg* 1947;125:129–141.
78. Linton RR, Jones CM, Volwiler W. Portal hypertension. The treatment by splenectomy and splenorenal anastomosis with preservation of the kidney. *Surg Clin N Am* 1947;27:1162–1170.
79. Marion P. Les obstructions portales. *Semaine Hôp Paris* 1953;29:2781–2790.
80. Clatworthy HW Jr, Wall T, Watman RN. A new type of portal-to-systemic venous shunt for portal hypertension. *Arch Surg* 1955;71:588–599.
81. Reynolds JT, Southwick HW. Portal hypertension. Use of venous grafts where side to side anastomosis is impossible. *Arch Surg* 1951;62:789–800.
82. Gliedman ML. Mesocaval shunts. *Mod Techn Surg Abdom Surg* 1982;14:1–13.
83. Gliedman ML. The mesocaval shunt for portal hypertension. *Am J Gastroenterol Surg* 1971;56:321–323.
84. Warren WO, Zeppa R, Foman JJ. Selective trans-splenic decompression of gastroesophageal varices by distal splenorenal shunt. *Ann Surg* 1967;166:437–455.
85. Davidson F, Denize A, Hurwitt ES, Laufman H. Reverse splenocaval anastomosis for prevention of postshunt ammonia intoxication. *Surg Gynecol Obstet* 1967;125:815–818.
86. Rowntree LG, Walters W, McIndoe AH. End result of tying of the coronary veins for prevention of hemorrhage from esophageal varices. *Proc Staff Meet Mayo Clin* 1929;4:263–264.
87. Phemister DB, Humphreys EM. Gastroesophageal resection and total gastrectomy in the treatment of bleeding varicose veins in Banti's syndrome. *Ann Surg* 1947;126:397–410.
88. Tanner NC. Gastroduodenal hemorrhage as a surgical emergency (discussion). *Proc R Soc Med* 1950;43:145–156.
89. Merendino KA, Dillard DH. The concept of sphincter substitution by an interposed jejunal segment for anatomic and physiologic abnormalities at the esophagogastric junction. *Ann Surg* 1955;142:486–509.
90. Koop CE, Roddy SR. Colonic replacement of distal esophagus and proximal stomach in the management of bleeding varices in children. *Ann Surg* 1958;147:17–25.
91. Berman JK, Koenig H, Muller LP. Ligation of the hepatic and splenic arteries in the treatment of portal hypertension. *Indiana Univ Bull* 1950;12:99.
92. Rienhoff WF Jr. Ligation of the hepatic and splenic arteries in the treatment of portal hypertension with report of six cases. *Bull Johns Hopkins Hosp* 1951;88:368–375.
93. Johnson G Jr, Womack NA, Gabriele OF, Peters RM. Control of the hyperdynamic circulation in patients with bleeding esophageal varices. *Ann Surg* 1969;169:661–671.
94. Sugiura M, Futagawa S. A new technique for treating esophageal varices. *J Thorac Cardiovasc Surg* 1973;66:677–685.
95. Smith AN, Preshaw RM, Bisset WH. The drainage of resistant ascites, by a modification of the Spitz-Holter valve technique. *J Roy Coll Surg Edinb* 1962;7:289–294.
96. Greenlee HB, Stanley MM, Reinhardt GF. Intractable ascites treated with peritoneovenous shunts (LeVeen). A 24- to 64-month follow-up of results in 52 alcoholic cirrhotics. *Arch Surg* 1981;116(5):518–24.

Editorial Comment

It would be difficult to add much to this superb review of the history of liver surgery. Where the past ends and the present begins is a peculiar dividing line but it might be well to add some comments on liver regeneration, particularly since any introduction to this subject invariably refers to the myth in which the Titans' punishment of Prometheus for stealing fire from Olympus involved the repetitive devouring of his liver by a **vulture** and the equally repetitive restoration. It seems unlikely, however, that the original construction of the myth was based on the recognition of the remarkable regenerative capacity of the liver but rather to familarity, even at that time, with the intermittent agony of the symptoms of biliary colic.

Regardless of the validity of the reference point to Prometheus, the investigation of this phenomenon, which is common to most mammalian species, has developed its own mythology as well as a hard core of incontrovertible and soundly based scientific observations.

Present concepts on hepatic regeneration will be covered later in this volume but the recent history of this fascinating subject seems to begin with two outstanding review articles in which Bucher (1,2) has summarized the morphologic, physiologic, and biochemical studies that have been done over the past half-century in this fascinating area, and which certainly provide a superb historical and scientific basis for subsequent work.

References

1. Bucher NLR. Regeneration of the mammalian liver. *Int Rev Cytol* 1963;15:245–300.
2. Bucher NLR. Experimental aspects of hepatic regeneration. *N Engl J Med* 1967;277:686–696, 738–746.

PART II
Basic Science Considerations

Chapter 2
Surgical Anatomy of the Liver

R. Y. CALNE

The liver is a challenging organ for the surgeon because it is a single, vital structure of high vascularity. It has a dual blood supply and its close relations to many other vital structures are relevant to most surgical procedures on the liver. The inferior vena cava runs through the liver, while the upper surface of the organ is in contact with the diaphragm and is closely related to the heart and lungs. Below the right lobe of the liver in the subhepatic Rutherford-Morrison space is a surgical area of extreme importance in which many pathologic conditions can occur (Fig. 2.1). Within a radius of 3 centimeters lie the gallbladder, right lobe of the liver, right adrenal gland, right kidney and renal vessels, the first and second parts of the duodenum, the head of the pancreas, the common bile duct, portal vein and hepatic artery, the inferior vena cava, and the heptic flexure of the colon. Trauma in any of these sites will be adjacent to or involve the right lobe of the liver. The neighbors of the left lobe are the intra-abdominal esophagus, the stomach, the vagi, the lesser sac, the aorta, and the pancreas.

Assessment of Hepatic Anatomy

The surgeon frequently has to make an assessment of the liver by indirect means. The organ is irregularly shaped, resembling a pear lying on its side cut obliquely in the longitudinal plane. Normally, it fills the right hypochondrium and extends into the left. It cannot be felt on abdominal examination unless it is enlarged because of the costal margin but since it moves with respiration and is dull to

The figures are reproduced with permission from the author. They were originally published in. *A Colour Atlas of Surgical Anatomy of the Abdomen in the Living Subject*. Wolfe Medical. London, United Kingdom. 1988.

percussion, clinical examination can often give an indication of the size of the liver. Palpation and percussion will determine if it is particularly small, large, or contains abnormal projections.

At laparotomy the liver may require assessment without visualization or with a very restricted view of the anterior surface of the right lobe. If the surgeon's hand is passed along the surface of the greater omentum upward toward the transverse colon and over the transverse colon to the stomach and lesser omentum it will then be directed to the liver. Various parts can be felt without any dissection, namely, the gallbladder, anterior diaphragmatic surfaces of the right and left lobes, and the inferior posterior surface of both lobes shelving upward to the posterior abdominal wall. Between the duodenum and caudate process of the caudate lobe lies the free edge of the lesser omentum containing the main hepatic artery, portal vein, and bile duct, together with lymphatic ducts and draining lymph nodes and a surprisingly extensive network of autonomic nerves. The hand passing over the anterior diaphragmatic surface of the right lobe cannot go beyond the falciform ligament medially and the coronary and right triangular ligaments above and laterally. The inferior shelving surface of the right lobe can only be palpated as far as the reflection of the peritoneum where the bare area begins above and the peritoneum passes into the inferior vena cava medially. Deep to the peritoneum in the right subhepatic space lies the upper pole of the right kidney, and between it and the vena cava lies the right adrenal gland with its large single vein, usually going directly into the vena cava. The gallbladder lying in its fossa in the right lobe marks the true anatomic division between the right and left lobes that passes through the gallbladder fossa toward the inferior vena cava (Fig. 2.2). Between the gallbladder and the fissures for the falciform ligament and ligamentum venosum is the quadrate lobe of the liver in front and the caudate lobe behind. A finger can be passed above the duodenum, between it and the caudate process posterior to the free edge of the lesser omentum in front of the inferior vena cava. This is the opening to the lesser sac called the aditus. The finger exploring the lesser sac can detect pathology in the pancreas, celiac artery, and splenic vessels. Passing from the anterior surface of the stomach along the lesser omentum to the fissure in the liver for the obliterated ligamentum venosum of embryologic importance, the hand will pass upwards to the inferior surface of the left lobe. As the hand passes laterally, the left lobe lies to the right and above the anterior surface of the spleen. Within the lesser sac the left triangular ligament prevents passage of the hand across the upper surface of the left lobe of the liver. If the left triangular ligament is divided, a normal left lobe can be turned anteriorly and to the right, exposing the esophageal hiatus, the abdominal vagi, and the lesser curve of the stomach. Even without dividing the left triangular ligament, careful palpation of the liver, as described above, gives the surgeon a good idea as to the consistency and configuration of the organ. Malignant lesions on the surface are felt, and frequently deposits can be detected within the liver parenchyma that do not appear on the surface due to the soft, blancmangelike consistency of the normal liver parenchyma. In cirrhosis and right-sided heart failure, the liver is hard. In advanced cirrhosis, the liver may be small and extremely nodular.

The falciform ligament and the fissure for the ligamentum venosum constitute the important surgical division between the lateral and medial segments of the left lobe. The caudate lobe lies mainly in the medial segment of the left lobe posteriorly. It is called the caudate lobe because of its tail-like process, which lies behind the portal vein at the upper border of the aditus to the lesser sac.

Surgical Considerations

The lobar anatomy described above is easily defined and is important surgically. There is, however, an extremely detailed description of intrahepatic lobular anatomy, which may be of importance to the academic anatomist but has little surgical relevance. This is because the vascular arrangements of the liver only allow exploitation of the grosser anatomic information, and variations in the intrahepatic relations of vessels are common. The gallbladder is a muscular pear-shaped structure lying embedded to a varying degree in the undersurface of the liver in the gallbladder fossa. The fundus of the gallbladder is anterior and directed to the right and the body of the organ passes toward the hilum of the liver where it is widened at Hartmann's pouch, which leads to the cystic duct. The cystic duct joins the common hepatic duct to form the common bile duct. Usually this junction is 1 or 2 cm from the hilum of the liver but it can be considerably lower; the cystic duct may run behind the common duct to just above the duodenum or may even have a common opening with the common hepatic duct at the ampulla of Vater. This variation is extremely important if any procedure is devised aimed at utilizing the cystic duct as a bile conduit. The point of junction of the cystic duct to the main biliary duct drainage system must be defined in such cases. Within the cystic duct is a spiral fold of mucosa, the valve of Heister, which allows passive flow of bile into the gallbladder. When the sphincter of Oddi at the duodenum is closed, the gallbladder will fill with bile. The mucosa of the gallbladder, which is highly vascular, concentrates the bile up to 10 times the original concentration of that secreted from the liver. Fatty food entering the duodenum liberates the hormone cholecystokinin, which passes into the portal venous system from the duodenal mucosa. Together with vagal activity, cholecystokinin is responsible for contraction of the gallbladder, which automatically causes the spiral valve to open and bile to pass into the duodenum to aid in digestion. Vagotomy renders the gallbladder atonic, enlarged, and prone to stone formation within it. The veins of the gallbladder pass either directly into the liver through the gallbladder bed or alongside the cystic duct to the portal vein at the liver hilum. Small arteries accompany these veins in addition to the main cystic artery, which is usually a branch of the right hepatic passing to Hartmann's pouch behind and above the cystic duct. Many variations of biliary drainage have been described but with the exception of the site of entry of the cystic duct mentioned above, most of them are extremely rare; for example, the right main hepatic duct may pass directly into the gallbladder. The surgeon should, however, be aware that virtually any abnormality is possible. Thus, when the surgeon is dissecting near the extrahepatic biliary drainage system, should he or she find a strange anatomic variant, this must be recognized for what it is and managed accordingly.

Most of the liver surface is covered with visceral peritoneum, which is fused with the fibrous covering of the liver called Glisson's capsule. In the embryo the left umbilical vein passes in the ligamentum teres to the liver in the mid-line. This is the anatomic junction of the medial lateral segments of the left lobe. The ligamentum teres is covered by peritoneum and forms the free edge of the falciform ligament, which continues over the diaphragmatic surface of the left lobe, posteriorly where the leaves of peritoneum of the falciform ligament diverge on the diaphragmatic surface of the liver. On the right side the peritoneum forms the coronary ligament and on the left side, the left triangular ligament. The lesser omentum contains, besides the important structure in its free edge, the hepatic branches of the anterior and posterior vagus nerves, and sometimes an anomalous left hepatic artery arising from the left gastric artery.

The nerve supply of the liver comes from the celiac plexus, from which nerve fibers arising from the semilunar-shaped celiac ganglion surround the celiac arterial trunk. This is mainly a sympathetic plexus but also contains important contributions from the vagi. Thus, the liver, with its extensive nervous supply from both vagi and sympathetics, might be expected to respond actively to nervous stimuli and this may well be the case. It is of interest, however, that all the nerves to the liver can be cut, for example, in a liver transplant operation, and this has very little effect on liver function, at least in the gross sense of clinical biochemical measurements.

Hepatic arterial anatomy is extremely important. The celiac artery passing from the aorta anteriorly trifurcates into (1) a left gastric branch which passes to the lesser curve of the stomach; (2) an undulating splenic arterial branch passing along the upper border of the pancreas posteriorly, lying alongside and above the splenic vein supplying the pancreas and the spleen; and (3) the third and largest branch, the common hepatic artery, which gives off a small tributary to the pancreas, in addition to a small branch to the pyloric antrum of

the stomach, the right gastric. The main artery then loops forward and cephalward within the leaves of the lesser omentum, giving off a caudal gastroduodenal branch supplying the duodenum and pancreas. The hepatic artery continues up toward the hilum of the liver dividing at a variable point into right and left branches (Fig. 2.3). Usually the artery is the most proximal major division, followed by the portal vein, while the highest of the three structures is the junction of the right and left hepatic ducts to form the common hepatic duct. In 17% of patients the main arterial blood supply to the right lobe of the liver arises from a branch of the superior mesenteric artery. This usually passes posterior to the portal vein and will be missed unless a special search is made, which is an important step if arterial ligation is planned for bleeding from the right lobe of the liver or to devascularize malignant deposits in the right lobe. Occasionally the superior mesenteric right hepatic branch passes in front of the portal vein where it is more easily identified. As already mentioned, in 23% of patients the left gastric artery provides the main left hepatic artery, passing in the lesser omentum. When either of these anomalous branches are present there may or may not be a normal hepatic arterial anatomy in addition but, if one of the anomalous branches is present, the caliber of the vessels will be smaller than normal and this may alert the surgeon to the possibility of additional abnormal vessels.

The upper surface of the right lobe is firmly adherent to the diaphragm. If one continues following the course of the coronary ligament to the right of the mid-line, it eventually turns back on itself as the right triangular ligament and then runs posteriorly away from the anterior leaf to behind the vena cava near the diaphragm, leaving a triangular portion of the right posterior diaphragmatic surface of the liver in direct contact with the diaphragm. This is called the bare area of the liver since it has no peritoneal covering. Some lymphatics and blood vessels pass directly from the bare area of the liver through the diaphragm into the chest, anastomosing with pleural vessels (Fig. 2.4).

The inferior vena cava is intimately related to the liver. After receiving the two main renal veins it reaches the undersurface of the liver and lies in a cleft between the right and left lobes in the saggital plain (Fig. 2.5). It receives the right adrenal vein posteriorly on the right side, and a variable number of lumbar veins and sometimes accessory hepatic veins enter anteriorly. Especially common is a vein draining into the anterior surface of the vena cava from the caudate lobe. This may be the only lobe with venous drainage in a patient with Budd-Chiari syndrome, where the rest of the liver becomes congested and eventually nonfunctional. In such cases the caudate lobe provides the patient with the sole remaining hepatic function and may hypertrophy considerably. The inferior vena cava ends its intra-abdominal course by passing through the diaphragm, at the back of the ninth thoracic vertebra. Just at this point it receives the main right, left and median hepatic veins, and three phrenic veins, right and left, which are easily seen and well described in anatomy texts, along with a constant posterior phrenic vein that passes on the surface of the right crus. This vein is important surgically but has escaped the attention of most conventional anatomists (Fig. 2.6).

Microscopic Anatomy

Microscopically the liver consists of lobules, each surrounded by a thin layer of fibrous tissue. Between the lobules are the portal triads conveying radicles of the hepatic artery, portal vein, and bile duct. There are important connections between the hepatic artery and portal vein. If the hepatic artery is ligated proximally, and cut on the cephalward side, blood flow will be seen coming in a retrograde direction via anastomoses from the portal vein, and vice versa. The main blood flow of both the portal vein and the hepatic artery is through the vascular sinusoides of the lobule to the central veins, and these are tributaries of the main hepatic veins. Bile secreted by the hepatocytes passes into the biliary canaliculi that lead to small tributaries of lobular ducts, and these eventually join the main bile duct system. Sinusoids are partially lined by monocytic-derived Kupffer's cells, which have important phagocytic activity removing particulate matter from the portal blood.

Liver Resections

The main vascular and biliary intrahepatic anatomy is extremely important because of surgical considerations, especially in hepatic resections. As already mentioned, the hepatic artery and portal vein usually bifurcate within the free edge of the lesser omentum. The hepatic artery division is further away from the liver than the portal vein. The junction of the right and left hepatic ducts is usually highest in the hilum of the liver. Radicals of these three structures then pass into the right and left lobes, fanning out from the hilum and dividing into major and minor branches. The hepatic venous tributaries pass upward and posteriorly at right angles to the hepatic artery, portal vein, and bile ducts. This relationship, which is likened by Fagreus to crossing of extended fingers of both hands (Fig. 2.7), has important surgical considerations because if the hepatic parenchyma is divided, it is usually necessary to suture-ligate the vessels. Ordinary ties tend to slip off the vessels because of their orientation to each other. There are three main hepatic veins, right, left, and median sagittal. In 60% of patients the median sagittal vein joins the left but in 40% it enters the vena cava independently. The hepatic veins have very short extrahepatic courses, joining the vena cava at approximately 45°. They are vulnerable to trauma because the large and heavy liver tends to tear at its connections with the diaphragm and such tears may enter the hepatic veins where they join the vena cava. It is extremely difficult to gain access to this area quickly. Dissection of the torn hepatic veins in a shocked patient may result in suction of air into the right side of the heart with fatal consequences. It is important for the anesthetist to maintain positive venous pressure so that instead of air being sucked in there will be loss of blood, which can be replaced through the defect.

Although local suture and wedge resections of liver are possible, the main operations for severe trauma and localized cancer are right lobectomy; right lobectomy with removal of the left medial lobe, sometimes called trisegmentectomy; left lateral segment removal; and left lobectomy with removal of both main left segments. Consideration of the vascular anatomy explains the rationale of these operations (Fig. 2.8). Other major resections are seldom possible without damaging central vital vessels or bile ducts. The lymphatic drainage of the liver is into lymph nodes in the hilum first and then into nodes in the lesser omentum along the hepatic and celiac arteries, then to the preaortic nodes, and finally into the thoracic duct.

In the past 15 years 33 patients have been admitted to Addenbrooke's Hospital with severe liver injuries, that is Grade III to IV, Grade III being

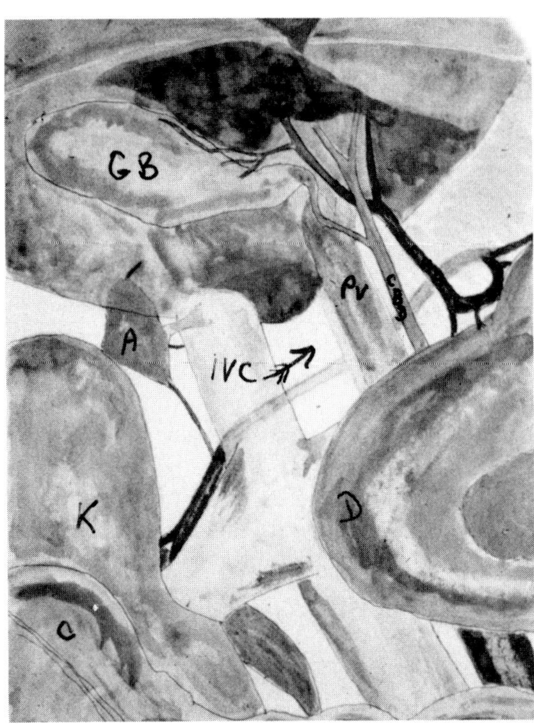

Figure 2.1 Diagram of the subhepatic passage of Rutherford Morison. Shows the proximity of important structures to the aditus of the lesser sac between the inferior vena cava (IVC) and the free edge of the lesser omentum, containing portal vein (PV), common bile duct (CBD), and common hepatic artery (CHA). The right adrenal gland (A) is shown draining through its single vein into the inferior vena cava. The right kidney and renal vessels are shown (K), as are the hepatic flexure of colon (C) and the duodenum (D). The gall bladder (GB) is shown above with its arterial supply, the cystic artery coming from the right hepatic artery.

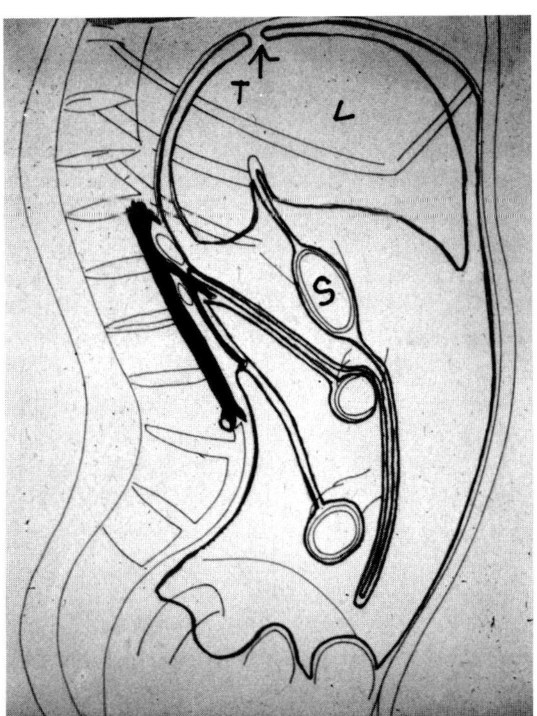

Figure 2.2 Diagram to show the peritoneal attachments of the liver and bowel, taking in a sagittal section. The peritoneum surrounding the stomach (S) extends as the lesser omentum to the fissure for the ligamentum venosum. There is visceral peritoneum covering the liver (L) and the peritoneum is reflected onto the diaphragm by the anterior and posterior leaves of the left triangular ligament (T).

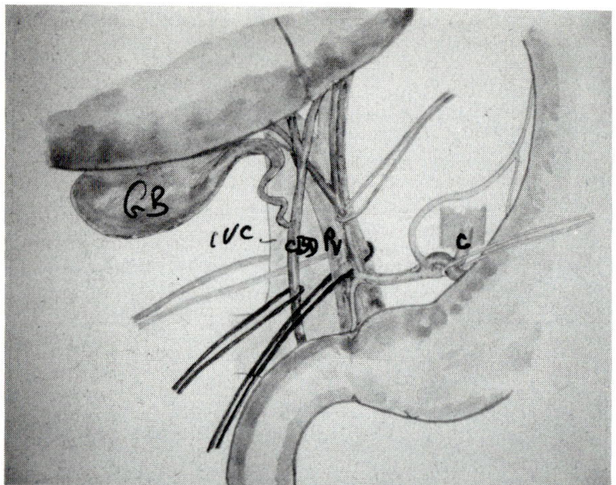

Figure 2.3   Diagram showing the disposition and relationship of the structures in the lesser omentum lying in front of the inferior vena cava (IVC) from which they are separated by the opening into the lesser sac, the aditus. The coeliac artery (C) is shown coming from the aorta and dividing into splenic, left gastric, and common hepatic. The common hepatic gives off the gastroduodenal and then turns upwards towards the liver, its major division is proximal to that of the portal vein (PV), which usually divides proximal to the junction of the right and left hepatic ducts to form the common bile duct (CBD), although they are shown at the same level in this diagram. The gall bladder (GB), cystic artery, and cystic ducts are also shown.

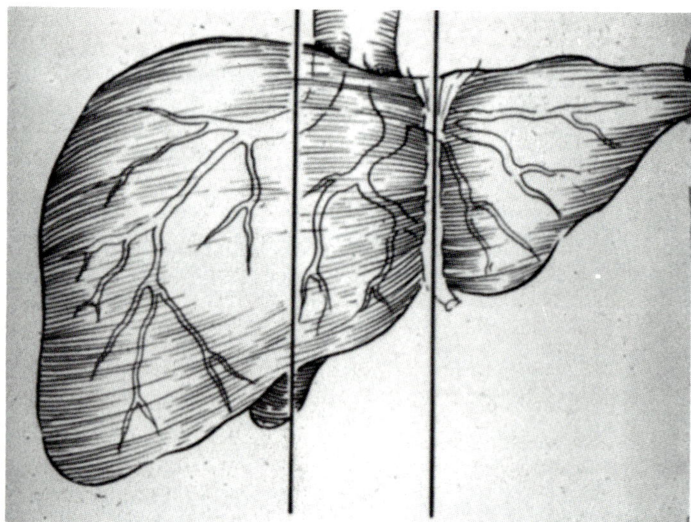

A

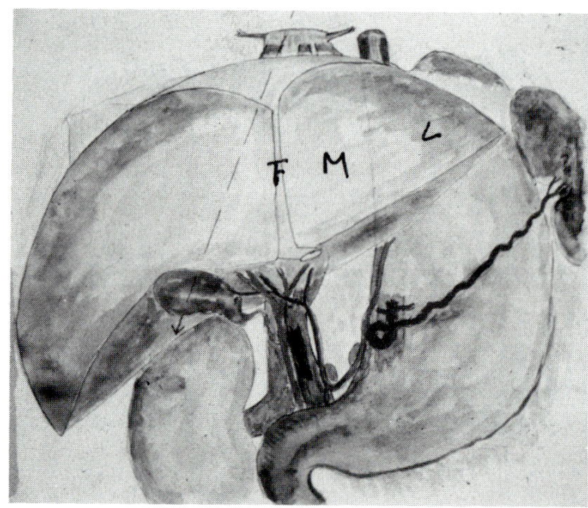

B

Figure 2.5   A. Diagram to show the main segmental anatomy of the liver from the surgical point of view. The plane between the anatomical right and left lobes extends obliquely from the gallbladder bed to the inferior vena cava. The right lobe of the liver is to the right of this plane, and the left lobe to the left. B. The left lobe is subdivided into lateral segments (L) and medial segments (M), separated by the falciform ligament (F).

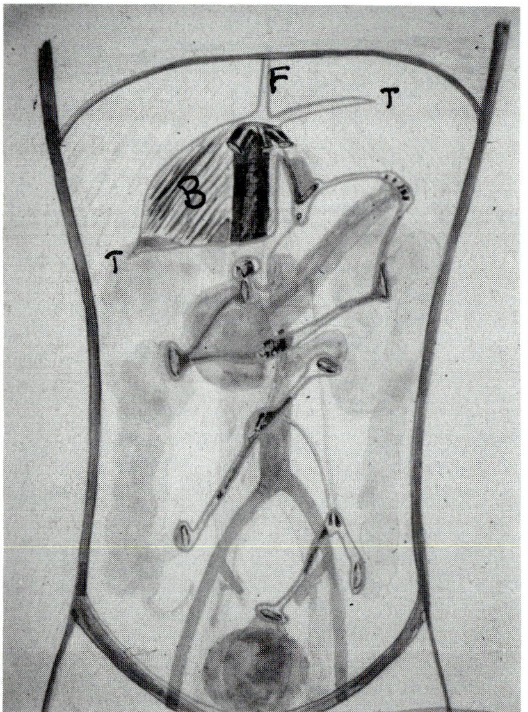

Figure 2.4   Shows the peritoneal reflections from the posterior abdominal wall. In the upper part of the diagram can be seen the reflections of the right and left triangular ligaments (T), the bare area (B), the inferior vena cava (IVC), the three hepatic veins joining it, and the falciform ligament (F).

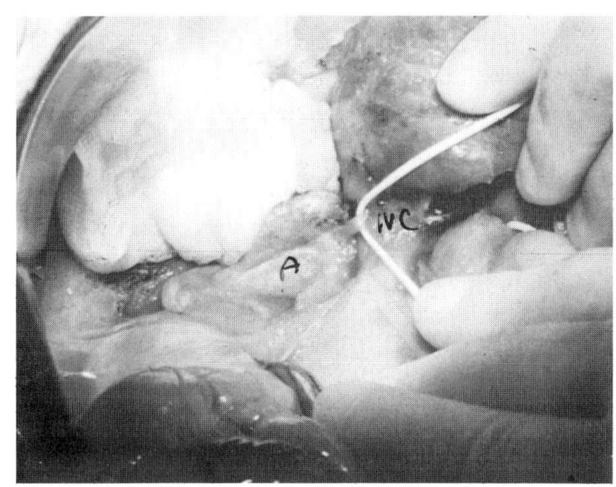

Figure 2.6 Photograph showing the right adrenal gland, displayed after elevation of the right lobe of the liver during dissection for hepatectomy in a transplant operation. The white rubber sling passes beneath the right adrenal vein, which drains directly into the inferior vena cava (IVC).

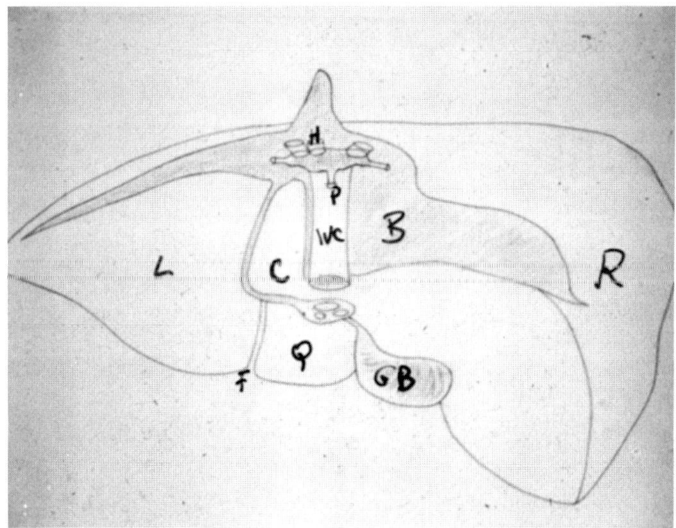

Figure 2.7 Diagram of the liver viewed posteriorly, showing the inferior vena cava in the center (IVC), with three hepatic veins (H) entering it, and also three phrenic veins, right, left, and posterior (P). The gallbladder (GB) with cystic duct is indicated. Between the gallbladder and the falciform ligament (F) is the quadrate lobe of the liver, and behind the quadrate lobe is the caudate lobe (C) and both parts of the left lobe (L). The bare area (B) is part of the right lobe (R).

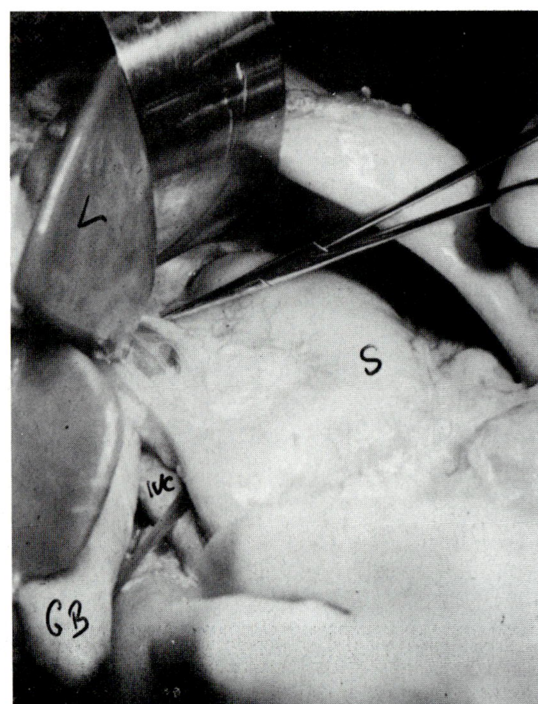

Figure 2.8 Appearance of the liver with the left lobe (L) turned upwards and to the right, after division of the right triangular ligament. The gallbladder (GB) is pointing downwards. There is a sling around the inferior vena cava (IVC). The stomach (S) is shown to the right, and the forceps points to an anomalous left hepatic artery arising from the left gastric artery.

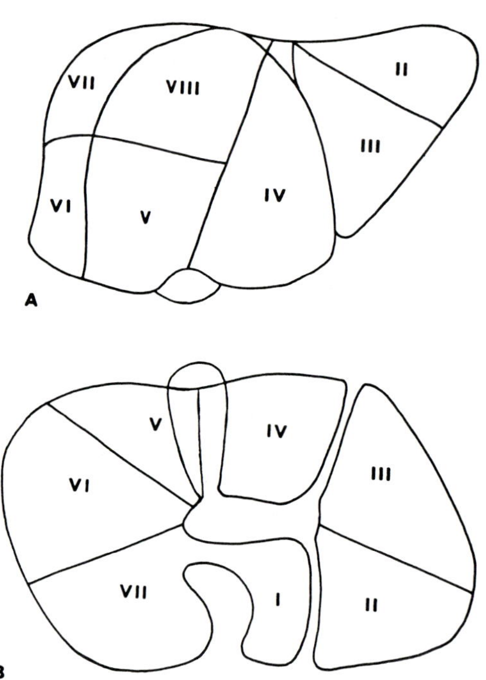

Figure 2.9 Anatomical segments of the liver as described and numbered by Couinaud.

parenchymal liver damage with serious bleeding from intrahepatic arteries and/or veins causing surgical shock and threatening life, and Grade IV having similar damage to Grade III with, in addition, a tear of the inferior vena cava or major hepatic vessels. A policy of management has been developed in which the minimum surgery has been performed that has been necessary to control bleeding. There were twenty-four male and nine female patients with an average age of 25. Seventeen were motorcyclists, one a cyclist, eight were occupants of motor vehicles, and five were pedestrians, including one who was hit on the right costal margin by a hockey ball. Two suffered from open injuries, one a stab injury, the other a gunshot wound. There were six deaths, 18%, including two out of 16 patients with Grade III trauma and four out of seven with Grade IV. Three were pedestrians, one a motorcyclist and two were occupants of motor vehicles. Two were over 70 years of age.

Patient Transfer

Thirteen of the patients were initially admitted to local hospitals where resuscitation, laparotomy, and packing were performed. The patients were then transported to Addenbrooke's Hospital where management was continued. All patients survived and were discharged with normal or near normal liver function.

Conservative Management

Four patients were treated conservatively. Two underwent no operative procedure. Their management was based on serial CT scans. One developed a late liver abscess that required needle drainage under radiologic control. These three patients all recovered fully. The fourth patient treated conservatively was one of the six fatalities with multiple injuries, including fractures of the femur, acetabulum, tibia, fibula, patella and radial head. The cause of death was renal failure combined with shock-lung. All ten patients whose injury was confined to the liver survived. Extrahepatic injuries, often severe, complicated management. In eight patients hepatic lobectomy was performed. There was one death from this group. Other surgical procedures included removal of hematomas, simple suturing, and debridement of the liver, and in five cases the right branch of the hepatic artery was ligated without resection. Two of these five patients died; one patient died from primary hemorrhage after unsuccessful attempts had been made to suture bleeding vessels, including the vena cava. In one patient the vena cava was sutured with survival.

The policy outlined above has resulted in full recovery in many patients with very severe liver injuries. There is, however, no room for complacency. Each patient should be assessed carefully both clinically and with CT scanning. Then the management involves performing the minimum procedure that will maintain the patient in reasonable condition.

Editorial Comment

Supplementing this excellent anatomic review based on the personal observations and experience of Professor Calne, a useful addition is shown in Figure 2.9, based on the work of Couinaud (1), which outlines a specific segmental anatomy plan that could be very useful to surgeons as a basis for understanding the hepatic arterial, portal venous, hepatic venous, and biliary anatomy of the liver.

In addition, the reader is referred to two excellent articles by Bismuth appearing in the *World Journal of Surgery* (2,3).

References

1. Couinaud, C. Le Foie. Etudes anatomiques et chirureicales. Paris: Masson, 1957.
2. Bismuth H. Surgical anatomy and anatomical surgery of the liver. *World J Surg* 1982;6:3–9.
3. Bismuth H, Houssin D, Castaing H. Major and minor segmentectomies "reglées" in liver surgery. *World J Surg* 1982;6:10–24.

Chapter 3
Liver Function

SHEILA SHERLOCK

Conventional tests are used to screen for unsuspected liver disease, to confirm its presence, and to estimate severity, assess prognosis, and evaluate therapy, (Table 3.1). Their use is being gradually reduced by more specific methods such as viral hepatitis markers and immunologic tests, such as the mitochondrial antibody for primary biliary cirrhosis, and by more accurate anatomic localization by ultrasonography and computed tomography (CT) scanning (1).

Serum Enzymes

Alkaline Phosphatase

The level rises in cholestasis, and to a lesser extent when liver cells are damaged. The increased serum alkaline phosphatase is of hepatic origin, as the alkaline phosphatase of bile is derived from the liver. Serum hepatic alkaline phosphatase may be distinguished from bone alkaline phosphatase by fractionation into isoenzymes, but this is not a routine method. Hepatic alkaline phosphatase is heat-stable whereas that from bone is heat-labile.

Raised levels are sometimes observed with primary or secondary tumors, even without jaundice or involvement of bone. Increased values are also found with other space-occupying lesions, such as amyloid, abscess, leukemia, or granulomas. Nonspecific mild evaluations are seen in a variety of conditions including Hodgkin's disease and heart failure. Isoenzymes are more specific but are not routinely performed.

Serum Gamma-Glutamyl Transpeptidase

Serum values are increased in both cholestasis and hepatocellular disease. Levels parallel serum alkaline phosphatase in cholestasis and may be used to confirm that a raised serum phosphatase is of hepatobiliary origin. Levels are increased with hepatic metastases, but not consistently.

Serum levels are raised in patients with alcohol abuse without liver disease. Increases may be due to microsomal enzyme-induction by alcohol. Unfortunately many factors influence the level so that increases are nonspecific.

Liver Plasma Proteins

The liver synthesizes numerous proteins (Table 3.2). They are produced by the hepatocyte being synthesized on polyribosomes bound to the rough endoplasmic reticulum, from which they are discharged into the plasma (2). A reduction in concentration usually reflects decreased hepatic synthesis although changes in plasma volume and losses, for example, into gut or urine, may contribute. Some liver-produced proteins are acute-phase reactants and rise in response to tissue injury such as inflammation. These include fibrinogen, haptoglobin, alpha$_1$-antitrypsin, C3 component of complement, and ceruloplasmin. An acute-phase response may contribute to well-maintained or even increased serum concentration of these proteins even with hepatocellular disease.

Ten grams of *albumin* are synthesized by the normal liver daily, whereas patients with cirrhosis can only synthesize about 4 g. In liver disease, the fall in serum albumin concentration is slow, for the half-life of albumin is about 22 days. Thus a patient with fulminant liver failure may die with a normal serum albumin value. A patient with decompensated cirrhosis would be expected to have a low level.

Haptoglobin is a glycoprotein composed of two types of polypeptide chains, alpha and beta, which are covalently associated by disulfide bonds (3).

Table 3.1. Essential Serum Methods in Hepatobiliary Disease

Test	Normal Range	International L	Value
Bilirubin			
Total	0.3–1.0 mg/dl	5–17 mmol	Diagnosis jaundice. Assess severity.
Conjugated	0.3 mg/dl	5 mmol	Gilbert's disease, hemolysis
Alkaline phosphatase	3–13 mg/dl		Diagnosis jaundice, hepatic
	1.5–4.0 Bodansky/dl	21–100	infiltrations
Aspartate transaminase		5–15	Early diagnosis hepatocellular
(AST SGOT)			disease, follow progress
Alanine transaminase		5–30	ALT relatively lower than AST in
(ALT SGPT)			alcoholism
Gamma-glutamyl		7–30	Diagnosis alcohol abuse, marker
transpeptidase		10–48	biliary phosphatase
Albumin	3.5–5.0 g/dl	35–50 g	Assess severity
Gammaglobulin	0.5–1.5 g/dl	5–15 g	Diagnosis chronic hepatitis and
			cirrhosis, follow course
Prothrombin time	10–14 sec		After vitamin K, assess severity
(PTT)			

Abbreviations: ALT, alanine aminotransferase; AST, aspartate aminotransferase.

Haptoglobin is largely synthesized by the hepatocyte. Hereditary deficiencies are frequent in U.S. blacks. Low values are found in severe chronic hepatocellular disease and in hemolytic crises.

Ceruloplasmin is the only copper-containing protein plasma and is responsible for the oxidase activity. A low concentration is found in 95% of those who are homozygous and in about 10% of those heterozygous for Wilson's disease (4). Ceruloplasmin increases to normal if a patient with Wilson's disease has a hepatic transplant. It is mandatory to estimate ceruloplasmin in all patients with chronic active hepatitis so that Wilson's disease, treatable with penicillamine therapy, may be excluded. However, low values are also found in very severe decompensated cirrhosis that is not due to Wilson's disease. High values are found in

Table 3.2. Plasma Proteins Synthesized by Hepatocytes and B-Lymphocytes

Plasma proteins synthesized by the hepatocyte
  Albumin
  Fibrinogen[a]
  Alpha$_1$-antitrypsin[a]
  Haptoglobin[a]
  Ceruloplasmin[a]
  Transferrin
  Prothrombin
  C3 and fetoprotein component of complement

Plasma proteins synthesized by B-lymphocytes
  IgG
  IgA
  IgM

[a]Acute-phase protein.

pregnancy, following estrogen therapy, and with large bile duct obstruction.

Transferrin is the main iron transport protein. Patients with treated idiopathic hemochromatosis show a consistent abnormality in hepatic iron uptake from transferrin (5), suggesting a cellular abnormality or iron uptake. The plasma transferrin is more than 90% saturated with iron in patients with untreated idiopathic hemochromatosis.

The C3 component of complement tends to be reduced in cirrhosis, normal in chronic active hepatitis, and increased in compensated primary biliary cirrhosis. Low values in fulminant hepatic failure reflect reduced hepatic synthesis and increased consumption due to activation of the complement system (6). Transient reductions are found in the early "immune complex" stage of acute hepatitis B.

Alpha-fetoprotein is a normal component of plasma proteins in human fetuses older than 6 weeks, and reaches maximum concentration at between 12 and 16 weeks of fetal life. A few weeks after birth it disappears from the circulation but reappears in the blood of patients with primary liver cancer and can be shown in the tumor (7). Raised values are also found with embryonic tumors of ovary and testis, with hepatoblastoma, and sometimes with carcinomas of the gastrointestinal tract with hepatic secondaries. Raised values are also found in hepatitis B-antigen-negative chronic active hepatitis and during acute viral hepatitis, where they may indicate hepatocellular regeneration. However, very high values with a positive test by immunodiffusion are virtually confined to primary liver cancer. In a hepatitis B surface antigen (HBsAg)-positive patient, rising values are of particular significance as an indicator of the development of carcinoma.

Amino Acids

A generalized or selective amino aciduria is a feature of hepatocellular disease. In patients with severe liver disease the usual picture is an increase in the plasma concentration of the aromatic amino acids, tyrosine, phenylalanine, and methionine, and a reduction in the branched-chain amino acids, valine, leucine, and isoleucine (8). The changes are explained by impaired hepatic function, portal systemic shunting of blood, and hyperinsulinemia and hyperglucagonemia. Patients with minimal liver disease also show changes, particularly a reduction in plasma proline, perhaps reflecting increased collagen production. There is no difference in the ratio between branched-chain and aromatic amino acids whether or not the patients show hepatic encephalopathy. Factors include hepatobiliary disease, concomitant drug administration, for instance, with barbiturates, and, in addition, there is a wide normal range (9). Its main use seems to be in children with suspected biliary tract disease. Screening serum gamma-glutamyl transpeptidase (γ-GT) levels may have led to more alcohol abusers being identified, although in one-third of these patients the serum level does not rise. The findings of increased levels, however, often lead to overinvestigation of an innocent who has never taken alcohol or a social drinker who has never abused alcohol.

Serum Transaminases (Aminotransferases)

Glutamic oxaloacetic transaminase (GOT) or aspartate transaminase aminotransferase is a mitochondrial enzyme present in large quantities in heart, liver, skeletal muscle, and kidney, and the serum level increases whenever these tissues are acutely injured, presumably due to release from damaged cells.

Glutamic pyruvic transaminase (GPT) or alanine aminotransferase is a cytosolic enzyme present in the liver. The absolute amount is less than GOT but a greater proportion is present there compared with heart and skeletal muscles so that a serum increase is more specific for liver damage than is GOT.

Transaminase determinations are useful in the early diagnosis of virus hepatitis. Measurements must be made early because normal values may be reached within a week of the onset. The patient may develop fatal acute hepatic necrosis in spite of falling transaminase values. Serial estimations are essential. Transaminase determinations are also useful in screening for liver injury due to drugs.

Routine screening may show unexpectedly raised transaminase levels often due to alcohol abuse, obesity, or heart failure. Very high levels are unusual in alcoholic liver disease. A high ratio of serum glutamic oxaloacetic transaminase (SGOT) to serum glutamic pyruvic transaminase (SGPT) (greater than 2) may be useful in diagnosing alcoholic hepatitis and cirrhosis (10). Results vary in cirrhosis, being particularly high in chronic active hepatitis. Other increases, usually less than five times the upper limit of normal, are noted in cholestasis and primary or secondary hepatic tumors.

Quantitative Assessment of Hepatic Function

Chronic liver diseases pass through a long period of minimum nonspecific symptoms ("compensated") until the final stage of ascites, jaundice, encephalopathy, and precoma ("decompensated"). Serial estimates of quantitative liver function in the early stages would be helpful both in monitoring treatment and in prognosis, but of no value in diagnosis. Such tests, however, suffer from the drawback of complexity so that they are now largely confined to clinical research.

Galactose Elimination Capacity

Galactose is pharmacologically safe and can be injected intravenously in a dose sufficient to saturate the enzyme system responsible for its elimination (11). The rate-limiting step is the initial phosphorylation by galactokinase. Account must be taken of the substantial fraction of the dose eliminated extrahepatically. This test seems to reflect hepatocellular function fairly accurately.

Breath Tests

Aminopyrine is oxidized (demethylated) by the cytochrome P-450 (microsomal) system in two steps to aminoantipyrine. It has many of the characteristics of an ideal breath test substance for the measurement of hepatic function (12–14). The aminopyrine is labeled with $^{14}CO_2$ and given by mouth. Samples are collected from the breath for intervals over 2 hours. Disappearance correlates with that from the plasma (15). The test reflects the residual functional microsomal mass and hence viable hepatic tissue. It is therefore of value in prognosis and to assess therapy rather than for screening or diagnosis. It may be useful to assess the effect of drugs on the hepatic microsomal enzyme function. Caffeine, galactose, and phenacetin have also been suitably labeled and used as breath test substances. However, all breath tests are complex and costly. They are unlikely to achieve general popularity.

Excretory Capacity

The old intravenous bromsulphalein (BSP) disappearance technique allowed an estimate of the storage capacity of the hepatocyte (BSP, TS) and its excretory function (BSP, T_m). It was abandoned, however, because of its complexity, its cost, and the untoward reactions to BSP (16).

Bile Acids

Bile acids are synthesized only in the liver, 250 to 500 mg being produced and lost in the feces daily. The primary bile acids, cholic acid and chenodeoxycholic acid, are formed from cholesterol (Fig. 3.1). Synthesis is controlled by the amount of bile acid returning to the liver in the enterohepatic circulation (Fig. 3.2). On contact with colonic bacteria the primary bile acids undergo 7-dehydroxylation with the production of the secondary bile acids, deoxycholic, and a very little lithocholic

acid. Tertiary bile acids, largely urosdeoxycholic acid, are formed in the liver by epymerization of secondary bile acids.

The bile acids are conjugated in the liver with the amino acids glycine or taurine forming bile salts. Sulfation and glucuronidation are additional detoxifying mechanisms that may be increased in cirrhosis or cholestasis (17). Bacteria can hydrolyze bile salts to bile acid and glycine or taurine. Bile salts are excreted into the biliary canaliculus against an enormous concentration gradient between liver and bile. Excretion depends on a carrier-mediated, active transport system. The bile salts enter into micellar association with cholesterol and phospholipids. In the upper small intestine the bile salt micelles are too large and too polar to be absorbed. They are intimately concerned with the digestion and absorption of lipids. When the terminal ileum and proximal colon are reached, absorption takes place by a transport process found only in the ileum. Nonionic passive diffusion occurs throughout the whole intestine and is most efficient for unconjugated dihydroxyglycine conjugates. The absorbed bile salts enter the portal venous blood and reach the liver, where they are taken up with great avidity by the hepatocytes. Synthesis is under negative feedback control. In the liver cell, they are reconjugated and re-excreted into the bile. Lithocholic acid is not re-excreted. The enterohepatic circulation of bile salts takes place 5 to 15 times daily. Because absorption efficiency differs, the individual bile acids have different synthesis and fractional turnover rates.

Changes in Disease

Bile salts increase the biliary excretion of water, lecithin, cholesterol, and conjugated bilirubin. Altered biliary excretion with defective biliary micelle

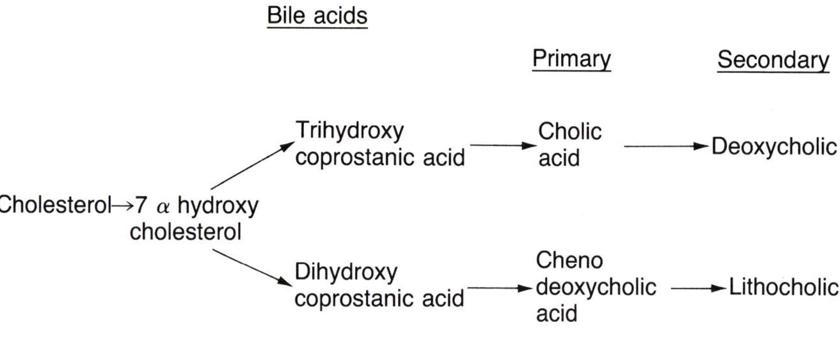

Figure 3.1. Production of primary and secondary bile acids. (Reproduced by permission from Sherlock S: *Diseases of the Liver and Biliary System*, 7th ed. Oxford: Blackwell Scientific Publications, 1985, p. 21.)

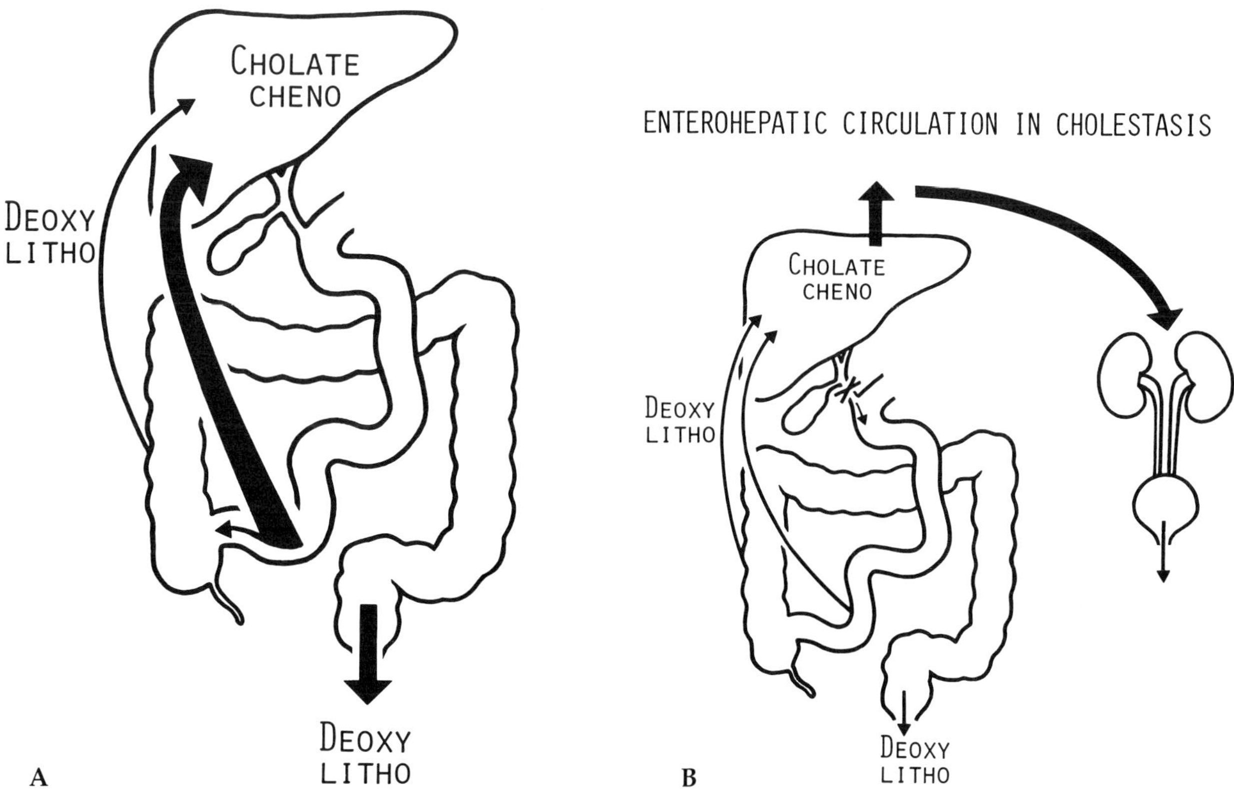

Figure 3.2. Enterohepatic circulation of bile acids in normal subjects (*a*) and in cholestasis (*b*). (Reproduced by permission from Sherlock S: *Diseases of the Liver and Biliary System*, 7th ed. Oxford: Blackwell Scientific Publications, 1985, p. 21.)

formation is important in the pathogenesis of gallstones and in the steatorrhoea of cholestasis. Bile salts help to emulsify dietary fat and probably play a part in the mucosal phase of absorption. Diminished secretion leads to steatorrhoea. They assist pancreatic lipolysis and release gastrointestinal hormones.

The postulated role of bile salts in causing the pruritus of cholestasis has never been satisfactorily confirmed. They may be responsible for target cells in the peripheral blood of jaundiced patients and for the secretion of conjugated bilirubin in urine. Removal of the terminal ileum interrupts the enterohepatic circulation and allows large amounts of primary bile acids to reach the colon and be dehydroxylated by bacteria, thus reducing the body's bile salt pool. The altered bile salts in the colon excite profound electrolyte and water loss with diarrhea.

Lithocholic acid is only slightly absorbed and is mostly excreted in the feces. It is cirrhogenic in animals and can be used to produce experimental gallstones. Taurolithocholic acid can cause intrahepatic cholestasis, perhaps by interfering with the bile salt–independent fraction of bile flow.

In cholestasis, bile acids are excreted in the urine by active transport and passive diffusion. They tend to be sulfated and these conjugates are actively secreted by the renal tubule (17).

Serum Bile Acids

Gas-liquid chromatography allows individual bile acids to be distinguished, but the method is time-consuming and the equipment expensive. Enzymatic assays are based on the use of bacterial 3-hydroxysteroid dehydrogenase. The use of a bioluminscence assay, capable of detecting bile salts in the picomole range, has brought the sensitivity of enzymatic techniques to that of radioimmunoassays (18). The method is simple and inexpensive. Radioimmunoassay techniques can measure individual bile acids (19) and commercial kits are available.

The concentration of total serum bile acids indicates the fraction that is absorbed from the intestine, but escapes extraction on its first passage through the liver. Intestinal load is more important than hepatic extraction in regulating peripheral serum bile acid levels. Raised levels of serum bile acids are specific for liver disease (20). Sensitivity of serum bile acids is less than originally thought in detecting hepatocellular damage in viral hepatitis or chronic liver disease. It is, however, better than the serum albumin or the prothrombin time because the value depends on hepatic injury, excretory function, and portal systemic shunting (21). The addition of a two-hour postprandial level to the fasting serum bile acid value adds little in sensitivity (22).

Bilirubin Metabolism and Jaundice

Bilirubin is the end-product of heme which is derived from hemoglobin and from myoglobin and many respiratory enzymes (Fig. 3.3). Approximately 6 g hemoglobin is broken down daily and 30 mg bilirubin is formed. Production takes place in reticuloendothelial cells.

About 20% of circulating bilirubin is not formed from the heme of mature erythrocytes. A small proportion comes from immature cells in spleen and bone marrow, and this component is increased in hemolytic states. The remainder is formed in the liver from heme cytochromes and unknown sources. This component is increased in pernicious anemia, congenital erythropoietic porphyria, and the Crigler-Najjar syndrome.

Unconjugated bilirubin is transported in the plasma tightly bound to albumin. A very small amount is dialyzable, but this can be increased by substances such as fatty acids and organic anions, which compete with bilirubin for albumin binding. The liver extracts such organic anions as fatty acids, bile acids, and nonbile acid cholephils, such as bilirubin, despite tight albumin binding (23). This results from interaction with the liver cell plasma membrane, perhaps involving a specific albumin receptor. Candidate carrier proteins have been isolated. Binding proteins, ligands, may be

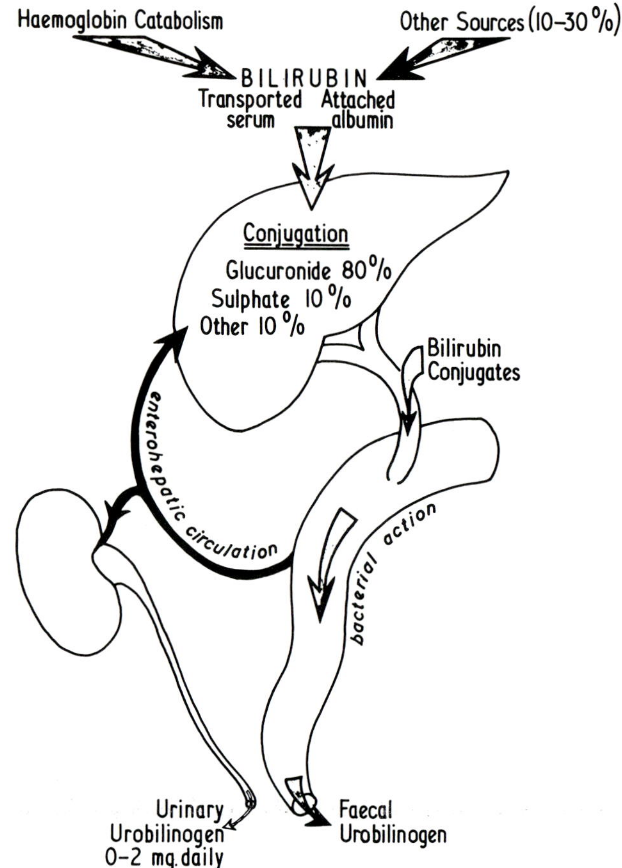

Figure 3.3. The metabolism of bilirubin. (Reproduced by permission from Sherlock S: *Diseases of the Liver and Biliary System*, 7th ed. Oxford: Blackwell Scientific Publications, 1985, p. 199.)

concerned with the transport of bilirubin from the plasma membrane to the endoplasmic reticulum.

Unconjugated bilirubin is nonpolar (lipid-soluble). It is converted to a polar (water-soluble) compound by conjugation and this allows its excretion into the bile. This involves an enzyme of the microsomal fraction called bilirubin uridine diphosphate (UDP) glucuronyl transferase, which converts the unconjugated bilirubin to the conjugated bilirubin monoglucuronide. Reduced concentrations of the enzyme are of importance in the neonate and in Gilbert's and Crigler-Najjar's hyperbilirubinemias.

The major bilirubin conjugate in human bile is the diglucuronide. The mechanisms and the site for the conversion of the mono- to the diglucuronide is still uncertain (24). It has always been unclear why in the late stages of cholestatic or hepatocellular jaundice, despite high serum bilirubin levels, none can be detected in the urine. This is apparently due to a third type of bilirubin, a bilirubin fractionated in van den Bergh's reaction. It is monoconjugate covalently bound to albumin and has a half-life of 3 weeks (25). It would not be filtered by the glomerulus and hence would not reach the urine. This lessens the practical application of urinary bilirubin tests. The third type of bilirubin accounts for the slow fall in jaundice after relief of biliary obstruction. Biliary canalicular excretion of bilirubin is thought to be an energy-requiring process that transports conjugated bilirubin across the canalicular surface of the hepatocyte into bile against a concentration gradient. Biliary excretion of glucoronide is the rate-limiting factor in the transport of bilirubin from plasma to bile. Secretion of the conjugated pigments involves a carrier-mediated active transport system. There are at least two independent mechanisms for biliary secretion of organic anions, one for bile salts and the other for other organic anions, including bilirubin. This is exemplified by the Dubin-Johnson syndrome, where there is a defect in the excretion of conjugated bilirubin while bile salt excretion is usually normal.

Classification of Jaundice

Jaundice might arise in four different ways. First, there may be increased bilirubin load on the liver cell. Second, there may be a disturbance in uptake and transport of bilirubin within the hepatocyte. Third, there may be defects in conjugation. Finally, the defect may be in the canalicular domain of the liver cell membrane with impaired excretion into the bile or there may be an obstruction to the large bile channels, thus preventing bilirubin from reaching the intestines. A simple classification is into three predominant types, prehepatic, hepatic, and cholestatic (Fig. 3.4). There is much overlap between them, and particularly between the hepatic and cholestatic varieties.

Total serum bilirubin levels are increased with normal transaminases, alkaline phosphatase, and proteins. The circulating serum bilirubin is largely unconjugated. Bilirubin cannot be detected in the urine. The cause may be hemolysis or a familial disturbance of bilirubin metabolism.

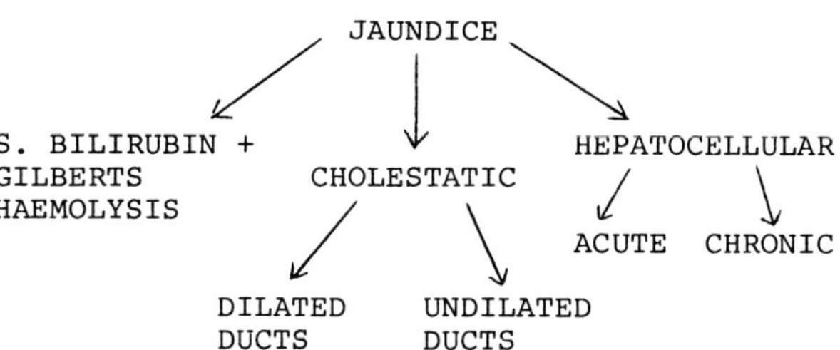

Figure 3.4. Classification of jaundice. (Reproduced by permission from Sherlock S: *Diseases of the Liver and Biliary System.* Oxford: Blackwell Scientific Publications, 1985, p. 202.)

Jaundice is accompanied by fatigue and malaise with varying degrees of hepatic failure, evidenced by encephalopathy, ascites, hypotension, and reduced synthesis of coagulation factors. Serum biochemistry shows increases in transaminases. Serum albumin levels are reduced in the long-standing case.

This is due to failure of adequate amounts of bile to reach the duodenum. Pruritus is prominent and the patient becomes increasingly pigmented. The serum shows increases in conjugated bilirubin, alkaline phosphatase, total cholesterol, and conjugated bile acids. Steatorrhoea is responsible for weight loss and malabsorption of the fat-soluble vitamins A, D, E, and K.

Investigation of the Jaundiced Patient

The importance of an accurate history and physical examination with routine testing of the urine and inspection of the feces cannot be overemphasized (Table 3.3). This routine is followed by basic biochemical tests, hemoglobin, white cell, and platelet counts, and a prothrombin time. A chest film is mandatory. Tests for hepatitis B [HBsAg and IgM anti-hepatitis B core (HB$_c$)] are helpful not only to diagnose a hepatitis B–related disease, but to alert health care staff of the risk of contracting the disease. Acute hepatitis A is diagnosed by the IgM anti-hepatitis A virus (HAV). There is no test for non-A, non-B hepatitis.

It is should now be clear whether the patient's jaundice is of prehepatic, hepatic, or cholestatic type. In the cholestatic patient, clinical or biochem-

Table 3.3. General Features of the Common Types of Jaundice.

	Gallstones in Common Bile Duct	Carcinoma Ampullary Region	Acute Virus Hepatitis	Cholestatic Drug Jaundice
Antecedent history	Dyspepsia, previous attack	Nil	Contacts, injections, transfusion, or nil	Taking drug
Pain	Constant epigastric, biliary colic, or none	Constant epigastric, back, or none	Ache over liver or none	None
Pruritus	+	+	Transient	+
Rate of development of jaundice	Slow	Slow	Rapid	Rapid
Type of jaundice	Fluctuant or persistent	Usually but not always progressive	Rapid onset, slow fall with recovery	Variable, usually mild
Weight loss	Slight to moderate	Progressive	Slight	Slight
Examination				
Diathesis	Frequently woman, obese	>40 yr	Usually young	Often older woman, psychotic
Depth of jaundice	Moderate	Deep	Variable	Variable, rash sometimes
Ascites	0	Rarely with metastases	If severe and prolonged	0
Liver	Enlarged, slightly tender	Enlarged, not tender	Enlarged and tender	Slightly enlarged
Palpable gallbladder	0	+ (sometimes)	0	0
Tender gallbladder area	+	0	0	0
Palpable spleen	0	Occasionally	About 20%	0
Temperature	↑	Not usually	↑ Onset only	↑ Onset
Laboratory investigations				
Leucocyte count	↑ or normal	↑ or normal	↓	Normal
Differential leucocytes	Polymorphs ↑	−	Lymphocytes ↑	Eosinophilia at onset
Feces				
Color	Intermittently pale	Acholic	Variable, light → dark	Pale
Occult blood	0	+	0	0
Urine: urobilin(ogen)	+	Absent	− Early + Late	− Early + Late
S. bilirubin (mg/dl)	Usually 3–10	Steady rise to 15–30	Varies with severity	Variable
S. alkaline phosphatase KA (u/dl)	>30	>30	<30	>30
S. aspartate transaminase (U)	<100	<100	>100 (early)	<100
S. total cholesterol (mg/dl)	Variable	Variable	<300	>300
Radiology				
Plain film abdomen	Gallstones 10%	Hepatomegaly	Hepatomegaly, slight	Hepatomegaly, slight
CT and ultrasound	Gallstones	Dilated ducts	Splenomegaly	Normal

(Reproduced by permission from Sherlock S: *Diseases of the Liver and Biliary System*, 7th ed. Oxford: Blackwell Scientific Publications, 1985.)

ical clues are not infallible and, consequently, neither is clinical evaluation. A small proportion of patients with extrahepatic obstruction are incorrectly diagnosed as having intrahepatic cholestasis, whereas a larger proportion of patients with intrahepatic disease are thought to have extrahepatic obstruction (26). Clinical evaluation is quite sensitive as defined by the number of true-positive tests expressed as a percentage of total true-positive plus false-negative ones.

Various algorithms (Fig. 3.5) are laid down for the investigation of the cholestatic patient. The

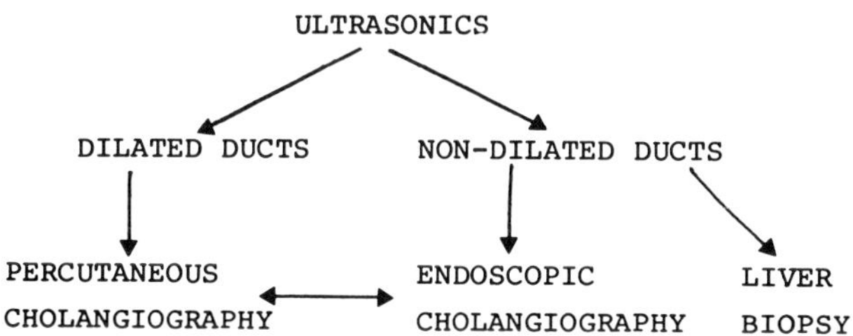

Figure 3.5. Diagnosis of cholestasis. (Reproduced by permission from Sherlock S: *Diseases of the Liver and Biliary System.* Oxford: Blackwell Scientific Publications, 1985, p. 227.)

sequence employed depends on the clinical impression, the facilities available, and the risk of each investigation. Cost plays a part (26,27).

Most physicians would agree that the first procedure in distinguishing hepatocellular from surgical "main duct obstructive jaundice" is electronically activated, linear array, real-time ultrasonography (28,29). This takes little time and may be performed by the clinician in the outpatient clinic. Knowledge of how to do a real-time ultrasound examination may be of more use to a hepatologist than knowing how to use the stethoscope, although both skills are desirable. Generalized intrahepatic biliary dilatation can be diagnosed. However, delineation of the distal extrahepatic ducts is rather difficult due mainly to intestinal gas. Hepatocellular jaundice is usually associated with a collapsed gallbladder with a thickened wall. Primary liver cancer, cholangiocarcinoma of the hilum, and carcinoma of proximal bile duct, gallbladder, and head of pancreas may be diagnosed with over 90% certainty. The procedure, however, must be followed by further delineation of the biliary system by direct cholangiography. Endoscopic retrograde cholangipancreatography (ERCP) or percutaneous transhepatic cholangiography (PTC) are sensitive and specific in detecting extrahepatic obstruction. A normal cholangiogram effectively rules it out. Site and etiology are correctly defined in over 90% of patients studied (30). Both methods have low but significant complication rates. ERCP is expensive and requires more skill than PTC, but provides more diagnostic information. The method chosen should be one that will be useful diagnostically and might be helpful therapeutically. Thus ERCP might precede endoscopic retrograde

sphincterotomy for common bile duct stone removal, and PTC is the choice when stenting of a malignant biliary stricture is being considered.

Cholestasis and the Secretion of Bile

Cholestasis is defined as failure of bile secretion by the hepatocyte. To the clinician it implies green jaundice with relative well-being, pruritus, dark bilirubin-containing urine, and pale fatty stools. To the clinical chemist, it implies a pile-up of all biliary substances in the blood; in particular, serum bile acid levels are increased. To the morphologist, it means visible stagnation of bile pigment in hepatocytes, bile canaliculi, and Kupffer cells. Bile is formed by several different energy-dependent transport processes (Fig. 3.6). Bile salts passing into the biliary canaliculus are the most important factors promoting bile flow. This *bile salt–dependent* active secretion carries with it bile pigments, organic anions, and water. The bile salts are steroids and could also change flow by altering the function of the canalicular membrane. *Bile salt–independent* flow is linked to active sodium transport, and a sodium Na^+, K^{2+} ATPase ion pump is the driving force. It is located on the basal-lateral surface of the hepatocyte. The cytoskeleton also plays an important part in bile secretion. Actin microfilaments are important in cell movement and cell shape. Microtubular systems may help transmit biliary lipids (cholesterol and phospholipid) to the canalicular membrane.

Ductular bile flow modifies canalicular flow by adding an inorganic electrolyte solution consisting mostly of sodium bicarbonate and sodium chlo-

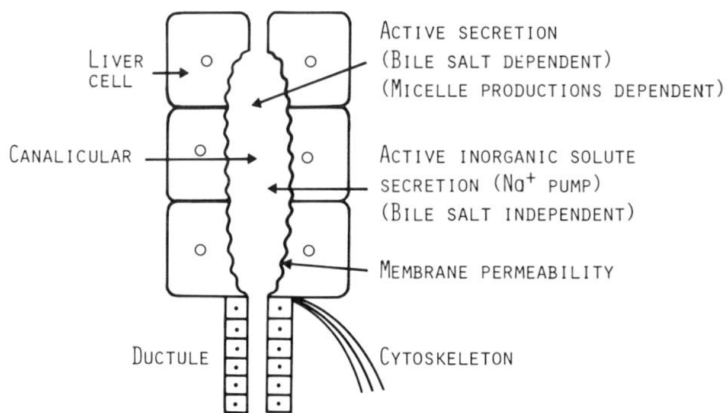

Figure 3.6. Mechanisms of bile formation. (Reproduced by permission from Sherlock S: *Diseases of the Liver and Biliary System.* Oxford: Blackwell Scientific Publications, 1985, p. 218.)

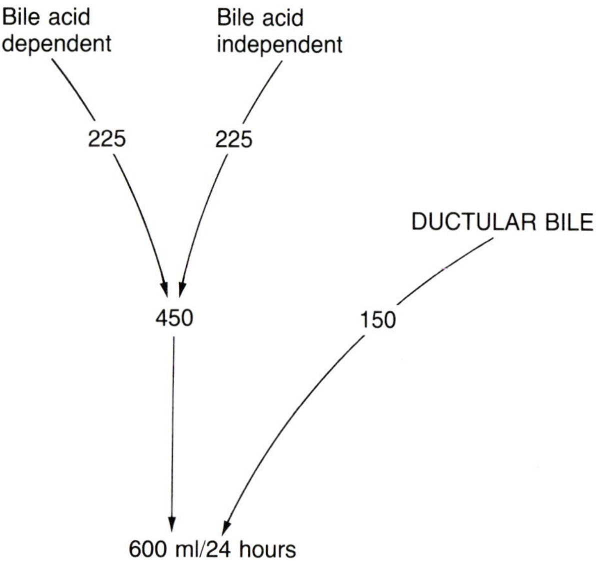

Figure 3.7. Twenty-four-hour volumes of bile in humans. (Reproduced by permission from Sherlock S: *Diseases of the Liver and Biliary System*, 7th ed. Oxford: Blackwell Scientific Publications, 1985, p. 218.)

ride. A limited amount of water and sodium chloride may be absorbed. Ductular bile flow is largely controlled by secretin. Gallbladder contraction is controlled by cholecystokinin. Ductular flow may serve to flush salts from the lower end of the common bile duct following gallbladder contraction. In humans, total bile flow is about 600 ml/24 hr, of which 225 ml is bile acid–dependent, 225 ml bile acid–independent, and 150 ml ductular (Fig. 3.7).

Intrahepatic cholestasis is initiated by failure of the Na^+, K^+ ATPase ion pump, dysfunction of the canalicular membrane with its chemical and physical characteristics, or dysfunction of the cytoskeleton and the tight junctions (Fig. 3.8). It is difficult to know which lesion is primary or secondary, or why it persists in some patients and subsides rapidly in others. The causes are numerous and include viral hepatitis, primary biliary cirrhosis, alcohol, and various drugs such as the promazines and sex hormones.

The Immune System and the Liver

Reticuloendothelial Phagocytic Activity

The hepatic reticuloendothelial system includes Kupffer cells and other sinusoidal cells (32). Pha-

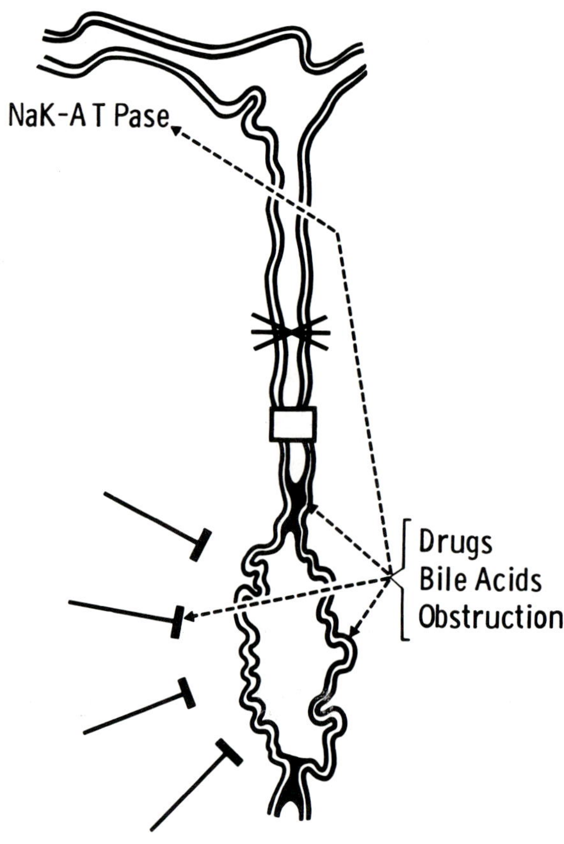

Figure 3.8. Cholestatic drugs or bile acids and biliary obstruction cause cholestasis by interfering with the Na^+-K^+-ATPase, located on the sinusoidal pole of the hepatocyte, the cytoskeleton, the canalicular membrane, and the tight junction between canaliculus and sinusoid. (Reproduced by permission from Sherlock S: *Diseases of the Liver and Biliary System*, 7th ed. Oxford: Blackwell Scientific Publications, 1985, p. 216.)

goctic function is impaired in cirrhosis despite compensatory overactivity of the reticuloendothelial system in other organs such as bone marrow and spleen (33) (Fig. 3.9).

Acute bacterial infections are common in cirrhosis. This has been related to defective leukocyte chemotaxis, low levels of serum complement, and impaired cell-mediated immunity, but depressed reticuloendothelial function plays a major role (34). Bacterial infections are particularly common in decompensated cirrhosis, where reduced reticuloendothelial system phagocytic activity may even be related to prognosis.

Kupffer cells play an important part in the reg-

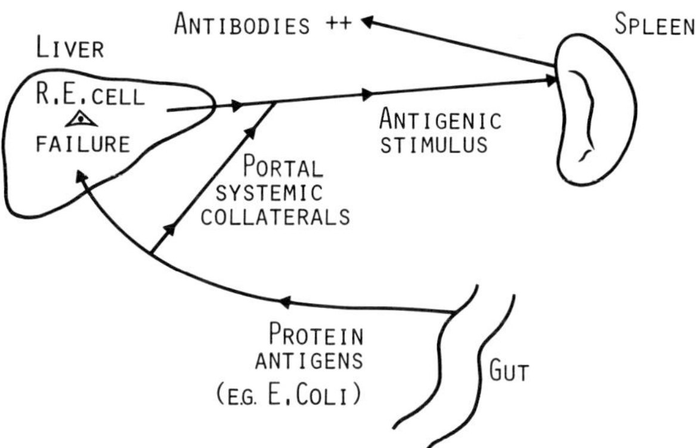

Figure 3.9. Mechanism of increased antibody levels in cirrhosis. (Reproduced by permission from Sherlock S: *Diseases of the Liver and Biliary System*, 7th ed. Oxford: Blackwell Scientific Publications, 1985, p. 341.)

ulation of immune responses to gut-derived antigens. Patients with chronic liver disease, notably chronic active hepatitis, have high-titer antibodies to the gut-associated bacteria *Escherichia coli* and bacteroides but not to non-gut-associated bacteria, such as *Hemophilus influenzae* (35). The high titers may be explained by failure of Kupffer's cells in the diseased liver to degrade antigens absorbed from the gut. This derangement of normal Kupffer's cell function is thought to be at least partially responsible for the hypergammaglobulinemia found in patients with chronic liver disease (36).

Autoantibodies

These are non organ-specific and cannot be casually implicated with any individual liver disease. Their appearance contributes to evidence of an immunoregulatory defect (37).

SMOOTH MUSCLE ANTIBODY

The reaction is heterogeneous and depends on different components of the cellular cytoskeleton. In autoimmune chronic active hepatitis, positive results are almost always due to antiactin. Low titers in various forms of viral hepatitis are due to a heterogeneous group of cytoskeleton proteins termed intermediate filaments.

NUCLEAR ANTIBODIES

Nuclear antibodies, as seen in systemic lupus erythematosus, are usually detected in autoim-

mune chronic active hepatitis; a cutoff is a titer of 1 in 20 or greater. Antibodies to double-stranded DNA are rarely found—in about 10% of patients. However, positive smooth muscle antibody (SMA) or a nuclear antibody are acceptable for the diagnosis of chronic active hepatitis of immune-type.

MITOCHONDRIAL ANTIBODIES

Mitochondrial antibodies (M-antibodies) reacting against the inner cristae of mitochondrial membranes are virtually constant in patients with primary biliary cirrhosis (PBC) if an adequate technique is used (38). Specificity is gained at titers of 1 in 80. Few diseases, other than Sjögren's disease, give positive titers. There are various subgroups of M-antibody reactive with different components of mitochondrial membranes (39). The characteristic one for PBC is known as M2 and can be differentiated from the various other types, one of which (M4) is found in a mixed syndrome with overlapping features of chronic active hepatitis and PBC.

Liver-Specific Antigens

Identification of the liver-specific antigen that initiates immunologic liver injury has been fraught with difficulty (37). The first candidate, liver-specific lipoprotein (LSP) proved unspecific, while the next, liver membrane antigen (LMAg), was associated with high antibody levels in the serum of patients with autoimmune chronic active hepatitis and low levels in other forms of inflammatory liver disease, including acute hepatitis A. The antibody reaction seemed related to persisting inflammation and necrosis, rather than to a specific etiology. Moreover, the hepatic membrane contains multiple immunoreactive components which might be responsible. There is urgent need for extraction and biochemical characterization of liver cell plasma membrane constituents (37).

Immunoregulation

This is disturbed in autoimmune chronic active hepatitis. Monoclonal demonstration of serum T cells shows overrepresentation of helper subsets, compared with suppressor (40). In the HB$_s$Ag-positive patient, the reverse is seen, the suppressors being in excess. Studies on the mononuclear cell infiltrate in chronic active hepatitis show that T cells predominate in all the specimens of liver biopsies studied. The T4/T8 cell ratio is higher in the HB$_s$Ag-negative patient than in the HBsAg-positive one (41). Much, however, needs to be done to understand the effective mechanisms initiating immunologic injury in primary biliary cirrhosis and chronic active hepatitis, and in identifying what determines tolerance.

References

1. Sherlock S. *Diseases of the Liver and Biliary System*, 8th ed. Oxford: Blackwell Scientific Publications. In press.
2. Tavill AS, The synthesis and degradation of liver produced proteins. *Gut* 1972; 13:225–241.
3. Putnam FW, *The Plasma Proteins*, 2nd ed. New York: Academic Press, 1972
4. Scheinberg IH, Sternlieb I. *Wilson's Disease*, Philadelphia: WB Saunders, 1983.
5. Batey RG, Pettit JE, Nicholas AW, Hoffbrand AV. Hepatic iron clearance from serum in treated hemochromatosis. *Gastroenterology* 1978; 75:856–859.
6. Potter BJ, Trueman AM, Jones EA. Serum complement in chronic liver disease. *Gut* 1973; 14:451–456.
7. Alpert E. Human alpha-fetoprotein (AFP). In: Popper H, Schaffner F, eds. *Progress in Liver Diseases*, vol. 5. New York: Grune & Stratton, 1976.
8. Morgan MY, Marshall AW, Milsom JP, Sherlock S. Plasma amino-acid patterns in liver disease. *Gut* 1982; 23:362–370.
9. Penn R, Worthington DJ. Is serum gamma glutamyl-transferase a misleading test? *Br Med J* 1983; 286:531–535.
10. Cohen JA, Kaplan MM. The SGOT/SGPT ratio—an indicator of alcoholic liver disease. *Dig Dis Sci* 1979; 24:835–838.
11. Bircher J. Quantitative assessment of deranged hepatic function: A missed opportunity. *Semin Liv Dis* 1983; 3:275–284.
12. Galizzi J, Long RG, Billing BH, Sherlock S. Assessment of the (14C)-amino-pyrine breath test in liver disease. *Gut* 1978; 19:40–45.
13. Monroe PS, Baker AL, Schneider JF, Krager PS, Klein PD, Schoeller D. The aminopyrine breath test and serum bile acids reflect histologic severity in chronic hepatitis. *Hepatology* 1982;2:317–322.
14. Baker AL, Kotake AN, Schoeller DA. Clinical utility of breath tests for the assessment of hepatic function. *Semin Liv Dis* 1983; 3:318–329.
15. Bircher J, Kupfer A, Gikalov I, Presig R. Aminopyrine demethylation measured by breath analysis in cirrhosis. *Clin Pharmacol Ther* 1976; 20:484–492.
16. Hacki W, Bircher J, Presig R. A new look at the plasma disappearance of sulfobromopthalein (BSP): Correlation with the BSP transport maximum and the hepatic plasma flow in man. *J Lab Clin Med* 1976; 88:1019–1031.
17. Summerfield JA, Cullen, Barnes S, Billing BH. Evidence for renal control of urinary excretion of bile acids and bile acid sulphates in the cholestatic syndrome. *Clin Sci Mol Med* 1977; 52:51–65.
18. Roda A, Kircka LJ, De Luca M, Hofmann AF. Bioluminescence measurement of primary bile acids using immobilized 7-alpha-hydroxysteroid dehydrogenase: Application to serum bile acids. *J Lipid Res* 1982; 23:1345–1361.
19. Baqir Y, Ross EP, Bouchier IAD. Homogenous enzyme immunoassay of chenodeoxycholate conjugates in serum. *Ann Biochem* 1979; 93:361–365.
20. Ferraris R, Colombatti G, Fiorentini MT, Carosso R, Arossa W, De La Pierre M. Diagnostic value of serum bile acids and routine liver function tests in hepatobiliary disease: Sensitivity, specificity and predictive value. *Dig Dis Sci* 1983; 28:129–136.
21. Hofmann AF. The aminopyrine demethylation breath test and the serum bile acid level: Nominated but not yet elected to join the common liver tests. *Hepatology* 1982; 2: 512–517.
22. Berry W, Richen J. Bile acid metabolism: Its relation to clinical disease. *Semin Liv Dis* 1983; 3:330–340.
23. Stremmel W, Tavoloni N, Berk PD. Uptake of bilirubin by the liver. *Semin Liv Dis* 1983; 3:1–10.
24. Chowdhury JR, Chowdhury NR. Conjugation and excretion of bilirubin. *Semin Liv Dis* 1983; 3:11–23.
25. Weiss JS, Gautam A, Lauff JJ, Sundberg MW, Jatlow P, Boyer JL, et al. The clinical importance of a protein-bound fraction of serum bilirubin in patients with hyperbilirubinaemia. *N Engl J Med* 1983; 309:147–150.
26. Scharschmidt BF, Goldberg HI, Schmid R. Current concepts in diagnosis. Approach to the patient with cholestatic jaundice. *N Engl J Med* 1983; 308:1515–1519.
27. Richter JM, Silverstein M, Shapiro R. Suspected obstructive jaundice: A decision analysis of diagnostic strategies. *Ann Intern Med* 1983; 99:46–51.
28. Okuda K, Tsuchiya Y, Saotome N, Ohnishi K. How to investigate cholestasis: Utility of ultrasound as the first imaging study. *Semin Liv Dis* 1983; 3:308–317.
29. Matzen P, Malchow-Moller A, Brun B, Gronvalls S, Haubek A, Henriksen JH, et al. Ultrasonography, computed tomography and cholescintigraphy in suspected obstructive jaundice—a prospective comparative study. *Gastroenterology* 1983; 84:1492–1497.
30. Vennes JA, Bone JH. Approach to the jaundiced patient. *Gastroenterology* 1983; 84:1615–1618.
31. Popper H. Cholestasis: The future of a past and present riddle. *Hepatology* 1981; 1:187–191.
32. Knook DL, Wisse K. *Sinusoidal Liver Cells*. Amsterdam: Biomedical Press, 1982.
33. Thomas HC, MacSween RNM, White RG. Role of the liver in controlling the immunogenicity of commensal bacteria in the gut. *Lancet* 1973; 1:1288–1291.
34. Rimola A, Soto R, Bory F, Arroyo V, Piera C, Rodes J. Reticuloendothelial system phagocytic activity in cirrhosis and its relation to bacterial infections and prognosis. *Hepatology* 1984; 4:53–58.
35. Triger DR, Alp MH, Wright R. Bacterial and dietary antibodies in liver disease. *Lancet* 1972; 1:60–61.
36. Hodges JR, Wright R. Normal immune mechanisms in the gut and liver. *Clin Sci* 1982; 63:339–347.
37. Mackay IR. Immunological aspects of chronic active hepatitis. *Hepatology* 1983; 3:724–728.
38. Munoz LE, Thomas HC, Scheuer PJ, Doniach D, Sherlock S. Is mitochondrial antibody diagnostic of primary biliary cirrhosis? *Gut* 1981; 22:136–138.
39. Berg PA, Klein R, Lindenborn-Fotinos J, Kloppel G. AT-Pase associated antigen (M2): Marker antigen for serological diagnosis of primary biliary cirrhosis. *Lancet* 1982; 2: 1423–1426.
40. Thomas HC, MacSween RNM, White RG. Role of the liver in controlling the immunogenicity of commensal bacteria in the gut. *Lancet* 1973; 1:60–61.
41. Colucci IG, Colombo M, Del Ninno E, Paronetto F. In situ

characterization by monoclonal antibodies of the mononuclear cell infiltrate in chronic active hepatitis. *Gastroenterology* 1983; 85:1138–1145.

Editorial Comment

There is little one could add to expand or embellish this excellent article on liver function by Professor Dame Sherlock, but some recent data on amino acid clearance as an indication of hepatic function as related to operative mortality have been published by a group in the Department working with Dr. G. H. Clowes. A summary by Dr. Clowes of these data follows in lieu of any other comment by the editor. There is some duplication in the discussion of hepatic function, which serves as prologue to Dr. Clowes' findings and complements the material presented in the previous chapter. Special material on amino acid clearance during liver transplantation is provided separately after Chapter 23 by Dr. Roger Jenkins.

Chapter 3A
Amino Acid Clearance in Liver Disease: Indicator of Hepatocyte Function, Prognosis, and Selection of Treatment

GEORGE II. A. CLOWES, Jr.

Health and, in fact, life itself depend upon the numerous metabolic processes of the liver. Following injury or the onset of infection, both hazards of surgery, the balance between survival and death is determined by the adequacy of a series of major defensive responses. Among those of greatest importance are (1) hemostasis, (2) activation of the immune system, (3) transport of substrates and metabolites by the integrated organ systems, and (4) wound healing. Each requires sufficient cellular energy production as well as synthesis of many special proteins.

At the center of this vast complex of metabolic processes lies the liver, perfused both by arterial and portal venous blood. In addition to its absolutely essential role of constantly regulating supplies of energy fuel substrates to all tissues, the liver has certain specific synthetic, secretory, and immunologic functions. All are needed for homeostasis in normal life. To a far greater extent, the reserve capacity of each is called upon to mount the defensive responses necessary to survival. Just as in septic or injured patients with normal liver activity, those with hepatic failure must mount the same series of defensive responses to survive. Thus, insufficiency of any hepatic function caused by cirrhosis or other liver disease may prejudice the balance between survival and death. This concept is summarized in Figure 3A.1.

The high morbidity and mortality rates of cirrhotic surgical patients are well known (1). Death, if not from hemorrhage or coagulation defects, is usually caused by overwhelming infection often accompanied by progressive multisystem failure or septic shock (2–6). Thus, means for assessing the liver's ability to respond adequately to satisfy the many metabolic demands associated with stress become matters of concern to physicians and surgeons who are caring for patients with significant liver failure. Numerous tests have been devised to measure the extent to which various "liver functions" may be impaired. Values obtained by these methods and their clinical significance are presented Chapter 3. However, relatively little success has attended efforts to measure in the clinical setting the reserve metabolic capacity of the liver under conditions of infection, trauma, or liver failure. Because of the liver's central role in mounting the metabolic defensive responses involving mobilization and utilization of amino acids (AAs), it is the purpose of this chapter to demonstrate how variations in AA metabolism, measured by clearance rates, can serve as indicators of hepatocyte function, prognosis, and aid in selection of therapy for patients with cirrhosis or other hepatic diseases.

A brief review of hepatic physiology is presented to emphasize the importance of AA metabolism in the closely interrelated functions of protein synthesis and energy production in all aspects of survival and recovery. Because of certain similarities, the characteristic alterations of AA metabolism observed in the presence of invasive infection or liver dysfunction are reviewed. Their clinical significance will become apparent when values from patients who survived are compared to those who subsequently died. Furthermore, the degree to which AA metabolism differs from normal can be employed to assess the risk to cirrhotic patients following general surgical procedures, various types of portacaval shunts, or liver resections (3,4). Finally, another group of patients,

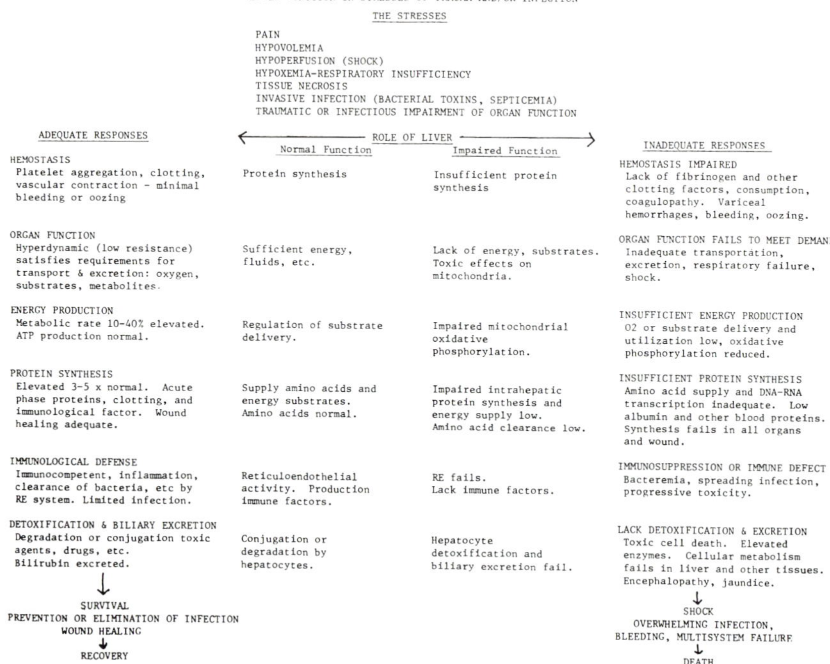

Figure 3A.1. The stresses and major responses to trauma and infection, both hazards of surgery, are presented diagramatically. If each response is adequate to counteract or prevent the cellular and tissue damage done by one or another stress, the patient survives to recover. Various liver functions play important roles in mounting adequate responses. Failure of any major liver function can impair one or more of the responses to stress, in which case the result is apt to be loss of immunocompetence, infection, multisystem failure, and death.

whose tests of AA utilization reveal liver impairment of such severity that the risk of mortality precludes any of the standard operations, can then be considered as candidates for hepatic transplantation (7).

Hepatic Physiology

The principal functions of the liver are performed by two cell types: *parenchymal cells* (hepatocytes) and *macrophages* (Kupffer's cells). Circulation is provided both by the arterial and portal system. Arterial blood from the hepatic artery passes through arterioles and capillaries to enter the sinusoids. Virtually all of the portal venous blood from the spleen, pancreas, and gut enters the sinusoids. Venules drain the sinusoids into the hepatic veins, which in turn empty into the vena cava.

The metabolic activities of the *hepatocytes*, summarized in Figure 3A.2, may be grouped under five major heads: (1) Provision of energy fuel substrates. Glucose is produced from fructose, galactose, lactate, and the carbon skeletons of deaminated amino acids. Small quantities of glucose are derived from glycerol. Fat, cholesterol, and lipoproteins are synthesized from glucose and from AA carbon skeletons; (2) Regulation of blood

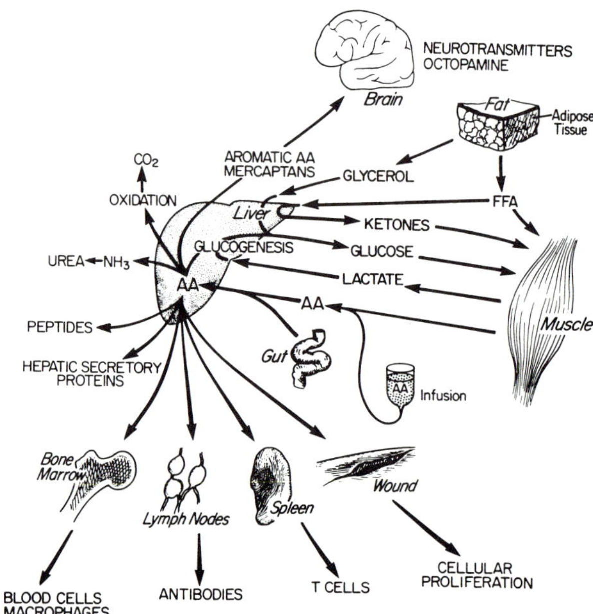

Figure 3A.2. The central role of the liver in regulating distribution of fat, carbohydrate, and AAs, the substrates for oxidative energy production by cells throughout the body are presented. Also illustrated are the various routes whereby AAs are employed by the liver and other central tissues in mounting immunologic or other defensive responses.

AA concentration, accomplished by deamination and degradation of excess AAs not required for peptide or protein synthesis; (3) Synthesis of hepatic secretory and structural proteins; (4) Secretion of bile acids and production of bilirubin for excretion into the bile canaliculi (8); (5) Detoxification of drugs and toxic substances of exogenous or endogenous origin by conjugation or degradation. Of the latter two functions, nothing further will be said in this chapter. Rather, the objective is to deal with the role of the liver in energy and protein metabolism as they pertain to immunocompetence and organ function in survival.

The *hepatic macrophages* are specialized endothelial cells located within the sinusoids. They constitute, with the splenic macrophages, approximately 85% to 95% of the reticuloendothelial (RE) system (9,10). These cells rapidly remove blood-borne bacteria and endotoxin from the portal circulation. The RE system is the last defense against widespread dissemination of microorganisms by bacteremia when inflammatory processes anywhere in the body have failed to limit microbial invasion. Phagocytosis by Kupffer's cells as by other macrophages depends upon both energy for synthesis of lysozymes and other proteins as well as for activation of superoxide radicals for bacterial killing (11,12). In particular, the Kupffer's cells require for phagocytosis of particulate matter the presence of fibronectin, a large alpha-$_2$-glycoprotein, which is synthesized by hepatocytes, fibroblasts, and vascular endothelial cells (13). In cirrhosis or sepsis, fibronectin concentration in the blood may be low, and thereby, impede the phagocytic process. Hofeler and Klingemann (14) found plasma fibronectin to be significantly depleted in acute hepatic failure and in all but the earliest stages of cirrhosis. As shown by their data presented in Table 3A.1, normal fibronectin concentration was 259 $\pm$ 34 mg/l compared to 167 $\pm$ 76 mg/l in advanced cirrhotics.

Experimentally, clearance of bacteria injected into the bloodstream occurs within 4 to 5 minutes. Although preserved until late in the progress of liver failure, the process may be significantly slowed due to reduced blood flow and oxygen supply. Impaired production of energy [adenosine triphosphate (ATP) and energy-rich phosphate bonds ($\sim$P)] in the Kupffer's cells (15) may contribute to inadequate lysosomal enzyme and superoxide production. Alternatively blockage of RE

Table 3A.1. Plasma Fibronectin

Patient Group	No.	Mg/L	Significance from Normal
Healthy	35	259 ± 34	
Cirrhosis			
Stage I	10	238 ± 34	NS
Stage II	10	217 ± 35	P <0.005
Stage III	25	167 ± 76	P <0.005
Acute hepatic failure	6	133 ± 87	P <0.005

Adapted by permission from Hofeler H, Klingemann HG. *J Clin Biochem* 1984; 22:15–19.
Abbreviations = NS, not significant.

phagocytic activity by particulate or other matter previously engulfed into phagosomes slows phagocytic disposal of bacteria and other matter.

The great permeability of sinusoidal endothelium readily allows exchange between hepatocytes, the interstitial fluid, and the blood plasma. The normal sinusoidal pressure being 2 to 4 mmHg, only slightly greater than inferior vena caval pressure, most of the secretory proteins and plasma proteins normally diffuse back into the sinusoids and veins. The remainder are transferred to the blood by lymphatic drainage from the liver. However, an elevation of hepatic sinusoidal pressure, whether caused by intrinsic venular or extrinsic venous obstruction, results in a significant increase of hepatic lymph flow. Ascitic fluid then leaks from the liver capsule into the peritoneum. Thus, in cirrhosis removal of ascitic fluid may result in large losses of hepatic secretory and other water soluble blood proteins.

Total hepatic blood flow and the proportions delivered by the portal and arterial systems vary widely. Under normal fed conditions, the hepatic arterial flow is 25% to 30% of the total blood entering the liver, but the arterial blood supplies more than 50% of the oxygen (16,17). Feeding or fasting, metabolic demands, and the presence of shock or vasoconstriction significantly alter the hepatic perfusion rate. For example, splanchnic and, therefore, portal blood flow is significantly reduced in the presence of vasoconstriction, whether induced by sympathetic activity in the presence of hypovolemic shock or by vasoactive drugs such as vasopressin. In general, liver blood flow of both arterial and splanchnic origin is governed by autoregulation, which in turn depends upon oxygen requirements for cellular metabolic work. Normal liver flow ranges from 30% to 40%

of cardiac output. Thus, hepatic blood flow is dependent upon energy requirements for metabolic activities within the liver. Autonomic nerves, hormones, and substrates produced by the activated immune system all are involved in establishing both the level of cellular work and the circulatory response. Another complete set of metabolic feedback mechanisms is related to the concentrations of carbohydrates, lipids, proteins, and AAs in the blood plasma or extracellular water. In the presence of liver disease, cellular destruction and elevated resistance to flow caused by sinusoidal or venular obstruction may be the limiting factor to hepatic oxygen consumption and metabolic activity.

Hepatic Roles in Energy and Protein Metabolism

The intermittent food intake characteristic of humans and many animals requires between feedings a continuous supply of fuel substrates for conservation of biologically useful energy by oxidative phosphorylation. Amino acids for protein synthesis must be readily available. Each substrate, including AAs, must be derived during a fast from endogenous sources. The supply of each much be matched to the need for cellular oxidative phosphorylation to produce ATP and other substances containing energy-rich phosphate bonds ($^\sim$P). These bonds are the biologic media of energy exchange for performance of cellular work. The production of each energy-rich phosphate bond represents 7 kcal. It is estimated that the total expenditure of energy for production of ATP and other $^\sim$P bonds amounts to 89 W/min in a 70–kg man. Since there are no reserve stores of ATP or other $^\sim$P, it is necessary for the mitochondria of all cells to continuously produce these substances at a considerable expenditure of energy.

Glucose (4 kcal/g) and fat (9 kcal/g) are the principal fuels employed by cells throughout the body. Amino acids derived from irreversibly degraded proteins (4 kcal/g) under certain circumstances serve as sources of energy either by direct oxidation of their carbon skeletons or by conversion to glucose.

Glucose

Specifically, the liver contributes to glucose metabolism: (1) by conversion of galactose and fructose absorbed from the gastrointestinal tract to glucose, (2) by the synthesis of glucose from lactate or carbon skeletons of AAs, a process referred to as "gluconeogenesis," and (3) by the synthesis and storage of glycogen for ultimate degradation and release of glucose to the bloodstream.

The blood glucose concentration normally is maintained within relatively narrow limits, 75 to 120 mg/dl and the average normal adult requires 150 to 170 g of glucose per day. Varying rates of glucose transport and oxidation in all tissues are balanced by varying rates of hepatic glycogenolysis and gluconeogenesis to ensure euglycemia. Thus, extremes of hypoglycemia and the hyperosmolarity of hyperglycemia are avoided. In the fed state, elevation of blood glucose stimulates insulin secretion from pancreatic beta cells. Insulin at a blood concentration above 25 to 30 μU/ml promotes glucose transport into cells and hepatic glycogen storage (18). During fasting, insulin blood levels below this value permit glycogenolysis and the release of glucose from the liver into blood.

Gluconeogenesis is an energy dependent process whereby glucose is synthesized in the liver from pyruvate, lactate, and tricarboxylic cycle intermediates. The common pathway is oxalacetate, phosphoenolpyruvate, fructose 1,6-diphosphate, fructose 6-phosphate to glucose 6-phosphate, and thence to glycogen. Each step is catalyzed by specific enzymes. Six ATP molecules or 42 kcal are required to produce one molecule of glucose. Gluconeogenesis is induced by an elevation of hepatocyte intracellular cyclic adenosine monophosphate (cAMP) in response to glucagon. As the concentration of certain AAs, especially alanine, rises in the blood, secretion of glucagon from the pancreatic alpha islet cells is stimulated (19). Induction of hepatic gluconeogenesis by elevation of intracellular cAMP is the principal function of glucagon at blood levels of 200 μU/ml or more. The process requires the presence of cortisol.

Carbohydrates are stored in hepatocytes as glycogen, permitting the liver to take up glucose in excess of that required to maintain a normal blood glucose concentration. Glucose is polymerized via uridine diphosphoglucose to large glycogen molecules with an average molecular weight of 5,000,000 that are stored as granules. Thus, the osmolarity of intracellular fluid is not affected. Two ATP molecules drive the process of converting 1.0

mol of glucose to the glucose unit of glycogen. *Glycogenolysis* occurs by separation of each successive glucose molecule in each glycogen branch by phosphorylation catalyzed by phosphorylase. The branching point of the glycogen molecule is hydrolyzed by the enzyme amylo–1,6–glucosidase, making successive polysaccharide chains available for degradation to glucose–6–phosphate.

Glycogen synthesis or its breakdown are closely related to concentrations of glucose 6-phosphate and the components of the tricarboxylic cycle. In the presence of an excess in any of these components, glycogen synthase is activated.

Early in a normal fast, only 25% of the glucose supply is produced by hepatic gluconeogenesis. The remainder is derived from hepatic glycogen stores. Glucose–6–phosphate is converted to glucose for release into the blood by glucose–6–phosphatase. This enzyme is uniquely required for this purpose. It is present almost entirely in the liver. Whereas muscle cells store glycogen, the absence of glucose–6–phosphatase prevents direct glucose release from this tissue. In muscle, glycogen can only be employed locally for energy production by glycolysis. The lactate produced by this process diffuses out of muscle cells to be recycled to glucose in the liver via the Cori Cycle (see Fig. 3A.2). Thus, in the postabsorptive state, after cessation of food intake, maintenance of blood glucose at concentrations in excess of 90 mg/dl is dependent upon the liver store of glycogen. However, the amount of hepatic glycogen in a well-fed individual is adequate to satisfy body glucose requirements for no more than 15 to 20 hours. Thereafter, such glucose as is required is produced by hepatic gluconeogenesis from lactate and amino acid carbon skeletons.

Alterations of carbohydrate metabolism vary in liver disease, according to the severity of hepatocyte impairment. Profound hypoglycemia is characteristic of acute liver necrosis following ischemia or acute hepatitis when ureagenesis and gluconeogenesis cease in the hepatocytes. Such patients present with blood glucose concentrations ranging from 20 to 40 mg/dl. They may be supported for a week or more by continuous glucose infusions. If hepatocyte function fails to return, inability to clear amino acids causes the total blood arterial concentration of AAs to reach extraordinary values, as high as 6000 to 6500 μM/l, approximately three times normal. Blood protein concentrations inexorably decline. Blood lactate under these circumstances attains values in excess of five times normal as the intrahepatic redox potential falls.

Fat, Triglycerides, Fatty Acids

The principal liver reactions in regard to fat metabolism are summarized as follows: (1) degradation of fatty acids into smaller fragments (ketones) by beta-oxidation, which not only furnishes energy to the liver itself, but also supplies a ketone fuel readily oxidized by almost all tissues; (2) synthesis of triglycerides from excess glucose and to a lesser extent from the carbon skeletons of deaminated amino acids.

Fatty acids, stored as triglycerides in adipose tissue, are mobilized in the presence of low blood insulin, <25 μU/ml, during normal starvation. In shock or severe stress, they may be released in response to elevated blood alpha adrenergic catecholamine stimulation. Plasma lipase promptly hydrolyzes triglycerides to release *free fatty acids*. In blood, free fatty acids are transported bound to albumin by noncovalent bonds. Entry of free fatty acids into the hepatocyte cytosol and thence to the mitochondria depends upon carnitine as a carrier (20). The fatty acid is degraded by sequential removal of two carbon fragments. The acetyl-coenzyme A (acetyl-CoA) molecules condense to form acetoacetic acid, much of which is converted to beta hydroxybutyric acid. This ketone is readily oxidized during starvation by cells of most tissues. Glycerol released during hydrolysis of fat is converted in the liver to glucose. However, this process produces less than 10% to 15% of required glucose under normal fasted or starved conditions.

In liver failure, as energy production fails due to mitochondrial injury or oxygen deprivation, the conversion of pyruvate to acetyl-CoA for entry into the Krebs cycle is inhibited. Lactic acid accumulates. The oxidation-reduction (redox) potential falls as the nicotinamide-adenine dinucleotide (oxidized form)/nicotinamide-adenine dinucleotide (reduced form) (NAD^+/NADH) ratio declines. Since pyruvate and lactate are both highly diffusible, the lactate/pyruvate ratio in blood reflects changes in cellular NAD^+/NADH ratio. More specifically in the liver, where ketones are produced by beta oxidation, another measure of declining hepatic redox potential is the ratio of acetoacetate to beta-hydroxybutyrate in the plasma. Ozawa (22) found this ratio to correlate closely with the hepatic energy charge [ATP + 1/2 adenosine diphosphate (ADP)/adenosine triphosphate (ATP) + ADP + adenosine monophosphate (AMP)]. Patients with acetoacetate/beta–hydroxybutyrate ratios below 0.25 all died in liver failure, usually with circulatory shock or overwhelming infections.

Triglycerides are produced principally in the liver whenever the available carbohydrate supply exceeds that which can be converted to glycogen for storage. The carbon skeletons of many deaminated AAs also can be converted into acetyl-CoA, which may then be synthesized into triglycerides. This process also may be seriously impaired in the presence of severe liver failure. The triglycerides are transported from the liver as very low density lipoproteins to be stored in adipose tissue. In the absence of adequate hepatic protein synthesis, an excess of caloric intake, whether by vein or by the enteric route, causes the triglyceride to be deposited in hepatocytes. The result is fatty liver, which if sufficiently severe further impairs hepatic function, and in extreme cases causes death.

Approximately 90% of phospholipids, which serve as components of membranes, and lipoproteins are synthesized in the liver. The important blood lipids include cholesterol, cholesterol esters, triglycerides, and phospholipids. Cholesterol, chemically, is relatively nonreactive. It is the principal sterol that plays a major role in modulating the fluidity of membranes. Essential for growth and activity of normal cells, cholesterol may be absorbed from diet or synthesized in the liver and gut. All blood lipids are insoluble in water and are carried by lipoproteins. Mostly synthesized in the liver, lipoproteins are complexes of polypeptides (apoproteins) bound to lipids (23). They appear as classes characterized by their density, when subjected to ultracentrifugation: chylomicrons, very low density lipoproteins (VLDL), low density lipoproteins (LDL), and high density lipoproteins (HDL).

Plasma lipids are usually elevated to obstructive liver disease such as primary biliary cirrhosis. Xanthomas characteristically appear on hands, feet, certain joints, and around the eyes (24).

Amino Acids and Proteins

Normally, amino acids (AA) derived from protein digestion in the gut are absorbed to satisfy needs for protein synthesis. Excess quantities are removed by pathways of deamination and degradation. Their carbon skeletons are then either oxidized or converted to glucose. The latter reactions occur almost entirely in the liver.

In daily life, and for that matter, during illness, small proportions of protein in virtually all tissues and in body fluids are constantly being hydrolyzed to release AAs. The majority of the AAs released are promptly employed to resynthesize the same protein. This process, known as *protein turnover*, is a means whereby tissues are modified to meet stresses such as muscle hypertrophy in response to exercise. Turnover is also a mechanism for furnishing supplies of AAs for energy production or for synthesis of required proteins at times when an exogenous supply via the gut may be inadequate.

During normal fasting or starvation, visceral protein is degraded, while muscle protein is preserved. Under the stresses of trauma or infection, the reverse occurs, and muscle protein degradation with AA release from the periphery proceeds at rates three to five times normal (25–28). A pattern of AA mobilization exists in noninfected patients with cirrhosis that, in many respects, resembles that observed during infection in patients with normal liver function (29). This sequence is summarized in Figure 3A.2.

Catabolism, the biochemical mechanism by which amino acids are irreversibly degraded to permit their carbon skeletons to be oxidized or converted to glucose, occurs in stages. The first step in any tissue is enzymatic removal and transfer of the alpha-amino group to another molecule by one or more enzymes known as transferases. Commonly, the amino group is transferred to the alpha-carbon of a ketoacid, such as alpha-ketoglutarate to form glutamate. Glutamate can accept another amino group to become glutamine. In muscle and many other tissues, the amino group of leucine is transferred to pyruvate derived from glucose to produce alanine (30). Under conditions of normal fasting and stress, the release of both alanine and glutamine from muscle exceeds their molecular proportion in the composition of muscle protein. Conversely, those AAs that the muscle is capable of oxidizing (branched-chain AAs, asparagine, aspartate, and glutamate) are released in proportionally lesser quantities (26). Alanine and glutamine are transferred to the liver for gluconeogenesis or oxidation.

UREA SYNTHESIS

Ammonia derived by amino acid degradation in tissues or produced by bacteria in the gut is detoxified for excretion as urea in the urine. Urea synthesis is an energy-dependent chemical process limited to the liver and to a small extent (10% to 20%) in the kidney. The alpha-amino nitrogen atoms separated from the AAs are combined with carbon dioxide to enter a cyclic process requiring ATP 4.0 mol to produce 1.0 mol of urea. Thus, ureagenesis fails in hepatocytes when they are sufficiently damaged to impair mitochondrial production of $\sim$P by oxidative phosphorylation.

The initial step in ureagenesis is the formation of an unstable compound, carbamoyl phosphate. The enzyme ornithine transcarbamoylase, in turn, transfers the carbamoyl group to ornithine, to produce citrulline. Citrulline leaves the mitochondrion to enter the cytosol, where the remaining portion of the urea cycle occurs. A second amino group from aspartate condenses with the carbamoyl carbon of citrulline to form argininosuccinate. This is cleaved to form arginine and fumarate. Arginine then is split to yield urea and regenerated ornithine, which permits the cycle to continue. Urea, a highly diffusible substance, is released for excretion in the urine.

PROTEIN EXPENDITURE

Approximately 300 to 400 g of protein turns over daily in a normal person (31). As much as 25% of the available AAs undergo oxidative degradation or conversion to glucose primarily in the liver. The deficit is replaced by intestinal absorption of approximately 90 g of AAs from digested dietary protein. The remaining 75% of AAs are restored to protein by resynthesis. In the normal fed state, between 10 and 20 g of urea nitrogen from degraded amino acids are excreted daily. Experimental evidence indicates that in the fed state more than 50% of ingested amino nitrogen is converted to urea, while 20% to 25% of absorbed AAs are released into the bloodstream and the remainder are employed for hepatic protein synthesis (32). When adaptation to starvation takes place, lipolysis occurs as blood glucose and insulin decline.

Ketones are formed by beta-oxidation in the liver. Ketones serve as energy fuel for almost all tissues. The quantity of urea nitrogen is reduced to approximately 6 g daily, which corresponds to about 35 g of degraded protein (21).

PROTEIN SYNTHESIS

In the normal process of protein synthesis, the liver is the most active organ. In addition to the use of AAs for protein synthesis during turnover, the daily production of new protein is approximately 50 g by the liver. Among the important secretory or export proteins produced in the liver are prealbumin, albumin, fibrinogen, transferrin and other transport proteins, ceruloplasmin, haptoglobin, and lipoproteins, as well as alpha-globulins. Others include antiprotease proteins such as alpha$_2$-macroglobulin and alpha$_1$-antitrypsin. These secretory proteins represent approximately 20% to 40% of hepatic protein synthesis. Production of albumin, about 120 to 200 mg/kg/day, is in part regulated by colloid osmotic pressure.

In the liver, protein synthesis proceeds as in cells of other organs. A strand of linear messenger RNA (mRNA) is transcribed from DNA in the nucleus of hepatocytes. The genetic message of RNA is translated on polyribosomes, where structural or constituent protein synthesis occurs. Export or secretory proteins are synthesized on the rough endoplasmic reticulum. The synthetic process takes place in stages of initiation, elongation, and termination. All AAs to be incorporated, guanosine triphosphate (GTP), potassium, and magnesium ions, as well as energy supplied by adenosine triphosphate (ATP), are required for completion of protein synthesis. GTP (1.0 mol) and ATP (4.0 mol), which is the equivalent of 28 kcal, are necessary to incorporate 1.0 mol of AA into a peptide or protein chain. The amount of protein produced by the liver in a day is approximately 0.01 mol. The proteins on average are 500 AAs long, which requires approximately 140 kcal. Polypeptide chain elongation continues until a "nonsense" codon terminates the signal. The polypeptide chain is either released via the Golgi apparatus or incorporated into cellular structure. Additionally, in the Golgi apparatus, the carbohydrate moiety of glycoproteins is added by specific glycosyltransferases. The carbohydrate portion of such a molecule is of importance in governing the interaction of glycoproteins with specific cell membrane receptors. Regulation of protein synthesis in the liver may occur at the following sites: gene rearrangement, processing of mRNA from the nucleus to the cytoplasm, transcription, and translation of mRNA.

In health, AA supply plays a major role in determining the rate of hepatic protein synthesis of secretory proteins found in the plasma (33). Fasting or starvation may inhibit synthesis by reducing the energy supply (ATP and GTP) that is required for this process to occur. Under normal conditions, refeeding reactivates transport of mRNA from the nucleus to the cytoplasm. Plasma osmotic pressure, in great measure associated with albumin concentration, also significantly influences the rate of hepatic protein synthesis. In cells directed to produce a particular protein such as albumin, de novo synthesis may rise two to three times when diet is restored.

EFFECTS OF CIRRHOSIS ON AMINO ACID MOBILIZATION AND PROTEIN SYNTHESIS

The economic pattern of protein conservation typical of normal people adapted to starvation contrasts with the accelerated rates of amino acid mobilization and utilization observed in cirrhotic and septic patients. The normal fasted person needs only to mobilize and employ AAs at a slow rate of no more than 30 to 50 g/day to satisfy requirements for gluconeogenesis. In many respects, the patterns of AA metabolism in noninfected patients with moderately severe liver disease resembles those observed in clinical sepsis. During a fast, AAs are mobilized from peripheral tissues in both cirrhotics and septic patients at rates two to four or even five times normal. Since there are no nonfunctional proteins in the body that might correspond to adipose tissue as a source of fat or glycogen as a source of glucose, degradation rates of amino acids and proteins can be of great importance to body economy in the presence of injury or infection. Muscle constitutes more than 40% of the lean body mass (34) and appears to serve as a principal reservoir of protein available for degradation to furnish AAs in cirrhosis or following injury and the onset of infection. If prolonged in cirrhosis, a state of severe protein malnutrition may supervene. Muscle wasting is characteristic of the patient with advanced cirrho-

sis, as well as in the post-traumatic and septic states, especially in circumstances when the exogenous protein intake is limited.

Experimental evidence supports these clinical observations on the source and use of AAs under stresses of trauma, sepsis, and cirrhosis. Lust (35), Levenson (36), and more recently Ryan (37) and Lindberg (17) observed that in normal fasted animals, small quantities of AAs required for gluconeogenesis and protein turnover are derived by breakdown of protein in visceral tissues. Muscle is preserved. On the other hand, muscle protein becomes a major source of amino acids in starved septic or traumatized animals. Recent experiments in the author's laboratory, employing rats with induced cirrhosis, also have revealed a significant increase (two to three times normal) of net degradation of muscle protein.

In both moderately advanced cirrhotics and in septic patients, approximately 30% to 40% of the AAs taken up by the liver are oxidized or converted to glucose. The remainder are employed for hepatic protein synthesis. Twenty to 30% of total hepatic protein synthesis are secretory proteins, which appear in the plasma.

As the severity of liver injury progresses in cirrhosis, the pattern of structural and secretory protein synthesis changes. Many secretory proteins measured in blood plasma fall below normal. Production of prealbumin declines. Prealbumin has a short half-life of 2 to 3 days in contrast to 2 to 3 weeks for albumin. In fact, the ratio of prealbumin to albumin is an indicator of progressively impaired hepatic protein synthesis. Production of clotting factors is reduced. The typical "acute-phase" reaction, with the exception of increased C_3 and ceruloplasmin release, is usually not present as it is in sepsis. Alpha$_2$-macroglobulin secretion is accelerated in virtually all types of cirrhosis (38). Gamma globulins increase in the blood plasma. These changes are reflected in the blood concentrations of various groups of blood proteins presented in Table 3A.2 (38). With the exception of acute hepatic necrosis, in which protein synthesis virtually stops, the greater the cirrhotic damage, the greater the production of immunoglobulin M (IgM) and other large proteins.

In noninfected preoperative patients with moderately advanced cirrhosis in the fasted state, the average muscle protein degradation and peripheral release of AAs occurs at rates very similar to

Table 3A.2. Changes in the Blood Concentrations of Various Groups of Blood Protein[a]

	Levels of Some Serum Protein Parameters in Liver Diseases						Acute-phase Proteins, TIBC, and α_2-Macroglobulin in Liver Diseases					
	Albumin (g/L)	Pre-albumin (mg/L)	Retinol-binding protein (mg/L)	α-Lipo-protein (% of normal)	Normo-test (%)	Thrombo-test (%)	α_1-anti-trypsin (g/L)	Hapto-globin (g/L)	Cerulo-plasmin (g/L)	C_3 (% of normal)	TIBC (mg Fc/L)	α_2-macro-globulin (g/L)
Reference group	38.4	340	55	100.0	100.0	95.0	2.22	1.06	0.28	100.0	3.30	1.99
Hepatitis												
Acute viral	32.9*	89*	22*	29.0*	57.1*	49.9*	3.20*	0.33*	0.32	91.9	3.36	2.56**
Acute toxic	25.5*	178*	51	58.7*	59.8*	33.0*	3.99*	1.42***	0.35**	131.0***	2.39*	2.00
Active chronic	28.7*	111*	21*	43.2*	56.7*	45.7*	3.50*	0.53*	0.25	75.5*	3.05	2.86*
Chronic persistent	35.6	226*	41*	77.0*	88.4	82.7	3.11*	0.83	0.31	98.6	3.39	2.83*
Cirrhosis												
Cryptogenic	27.3*	121*	23*	53.3*	69.5*	68.8**	3.40*	0.67*	0.31	83.1***	2.79*	2.46*
Primary biliary	30.9*	141*	38*	69.1*	99.2	89.6	3.52*	1.28	0.47*	121.0***	3.62	2.96*
Alcoholic	30.4*	164*	35*	44.6*	65.5*	47.6*	3.96*	1.17	0.32	111.5	2.66*	3.14*
Steatosis	37.9	326	106*	87.9*	104.8	136.0	3.51*	1.59*	0.27	96.9	3.05	2.68***
Hepatic tumors	25.7*	127*	43	45.1*	81.2*	58.9*	6.33*	2.62*	0.49*	140.5*	2.96***	2.43***

[a]Statistical significance between each group and the reference group was calculated by Student's *t*-test, and the symbols indicate: *p $\leq$ 0.001, **p $\leq$ 0.01, *** p $\leq$ 0.05, no symbol = $p > 0.05$.
Adapted by permission from Skrede S, Blomhoff JP, Elgjo K, et al. *Scand J Clin Lab Invest* 1975; 35:399–406. *Abbreviations*: TIBC, total iron binding capacity.

those observed in sepsis (4,29). Of course, the ability to clear AAs in patients with severe liver failure is dependent upon the degree of hepatic dysfunction. Employing [U-^{14}C] tyrosine as a tracer, O'Keefe et al. (39,40) have demonstrated increased flux and reduced oxidation of tyrosine in patients with severe liver disease, probably due to partial defects in hepatic enzymes that participate in the process (41). More recently, Shanbhogue et al. (42) investigated protein turnover in patients with endstage liver disease, comparing them to normal patients awaiting elective operations. Plasma enrichment by infusion of ^{13}C leucine, D-5 phenylalanine, and [U-^{14}C] tyrosine disclosed that tyrosine flux in patients with severe liver dysfunction was 3242 ± 811 versus 2899 ± 688 μmol/hr in control subjects, while values for tyrosine oxidation were 328 ± 179 versus 422 ± 185 μmol/hr, respectively. Significant differences in leucine flux and oxidation did not exist between the control and cirrhotic groups. This finding indicates that clearance of tyrosine is a function of hepatocytes, whereas leucine is oxidized and cleared by all tissues.

Observations by the author and colleagues (3,4) have shown that the mobilization of AAs from peripheral tissues in cirrhotic patients range from 401 to 126 μmol/m^2/min depending upon the severity of the disease. These values are of the same order of magnitude observed in septic patients.

Thus, the normal starved individual tends to sacrifice visceral proteins and to preserve muscle tissue to satisfy the needs for AAs, while the fasted septic or cirrhotic patients (29,42), in whom rapid muscle wasting and weakness are prominent, mobilize amino acids by muscle protein degradation.

What the mediators and mechanisms may be that induce the accelerated rates of amino acid transfer from peripheral to central tissues in cirrhosis or other liver disease is not clear. It is evident in the presence of infection and inflammation that agents elaborated by activated macrophages, probably in concert with the "counterregulatory" hormones (catecholamines, glucagon, and cortisol), stimulate the characteristic changes of the "acute phase response" in protein and AA metabolism (29,43). Among the important monokines involved in these reactions are interleukin-1 (IL-1) (44), proteolysis inducing factor (PIF), the small active circulating cleavage product of IL-1 (45), and tumor necrosis factor (TNF) (46,47). Each has been demonstrated by clinical or experimental observations to accelerate release of amino acids from muscle and to induce hepatic protein synthesis in a fashion similar to the pattern in sepsis (48,44).

The relationship of these mediators to the pattern in liver failure is not well understood. It is tempting to argue that stimulation of macrophages (Kupffer's cells) in the liver might produce monokines capable of altering metabolism and activating the immune system. However, Kupffer's cells alone or in liver slices, stimulated by endotoxin, have failed to produce a mediator with the properties of the monokines listed above. Isolated hepatocytes co-cultured with Kupffer's cells in the presence of complement or endotoxin exhibit a biphasic response. Such stimulated preparations ultimately synthesize less protein (49,50). Either the Kupffer's cells do not release monokine-like substances or powerful inhibitors are produced at the same time (51). As will be shown below, the livers of cirrhotic patients appear to be maximally stimulated to clear AAs, whether by accelerated protein synthesis or by other routes. Thus, it is evident that release of AAs from peripheral tissues, principally by muscle protein degradation, is greatly accelerated in cirrhosis. Those cirrhotic patients whose liver can clear the abnormally high influx of AAs at rates similar to septic patients are prone to survive. Those who fail to mobilize and employ AAs at accelerated rates usually die postoperatively of overwhelming infection and multisystem failure (4).

Measurements of Amino Acid Clearance

Patterns of AA mobilization, transfer, and utilization may be assessed by several different methods.

First, by plasma enrichment with stable or unstable isotopes of one or more AAs, it is possible to determine rates of flux, clearance, oxidation, and incorporation into protein of one or more labeled AAs (39,42,52). The results of such studies, as described above, are probably more accurate than those obtained by measurements of amino acid clearance. However, studies with isotopes require infusions and frequent blood sampling to be certain that a steady state has been reached. Furthermore, measurements of isotope content in blood, urine, and expired gas is time-consuming. Although valuable for study of the metabolic alterations of liver disease, this methodology in its present state is not practical for routine assessment of liver functions.

Second, the plasma concentration of AAs is a function of rates of release and removal of AA from blood plasma, and can be of value as a qualitative indicator of liver failure (53,54). A third method of measuring AA mobilization, transfer, and utilization is by assessing release rates of AAs from muscle protein by measuring (1) the product of arteriovenous difference and plasma flow rate across an extremity (26), or (2) the urinary excretion rate of 3-methyl histidine (3-MEH) (55–57).

A fourth method is by measuring the plasma clearance rates of AAs by assessing the rate of AA uptake in the liver and other central tissues (1) during a state of equilibrium in the postabsorptive state in fasted individuals, (2) during infusion of a known AA solution at a known rate when equilibrium has been established (29), and (3) by assessing the rate of return of AA plasma concentration following intravenous injection of a 100-ml bolus of 10% AA solution (58).

Amino Acid Plasma Concentrations

Amino acids are quite freely diffusible between body water compartments except at the blood–brain barrier. In the normal cerebrospinal fluid, the ratio of AAs to those in the blood plasma ranges from −0.9 for glutamine, to 0.17 for tyrosine or methionine, to as low as 0.10 for leucine and other branched–chain AAs (59). Vinnars (60) and Askanazi (61) found after trauma or in the presence of sepsis that the intracellular muscle concentration of amino acids rises to approximately 8% above normal. However, this is a small gradient, permitting AAs mobilized from degraded muscle protein to diffuse into the extracellular water. In dogs, simultaneous measurements of AA concentrations in femoral venous blood plasma and in lymph from the femoral lymphatics reveal a remarkable similarity. Thus, the blood plasma concentrations are representative of the whole body extracellular AA pool. The AA content of arterial or venous whole blood may be 5% higher than plasma, since red cells normally transport AA in quantities slightly more than plasma alone (62).

Heparinized blood samples, deproteinized by TCA precipitation, are employed for measurements of plasma or whole blood AA concentrations. Either high performance liquid chromatography (HPLC) or AA analyzers designed specifically for the purpose are employed. Recently, a method has been reported for determining total AA concentrations by fluorometry, which is stated to correlate well with total AA concentrations measured by an AA analyzer (63).

In the author's laboratory, a rapid method recently has been developed to estimate total AA concentration in blood plasma samples. Ultrafiltration and the ninhydrin reaction are employed. To remove the large protein molecules greater than 100 kd, the plasma sample is first passed through a polysulfone ultrafiltration disk (100 K, 44.5 mm: Millipore Corp., Milford, MA). The filtrate from this step is then passed through a second ultrafiltration disk with a pore size designed to allow passage of molecules up to 1.0 kd (1 K polycellulose, 44.5 mm; Millipore). The ninhydrin reagent kit (Ready-Nin, Beckman Instruments, Palo Alto, CA) is a solution in methyl cellosolve with sodium acetate buffer and titanous chloride at pH 5.6 ± 0.1. Equal parts of the ninhydrin solution and the second plasma filtrate are mixed. After shaking and heating to 100°C, followed by cooling in the dark, the absorbances of the diluted solution are read at 570 nm (64). A standard curve of absorbance is constructed from dilutions of a solution containing essential AAs in physiologic proportions. Total plasma AA values measured by this method have been found to correlate well with measurements of total AA concentrations obtained from the AA analyzer (r = 0.756, P < 0.001). Although this system gives no values for individual AAs, it is capable of delivering results in the clinical situation within a fraction of the time required for the usual analysis employing a standard AA analyzer.

Production or Release Rate of Amino Acids from the Peripheral Tissues

The release rate, from an extremity, of a given AA or the sum total of all AAs can be determined by the product of arterial-venous concentration difference (ΔA-V) times the plasma flow rate in the vein from which the sample is taken. Since the muscle mass of the lower extremity is the greatest in the body, approximately one-fifth of all skeletal muscle (65), samples from the femoral vein are usually employed. Ten milliliters of blood is collected in heparinized plastic tubes simultaneously from any artery and from a femoral vein. The blood samples are promptly cooled and transported to the laboratory for plasma AA analysis.

Blood flow in a lower extremity in 64 patients, of whom 24 had cirrhosis, was measured by dilution of indocyanine green dye, which was injected into a foot vein at a constant rate (26). To avoid complications of vasoconstriction, none of the patients tested was in shock. An excellent correlation ex-

isted between leg blood flow and the cardiac output in normal, septic, and cirrhotic patients, provided cardiac index was in excess of 2.8 l/m²/min (r = 0.716, P < 0.01). The mean value of leg blood flow was 5.13 ± 0.45% of cardiac output. Finley et al. (66) and Wright et al. (67), employing radioactive xenon clearance, and Wilmore et al. (68), using plethysmography, all arrived at similar relationships. Therefore, it is possible to estimate leg blood flow as approximately 5% of cardiac index without introducing unreasonable errors.

3-methyl histidine (3-MEH) is an amino acid synthesized by muscle tissue by methylation of histidyl residues (57) and is incorporated into muscle protein. However, following muscle protein degradation, 3-MEH is not reincorporated into muscle protein as other amino acids are. Experimental evidence and clinical observation suggest that 3-MEH is excreted almost in toto following its release into the plasma (55). 3-MEH has been used to measure rates of muscle protein degradation. However, 3-MEH is not entirely satisfactory for this purpose. It does not indicate what proportion of the AAs derived from degraded muscle protein are employed locally in the muscle protein resynthesis, which is part of the "protein turnover" process. Therefore, it is probably not an exact measure of the muscle net protein degradation rate. Furthermore, there is evidence that muscle other than skeletal muscle may contribute 3-MEH, especially in states of protein depletion (69).

Amino Acid Uptake by Liver and Other Central Tissues

Desirable as it might be to measure the blood or plasma flow rate and arteriovenous differences of amino acids across the liver, as was done in animals by Lindberg (70) and Immamura (16), this is not practical in the clinical setting. Neither it is possible to determine flow rates and arteriovenous differences across the individual vascular beds of the important visceral organs. Therefore, one must be content with an estimation of the net uptake or release of AAs by the "central organs" shown in Figure 3A.2. These include not only the liver, but also the spleen, bone marrow, lymph nodes, as well as the wound, all of which employ AAs to synthesize proteins important to immunocompetence, organ function, and healing. The gut is a part of this complex of central organs. In the fed

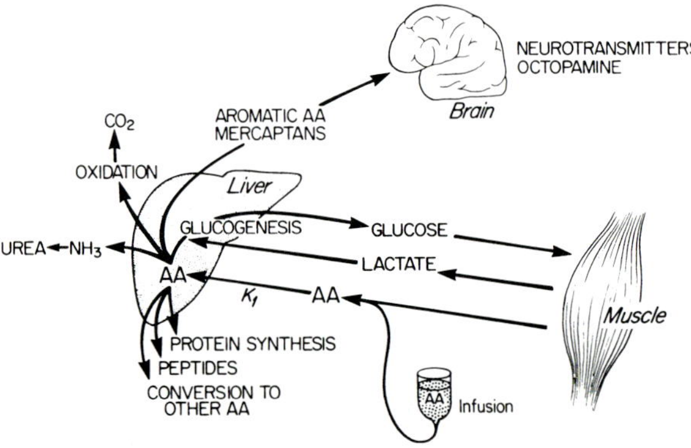

Figure 3A.3. This diagram presents the concept of amino acid transfer in the fasted state from endogenous peripheral tissues (principally from muscle protein degradation) and from an exogenous source of AA solution (of known composition at a known rate of infusion) to liver and other central tissues. At the *top*, the means for calculating the CPCR-AA are summarized. ΔA-FVAA.

state, it absorbs AAs from intestinal contents for delivery into the plasma AA pool. However, during starvation, particularly in sepsis or liver failure, the structural proteins of the intestinal mucosa tend to be degraded for release of AAs. It is not possible without measurements of portal vein AA concentration to estimate the uptake or release of AAs from the gut, but it is possible to estimate the total net AA exchange by all visceral tissues.

The "Central Plasma Clearance Rate of Amino Acids" (CPCR-AA) was developed for this purpose. The concept is illustrated in Figure 3A.3. Since no applicable method has been devised to measure the rate of AAs absorption from the gut after feeding, it is necessary to measure the CPCR–AA in the fasted state, preferably after 12 hours of food withdrawal. Assuming a state of equilibrium in the postabsorptive state, the rate of AA entry from peripheral tissues into the blood (K_1) must be equal to the net rate of their extraction by the liver and all other central tissues. In the absence of enteric feeding, the total peripheral entry rate (K_1) equals the peripheral production, principally from muscle (26).

If clearance is to be measured during intravenous administration of AAs, the composition of the solution and concentrations of each AA must

be known. The solution must also be infused at a known rate into a vein, other than that being sampled for arteriovenous difference, in order to calculate the rate of entry of each AA into the plasma pool. Four to six hours of infusion allows equilibrium between intake and clearance to occur.

Thus, calculation of CPCR-AA is as follows: The release rate of AAs from peripheral tissues, principally from muscle, is measured in one leg.

1. Femoral vein plasma flow =
   cardiac index × 0.05 × (1 − hematocrit).

Since the skeletal muscle of the lower extremity is approximately one-fifth of the total body muscle mass (65), the value for the release rate of amino acids from the peripheral tissues can be expressed by the formulas:

2. Total peripheral production rate
   (μmol/m^2/min) =
   arterial-femoral venous difference
   ($\Delta A - FV$) × leg plasma flow × 5

3. Amino acid entry rate (K_1) (μmol/m^2/min) =
   peripheral production rate + AA infusion rate

Assuming a state of equilibrium, the peripheral entry rate of AAs is equal to the central extraction rate. If the total pool of each AA in the extracellular water is reflected by the concentration of a given AA, its peripheral entry rate divided by its plasma concentration must equal the percent of the total pool cleared by the central tissues per unit of time per square meter of body surface area. Thus,

4. Percent of extracellular AA pool
   cleared/m^2/min =

$$\frac{K^1 \; (\mu\text{mol/m}^2/\text{min})}{\text{Arterial plasma concentration } (\mu\text{mol/1}) \times \text{estimate of total ECW}}$$

Extracellular water (ECW), which includes both tissue and plasma extracellular water, has been measured by Moore and others (71) by isotope dilution. Formula and nomograms have been constructed to estimate ECW. However, in the presence of edema and ascites during liver disease, such estimates may have large errors. Therefore, it is more convenient to base calculations of clearance on the amount of plasma cleared of amino acids by the central tissues in a given unit of time.

Central Plasma Clearance Rate of Amino Acids

Although the blood flow to the liver and other central tissues, which are actively extracting AAs, amounts to more than 50% of cardiac output, it is unlikely that any quantity of plasma is entirely cleared of AAs during its passage through them. Nevertheless, it is a convenient concept to consider the rate of AA extraction from plasma by these tissues, as the quantity of plasma from which any AA or all AAs would be completely removed at a known plasma concentration per unit of time. Thus, CPCR-AA, ml/m^2 of body surface/min is given by the formula

5. CPCR-AA (ml/m^2/min) =

$$\frac{K_1 \ (\mu mol/m^2/min) \times 1000}{arterial\ concentration\ (\mu mol/l)}$$

Significance of Values Obtained by Measurement of Amino Acid Clearance

As described above, three values indicating the state of AA metabolism are obtained when CPCR-AA is measured clinically, either in the fasted state or during intravenous infusion of a solution containing AAs. Each is of importance in assessing the state of liver function. They include: (1) arterial blood plasma AA concentrations (Conc. AA), (2) entry rate (K_1) of AA into the blood plasma pool [peripheral production rate (PPR-AA) plus AA infusion rate], and (3) the rate of plasma clearance of AA by the liver and other central tissues (CPCR-AA).

Effects of Hepatocyte Injury

Before undertaking a description of the alterations of amino acid metabolism characteristic of patients with cirrhosis, it is proposed to examine the effects of liver injury upon the usual metabolic responses to infection.

In Figure 3A.4 are presented for comparison data obtained from (1) normal postabsorptive individuals, (2) fasted septic patients with apparently normal liver function, and (3) fasted septic patients with evidence of hepatic insufficiency (serum bilirubin in excess of 2.5 mg/dl) (54,72). Histologically, the livers of patients with peritonitis are apt to reveal hepatocyte, cellular, and organella swelling (73).

The normal postabsorptive person releases AAs peripherally at a mean rate of but 124 μmol/m^2/

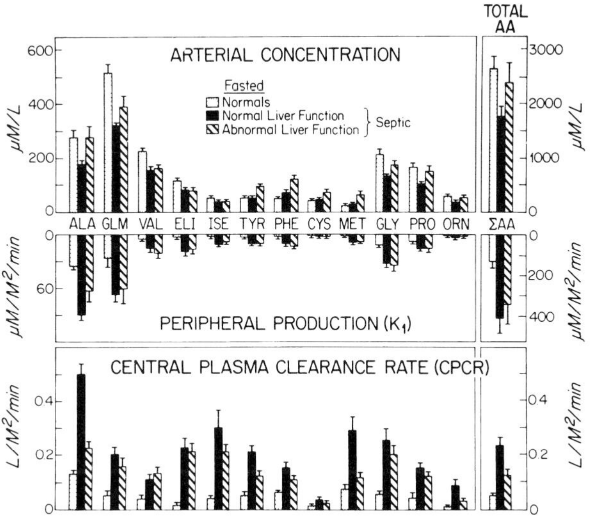

Figure 3A.4. The effects of liver injury during sepsis are illustrated by a comparison of AA concentrations, peripheral production rates, and CPCR-AA in fasted normal individuals, septic patients with normal liver function, and septic patients with evidence of hepatic failure. Note in the septic patients with liver failure the elevated concentrations and reduced clearance rates, particularly of aromatic AA, sulfur-containing AA, as well as alanine, glutamine, glycine, proline, and ornithine. This group of AAs are metabolized primarily in hepatocytes. These abnormalities are indicators of reduced hepatocyte function. ALA, alanine; CYS, cystine; GLM, glutamine; GLY, glycine; ISE, isoleucine; MET, methionine; ORN, ornithine; PHE, phenylalanine; PRO, proline; TYR, tyrosine; VAL, valine.

min, and only 46 ml plasma/m^2/min is cleared. This small AA supply satisfies the needs for gluconeogenesis and protein turnover in the normal fasted state.

The concentrations of AAs in septic patients with normal livers are equal to or less than those observed in the fasted normal individuals. The only exception is phenylalanine. The normal total AA concentration is 2650 μmol/l, compared to 1820 μmol/l in the septic group with normal livers. This is true despite the fact that peripheral release of AAs into the plasma is three times that of the normal, and the calculated CPCR-AA is approximately five times normal, 225 ± 18 versus 42 ± 7 ml/m^2/min (P < 0.001). Septic patients with evidence of liver failure have higher total blood AA concentrations (2430 μmol/l) and lower CPCR-AA (153 ± 29 ml/m^2/min) (P < 0.05) than septic patients with normal livers.

Fischer et al. (74) and others (42) pointed out that the total concentration of AAs, as well as those of certain specific AAs, tend to rise above

Table 3A.3. Normal Amino Acid Values in Ten Postabsorptive Patients Fasted 12 hr or More[a]

	Arterial Plasma Concentration ($\mu mol/L$)	Peripheral Production ($\mu mol/m^2/min$)	Central Plasma Clearance Rate ($ml/m^2/min$)
Gluconeogenic			
Alanine	278 ± 26	35 ± 4	131 ± 12
Glutamine	515 ± 32	27 ± 9	53 ± 10
Glutamic acid	95 ± 11	−16 ± 1.5	−174 ± 0.03
Branched-Chain			
Valine	224 ± 13	6 ± 2.5	37 ± 12
Leucine	117 ± 22	4 ± 2	10 ± 6
Isoleucine	54 ± 3	2 ± 2	34 ± 12
Aromatic			
Tyrosine	56 ± 4	3 ± 0.6	48 ± 10
Phenylalanine	49 ± 3	3 ± 1	55 ± 6
Tryptophan	43 ± 3	2 ± 1	27 ± 9
Sulfur AA			
Cystine	45 ± 6	0.6 ± 0.6	12 ± 7
Methionine	22 ± 2	1.6 ± 0.6	72 ± 20
Miscellaneous			
Glycine	213 ± 21	11 ± 3	52 ± 12
Proline	169 ± 12	8 ± 3	44 ± 16
Lysine	162 ± 13	10 ± 4	59 ± 17
Threonine	132 ± 13	7 ± 2	54 ± 8
Serine	106 ± 10	0.6 ± 1.6	6 ± 12
Arginine	79 ± 9	9 ± 2	114 ± 17
Histidine	81 ± 6	4 ± 2	56 ± 15
Ornithine	60 ± 4	0 ± 1	0 ± 51
Taurine	60 ± 10	1 ± 1	18 ± 14
Asparagine	40 ± 3	4 ± 2	103 ± 22
Aspartate	8 ± 6	−0.5 ± 0.5	−43 ± 35
Citrulline	36 ± 6	0.0 ± 0.6	0 ± 12
Hydroxyproline	19 ± 2		
Total amino acids	2663 ± 221	124 ± 38	46 ± 8

[a]Values ± standard errors.

normal as the severity of liver dysfunction increases. Since blood concentrations of any or all AAs reflect the rates of their production versus their rates of removal, it is not surprising that the aromatic AAs (tyrosine, phenylalanine), the sulfur-containing AAs (cystine and methionine), and certain others, including alanine, glycine, and ornithine, are higher in the patients with more severely damaged livers.

Each of these AAs is specifically cleared by the hepatocytes. In septic patients with liver damage, the derived CPCR-AA values reflect a significantly reduced ability to clear the same AA, the concentrations of which were elevated. On the other hand, all other AAs, including the branched-chain group, which are metabolized by tissues throughout the body, are cleared at higher rates. Although the total CPCR-AA value for the septic group with liver failure is twice that observed in normal fasting, it is only half the rate at which AAs would be employed ideally for synthesis of "acute-phase" and other proteins required for survival (3). From the data in Figure 3A.4, it is apparent that hepatocyte damage impairs the ability of the central tissues, particularly the liver, to utilize AAs made available to it by hydrolysis of muscle protein. Although plasma concentrations of specific AAs reflect reduced liver metabolism (P < 0.05), the CPCR-AA is a far more sensitive index of impaired hepatocyte function (P < 0.005), as shown by the columns on the right of Figure 3A.4.

Cirrhosis

Amino acid measurements from a series of fasted normal volunteers are presented in Table 3A.3. These will serve for comparison with the preoperative AA values from 95 fasted cirrhotic patients without evidence of infection, which are presented in Table 3A.4. Survivors are compared with those

Table 3A.4. Preoperative Amino Acid Values in Fasted Noninfected Cirrhotic Patients[a]

	Arterial Plasma Concentration ($\mu mol/L$)		Peripheral Production ($\mu mol/m^2/min$)		Central Plasma Clearance Rate ($ml/m^2/min$)	
	Survivors	Deaths	Survivors	Deaths	Survivors	Deaths
Gluconeogenic						
Alanine	251 ± 24	322 ± 30*	61 ± 11	46 ± 9	243 ± 71	143 ± 32**
Glutamine	578 ± 61	517 ± 78	85 ± 12	4 ± 5*	147 ± 73	80 ± 36**
Glutamic acid	64 ± 22	24 ± 5*	−4 ± 3	−3 ± 2	−63 ± 56	−125 ± 91
Branched-Chain AA						
Valine	137 ± 16	178 ± 17	27 ± 6	13 ± 3	197 ± 29	73 ± 120
Leucine	82 + 8	98 ± 10	16 ± 4	16 ± 5	195 ± 38	163 ± 83
Isoleucine	41 ± 6	43 ± 4	10 + 7	8 ± 1	244 ± 25	186 ± 42
Aromatic						
Tyrosine	63 ± 10	108 ± 14*	11 ± 2	7 ± 1	185 ± 56	65 ± 16**
Phenylalanine	62 ± 7	110 ± 11*	9 ± 1	11 ± 4	145 ± 33	100 ± 41
Tryptophan	35 ± 8	30 ± 7	4 ± 2	2 ± 3	114 ± 50	67 ± 36
Sulfur AA						
Cystine	48 ± 4	60 ± 8*	4 ± 1	5 ± 3	83 ± 44	83 ± 72
Methionine	27 ± 3	67 ± 15*	6 ± 1	7 ± 2	222 ± 57	104 ± 21**
Miscellaneous						
Glycine	157 ± 9	218 ± 15*	31 ± 4	24 ± 4	197 ± 36	110 ± 24*
Proline	145 ± 17	132 ± 12	23 ± 3	17 ± 5*	159 ± 42	129 ± 19
Lysine	154 ± 11	215 ± 24	28 ± 5	36 ± 13	182 ± 31	167 ± 39
Threonine	95 ± 8	131 ± 15	25 ± 3	21 ± 5	120 ± 80	40 ± 60
Serine	80 ± 7	90 ± 12	18 ± 2	12 ± 4*	60 ± 30	80 ± 30
Arginine	58 ± 8	69 ± 13	18 ± 4	11 ± 11	302 ± 45	159 ± 33**
Histidine	54 ± 4	80 ± 8	9 ± 3	15 ± 8	181 ± 38	144 ± 46
Ornithine	45 ± 4	64 ± 8*	6 ± 1	5 ± 5	160 ± 46	76 ± 21**
Taurine	38 ± 6	53 ± 22	5 ± 3	−3 ± 4	240 ± 40	−80 ± 50*
Asparagine	37 ± 4	51 ± 6*	10 ± 2	10 ± 2	270 ± 38	132 ± 32*
Aspartate	6 ± 1	8 ± 1	0.8 ± 0.3	0.5 ± 0.8	240 ± 60	50 ± 70**
Citrulline	19 ± 3	19 ± 3	2 ± 1	2 ± 1	230 ± 40	142 ± 116
Hydroxyproline	8 ± 2	15 ± 3*	4 ± 1	2 ± 1	120 ± 80	40 ± 60
Total amino acids	2227 ± 110	2718 ± 199*	390 ± 38	283 ± 43*	191 ± 22	102 ± 13**

[a]Values ± standard error.
*Significant difference survivors from subsequent deaths ($p < 0.05$ or less).
**$P < 0.001$.

who subsequently died postoperatively. In the latter group, concentrations of alanine, tyrosine, phenylalanine, cystine, methionine, glycine, ornithine, and hydroxyproline, as well as total AA concentration, are elevated to a modest extent above those of the survivors (P < 0.05). However, CPCR-AA for these particular AAs and for total AA are reduced to a highly significant degree from the patients who recovered. The sum total CPCR-AA for the survivors is 191 ± 22 ml/m²/min, compared to 102 ± 13 ml/m²/min in nonsurvivors (P < 0.001).

Prognostic Value of CPCR-AA in Relation to Various Surgical Operations

The preoperative CPCR-AA values from studies of 114 cirrhotic patients are presented in Table 3A.5, with other observations pertinent to assessment of liver function. Of this series, 19 patients were infected at the time of study. Infection was present principally in those who required emergent portacaval shunts for recurrent bleeding (39%) or general surgical procedures (53%) for peritonitis, obstruction, or amputations for gangrene. All who underwent portacaval shunts or sclerotherapy had been subject to variceal bleeding, but at the time AA measurements were made, bleeding had been brought under control and the hemodynamic state had been restored. None were in shock.

The diagnosis of cirrhosis was confirmed in all but six patients histologically, either by preoperative needle biopsies or operative biopsies. Alcoholic cirrhosis was present in 75% and posthepatitis cirrhosis in 15% of the patients.

The mean cardiac index of the entire group was 3.3 ± 0.3 l/m²/min at the time of study. No significant difference existed between survivors and

Table 3A.5. Preoperative Values of Cirrhotic Surgical Patients Who Survived or Died Postoperatively Following Various Surgical Procedures

	No.	Alcoholic Cirrhosis (%)	Infected (%)	Serum Bilirubin (mg/dl)	Prothrombin Time (sec)	Ascites (%)	Encephalopathy (%)	CPCR-AA (ml/m²/min)
Portacaval shunts								
Survived	26	73	7	2.4 ± 0.5	13 ± 0.5	82	32	267 ± 55
Died	18	84	33	7.8 ± 2.6	15 ± 0.4	79	57	93 ± 11
Warren shunts								
Survived	15	70	0	2.2 ± 0.6	14 ± 0.5	38	27	165 ± 27
Died	4	75	0	2.4 ± 0.7	14 ± 0.5	100	25	79 ± 16
Liver resection[a]								
Survived	8	50	0	2.0 ± 0.4	13 ± 0.4	25	0	190 ± 28
Died	3	67	0	4.9 ± 2.3	16 ± 0.3	66	0	106 ± 21
Sclerotherapy								
Survived	7	100	12	4.1 ± 1.7	14 ± 0.9	71	57	138 ± 25
Died	7	86	18	15.4 ± 4.7	17 ± 0.8	83	83	75 ± 9
Other surgery[b]								
Survived	14	71	43	1.9 ± 0.5	14 ± 0.5	43	50	208 ± 45
Died	12	83	50	8.9 ± 2.5	17 ± 1.2	58	42	91 ± 17
Total patients								
Survived	70	72 ± 8	12 ± 9	2.5 ± 0.9	13.6 ± 0.3	51 ± 12	33 ± 11	204 ± 17
Died	44	79 ± 8	20 ± 11	7.8 ± 2.5	15.8 ± 0.7	77 ± 8	41 ± 16	89 ± 8
Total patient studies:	114							

[a]Hepatoma 63%, metastatic tumor, 37%.
[b]Intra-abdominal 58%, amputation 23%, other 19%.

deaths in any group. Certain other important clinical findings are presented in Table 3A.5. Ascites and encephalopathy were present in greater percentages among the seriously ill patients treated by sclerotherapy. With the exception of the group who underwent elective Warren distal splenorenal shunts, the incidence of ascites and encephalopathy in the remaining patients was not significantly different between survivors and those who subsequently died.

The results are summarized not only according to postoperative survival or death, but are differentiated for each of the five types of surgical treatment. Four patients who died in the perioperative period of technical or other causes unrelated to metabolism or infection were eliminated. The 44 postoperative deaths all occurred 5 days or more following surgery and were associated with infection in all instances. Twenty patients died in multisystem failure, 2 had uncontrollable coagulopathy, 10 died in septic shock, and the remainder of various infectious complications.

Among the so-called routine "liver function tests," serum bilirubin was significantly greater in those who died: 7.8 ± 2.5 versus 2.5 ± 0.9 mg/dl ($P < 0.01$). Elevation of prothrombin time was marginally greater in the patients who died ($P < 0.05$). Although preoperative blood albumin concentra-

tion was slightly lower in the deaths, 2.8 ± 0.3 versus 3.1 ± 0.2, the difference was not significant. The blood enzymes (aspartate amino transferase, lactate dehydrogenase, and alkaline phosphatase), which usually indicate the presence of cellular damage or destruction, were not discriminators of survival or death.

Examination of the preoperative CPCR-AA values in the final column of Table 3A.5 reveals that highly significant differences exist between the survivors and those who died postoperatively in each group. The overall mortality was 38%. The CPCR-AA of those who recovered was 204 ml/m²/min, compared to 89 ± 8 ml/m²/min in the patients who died ($P < 0.001$).

Two groups of patients are of particular interest. Patients who recovered from Warren distal splenorenal shunts required less AA clearance (165 ± 27 ml/m²/min) than survival from other surgical procedures. Possibly this phenomenon is related to preservation of portal perfusion following the Warren shunt. The other group in which the survivors had remarkably low CPCR-AA values (138 ± 25 ml/m²/min) were the patients who were treated by sclerotherapy of esophageal and gastric varices. This finding probably is evidence of lack of infectious or traumatic stress. However, the hospital mortality in the 14 patients studied prior to

Table 3A.6. Comparison of Preoperative and Postoperative Amino Acid Metabolism in Survivors and Deaths

	Total Arterial Concentration (μmol/L)		Total Entry Rate (K_1) (μmol/m²/min)		CPCR-AA (ml/m²/min)	
	Preoperative	Postoperative	Preoperative	Postoperative	Preoperative	Postoperative
Survived	2311 ± 150	2349 ± 198	465 ± 41	489 ± 61	220 ± 26	212 ± 24
Died	2788 ± 155	3852 ± 688	271 ± 48	277 ± 43	97 ± 16	89 ± 12
Significance	$p < 0.025$	$p < 0.05$	$p < 0.01$	$p < 0.01$	$p < 0.001$	$p < 0.0005$

Adapted from Clowes GHA Jr, McDermott WV, Williams LF, et al. *Surgery* 1984; 96:675–685.

sclerotherapy was 50%, the highest for any form of treatment.

Looked at another way, a significant relationship exists between survival or death and the preoperative CPCR-AA value. The greater the CPCR-AA value in a cirrhotic patient, the less chance there was of death following the stresses of surgery. Whereas all patients with a preoperative total CPCR-AA greater than 200 ml/m²/min survived, those with values less than 100 ml/m²/min had a staggering 84% mortality.

Relationship of Preoperative to Postoperative Amino Acid Measurements

In Table 3A.6 are presented the results from a series of 30 patients in whom AA measurements were made in both the preoperative and postoperative periods. They underwent either portacaval shunt or general surgical procedures. The postoperative AA arterial concentrations remained unchanged in survivors, but rose in patients who would subsequently die. Despite very little change in the K_1 in the postoperative period, in both the survivors and deaths, CPCR-AA in the two groups remained almost unchanged postoperatively. The difference of CPCR-AA for survivors and patients who died also remained different to a highly significant degree ($P < 0.001$) in the postoperative period. Thus, it is evident that unless the liver is damaged by ischemia or other insult during surgery, hepatocyte function in cirrhotic patients remains relatively unchanged following an operation.

Effects of Parenteral Amino Acid Infusion

From data in Tables 3A.4 and 3A.6, and in Figure 3A.5, it is apparent that the K_1 in fasted cirrhotic patients is less in those who failed to survive than in the group who recovered. Furthermore, the blood concentrations of AAs is significantly higher ($P < 0.05$) and the calculated CPCR-AA values are less in the nonsurvivors ($P < 0.001$). However, the

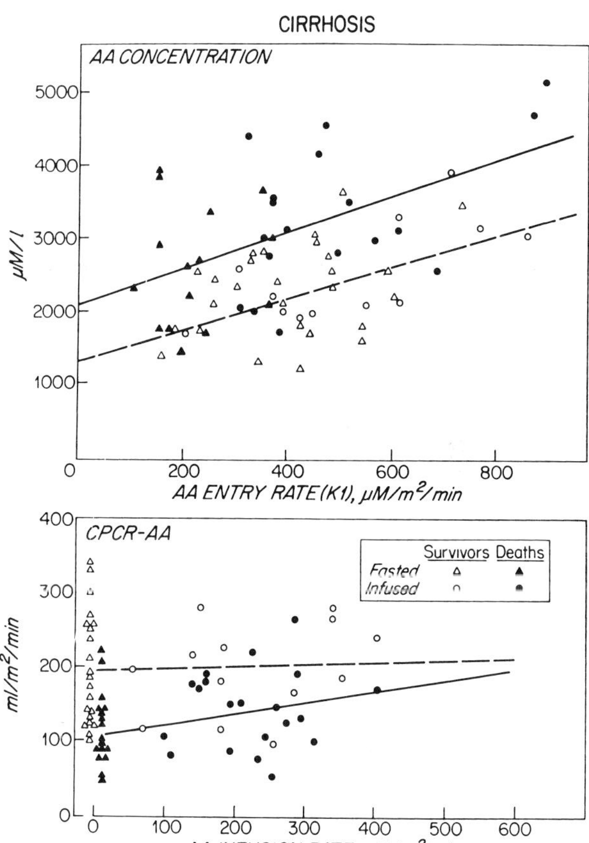

Figure 3A.5. Parenteral infusion of AA solution in cirrhotic patients increases the arterial concentration of AAs (*upper graph*) in both survivors and in those who subsequently died. However, as the rate of AA infusion increased, there was a slight but insignificant elevation of CPCR-AA in the death group, but no change occurred in the CPCR-AA of the survivors during AA infusion. The latter observation suggests that the clearance rate of AA is fully stimulated. Despite an elevation of AA plasma concentration by AA infusion, the CPCR-AA does not rise in this group of patients who recovered.

Table 3A.7. Amino Acid Metabolism in Fasting Patients Compared to Effects of Parenteral Alimentation in Cirrhotic Patients

	Arterial Concentration (μM/L)	AA Entry Rate into Plasma (K_1)		CPCR-AA (ml/m²/min)
		Infusion (μM/m²/min)	Peripheral Production (μM/m²/min)	
Fasted				
Survivors	2129 ± 125*'**	—	400 ± 33*'**	196 ± 17*
Deaths	2708 ± 164*'***	—	275 ± 27*'***	105 ± 20*'***
AA infusion				
Survivors	2585 ± 209*'**	226 ± 32	277 ± 51**	197 ± 18*
Deaths	3464 ± 253*'***	225 ± 17	245 ± 37	142 ± 13*'***

*P < 0.05 comparing survivors and deaths.
**P < 0.05 comparing fasted and AA-infused survivors.
***P < 0.05 comparing fasted and AA-infused deaths.

question remains as to whether parenteral infusion of AAs might favorably affect CPCR-AA. Cirrhotic patients were studied in the fasted state and also during a course of parenteral alimentation. Amino acid values obtained under both conditions are presented in Table 3A.7. In the fasted, noninfected, cirrhotic survivors, the arterial AA concentrations were lower than in patients who subsequently died, 2129 versus 2708 μmol/l (P < 0.01). Although AA concentrations rose in both groups during AA infusion, the actual increase was less in the surviving patients: 456 μmol/l compared to 756 μmol/l in the nonsurvivors. Despite a modest increase of approximately 25% in the K_1 or AA entry rate (peripheral production AA + infusion AA) in survivors, there was no change in CPCR-AA. Regardless of the rate of AA infusion, as shown in Figure 3A.5, total CPCR-AA did not increase; the AA concentration merely rose proportionately to the rate of AA entry into plasma. Thus, it appears that the system is maximally stimulated for uptake and clearance of AAs. On the other hand, a modest but significant 35% increase of CPCR-AA (P < 0.05) did occur during AA infusion into patients who later failed to recover. But this was at a cost of a mean arterial blood amino acid concentration of 3464 μmol/L, a 28% elevation over the value during fasting.

Although the usual seriously ill patient with advanced cirrhosis fails to respond to prolonged parenteral alimentation, occasional patients (approximately 8%) have shown improved CPCR-AA values in the course of 1 to 2 months. In a very few instances, not more than four in our experience, patients originally considered poor risks by CPCR-AA have progressively improved to the point that CPCR-AA was in the upper range, and they were safely operated upon. The important point is that the patients who responded favorably were all protein depleted with evidence of severe muscle wasting.

Tissue Metabolism

To establish whether a relationship exists between the rates of hepatic protein synthesis and the CPCR-AA, liver biopsies were obtained in 26 cirrhotic patients in whom CPCR-AA was measured just before the operation. The biopsies were immediately cooled in an ice bath for transport to the laboratory where each was promptly sliced to less than 0.5 mm thickness for incubation in Krebs-Henseleit bicarbonate buffer. Amino acids at physiologic concentrations were included in the medium. Incorporation of U-^{14}C tyrosine into protein was measured. In vitro synthesis rates of structural (tissue) protein, secretory protein in the medium, and total protein were measured. Rates of in vitro tyrosine incorporation into protein, conversion to glucose, and oxidation by livers or cirrhotic patients are presented in Table 3A.8 for comparison with mean values from liver biopsies of noninfected (control) patients and septic patients. It will be noted that both structural and secretory protein synthesis rates in livers of cirrhotic and septic patients were approximately twice those of the normal control group of patients who were neither infected nor injured. Of importance to establishing the relationship of CPCR-AA to protein synthesis is the correlation, presented in Figure 3A.6, be-

Table 3A.8. In Vitro Tyrosine Metabolism of Liver Biopsies (nmol/g/2 hr)[a]

	Normal (control)	Cirrhosis	Septic
Protein synthesis			
Structural	51 ± 4	115 ± 5	135 ± 7
Secretory	15 ± 3	26 ± 5	33 ± 6
Tyrosine			
Oxidation	30 ± 6	64 ± 14	50 ± 10
Gluconeogenesis	1.9 ± 0.5	3.2 ± 0.9	5.6 ± 1.2

[a]Mean ± standard error.

tween CPCR-AA measured immediately preoperatively and the rates of total in vitro hepatic protein synthesis in the same patients ($r = 0.76$, $P < 0.01$). A similar relationship had previously been observed in septic patients (29).

Although others (39,42), employing isotopically labeled AAs in vivo, have demonstrated important differences between normal control subjects and far advanced cirrhotics in protein-synthetic rates of the whole body, these data suggest that as the CPCR-AA declines with more severe disease, the capacity of the liver to synthesize proteins also declines. Furthermore, as previously described in Table 3A.2, the nature of the proteins secreted into the blood plasma by cirrhotic patients differ, not only from normal, but from those of the "acute-phase" proteins in the plasma of septic patients. Further validation of in vitro measurements of hepatic protein synthesis has been a demonstration by two-dimensional isoelectric focusing and

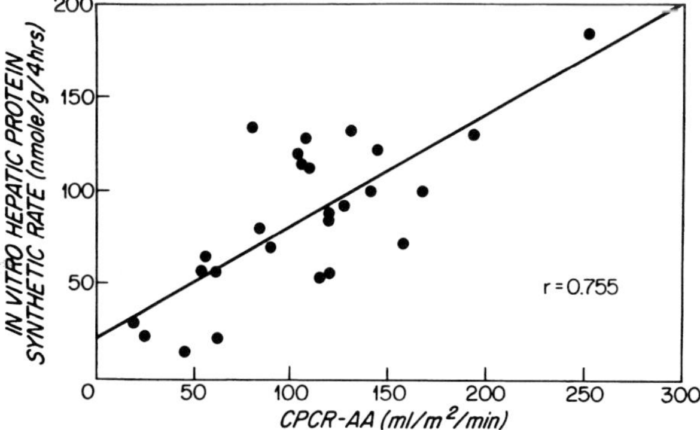

Figure 3A.6. The correlation between CPCR-AA values measured just before operation and the in vitro rates of protein synthesis in slices of liver biopsies obtained during surgery is highly significant ($r = 0.755$, $P < 0.001$). This finding suggests that CPCR-AA reflects the rate of employment of AA for protein synthesis.

electrophoresis of the similarity of proteins present in the plasma of a given patient and in the incubating medium of the liver biopsy from that same patient.* Furthermore, striking differences exist between the blood proteins of severe cirrhotic patients and those with less severe disease. These differences appear to be related inversely to the measured CPCR-AA values.

Encephalopathy

Coma in cirrhotic surgical patients has been recognized as a significant indicator of high mortality (74,75). Sometime ago, Fischer (76,77) suggested that high blood concentrations of aromatic and low levels of branched-chain AAs observed in advanced cirrhosis might cause an imbalance of passage across the blood–brain barrier. The resulting encephalopathy was thought to be caused by the production of octopamines and other false neurotransmitters from the excess aromatic AAs. Mercaptans, derived from methionine, short-chain fatty acids, and a variety of other agents associated with metabolic defects, are found in the plasma and cerebrospinal fluid of comatose patients. These substances, experimentally, can induce coma in animals (75). However, alterations of AA ratios are not always accompanied by encephalopathy or coma. The question remains whether failure of energy metabolism, reduced utilization of AAs, and inadequate synthesis of proteins essential for immunocompetence, maintenance of organ function, and survival may be the primary causes of death in comatose cirrhotic patients.

To assess the relationship of high mortality in coma to these factors, Loda et al. (48) undertook the study of 59 patients with advanced cirrhosis of various types, the majority having alcoholic cirrhosis. The state of encephalopathy of each patient was assessed according to the classification of Ritt et al. (78), which is based upon physiologic tests, neurologic examination, and electroencephalogram. The three groups and the results of studies made upon them are summarized in Table 3A.9.

The comatose patients are set apart from the alert and encephalopathic groups, not only by a much higher mortality, but by a variety of other factors. Whereas both the alert and encephalopa-

*Unpublished data of Calvin A. Saravis, Ph.D., produced in the author's laboratory.

Table 3A.9. Alert, Encephalopathic, and Comatose Cirrhotic Patients: Hemodynamic, Metabolic, and Coma-inducing Factors

	Alert (16)	*Encephalopathic (19)*	*Comatose (24)*
Ritt coma level	0	1–2	3–4
Cardiac index ($l/m^2/min$)	3.7 ± 0.2	4.7 ± 0.3[a]	4.7 ± 0.3
Systemic vascular resistance ($dyn/sec/cm^5$)	1263 ± 34	929 ± 72[a]	717 ± 48[b]
ΔArterial-mixed venous O_2 (vol%)	3.6 ± 0.3	3.8 ± 0.2	2.3 ± 0.1[b]
O_2 consumption ($ml/m^2/min$)	135 ± 10	159 ± 13	103 ± 7[b]
Ammonia ($\mu mol/L$)	108 ± 26	88 ± 28	95 ± 28
Ratio BCAA/aromatic AA	2.9 ± 0.2	1.8 ± 0.2[a]	1.5 ± 0.2
Octopamine ($\mu mol/ml$)	0.3 ± 0.1	1.2 ± 0.3[a]	6.7 ± 1.6[b]
α-Aminobutyric acid ($\mu mol/L$)	16.8 ± 3.1	17.5 ± 4.7	28.5 ± 4.1[b]
Total AA concentration ($\mu mol/L$)	2341 ± 230	2619 ± 197	4762 ± 56[b]
CPCR-AA ($ml/m^2/min$)	240 ± 30	300 ± 50	120 ± 20[b]
Mortality (%)	19	37	83

Abbreviations: BCAA, branched-chain amino acids.
[a]Significantly different from alert ($p < 0.01$).
[b]Significantly different from alert and encephalopathic ($p < 0.01$).

thic patients were hypermetabolic, the comatose group were well below normal. Despite high cardiac indices, arterial-mixed venous oxygen differences and oxygen consumption were significantly lower. This finding confirms previous observations by Siegel et al. (6), who found that low oxygen consumption in cirrhotic patients who would die probably is not caused by inadequate cardiac output, but rather is related to inadequate oxygen extraction and impaired oxidative metabolism. Further support for this concept was furnished by Ozawa et al. (22). A low ratio of blood acetoacetate to beta-hydroxybutyrate reflects the depression of redox potential and is accompanied by a reduction of cellular energy charge.

However, in hepatic failure of this severity, a number of defects exist that may contribute individually or in concert to death. Usually death is caused by lack of coagulation factors, overwhelming infection, and progressive multisystem failure (2,6,22). Principal among the metabolic defects that affect mortality (19% in alert patients, 37% in encephalopathic patients, and 83% in comatose patients) are inadequate energy production, inability to clear excess AAs, synthesis of false neurotransmitters, and neurotoxic agents (octopamine and alpha-amino-butyric acid). Loda et al. (48) found the whole body oxygen consumption to be only 103 ± 6.8 ml/m^2/min in comatose patients compared with values of 135 ± 10 in alert and 159 ± 12 ml/m^2/min in encephalopathic patients (P < 0.01). The CPCR-AA values of 120 ± 20 ml/m^2/min in coma, 240 ± 30 ml/m^2/min in alert, and 300 ± 50 ml/m^2/min in encephalopathic patients reveal AA clearance to be severely impaired in comatose patients who had the very high mortality. An inverse correlation existed between tyrosine plus phenylalanine plasma concentrations and whole body oxygen consumption (r = −0.56, P < 0.01), and with CPCR-AA (r = −0.61, P < 0.01). However, tyrosine and phenylalanine concentrations correlated directly with octopamine and alpha-amino-butyric acid (r = 0.64), both of which reach toxic levels in comatose patients. Thus, one may conclude not only that coma and encephalopathy are symptoms of hyperaminoacidemia in liver failure, but that death in such patients is principally caused by failure of energy metabolism and loss of hepatocyte ability to clear excess AAs or to employ them for synthesis of vital proteins. For these reasons, it may be of value to measure total oxygen consumption (VO$_2$) to supplement the prognostic value of CPCR-AA in seriously ill patients with liver failure.

Child's Classification and Prognosis

Based upon his clinical experience with cirrhotic surgical patients, Gardner Child (1) developed a system of three classes for determining surgical risk. The factors employed for gradation of severity were ascites, hypoalbuminemia, jaundice, and encephalopathy. In some measure, these parameters characterized the severity of hepatic physiologic and biochemical disorders, which have been reviewed above. The presence of ascites reflects abnormal lymph production caused by portal and sinusoidal hypertension. This factor indirectly in-

Table 3A.10. Survival Versus Death Comparing Preoperative CPCR-AA and Child's Classification (Excluding Transplant Candidates)[a]

	Child's Classification		
	A	*B*	*C*
I. Survived			
CPCR-AA	152 ± 23 (8)	192 ± 25 (19)	214 ± 47 (6)
(significance:			
I vs. II)	(NS)	($p < 0.001$)	($p < 0.05$)
II. Died CPCR-			
AA	96 ± 54 (2)	80 ± 12 (12)	101 ± 13 (13)

Abbreviations: NS, not significant.
[a]CPCR-AA units = $ml/m^2/min$.

fluences AA metabolism by the effects of reduced blood flow and oxygen delivery. Both may be caused by scarring and stenosis of the venous drainage from the capillaries and sinusoids. Hypoalbuminemia occurs with impairment of hepatic protein synthesis. As previously shown, protein synthesis correlates well with CPCR-AA. Encephalopathy is, in part, related to abnormalities of AA clearance and the production of octopamine and alpha-amino-butyric acid from excess tyrosine. Encephalopathy and coma are symptoms of severe disorders of AA and energy metabolism, which are clearly related to CPCR-AA. Finally, jaundice is caused by a defect in bile synthesis or excretion by the hepatocytes, and was the only so-called liver function test that was significantly different in survivors and patients who subsequently died (P < 0.05). Despite the value of Child's classification as a predictor of mortality, it fails to differentiate which member of any cirrhotic patient group will die. From the data in Table 3A.10, it is clear that in a group of 60 patients, for whom Child's classification was established, the mean CPCR-AA of those who survived shunt or general surgical procedures was 196 ± 25 $ml/m^2/min$, compared to 92 ± 21 $ml/m^2/min$ in those who died. Of even more importance to selection of patients, on a basis of risk, are the differences of CPCR-AA in the survivors and deaths in those classified as A, B, or C. For example, it is a surprise to find 6 patients who recovered in Child's class C with a CPCR-AA value of 214 ± 47 $ml/m^2/min$. In the same class, there were 13 patients who died with a mean preoperative CPCR-AA of only 101 ± 13 $ml/m^2/min$. Thus, AA clearance, as measured by these techniques, has proven to be an accurate predictor of hepatic function and reserve, and of the capacity of the

organism to withstand operations and other forms of stress.

References

1. Child CG III. *The Hepatic Circulation and Portal Hypertension*. Philadelphia: WB Saunders, 1954.
2. Cerra FB, Siegel JH, Border JR, Coleman B, McMenamy RH. The hepatic failure of sepsis: Cellular vs. substrate. *Surgery* 1979; 86:409–22.
3. Clowes GHA Jr, McDermott WV, Williams LF, Loda M, Menzoian JO, Pearl RH. Amino acid clearance and prognosis in cirrhotic surgical patients. *Surgery* 1984; 96:675–685.
4. Pearl RH, Clowes GHA Jr, Bosari S, et al. Amino acid clearance in cirrhosis: A predictor of postoperative morbidity and mortality. *Arch Surg* 1987; 122:468–473.
5. Pittiruti M, Siegel JH, Sganga G, et al. Increased dependence of leucine in posttraumatic sepsis: Leucine/tyrosine clearance ratio as an indicator of hepatic impairment in septic multiple organ failure syndrome. *Surgery* 1985; 98:378–387.
6. Siegel JH, Giovannini I, Coleman B, Cerra FB, Nespoli A. Pathologic synergy in cardiovascular and respiratory compensation with cirrhosis and sepsis. *Arch Surg* 1982; 117:225–238.
7. Jenkins RL, Clowes GHA Jr, Bosari S, Pearl RH, Khettry U, Trey C. Survival from hepatic transplantation: Relationship of protein synthesis to histological abnormalities in patient selection and postoperative management. *Ann Surg* 1986; 204:364–374.
8. Billing BH. Bilirubin metabolism. In: Schiff L, ed. *Diseases of the Liver*. Philadelphia: JB Lippincott, 1975, pp. 287–313.
9. Fauconneau G, Michel MC. The role of gastrointestinal tract in the regulation of protein metabolism. In: Munro HN, ed. *Mammalian Protein Metabolism*, vol. IV. New York: Academic Press, 1970.
10. Saba TM. Plasma fibronectin and hepatic Kupffer cell function. In: Popper H, Schaffner F, eds. *Progress in Liver Disease*, vol. III. New York: Grune & Stratton, 1982, pp. 109–131.
11. Lanser ME, Mao P, Brown GE, et al. Serum mediated depression of neutrophil chemiluminescence following blunt trauma. *Ann Surg* 1985; 202:111–117.
12. McCord JM. The superoxide free radical: Its biochemistry and pathophysiology. *Surgery* 1983; 94:412.
13. Saba TM, Jaffe E. Plasma fibronectin (opsonic glycoprotein): Its synthesis by vascular endothelial cells and role in cardiopulmonary integrity after trauma as related to reticuloendothelial function. *Am J Med* 1980; 68:577–594.
14. Hofeler H, Klingemann HG. Fibronectin and factor VIII-related antigen in liver cirrhosis and acute liver failure. *J Clin Chem Clin Biochem* 1984; 22:15–19.
15. Chaudry IH, Schleck S, Kovacs KF, Baue AE. Effect of prolonged starvation on reticuloendothelial function and survival following trauma. *J Trauma* 1981; 21:604–611.
16. Immamura M, Clowes GHA Jr, Blackburn GL, et al. Liver metabolism and gluconeogenesis in trauma and sepsis. *Surgery* 1975; 77:867–880.
17. Lindberg BO, Clowes GHA Jr. The effects of hyperalimentation and infused leucine on the amino acid metabolism in sepsis: An experimental study in vivo. *Surgery* 1981; 90:278–290.
18. Cahill GF Jr. Physiology of insulin in man. *Diabetes* 1971; 20:785–99.
19. Unger RH. Glucagon and the insulin/glucagon ratio in

diabetes and other catabolic illnesses. *Diabetes* 1971; 20: 834–838.

20. Owen OE, Felig P, Morgan AP, Wahren J, Cahill GF Jr. Liver and kidney metabolism during prolonged starvation. *J Clin Invest* 1969; 48:574–583.

21. Cahill GF Jr. Starvation in man. *N Engl J Med* 1970; 282: 668–675.

22. Ozawa K, Aoyama H, Yasuda K, et al. Metabolic abnormalities associated with postoperative organ failure: A redox theory. *Arch Surg* 1983; 118:1245–1251.

23. Jackson RL, Morrisett JD, Gotto AM Jr. Lipoprotein structure and metabolism. *Physiol Rev* 1976; 56:259–316.

24. Day RC, Harry DS, McIntyre N. Plasma lipoproteins and the liver. In: Wright R, Alberti KGMM, Karran S, Millward-Sadler GH, eds. *Liver and Biliary Disease.* Philadelphia: WB Saunders, 1979.

25. Beisel WR. Magnitude of the host nutritional responses to infection. *Am J Clin Nutr* 1977; 30:1236–1247.

26. Clowes GHA Jr, Randall HT, Cha C-J. Amino acid and energy metabolism in septic and traumatized patients. *JPEN* 1980; 4:195–205.

27. Long CL, Birkhahn RH, Geiger JW, Blakemore WS. Contribution of skeletal muscle protein in elevated rates of whole body protein catabolism in trauma patients. *Am J Clin Nutr* 1981; 34:1087–1093.

28. Pearl RH, Clowes GHA Jr, Hirsch EF, Loda M, Grindlinger GA, Wolfort S. Prognosis and survival as determined by visceral amino acid clearance in severe trauma. *J Trauma* 1985; 25:777–783.

29. Clowes GHA Jr, Hirsch E, George BC, Bigatello LM, Mazuski JE, Villee CA Jr. Survival from sepsis: The significance of altered protein metabolism regulated by proteolysis inducing factor, the circulating cleavage product of interleukin-1. *Ann Surg* 1985; 202:446–458.

30. Goldberg AL, Chang TW. Regulation and significance of amino acid metabolism in skeletal muscle. *Fed Proc* 1978; 37:2301–2307.

31. Young VR, Steffee WP, Pencharz PB, Winterer JC, Scrimshaw NS. Total human body protein synthesis in relation to protein requirements at various ages. *Nature* 1975; 253: 192–194.

32. Elwyn DH. The role of the liver in regulation of amino acid and protein metabolism. In: Munro HN, ed. *Mammalian Protein Metabolism,* vol. IV. New York: Academic Press, 1970; pp. 523–558.

33. Garrow JS. Nutrition and plasma proteins. In: Allison AC, ed. *Structure and Function of Plasma Proteins,* vol. I. New York: Plenum Press, 1974, pp. 283–304.

34. Cahill GF Jr, Aoki TT, Marliss EB. Insulin and muscle protein. In: Steiner DF, Freinkel N, eds. *Handbook of Physiology, Endocrine Pancreas.* Washington, DC: American Physiological Society, 1972, pp. 563–577.

35. Lust G. Effect of infection on protein and nucleic acid synthesis in mammalian organs and tissues. *Fed Proc* 1966; 25:1688–1694.

36. Levenson SM, Braasch JW, Mueller H, et al. In: Zimmerman L, Levine RL, eds. *Physiologic Principles of Surgery.* Philadelphia: W.B. Saunders, 1957, p. 1.

37. Ryan NT. Metabolic adaptations for energy production during trauma and sepsis. *Surg Clin N Amer* 1976; 56:1073–1090.

38. Skrede S, Blomhoff JP, Elgjo K, Gjone E. Serum proteins in diseases of the liver. *Scand J Clin Lab Invest* 1975; 35:399–406.

39. O'Keefe SJD, Abraham RR, El-Zayadi A, et al. Increased plasma tyrosine concentrations in patients with cirrhosis and fulminant hepatic failure associated with increased plasma tyrosine flux and reduced hepatic oxidation capacity. *Gastroenterology* 1981; 81:1017–1024.

40. O'Keefe SJD, Abraham RR, Davis M, et al. Protein turnover in acute and chronic liver disease. *Acta Chir Scand* 1981; 507(Suppl):91–101.

41. Nordlinger BM, Fulenwider JT, Ivey GL, et al. Tyrosine metabolism in cirrhosis. *J Lab Clin Med* 1979; 94:833–840.

42. Shanbhogue RLK, Bistrian BR, Laksham K, et al. Whole body leucine, phenylalanine, and tyrosine kinetics in end-stage liver disease before and after transplantation. *Metabolism* 1987; 36:1047–1053.

43. Watters JM, Bessey PQ, Dinarello CA, Wolff SM, Wilmore DW. Both inflammatory and endocrine mediators stimulate host responses to sepsis. *Arch Surg* 1986; 121:179–190.

44. Dinarello CA. Interleukin-1. *Rev Infect Dis* 1984; 6:51–95.

45. Clowes GHA Jr, George BC, Villee CA Jr, Saravis CA. Muscle proteolysis induced by a circulating peptide in patients with sepsis or trauma. *N Engl J Med* 1983; 308:545–552.

46. Berger M, Wetzler EM, Wallis RS. Tumor necrosis factor is the major monocyte product that increases complement receptor expression on mature human neutrophils. *Blood* 1988; 71:151–158.

47. Tracey KJ, Beutler B, Lowry SF, et al. Shock and tissue injury induced by recombinant human cachectin. *Science* 1986; 234:470–474.

48. Loda M, Clowes GHA Jr, Nespoli A, Bigatello L, Birkett DH, Menzoian JO. Encephalopathy, oxygen consumption, visceral amino acid clearance and mortality in cirrhotic surgical patients. *Am J Surg* 1984; 147:542–550.

49. West MA, Keller GA, Cerra FB, Simmons RL. Mechanism of hepatic insufficiency in septic multiple system organ failure. *Surg Forum* 1984; 35:44–46.

50. West MA, Keller GA, Hyland BJ, Cerra FB, Simmons RL. Hepatocyte function in sepsis: Kupffer cells mediate a biphasic protein synthesis response in hepatocytes after exposure to endotoxin or killed Escherichia coli. *Surgery* 1985; 98:388–395.

51. Bosari S, Love W, Clowes GHA Jr, Albright J, George BC. In vitro liver and muscle protein metabolism in noninfected and infected normal and cirrhotic rats. *Surg Forum* 1987; 38:10–12.

52. Waterlow JC. Protein turnover with special reference to man: Review. *Q J Exp Physiol* 1984; 69:409–438.

53. Fischer JE, Bower RH. Amino acids in liver disease. In: Epstein M, ed. *The Kidney in Liver Disease.* New York: Elsevier Biomedical Press, 1983.

54. Freund H, Atamian S, Holroyde J, Fischer JE. Plasma amino acids as predictors of the severity and outcome of sepsis. *Ann Surg* 1979; 190:571–576.

55. Bilmazes C, Kein CL, Rohrbaugh DK, et al. Quantitative contribution of skeletal muscle to elevated rates of whole body protein breakdown in burned children as measured by 3-methylhistidine output. *Metabolism* 1978; 27:671–676.

56. Long CL, Birkhahn RH, Geiger JW, Schiller WR, Blakemore WS. Urinary excretion of 3-methylhistidine: An assessment of muscle protein catabolism in adult normal subjects and during malnutrition, sepsis, and skeletal trauma. *Metabolism* 1981; 30:765–776.

57. Young VR, Haverberg LN, Bilmazes C, et al. Potential use of 3-methylhistidine secretion as an index of progressive reduction in muscle protein catabolism during starvation. *Metabolism* 1973; 22:1429–1436.

58. Fath JJ, Ascher NL, Konstantinides FN, et al. Metabolism during hepatic transplantation: Indicators of allograft function. *Surgery* 1984; 96:664–673.

59. Davson H, Welch K, Segal MB. *The Physiology and Pa-*

thophysiology of the Cerebrospinal Fluid. New York: Churchill Livingstone, 1987, pp. 247–374.

60. Vinnars E, Bergstrom J, Furst P. Influence of the postoperative state on the intracellular free amino acids in human muscle tissue. *Ann Surg* 1975; 182:665–671.

61. Askanazi J, Carpentier YA, Michelsen CB, et al. Muscle and plasma amino acids following injury: Influence of intercurrent infection. *Ann Surg* 1980; 192:78–85.

62. Felig P, Wahren J, Raf L. Evidence of inter-organ amino acid transport by blood cells in humans. *Proc Natl Acad Sci USA* 1973; 70:1775.

63. Konstantinides FN, Fath JJ, White M, et al. OPA: An alternate to total free plasma amino acids by HPLC. *Fed Proc* 1985; 44:1213.

64. Blackburn S. Estimation of the amino acids from the column. In: *Amino Acid Determination: Methods and Techniques*. New York: Marcel Dekker, 1968, pp. 69–80.

65. Tavill AS. Protein metabolism and the liver. In: Wright R, Alberti KG-MM, Karran S, Millward-Sadler GH, eds. *Liver and Biliary Disease*. Philadelphia: WB Saunders, 1979, pp. 83–107.

66. Finley RJ, Inculet RI, Pace R, et al. Major operative trauma increases peripheral amino acid release during steady-state infusion of total parenteral nutrition in man. *Surgery* 1986; 99:491–500.

67. Wright CJ, Duff JH, McLean APH, et al. Regional capillary blood flow and oxygen uptake in severe sepsis. *Surg Gynecol Obstet* 1971; 132:637–644.

68. Wilmore DW, Aulick LH, Mason AD, Pruitt BA. Influence of the burn wound on local and systemic responses to injury. *Ann Surg* 1977; 186:444–458.

69. Lundholm K, Bennegard K, Eden E, Svaninger G, Emergy PW, Rennie MJ. Efflux of 3-methylhistidine from the leg in cancer patients who experience weight loss. *Cancer Res* 1982; 42:4807–4811.

70. Lindberg BO, Clowes GHA Jr. An experimental method for study of liver blood flow and metabolism in intact animals. *J Surg Res* 1981; 31:156–164.

71. Moore FD, Olesen KH, McMurrey JD, Parker HV, Ball MR, Boyden CM. *The Body Cell Mass and Its Supporting Environment*. Philadelphia: WB Saunders, 1963.

72. Freund HR, Ryan JA, Fischer JE. Amino acid derangements in patients with sepsis: Treatment with branched chain amino acid rich infusions. *Ann Surg* 1978; 188:423.

73. Teplitz C. The pathology and ultrastructure of cellular injury and inflammation in the progression and outcome of trauma, sepsis, and shock. In: Clowes GHA Jr, ed. *Trauma, Sepsis, and Shock: The Physiological Basis of Therapy*. New York: Marcel Dekker, 1988.

74. Fischer JE, Rosen HM, Ebeid AM, James JH, Keane JM, Soeters PB. The effect of normalization of plasma amino acids on hepatic encephalopathy in man. *Surgery* 1976; 80: 77–91.

75. Zieve L. The mechanism of hepatic coma. *Hepatology* 1981; 1:360–365.

76. Fischer JE. Baldessarini RJ. False neurotransmitters and hepatic failure. *Lancet* 1971; 1:75–80.

77. Nachbauer CA, Fischer JE. The failing liver. *Surg Clin North Am* 1981; 61:221.

78. Ritt DJ, Whelan G, Werner DJ, et al. Acute hepatic necrosis with stupor or coma: An analysis of 31 patients. *Medicine* 1969; 48:151–172.

Editorial Comment

All of us in the Deaconess environment who have been interested in the complex facets of liver disease with its metabolic abnormalities have been intrigued with the superb data that has been recently coming from Dr. Clowes' laboratory on AA clearance. A further extension of this work will appear following the chapter on "Liver Transplantation," but the data have been utilized widely by all of us in providing a remarkably accurate prediction in terms of the prognosis of patients with fulminant hepatic necrosis of varying etiologies, progressive terminal cirrhosis, portal hypertension with massive hemorrhage and as a guide to the progress of patients following varying types of surgery carried out in the presence of liver disease.

The short segment in this chapter on encephalopathy perhaps needs some comment. It should be emphasized that coma in cirrhotic surgical patients as referred to in this section designates only the form of central nervous system derangement so commonly seen with extensive hepatocellular damage from whatever cause and usually indicates a fatal outcome.

The metabolic data in this section do not, however, refer to the reversible central nervous system disorder that is not related to hepatocellular disorder directly but rather to the hemodynamically produced neurological syndrome that is best referred to as portal systemic encephalopathy.

The changes in these two states may appear somewhat similar clinically but quite different and the pathogenesis of these disorders, while still not entirely clarified are distinctly different.

This important metabolic distinction is discussed at some length in Chapter 17 on "Hepatic Encephalopathy."

Chapter 4
Surgical Pathology of the Liver

URMILA KHETTRY

The liver is an unpaired, complex organ that becomes involved by a variety of disease processes. Surgical specimens from the liver, for the diagnosis and/or treatment of these lesions include needle biopsies, wedge biopsies, lobectomies, and in certain centers (where liver transplantation is performed) total hepatectomies. Needle biopsy is by far the most commonly performed procedure on the liver and many different approaches can be employed: percutaneous, via a laparoscope, during laparotomy, and rarely transjugular (1). The biopsies performed under direct vision, namely, via a laparoscope or during laparotomy offer a distinct advantage over a "blind" percutaneous biopsy because the likelihood of finding a focal lesion is much increased. A wedge biopsy is also helpful in this respect and also in certain situations where a larger specimen offers a better chance of diagnosing a particular lesion. However, the danger of missing a deeper lesion does exist with this technique. Fine-needle aspiration biopsy, particularly under ultrasonic guidance, is becoming a popular diagnostic tool for hepatic masses. Lobectomy, segmentectomy, and hepatectomy (followed by transplantation) specimens are becoming increasingly available to surgical pathologists, but are still restricted to large centers where special surgical and ancillary skills are available.

In this chapter we will discuss the pathologic aspects of surgical and medical diseases of the liver followed by a review of the transplantation pathology. The surgical diseases of the liver include a number of tumor and tumorlike conditions (Table 4.1), for which resections are being performed with increasing frequency. The account of the vast array of medical diseases will be deliberately brief.

Normal Histology

The liver is composed of innumerable small subunits called hepatic lobules that are arranged in a hexagonal fashion (Fig. 4.1). A branch of the hepatic vein (central vein) occupies the center of the lobule and many portal areas are present along its periphery. Cords or plates of hepatocytes, normally one cell thick, radiate out from the central vein toward the portal areas. The plates are surrounded on the two sides by vascular channels called sinusoids, lined by endothelium and Kupffer cells. Disse's space containing reticulin fibers and Ito's cells (lipocytes) separates the endothelium from hepatocytes. The layer of hepatocytes next to the portal areas is termed the "limiting plate." The hepatocytes themselves are polygonal cells with well-defined borders; ample, eosinophilic, granular cytoplasms; and a central round nucleus with a prominent nucleolus. Bile canaliculi are located between adjacent hepatocytes and form an elaborate network. Bile drains from these canaliculi into the portal (interlobular) bile ducts via Hering's canals, which are located at the periphery of the lobule. The portal areas contain connective tissue, amid which are present the interlobular bile duct as well as branches of hepatic artery and portal vein. A lobule can be arbitrarily divided into three zones: centrilobular, midzonal, and periportal or peripheral.

Rappaport (2) has suggested the acinus concept, which is a more functional subunit with portal tract as its center. The simple liver acinus has three zones: zone 1 is nearest to the portal area and receives blood with maximum amounts of oxygen and other nutrients. The availability of blood and nutrients progressively decreases from zone 1 to zone 3. Thus, zone 3 or the area around the central

Table 4.1. Histologic Classification of Tumors of the Liver

Epithelial tumors
  Benign
    Hepatocellular adenoma
    Bile duct adenoma
    Bile duct cystadenoma
  Malignant
    Hepatocellular carcinoma
    Cholangiocarcinoma
    Combined hepatocellular and cholangiocarcinoma
    Bile duct cystadenocarcinoma
    Others
      Squamous cell carcinoma
      Mucoepidermoid carcinoma
      Undifferentiated carcinoma

  Mixed
    Hepatoblastoma
    Teratoma
    Carcinosarcoma or malignant mixed tumor

Nonepithelial tumors
  Benign
    Hemangioma
    Infantile hemangioendothelioma
    Others—lipoma, myelolipoma, etc.
  Malignant
    Hemangiosarcoma
    Hemangioendothelioma
    Malignant lymphoma and leukemia
    Embryonal rhabdomyosarcoma
    Leiomyosarcoma
    Fibrosarcoma

Metastatic tumors

Tumorlike lesions
  Cysts
  Bile duct hamartoma
  Mixed hamartoma
  Mesenchymal hamartoma
  Focal nodular hyperplasia
  Heterotopias
  Focal fatty change
  Pseudolipoma
  Inflammatory pseudotumor

vein is most susceptible to vascular or anoxic injury.

Surgical Diseases of the Liver

Epithelial Tumors

HEPATOCELLULAR ADENOMA

Hepatocellular adenoma is a benign tumor solely composed of hepatocytes with minimal nuclear variation and specifically lacking bile ductal elements (3). Before the introduction of oral contraceptives into general use, it was an extremely rare tumor. Since 1960, there has been an increase in its incidence, particularly in young women using oral contraceptive agents (4,5). Further proof of this association has come from various studies (6–10) showing regression of tumor following discontinuation of the drug. "Menstranol"-containing "pills" seem to be implicated in more cases than those containing other contraceptive steroids (7,11). Rare occurrences in infants, children, men, and women not on contraceptive agents has been recorded (12). A single case of familial occurrence has been reported (13).

These tumors may remain asymptomatic or present as a mass, or at times present with an acute abdomen resulting from the most fearsome complication of hemorrhage and rupture. Malignant transformation is highly unlikely with these tumors (5); however, Boyd and Mark (14) report a case in a man on anabolic steroids.

The gross appearance (Fig. 4.2) of hepatocellular adenomas varies, depending upon the complicating factors. These tumors are sharply demarcated, lobulated, somewhat soft, and tend to be larger (median diameter 13 centimeters) in women using contraceptive agents than those occurring in women not using these drugs (median diameter in 10 cm (3); 70% of the latter are solitary (15). No cirrhosis or other chronic diffuse abnormality is seen in the adjacent liver. A complete or incomplete fibrous capsule may be present. The tumors may protrude from the liver surface and about 2% may be pedunculated (15). Although no central stellate scar with radiating septa is seen, there may be fibrosis within the tumor as a result of previous intralesional hemorrhages. Dilatation and congestion of blood vessels within and outside the tumor is often quite striking. Therefore, percutaneous liver biopsy in these tumors is dangerous and of limited diagnostic yield.

Microscopically, the tumor is composed of a uniform, rather monotonous population of normal or enlarged hepatocytes with bland nuclei, lacking significant mitotic rate, arranged in sheets, cords, or acinar pattern accompanied by sinusoidal tissue (Fig. 4.3). A trabecular pattern is never seen. The cytoplasm may be acidophilic or clear. Portal triads, bile ducts, and central veins are absent in the tumor, but bile production may be seen. Droplets of alpha$_1$-antitrypsin have been demonstrated in many hepatocytes within the tumor in the absence of alpha$_1$-antitrypsin deficiency (16). Fibrosis with hemosiderin deposits may be found as a result of

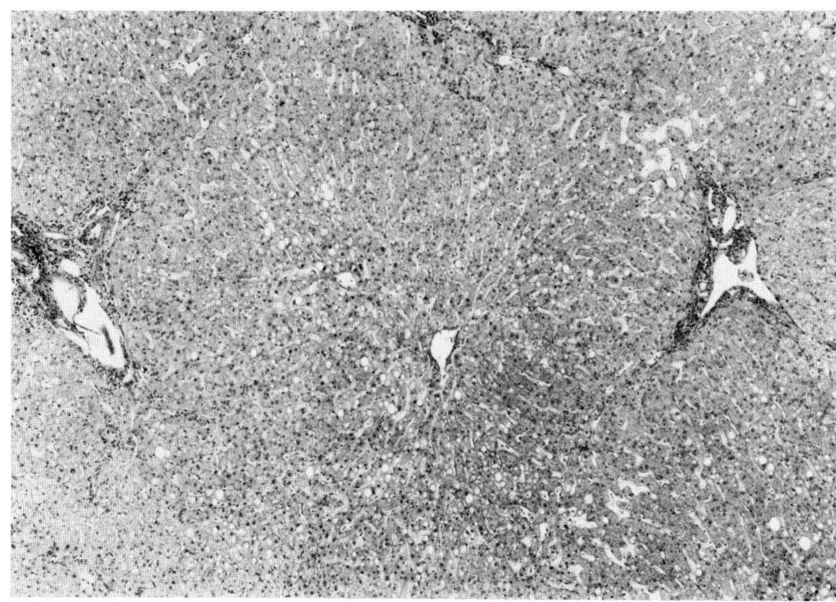

Figure 4.1. Low-power view of normal liver lobule showing a central vein with radiating cords of hepatocytes. Two portal triads are seen at the periphery of the lobule on either side (×180).

previous hemorrhage. Occasional tongues of neoplastic tissue may extend into the surrounding parenchyma. In cases where the tumor is resected without adequate margin, such extension may be responsible for recurrence.

Hepatic adenomas can be easily distinguished from focal nodular hyperplasia if strict criteria are adhered to, but differentiation from a well-differentiated hepatocellular carcinoma may pose a problem at times. Bland nuclear characteristics, lack of significant mitotic activity, and absence of a true trabecular pattern with no evidence of vascular invasion speak in favor of an adenoma in such cases.

BILE DUCT ADENOMA

These rare tumors occur singly just beneath the liver capsule and are composed of proliferating bile ducts in a fibrous stroma. Histologically, they are similar to von Meyenburg's complex; however, the bile duct elements are more numerous in adenomas (15,17). Occasionally they may be mistaken

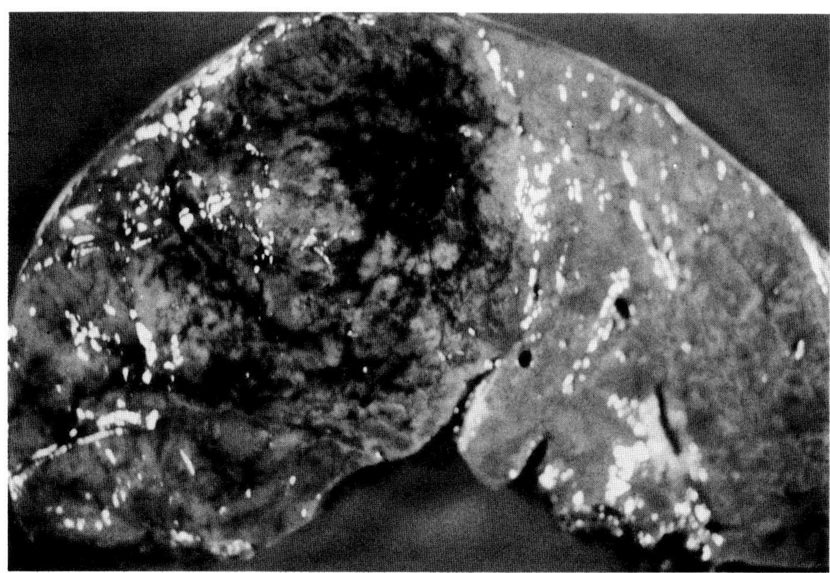

Figure 4.2. Hepatic adenoma (gross). A well-defined nodule with hemorrhagic cut surface.

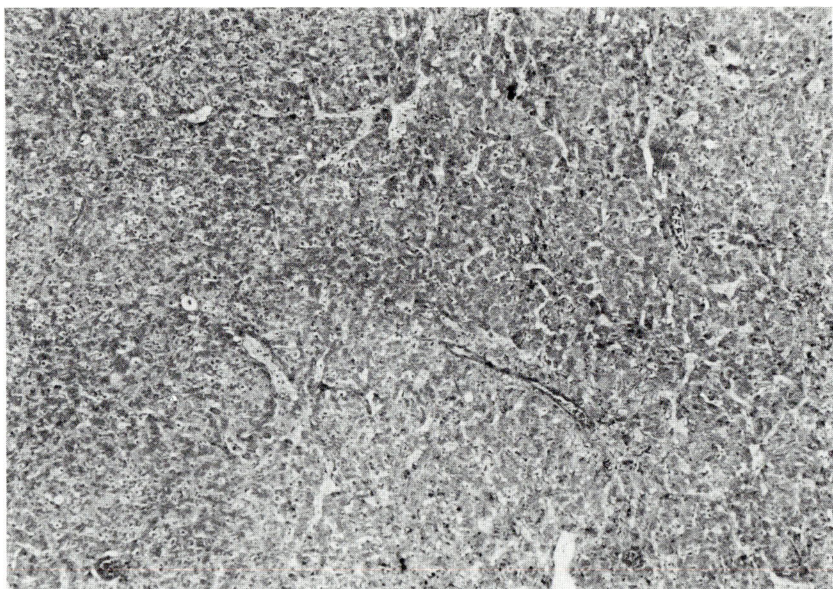

Figure 4.3. Photomicrograph of a hepatic adenoma. Irregular cords of benign-appearing hepatocytes are separated by sinusoids. No portal tracts or bile ducts are seen within the lesion (×180).

for a metastatic carcinoma by an inexperienced pathologist.

BILE DUCT CYSTADENOMA

These are benign cystic tumors, seen more frequently in women (18), and may be intra- or extrahepatic. Three-fourths of these tumors occur within the liver; the most frequent site in one study (19) was the anterior and the inferior surface of the right lobe.

These tumors (Fig. 4.4) are usually large, 10 cm or more in diameter (range 1.5–35 cm) (20), almost always multiloculated, and contain clear or yellow-green mucinous fluid. The lining epithelium is tall columnar, which may be thrown into papillary fronds (Fig. 4.5). The tumors rich in papillary projections need closer scrutiny with ample histologic sampling to rule out malignant change. The connective tissue under the epithelium is usually dense (21) and resembles ovarian stroma.

Incomplete excision may be followed by recur-

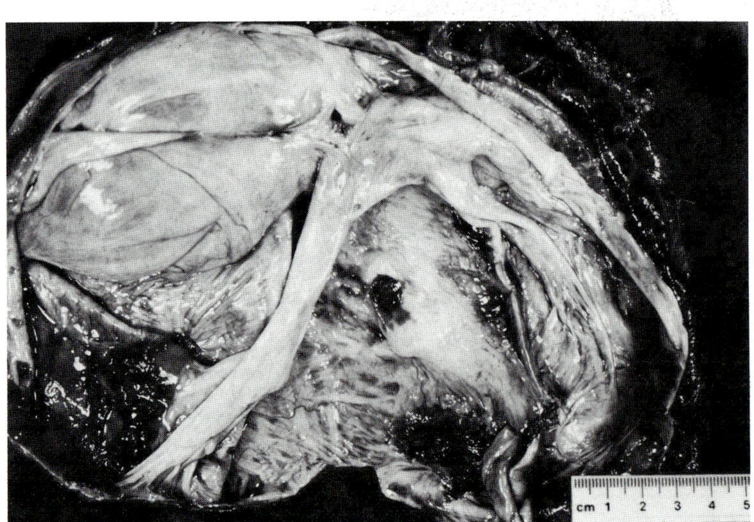

Figure 4.4. Bile duct cystadenoma (gross). Thin-walled cystic lesion has been opened to show the inner septa.

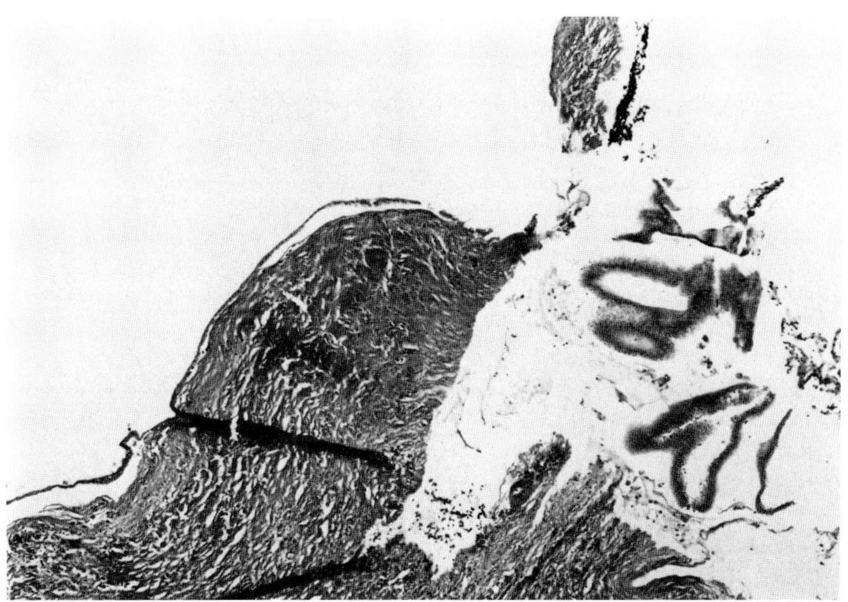

Figure 4.5. Photomicrograph of the same bile duct cystadenoma as shown in Figure 4.4. Fibrous-walled cyst has a cuboidal to columnar cell lining. In places (*right*) the epithelium is thrown into complex configurations, a feature distinguishing it from a congenital cyst (×180).

rence. The obvious differential diagnostic problem is a congenital simple cyst. The multilocular nature, the characteristic stroma, and most importantly the lining tall columnar epithelium with papillary formations are features of a cystadenoma (22,23). Rarely the cyst wall may be focally calcified. In such cases an erroneous diagnosis of a hydatid cyst may be made radiologically (20).

HEPATOCELLULAR CARCINOMA (HEPATOMA)

Hepatocellular carcinoma is a malignant tumor of the liver derived from hepatocytes. It is well established that environmental factors play a key role in the pathogenesis of this tumor. There is a striking variability in its incidence in the different parts of the world, the highest being in Asian and African countries.

Of the numerous etiologic factors implicated in the pathogenesis of this tumor, hepatitis B virus (HBV) infection, and cirrhosis of various types are the most important (24). Numerous serologic studies and tissue studies have provided the corroborative evidence (15). In a recent review by Chlebowski et al. (25), cirrhosis and hepatitis B surface antigen (HB$_s$Ag) were associated with 63% and 32% of the cases, respectively. Hepatocellular carcinoma developed in 24% of patients with postnecrotic cirrhosis in the series of Purtilo and Gottlieb (24), whereas in MacSween's study (26) the overall incidence of hepatocellular carcinoma in hepatic

cirrhosis was 12.3%. Wu and Lam (27) were able to demonstrate HB$_s$Ag in the cytoplasm of both malignant and nonmalignant hepatocytes. Hepatocellular carcinoma in cirrhotic patients manifests at a later age than in patients without cirrhosis (15). Men are affected more often than women.

Many studies have also implicated hormones, both anabolic and estrogenic steroids, in the development of hepatocellular carcinoma (28–30).

There is also one short report of a hepatocellular carcinoma occurring following the use of a nonsteroidal estrogenlike drug (31). In Goodman and Ishak's study (32) of hepatocellular carcinoma occurring in women, an absolute association between oral contraceptive use and incidence of hepatocellular carcinoma could not be demonstrated. Other associated factors include alpha$_1$-antitrypsin deficiency, hepatic irradiation, and various forms of chemicals (15,33).

Elevated alpha-fetoprotein levels can be detected in the serum of 40% to 90% of patients with hepatocellular carcinoma. Immunohistochemical studies on tissue sections can demonstrate its presence within the tumor cells. Slight elevations of alpha-fetoprotein may be seen in regenerative nodules (34). Interestingly, alpha-fetoprotein may not be elevated in hormone-induced hepatocellular carcinoma (14). Ordonez and Manning (35) studied alpha$_1$-antitrypsin and alpha$_1$-antichymotrypsin in hepatomas by immunocytochemical techniques. While 19 of 33 hepatocellular carci-

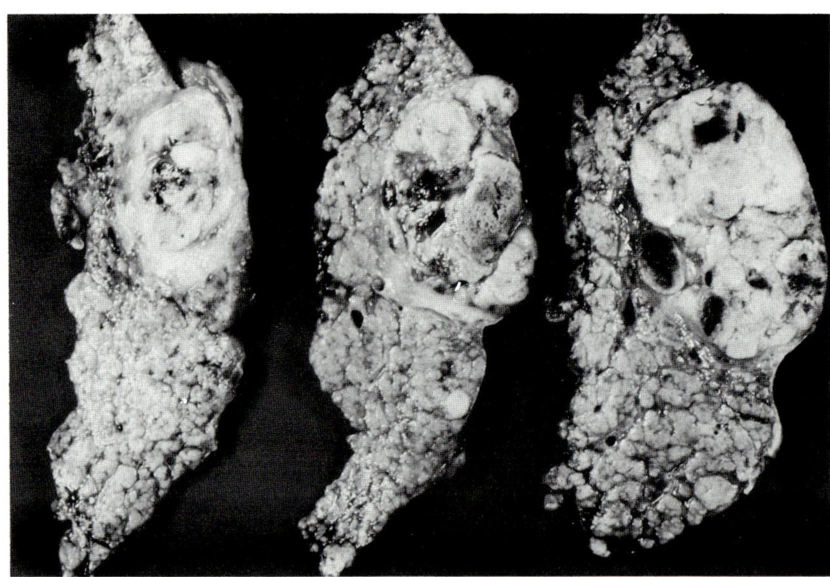

Figure 4.6. Hepatocellular carcinoma (gross). Partial hepatectomy specimen showing a lobulated unencapsulated mass with focally necrotic cut surface. Adjacent liver shows advanced cirrhosis.

nomas stained positive for alpha$_1$-antitrypsin (57.5%), all 33 tumors contained alpha$_1$-antichymotrypsin. It is interesting to note that all three cases of clear cell type were negative for alpha$_1$-antitrypsin. These two markers are generally associated with histiocytic malignancies and have not been widely used in cases of hepatic tumors. The diagnosis of hepatocellular carcinoma can be established by various biopsy techniques. In the series of Chlebowski et al. (25), the yield of positivity was as follows: blind percutaneous liver biopsy 83%, peritoneoscopy with directed biopsy 88%, and laparotomy 98%. In recent years, fine-needle aspiration biopsy performed under ultrasonic guidance is being used with increasing frequency to diagnose hepatic masses (36). Great success rates have been reported with minimal associated complications. However, in my experience, the success rate varies tremendously with the experience of the pathologist and is also case dependent. A well-differentiated tumor or an extremely poorly differentiated tumor may pose great problems. In the case of well-differentiated tumors, bland cytologic features may not permit an unequivocal diagnosis of malignancy, whereas in high-grade tumors the unequivocal diagnosis of malignancy can be made but their hepatocytic origin may not be easily ascertained.

Grossly, these tumors can be (1) massive, with or without small secondary nodules; (2) nodular with multiple growths; and (3) diffuse (15) (Fig. 4.6). These various types of gross appearance do not correlate with the different types of clinical presentations (37). The tumors may or may not be encapsulated or well circumscribed and tend to be softer than the normal liver. Rare variants with fibrosis and sclerosis are firm to hard. The color is usually tan but may be yellow (tumor rich in fat) or green (due to abundant bile production). Surface umbilication, common in metastatic carcinoma, is rarely seen. Tumor may be seen to invade the portal venous radicles or bile ducts (38).

The microscopic appearance of hepatocellular carcinoma is highly variable, ranging from well-differentiated tumors (Fig. 4.7) to markedly anaplastic tumors (Fig. 4.8). The well-differentiated tumors are difficult to distinguish from non-neoplastic liver tissue, whereas at the anaplastic poorly differentiated end of the spectrum hepatocytic features may be completely lost. The tumors can have different histologic patterns; the trabecular type is most common. A typical malignant cell has ample eosinophilic cytoplasm, a vesicular nucleus, and a prominent nucleolus. Bile production can be seen and, when present, is helpful to the pathologist (39). Intracytoplasmic globular inclusions or Mallory's hyalin may also be seen (40–42). At times, the tumor may have a prominent acinar pattern and may be mistaken for an adenocarcinoma. Lack of mucin production and cytologic details similar to those of hepatocytes help in the distinction. A closer examination of margins can be helpful; malignant hepatocytes

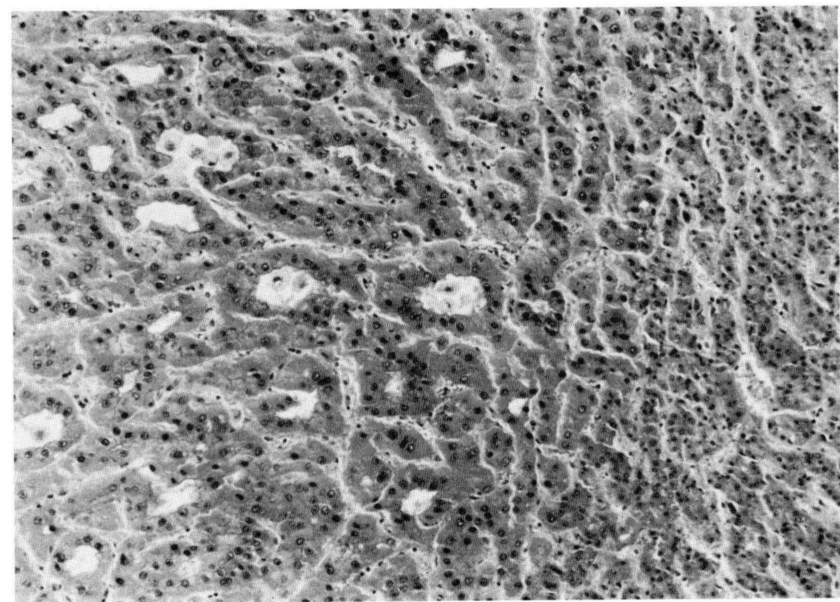

Figure 4.7. Photomicrograph of a well-differentiated hepatocellular carcinoma. Irregular cords of hepatocytes have rather bland cytologic features. Nucleoli are very prominent (×180).

often merge with the non-neoplastic hepatocytic cords, a finding that is virtually never duplicated by any other tumor. Rarely, a hepatocellular carcinoma may be composed of spindle cells or clear cells. Lai et al. (43) studied different histologic parameters, namely, cytologic differentiation, histologic architecture, degree of pleomorphism, bile production, other secretions, hyaline bodies, and giant cells; they found no correlation between any of these and the clinical outcome. Only the presence of clear cells in moderate to marked amounts correlated positively with survival. Others could not confirm this (44,45). We have observed a case of a young woman who had a large clear cell hepatocellular carcinoma (Fig. 4.9) with several satellite nodules in the opposite lobe of the liver. The woman is alive, well, and free of disease at the time of this writing, 12 years after the resection of

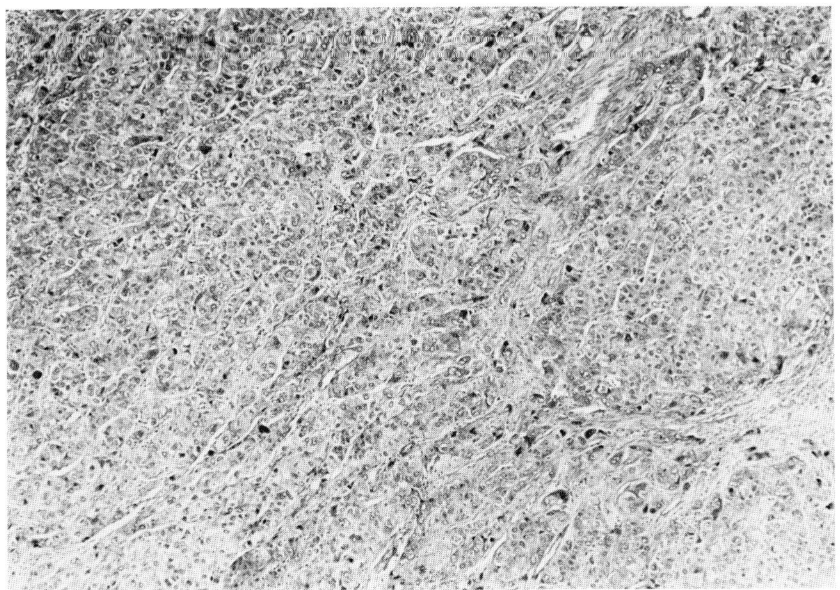

Figure 4.8. Photomicrograph of a high-grade hepatocellular carcinoma. Anaplastic cells with markedly pleomorphic nuclei have a trabecular pattern. In many poorly differentiated tumors, the trabecular pattern may be lost as well (×180).

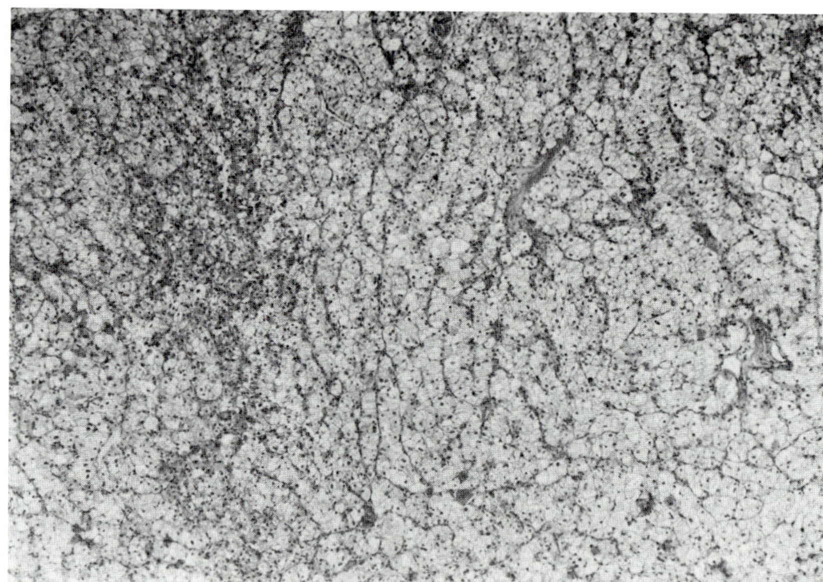

Figure 4.9. Photomicrograph of a clear cell hepatoma with a striking resemblance to renal cell carcinoma (×180).

the large mass. The satellite nodules seem to have regressed by clinical and radiologic assessments. Spontaneous regression of hepatocellular carcinoma has been reported (46,47). One could argue that our case was probably that of a clear cell hepatic adenoma, but focal invasion of portal venous radical (microscopic) present in our patient would speak against a benign tumor.

Two other variants of hepatocellular carcinoma must be distinguished because of their unique pathology and association with a long survival; these are the so-called "encapsulated hepatoma" and "fibrolamellar hepatoma." Okuda et al. (48) reported a series of 26 hepatocellular carcinomas that were surrounded by a grossly distinct capsule, a few millimeters to 1.0 cm thick. Patients in whom the diagnosis was made early had a prolonged clinical course. Such tumors comprised 10% of one series (15). The other type of hepatocellular carcinoma that is said to have a good prognosis is the fibrolamellar hepatoma (49,50). In one series (50) the mean survival, exclusive of operative deaths, was 68 months. Contrary to this, the results of a recent series (51) consisting of 16 patients of 133 with hepatocellular carcinomas did not agree with this. Fibrolamellar hepatoma appears to be a distinct clinicopathologic entity. It occurs almost exclusively in young individuals, mostly women, and in the absence of cirrhosis. Its histologic appearance is characteristic (Fig. 4.10). Large polygonal cells are separated by large areas of dense

lamellar fibrosis. The tumor cell nuclei are bland and mitoses are scarce. Ultrastructurally these polygonal cells are packed with mitochondria (52). The gross pattern of fibrosis (Fig. 4.11) in many instances is reminiscent of focal nodular hyperplasia with a dense acellular central area and radiating fibrous trabeculae. A suggestion has been made that fibrolamellar hepatoma may arise in focal nodular hyperplasia with variable malignant potential (53). In the series of Berman et al. (50), 3 of 12 patients had focal nodular hyperplasia in the adjacent liver. One of three of Farhi's (52) patients had an 0.5-cm focal nodular hyperplasia.

The typical clinical course of hepatocellular carcinoma is that of progressive deterioration with less than 6 months' survival following the diagnosis (54,55). The clinical course may be complicated by tumor rupture with hemoperitoneum, portal venous thrombosis, and rarely by certain systemic manifestations caused by biologically active substances produced by the tumor (56,57). A few reports of survival for extended periods of time can be found in the literature. Lai et al. (54) have noted survivals up to $4\frac{1}{2}$ years. Two long-term survivors have been observed by Penalba et al. (58) and Yoshida et al. (59).

CHOLANGIOCARCINOMA (INTRAHEPATIC BILE DUCT CARCINOMA)

This is a malignant tumor derived from bile ductal epithelium. These tumors can be extra- or intrahe-

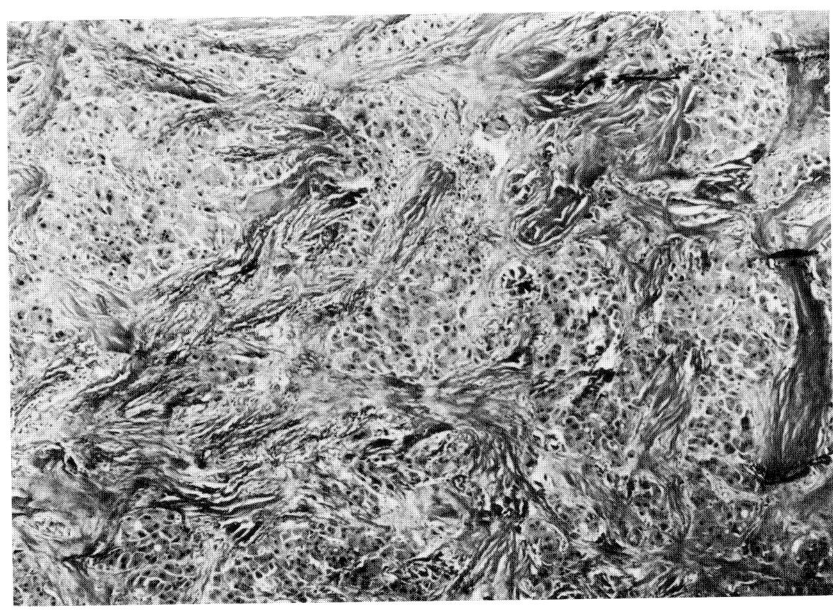

Figure 4.10. Photomicrograph of a fibrolamellar hepatoma. Large protoplasmic cell nests are separated by dense bands of collagen (×180).

patic. We will limit our discussion to the intrahepatic type, which differs from the extrahepatic type in the modes of clinical presentation, metastatic potential, surgical approach, and prognosis (15). When these tumors arise at the porta hepatis (bifurcation of hepatic ducts), the symptoms appear usually early. This variant is referred to as "Klatskin tumor" (60). The proximal tumors (intrahepatic) are rarely symptomatic early in their course and present as space-occupying lesions.

These tumors must be distinguished from hepatocellular carcinoma.

Cholangiocarcinoma is seen more commonly in the Orient, particularly in areas where the infestation with liver fluke is prevalent (61). In an autopsy series from Hong Kong (62) involving 50 cases, the incidence of *Clonorchis sinensis* was 82%. There is a slight male predominance and the tumor commonly occurs in the sixth or seventh decades of life. Usually there is no background hepatocytic

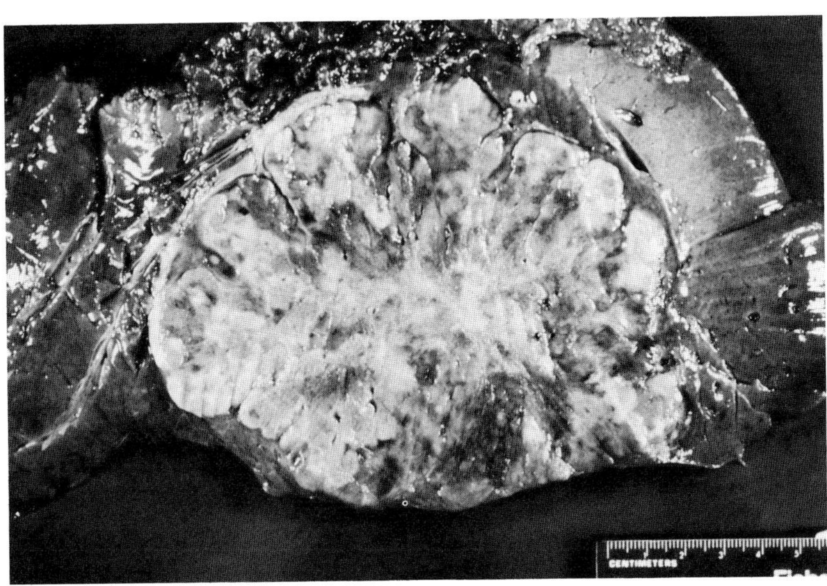

Figure 4.11. Gross photograph of a fibrolamellar hepatoma. The cut surface of the tumor is lobulated with a central area of dense fibrosis. Liver parenchyma adjacent to the tumor is unremarkable.

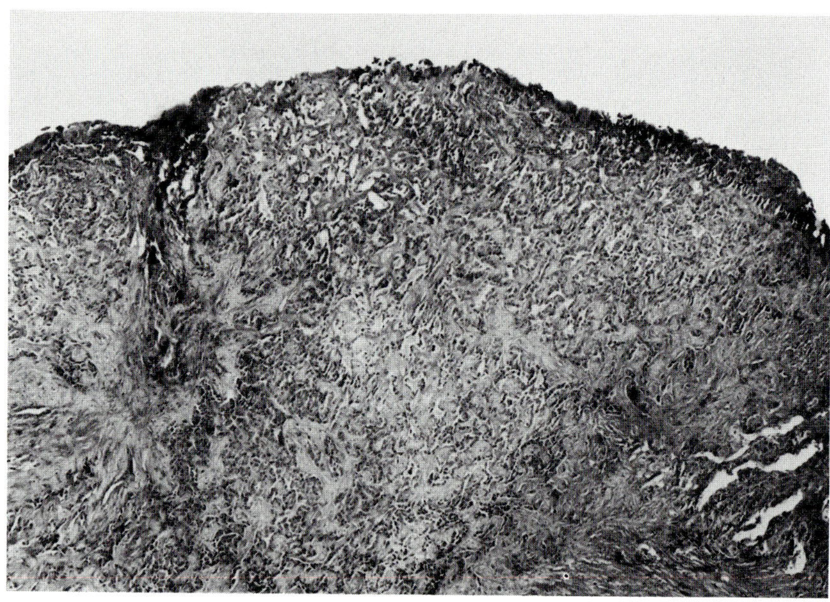

Figure 4.12. Photomicrograph of a cholangiocarcinoma; moderately differentiated adenocarcinoma has a dense fibrous stroma.

disease (63). This tumor is also seen in association with certain other extra- or intrahepatic diseases, namely, ulcerative colitis (15,61), congenital hepatic fibrosis (64), and cystic dilatation of the intrahepatic bile ducts (61,65–69). Average survival from the time of diagnosis is less than 1 year (15).

The gross appearance of these tumors is that of a yellow or white, hard, bulky mass that may be single, multiple, or diffuse. Unlike the hepatocellular carcinoma, tumor nodules under the capsule are umbilicated. Most of these tumors arise in the right lobe.

Histologically, these are adenocarcinomas of varying differentiation (Fig. 4.12). Intense desmoplasia is a characteristic feature. Elevated levels of alpha-fetoprotein are not observed in the serum nor can they be demonstrated on tissue sections by immunocytochemistry. Bile is never produced by the tumor; however, variable amounts of bile may be seen in the adjacent liver, particularly when large bile ducts are obstructed by the tumor. Mucin production is often seen. A papillary pattern is more common in cholangiocarcinoma than in hepatocellular carcinoma. Vascular invasion may be seen, but is not as common as in hepatocellular carcinoma. Spread by lymphatic routes is more common than in hepatocellular carcinoma (62). Histologically these tumors resemble those seen in the gallbladder and pancreas. Indeed, metastatic adenocarcinoma is the most difficult differential diagnosis to exclude.

A variant called "cholangiolocarcinoma" has an overall histologic pattern that resembles small bile ductules, namely, Hering's canals with low cuboidal cells, small nuclei, and clear cytoplasm. This distinction is rarely made in practice and is of no prognostic importance.

COMBINED HEPATOCELLULAR CARCINOMA AND CHOLANGIOCARCINOMA

Rarely, a malignant tumor of the liver can have features of both hepatocellular carcinoma and cholangiocarcinoma. These tumors comprise no more than 5% of primary liver carcinomas (70). A hepatocellular carcinoma with patchy "pseudoglandular" pattern should not be labeled as a combined tumor. Goodman et al. (70) have reported a series of 24 cases. Grossly, the tumors were large with a variegated cut surface. Histologically, they grouped the tumors into three types. (1) *Type I—collision tumors* consisting of two separate masses, one hepatocellular carcinoma and the other cholangiocarcinoma. Although contiguity could be demonstrated, no transition zone was apparent. (2) *Type II—transitional tumors* consisting of two contiguous masses with areas of hepatocellular carcinoma and adenocarcinoma as in type I, although a gradual transition from one to the other could be demonstrated. (3) *Type III fibrolamellar tumors* with an intimate intermingling of the two components through the mass. Seven of the eight cases had features of a fibrolamellar variant of hepatocellular carcinoma.

Type I and type II tumors occurred in older age groups as opposed to type III tumors, which were seen in younger patients. Patients with the first two types of tumors lived for less than 2 months following the diagnosis, whereas the average survival for patients with type III tumors was 14 months. The pattern of metastasis for all three types was similar and identical to that of other liver carcinomas.

BILE DUCT CYSTADENOCARCINOMA

This is a rare tumor of the liver. Most of the cases seem to arise within a cystadenoma, its benign counterpart (18,20,71). Cellular atypia with anaplasia, anisocytosis, anisokaryosis, and loss of polarity of the lining epithelium help to establish the diagnosis of malignancy. Invasion of surrounding parenchyma may or may not be seen. Also, these tumors may spread outside the liver but the overall survival is much better than that of cholangiocarcinoma (18). Radiologically, these tumors are impossible to distinguish from their benign counterpart (20). Iemoto et al. (72) have reported a case where a diagnosis of cystadenocarcinoma was made on an ultrasonically guided needle biopsy, a rather unique situation.

OTHERS

Primary *squamous cell carcinoma* of the liver has been reported (73,74), usually in association with cystic disease. *Mucoepidermoid carcinoma* most probably arising in bile ducts as a variant of cholangiocarcinoma has been reported as well (75).

Mixed Tumors

HEPATOBLASTOMA

Hepatoblastoma is a primary malignant tumor of the liver seen usually in children. However, rare examples of adult cases are reported (76,77). This tumor is more common in men (15) and may be associated with other congenital malformations (15,78,79). The histologic and cytologic characteristics of tumor cells resemble embryonal or fetal liver, and this feature must be recognized and distinguished from childhood hepatocellular carcinoma because of a more favorable prognosis of the

former (78,80). Elevated serum levels of alphafetoprotein may be observed. One example of hepatoblastoma producing ectopic gonadotropin has been reported (81). This tumor can metastasize, and favored sites are lung and abdominal lymph nodes.

These are usually large tumors composed of single or multiple nodules. The color and consistency are variable. The cut surface has a lobulated appearance with presence of fibrous septa.

Based on their microscopic appearance, these tumors can be divided into two types: pure epithelial and mixed epithelial-mesenchymal (18). The epithelial component can be either fetal or embryonal type depending on the degree of differentiation. The fetal type of cells are smaller than normal hepatocytes and contain bile, glycogen, and lipid in varying amounts. Bile canaliculi are present. The embryonal cells are much smaller with abundant mitoses and contain no secretory product. The proportion of these elements is variable and prognosis is dependent on the presence or absence of embryonal cells (82), being poorest for the tumors rich in them. A case of highly malignant mucoid anaplastic hepatoblastoma has been described (83). The mesenchymal component in the mixed tumors may be comprised of a variety of elements, namely, osteoid, cartilage, immature skeletal muscle, or primitive mesenchyme. The mesenchymal component has no bearing on prognosis (82). The epithelial component usually predominates in metastatic lesions. This tumor is thought to arise from multipotential blastema capable of both epithelial and mesenchymal differentiation (15). Ultrastructural studies support this concept (84,85).

OTHER MIXED TUMORS

Other mixed tumors of the liver that have been rarely reported are carcinosarcoma (15), teratoma (15) and malignant mixed tumor (86,87). Malignant mixed tumor and carcinosarcoma are terms probably used for the same tumor.

Nonepithelial Tumors

HEMANGIOMA

The cavernous hemangioma is the most common benign tumor of the liver. It is seen in all ages and in both sexes. Its incidence varies from 0.4% to

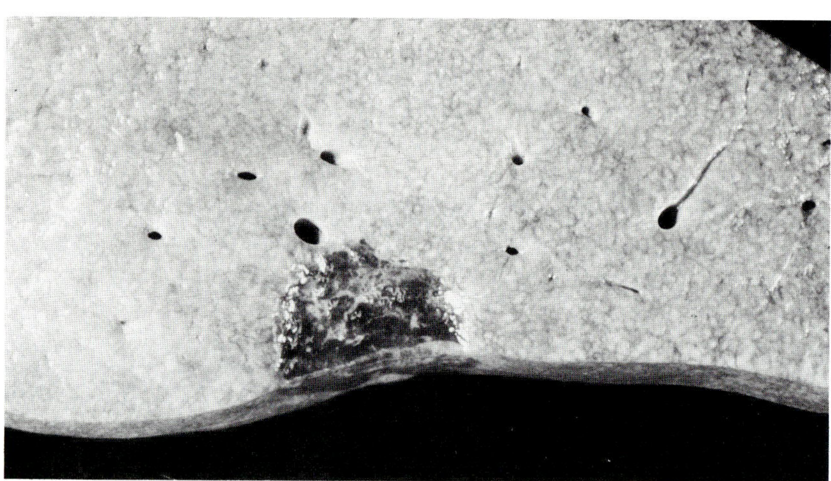

Figure 4.13. Hemangioma of the liver. Dark red-brown, well-circumscribed unencapsulated tumor is an otherwise normal liver.

7.3% (5). The vast majority of tumors are small, asymptomatic, and are found incidentally at laparotomy or at autopsy. Usually, these are single but may be multiple in about 10% of cases (5,88). Rarely a large tumor may present as a mass or an abdominal catastrophe resulting from rupture and hemoperitoneum (88,89). The gross appearance is that of a red to brown, usually well-circumscribed, spongelike mass (Fig. 4.13). On microscopic examination, varying-sized spaces lined by endothe-

lium and separated by dense fibrous septa are present (Fig. 4.14). Percutaneous needle biopsy or incisional biopsy may lead to massive hemorrhage and is therefore contraindicated.

INFANTILE HEMANGIOENDOTHELIOMA

This is a benign tumor of the liver presenting early during the neonatal period. The usual accompanying features are cardiac failure and cutaneous he-

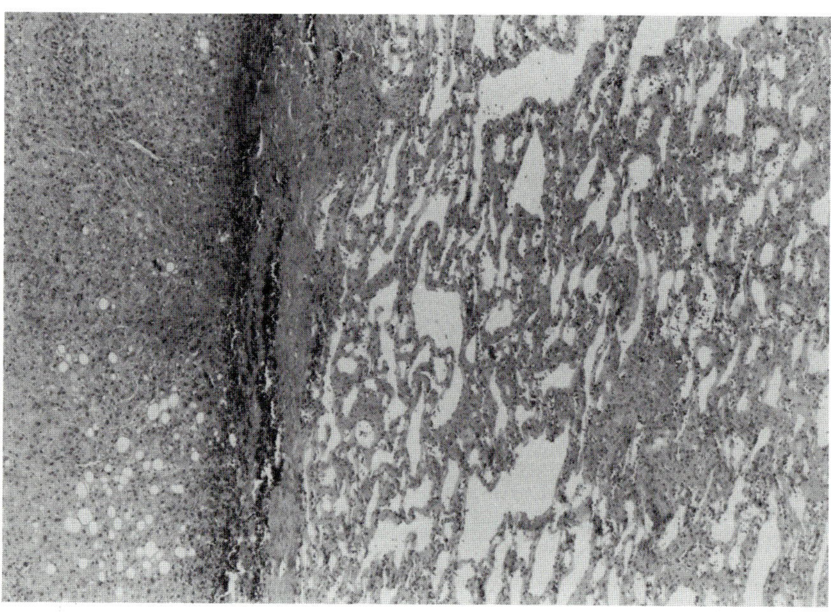

Figure 4.14. Photomicrograph of a hemangioma. Benign endothelium-lined anastomosing channels are characteristic of this tumor (×112).

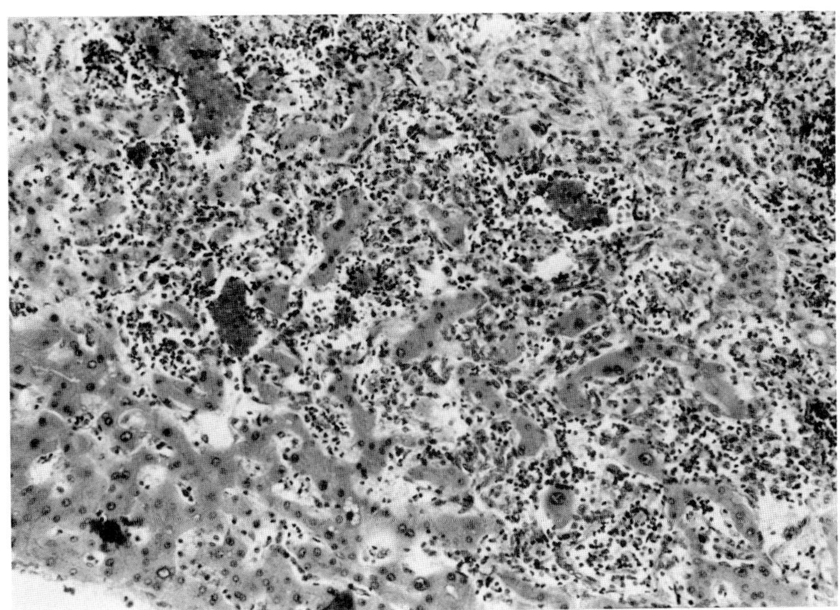

Figure 4.15. Hemangiosarcoma, photomicrograph. Highly anaplastic cells are infiltrating the liver parenchyma in a sinusoidal pattern (×450).

mangiomas (15,90). The presence or absence of cardiac failure and its severity dictates the clinical outcome.

These tumors may be solitary or multiple, large or small, gray-pink with deep purple spongy centers. Microscopically, proliferating small vascular spaces lined by plump endothelial cells are seen.

OTHERS

Benign mesenchymal tumors like lipoma and myelolipoma of the liver have been reported in the liver (91,92).

HEMANGIOSARCOMA

Hemangiosarcoma or angiosarcoma is an exceedingly rare, vasoformative tumor of the liver. It is associated with an extremely grim prognosis. Inorganic arsenicals, Thorotrast, vinyl chloride, and other carcinogens have been implicated in the induction of this tumor in humans (15,93). In a minority of cases association with androgenic anabolic steroids has also been proposed (93). One case associated with diethylstilbestrol exposure (94) and another arising in the background of hemochromatosis with cirrhosis (95) have also been reported.

The gross appearance is of one large solitary mass or multiple hemorrhagic nodules of varying sizes. At times, the entire liver could be transformed into a spongelike mass containing blood, and an erroneous diagnosis of peliosis hepatis may be made even by an experienced pathologist. Microscopic examination reveals a tumor forming blood vessels (Fig. 4.15). The degree of differentiation may vary and parts of the tumor may be totally anaplastic. Tumor spread along the sinusoids is pathognomonic (96). Kaposi's sarcoma, a malignant vascular tumor that has been seen with increasing frequency in recent years, may pose a difficult differential diagnostic problem. A detailed clinical history and strict adherence to the pathologic criteria should sort out these difficult cases.

EPITHELIOID HEMANGIOENDOTHELIOMA

Epithelioid hemangioendothelioma is a very rare hepatic tumor that can be seen in all ages and both sexes. Tumors with identical histology are seen elsewhere in the body as well. In a recent report (97), association with oral contraceptive agents has been proposed.

These tumors tend to grow in multiple foci and involve the liver extensively. On microscopic examination the tumor cells have an epithelioid appearance and they grow cohesively within the vascular system. The vascular system is often obliterated by these nodules of tumor cells. The angiogenic nature may not be easily discernible in some cases: factor VIII–related antigen is always positive in tumor cells (97,98) and is a helpful marker in problem cases. A recent excellent review by Ishak et al. (98) details the pathology and clinical features in 32 patients.

OTHERS

Leiomyosarcoma (99,100), fibrosarcoma (101), and rhabdomyosarcoma (15) may be seen originating in the liver.

Malignant lymphoma and leukemia can involve liver as a part of generalized process. Rarely, the liver may be the apparent primary and only site of involvement (102–105). Although a frozen section diagnosis may be difficult, in most cases it could be suggested, particularly if an imprint (touch preparation) of the tumor is made along with the tissue section.

Metastatic Tumors

The liver is the most frequent site of metastatic tumor in the body and a majority of these tumors reach the liver via the portal venous system (106). These foci of metastatic tumor may be solitary or multiple, discrete or confluent (Fig. 4.16). At times diffuse metastatic carcinomatosis may mimic cirrhosis clinically (107).

Partial hepatic resection for metastatic cancer is frequently performed, mostly for colorectal carcinoma (15,108). Although these resected specimens are not a diagnostic dilemma for the surgical pathologist, on rare occasions they may pose a problem, particularly when the histology is not inconsistent with a primary hepatic tumor and the clinical history is unusual. We have observed a solitary hepatic metastasis in a woman with bilateral breast carcinomas resected 17 and 22 years before. Histologically, hepatoma could not be easily excluded in the resected hepatic specimen. However, the very high estrogen receptor protein level was most helpful in making the correct diagnosis. It must be noted that low levels of estrogen receptor protein (less than 10 femtomoles per milligram cytosol protein) may be seen in hepatomas (109). In similar unusual cases, the pathologist must make full use of all the ancillary tools, namely, electron microscopy, immunocytochemistry, and so forth to arrive at the correct diagnosis.

Tumorlike Lesions

CYSTIC LESIONS OF THE LIVER

Hepatic cysts (Table 4.2) are uncommon; they may be congenital or acquired. Sanfellipo et al. (110) reported 150 cases of cystic disease of liver seen during an 18-year period. The incidence in their series was 17 per 10,000 abdominal explorations.

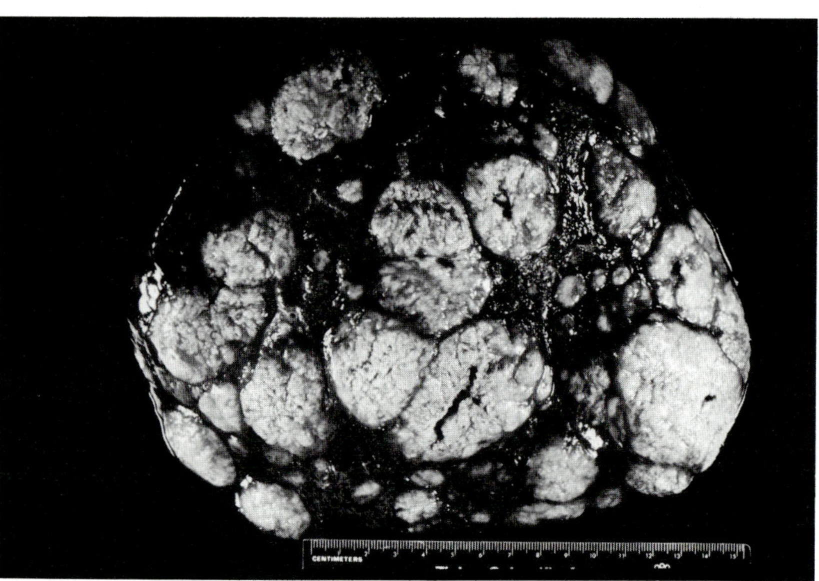

Figure 4.16. Liver with multiple nodules of metastatic colon carcinoma (autopsy specimen).

Table 4.2. Classification of Hepatic Cysts

Congenital
  Solitary
  Multiple
  Polycystic liver disease
Acquired
  Post-traumatic
  Inflammatory
    Pyogenic
    Parasitic
  Neoplastic
    Cystic tumors (cystadenoma and cystadenocarcinoma)
    Cystic degeneration of solid tumors (primary or
      metastatic)
    Dermoid cyst
  Miscellaneous
    ? Endometriotic cyst

The congenital cysts were more frequent in women while the acquired ones were more commonly seen in men. Most of the cysts were located in the right lobe of the liver.

The congenital cysts can be solitary or multiple; the most florid example of the latter being the polycystic disease of the liver. All congenital cysts are lined by low cuboidal epithelium resembling the epithelium of the biliary tract. Bile ducts can be seen in the fibrous wall of the cysts. Various theories regarding their origin have been proposed

(111). These cysts are usually asymptomatic but may be brought to attention because of complications such as rupture, hemorrhage, or infection.

Polycystic disease of the liver is an embryologic maldevelopment (20), not infrequently associated with polycystic disease of kidney (20,111,112). The liver in a full-blown case is massively enlarged and riddled with varying-sized cysts (Fig. 4.17). Liver transplantation is indicated in advanced polycystic disease.

Caroli's disease is another example of a congenital lesion in which cysts dominate the pathologic picture. The lesions here are derived from intrahepatic ductal system with alternate segments of stenosis and dilatation. Bile stasis, cholelithiasis, cholangitis, and abscess formation are major complications (20). A rare complication of all congenital cysts is the development of malignancy. Both adeno- and squamous cell carcinomas have been reported (69,73,74,113).

The acquired cysts of the liver may be post-traumatic, inflammatory, or neoplastic. Traumatic cyst is essentially a focal area of parenchymal rupture with accumulation of blood and/or bile. Inflammatory cysts can arise from both specific and nonspecific processes. Abscesses, bacterial or

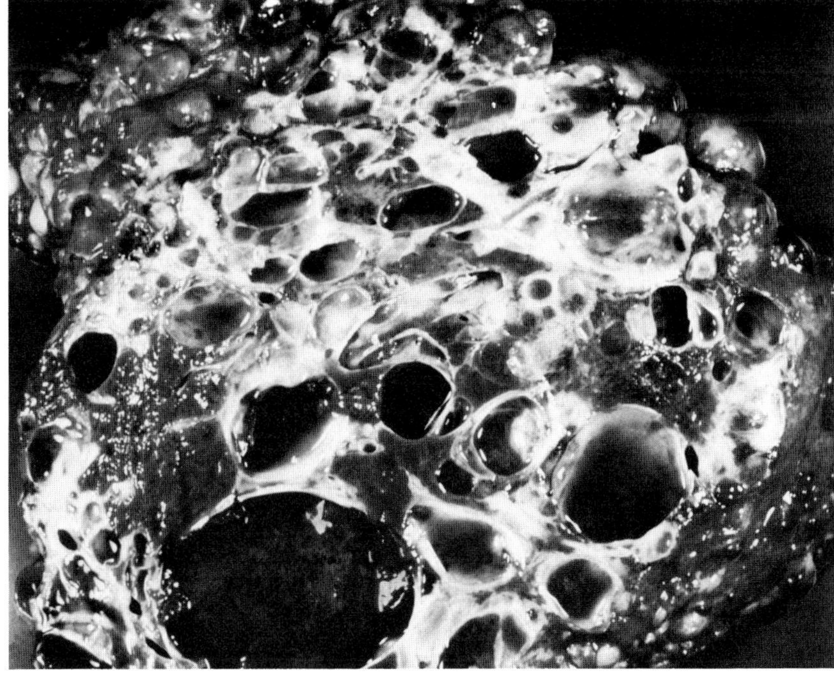

Figure 4.17. Polycystic liver removed at the time of orthotopic liver transplantation. The entire liver is replaced by thick- and thin-walled cysts.

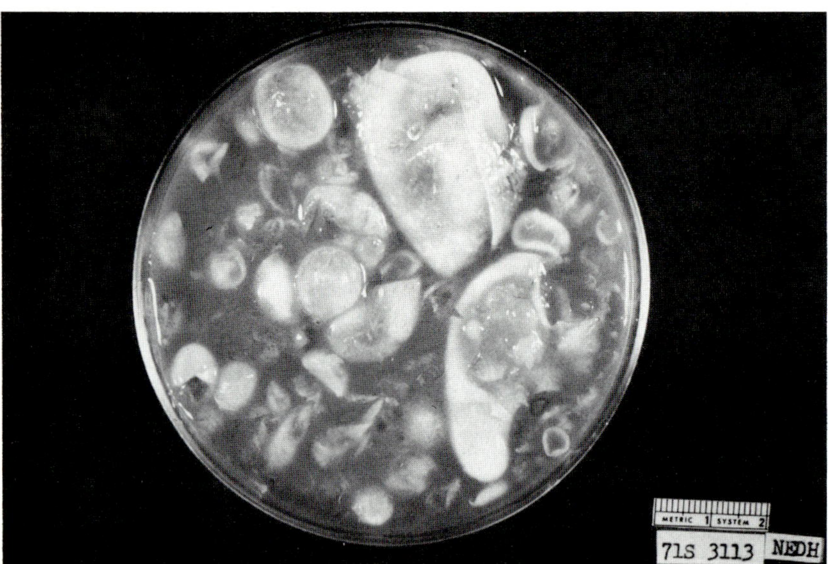

Figure 4.18. Intact and fragmented hydatid cysts of the liver removed surgically.

amoebic, can present as cysts. Hydatid cyst (Fig. 4.18) is the most common acquired cystic lesion of the liver worldwide (15,20). The cyst consists of a dense fibrous ectocyst derived from the host and an endocyst derived from the parasite. The cyst may be unilocular or multilocular; calcification may be present and indeed is a helpful radiologic sign. Aspiration of the cyst contents yields fluid containing the hydatid sand. The pathologic diagnosis is made by demonstrating scolices and hooklets in the hydatid sand, i.e., the sediment (Fig. 4.19). The hooklets are acid-fast, a feature that makes their detection easy, even in a specimen where the sediment is scant.

Rarely tumors, primary or metastatic (114), can undergo liquefactive degeneration and present as cystic masses. Cystic tumors have already been discussed.

Dermoid cysts or cystic teratomas similar to ones seen in the ovary may be rarely encountered in the

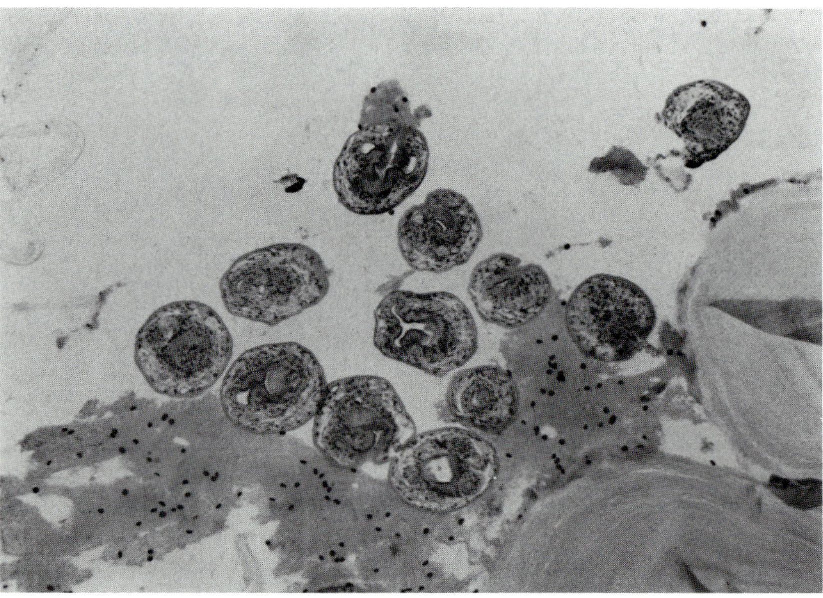

Figure 4.19. Hydatid sand containing cross-sections of scolices (×450). (Case contributed by Dr. K. Balogh, Department of Pathology, New England Deaconess Hospital.)

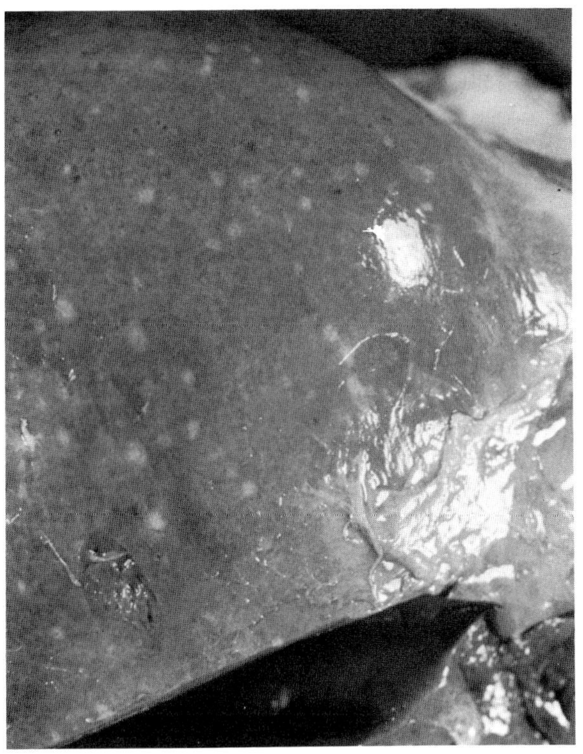

Figure 4.20. von Meyenburg's complexes (gross); autopsy liver. Small white-tan nodules are scattered all through the liver.

liver (20,115). Other examples of cysts that one might possibly encounter include endometriotic cyst seen on the surface of the liver in women with advanced endometriosis (20).

MULTIPLE BILE DUCT HAMARTOMAS

These are small innocuous lesions usually found incidentally either at autopsy or at laparotomy. Chung (116) found six cases out of 875 consecutive autopsies performed over $4\frac{1}{2}$ years. When discovered during surgery, these hamartomas need to be differentiated from metastatic carcinoma or disseminated granulomatous disease. There are many synonyms for this entity: cholangioadenoma, microhamartoma, or von Meyenburg's complexes. It is generally accepted that they represent developmental anomaly or hamartoma and not a true neoplasm. These may be related to the polycystic disease of liver (116). Grossly, gray-white firm nodules, 0.1 to 1.0 cm in diameter, are scattered all through the liver (Fig. 4.20). Microscopically, the nodular lesions are discrete and composed largely of bile ducts, ductules, and blood vessels embedded in a fibrocollagenous stroma (Fig. 4.21). Often the bile ducts are dilated, tortuous, and branching. They are lined by a single layer of cuboidal or low columnar cells. These ducts may contain amorphous bile-stained debris. Malignant transformation is extremely rare (117).

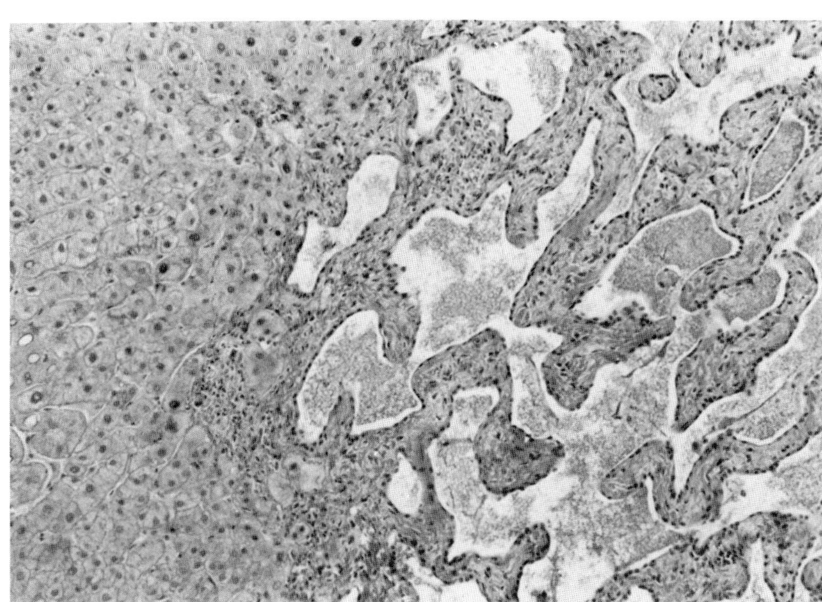

Figure 4.21. von Meyenburg's complexes. Embedded in fibrous stroma are interconnected ductlike structures lined by cuboidal epithelium ($\times$450).

Table 4.3. Diagnostic Features of Hepatic Cell Adenoma and Focal Nodular Hyperplasia

	Liver Cell Adenoma	*Focal Nodular Hyperplasia*
Clinical presentation	Symptomatic in most cases	Usually discovered incidentally
Capsule	Partial or complete	Well demarcated but unencapsulated
Size	Tend to be large	Usually smaller than adenomas
Consistency	Fleshy, soft	Firm to rubbery
Central scar	Not present	Always present
Radiating fibrous septa	Not usually seen but focal fibrosis may be present as a result of prior hemorrhage or infarct	Always present
Nodularity of parenchyma	Not seen	Present
Hemorrhage and/or necrosis on the cut surface	More common	Uncommon
Bile ducts	Not present within the mass	In fibrous septa and at periphery
Ductules	Not present within the mass	Present within the fibrous septa
Vascularity	Sinusoidal	Large veins and arteries present at periphery and fibrous septa
Vascular abnormalities	Not seen	Present
Bile stasis	Variable	Usually not seen
Glycogen	Normal or increased	Excessive
Ultrastructure	Normal	Simplified, with great reduction in structures and organelles

MIXED HAMARTOMA

This rare lesion is exclusively seen in infants. Grossly, a large (8- to 10-cm) firm tan-gray mass is present. Microscopically, it consists of hepatocytes, bile ductules, and vessels traversed by wide bands of collagen. Focal nodular hyperplasia may be in the differential diagnosis but is usually not difficult to distinguish.

MESENCHYMAL HAMARTOMA

Mesenchymal hamartoma is a rare benign lesion of unknown histogenesis (118,119) and is seen in very young children (usually less than 2 years of age) with no predilection for either sex. It presents as an abdominal mass. The patient is otherwise asymptomatic. The prognosis following surgical resection is excellent.

These are usually solitary and large with an irregular cystic appearance on the outer surface. On microscopic examination, the outstanding feature is the massively edematous connective tissue containing cystic spaces. Embedded in this stroma are bile ducts, hepatocytes, hematopoietic elements, and blood vessels.

FOCAL NODULAR HYPERPLASIA

Focal nodular hyperplasia is a space-occupying lesion of the liver, which has been called focal cirrhosis and hepatic hamartoma. Because of the uncertain etiology, the noncommittal term "focal nodular hyperplasia" is preferred over others. Various theories as regards to its histogenesis have been put forth. Some regard it as a hamartoma or a congenital malformation (120) while others think it represents a localized response or reparative process to an injury, probably vascular (20) in origin. Benz and Baggenstoss (121) suggested that these are regions that may have a predilection to injury because of congenitally abnormal blood supply and biliary drainage. Although more common in adults, it can be seen at any age. It is more frequently observed in women than in men.

Focal nodular hyperplasia is often confused with hepatic cell adenoma because of lack of uniform terminology, certain overlapping features, and particularly when only small nondiagnostic samples are available for study. The various differential diagnostic features are listed in Table 4.3. The data regarding the relationship of focal nodular hyperplasia to oral contraceptive agents are conflicting (5,9,10,122). Friedman et al. (123) have reported one case of simultaneous occurrence of focal nodular hyperplasia and hepatic cell adenoma. Although Ross et al. (124) have reported a case of focal nodular hyperplasia regression after discontinuation of oral contraceptives, one cannot be certain from their description that it was indeed a focal nodular hyperplasia. A case of focal nodular

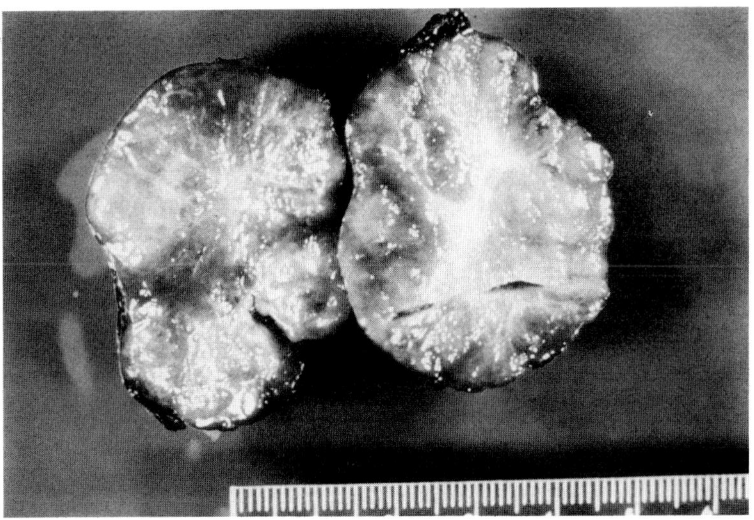

Figure 4.22. Focal nodular hyperplasia (gross). Well-demarcated nodule with a central stellate scar.

hyperplasia in an 11-year-old boy receiving synthetic anabolic androgens has been reported as well (125). Increased incidence of hemangiomas of the liver has been an associated finding. We have observed one such case.

The modes of presentation vary, in most cases being asymptomatic and incidentally discovered during unrelated laparotomy or at autopsy. In the Armed Forces Institute of Pathology (AFIP) series (5), only 20% of patients had signs and symptoms referrable to focal nodular hyperplasia. Patients on oral contraceptive agents may present with acute abdominal symptoms due to intralesional hemorrhage and/or rupture with hemoperitoneum (9,10). The natural history of focal nodular hyperplasia without surgery is not known; however, the recent report (53) suggesting fibrolamellar hepatoma as the malignant counterparts of focal nodular hyperplasia is interesting.

The gross appearance of focal nodular hyperplasia is of a discrete, well-circumscribed but not encapsulated, multinodular, cirrhoticlike mass in an otherwise normal liver (Fig. 4.22). In some series (120,126), lesions were evenly distributed between the left and right lobes of liver, while in another (5) the right lobe was favored. These lesions are usually solitary (80% of the cases), subcapsular, bulging from the surface and less than 5.0 cm in greatest dimension. The tumor is often lighter in color than the surrounding hepatic parenchyma and its consistency is firm or rubbery. The gross appearance of its cut surface, with a myxoid central or eccentric, depressed stellate scar and radiating fibrous tissue septa, is pathognomic in all cases.

On microscopic examination, nodules of cytologically normal hepatocytes are seen separated by fibrous tissue septa (Fig. 4.23). The hepatocytic nodules form disorderly thick cords and blend imperceptibly with the surrounding liver. Excessive cytoplasmic glycogen or Mallory's hyalin may be seen within their cytoplasm (127). The fibrous septa contain numerous bile ductules, blood vessels, and inflammatory infiltrate. Small aggregates of bile ductules can be seen within the hepatocytic nodules as well. The vessels within the fibrous septa display a variety of abnormalities: concentric or eccentric mural thickening, varying degrees of occlusion with fresh or organizing thrombi, or phlebitis and intimal proliferation. These changes may be primary or secondary. Their etiology is uncertain, but is probably not related to contraceptive steroids because they were seen before the introduction of oral contraceptive agents (128).

Ultrastructurally the different cellular components, that is, hepatocytes, biliary epithelium, Kupffer cells, etc., are quite similar to those in the adjacent normal parenchyma.

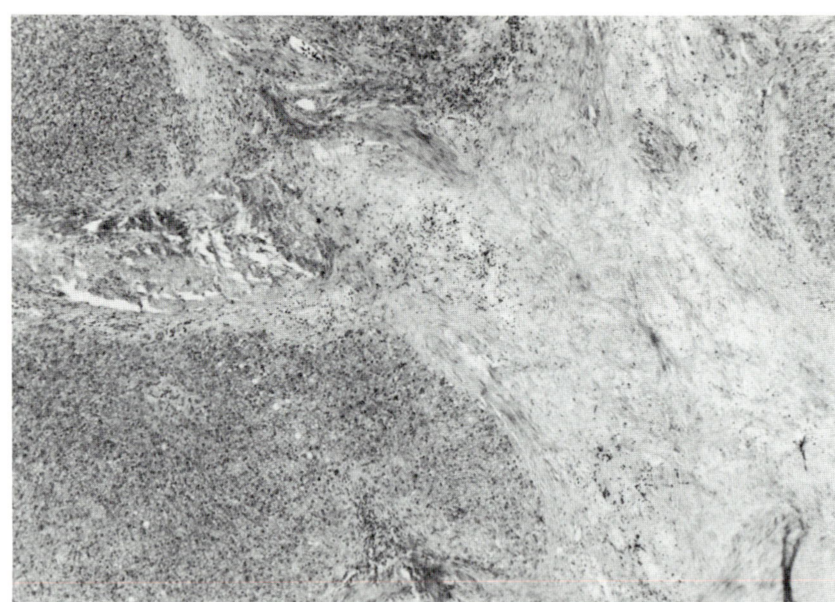

Figure 4.23. Photomicrograph of focal nodular hyperplasia. Nodules of hepatocytes are separated by dense fibrous tissue (×112).

Heterotopias is an adrenal or pancreatic tissue that may be seen within the liver (129). *Focal fatty change*, consisting of nodules or patchy areas composed solely of hepatocytes containing excessive amounts of fat, has been diagnosed by radiologic techniques. *Pseudolipoma* of Glisson's capsule (130) are small nodules of adipose tissue incorporated in the surface of the liver due to detachment of appendices epiploicae from the colon. *Inflammatory pseudotumor* is an extremely rare reported lesion (131,132) pathologically identical to the ones seen in other sites (e.g., lung). Other synonyms for this lesion are "plasma cell granuloma" or "postinflammatory tumor." These are localized proliferations of plasma cells and other inflammatory cells embedded in a fibrous stroma. Plasmacytoma is the main differential diagnostic problem.

Medical Diseases of the Liver

Hepatitis

The term "hepatitis" means hepatocellular injury with inflammation. Although many etiologic factors can be implicated in the pathogenesis of hepatitis, by far the most common causative agents belong to a group of viruses called "hepatitis viruses." There are at least three types of hepatitis viruses: type A; type B; and type non-A, non-B. Non-A, non-B hepatitis is largely diagnosed by exclusion (133) and probably includes more than one type of virus (134). The recently described "delta-agent" (135–137) will be described separately in this section.

All three types of viruses mentioned above produce a similar histologic picture with a few minor differences (138). Type A infection is generally mild with no tendency toward chronicity (139) whereas type B and type non-A, non-B can be a very severe acute illness and also can progress to a chronic stage (139). Several recent monographs and review articles have the detailed, up-to-date information regarding the epidemiology, serology, and clinical features of the various types of hepatitis (140–142).

Acute viral hepatitis can be caused by all three agents that have been mentioned. Hepatitis type A and HB_sAg and hepatitis B core antigens (HB_cAg) have been demonstrated in liver biopsies from patients with acute viral hepatitis (143). The clinical symptoms can vary from mild to severe.

In an established case, the constellation of pathologic findings is characteristic (133,144,145) (Fig. 4.24). The hepatic lobule is the seat of primary

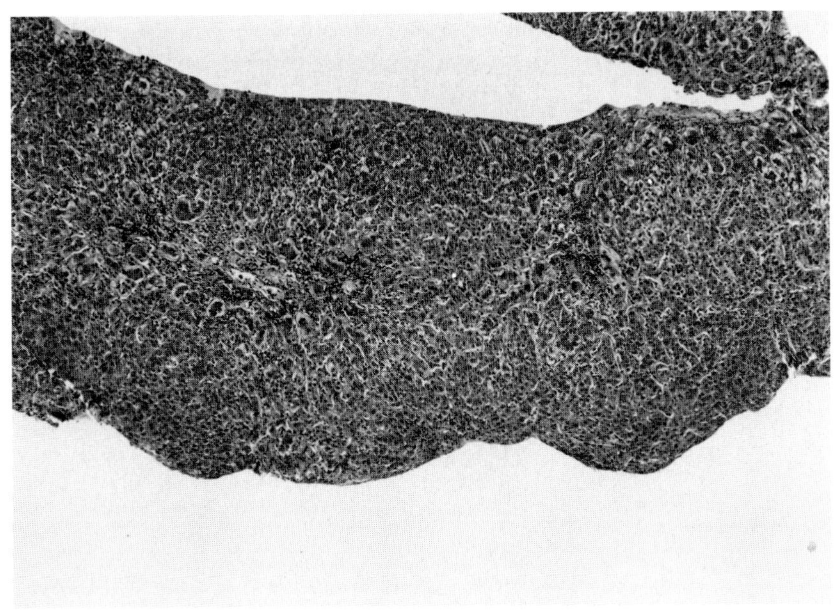

Figure 4.24. Acute hepatitis. There is disarray of lobular architecture with inflammatory infiltrate in both portal triads and liver lobule (×112). (Case contributed by Dr. K. Balogh, Department of Pathology, New England Deaconess Hospital.)

damage, with participation of portal areas and bile ducts to a lesser degree. The most striking microscopic change is the so-called "lobular disarray," namely, disturbed normal architectural pattern. This results from various changes (133,146,147) including degeneration and regeneration of hepatocytes, proliferation of Kupffer cells, and infiltration by inflammatory cells. Ballooning degeneration of hepatocytes with swelling and clearing of cytoplasm is seen all through the lobules but is more marked in the centrilobular zone (148). Fatty change is rare except in non-A, non-B hepatitis (142). "Acidophilic bodies" (Fig. 4.25), consisting of small, shrunken, deeply eosinophilic degenerating hepatocytes with absent or pyknotic nucleus, are scattered randomly through the parenchyma (148). Single or multiple cell dropout with resultant gaps in hepatocytic plates are also seen (148). Regener-

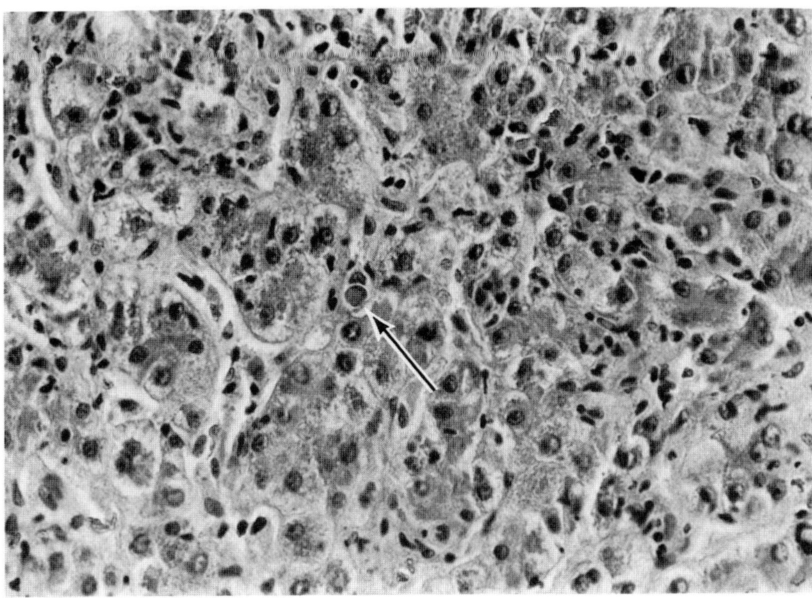

Figure 4.25. Acute hepatitis. An "acidophil body" (*arrow*) is seen. This high-power view also illustrates the lobular inflammation, Kupffer's cell hyperplasia, and total lack of normal lobular arrangement (×450). (Case contributed by Dr. K. Balogh, Department of Pathology, New England Deaconess Hospital.)

ative activity of hepatocytes, particularly near the portal areas, may be very prominent. Centrilobular cholestasis is also present in some cases.

Inflammatory infiltrate is seen in both lobular and portal areas. It consists of lymphocytes, macrophages, and a few neutrophils. In the lobules the inflammation is diffuse with focal accentuation in the areas of cellular dropout. Phlebitis of the central veins has been described (133). Kupffer cell hyperplasia is clearly evident. The cells in the portal infiltrate are the same as in the lobular infiltrate. All portal areas are affected and the limiting plates are not breached. Bile duct proliferation may be seen. In acute non-A, non-B hepatitis, the histologic findings may be somewhat atypical. The inflammatory response is usually less severe with a remarkable paucity of lymphocytes and a much larger (out of proportion) number of "acidophilic bodies."

During the resolving phase of a typical acute viral hepatitis, there is a decrease in the degenerative and regenerative changes with marked Kupffer cell hyperplasia. Lipofuscin deposition may be prominent (148).

Acute viral hepatitis may be associated with submassive confluent or bridging necrosis (146, 149,150), which results from continuous areas of hepatocytic dropout between contiguous central veins or between central veins and portal tracts (148) with collapse of reticulin network. This exaggerated histologic response is probably related to the difference in patients' immune response (146). The inflammatory infiltrate in the areas of bridging necrosis is prominent. At this stage healing may occur; however, further progression of the process is characterized by collapse of the reticulin framework (148). This is a severe form of hepatitis and can lead to hepatic failure or development of cirrhosis (149). At autopsy or during orthotopic liver transplantation, large regenerating nodules grossly mimicking hepatoma may be seen (151).

Massive hepatic necrosis occurs in the most fulminant form of acute hepatitis and is often fatal, with a mortality rate of 75% or more (148). In such instances, the entire liver lobule undergoes necrosis (150) with a marked mononuclear inflammatory response. The Kupffer cells are markedly hyperplastic and contain lipofuscin. The portal structures are spared and the bile ducts may show signs of proliferation. The portal inflammatory infiltrate often contains neutrophils. If the patient survives

the acute phase, recovery does occur. Early during the recovery phase, cholestasis may be seen. Reticulin collapse with distortion of the hepatic architecture and fibrosis are late features (142,147), seen after full recovery.

At times, acute viral hepatitis may produce a pronounced cholestatic picture (148,151) with feathery degeneration of centrilobular hepatocytes. Other findings of a typical acute viral hepatitis may also be seen and are of great help in distinguishing this syndrome from extrahepatic bile duct obstruction. This cholestatic form is most often seen with type A hepatitis (142,144) and may run a prolonged course before recovery.

CHRONIC HEPATITIS

Chronic hepatitis can be of viral or autoimmune origin. Similar features may also be seen in certain drug-induced liver injury or metabolic diseases like Wilson's disease and alpha$_1$-antitrypsin deficiency (133,148). Hepatic dysfunction has to be present for at least 6 months before the diagnosis of chronic hepatitis can be made (142,146,150, 152,153).

Chronic hepatitis can be of three types: chronic lobular, chronic persistent, and chronic active (154,155). Each of the three subtypes is associated with a distinctive histologic picture and prognosis.

CHRONIC LOBULAR HEPATITIS

This is the most mild form of chronic hepatitis and essentially represents protracted acute viral hepatitis (148). Although the clinical course can extend from 6 months to several years, complete clinical and histologic recovery is generally the rule. At the height of the process, mild hepatocytic ballooning, acidophilic bodies, and lobular inflammation is seen histologically. Portal inflammation may be present, usually to a mild degree (155). Kupffer cell hyperplasia may be prominent (153).

CHRONIC PERSISTENT HEPATITIS

This is another self-limited form of chronic hepatitis which can persist for years (145). Development of cirrhosis is not a threat (156,157). Histologically this form is characterized by inflammatory infiltrate in portal areas consisting of lymphocytes, plasma cells, and macrophages (144,

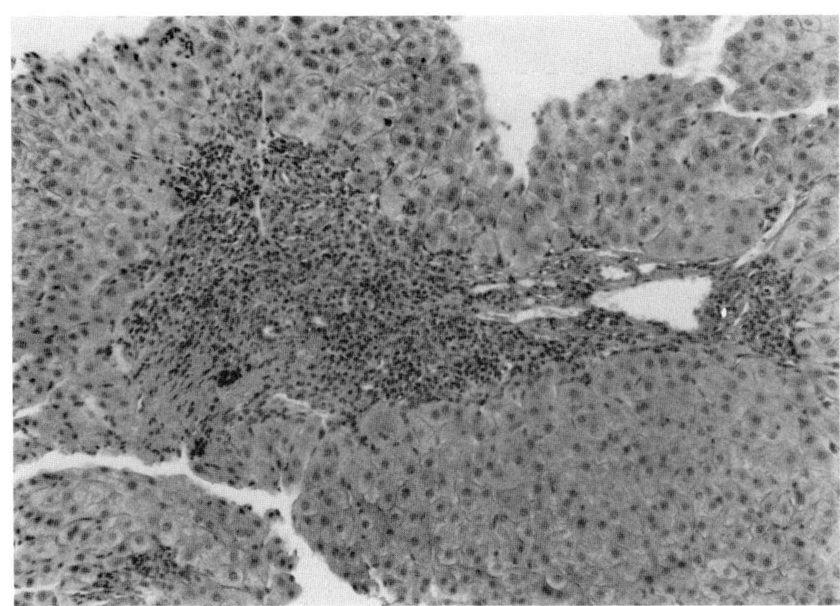

Figure 4.26. Chronic persistent hepatitis. Mononuclear infiltrate in expanded portal area (×180). Limiting plates are intact.

147,155) (Fig. 4.26). Proliferation of bile ductules is also seen. The portal infiltrate may rarely spill over to the periphery of the lobule but "piecemeal necrosis" of hepatocytes is not seen (148). The lobular changes of disarray and hepatocytic necrosis are minimal or absent (153).

CHRONIC ACTIVE HEPATITIS

The diagnosis of chronic active or chronic aggressive hepatitis carries the ominous potential of development of cirrhosis (147,148,156,157). The brunt of injury is borne by the portal triads and periportal hepatocytes (144,147). The portal tracts are variably expanded with inflammatory infiltrate consisting of lymphocytes, plasma cells, and macrophages. Plasma cells can be prominent, particularly in the "lupoid" or "autoimmune" form. The diagnostic hallmark of chronic active hepatitis is piecemeal necrosis (145,148,157,158) (Fig. 4.27), which by definition means destruction of limiting plate, that is, liver cells at the interface between parenchyma and connective tissue in association with an inflammatory infiltrate composed predominantly of lymphocytes and plasma cells. The hepatocytes of the limiting plate show degenerative changes, or "apoptosis" as proposed by some (159), and are surrounded by inflammatory cells and collapsed reticulin. The nature of "piecemeal necrosis" has intrigued many investigators. It is

clear that mononuclear cells mediate the necrosis of hepatocytes. In Kawanishi's electron microscopic studies (160), close apposition between small lymphocytes and hepatocytes was noted with associated degenerative changes in these hepatocytes. Many immunopathologic studies have attempted to characterize the infiltrative cells (156,161,195). In conclusion, it appears that T-cell-mediated cytotoxicity is the most important pathogenetic mechanism causing "piecemeal necrosis." However, in "autoimmune" chronic active hepatitis "antibody-dependent cellular cytotoxicity" plays a vital role. In addition to piecemeal necrosis, bridging necrosis and increased portal fibrosis may be seen as well (153). Bile ductal changes similar to those seen in primary biliary cirrhosis may be present, particularly in non-A, non-B hepatitis (142,155,162).

Type B hepatitis can be histologically distinguished from the other types of hepatitis by the presence of "ground-glass cells" and "sanded nuclei" (141,148). These two features are randomly scattered through the parenchyma. "Ground-glass cells" are hepatocytes that are enlarged and have eosinophilic cytoplasm resembling frosted glass (163). The cytoplasm of these cells stains positive with orcein or aldehyde fuchsin and with the immunoperoxidase technique HB$_s$Ag can be demonstrated in the cytoplasm. These cells are seen in abundance in chronic hepatitis B virus (144) carri-

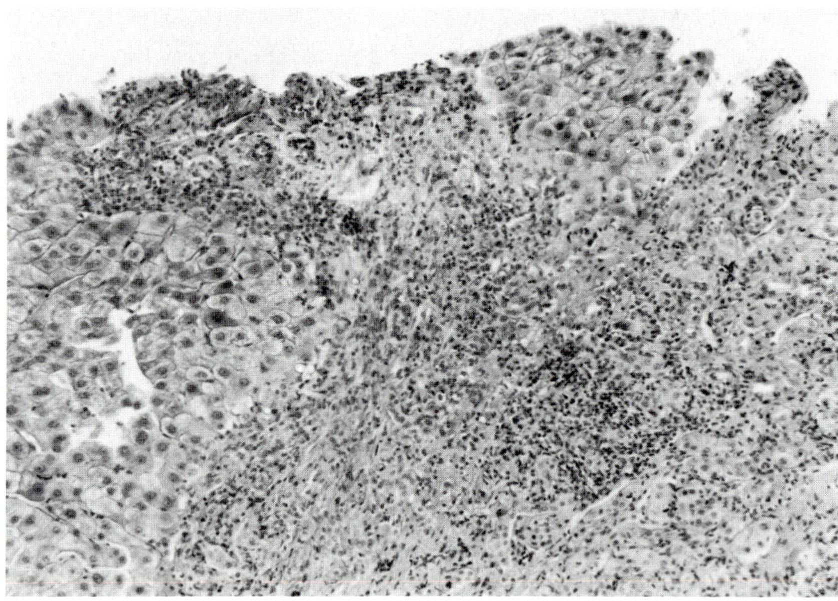

Figure 4.27. Chronic active hepatitis with marked portal mononuclear infiltrate and extension of inflammatory infiltrate into the lobule (piecemeal necrosis) (×180).

ers. "Sanded nuclei" are seen in the presence of HB$_c$Ag in the nucleus (141,148,164). By light microscopy these nuclei bear tiny, irregularly shaped inclusions, and by electron microscopy both HB$_s$Ag and HB$_c$Ag particles can be demonstrated in them.

In 1977, Rizzoto et al. (135) described the "delta-agent," which seemed to complicate the infection of hepatitis B virus. At present it is thought to represent a transmissible, defective virus that requires hepatitis B virus as a helper (165–167). The overall histologic pattern with "delta-agent" superinfection resembles more closely non-A, non-B hepatitis, cytopathic damage being more marked than cellular cytotoxicity (166,167). Predominant findings include eosinophilic degeneration of hepatocytes with formation of acidophile bodies, lobular infiltrating cells consisting mostly of macrophages, and portal mononuclear infiltrate.

Other viruses such as cytomegalovirus, herpes simplex, adenovirus, and Epstein-Barr (EB) virus can cause hepatitis as well (see Pathology of Liver Transplantation, page 72). Bacteria, fungi, and parasites are all capable of infecting the liver (142).

Alcoholic Liver Disease

Lesions of liver resulting from excessive use of alcohol, in the absence of any other etiologic agents, are grouped under alcoholic liver disease.

Liver biopsy specimens from these alcoholic patients have varied microscopic changes (168). Although these various histopathologic features are individually nonspecific, when seen together they are fairly characteristic of alcoholic liver disease. However, similar changes can be seen following an ileojejunal bypass, after intestinal resection, and in diabetics (151,169).

Fatty change (Fig. 4.28) of a mild, moderate, or severe degree is the earliest lesion (170) and is seen in approximately 90% of patients. Other causes of fatty liver are listed in Table 4.4. It is a reversible condition and disappears in about 6 to 8 weeks following withdrawal of alcohol (171). Microscopically, the individual hepatocytes become enlarged and contain intracytoplasmic fat droplets (172). These droplets appear as clear areas on routine histologic sections. Associated cholestasis and centrilobular lytic necrosis may be seen (168,170).

Two types of intracytoplasmic structures are seen fairly frequently in alcoholic liver disease (169,171): Mallory bodies and megamitochondria. Mallory bodies, also known as "alcoholic hyalin," are densely eosinophilic, somewhat twisted, rope-like structures that surround the nucleus as a complete or incomplete wreath (Fig. 4.29). Identical intracytoplasmic structures can be seen in Indian childhood cirrhosis, Wilson's disease, galactosemia, primary biliary cirrhosis, and other cholestatic syndromes. Therefore, noncommittal

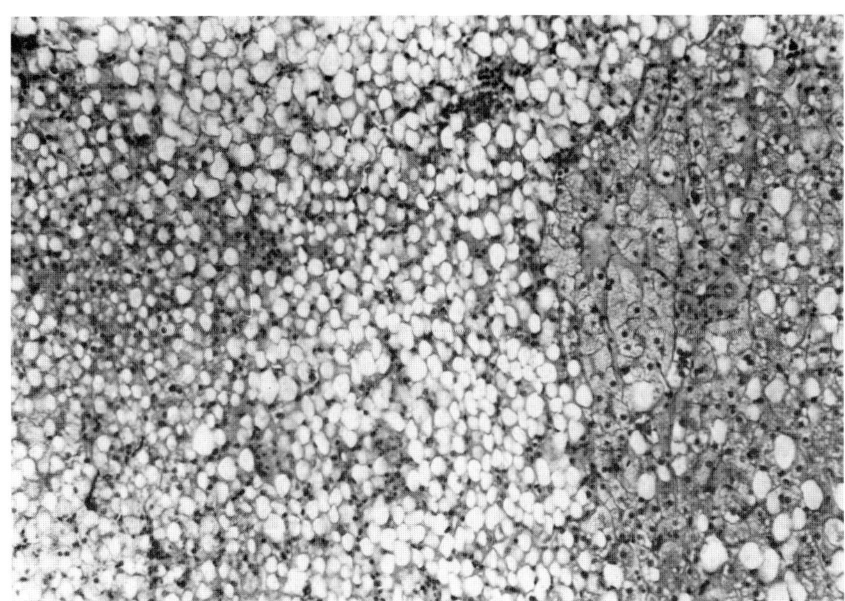

Figure 4.28. Fatty change with enlargement of hepatocytes; many contain clear intracytoplasmic spaces representing fat globules (×180).

terms like Mallory's body or Mallory's hyalin are preferred over alcoholic hyalin. Mallory bodies have been the subject of extensive research (173,174). It is generally accepted that they are of intermediate filament origin (174,175). Megamitochondria are enlarged, damaged mitochondria (confirmed by electron microscopy) (175,176) that resemble red blood cells and are present within the cytoplasm of hepatocytes, particularly in the centrilobular zones. They are spherical, eosinophilic hyaline bodies and can be readily distinguished from Mallory's hyalin.

Table 4.4. Etiologic Factors Associated with Fatty Liver

Alcoholism
Obesity
Intestinal bypass
Intestinal resection
Diabetes mellitus
Parenteral nutrition
Reye's syndrome
Fatty liver in pregnancy
Drug induced
  Tetracycline
  Methotrexate
  Steroids
  Hypervitaminosis A
Carbon tetrachloride toxicity
Kwashiorkor
Others
  Congenital metabolic disorders (Wilson's disease,
    galactosemia, etc.)
  Infections (viral, malaria)

An inflammatory response composed predominantly of neutrophils may be seen within the hepatic lobules. The neutrophilic aggregates may surround a degenerating hepatocyte or a hepatocyte containing a Mallory body. Kupffer cell hyperplasia is often seen. Scattered lipogranulomas in the portal areas are not uncommon.

Alcoholic hepatitis (172) is an ill-defined syndrome presenting clinically with anorexia, weight loss, jaundice, unexplained fever, and ascites. Progression to hepatic failure may be rapid. On liver biopsy, centrilobular hyaline necrosis of hepatocytes with sclerosis of central veins and abundant Mallory's hyalin is seen. Cholestasis and intralobular neutrophilic infiltrate may be very prominent in some cases. Edmondson (168,177) proposed the term "sclerosing hyaline necrosis" for this syndrome. In one study (178), the amount of Mallory's hyalin was found to be the best single indicator of the severity of alcoholic hepatitis. A chronic hepatitislike picture in alcoholics has also been reported (179). The pathogenetic mechanisms of this form of alcoholic liver disease are not quite clear. If the alcoholic liver damage is not arrested early, it progresses to fibrosis and eventually to cirrhosis. Excessive connective tissue is deposited typically around the central veins. Periportal fibrosis may or may not be present. Individual hepatocytes may be wrapped with fibrous

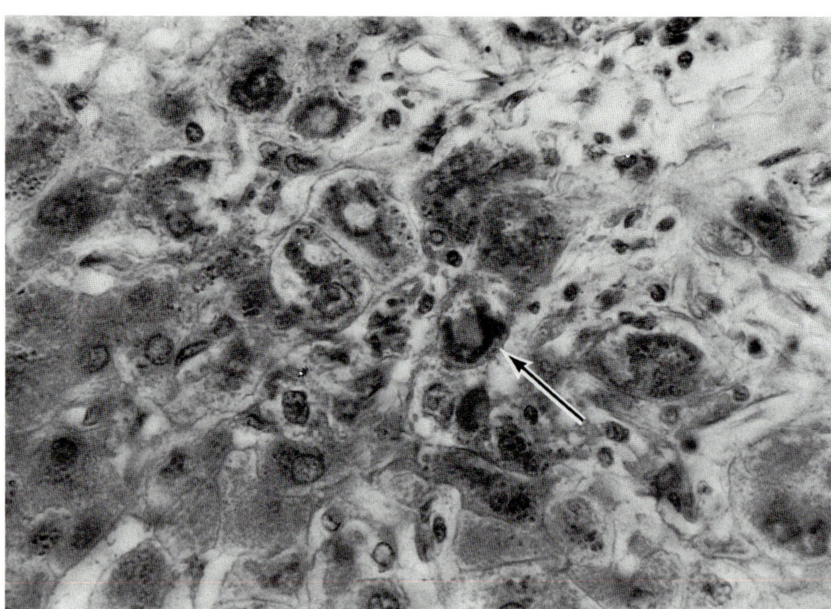

Figure 4.29. Mallory bodies. Hepatocytes contain intracytoplasmic granular, ropy, perinuclear, wreath-like structures (*arrow*) (×1800).

tissue and increased connective tissue deposition in the walls of sinusoids is typically also seen (151).

Cholestatic Liver Disease

Defective flow of bile results in its accumulation within hepatocytes, bile canaliculi, bile ducts, and Kupffer cells and leads to cholestatic liver disease. This accumulation of bile pigment within parenchymal structures presents microscopically as a yellow-green and homogeneous material. Distinction from hemosiderin and lipofuscin is essential to arrive at the correct diagnosis. Special stains are a reliable help in this regard.

Cholestatic liver diseases can be acute or chronic and a result of extra- or intrahepatic causes.

ACUTE EXTRAHEPATIC CHOLESTASIS

Acute extrahepatic cholestasis is due to arrested bile flow caused by mechanical obstruction of bile ducts (extrahepatic) secondary to calculus, tumor, stricture, parasites, and so forth. The presence of cholestasis is directly related to the degree of obstruction and is usually not significant unless the obstruction is marked. Histologically the centrilobular area is the first to be affected and shows intracanalicular cholestasis. The hepatocytes in this zone at times are enlarged, their cytoplasm appears foamy, fuzzy, and shows the so-called

"feathery degeneration" (180) (Fig. 4.30). The portal tracts are expanded by edema and an inflammatory infiltrate rich in neutrophils. Cholangiolar proliferation may be present. Acute inflammation of varying degrees involving bile ducts (acute cholangitis) is often present along with bile plugs in these ducts.

ACUTE INTRAHEPATIC CHOLESTASIS

Acute intrahepatic cholestasis with bile plugs in canaliculi can be seen in many nonobstructive conditions, namely alcoholic liver disease, drug-induced hepatotoxicity, viral hepatitis, and various metabolic disorders (151). In alcoholics a component of extrahepatic obstruction may be secondary to pancreatitis. A variety of drugs can be associated with intrahepatic cholestasis (181), which may be associated with mild to severe hepatocellular damage and a periportal infiltrate of eosinophils.

CHRONIC EXTRAHEPATIC CHOLESTASIS

Chronic extrahepatic cholestasis may show similar microscopic changes as acute extrahepatic cholestasis; the overall picture, however, is more striking. The "feathery degeneration" of hepatocytes, the amount of bile retention, and the proliferation of bile ductules are much more marked and also associated with bile lakes. Increased portal fibrosis

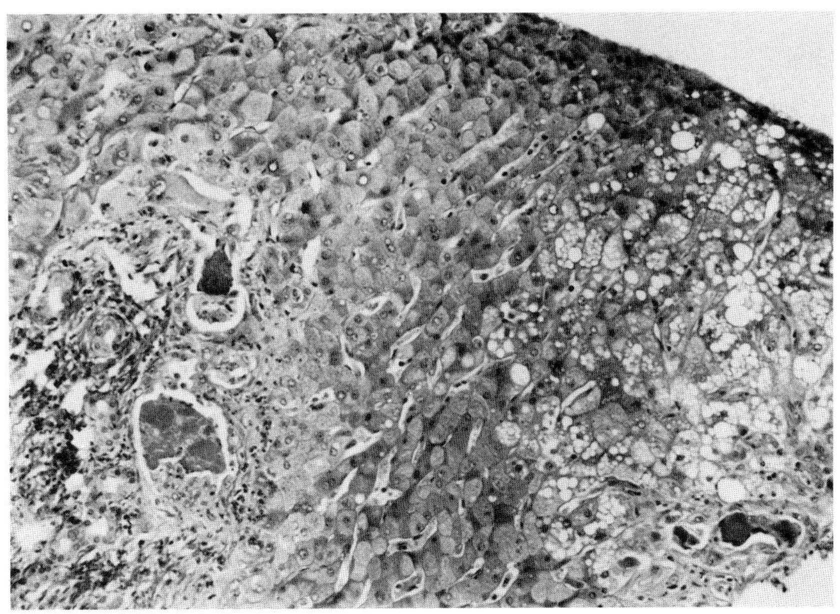

Figure 4.30. Liver biopsy shows obstructive changes and acute cholangitis. Portal tract (*left*) has bile plugs within the bile ducts with injured ductal epithelium. Inflammatory infiltrate, consisting predominantly of neutrophils, is seen within and around the bile ducts. Centrilobular hepatocytes (*right*) show the so-called "feathery degeneration" (×450).

can lead to secondary biliary cirrhosis in long-standing cases.

Extrahepatic biliary atresia of childhood and sclerosing cholangitis are two examples of chronic disorders that give rise to cholestatic picture on liver biopsy. In extrahepatic biliary atresia, in addition to the findings described above, focal giant cell transformation of hepatocytes may be seen.

Sclerosing cholangitis can be primary or secondary to inflammation and/or surgical manipulation of the biliary tract. The primary type is at times associated with other diseases, such as ulcerative colitis or retroperitoneal fibrosis (151,181,182). The involvement of the biliary tract in primary sclerosing cholangitis may be complete or partial (involvement of either the extrahepatic or the intrahepatic portions). The affected ducts are thick and cordlike with markedly narrowed lumina. Distinction from sclerosing carcinoma may be difficult at times and a biopsy may be essential to rule it out. Cholestasis and other histologic findings can vary from mild to marked, depending on the degree of obstruction. Concentric fibrosis is seen around the interlobular bile ducts (Fig. 4.31) when the process involves the intrahepatic ducts. This periductal fibrosis greatly narrows the ductal lumen and eventually causes its complete disappearance and replacement by a fibrous nodule. In late stages of primary sclerosing cholangitis the number of bile ducts is markedly decreased.

CHRONIC INTRAHEPATIC CHOLESTASIS

Primary biliary cirrhosis or chronic nonsuppurative destructive cholangitis typically presents a picture of chronic intrahepatic cholestasis. Predominantly seen in women of the reproductive age group (183), primary biliary cirrhosis has been an enigma to hepatologists and immunologists alike. A vast literature is available on the probable pathogenetic mechanisms of this disorder (183–188,195).

A definite histopathologic diagnosis may be difficult to make in early stages but distinction from biliary obstruction is rarely the problem. A good correlative clinical history is helpful (189). The primary site of injury is the small interlobular bile duct (190). An inflammatory infiltrate composed predominantly of lymphocytes and plasma cells is seen in portal areas, with a particular tendency to involve the bile ducts (183) (Fig. 4.32). The infiltrate is seen within the walls of the ducts with destruction of epithelial lining and disruption of basement membrane. This is the most pathognomonic stage and has been referred to as "chronic nonsuppurative destructive cholangitis" (191). Atypia of epithelial cells with hyperchromasia of nuclei may be seen. The affected ducts are greatly distorted, showing angulated and pointed edges. Epithelioid granulomas (see Fig. 4.32) or collections of histiocytes are often seen surrounding these abnormal ducts, but may also be seen in the

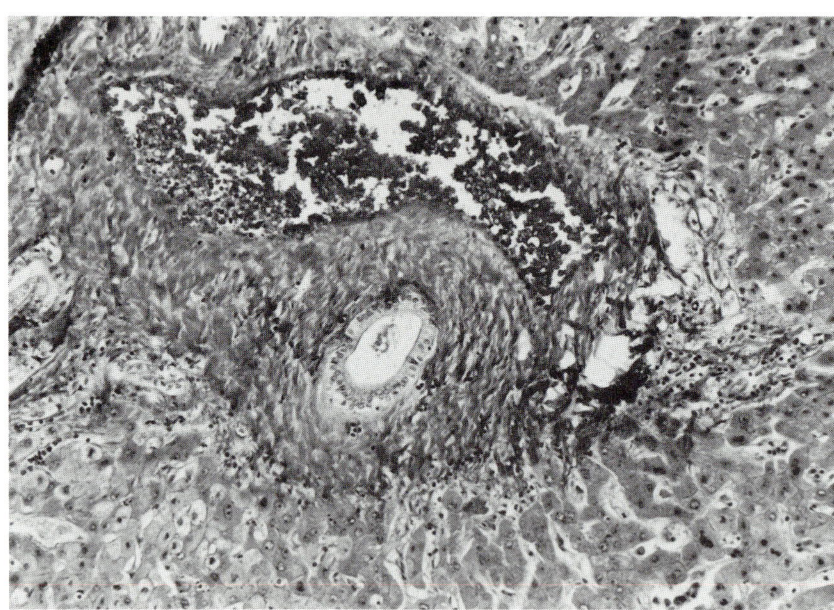

Figure 4.31. Primary sclerosing cholangitis. Bile duct in a portal triad has concentric fibrosis (×450).

hepatic lobules. Scattered lymphoid follicles with germinal centers are present as well (190,191). All these findings do not involve every portal tract to the same extent. In advanced cases, interlobular bile ducts are greatly reduced in number. Cholangiolar proliferation, however, may be seen and should not be confused with bile ductular proliferation. Peripheral cholestasis with increased amounts of copper deposition (192) are other associated findings. Mallory's hyalin may be seen in periportal hepatocytes (151). Hepatic lobules are usually not involved by the inflammatory process; however, in some advanced cases piecemeal necrosis may be seen. Increased portal fibrosis and cirrhosis occur late in the course of disease. Development of hepatocellular carcinoma is an extremely rare but reported complication (193).

Histopathologically primary biliary cirrhosis can

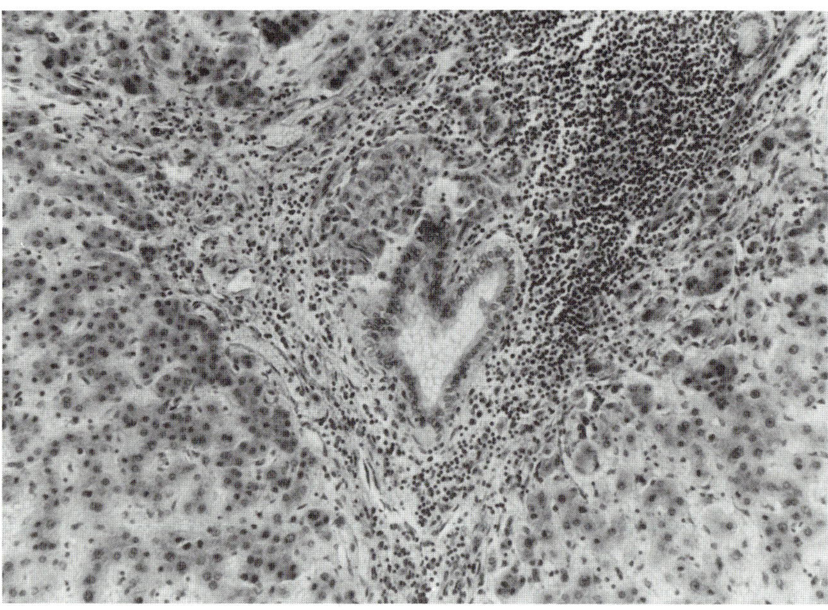

Figure 4.32. Primary biliary cirrhosis. Injured atypical bile duct surrounded by inflammatory infiltrate and epithelioid granuloma (×450).

be divided into four stages (191,194). One must remember, however, that these stages overlap considerably and the pathognomonic duct lesion may be seen very late, even in the presence of well-established cirrhosis (183).

Stage 1: *florid duct lesion* in which the pathognomonic lesion of "nonsuppurative destructive cholangitis" is present with inflammation and edema of the portal tracts.

Stage 2: *ductular proliferation* in which changes seen in stage 1 are much more intense, and in addition marked ductular proliferation is seen.

Stage 3: *scarring* in which there is decrease in the intensity of the inflammatory infiltrate, but formation of early fibrous septa is evident. Interlobular bile ducts are decreased in number.

Stage 4: *cirrhosis* in which progressive formation of fibrous septa is accompanied by development of the regenerative nodules and marked paucity of bile ducts. The various histopathologic stages may remain static for long periods of time (189). It must be noted that cirrhosis appears quite late.

Chronic cholestatic viral hepatitis, drug-induced cholestasis, and sarcoidosis can sometimes mimic primary biliary cirrhosis. A complete clinical evaluation including the various laboratory tests and liver biopsy interpretation can help arrive at the correct diagnosis.

Vascular Disorders of the Liver

HEPATIC CONGESTION

This is the most frequent vascular abnormality of the liver, heart failure being the most common etiologic factor. Grossly, in advanced cases, the liver has a "nutmeg" appearance. Dilatation with congestion of central veins and centrilobular sinusoids is the typical microscopic finding. In addition to this, atrophy and necrosis of centrilobular hepatocytes with focal hemorrhage may be seen in long-standing cases, which eventually results in central fibrosis. "Cardiac cirrhosis" is a term, probably an incorrect one, applied to this last condition.

SHOCK LIVER

In cases of prolonged shock or severe acute congestive heart failure, centrilobular sinusoidal congestion with striking degeneration of hepatocytes is seen (151). A neutrophilic inflammatory reaction is seen if the patient survives the acute phase. "Ischemic hepatitis" is also a term applied to this lesion with a clinical picture that could be confused with viral hepatitis (196). During the recovery phase, areas of cell dropout and lipofuscin-laden macrophages are seen.

PERIPORTAL SINUSOIDAL DILATATION

This has been reported in women using oral contraceptive pills (197). Dilatation of periportal sinusoids is seen involving all lobules. At times, the midzone may be involved as well. Liver plates appear thinned out and atrophic.

PELIOSIS HEPATIS

Peliosis hepatis is an extreme degree of sinusoidal dilatation with formation of blood lakes of varying sizes. These blood-filled spaces may be partially lined by endothelium. The pathogenesis of this change is not entirely clear. In the past, it used to be a complication of debilitating illnesses such as tuberculosis. In the mid-1970s, an association with anabolic steroid therapy has been noted (198,199).

VASCULAR THROMBOSIS AND OCCLUSION

Thrombosis and occlusion can involve the portal vein and its branches, the hepatic artery and its branches, the inferior vena cava, the hepatic veins, or the sublobular venules.

Thrombosis of the portal vein is usually secondary to other processes, namely, tumor, cirrhosis, surgery, adjacent inflammation, etc. Rarely true infarcts can result from portal venous thrombosis; the more common lesion seen in these cases are Zahn's infarcts. These are circumscribed areas of hepatocellular atrophy with sinusoidal dilatation and congestion (151,200).

Occlusion of the hepatic artery generally results in hepatic infarcts. The cause of the occlusion can be varied, namely, surgical ligation, thrombosis, aneurysm, or arteritis. An infarct of the liver, unlike the changes in "shock liver," follows no architectural boundaries. Liver lobules together with the portal tracts in the involved area undergo coagulative necrosis. Recovery is associated with histologic evidence of organization and later fibrosis.

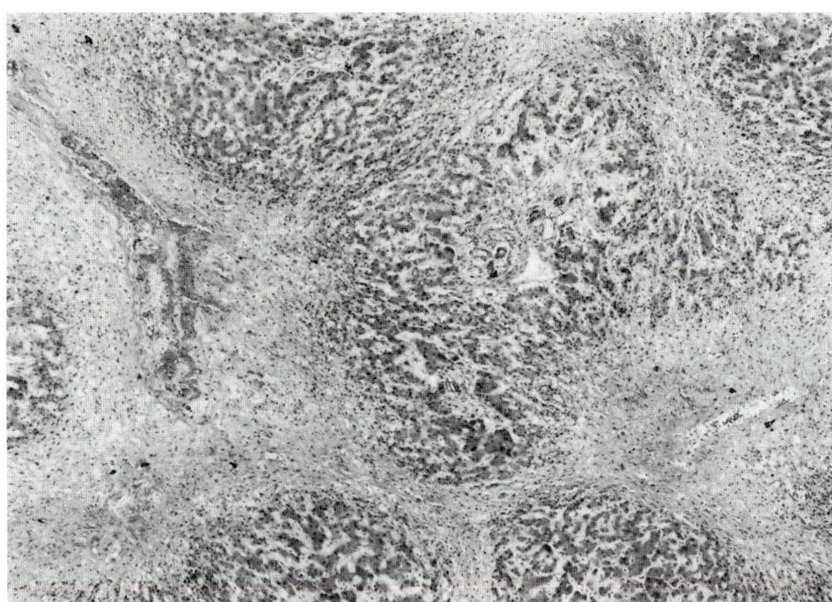

Figure 4.33. Budd-Chiari syndrome. Photomicrograph of the liver at autopsy showing centrilobular necrosis with hemorrhage and congestion. Organizing thrombus is seen in a central vein (*left*) (×180).

Thrombosis of hepatic veins and/or inferior vena cava results in the so-called "Budd-Chiari syndrome" (Fig. 4.33). The etiology of this lesion is multifactorial and includes coagulation disorders, tumor invasion, inflammation, and drugs such as contraceptive agents (151,200). The most prominent histologic finding on liver biopsy is severe sinusoidal dilatation and congestion of hepatocytes in the centrilobular areas. Associated hepatocytic atrophy may be seen. Distinction from congestive heart failure may be difficult on liver biopsies. In chronic long-standing cases centrilobular fibrosis with periportal regeneration and attempted nodule formation is seen (200).

Veno-occlusive disease is an extremely rare disorder characterized by marked narrowing of central and sublobular veins. Pyrrolizidine alkaloids (201) and chemotherapeutic agents have been implicated in the pathogenesis of this lesion. It is a noted complication in bone marrow transplant recipients (202). Microscopically early lesions are characterized by central and sublobular venous intimal swelling with subendothelial reticulin deposition resulting in compromise of vascular lumen. As the lesion progresses, fibrosis with hyalinization of the vessel wall occurs. Superimposed thrombosis is rarely seen.

Metabolic Diseases

The metabolic diseases involving the liver include a variety of storage disorders and lesions associated with deposition of different substances. The list of these diseases is a long one and the reader is referred to one of the major texts in hepatopathology (203–205). We will limit ourselves to the discussion of just a few selected disorders.

HEMOCHROMATOSIS

Idiopathic or primary hemochromatosis results from increased deposition of iron in the hepatocytes, Kupffer cells, and even bile ductal epithelium (Fig. 4.34). Initially the periportal hepatocytes are involved but with progression of the disease, the entire lobule is affected (206). Associated portal fibrosis and cirrhosis are part of the disorder. Development of hepatocellular carcinoma is not infrequent. Iron pigment may be deposited in other parts of the body as well.

Increased iron deposition in the liver may also occur following repeated blood transfusions, dietary overload, and some hematologic disorders (151,205). A syndrome of idiopathic neonatal iron storage involving the liver, pancreas, heart, and endocrine and exocrine glands has been reported (207).

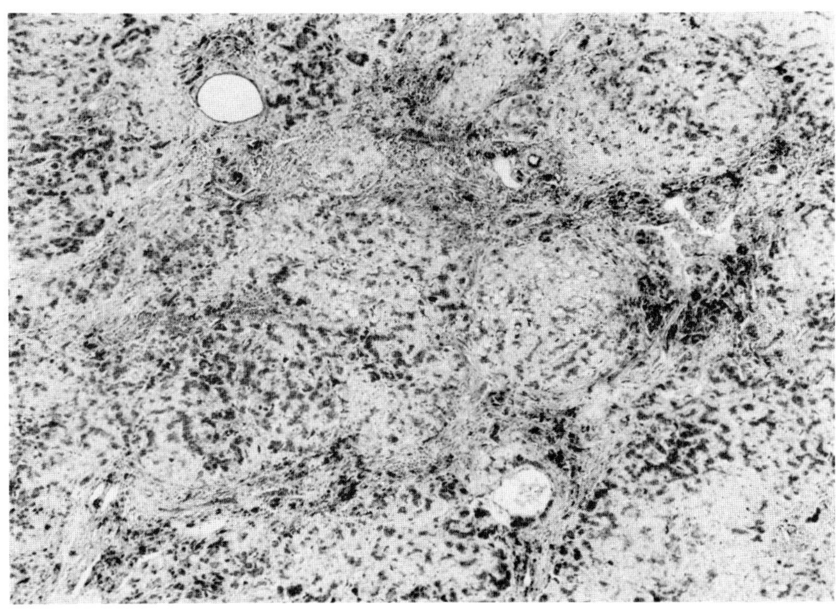

Figure 4.34. Hemochromatosis. Marked iron deposition (dark granular material) and cirrhosis with pseudolobule formation (×180).

WILSON'S DISEASE

This disease with autosomal recessive inheritance (203) is characterized by increased accumulation of copper in the tissues, liver being one of the earliest sites of involvement. Unfortunately the microscopic findings are not specific (208) and therefore, good clinical correlation is of utmost importance. Fatty change is the earliest light microscopic lesion that may or may not be accompanied by foci of hepatocellular necrosis. Later in the course of the disease, a picture similar to chronic active hepatitis develops. Periportal copper deposition is a helpful differential diagnostic feature at this stage (208). Micro- and macronodular cirrhosis is the final outcome. In some cases periseptal "Mallory bodies" may be seen (208). Large amounts of copper are deposited in these livers and special histologic processing is usually needed to document it (151,203).

ALPHA$_1$-ANTITRYPSIN DEFICIENCY

Alpha$_1$-antitrypsin is a protease inhibitor produced in the hepatocytes. An inherited deficiency of this enzyme is associated with hepatic pathology in about 10% of patients (203) homozygous for genotype PiZZ. A variety of histologic changes have been described, ranging from a picture similar to "neonatal hepatitis," or paucity of intrahepatic bile ducts, to full-blown cirrhosis (209). The most striking histologic finding in liver biopsies of these patients is the presence of round periodic acid-Schiff (PAS)-positive droplets within the hepatocytes, which have been shown to contain alpha$_1$-antitrypsin by immunocytochemistry (209, 210). Hepatocellular carcinoma may develop in some cases of cirrhosis secondary to this disorder.

Cirrhosis and Fibrosis

Cirrhosis may be defined as diffuse fibrosis of liver parenchyma with regenerative nodule formation (Fig. 4.35). It is more than just simple scarring. The structural changes are irreversible and represent the end-stage of a variety of liver diseases (151). In the past, the commonly used classifications combined the morphologic, etiologic, and pathogenetic terms, which resulted in some confusion; more recently, the trend is toward using a classification based either on morphology or etiology (Tables 4.5, 4.6).

Morphologically, cirrhosis can be of two major types (151,211), micronodular and macronodular. Transitional forms or mixed forms may be seen in which there are approximately equal numbers of small and large nodules (151). In micronodular cirrhosis, the majority of the nodules measure 3

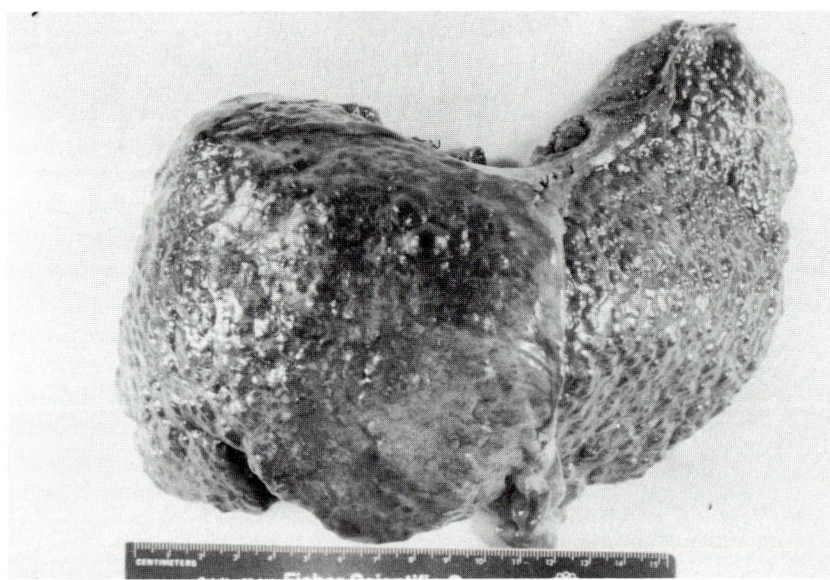

Figure 4.35. Cirrhosis (gross). Varying-sized regenerative nodules are separated by fibrous bands.

mm or less in diameter, while in macronodular type the nodules vary in size and may be large (212). Distinction between the two types may be difficult on liver biopsy specimens (151) and is best made on gross examination of the liver. The micronodular form may change to the macronodular type with passage of time because of necrosis and overgrowth of the regenerating nodules.

A micronodular pattern is seen in alcoholics and in patients with venous outflow tract or biliary obstruction, hemochromatosis, Indian childhood cirrhosis, and cirrhosis associated with poor nutrition (213). The fibrous septa in the micronodular type of cirrhosis are usually thin and of even width. The histology of the nodules and the fibrous septa vary with the different etiologic factors (Table 4.7). Development of hepatocellular carcinoma is much less frequent in this morphologic category of cirrhosis (214).

The macronodular type of cirrhosis results from multilobular necrosis with collapse and subsequent regeneration. Another mechanism by which macronodules can be formed is by enlargement of nodules in the micronodular type of cirrhosis. The

fibrous septa are of varying width and can be very broad. Grossly the liver is greatly distorted. This is the common pattern of cirrhosis that develops in patients with chronic active hepatitis.

A classification of cirrhosis by etiology into three

Table 4.6. Classification of Cirrhosis by Etiology

Established etiologic associations
Viral hepatitis
Alcoholism
Metabolic diseases
Hemochromatosis
Wilson's disease
Alpha$_1$-antitrypsin deficiency
Cystic fibrosis
Others
Biliary disease
Primary biliary cirrhosis
Secondary biliary cirrhosis
Venous outflow obstruction
Budd-Chiari syndrome
Veno-occlusive disease
Drugs and toxins
Intestinal bypass for obesity
Others
Debatable etiologic factors
Autoimmunity
Toxins
Parasitic diseases
Malnutrition
Cirrhosis of unknown etiology
Cryptogenic
Indian childhood cirrhosis

Table 4.5. Classification of Cirrhosis Based on Morphology

Micronodular
Macronodular
Mixed forms

Table 4.7. Pathologic Characteristics of Cirrhosis According to Etiology

	Viral Hepatitis	Alcoholic	Hemo-chromatosis	Wilson's Disease	Biliary Primary/Secondary		Venous Outflow Obstruction
Nodule size	Micro or macro	Micro	Micro	Macro	Micro	Micro	Micro
Fatty change	−	+	±	±	−	−	−
Lipogranuloma	−	±	−	−	−	−	−
Lobular pattern	−	−	+	−	−	+	+
Pericellular fibrosis	−	+	−	−	−	−	−
Mallory's hyalin	−	+ (Centrilobular and panlobular)	−	± Periseptal	± Periseptal	± Periseptal	−
Copper	±	−	−	+	+	±	−
Excessive iron deposition	−	±	+	−	−	−	−
Cholestasis	±	±	−	±	+	+	−
Bile duct proliferation	+	+	±	±	− (Late stages)	+	−
Inflammation	±	±	−	−	+	−	−
Granuloma	−	−	−	−	±	−	−
HB$_s$AG, HB$_c$AG	+ (If HBV associated)	−	−	−	−	−	−

+ = present; − = absent; ± = may or may not be present.

categories (see Table 4.6) has been proposed by Anthony et al. (212).

Although the gross appearance of a cirrhotic liver is quite characteristic, the histologic diagnosis may not be easily made at times. These difficulties can be minimized if certain facts are remembered. Micronodular cirrhosis is not difficult to diagnose on biopsy material because multiple small nodules may be present in the specimen with intervening fibrous tissue septa. On the other hand, the macronodular type may not be so easy to recognize if the biopsy is from the interior of one single large nodule. An open wedge biopsy must be deep enough, that is, more than 2 mm, to avoid confusion with subcapsular fibrosis, a feature seen in many normal livers (151,215). Fragmentation of the biopsy specimen (particularly needle) with rimming of these fragments by fibrous tissue is another helpful feature in favor of cirrhosis. The degree of activity, namely, extent of ongoing hepatocytic necrosis, severity of inflammatory infiltrate, and Kupffer cell hyperplasia in a cirrhotic process, must be assessed histologically, as it does seem to correlate well with the clinical progression of liver damage and therefore with the prognosis (211).

The concept of liver cell dysplasia has become popular in recent years and is regarded as a possible precursor of hepatocellular carcinoma (216,217).

Other hepatic lesions associated with fibrosis include congenital hepatic fibrosis, cystic disease of the liver, and hepatoportal sclerosis. In these lesions the fibrosis is nonprogressive. Cystic disease of liver has already been discussed in Surgical Diseases of the Liver (page 40). Congenital hepatic fibrosis is characterized by portal fibrosis containing dilated bile ducts. This fibrous tissue proliferation forms anastomosing septa dividing the normal liver parenchyma into nodules and thus resembling cirrhosis on gross appearance. However, true regenerative nodule formation is never seen. Hepatoportal sclerosis or noncirrhotic portal fibrosis clinically presents with portal hypertension and its associated complications. However, the microscopic findings are rather nebulous. Mild to moderate portal fibrosis with mild disturbance of the basic hepatic architecture is all one sees in most patients.

Nodular Regenerative Hyperplasia

Nodular regenerative hyperplasia of the liver is a poorly understood entity that may be grossly con-

Table 4.8. Conditions Associated with Nodular Regenerative Hyperplasia

Immune complex diseases
   Rheumatoid arthritis
   Felty's syndrome
   Scleroderma and CRST syndrome
   Mixed cryoglobulinemia
   Subacute bacterial endocarditis
   Tuberculosis

Monoclonal gammopathies
   Waldenström's macroglobulinemia
   Chronic lymphocytic leukemia with plasmacytoma
   Multiple myeloma and plasma cell dyscrasias
   Monoclonal gammopathy

Myeloproliferative disorders
   Polycythemia vera
   Myelofibrosis
   Primary thrombocythemia

Modified from Wanless IR, Solt LC, Kortan P. Nodular regenerative hyperplasia of the liver associated with macroglobulinemia; a clue to the pathogenesis. *Am J Med* 1981; 70:1203–1209. (Ref 221).

fused with cirrhosis and is associated with a variety of systemic disorders (Table 4.8). Various terms have been used in the literature for this change, such as adenomatous hyperplasia (218), nodular transformation (219), and so forth.

It presents clinically with signs and symptoms of portal hypertension. Rarely, it may be encountered at autopsy as an incidental finding, particularly when the liver is only partially involved.

The gross appearance is characterized by transformation of hepatic parenchyma into varying-sized nodules with little or no fibrosis. Microscopically, there are nodules of hyperplastic hepatocytes with preservation of basic architectural framework. No cirrhosis or hepatocellular damage is seen. Accurate interpretation may be difficult without an open biopsy (220,221).

Pathology of Liver Transplantation

Orthotopic liver transplantation (OLT) in humans is being carried out with increasing frequency in recent years. Many centers have sprung up across the United States and also in the other parts of the world. The survival figures are constantly improving (222) as the surgical techniques are being refined and better immunosuppressive agents are becoming available (223).

For the pathologist, OLT has brought along a unique opportunity to study a variety of disease

Table 4.9. Indications for Liver Transplantation

Biliary atresia
Cirrhosis (all types with possible exception of alcoholic)
Tumors involving liver only
Chronic hepatitis
Primary biliary cirrhosis
Massive hepatic necrosis
Sclerosing cholangitis
Metabolic disorders
Budd-Chiari syndrome
Congenital hepatic fibrosis

processes that were not seen before. As the procedure itself has evolved with the constantly changing clinical concepts, so have the pathologic lesions associated with it. The literature on the pathology of OLT is scanty and conflicting (224–226). Initially, most of the patient-management decisions were made on clinical grounds alone, but more recently, the clinical staff in some centers, including our institution, are actively seeking information from liver biopsies on a routine basis.

For a long time, the pathologic studies were limited to autopsy material, with the exception of a few biopsies and a rare transplant hepatectomy specimen (227).

Although some analogies can be drawn from the vast experience with the kidney transplants, for the most part, liver transplantation and its associated complications differ greatly from other organ grafting.

OLT is performed in children and in adults for numerous indications (Table 4.9). The pathologic lesions and complications following liver transplants can involve not only the liver, but other organ systems as well. We will limit our discussion to the pathologic lesions seen in the graft itself, resulting in graft failure in most cases (Table 4.10).

Perioperative Period

The changes seen in the liver biopsies performed before, during, and soon after transplantation essentially reflect the damage caused by varying degrees of ischemia warm or cold.

Most of these changes are reversible and recovery occurs within 3 weeks (226). Snover et al. (226) studied liver biopsies taken at the time of insertion of the liver, which showed generalized hepatocellular swelling. Our experience with similar pretransplant biopsies has been identical to theirs. Our surgical team has also performed biopsies "1

Table 4.10. Pathologic Lesions Involving the Graft Following OLT

Perioperative period
  Ischemic damage of various degrees
Postoperative period (early and late)
  Lesions caused by technical problems
    Vascular
    Biliary tract
  Infection
    Bacterial
    Fungal
    Viral
  Rejection reaction
    Acute
    Chronic
  Functional cholestasis
  Recurrence of original disease
    Tumor
    Primary biliary cirrhosis
    Chronic active hepatitis
    Budd-Chiari syndrome
  Transplanted disorders
  Drug toxicity
    Azathioprine
    Cyclosporin A
    Others
  Others
    Development of lymphoma
    Calcifications

---

hour" after the hepatic artery anastomosis, and these have shown aggregates of polymorphonuclear leukocytes within the liver lobules without hepatocytic destruction, a change, we think, related to the operative manipulations. In one case, we did find patchy areas of centrilobular hepatocytic necrosis, which correlated with poor graft function in the immediate postoperative period. Eggink et al. (225), on the other hand, report no abnormalities in any of their "1-hour" post-transplantation biopsies.

Postoperative Period—Early and Late

TECHNICAL PROBLEMS

During the early phases of OLT, technical problems were the foremost cause of graft failure (227,228), but as the surgical skills have been refined, these problems have slipped lower on the list.

The technical failures include vascular and/or perfusion problems and those of the biliary tract.

VASCULAR AND/OR PERFUSION PROBLEMS

These result in ischemic damage to the graft; various types of ischemic injuries in the peritrans-

plant period have already been alluded to. Ischemic damage in the postoperative period can result from thrombosis of the hepatic artery or portal vein, or are due to vascular compromise from other causes such as compression by an enlarged caudate lobe, and the like (224,229). We have observed a case of fungal arteritis involving the hepatic artery with resultant occlusive thrombosis and necrosis of the graft. Thrombosis of the inferior vena cava is uncommon and has been reported in a case of recurrent Budd-Chiari syndrome in the transplanted liver. In our series of 39 OLTs in 35 patients, there have been two cases of marked ischemic damage with total necrosis of the graft necessitating retransplantation 3 to 4 days after the first transplantation. Two other patients suffered ischemic damage to the graft, but in these cases the graft function improved after an initial lag phase.

Regardless of the time interval between surgery and vascular insults, we always found similar pattern in biopsies of such livers. In the early phase, centrilobular (Rappaport zone 3) necrosis is seen along with hemorrhage in the same area. At this stage, the process may be still reversible and if controlled, the new liver is left with mild centrilobular scarring. During the recovery phase, tremendous regeneration of the hepatocytes is seen along with multinucleation and abundant mitoses. If the basic problem is not controlled, the area of necrosis enlarges and involves the remainder of the lobule; massive irreversible hepatic necrosis ensues (Fig. 4.36). The portal structures are relatively well preserved, and indeed, the bile ducts may show attempted regeneration. Death usually results if there is no second transplantation in time. Therefore, this end-stage lesion is only seen in transplant hepatectomy specimens or at autopsy.

BILIARY TRACT COMPLICATIONS

The biliary tract has been called the "Achilles heel" of liver transplantation (228–230). In the two major series (222,231), there has been a high risk of biliary anastomosis breakdown with or without obstruction and ascending cholangitis. Some patients also had the problem of developing amorphous sludge in the biliary tree; this occurred both early and late in the postoperative period. Excellent examples have been illustrated in the literature (227,233). This problem is no longer encoun-

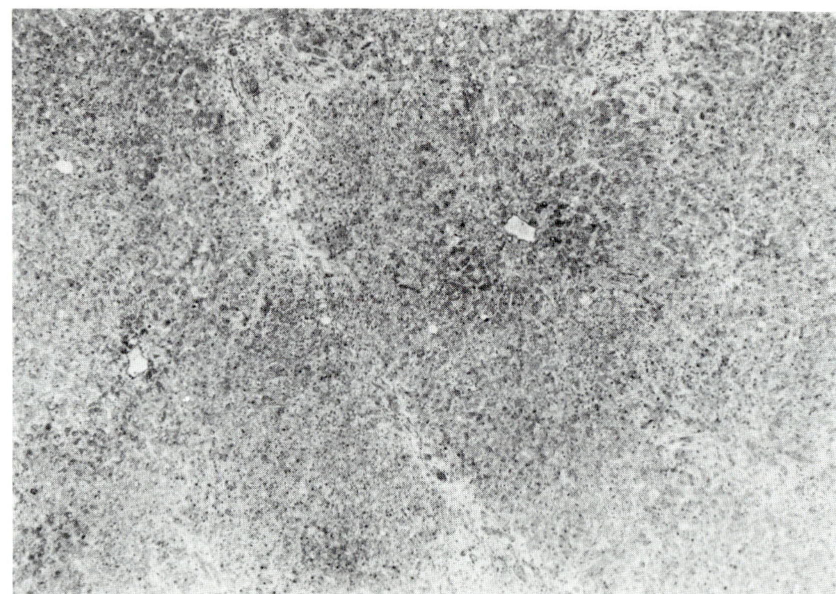

Figure 4.36. Massive ischemic damage. A liver graft with diffuse coagulative necrosis of the hepatocytes (×112).

tered since the biliary tree has been flushed routinely during harvesting of the liver.

All biliary tract complications are associated with histopathologic changes of obstruction with or without cholangitis. At times, distinction from rejection is difficult (232). Typically, early obstruction is characterized by centrilobular intracanalicular cholestasis with enlargement and ballooning of hepatocytes in this zone. The same feature may also be seen for a few days postoperatively in biopsies from livers with mild ischemic damage, when the excretion of bile is not very efficient. Clinical correlation is of utmost importance in these cases. When the obstruction becomes more severe, the pathologic findings are pathognomonic. Large bile lakes are formed; the entire liver lobule may show cholestasis with large bile plugs within the interlobular bile ducts. The hepatocytes, particularly in the centrilobular areas, undergo the so-called "feathery degeneration." These obstructive changes are often associated with cholangitis (see Fig. 4.30); bile ducts in the portal areas are proliferative with numerous neutrophils and other leukocytes inside their lumen and also in the adjacent portal tissue. This lesion may be easily confused with rejection.

INFECTION

Infection has been an important cause of graft failure and death of patients in two reported major series (229,231,233). This has certainly been true in our patients as well. Generalized infection, particularly with lung involvement, is usually the case. We will limit ourselves to the study of infections involving the graft only. Clinically, infection of the graft is difficult to diagnose and to distinguish from other causes of graft failure, particularly rejection—a most important differential diagnosis indeed.

Infections involving the graft could be bacterial, viral, or fungal. Bacterial infection of the biliary tract causes cholangitis. Abscesses can occur as a part of cholangitis, systemic disease, or as infection of an infarcted area. Fungal infections usually occur late in the course and may be part of a generalized process. Viral infection of the hepatic graft, particularly with cytomegalovirus (CMV), is the most frequent cause of graft infection in our cases and in other series as well (224,228). In a typical case there are small foci of neutrophils scattered throughout the hepatic parenchyma. These microabscesses are usually seen around enlarged hepatocytes, which contain the characteristic intranuclear "owl eye"–type CMV inclusion bodies (Fig. 4.37). The cytoplasm of these hepatocytes also contains fine, granular, virus-related particles. Sometimes step sections are needed to demonstrate the presence of these intranuclear and cytoplasmic inclusions. CMV inclusions can also be seen in the epithelium of the bile ducts and

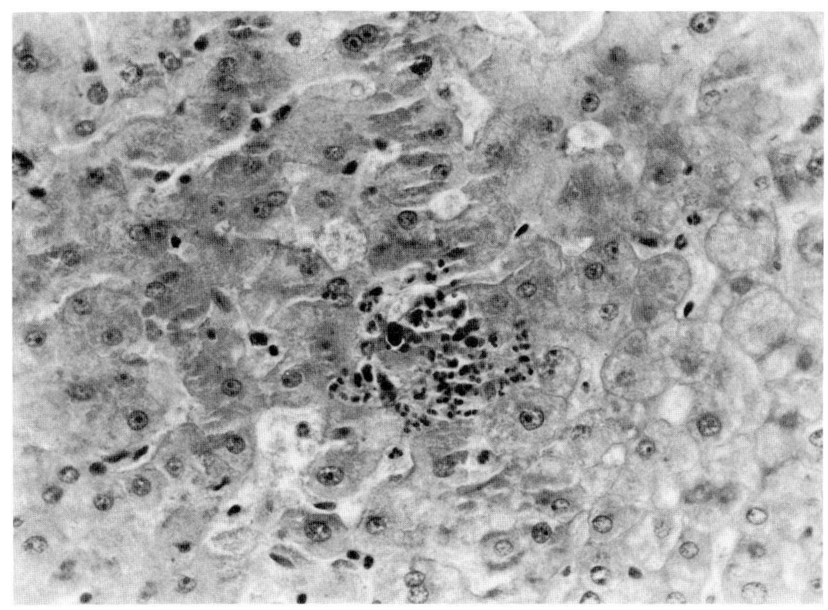

Figure 4.37. Cytomegalovirus hepatitis. Collection of neutrophils and lymphocytes surrounds an enlarged hepatocyte with a large homogeneous intranuclear inclusion (×450).

in the endothelium of veins and arteries, as well as in the sinusoidal lining cells (224). The involvement can vary from mild to marked. At times, even with the presence of a typical clinical syndrome including diagnostic serology, CMV inclusions cannot be observed (234). Immunoperoxidase stain to facilitate detection of CMV antigen has been used, but is of limited value (234). Mild lymphocytic infiltrate of portal areas with lymphocytic beading of sinusoids and focal granulomatous reaction are associated features that are shared with EB virus hepatitis (234,235) and also certain drugs (236). Diagnosis of EB virus hepatitis rests upon serologic evidence.

Herpes simplex hepatitis can also occur in the graft (224). Large confluent areas of necrosis, without respecting the architectural boundaries, rimmed by inflammatory infiltrate containing neutrophils and typical "ground-glass" intranuclear inclusions (Cowdry type A), are the microscopic hallmarks of herpetic hepatitis (Fig. 4.38).

HBV may infect a graft or can recur in it. The usual histologic changes that are dependent upon a competent immune system for their development may not be seen in these patients and therefore the diagnosis may be missed. In the Pittsburgh series (224), there were two cases of recurrent hepatitis type B infection with typical histologic features.

REJECTION

Rejection of hepatic allografts is now the cause of one of the major graft syndromes in the postoperative period since the technical problems have been greatly reduced. However, it is generally agreed that liver grafts are rejected less aggressively than other organ transplants (223). The true incidence of rejection is extremely difficult to assess.

The clinical picture of rejection of liver allograft is modified by immunosuppressive therapy. However, unmodified rejection has been reported (232) in a patient who underwent OLT for subacute hepatic necrosis following viral hepatitis and in whom the immunosuppressive therapy was withheld. The patient had a vigorous rejection reaction and died on the seventh postoperative day; microscopically intense mononuclear infiltrate was seen involving portal triads and all vascular endothelium.

Hepatic allograft rejection modified by immunosuppression has been subclassified into two types (237): acute cellular and chronic vascular. We have not found this subdivision to be of much help since both types may be present simultaneously. Hyperacute rejection mediated by humoral mechanisms, as seen in renal transplants, is not seen with hepatic transplants (231).

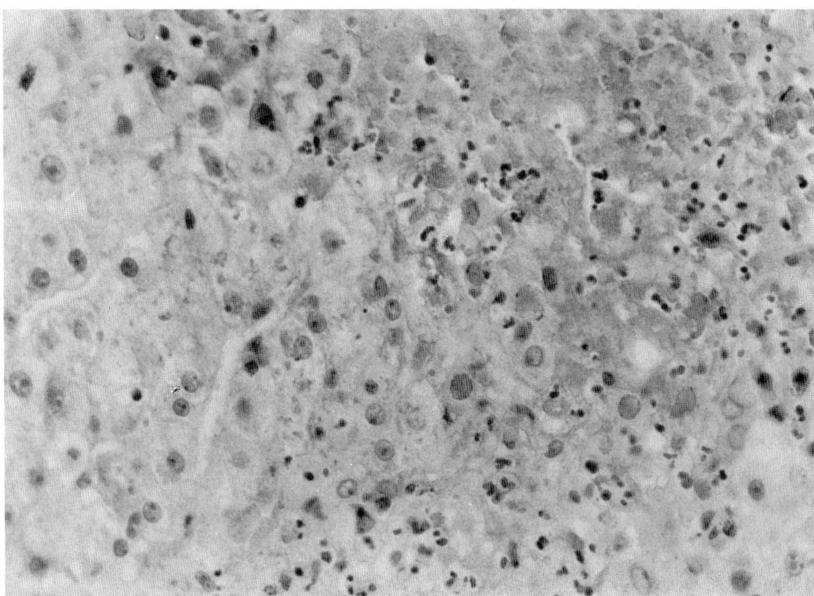

Figure 4.38. Herpes simplex hepatitis. An area of necrosis is rimmed by hepatocytes containing intranuclear inclusions. Cells are not enlarged. Nuclei have a homogeneous inner structure (×450).

Acute cellular rejection occurs early (within 2 months) in the postoperative period. In the Pittsburgh series (224) of 62 patients, it was never seen before 6 to 7 days after the transplant. A liver biopsy (Figs. 4.39, 4.40) shows mononuclear infiltration of portal triads, which may be patchy at first (224–226,229,232,238). A few neutrophils and eosinophils may be present as well. The infiltrate has a tendency to be related to portal venous branches and also to surround the bile ducts (see Figs. 4.39, 4.40). Liver lobules may be spared in early stages; however, mild to moderate cholestasis in the centrilobular zones is not unusual. With the progression of the rejection process, the portal infiltrate becomes more intense and may occasionally involve the periphery of the hepatic lobule associated with piecemeal necrosis (224). The pathognomonic histologic sign of rejection, namely,

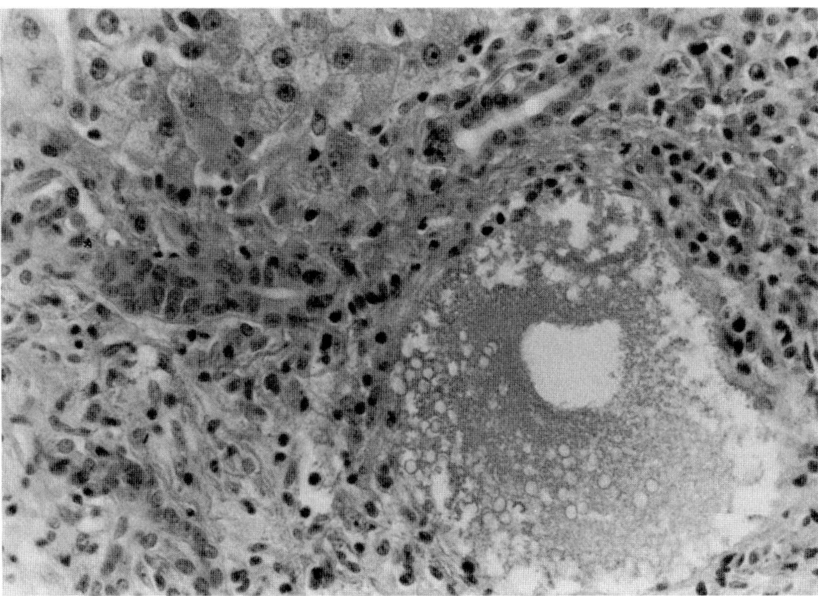

Figure 4.39. Cellular rejection reaction in a liver graft. Mononuclear infiltrate is seen in a portal area with lymphocytes beneath the portal venous endothelium (×450).

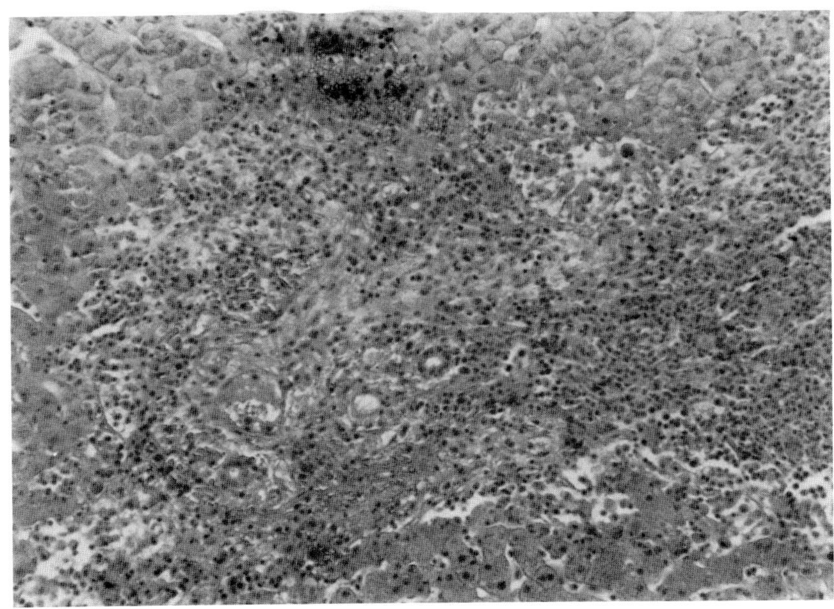

Figure 4.40. Cellular rejection reaction in a liver graft. Marked portal mononuclear infiltrate with expansion of the triad. The infiltrate surrounds the bile ducts (×180).

lymphocytic endothelialitis (mononuclear cells underneath the venous endothelium) is easily found (226). Early rejection episodes (occurring within 2 months of transplant) had the most intense infiltrate in the Pittsburgh series (224) whereas the subsequent episodes were generally less severe (224). Varying degrees of bile duct damage are also seen with paranuclear vacuolization of the epithelium, irregularity and loss of polarity of the epithelial cells, atypia of nuclei, nuclear pyknosis, and increased mitotic rate. Disruption of ductal basement membrane may also occur. By electron microscopy (239) striking degenerative changes are seen in the nuclei and cellular organelles of the bile duct epithelium. Similar changes have been reported in chronic graft-versus-host disease (226, 240). In advanced lesions, mononuclear cells are present in the center of the lobule as well, with or without hepatocytic necrosis. Cholestasis may be marked. A group from the Netherlands has reported four distinct graft syndromes (225), namely, rejection, cholangitis, viral infection, and pure cholestasis, that they were able to recognize easily. According to them, the rejected grafts had a picture similar to idiopathic autoimmune chronic liver disease with no bile duct changes; a finding that has been refuted by all other groups.

With increased immunosuppression, healing does occur in most cases (224,241). The cellular infiltrate decreases in intensity and ultimately may completely disappear. Mild central and portal venous scars may be left (224). Snover et al. (226) found two other histologic changes following immunosuppressive therapy: one simulating cholangitis with obstruction, and the other with an increased number of eosinophils raising the question of drug reaction. Both of these reaction patterns responded to a further boost in immunosuppression. Acute arterial lesions (vasculitis with fibrinoid necrosis) within the first 2 months were observed by Demetris et al. (224) but this has not been reported by others.

Immunologic studies on hepatic allograft rejection in humans are scarce. Andres et al. (242) studied immunoglobulin and complement deposition in rejected hepatic allografts, and their data are essentially inconclusive. Using monoclonal antibodies, in situ analysis (161,243) of the mononuclear cells has revealed the infiltrates to be rich in T lymphocytes and has shown a particular preponderance of the suppressor/cytotoxic T cells in the areas of piecemeal necrosis. Takács et al. (244) have reported expression of class II histocompatibility antigen (HLA-DR) on the bile duct cells in one rejected hepatic allograft. From these limited data it appears that acute hepatic allograft rejection is a cell-mediated immune injury directed against bile duct epithelium and/or vascular endothelial antigens. Hepatocytes seem to be spared.

Chronic rejection has been the single most com-

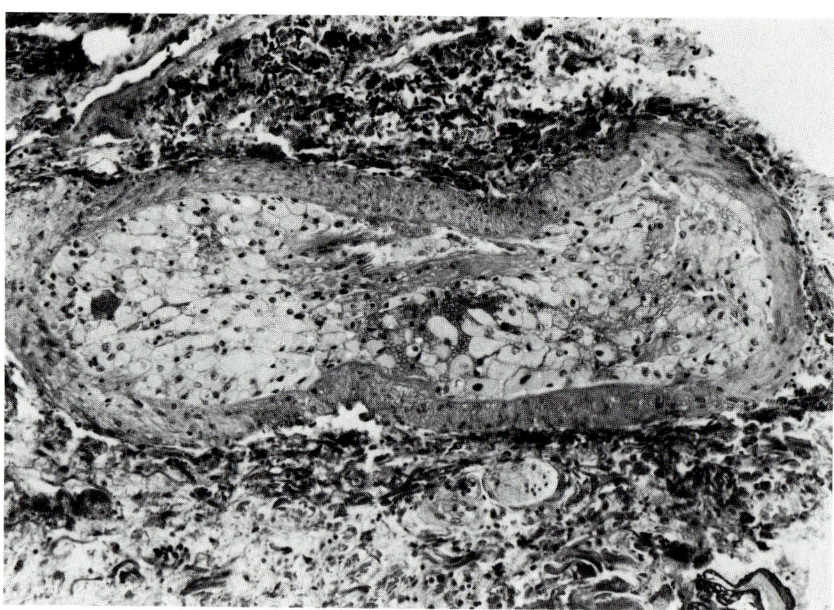

Figure 4.41. Chronic rejection. A branch of the hepatic artery at the hilum of a transplant hepatectomy specimen has marked subendothelial accumulation of foam cells ($\times$1800).

mon cause of late death (241). It usually starts with an episode of acute rejection and relentlessly progresses to a chronic phase unresponsive to any form of therapy. A progressively increasing cholestasis is seen on liver biopsies; the characteristic microscopic lesion is accumulation of foamy macrophages in the subendothelial layer of blood vessels (224,229,231,237). This change is usually present in medium- to large-sized hilar vessels but may also be seen in the branches of hepatic artery in a portal tract. As is evident from the illustration (Fig. 4.41), this lesion causes narrowing of the lumen, at times greatly compromising the blood flow. Fibroproliferative endoarteritis involving medium-sized arteries has also been reported (226). The changes in the small vessels are much more subtle and include sclerosis, intimal proliferation, and reduplication of the elastic lamina. Endothelialitis is not seen.

The bile ducts may be greatly reduced in number (227,238) or may be rapidly destroyed with little inflammatory infiltrate; this constitutes the so-called "vanishing bile duct syndrome" (230), as a part of chronic rejection. With the disappearance of bile ducts, other portal structures may also shrink and ultimately disappear. The diagnosis of chronic rejection may be difficult on a liver biopsy if not enough attention is paid to the decreased number of bile ducts. Cholestasis is generally marked. Hepatic fibrosis and cirrhosis (224,229) may be seen very late.

FUNCTIONAL CHOLESTASIS

"Functional cholestasis" in liver allografts, as reported by Demetris et al. (224), is similar to the fourth group of graft syndromes of Eggink et al. (225), and consists of "pure parenchymal cholestasis." Moderate to severe centrilobular hepatocellular and intracanalicular cholestasis with minimal or absent portal inflammation is the characteristic finding. The exact etiology of this lesion is not clear; all patients in the Pittsburgh series (224) had elevated serum bilirubin and coagulopathy but no evidence of bile duct obstruction.

Recurrence of the Original Liver Disease

Recurrence of the original disease in the graft is a potential threat and is most common in patients who undergo OLT for malignant liver tumors. Primary hepatic tumors as an indication for OLT is a highly controversial issue. An English group (232) favors performing transplant in these cases, whereas Starzl in the United States (229,231,245) considers it no longer a valid indication because of the high recurrence rate of the tumor. In the English series (232,233), most patients died of recurrent tumor between 6 and 18 months following transplantation. It is noteworthy that the results are good with the "fibrolamellar" type of hepatoma, which may be late in spreading (223, 231).

Neuberger et al. (246) have reported three patients who underwent OLT for primary biliary cirrhosis and in whom the diagnosis of recurrent primary biliary cirrhosis was made 3, $3\frac{1}{4}$, and $3\frac{1}{2}$ years following transplantation. The histologic findings in the liver biopsies were striking: a mixed cellular infiltrate in portal areas and a reduced number of bile ducts. In one case, a portal granuloma was seen. Neuberger and colleagues' contention that reappearance of antimitochondrial antibodies (AMA) many months following transplantation was significant and helped in making the diagnosis, has been challenged by Weaver et al. (247). It must be noted that all reported histologic findings, with the exception of a poorly developed granuloma, can also be seen in a rejection reaction (238,240,248). Suffice it to say that nonsuppurative destructive cholangitis is one of the generic ways liver responds to a variety of injurious processes, and that we will have to await development of more specific tests to distinguish between recurrence of primary biliary cirrhosis and late chronic rejection in a hepatic allograft.

As has been mentioned already, chronic active hepatitis with positive antigen/s status can quite likely recur in a hepatic allograft (228,231).

Seltman et al. (249) have reported a tragic case of recurrent Budd-Chiari syndrome in a young woman. In addition to vena caval and intrahepatic venous thrombosis, extensive thrombosis was also seen in many organs at autopsy.

TRANSPLANTED DISORDERS

Although there is no literature available on this problem in relation to liver transplants, the potential does exist for transplanting an infection or tumor via the graft.

DRUG TOXICITY

Drug toxicity as a cause of graft dysfunction, albeit uncommon, can be seen. Imuran (azathioprine) has been implicated in at least one reported case (245). Toxicity with Imuran is enhanced in the presence of active liver disease. Intrahepatic cho-

lestasis without cellular infiltration is the most common microscopic change, but other complicating factors may be present and can distort the histologic picture.

Cyclosporin A (CyA) is another potentially hepatotoxic drug that can cause frank jaundice in some cases. The exact histopathologic features of CyA toxicity have not been described as yet, but according to one report (250) a striking increase in eosinophils was seen in the portal infiltrate following CyA therapy. It is not clear from that report whether this change was in any way dose-related or was seen only in cases of toxicity. Among our own cases (unpublished observation), one patient had progressively profound jaundice with marked centrilobular cholestasis on multiple liver biopsies. Clinically there was no explanation for this syndrome. The process began to resolve and ultimately did clear completely when the CyA dosage was decreased. Therefore, in retrospect, we think that it represented CyA toxicity.

In this context, one must remember the other potentially hepatotoxic drugs that a patient may be taking for various reasons, and that could cause graft dysfunction. Some of the drugs (e.g., Dilantin) (236) can cause a histologic picture of hepatitis and may pose great differential diagnostic problems.

OTHERS

Development of reticulum cell sarcoma (autopsy-proven primary) in the donor liver within 6 months following transplant has been reported in one case by Williams et al. (232). A review of donor's autopsy did not reveal any evidence of lymphoma.

References

1. Bull HJM, Gilmore IT, Bradley RD, et al. Experience with transjugular liver biopsy. *Gut* 1983; 24:1057–1060.
2. Rappaport AM. The microcirculatory acinar concept of normal and pathological hepatic structure. *Beitr Pathol* 1976; 157:215–243.
3. Fechner RE. Benign hepatic lesions and orally administered contraceptives. A report of seven cases and critical analysis of the literature. *Hum Pathol* 1977; 8:255–268.
4. Baum JK, Holtz F, Bookstein JJ, Klein EW. Possible association between benign hepatomas and oral contraceptives. *Lancet* 1973; 2:926–929.
5. Ishak KG, Rabin L. Benign tumors of the liver. *Med Clin North Am* 1975; 59:995–1013.
6. Andersen PH, Packer JT. Hepatic adenoma, observations after estrogen withdrawal. *Arch Surg* 1976; 111:898–900.

7. Kay S. Nine year follow-up of a case of benign liver cell adenoma related to oral contraceptives. *Cancer* 1977; 40: 1759–1760.

8. Ramseur WL, Cooper MR. Asymptomatic liver cell adenomas. Another case of resolution after discontinuation of oral contraceptive use. *JAMA* 1978; 239:1647–1648.

9. Mays ET, Christopherson W. Hepatic tumors induced by sex steroids. *Semin Liver Dis* 1984; 4:147–157.

10. Christopherson WM, Mays ET, Barrows G. A clinicopathologic study of steroid-related liver tumors. *Am J Surg Pathol* 1977; 1:31–41.

11. Edmondson HA, Reynolds TB, Henderson B, Benton B. Regression of liver cell adenomas associated with oral contraceptives. *Ann Intern Med* 1977; 86:180–182.

12. Wheelar DA, Edmundson HA, Reynolds TB. Spontaneous liver cell adenoma in children. *Am J Clin Pathol* 1986; 85:6–12.

13. Foster JH, Donohue TA, Berman MM. Familial liver cell adenomas and diabetes mellitus. *N Engl J Med* 1978; 299: 239–241.

14. Boyd PR, Mark GJ. Multiple hepatic adenomas and a hepatocellular carcinoma in a man on oral methyl testosterone for eleven years. *Cancer* 1977; 40:1765–1770.

15. Blaustein PA. Surgical diseases of the liver. In: Silverberg SG, ed. *Principles and Practice of Surgical Pathology*. New York: John Wiley & Sons, 1983, pp. 995–1015.

16. Palmer PE, Christopherson WM, Wolfe HJ. Alpha₁-antitrypsin, protein marker in oral contraceptive-associated hepatic tumors. *Am J Clin Pathol* 1977; 68:736–739.

17. Gibson JB, Sobin LH. *Histological Typing of Tumors of the Liver, Biliary Tract and Pancreas*. International Histological Classification of Tumours, No. 20. Geneva: World Health Organization, 1978, p. 19.

18. Ishak KG, Willis GW, Cummins SD, Bullock AA. Biliary cystadenoma and cystadenocarcinoma, report of 14 cases and review of the literature. *Cancer* 1977; 38:322–338.

19. Short WF, Nedwich A, Levy HA, Howard JM. Biliary cystadenoma. *Arch Surg* 1971; 102:78–80.

20. Scully RE, Mark EJ, McNeely BU. Case Records of the Massachusetts General Hospital. Case 46-1985, *N Engl J Med* 1985; 313:1275–1282.

21. Wheeler DA, Edmondson HA. Cystadenoma with mesenchymal stroma (CMS) in the liver and bile ducts. A clinicopathologic study of 17 cases, 4 with malignant change. *Cancer* 1985; 56:1434–1445.

22. Edmondson HA. Bile duct cystadenoma and papilloma. In: *Tumors of the Liver and Intrahepatic Bile Ducts. Atlas of Tumor Pathology*, Fasc. 25. Washington, D. C.: Armed Forces Institute of Pathology, 1958, pp. 24–27.

23. Marsh JL, Dahms B, Longmire Jr WP. Cystadenoma and cystadenocarcinoma of the biliary system. *Arch Surg* 1974; 109:41–43.

24. Purtilo DT, Gottlieb LS. Cirrhosis and hepatoma occurring at Boston City Hospital (1917–1968). *Cancer* 1973; 32: 458–462.

25. Chlebowski RT, Tong M, Weissman J, et al. Hepatocellular carcinoma; diagnostic and prognostic features in North American patients. *Cancer* 1984; 53:2701–2706.

26. MacSween RMN. A clinicopathological review of 100 cases of primary malignant tumours of the liver. *J Clin Pathol* 1974; 27:669–682.

27. Wu PC, Lam KC. Cytoplasmic hepatitis B surface antigen and the ground-glass appearance in hepatocellular carcinoma. *Am J Clin Pathol* 1979; 71:229–234.

28. Pryor AC, Cohen RJ, Goldman RL. Hepatocellular carcinoma in a woman on long-term oral contraceptives. *Cancer* 1977; 40:884–888.

29. Glassberg AB, Rosenbaum EH. Oral contraceptives and malignant hepatoma. *Lancet* 1976; 1:479.

30. Bernstein MS, Hunter R, Yachnin S. Hepatoma and peliosis hepatitis developing in a patient with Fanconi's anemia. *N Engl J Med* 1971; 284:1135–1136.

31. Thalassinos NC, Lymberatos C, Hadjioannou J, Gardikas C. Liver cell carcinoma after long-term oestrogen-like drugs. *Lancet* 1974; 2:270.

32. Goodman ZD, Ishak KG. Hepatocellular carcinoma in women: Probable lack of etiologic association with oral contraceptive steroids. *Hepatology* 1982; 2:440–444.

33. Moore TA, Ferrante WA, Crowson TD. Hepatoma occurring two decades after hepatic irradiation. *Gastroenterology* 1976; 71:128–132.

34. Nagasue N, Akamizu H, Yukaya H, Yuuki I. Hepatocellular pseudotumor in the cirrhotic liver. *Cancer* 1984; 54: 2487–2494.

35. Ordonez NG, Manning JT. Comparison of alpha₁-antitrypsin and alpha₁-antichymotrypsin in hepatocellular carcinoma: An immunoperoxidase study. *Am J Gastroenterol* 1984; 79:959–963.

36. Tatsuta M, Yamamoto R, Kasugai H, et al. Cytohistologic diagnosis of neoplasms of the liver by ultrasonically guided fine-needle aspiration biopsy. *Cancer* 1984; 54: 1682–1686.

37. Nagasue N, Yukaya H, Hamada T, et al. The natural history of hepatocellular carcinoma, A study of 100 untreated cases. *Cancer* 1984; 54:1461–1465.

38. Scully RE, Galdabini JJ, McNeely BU. Case records of the Massachusetts General Hospital. Case 9-1979. *N Engl J Med* 1979; 300:484–489.

39. Parker Jr JC, Dahlin DC, Stauffer MH. Malignant hepatoma: Evaluation of surgical (including needle biopsy) material from 69 cases. *Mayo Clin Proc* 1970; 45:25–35.

40. Cohen C. Intracytoplasmic hyaline globules in hepatocellular carcinomas. *Cancer* 1976; 37:1754–1758.

41. Norkin SA, Campagna-Pinto D. Cytoplasmic hyaline inclusions in hepatoma. *Arch Pathol* 1968; 86:25–32.

42. Keeley AF, Iseri OA, Gottlieb LS. Ultrastructure of hyaline cytoplasmic inclusions in a human hepatoma: Relationship to Mallory's alcoholic hyalin. *Gastroenterology* 1972; 62:280–293.

43. Lai CI, Wu PC, Lam KC, Todd D. Histologic prognostic indicators in hepatocellular carcinoma. *Cancer* 1979; 44: 1677–1683.

44. El-Domeiri AA, Huvos AG, Goldsmith HS, Foote FW Jr. Primary malignant tumors of the liver. *Cancer* 1971; 27:7–11.

45. Buchanan TF Jr, Huvos AG. Clear cell carcinoma of the liver. *Am J Clin Pathol* 1974; 61:529–539.

46. Lam KC, Ho JCI, Yeung RTT. Spontaneous regression of hepatocellular carcinoma, a case study. *Cancer* 1982; 50: 332–336.

47. Gottfried EB, Steller R, Paronetto F, Lieber CS. Spontaneous regression of hepatocellular carcinoma. *Gastroenterology* 1982; 82:770–774.

48. Okuda K, Musha H, Nakajima Y, et al. Clinicopathologic features of encapsulated hepatocellular carcinoma. *Cancer* 1977; 40:1240–1245.

49. Craig JR, Peters RL, Edmundson HA, Omata M. Fibrolamellar carcinoma of the liver: A tumor of adolescents and young adults with distinctive clinico-pathologic features. *Cancer* 1980; 46:372–379.

50. Berman MM, Libbey NP, Foster JH. Hepatocellular carcinoma, polygonal cell type with fibrous stroma—an atypical variant with a favorable prognosis. *Cancer* 1980; 46:1448–1455.

51. Nagorney DM, Adson MA, Weiland LH, et al. Fibrolamellar hepatoma. *Am J Surg* 1985; 149:113–119.

52. Farhi DC, Shikes RH, Silverberg SG. Ultrastructure of fibrolamellar oncocytic hepatoma. *Cancer* 1982; 50:702–709.

53. Vecchio FM, Fabiano A, Ghirlanda G, et al. Fibrolamellar carcinoma of the liver: The malignant counterpart of focal nodular hyperplasia with oncocytic change. *Am J Clin Pathol* 1984; 81:521–526.

54. Lai CL, Lam KC, Wong KP, et al. Clinical features of hepatocellular carcinoma: Review of 211 patients in Hong Kong. *Cancer* 1981; 47:2746–2755.

55. Kishi K, Shikata T, Hirohashi S, et al. Hepatocellular carcinoma, a clinical and pathologic analysis of 57 hepatectomy cases. *Cancer* 1983; 51:542–548.

56. Primack A, Wilson J, O'Connor GT, et al. Hepatocellular carcinoma with the carcinoid syndrome. *Cancer* 1971; 27:1182–1189.

57. Barsky SH, Linnoila I, Triche TJ, Costa J. Hepatocellular carcinoma with carcinoid features. *Hum Pathol* 1984; 15:892–894.

58. Penalba C, Larouze B, Mechali D, et al. Prolonged survival with hepatocellular carcinoma. *Gastroenterology* 1982; 83:1159.

59. Yoshida T, Okazaki N, Yoshino M, et al. Minute hepatocellular carcinoma without appreciable change in size for seven years: A case report. *Cancer* 1982; 49:1491–1495.

60. Klatskin G. Adenocarcinoma of the hepatic duct at its bifurcation within the porta hepatis. *Am J Med* 1965; 38:241–256.

61. Stenger RJ. Liver tumors. In: *Interpretation of Liver Biopsies. Biopsy Interpretation Series*. New York: Raven Press, 1983, pp. 131–147.

62. Chou ST, Chan CW. Mucin-producing cholangiocarcinoma: An autopsy study in Hong Kong. *Pathology* 1976; 8:321–328.

63. Okuda K, Kubo Y, Okazaki N, et al. Clinical aspects of intrahepatic bile duct carcinoma including hilar carcinoma, a study of 57 autopsy-proven cases. *Cancer* 1977; 39:232–246.

64. Daroca PJ Jr, Tuthill R, Reed RJ. Cholangiocarcinoma arising in congenital hepatic fibrosis. A case report. *Arch Pathol* 1975; 99:592–595.

65. Landais P, Grunfeld JP, Droz D, et al. Cholangiocellular carcinoma in polycystic kidney and liver disease. *Arch Intern Med* 1984; 144:2274–2276.

66. Gallagher PJ, Millis RR, Mitchinson MJ. Congenital dilatation of the intrahepatic bile ducts with cholangiocarcinoma. *J Clin Pathol* 1972; 25:804–808.

67. Imamura M, Miyashita T, Tani T, et al. Cholangiocellular carcinoma associated with multiple liver cysts. *Am J Gastroenterol* 1984; 79:790–795.

68. Phinney PR, Austin GE, Kadell BM. Cholangiocarcinoma arising in Caroli's disease. *Arch Pathol Lab Med* 1981; 105:194–197.

69. Azizah N, Paradinas FJ. Cholangiocarcinoma coexisting with developmental liver cysts: A distinct entity different from liver cystadenocarcinoma. *Histopathology* 1980; 4:391–400.

70. Goodman ZD, Ishak KG, Langloss JM, et al. Combined hepatocellular cholangiocarcinoma. A histologic and immunohistochemical study. *Cancer* 1985; 55:124–135.

71. Woods GL. Biliary cystadenocarcinoma: Case report of hepatic malignancy originating in benign cystadenoma. *Cancer* 1981; 47:2936–2940.

72. Iemoto Y, Kondo Y, Nakano T, et al. Biliary cystadenocarcinoma diagnosed by liver biopsy performed under ultrasonographic guidance. *Gastroenterology* 1983; 84:399–403.

73. Bloustein PA, Silverberg SG. Squamous cell carcinoma originating in an hepatic cyst. *Cancer* 1976; 38:2002–2005.

74. Greenwood N, Orr W McN. Primary squamous cell carcinoma arising in a solitary non-parasitic cyst of the liver. *J Pathol* 1972; 107:145–148.

75. Pianzola LE, Drut R. Mucoepidermoid carcinoma of the liver. *Am J Clin Pathol* 1971; 56:758–761.

76. Carter R. Hepatoblastoma in the adult. *Cancer* 1969; 23:191–197.

77. Meyer P, LiVolsi VA, Cornog JL. Hepatoblastoma associated with an oral contraceptive. *Lancet* 1974; 2:1387.

78. Ishak KG, Glunz PR. Hepatoblastoma and hepatocarcinoma in infancy and childhood. Report of 47 cases. *Cancer* 1967; 20:396–422.

79. Geiser CF, Baez A, Schindler AM, Shih VE. Epithelial hepatoblastoma associated with congenital hemihypertrophy and cystathioninuria: Presentation of a case. *Pediatrics* 1970; 46:66–73.

80. Lack EE, Neave C, Vawter GF. Hepatocellular carcinoma. Review of 32 cases in childhood and adolescence. *Cancer* 1983; 52:1510–1515.

81. McArthur JW, Toll GD, Russfield AB, et al. Sexual precocity attributable to ectopic gonadotropin secretion by hepatoblastoma. *Am J Med* 1973; 54:390–403.

82. Kasai M, Watanabe I. Histologic classification of liver-cell carcinoma in infancy and childhood and its clinical evaluation. A study of 70 cases collected in Japan. *Cancer* 1970; 25:551–563.

83. Joshi VV, Kaur P, Ryan B, et al. Mucoid anaplastic hepatoblastoma. A case report. *Cancer* 1984; 54:2035–2039.

84. Silverman JF, Fu YS, McWilliams NB, Kay S. An ultrastructural study of mixed hepatoblastoma with osteoid elements. *Cancer* 1975; 36:1436–1443.

85. Gonzalez-Crussi F, Manz HJ. Structure of a hepatoblastoma of pure epithelial type. *Cancer* 1972; 29:1272–1280.

86. Ladaga L, Kay S, Melcher M, King JN. Combined epithelial and sarcomatous elements in a liver cancer associated with oral contraceptive use. *Am J Surg Pathol* 1979; 3:185–190.

87. Kishimoto Y, Hijiya S, Nagasako R. Malignant mixed tumor of the liver in adults. *Am J Gastroenterol* 1984; 79:229–235.

88. Ecker JA, Doane WA. Massive cavernous hemangioma of the liver. *Am J Gastroenterol* 1969; 52:25–36.

89. Adam YG, Huvos AG, Fortner JG. Giant hemangiomas of the liver. *Ann Surg* 1970; 172:239–245.

90. Blumenfeld TA, Fleming ID, Johnson WW. Juvenile hemangioendothelioma of the liver. Report of a case and review of the literature. *Cancer* 1969; 24:853–857.

91. Ramchand S, Ahmed Y, Baskerville L. Lipoma of the liver. *Arch Pathol* 1970; 90:331–333.

92. Rubin E, Russinovich NAE, Luna RF, et al. Myelolipoma of the liver. *Cancer* 1984; 54:2043–2046.

93. Falk H, Popper H, Thomas LB, Ishak KG. Hepatic angiosarcoma associated with androgenic-anabolic steroids. *Lancet* 1979; 2:1120–1122.

94. Hoch-Ligeti C. Angiosarcoma of the liver associated with diethylstilbestrol. *JAMA* 1978; 240:1510–1511.

95. Sussman EB, Nudick I, Gray GF. Hemangioendothelial sarcoma of the liver and hemochromatosis. *Arch Pathol* 1974; 97:39–42.

96. Ludwig J, Hoffman HN II. Hemangiosarcoma of the

liver. Spectrum of morphologic changes and clinical findings. *Mayo Clin Proc* 1975; 50:255–263.

97. Dean PJ, Haggitt RC, O'Hara CJ. Malignant epithelioid hemangioendothelioma of the liver in young women: Relationship to oral contraceptive use. *Am J Surg Pathol* 1985; 9:965–704.

98. Ishak KG, Sesterhenn IA, Goodman ZD, et al. Epithelioid hemangioendothelioma of the liver: A clinicopathologic and follow-up study of 32 cases. *Hum Pathol* 1984; 15:839–852.

99. Masur H, Sussman EB, Molander DW. Primary hepatic leiomyosarcoma: A report of two cases. *Gastroenterology* 1975; 69:994–997.

100. Chen KTK. Hepatic leiomyosarcoma. *J Surg Oncol* 1983; 24:325–328.

101. Alrenga DP. Primary fibrosarcoma of the liver, Case report and review of the literature. *Cancer* 1975; 36:446–449.

102. Ryan J, Straus DJ, Lange C, et al. Primary lymphoma of the liver. *Cancer* 1988; 61:370–375.

103. Torres A, Bollozos GD. Primary reticulum cell sarcoma of liver. *Cancer* 1971; 27:1489–1492.

104. Daniel SJ, Attiyeh FF, Dire JJ, et al. Primary lymphoma of the liver treated with extended left hepatic lobectomy. *Cancer* 1985; 55:206–209.

105. Osborne BM, Butler JJ, Guarda LA. Primary lymphoma of the liver. Ten cases and a review of the literature. *Cancer* 1985; 56:2902–2910.

106. Edmundson HA. Metastatic tumors. In: *Tumors of the Liver and Intrahepatic Bile Ducts. Atlas of Tumor Pathology, Fasc. 25.* Washington, D.C.: Armed Forces Institute of Pathology, 1958, pp. 179–190.

107. Borja ER, Hori JM, Pugh RP. Metastatic carcinomatosis of the liver mimicking cirrhosis. Case report and review of the literature. *Cancer* 1975; 35:445–449.

108. Adson MA, van Heerden JA, Adson MH, et al. Resection of hepatic metastases from colorectal cancer. *Arch Surg* 1984; 119:647–651.

109. Nagasue N, Ito A, Yukaya H, Ogawa Y. Estrogen receptors in hepatocellular carcinoma. *Cancer* 1986; 57:87–91.

110. Sanfelippo PM, Beahrs OH, Weiland LH. Cystic disease of the liver. *Ann Surg* 1974; 179:922–925.

111. Hadad AR, Westbrook KC, Graham GG, et al. Symptomatic non-parasitic liver cysts. *Am J Surg* 1977; 134:739–744.

112. Howard RJ, Hanson RF, Delaney JP. Jaundice associated with polycystic liver disease. *Arch Surg* 1976; 111:816–817.

113. Bloustein PA. Association of carcinoma with congenital cystic conditions of the liver and bile ducts. *Am J Gastroenterol* 1977; 67:40–46.

114. Dent GA, Feldman JM. Pseudocystic liver metastases in patients with carcinoid tumors: Report of three cases. *Am J Clin Pathol* 1984; 82:275–279.

115. Edmundson HA. Teratoma. In: *Tumors of the Liver and Intrahepatic Bile Ducts. Atlas of Tumor Pathology,* fasc. 25. Washington, D.C.: Armed Forces Institute of Pathology, 1958, pp. 158–159.

116. Chung EB. Multiple bile duct hamartomas. *Cancer* 1970; 26:287–296.

117. Homer LW, White HJ, Read RC. Neoplastic transformation of von Meyenburg complexes of the liver. *J Pathol Bacteriol* 1968; 96:499–502.

118. Dehner LP, Ewing SL, Sumner HW. Infantile mesenchymal hamartoma of the liver. *Arch Pathol* 1975; 99: 379–382.

119. Sutton CA, Eller JL. Mesenchymal hamartoma of the liver. *Cancer* 1968; 22:29–34.

120. Fechner RE, Roehm Jr OF. Angiographic and pathologic correlations of hepatic focal nodular hyperplasia. *Am J Surg Pathol* 1977; 1:217–224.

121. Benz FJ, Baggenstoss AH. Focal cirrhosis of the liver: Its relation to so-called hamartoma (adenoma; benign hepatoma). *Cancer* 1953; 6:743–755.

122. Ishak KG. Hepatic lesions caused by anabolic and contraceptive steroids. *Semin Liver Dis* 1981; 1:116–128.

123. Friedman LS, Gang DL, Hedberg SE, Isselbacher KJ. Simultaneous occurrence of hepatic adenoma and focal nodular hyperplasia: Report of a case and review of the literature. *Hepatology* 1984; 4:536–540.

124. Ross D, Pina J, Mirza M, et al. Regression of focal nodular hyperplasia after discontinuation of oral contraceptives. *Ann Intern Med* 1976; 85:203–204.

125. Alberti-Flor JJ, Iskandarini M, Jeffers L, et al. Focal nodular hyperplasia associated with the use of a synthetic anabolic androgen. *Am J Gastroenterol* 1984; 79:150–151.

126. Knowles DM, Wolff M. Focal nodular hyperplasia of the liver. A clinicopathologic study and review of the literature. *Hum Pathol* 1976; 7:533–545.

127. Ruebner BH, Montgomery CK. Space occupying lesions of the liver. In: *Pathology of the Liver and Biliary Tract.* New York: John Wiley & Sons, 1982, pp. 233–286.

128. Edmondson HA. Focal nodular hyperplasia. In: *Tumors of the Liver and Intrahepatic Bile Ducts. Atlas of Tumor Pathology,* fasc. 25. Washington, D.C.: Armed Forces Institute of Pathology, 1958, pp. 193–194.

129. Anthony PP. Hepatic neoplasms. In: MacSween RNM, Anthony PP, Scheuer PJ, eds. *Pathology of the Liver.* Edinburgh: Churchill Livingstone, 1979, pp. 387–413.

130. Persaud V. Pseudolipoma of Glisson's capsule. *Arch Pathol* 1969; 88:555–556.

131. Someren A. "Inflammatory pseudotumor" of liver with occlusive phlebitis. Report of a case in a child and review of the literature. *Am J Clin Pathol* 1978; 69:176–181.

132. Chen KTK. Inflammatory pseudotumor of the liver. *Hum Pathol* 1984; 15:694–696.

133. Phillips MJ, Poucell S. Modern aspects of the morphology of viral hepatitis. *Hum Pathol* 1981; 12:1060–1084.

134. Tabor E. The three viruses of non-A, non-B hepatitis. *Lancet* 1985; 1:743–745.

135. Rizzeto M, Canese MG, Arico S, et al. Immunofluorescence detection of a new antigen/antibody system (delta/anti-delta) associated with hepatitis B virus in liver and serum of HBsAg carriers. *Gut* 1977; 18:997–1003.

136. Rizzetto M, Hoyer BH, Purcell RH, Gerin JL. Hepatitis delta virus infection. In: Vyas GN, Dienstag JL, Hoofnagle JH, eds. *Viral Hepatitis and Liver Disease.* New York: Grune & Stratton, 1984, pp. 371–378.

137. Hoofnagle JH. Type A and type B hepatitis. *Lab Med* 1983; 14:705–716.

138. Uchida T, Kronborg I, Peters RL. Acute viral hepatitis: Morphologic and functional correlations in human livers. *Hum Pathol* 1984; 15:267–277.

139. Knodell RG, Conrad ME, Ishak KG. Development of chronic liver disease after acute non-A, non-B posttransfusion hepatitis. Role of gamma globulin prophylaxis in its prevention. *Gastroenterology* 1977; 72:902–909.

140. Stenger RJ. Viral hepatitis. In: *Interpretation of Liver Biopsies. Biopsy Interpretation Series.* New York: Raven Press, 1983, pp. 27–38.

141. Bianchi L, Zimmerli-Ning M, Gudat F. Viral hepatitis. In: MacSween RNM, Anthony PP, Scheuer PJ, eds. *Pathology of the Liver.* Edinburgh: Churchill Livingstone, 1979, pp. 164–191.

142. Ruebner BH, Montgomery CK. Hepatitis. In: *Pathology of the Liver and Biliary Tract.* New York: John Wiley & Sons, 1982, pp. 33–59.

143. Mathiesen LR, Fauerholdt L, Moller AM, et al. Immunofluorescence studies for hepatitis A virus and hepatitis B surface and core antigen in liver biopsies from patients with acute viral hepatitis. *Gastroenterology* 1979; 77:623–628.

144. Ishak KG. Light microscopic morphology of viral hepatitis. *Am J Clin Pathol* 1976; 65:787–827.

145. Popper H. Clinical pathologic correlation in viral hepatitis. The effect of the virus on the liver. *Am J Pathol* 1975; 81:609–628.

146. Boyer JL. The diagnosis and pathogenesis of clinical variants in viral hepatitis. *Am J Clin Pathol* 1976; 65:898–908.

147. Peters RL. Viral hepatitis: A pathologic spectrum. *Am J Med Sci* 1975; 270:17–31.

148. MacSween RNM. Pathology of viral hepatitis and its sequelae. *Clin Gastroenterol* 1980; 9:23–45.

149. Boyer JL, Klatskin G. Pattern of necrosis in acute viral hepatitis. Prognostic value of bridging (subacute hepatic necrosis). *N Engl J Med* 1970; 283:1063–1071.

150. Bianchi L, deGroote J, Desmet VJ, et al. Morphological criteria in viral hepatitis. Review by an international group. *Lancet* 1971; 2:333–337.

151. Ishak KG, Stromeyer FW. Medical diseases of the liver. In: Silverberg SG, ed. *Principles and Practice of Surgical Pathology*, vol. 2. New York: John Wiley & Sons, 1983, pp, 937–994.

152. Conn HO. Chronic hepatitis: Reducing an iatrogenic enigma to a workable puzzle. *Gastroenterology* 1976; 70: 1182–1184.

153. Ludwig J. A review of lobular, portal, and periportal hepatitis. Interpretation of biopsy specimens without clinical data. *Hum Pathol* 1977; 8:269–276.

154. Scheuer PJ. Liver biopsy in chronic hepatitis 1968–1978. *Gut* 1978; 19:554–557.

155. Lefkowitch JH. Liver biopsy interpretation in chronic hepatitis. In: Fenoglio C, Wolff M, eds. *Progress in Surgical Pathology*, vol. 3. New York: Masson, 1981, pp. 221–232.

156. Alexander G, Williams R. Characterization of the mononuclear cell infiltrate in piecemeal necrosis. Editorial. *Lab Invest* 1984; 50:247–249.

157. Sherlock S, Niazi SP, Fox RA, Scheuer PJ. Chronic liver disease and primary liver cell cancer with hepatitis-associated (Australia) antigen in serum. *Lancet* 1970; 1: 1243–1247.

158. Colucci G, Colombo M, Del Ninno E, Paronetto F. In situ characterization by monoclonal antibodies of the mononuclear cell infiltrate in chronic active hepatitis. *Gastroenterology* 1983; 85:1138–1145.

159. Kerr JFR, Searl J, Halliday WJ, et al. The nature of piecemeal necrosis in chronic active hepatitis. *Lancet* 1979; 2:827–828.

160. Kawanishi H. Morphologic association of lymphocytes with hepatocytes in chronic liver disease. *Arch Pathol Lab Med* 1977; 101:286–290.

161. Si L, Whiteside TL, Van Thiel DH, Rabin BS. Lymphocyte subpopulations at the site of "piecemeal" necrosis in end stage chronic liver diseases and rejecting liver allografts in cyclosporine-treated patients. *Lab Invest* 1984; 50: 341–347.

162. Poulsen H, Christoffersen P. Abnormal bile duct epithelium in chronic aggressive hepatitis and cirrhosis. A review of morphology and clinical biochemical and immunologic features. *Hum Pathol* 1972; 3:217–225.

163. Hadziyannis S, Gerber MA, Vissoulis C, Popper H. Cytoplasmic hepatitis B antigen in "ground-glass" hepatocytes of carriers. *Arch Pathol* 1973; 96:327–330.

164. Bianchi L, Gudat F. Sanded nuclei in hepatitis B eosinophilic inclusions in liver cell nuclei due to excess in hepatitis B core antigen formation. *Lab Invest* 1976; 35:1–5.

165. Stocklin E, Gudat F, Krey G, et al. Delta antigen in hepatitis B: Immunohistology of frozen and paraffin-embedded liver biopsies and relation to HBV infection. *Hepatology* 1981; 1:238–242.

166. Popper H. Pathologic observations on delta infection. In: *Viral Hepatitis and Liver Disease.* New York: Grune & Stratton, 1984, pp. 381–384.

167. Popper H, Thung SN, Gerber MA, et al. Histologic studies of severe delta agent infection in Venezuelan Indians. *Hepatology* 1983; 3:906–912.

168. Edmondson HA. Pathology of alcoholism. *Am J Clin Pathol* 1980; 74:725–742.

169. Ruebner BH, Montgomery CK. Alcoholic liver injury. In: *Pathology of the Liver and Biliary Tract.* New York: John Wiley & Sons, 1982, pp. 95–105.

170. Edmondson HA, Peters RL, Frankel HH, Borowsky S. The early stage of liver injury in the alcoholic. *Medicine* 1967; 46:119–129.

171. Christoffersen P, Poulsen H. Alcoholic liver disease. In: MacSween RNM, Anthony PP, Scheuer PJ, eds. *Pathology of the Liver.* Edinburgh: Churchill Livingstone, 1979, pp. 232–247.

172. Baptista A, Bianchi L, deGroote J, et al. Alcoholic liver disease: Morphological manifestations. Review by an international group. *Lancet* 1981; 2:707–711.

173. Yokoo H, Minick OT, Batti F, Kent G. Morphologic variants of alcoholic hyalin. *Am J Pathol* 1972; 69:25–40.

174. French SW. The Mallory body: Structure, composition and pathogenesis. *Hepatology* 1981; 1:76–83.

175. Sherlock S. Patterns of hepatocyte injury in man. *Lancet* 1982; 1:782–786.

176. Yokoo H, Singh SK, Hawasli AH. Giant mitochondria in alcoholic liver disease. *Arch Pathol Lab Med* 1978; 102:213–214.

177. Edmondson HA, Peters RL, Reynolds TB, Kuzma OT. Sclerosing hyaline necrosis of the liver in the chronic alcoholic. *Ann Intern Med* 1963; 59:646–673.

178. Boitnott JK, Maddrey WC. Alcoholic liver disease: I. Interrelationships among histologic features and the histologic effects of prednisolone therapy. *Hepatology* 1981; 1:599–612.

179. Goldberg SJ, Mendenhall CL, Connell AM, Chedid A. "Nonalcoholic" chronic hepatitis in the alcoholic. *Gastroenterology* 1977; 72:598–604.

180. Gall EA, Dobrogorski O. Hepatic alterations in obstructive jaundice. *Am J Clin Pathol* 1964; 41:126–139.

181. Ruebner BH, Montgomery CK. Hyperbilirubinemia and cholestasis. In: *Pathology of the Liver and Biliary Tract.* New York: John Wiley & Sons, 1982, pp. 117–140.

182. Chapman RWG, Arborgh BAM, Rhodes JM, et al. Primary sclerosing cholangitis: A review of its clinical features, cholangiography, and hepatic histology. *Gut* 1980; 21:870–877.

183. Scheuer PJ. Primary biliary cirrhosis: Diagnosis and pathogenesis. *Postgrad Med* 1983; 59:106–115.

184. Thomas HC, Potter BJ, Sherlock S. Is primary biliary cirrhosis an immune complex disease? *Lancet* 1977; 2: 1261–1264.

185. Thomas HC, Epstein O. Pathogenic mechanisms in primary biliary cirrhosis. *Springer Semin Immunopathol* 1980; 3:375–384.

186. Baggenstoss AH, Foulk WT, Butt HR, Bahn RC. The pathology of primary biliary cirrhosis with emphasis on histogenesis. *Am J Clin Pathol* 1964; 42:259–276.

187. Ballardini G, Bianchi FB, Doniach D, et al. Aberrant expression of HLA-DR antigens on bile duct epithelium in primary biliary cirrhosis: Relevance to pathogenesis. *Lancet* 1984; 2:1009–1013.

188. Berg PA, Baum H. Serology of primary biliary cirrhosis. *Springer Semin Immunopathol* 1980; 3:355–373.

189. Long RG, Scheuer PJ, Sherlock S. Presentation and course of asymptomatic primary biliary cirrhosis. *Gastroenterology* 1977; 72:1204–1207.

190. Nakanuma Y, Ohta G. Histometric and serial section observations of the intrahepatic bile ducts in primary biliary cirrhosis. *Gastroenterology* 1979; 76:1326–1332.

191. Rubin E, Schaffner F, Popper H. Primary biliary cirrhosis. *Am J Pathol* 1965; 46:387–407.

192. Fleming CR, Dickson ER, Baggenstoss AH, McCall JT. Copper and primary biliary cirrhosis. *Gastroenterology* 1974; 67:1182–1187.

193. Krasner N, Johnson PJ, Portmann B, et al. Hepatocellular carcinoma in primary biliary cirrhosis: Report of four cases. *Gut* 1979; 20:255–258.

194. Scheuer PJ. Primary biliary cirrhosis. *Proc R Soc Med* 1967; 60:1257–1260.

195. Eggink HF, Houthoff HJ, Huitema S, et al. Cellular and humoral immune reactions in chronic active liver disease. I. Lymphocyte subsets in liver biopsies of patients with untreated idiopathic autoimmune hepatitis, chronic active hepatitis B and primary biliary cirrhosis. *Clin Exp Immunol* 1982; 50:17–24.

196. Bynum TE, Boitnott JK, Maddrey WC. Ischemic hepatitis. *Dig Dis Sci* 1979; 24:129–135.

197. Winkler K, Poulsen H. Liver disease with periportal sinusoidal dilatation. A possible complication to contraceptive steroids. *Scand J Gastroenterol* 1975; 10:699–704.

198. Nadell J, Kosek J. Peliosis hepatis, twelve cases associated with oral androgen therapy. *Arch Pathol Lab Med* 1977; 101:405–410.

199. Taxy JB. Peliosis, a morphologic curiosity becomes an iatrogenic problem. *Hum Pathol* 1978; 9:331–340.

200. Bras G, Brandt KH. Vascular disorders. In: MacSween RNM, Anthony PP, Scheuer PJ, eds. *Pathology of the Liver.* Edinburgh: Churchill Livingstone, 1979, pp. 315–334.

201. Stillman AE, Huxtable R, Consroe P, et al. Hepatic veno-occlusive disease due to pyrrolizidine (senecio) poisoning in Arizona. *Gastroenterology* 1977; 73:349–352.

202. Shulman HM, McDonald GB, Matthews D, et al. An analysis of hepatic veno-occlusive disease and centrilobular hepatic degeneration following bone marrow transplantation. *Gastroenterology* 1980; 79:1178–1191.

203. Ruebner BH, Montgomery CK. Metabolic diseases associated with hepatocellular necrosis, diseases with abnormal hepatic storage product and hepatic pigments. In: *Pathology of the Liver and Biliary Tract.* New York: John Wiley & Sons, 1982, pp. 157–195.

204. Ishak KG, Sharp HL. Metabolic errors and liver disease. In: MacSween RNM, Anthony PP, Scheuer PJ, eds. *Pathology of the Liver.* Edinburgh: Churchill Livingstone, 1979, pp. 88–147.

205. Kent G, Bahu RM. Iron overload. In: MacSween RNM, Anthony PP, Scheuer PJ, eds. *Pathology of the Liver.* Edinburgh: Churchill Livingstone, 1979, pp. 148–163.

206. Kent G, Popper H. Liver biopsy in diagnosis of hemachromatosis. *Am J Med* 1968; 44:837–841.

207. Goldfischer S, Gritsky HW, Change CH, et al. Idiopathic neonatal iron storage involving the liver, pancreas, heart, and endocrine and exocrine glands. *Hepatology* 1981; 1: 58–64.

208. Stromeyer FW, Ishak KG. Histology of the liver in Wilson's disease, a study of 34 cases. *Am J Clin Pathol* 1980; 73:12–24.

209. Sharp HL. The current status of alpha₁-antitrypsin, a protease inhibitor, in gastrointestinal disease. *Gastroenterology* 1976; 70:611–621.

210. Palmer PE, Wolfe HJ, Dayal Y, et al. Immunocytochemical diagnosis of alpha₁-antitrypsin deficiency. Review of eight cases. *Am J Surg Pathol* 1978; 2:275–281.

211. Popper H. Pathologic aspects of cirrhosis. A review. *Am J Pathol* 1977; 87:227–264.

212. Anthony PP, Ishak KG, Nayak NC, et al. The morphology of cirrhosis. *J Clin Pathol* 1978; 31:395–414.

213. Scheuer PJ. Cirrhosis. In: MacSween RNM, Anthony PP, Scheuer PJ, eds. *Pathology of the Liver.* Edinburgh: Churchill Livingstone, 1979, pp. 258–271.

214. Shikata T. Primary liver carcinoma and liver cirrhosis. In: Okuda K, Peters RL, eds. *Hepatocellular Carcinoma.* New York: John Wiley & Sons, 1976, pp. 53–71.

215. Petrelli M, Scheuer PJ. Variation in subcapsular liver structure and its significance in the interpretation of wedge biopsies. *J Clin Pathol* 1967; 20:743–748.

216. Anthony PP, Vogel CL, Barker LF. Liver cell dysplasia: A premalignant condition. *J Clin Pathol* 1973; 26:217–223.

217. Akagi G, Furuya K, Kanamura A, et al. Liver cell dysplasia and hepatitis B surface antigen in liver cirrhosis and hepatocellular carcinoma. *Cancer* 1984; 54:315–318.

218. Gindhart TD, Cimis RJ, Mosenthal WT, Longnecker DS. Adenomatous hyperplasia of the liver. *Arch Pathol Lab Med* 1979; 103:34–37.

219. Mones JM, Saldana MJ, Albores-Saavedra J. Nodular regenerative hyperplasia of the liver. *Arch Pathol Lab Med* 1984; 108:741–743.

220. Stromeyer FW, Ishak KG. Nodular transformation (nodular "regenerative" hyperplasia) of the liver. A clinicopathologic study of 30 cases. *Hum Pathol* 1981; 12:60–71.

221. Wanless IR, Solt LC, Kortan P. Nodular regenerative hyperplasia of the liver associated with macroglobulinemia; a clue to the pathogenesis. *Am J Med* 1981; 70:1203–1209.

222. Calne RY, Williams R, Lindop M, et al. Improved survival after orthotopic liver grafting. *Br Med J* 1981; 283: 115–118.

223. Anonymous: Transplantation overview, liver grafting. *Transplantation* 1983; 35:109–111.

224. Demetris AJ, Lasky S, Van Thiel DH, et al. Pathology of hepatic transplantation. A review of 62 adult allograft recipients immunosuppressed with a cyclosporine/steriod regimen. *Am J Pathol* 1985; 118:151–161.

225. Eggink HF, Hofstee N, Gips CH, et al. Histopathology of serial graft biopsies from liver transplant recipients. *Am J Pathol* 1984; 114:18–31.

226. Snover DC, Sibley RK, Freese DK, et al. Orthotopic liver transplantation: A pathological study of 63 serial liver biopsies from 17 patients with special reference to the diagnostic features and natural history of rejection. *Hepatology* 1984; 4:1212–1222.

227. Fennell RH Jr, Roddy HJ. Liver transplantation. The pathologist's perspective. *Pathol Annu* 1979; 14:155–182.

228. Starzl TE, Koep LJ, Halgrimson CG, et al. Fifteen years of

clinical liver transplantation. *Gastroenterology* 1979; 77: 375–388.

229. Starzl TE, Porter KA, Brettschneider L, et al. Clinical and pathologic observations after orthotopic transplantation of the human liver. *Surg Gynecol Obstet* 1969; 128:327–339.

230. Portmann B, Neuberger JM, Williams R. Intrahepatic bile duct lesions. In: Calne RY, ed. *Liver Transplantation*. New York: Grune & Stratton, 1983, pp. 279–287.

231. Starzl TE, Iwatsuki S, Van Thiel DH, et al. Evolution of liver transplantation. *Hepatology* 1982; 2:614–636.

232. Williams R, Smith M, Shilkin KB, et al. Liver transplantation in man: The frequency of rejection, biliary tract complications, and recurrence of malignancy based on an analysis of 26 cases. *Gastroenterology* 1973; 64:1026–1048.

233. Wight DGD. Pathology of liver transplantation (other than rejection). In: Calne RY, ed. *Liver Transplantation*. New York: Grune & Stratton, 1983, pp. 289–316.

234. Snover DC, Horwitz CA. Liver disease in cytomegalovirus mononucleosis: A light microscopical and immunoperoxidase study of six cases. *Hepatology* 1984; 4:408–412.

235. Wadsworth RC, Keil PG. Biopsy of the liver in infectious mononucleosis. *Am J Pathol* 1952; 28:1003–1025.

236. Mullick FG, Ishak KG. Hepatic injury associated with diphenylhydantoin therapy. A clinicopathologic study of 20 cases. *Am J Clin Pathol* 1980; 74:442–452.

237. Wight DGD. Pathology of rejection. In: Calne RY, ed. *Liver Transplantation*. New York: Grune & Stratton, 1983, pp. 247–277.

238. Vierling JM, Fennell RH Jr. Histopathology of early and late human hepatic allograft rejection: Evidence of progressive destruction of interlobular bile ducts. *Hepatology* 1985; 5:1076–1082.

239. Fennell RH Jr, Vierling JM. Electron microscopy of rejected human liver allografts. *Hepatology* 1985; 5:1083–1087.

240. Fennell RH Jr. Ductular damage in liver transplant rejection. Its similarity to that of primary biliary cirrhosis and graft-versus-host disease. *Pathol Annu* 1981; 16:289–294.

241. Starzl TE, Klintmalm GBG, Iwatsuki S, Fernandez-Bueno C. Past and future prospects of orthotopic liver transplantation. *Arch Surg* 1981; 116:1342–1343.

242. Andres GA, Accini L, Ansell ID, et al. Immunopathologic studies of orthotopic human liver allografts. *Lancet* 1972; 1:275–279.

243. Eggink HF, Houthoff HJ, Huitema S, et al. In situ analysis of mononuclear cell infiltrate in liver biopsies of patients with orthotopic liver transplantation. In: Peeters H, ed. *Protides of Biological Fluids, proceeding of the 30th Colloquium*. Oxford: Pergamon Press, 1982, pp. 441–444.

244. Takacs L, Szende B, Monostori E, et al. Expression of HLA-DR antigens on bile duct cells of rejected liver transplant. *Lancet* 1983; 2:1500.

245. Starzl TE, Porter KA, Putnam CW, et al. Orthotopic liver transplantation in 93 patients. *Surg Gynecol Obstet* 1976; 142:487–505.

246. Neuberger J, Portmann B, MacDougall BRD, et al. Recurrence of primary biliary cirrhosis after liver transplantation. *N Engl J Med* 1982; 306:1–4.

247. Weaver GA, Franck WA, Streck WF. Recurrence of primary biliary cirrhosis after liver transplantation. *N Engl J Med* 1982; 306:1235–1236.

248. Fennell RH Jr, Shikes RH, Vierling JM. Relationship of pretransplant hepatobiliary disease to bile duct damage occurring in the liver allograft. *Hepatology* 1983; 3:84–89.

249. Seltman HJ, Dekker A, Van Thiel DH, et al. Budd-Chiari syndrome recurring in a transplanted liver. *Gastroenterology* 1983; 84:640–643.

250. Starzl TE, Klintmalm GBG, Porter KA, et al. Liver transplantation with use of cyclosporin A and prednisone. *N Engl J Med* 1981; 305:266–269.

Editorial Comment

After a brief but very nice introductory section that blends the structure and function of the normal liver in a helpful informative way, this chapter covers extensively the number of pathological conditions that may effect the liver. These include neoplastic, infectious, inflammatory, toxic, obstructive, and hemodynamic disorders, all of which have distinctive if frequently subtle variances in the pathological presentation by microscopic exam.

Dr. Khettry has stayed well within the boundaries prescribed for this particular section. The relations of the pathology with various etiological factors are accurate and sufficient, although if some readers feel these correlations are too succinct, more specific detail on etiology and epidemiology of the various disorders of the liver may be found elsewhere in the book. If Dr. Khettry had attempted to do an effective report on the epidemiology and etiology of primary hepatocellular carcinoma, the chapter could easily have been a textbook in itself. As it is, her ability to confine her material without losing the broader picture has presented us with an excellent section of particular use to the surgeon whose interest may be in the liver, but whose expertise is likely to be limited enough to require frequent reference to the details to be found in this chapter. For the surgeon in particular, this is a superb contribution.

Chapter 5
Metabolic Liver Diseases

SANJEEV ARORA
MARSHALL M. KAPLAN

Hemochromatosis

Disorders of iron overload can be divided into the following categories:

1. Inherited
   a. Idiopathic primary hemochromatosis
2. Secondary
   a. Atransferrinemia
   b. Thalassemia major
   c. Zellweger's cerebrohepatorenal syndrome
3. Acquired
   a. Alcoholic cirrhosis
   b. Transfusion siderosis
   c. Increased intake of iron supplements
   d. Porphyria cutanea tarda

In this chapter we will focus on idiopathic primary hemochromatosis. Hemochromatosis is an iron storage disorder in which inherited defects in iron metabolism result in iron absorption inappropriate to the level of body stores. The average adult man can excrete up to 1 milligram of iron per day, and the menstruating woman up to 1.5 mg/day. In the normal individual, intestinal iron absorption is carefully regulated to match iron excretion.

In idiopathic hemochromatosis this regulation is lost, and there is a longstanding inappropriately high intestinal absorption that leads to excess iron stores. Patients with symptomatic disease may have 20 to 40 grams of total body iron stores in contrast to 1 g in normal subjects (1). The increased deposition of iron in cells leads to organ failure in the form of cirrhosis, diabetes, and cardiac failure. The mode of inheritance of idiopathic hemochromatosis is autosomal recessive (2). The gene for idiopathic hemochromatosis is located on the short arm of chromosome 6. It is in close proximity and tightly linked to the human leukocyte antigen

(HLA) HLA-A locus. The frequency of the idiopathic hemochromatosis gene in the general population has been computed to be as high as 5.6%. This would indicate a disease frequency of 0.3% based on an autosomal-recessive mode of inheritance. There have been several reports of families with a vertical pattern of inheritance, which was considered to represent an autosomal-dominant transmission. This pattern of vertical disease transmission is now known to be a result of homozygous-heterozygous matings (3). This is not a very rare occurrence because of the relatively high prevalence of the hemochromatosis gene in Caucasian populations.

There is a high frequency of HLA antigens A_3, B_7, and B_{14} in patients with hemochromatosis (Table 5.1). However, their presence cannot be used to diagnose or exclude the disease (4).

HLA A_3 and HLA B_{14} occur together very rarely in the normal population, -0.2%; thus, they are 99.8% specific for the diagnosis of hemochromatosis. The test, however, lacks sensitivity since only 16% of patients with hemochromatosis will have A_3 and B_{14}. Because of low probability in identifying an index case of hemochromatosis by HLA typing, it is not recommended as a screening procedure but is very useful in family screening. Homozygous siblings of hemochromatosis patients have two HLA haplotypes identical to those of the proband, and the heterozygotes have only one HLA haplotype identical to the proband. Homozygotes present with the clinical symptoms and signs as described later. However, the clinical expression of the disease varies with age, sex, or chronic blood loss. Females have a lower prevalence of symptomatic disease. This has been attributed to chronic menstrual blood losses and a lower intake of dietary iron. About 30% of heterozygotes

Table 5.1. HLA Typing in Hemochromatosis[a]

HLA Type	Frequency in Hemochromatosis (%)	Frequency in Normal Population (%)
A_3	71	28
B_7	46	28
B_{14}	18	6
$A_3 B_7$	38	6
$A_3 B_{14}$	16	0.2

[a] See Rudy et al. 1983, (4).

have slightly increased iron absorption and small increases in iron stores. However, progressive iron overload with symptomatic hemochromatosis does not occur.

Pathophysiology

The exact metabolic defect responsible for the increased absorption of iron is unknown. The three major hypotheses are

1. Primary intestinal mucosal defect.
2. Primary increase in hepatic iron uptake (reticuloendothelial system).
3. Abnormal metabolism of iron.

There is also a controversy as to the mechanism by which iron exerts its toxic affect. One possible explanation is that hemosiderin destabilizes the lysozome and thus damages the cell. A second mechanism proposes that intrahepatic iron produces peroxidative damage to the polyunsaturated fatty acids of membrane phospholipids.

Pathology

The liver is usually enlarged and reddish-brown in color. Hemosiderin deposits are found in most hepatocytes, particularly those on the periphery of regenerative nodules. Bile duct epithelial cells and mesenchymal cells in the fibrous septa also contain iron. Kupffer's cells are usually not heavily loaded with iron since transferrin bound iron is taken up selectively by hepatocytes and not by reticuloendothelial cells. Piecemeal necrosis and other inflammatory changes are usually minimal or absent. Liver biopsies have been used for monitoring treatment programs. They are useful but not indispensible. Near the end of a successful program of

iron depletion the liver biopsy shows a characteristic and fairly specific pattern of iron distribution; namely, the presence of iron in bile duct epithelial cells but not in hepatocytes.

The degree of stainable iron on liver biopsies has been arbitrarily graded 0 to 4. In patients with symptomatic hemochromatosis, the level of stainable iron is grade 3 to 4 (5). There may be some overlap with other diseases that cause an increase in hepatic iron, for example, alcoholism. This may make it difficult to distinguish hemochromatosis in a young subject from the hemosiderosis associated with alcoholism. The heaviest accumulation of iron in hemochromatosis occurs in the liver and the pancreas. Hemosiderin is present to a large extent in the acinar cells of the pancreas and to a lesser extent in the islets of Langerhans. Other places of deposition of iron are the conduction system of the AV node of the heart, and the pituitary, adrenal, thyroid, and parathyroid glands.

Clinical Features

Symptoms of hemochromatosis occur primarily in men, with a male/female ratio of 5–1. Symptoms usually begin in the fifth decade of life, although they may be present as early as the second or third decade. The most common initial symptoms are weakness, lethargy, loss of libido, sexual impotence, arthralgias, and abdominal pain. Other less common symptoms are amenorrhea and dyspnea on exertion.

Evaluation may reveal the classic triad of pigmentation of skin, hepatomegaly, and diabetes. Testicular atrophy is common, due to pituitary dysfunction rather than increased iron deposition in the testes. The patient may have loss of body hair, splenomegaly, jaundice, peripheral edema, or ascites. The skin is either bronze or blue-grey in color. This is due primarily to increased melanin pigment in the skin. The joint disease may also involve the proximal interphalangeal joints, wrist, hips, and knees.

The liver function tests usually reveal minor elevations in aminotransferases (transaminases), usually two to four times normal. The alkaline phosphatase is elevated in about 20% of the cases and is often between 225 and 300 units. Hypoalbuminemia and hypoprothrombinemia develop late in the course of the disease. Carbohydrate intolerance occurs in approximately 80% of patients and overt diabetes mellitus in 60%. Complications of diabetes such as neuropathy, retinopathy, and peripheral neuropathy may occur. Severe heart failure may occur but is uncommon. Cardiac arrhythmias are more common and are present in 15% of patients.

About 50% of patients develop a characteristic arthropathy, characterized by involvement of the metacarpophalangeal joint of the index finger. The joint disease may also involve the proximal interphalangeal joints, wrists, hips, and knees. The synovium has deposits of iron and calcium pyrophosphate.

Cirrhosis of the liver is usually present when hemochromatosis is diagnosed. In one recently reported large study, 70% of the patients had cirrhosis at the time of diagnosis. However, the prevalence of cirrhosis in patients diagnosed after 1976 was only 50% (6). This change probably reflects the impact of early diagnosis and screening procedures on the natural history and clinical presentation of this disease. Patients with hemochromatosis have a high incidence of hepatocellular carcinoma. The relative risk is 219 (6). Previous observations suggest that treatment of hemochromatosis does not diminish the incidence of hepatocellular carcinoma once cirrhosis has developed. Early diagnosis, before the development of cirrhosis, however, may prevent the development of hepatocellular carcinoma since there are no reports of the development of liver cancer in a noncirrhotic patient with hemochromatosis (6).

Diagnosis

The diagnosis of hemochromatosis is made on the basis of clinical features together with laboratory evidence of increased iron stores. The major diagnostic problem is to distinguish patients with idiopathic hemochromatosis from those with iron overload secondary to other types of cirrhosis. The results of iron storage tests are given in Table 5.2.

Serum iron is usually high in patients with hemochromatosis, yet the test is not very useful because it lacks sensitivity and specificity. The false-positive rate is 10% and the false-negative rate 24% (7).

Transferrin saturation, on the other hand, is the earliest and most sensitive indicator of iron overload (8). Virtually all patients with hemochroma-

Table 5.2. Iron Stores in Familial Hemochromatosis

	Normal Range	*Hemochromatosis*
Serum iron	50–150 μg/dl	>200 μg/dl
Transferrin saturation	25–50%	>50%
Serum ferritin	10–200 μg/L	>1000 μg/L
Hepatic iron	168–1843 μg/g dry weight	>2000 μg/g dry weight

Abbreviations: dl, deciliter; L, liter.

tosis under the age of 20 have a transferrin saturation exceeding 50%. Though the test is very sensitive it lacks specificity (false-positive rate 33%) (7). Serum ferritin concentration is the best reflection of the total body and hepatic iron stores but is not specific for this. Serum ferritin may be elevated in the absence of iron overload in lymphomas, lymphocytic leukemia, hyperthyroidism, and acute and chronic hepatocellular necrosis.

If both serum ferritin and transferrin saturation are elevated, a liver biopsy is indicated to assess histology and quantify liver stores. On the other hand, if both serum ferritin and transferrin saturation are normal, the probability of hemochromatosis is near zero and no further testing is necessary. Chelation tests, such as measurement of urinary iron excretion following an injection of desferroxamine, are cumbersome and do not contribute much to the evaluation. These tests have lately been discarded (9).

A major diagnostic problem is to distinguish patients with alcoholic liver disease and iron overload from homozygotes with early iron overload. There appears to be a high incidence of excessive alcohol intake in patients with genetic hemochromatosis, and therefore it is important to distinguish genetic hemochromatosis in an alcoholic from alcoholic liver disease with increased stainable iron.

Stainable iron in alcoholic liver disease with hemosiderosis may be similar to that in genetic hemochromatosis. Measurement of serum ferritin and transferrin saturation are helpful. However, there may be considerable overlap in their values. Recent studies have shown that measurement of hepatic iron may be the best way to distinguish between alcoholic liver disease and genetic hemochromatosis.

Patients with alcoholic liver disease rarely have hepatic iron levels over 10 mg/g of dry weight. In a more recent study by Bassett et al., none of the patients with alcoholic liver disease exceeded a level of 5.6 mg/g dry weight (10). In contrast, histologic damage to the liver occurred only after hepatic iron exceeded 22.4 mg/g of dry weight of liver tissue 400 micromoles per gram. This suggests that there may be a toxic threshold for hepatic iron, above which cirrhosis develops (10). Patients with alcoholic liver disease whose hepatic iron levels are over 10 mg/g of dry weight of liver should be assumed to have genetic hemochromatosis.

Homozygotes, when tested at an early age in the precirrhotic stage, may have hepatic iron levels well below 10 mg/g dry liver tissue. It has been suggested that these patients can be recognized by means of a hepatic iron index calculated as

$$\frac{\text{hepatic iron } (\mu\text{mol/g})}{\text{age of the patient in years}}$$

In the study by Bassett et al., every patient with genetic hemochromatosis had a hepatic iron index above 2, while all normal subjects and those with alcoholic liver disease had an index below 2 (10, 11).

Computed tomography scan has been shown in some studies to provide a quantitative index of hepatic iron stores. A good correlation has been described between hepatic iron stores and computed tomography (CT) attenuation values. The problem with the test is that spuriously low values may occur if there is concomitant presence of fat in the liver.

The determination of magnetic susceptibility of the liver and magnetic resonance imaging (MRI) are other noninvasive techniques that can assess hepatic iron stores (12,13). These techniques are presently expensive and have a limited role in the diagnosis and management of patients.

Family Screening

HLA typing can be used to predict the risk of hemochromatosis in the siblings of the proband. The family members should be screened with measurement of serum ferritin and transferrin saturation. If either is abnormal, a liver biopsy should be performed. Even if the serum ferritin and transferrin saturation are normal, the tests should be repeated after two years since the patients may develop iron overload over time.

Treatment and Prognosis

Excess iron is removed by weekly phlebotomy of 500 ml (250 mg iron). Phlebotomies may be continued safely until the hematocrit falls below 35% and fails to rise above this level after 2 weeks. This indicates the desired iron depletion. It may take up to 2 years to deplete the iron stores. Serum ferritin can be tested serially to evaluate iron stores. Most of the signs and symptoms of hemochromatosis improve after depletion of excess iron stores. The exceptions are arthritis, diabetes, and testicular atrophy.

Patients without cirrhosis at the onset of treatment have a life expectancy not different from that of age- and sex-matched normal population (6). The presence of cirrhosis or diabetes at the time of diagnosis worsens the prognosis. Inability to deplete the iron stores within $1\frac{1}{2}$ years of treatment is also considered to be a bad prognostic sign.

Desferroxamine given by subcutaneous infusion may be useful in patients who are anemic and do not tolerate phlebotomy.

Wilson's Disease

Wilson's disease is an inborn error of copper metabolism that is characterized by increased copper stores throughout the body. The organs most commonly involved are the liver, central nervous system, cornea, lens, and kidney. The disease is named after Samuel Alexander Kinnier Wilson (14), who in 1912 accurately described the disease as a rare familial disorder that was progressive and invariably fatal. He observed that it affected young people and was manifested by involuntary movements, spasticity, dysphagia, dysarthria, and transient mental symptoms along with cirrhosis of the liver.

The disease has an autosomal-recessive mode of inheritance and occurs in patients that are homozygous for the gene. Previous estimates of the prevalence of Wilson's disease were considerably lower than current estimates, probably because of the limited awareness of the presence of the disease and difficulties in making the diagnosis. Data from 1984 suggest a worldwide prevalence of Wilson's disease to be about 30 per million (15). Based on these estimates there would be one heterozygous carrier in 90 persons with a gene frequency of 1 in 180 persons. The estimates of gene frequency have not been directly verified because of our inability to accurately detect heterozygotes by available tests. As would be expected, ethnic groups with a high degree of consanguinity, such as Yemenite Jews and Iranian village communities, have a high prevalence of Wilson's disease.

The abnormality in copper metabolism initially results in a high concentration of copper in the liver, often as much as 1000 micrograms per gram dry weight. The normal is less than 50 μg/g dry weight. Liver injury starts early in childhood. However, clinical hepatic dysfunction almost never occurs before the age of 5 years. After the liver is saturated with copper, the metal is released into the blood stream and accumulates in other organs. Normal people absorb less than 50% of the copper in their diet. Urinary excretion is negligible. Approximately the same amount of copper that is absorbed is excreted into the bile and then into feces. Current evidence suggests that patients with Wilson's disease do not have increased absorption of copper. In contrast, it appears that there is decreased biliary excretion of copper leading to its accumulation in the liver. The site of the excretory defect may be the hepatocyte lysosome.

Accumulation of copper in the cells can cause damage by combining with the sulfhydryl, carbonyl, or amino groups and then interfering with cell metabolism. Excess copper may also directly stimulate fibrogenesis. After large amounts of copper have accumulated in the liver, there is usually a gradual release of copper from the liver. Copper then diffuses into the brain, eye, and other organs. Infrequently, in the setting of acute hepatic necrosis, large amounts of copper may be released into the blood stream and cause acute hemolysis. Alternatively, the release of copper from the damaged liver may occur in an individual whose liver disease is silent, both clinically and biochemically. The only evidence of liver damage at this stage may be cirrhosis demonstrated by biopsy.

Histopathology

The histopathologic changes in Wilson's disease are variable. There may be nonspecific changes, or changes consistent with acute hepatitis, chronic active hepatitis, or cirrhosis.

In the early stages of disease before cirrhosis has developed, there is moderate to marked fatty change and focal liver cell necrosis (16). The peri-

portal hepatocytes commonly have glycogenated nuclei. There is a gradual progression of periportal fibrosis. Over time the patient may develop histologic changes suggestive of chronic active hepatitis. Helpful but not pathognomonic features include an increased quantity of stainable cooper in periportal hepatocytes, steatosis, glycogenated nuclei, and Mallory's bodies. Eventually cirrhosis develops. It is usually macronodular.

Initially copper is present diffusely in the cytoplasm of the hepatocytes (17). Later, but still in the early symptomatic stage, the metal spreads into the lysosomes. In advanced disease the copper is usually confined to the lysosomes. Cytoplasmic copper is believed to be the form that damages hepatocytes. If liver biopsy is done in early stages of Wilson's disease, when copper is diffusely distributed throughout the liver cell cytoplasm, insensitive copper stains such as rhodamine may be negative. However, more sensitive stains such as the Timm's silver sulfide stain usually detect the copper (15). In contrast, in the later stages of the disease, although total hepatic copper levels may be lower than in the early stages, it is easier to detect the copper histologically since it is concentrated in the lysosome. The most unique ultrastructural change in Wilson's disease is noted in liver cell mitochondria. They are enlarged, heterogeneous, and have increased matrix density. There is also separation of the inner and outer membranes of the mitochondria and inclusion bodies in the mitochondrial matrix.

Clinical Features

The liver is the initial target in Wilson's disease. There may be a wide variability in clinical presentation and histologic changes. Even siblings may have different hepatic and neurologic presentations. Clinical hepatic disease has not been seen before the age of 5, although hepatic copper levels may be very high at this time. The disease may present as acute hepatitis, fulminant hepatitis, chronic active hepatitis, or cirrhosis. Some patients are asymptomatic and are recognized because of abnormal liver function tests. The usual age of presentation of liver disease is between 8 and 12 years (18). It is extremely unlikely for liver disease to present after the age of 35, although one patient with cirrhosis was first diagnosed after the age of 50 years (19).

About a fourth of the patients with liver disease will present with malaise, anorexia, lassitude, and jaundice, and will appear to have acute viral hepatitis. This episode is usually self-limited, resolves completely, and may be mistaken for viral hepatitis or infectious mononucleosis. The presence of persistent unconjugated hyperbilirubinemia due to ongoing hemolysis or hypouricemia due to renal tubular damage should alert the physician to consider Wilson's disease. Rarely, the first presentation of Wilson's disease may resemble fulminant hepatitis. There is worsening encephalopathy, coagulopathy, renal failure, and usually a fatal outcome.

A more common presentation mimics chronic hepatitis. In addition to the symptoms of hepatitis described above, there may be stigmata of chronic liver disease such as delayed puberty, testicular atrophy, gynecomastia, ascites, edema, splenomegaly, esophageal varices, and hypoalbuminemia.

Approximately 40% of patients with Wilson's disease present with psychiatric or neurologic symptoms, usually in their teens or twenties. Although these patients may not have clinically evident liver disease, they always have cirrhosis. The most common age for this type of presentation is 14 or 15 years, although in rare instances it can occur up to the age of 40 (20). The two most common neurologic symptoms are tremors and rigidity. Other manifestations include clumsiness of gait, slurring of speech, drooling, uncontrollable grinning (risor sardonicus), and seizures. There is a notable absence of sensory impairment in patients with Wilson's disease, except for the presence of recurrent headaches in some patients. A small percentage of patients may present with psychiatric problems such as dementia, psychosis, neurosis, and emotional instability. Wilson's disease should always be included in the differential diagnosis of young patients with psychiatric disease.

All patients with neuropsychiatric Wilson's disease have Kayser-Fleischer rings. The rings are greenish-brown in color and start as a small crescent at the top of the corneal limbus. This is followed by involvement of the inferior corneal quadrant. These two crescents gradually merge to form complete rings. A slit lamp examination confirms that the pigment is localized to Descemet's membrane. Complete and broad rings signify longstanding disease. Not all patients with hepatic disease alone have Kayser-Fleischer rings.

Patients with Wilson's disease may also develop cataracts due to deposition of copper in the anterior and posterior lens capsule. These cataracts, called "sunflower cataracts" because of the shape of the opacity, rarely interfere with vision.

There is often evidence of renal tubular dysfunction: uricosuria, phosphaturia, glucosuria, bicarbonaturia, and aminoaciduria. There is also a high incidence of urinary calculi, probably secondary to hypercalciuria. Numerous bone abnormalities have been observed in patients with Wilson's disease. These include osteoporosis, osteomalacia, spontaneous fractures, osteoarthritis, kyphoscoliosis, and osteochondritis dessicans.

Diagnosis

Determination of the serum ceruloplasmin, an acute-phase reactant, is one of the most valuable tests in making a diagnosis of Wilson's disease. Ceruloplasmin, a blue serum alpha$_2$ globulin (molecular weight 132,000) contains 0.3% copper. Its concentration is either low or undetectable in 95% of patients with Wilson's disease. However, 20% of healthy heterozygotes also have low ceruloplasmin levels (21). Serum ceruloplasmin levels can increase in response to estrogens, pregnancy, inflammatory diseases, or other liver diseases. Ceruloplasmin does not play a role in the pathogenesis of Wilson's disease. Some Wilson's disease patients have normal ceruloplasmin levels and some healthy heterozygotes have low levels. Moreover, a subset of Wilson's disease patients have a paradoxical increase in serum ceruloplasmin levels as their liver disease worsens. This may reflect the fact that ceruloplasmin is an acute-phase reactant.

Twenty-four-hour urinary copper determination is a useful test. Values usually exceed 100 μg/24 hr in patients with Wilson's disease, with normal levels less than 20 μg/24 hr. Meticulous care must be taken that copper-free containers are used. Occasionally the ability of D-penicillamine to increase urinary copper excretion to 1000 μg/24 hr or more provides confirmatory evidence in a patient whose 24-hour urinary excretion results are in an equivocal range.

A liver biopsy should routinely be done in order to obtain histology and to quantify hepatic copper concentration. Copper concentration greater than

200 μg/g dry weight liver is usually seen in Wilson's disease. Normal is less than 50 μg/g dry weight liver. Patients with other chronic cholestatic liver diseases such as primary biliary cirrhosis, chronic active hepatitis, and childhood cirrhosis of India may have elevated hepatic and urinary copper values similar to those seen in patients with Wilson's disease. However, serum ceruloplasmin levels are usually elevated rather than low in these other conditions. In rare instances Kayser-Fleischer rings may be seen in these disorders.

Without exception all patients in whom the diagnosis of Wilson's disease is considered should have a slit lamp examination to detect Kayser-Fleischer rings. The absence of these rings, confirmed by an experienced ophthamologist, will exclude the diagnosis of Wilson's disease in a patient with neurologic disease. Documentation of the size and width of the rings is useful for following patients since effective therapy decreases the size of the rings. The absence of Kayser-Fleischer rings in a patient with liver disease only does not rule out Wilson's disease.

Management

The drug of choice for the management of Wilson's disease is D-penicillamine. It binds copper stoichiometrically so that the amount of urinary copper increases with increasing doses of D-penicillamine. Initially a cupriuresis of about 2000 μg/day is desired. This falls as the copper stores are depleted. The initial starting dose of D-penicillamine ranges from 1000 to 1500 mg/day in three or four divided doses. This may occasionally have to be increased if the response is inadequate. The drug should preferably be taken on an empty stomach either 30 minutes before or 2 hours after a meal. The dose of the drug may be reduced once clinical benefit is seen and adequate cupriuresis obtained. A maintenance dose of 500 to 1000 mg/day may suffice. Patients should be advised to avoid foods rich in copper such as liver, shellfish, nuts, dried fruits, chocolate, cocoa, and mushrooms. About 20% of patients develop some side effect in the first few weeks of D-penicillamine treatment. These are allergic in nature and consist of rash, fever, thrombocytopenia, granulocytopenia, or agranulocytosis. It is important to check baseline values before treatment in order to distinguish the cytopenias secondary to cirrhosis from those of drug toxicity.

Patients with one or more of these side effects may be desensitized by stopping D-penicillamine until all hypersensitivity manifestations have cleared and then reinstituting the drug at low doses such as 25 mg/day. The dose is gradually increased by doubling it every 2 weeks. Steroids may be used temporarily at the time of restarting the D-penicillamine, although its necessity is uncertain. Patients should be followed closely during the first few weeks of treatment with D-penicillamine. Side effects should be watched for and the responses to treatment verified. In a minority of patients, the liver disease may worsen before it improves. A complete blood count, platelet count, and urinalysis should be done at each visit.

Some patients who tolerate D-penicillamine early in their course may develop toxicity later. Serious late complications include nephrotic syndrome, Goodpasture's syndrome, a systemic lupuslike illness, and myasthemia gravis. Bone marrow suppression with thrombocytopenia and agranulocytosis may also occur late in the course of treatment. High doses of penicillamine, usually 2 g or more, for extended periods may cause the characteristic skin lesion called penicillamine dermopathy. Large doses of penicillamine interfere with the cross-linking of elastin and collagen and result in sensitivity of the skin to minor trauma. This may cause bleeding into the subcutaneous tissues and lead to well-demarcated brownish blotches on the skin with small white papules in them (22).

Severe kidney or bone marrow toxicity may require that penicillamine be discontinued. Triethylene tetramine dihydrochloride (Trien) has been used as a second-line drug in patients with Wilson's disease who are unable to tolerate penicillamine (23,24). Trien has a good safety profile, but is not as effective as penicillamine.

A new treatment currently being evaluated is oral zinc. Zinc inhibits copper absorption and increases its fecal excretion (25). How this occurs is under investigation. Excess dietary zinc can sustain a negative copper balance in patients with stable Wilson's disease who have previously been treated with penicillamine (26). It is not known if zinc is effective as initial therapy for patients with newly diagnosed Wilson's disease.

Most patients with Wilson's disease are young and do not have a full understanding of their disease. The importance of uninterrupted drug therapy should be repeatedly emphasized to the patient and the family. Stoppage of therapy for as little as 9 months may result in the return of symptomatic disease and in rare instances, the return may be very severe.

Medical therapy is usually not effective in patients who present with fulminant hepatitis. These patients should be considered for liver transplantation (27). Successful surgery will be lifesaving and may result in a metabolic cure. Patients with far-advanced liver disease that is unresponsive to penicillamine therapy should also be considered for liver transplantation.

With adequate treatment virtually all patients with asymptomatic Wilson's disease and the majority of patients with symptomatic disease will enjoy good health and normal longevity. A few patients with advanced dystonic neurologic disease or far-advanced liver disease do not benefit from medical management.

Alpha$_1$-Antitrypsin Deficiency

Alpha$_1$-antitrypsin (α_1-AT) is a major serum protease inhibitor synthesized primarily by hepatocytes. It acts to protect tissue against injury caused by activated proteinases such as trypsin and elastase (28). Normally there is a careful balance between tissue proteinases and proteinase inhibitors. α_1-antitrypsin is a low-molecular-weight glycoprotein that migrates in the alpha$_1$ (α_1)-region on serum protein electrophoresis and accounts for about 90% of the α_1-globulin fraction in the serum. α_1-AT is an acute-phase reactant; thus its levels in body fluids increase in response to injury. This increase is believed to represent a protective measure against cellular proteinases that are released during inflammation, for example, by polymorphonuclear cells. One cause of neonatal hepatitis and childhood cirrhosis is a deficiency of α_1-AT. The identical deficiency is seen in adults with early-onset pulmonary emphysema. Many patients with emphysema have been found to have asymptomatic cirrhosis.

α_1-AT exists in the serum as a polymorphic glycoprotein, and more than 30 different phenotypic forms have been described. These protease inhibitor (Pi) variants are named alphabetically according to their relative mobility on acid starch gel. For example, PiMM migrates faster than PiZZ. Our present techniques to distinguish the variants are based on isoelectric focusing. The normal phenotype is PiMM. It is present in about 70% of individuals. The slowest migrating, that is, the most cathodal variant, PiZZ, is of importance with regard to liver and pulmonary disease. Individuals who are homozygous for PiZZ have serum α_1-AT levels that are less than 2 mg/ml. This is 10% to 20% of normal levels. PiZZ individuals are clearly at risk for developing childhood liver diseases and early-onset pulmonary emphysema. It is a matter of debate whether some intermediate genotypes MZ, MS, and SZ are ever associated with disease. The incidence of PiZZ variant, henceforth called α_1-AT deficiency, is approximately 1 in 2000 to 4000 live births. PiZZ differs from PiMM by replacement of a glutamic acid residue with a lysine at residue 342, and by the lack of a normal complement of sialic acid compared with PiMM. This change reflects a guanine to adenine transition at the corresponding location in the gene. The above alterations in the molecule appear to interfere with the uptake of the α_1-AT into the Golgi apparatus and its subsequent secretion from the hepatocyte. The exact pathogenesis of α_1-AT deficiency liver disease is not known. It is possible that retention of α_1-AT in the liver may cause hepatocellular injury. This is unlikely. All patients with α_1-AT deficiency retain α_1-AT in the liver, but most do not develop liver disease. Rather, α_1-AT deficiency may act as a permissive factor in the development of liver disease. A current hypothesis proposes that the lack of antiprotease activity in serum allows hepatic damage to occur and be perpetuated whenever inflammatory cells are activated in the liver and release elastase and proteases.

Pathology

The liver biopsy in α_1-AT deficiency shows the presence of periodic acid-Schiff (PAS)-diastase-positive globules in periportal hepatocytes and occasionally in bile duct epithelial cells. Examination of the liver with transmission electron microscopy reveals a finely amorphous material located within the lumen of dilated smooth and rough endoplasmic reticulum. The inclusion bodies are usually 1 to 8 micrometers in diameter but may be considerably larger, and react with antibodies to α_1-AT. Using sensitive immunologic techniques, PAS-positive inclusion bodies can be found in the vast majority of patients with the PiZZ genotype.

However, only a small fraction, approximately 20% of these, develop neonatal hepatitis or childhood cirrhosis, although up to 66% may have abnormal biochemical tests of liver function. Patients with cholestasis show mild degenerative changes in hepatocytes and occasionally ductular proliferation. Some patients may have portal expansion, fibrosis, and a paucity of bile ducts. This is associated with a markedly worse prognosis (29).

Clinical Features

The best data are from a large prospective study in Sweden. Between 1972 and 1974, 100,000 newborns were screened for α_1-AT deficiency and 120 were found with PiZZ (30,31). Of the 120 newborns with PiZZ, only 12% had cholestasis and an additional 7% had clinical evidence of liver disease in infancy. On follow-up of the other patients, another 47% had elevations of aminotransferases at 3 months, which persisted on later follow-up. Therefore, only 34% of all the newborns with PiZZ had no clinical or biochemical evidence of liver disease.

At 6 months of age, the infants with clinically apparent liver disease appeared to have recovered from the liver disease. However, two of the children with neonatal cholestasis had liver cirrhosis by age 4. This study provided an estimate of clinically important liver disease in infancy, but probably underestimated the total extent of liver disease since liver biopsies were not done on children with neonatal cholestasis whose liver function tests (LFTs) improved. Other studies have shown that three-quarters of PiZZ patients who develop clinically apparent liver disease presented with cholestasis during infancy.

Of all infants with neonatal cholestasis, only 25% recover without chronic liver disease, although in the vast majority of these patients the serum bilirubin returns to normal in the first 6 months of life. Of all children presenting with cholestasis about 25% continue to have abnormal liver function tests; develop portal hypertension, coagulopathy, ascites; and die of complications of liver disease during the first 10 years of life. Another 25% of patients have a slower progression of chronic liver disease and die between the ages of 10 and 20 years. Another 25% have minimal hepatocellular dysfunction and live normally into

adulthood. These patients, however, develop fibrosis on liver biopsy and may develop cirrhosis in later life. The final 25% recover completely (32). The clinical course of liver disease is similar in siblings in families where more than one child had α_1-AT deficiency.

The hepatic manifestations depend on the age at presentation. In the neonatal period, α_1-AT deficiency presents as acute hepatitis or a cholestatic syndrome with jaundice and moderately elevated serum aminotransferases. The alkaline phosphatase may be greater than four times normal. In many of these infants the bilirubin returns to normal by 3 to 6 months. Many of these infants present in early childhood or adolescence with manifestations of cirrhosis including splenomegaly, hepatomegaly, ascites, coagulopathy, and variceal bleeding. Because there is a wide spectrum of disease from benign to rapidly fatal, several authors have attempted to define prognostic factors. A poor prognosis is suggested by a persistent marked elevation in aminotransferases or conjugated bilirubin, splenomegaly, ascites, and persitent firm hepatomegaly (29). Infants who have a paucity of interlobular bile ducts on liver biopsy have a poor outlook. One must be cautious in reading this change unless there is a large biopsy specimen with many portal tracts. Other changes associated with a poor prognosis are marked portal fibrosis and ductular proliferation.

The liver disease in adults with α_1-AT deficiency is much more insidious than it is in childhood. In one study at least 19% of patients over the age of 50 had cirrhosis. This number is probably an underestimate of the true prevalence of α_1-AT deficiency liver disease in adults. Some of these patients may develop progressive liver disease and die of liver failure. There is an increased incidence of hepatocellular carcinoma in adults with α_1-AT deficiency, although the exact incidence is not known. A study done in 1986 has shown that patients may have a 20-fold increased risk for hepatocellular carcinoma. Men appear to be at higher risk than women (33).

Diagnosis

The diagnosis of α_1-AT deficiency should be suspected in all individuals with neonatal hepatitis and juvenile cirrhosis, and in adults with early-onset emphysema. It should be considered in adults with abnormal LFTs or cirrhosis of unknown etiology.

α_1-AT normally makes up 90% of the serum α_1-globulin on serum protein electrophoresis. If this band is missing or present in unusually low concentration, the diagnosis of α_1-AT deficiency is suggested. More accuracy is achieved by quantifying the α_1-AT with antigen-antibody diffusion methods, utilizing Mancini's plates or rocket immunoelectrophoresis. Confirmation of the diagnosis is usually done by Pi typing. A number of methodologies exist. However, isoelectric focusing is the preferred method. Liver biopsy shows the changes previously described.

Management

There is no known treatment for the liver disease associated with α_1-AT deficiency. Danazol, a 17-α substituted alkyl steroid, has been shown to increase serum antitrypsin levels up to 37% in PiZZ individuals. There is, however, no evidence of its clinical value. Its use has largely fallen out of favor because of a theoretical risk of exacerbating the liver disease.

A concentrate of α_1-AT has been produced from the Cohn fraction IV-I and clinical trials are currently underway at the National Institutes of Health (34). The therapeutic end-point is an increase in plasma antielastase activity, although the efficacy of this treatment is unknown.

A gene for human antitrypsin has been expressed in yeast recently and commercial qualities of α_1-AT are now available for testing (35).

Liver transplantation has been performed in children with end-stage α_1-AT deficiency liver disease and is now the treatment of choice (36). It corrects both the liver disorder and the underlying metabolic abnormalities.

Prenatal diagnosis of α_1-antitrypsin deficiency PiZZ is possible. This was previously done by Pi typing of blood samples obtained by fetoscopy. However, this technique entails significant risk. Prenatal diagnosis of α_1-AT deficiency is now possible by direct analysis of the mutation site in the gene. Despite the possibility of the prenatal diagnosis, there are little data to justify abortion because of the inability to predict which children will have the liver disease.

Gaucher's Disease

Gaucher's disease is an inherited disorder of glycolipid metabolism characterized by the accumulation of glucoceboside in various organs of the body. The disease affects all ages and is inherited as an autosomal-recessive trait. The disorder has been divided into three clinical types according to the age at onset and the presence or absence of neurologic involvement. Type I is the adult form, also called the chronic non-neuronopathic form because of the notable absence of neurologic disease. Type II is the infantile form, also called the acute neuronopathic form because of the presence of rapidly progressive neurologic disease causing death by the age of 3 years. Type III is the juvenile form, also called subacute neuronopathic form, in which neurologic disease occurs later than in type II and is less severe and more slowly progressive.

All patients with Gaucher's disease have reduced activity of the enzyme glucocerebrosidase in their body tissues. This enzyme catalyzes the following reaction: glucocerebroside + H_2O (glucocerebrosidase) $\rightarrow$ ceramide + glucose. Reduced activity of this enzyme results in the accumulation of the substrate glucocerebroside in various organs throughout the body.

Pathology

The characteristic histologic finding is the presence of large lipid-containing cells in the reticuloendothelial system. The cells are 20 to 100 μm in diameter with an eccentric nucleus. Because of the presence of the glucocerebroside, the cytoplasm may have a "wrinkled tissue paper" or "crumpled silk" appearance (37). These cells can be seen in the liver, spleen, lymph nodes, lungs, and bone marrow. The Gaucher's cells stain positively for acid phosphatase and have spindle-shaped inclusion bodies in the cytoplasm. The Gaucher's cell is an altered macrophage, which is derived from the histiocytes in the spleen and the Kupffer's cells in the liver.

There is accumulation of large amounts of glucocerebroside in the spleen, which usually causes moderate to massive splenomegaly. There is a considerable amount of splenic fibrosis and distortion of the normal architecture. However, splenic rupture is uncommon. Almost all patients with Gaucher's disease have histologic evidence of liver involvement. In a majority of the patients the largest numbers of lipid-laden storage cells are seen in the central and pericentral regions of the liver (zone 3). These cells may cause compression of the central veins. Smaller numbers of Gaucher's cells may be seen in the portal and periportal zone (zone 1). Often there is evidence of fibrosis around the storage cells. Less commonly, thick fibrous bands are seen extending from central veins to other central veins or portal triads leading to cirrhosis (38). There is minimal evidence of hepatic injury or necrosis. Other organs involved in Gaucher's disease are the bones, lymph nodes, kidneys, heart, lungs, and eyes.

Clinical Features

TYPE I DISEASE

Type I Gaucher's disease affects all ethnic groups. However, Askenazic Jews have the highest incidence. The disease may present at any time, from infancy to the eighth decade of life. The most common presentation is massive splenomegaly. Other patients may have thrombocytopenia, anemia, or leukopenia secondary to hypersplenism. The majority of patients eventually need splenectomy for the hematologic complications, and rarely for discomfort caused by the massive spleen.

Most patients have hepatomegaly at the time of diagnosis. Many patients exhibit mild to moderate elevation in aminotransferases or alkaline phosphatase. However, it is not inconsistent to have normal liver function tests in the presence of moderate hepatomegaly. Hepatic failure or complications of cirrhosis are uncommon. A small percentage of patients have diffuse infiltration of the liver, marked fibrosis, and progress to have portal hypertension, variceal bleeding, and ascites (38–40). The severity of the liver involvement tends to parallel the severity of involvement of the other organ systems. A technetium liver-spleen scan usually shows evidence of hepatosplenomegaly and decreased hepatic uptake of isotope.

Patients eventually develop bone complications in the form of aseptic necrosis of the hip or fractures of vertebrae or long bones. Severe bone pain may occur in the absence of fractures. X-ray films reveal expansion of the cortex of bones, cystlike cavities in long bones, osteopenia, or erosions of bone. Pulmonary involvement may manifest as recurrent pulmonary infections and pulmo-

nary hypertension. Involvement of the heart may cause restrictive pericarditis or restrictive cardiopmyopathy.

TYPE II DISEASE

The disease presents during the first $1\frac{1}{2}$ years of life, usually with hepatosplenomegaly. This is soon followed by progressive neurologic impairment leading to spasticity. There is involvement of cranial nerve nuclei and extrapyramidal tracts, which leads to death before the age of 3 years.

TYPE III DISEASE

These patients appear to have a course intermediate between type I and type II disease. Hepatosplenomegaly often appears first. At this stage the patients may be considered to have type I Gaucher's disease. Later neurologic disease develops in the form of slowly progressive spasticity, ataxia, and cranial nerve paralysis.

DIAGNOSIS

Both in infancy and adulthood the diagnosis of Gaucher's disease is usually suspected by the finding of hepatosplenomegaly. Less commonly, patients may present with thrombocytopenia secondary to hypersplenism, or with bone pain or pathologic fractures secondary to bone involvement. The plasma level of nontartrate inhibitable acid phosphatase is often elevated. Examination of the bone marrow usually reveals large numbers of Gaucher's cells. A liver biopsy shows the lipid-laden cells. The diagnosis can be confirmed by measuring the amount of glucocerebroside in liver tissue.

The best way to confirm the diagnosis is to measure the glucocerebrosidase activity in the peripheral blood leukocytes. Cultured fibroblasts obtained by a skin biopsy may also be used for this purpose. Measurement of glucocerebrosidase activity in leukocytes and cultured skin fibroblasts can also be used to detect heterozygotes. This information enables the physician to perform genetic counseling for couples who are heterozygotes.

TREATMENT

The management of Gaucher's disease involves supportive care and the treatment of complications. Symptomatic thrombocytopenia and anemia are usually improved by splenectomy. Attempts have been made to infuse human placental glucocerebrosidase intravenously to correct the metabolic abnormality. Such intervention can decrease the amount of glucocerebroside in the liver and that associated with the erythrocytes (41). The long-term influence of replacement therapy on the natural history of the disease is not known.

Niemann-Pick Disease

Niemann-Pick disease (NPD) is a lipid storage disorder that is characterized by the accumulation of sphingomyelin (ceramide phosphoryl choline) and other lipids throughout the body. All patients with this disorder have hepatosplenomegaly and foam cells in the bone marrow, and most present with progressive nervous system dysfunction (42).

There are five types of disease, labeled A, B, C, D, and E, which are distinguished by their clinical characteristics and pattern of enzyme abnormalities. These types range in severity, type A being associated with the most severe from of disease and type E causing only asymptomatic hepatosplenomegaly. The metabolic defect in NPD is a marked deficiency of the enzyme sphingomyelinase. This enzyme catalyzes the hydrolytic cleavage of sphingomyelin into ceramide and phosphoryl choline.

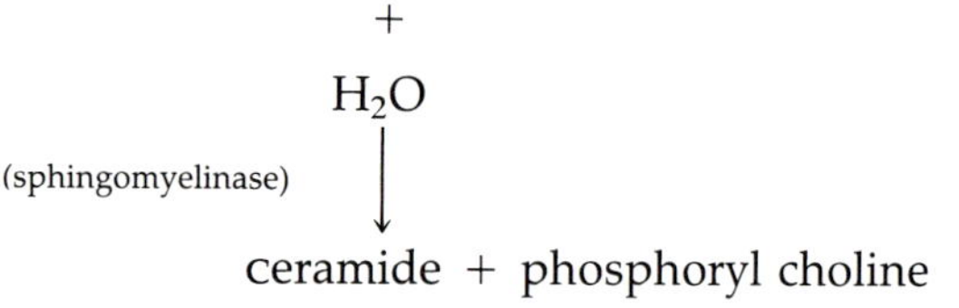

(ceramide phosphorylcholine) sphingomyelin

\+

H_2O

(sphingomyelinase)

↓

ceramide + phosphoryl choline

In NPD the deficiency of sphingomyelinase is associated with the accumulation of large amounts of sphingomyelin in the tissues (43). The level of sphingomyelinase in patients with type A disease is less than 10% of normal in liver tissue and about 4% of normal in leukocytes and cultured skin fibroblasts. As a result the amount of sphingomyelin in tissue is greatly increased. For example, in the spleen of patients with type A NPD, sphingomyelin may be increased to 370 mg/g of dry weight in comparison to a normal value of 15 mg/g of dry weight. Patients with type B disease also have very

low levels of sphingomyelinase. However, these are slightly higher than the levels seen in type A. Type B patients may have 250 to 280 mg/g dry weight of sphingomyelin in the spleen. Type C patients have 38% to 63% of sphingomyelinase activity in their fibroblasts and may have normal activity in the liver and spleen. The level of sphingomyelin in their spleen, however, is increased and has been reported to be between 25 and 225 mg/g of dry weight. Patients with type D NPD have more modest increases in the amount of sphingomyelin in the organs but do not have any demonstrable sphinomyelinase deficiency. The enzymatic defect in this type of NPD remains unresolved. Patients with type E NPD disease have moderate increases in sphingomyelin in one or more organs, but do not have evidence of familial involvement and this disorder has not been shown to be of genetic origin. All other types of NPD, that is, types A, B, C, and D, are transmitted as an autosomal-recessive trait. Affected siblings in a family always have the same type of disorder.

Clinical Features

TYPE A NPD

This variant accounts for the vast majority of patients with NPD. Most of the patients are Ashkenazic Jews. The disease presents early in infancy with hepatosplenomegaly and central nervous system involvement. The infants develop malnutrition due to feeding difficulties. The combination of hepatosplenomegaly with generalized emaciation produces protuberant abdomens and thin extremities. About half the infants have a cherry-red spot in the macular region of the eye. They may also develop corneal or retinal opacification. There is gradual loss of intellectual capacity, motor function, and muscle tone. The disease is fatal by age 3 to 4 years.

TYPE B NPD

The distinguishing feature of this variant is the notable absence of central nervous system impairment. The children present with splenomegaly followed by liver enlargement. Apart from organomegaly they may reach adulthood in good health. Patients also have diffuse lung infiltration with sphingomyelin. This presents as dyspnea on exertion and recurrent pulmonary infections.

TYPE C NPD

These children are asymptomatic in the first 1 or 2 years of life. They later develop slowly progressive neurologic damage with less dramatic hepatosplenomegaly. Death usually occurs between 5 and 15 years of age.

TYPE D NPD (NOVA SCOTIA VARIANT)

The ancestry of patients with this disorder has been traced to a couple born in Nova Scotia in the 1600s. Patients present with hepatosplenomegaly and neurologic abnormality early in childhood, between ages 2 and 4 years.

TYPE E NPD

These patients present in adult life with moderate hepatosplenomegaly without neurologic impairment. They do not have familial involvement.

Pathology and Organ Involvement

The characteristic NPD cell is large, 20 to 90 μm in diameter, and foamy in appearance. The cytoplasm is filled with small lipid droplets, which give a mulberry appearance to the cells.

The spleen is the most extensively involved organ and is infiltrated by masses of foam cells. The resulting hypersplenism may cause anemia and thrombocytopenia. The liver is usually $1\frac{1}{2}$ times normal size and is largest in type B NPD. Biochemical tests of liver function are usually normal, except for type B NPD, in which elevated serum aminotransferases, bilirubin, and alkaline phosphatase may occur. The bone marrow is infiltrated with foam cells in all types of NPD. Other organs involved are the lung and heart. The small intestine, adrenals, gonads, thyroid, pituitary, and pancreas may be involved but there is no apparent impairment of function.

The predominant region of the brain involved is the cerebral cortex in types A and C. However, other areas such as the basal ganglia, spinal cord, and autonomic ganglia may be involved.

Diagnosis

The diagnosis is made by the finding of hepatosplenomegaly, other clinical features such as the cherry-red spot in the macula, and the presence of lipid-laden cells in the bone marrow. Confirmation can be obtained by commercially available assays of sphingomyelinase activity (44). The levels of sphingomyelin in tissues can also be measured if needed. Heterozygotes can be identified since they have 54% to 64% of sphingomyelinase activity in their circulating leukocytes and decreased enzyme activity in fibroblasts grown in tissue culture of skin biopsy specimens.

Prenatal diagnosis of NPD is a well-established procedure in which the diagnosis is made by assaying the sphingomyelinase activity in the cultured fetal cells obtained by amniocentesis (45).

Treatment

There is no known treatment for NPD. Splenectomy may relieve the thrombocytopenia. Pulmonary infections need to be aggressively treated. Enzyme replacement is a therapeutic modality that has to be explored in animal models of NPD.

Glycogen Storage Diseases

There are at least 10 different types of glycogen storage diseases. All involve the liver and cause hepatomegaly except for type V (muscle phosphorylase deficiency) and type VII (phosphofructokinase deficiency), which involve only skeletal muscle. The glycogen storage diseases are characterized by deficiencies in enzymes involved in the degradation or synthesis of glycogen. Most glycogenosis are accompanied by an excess accumulation of glycogen in the liver or muscle. All of the hepatic glycogenosis have a derangement in glucose homeostasis and have a limited ability to mobilize glucose from hepatic glycogen stores. Since hepatic glycogen serves as a major carbohydrate reserve, these conditions are usually associated with varying degrees of fasting hypoglycemia. Type I glycogen storage disease, Von Gierke's disease, was the first inherited disease that was shown to be caused by the deficiency of a specific enzyme, in this case glucose-6-phosphatase (46). This was followed by the discovery of several other enzyme defects in glycogen metabolism and the introduction of a numbering system. For this discussion we limit ourselves to the most commonly encountered disorder of glycogen metabolism, type I glycogen storage disease.

This disease has an autosomal-recessive pattern

of inheritance and is characterized by a combination of fasting hypoglycemia, hyperlipidemia, hyperuricemia, systemic acidosis, hepatomegaly, and renal enlargement. The hepatomegaly is present at birth and persists throughout life. Splenomegaly is uncommon. The children are of short stature and often have osteoporosis, which is probably secondary to the chronic acidosis. The extent of hypoglycemia varies but fasting for 3 hours will invariably cause the blood glucose to drop below 70 mg/dl. Blood glucose levels of 5 to 10 mg% have been seen (47). Such severe hypoglycemia may percipitate convulsions. However, some patients are asymptomatic, a finding which suggests that the brain may be able to utilize other substrates for energy production. The hormonal responses to hypoglycemia are normal. There is a rise in the serum level of glucagon in response to hypoglycemia, but the increase in blood glucose after intravenous infusion of glucagon or epinephrine is blunted. The hypoglycemia results in active glycogenolysis and gluconeogenesis. Since there is an absence of glucose-6-phosphatase, glucose cannot be generated from glycogenolysis or gluconeogenesis and there is an excess production of glycerol, acetyl coenzyme A, and increased levels of reduced nicotinamide adenine dinucleotide (NADH) and nicotinamide-adenine dinucleotide phosphate (reduced form) (NADPH). This results in an increased rate of cholesterol and triglyceride synthesis. The serum levels of free fatty acids are also increased as a direct metabolic consequence of hypoglycemia. As a consequence of the sustained hypercholesterolemia, these patients develop xanthomas on the extensor surfaces of the arms and legs.

The hyperuricemia may result in gouty tophi. Other complications of gout usually develop in patients who reach puberty. These patients also have defective hemostasis due to abnormal platelet aggregation and adhesion. Clinically significant bleeding may occasionally occur. A large number of patients develop hepatic adenomas (48). Hepatocellular carcinoma has been found in some of these nodules.

Diagnosis

The preferred method of diagnosis is the demonstration of a deficiency of glucose-6-phosphatase in liver tissue obtained by open biopsy, a process that allows adequate tissue to permit the necessary enzyme assays. Some authors advocated percutaneous needle biopsy of the liver in order to prevent complications of anaesthesia and surgery (49). If the metabolic derangements are not corrected prior to anaesthesia, intractable acidosis can occur (50). The liver cells demonstrate prominent nuclear glycogenosis and marked macrovesicular fatty infiltration. There is little or no fibrosis.

Treatment

The most effective treatment for type I glycogen storage disease is continuous intragastric feeding. This has to be maintained during the night along with frequent high-carbohydrate meals during the day. This results in a growth spurt along with correction of the hyperlipidemia, acidosis, and hyperuricemia (51). Portosystemic shunting is also effective treatment, although it is not usually as effective as continuous intragastric feeding (52). A comprehensive review of the rationale and results is provided in Chapter 7, *this volume*. Liver transplant has been done successfully in individuals who were unable to be maintained on medical therapy.

References

1. Bomford A, Williams R. Long term results of venesection therapy in idiopathic hemochromatosis. *Q J Med* 1976; 45: 611–623.
2. Simon M, et al. Idiopathic hemochromatosis: Demonstration of recessive transmission and early detection by family HLA typing. *N Engl J Med* 1977; 297:1017–1021.
3. Bassett ML, et al. Idiopathic hemochromatosis: Demonstration of homozygous-heterozygous mating by HLA typing of families. *Hum Genet* 1982; 60:352–356.
4. Rudy DR, et al. Idiopathic hemochromatosis. *Am Fam Physician* 1983; 28(5):176–183.
5. Edwards C, et al. Homozygosity for hemochromatosis: Clinical manifestations. *Ann Intern Med* 1980; 93:519–525.
6. Niederau C, et al. Survival and cause of death in cirrhotic and in noncirrhotic patients with primary hemochromatosis. *N Engl J Med* 1985; 313(20):1256–1262.
7. Halliday JW, et al. Serum ferritin in diagnosis of hemochromatosis. *Lancet* 1977; 2:621–623.
8. Gollan JL. Diagnosis of hemochromatosis. *Gastroenterology* 1983; 84(2):418–421.
9. Bassett ML, et al. Genetic Hemochromatosis. *Semin Liver Dis* 1984; 4(3):217–222.
10. Bassett ML, et al. Value of hepatic iron measurements in early hemochromatosis and determination of the critical iron level associated with fibrosis. *Hepatology* 1986; 6(1):24–29.
11. Tavill AS, Bacon BR. Hemochromatosis: How much iron is too much? *Hepatology* 1986; 6(1):142–145.
12. Brittenham GM, et al. Magnetic susceptibility measurement of human iron stores. *N Engl J Med* 1982; 307:1671–1675.

13. Stark DD, et al. Magnetic resonance imaging and spectroscopy of hepatic iron overload. *Radiology* 1985; 154:137–142.

14. Wilson SAK. Progressive lenticular degeneration: A familial nervous disease associated with cirrhosis of the liver. *Brain* 1912; 34:295–507.

15. Scheinberg IH, Sternlieb I. Wilson's disease. In: *Major Problems in Internal Medicine*, vol. 23. Philadelphia: WB Saunders, 1984.

16. Stromeyer FW, Ishak KG. Histology of the liver in Wilson's disease. A study of 34 cases. *Am J Clin Pathol* 1980; 73:12–24.

17. Goldfischer S, Sternlieb I. Changes in the distribution of hepatic copper in relation to the progression of Wilson's disease. *Am J Pathol* 1968; 53:883–901.

18. Walshe JM. The liver in Wilson's disease. In: Schiff L, Schiff ER, eds. *Diseases of the Liver*, 5th ed. Philadelphia: JB Lippincott, 1982, pp. 1043–1059.

19. Fitzgerald MA, et al. Wilson's disease (hepatolenticular degeneration) of late adult onset: Report of case. *Mayo Clin Proc* 1975; 50:438–442.

20. Walshe JM. Copper: Its role in the pathogenesis of liver disease. *Seminars Liver Dis* 1984; 4(3).

21. Gibbs K, Walshe JM. A study of ceruloplasmin concentration found in 75 patients with Wilson's disease, their kinships and various control groups. *Q J Med* 1979; 48:447–463.

22. Nimmi ME. Mechanism of inhibition of collagen cross linking by penicillamine. *Proc R Soc Med* 1977; 70(Suppl 3):65–72.

23. Walshe JM. Treatment of Wilson's disease with trientine (triethylene tetramine) dihydrochloride. *Lancet* 1982; 1:643–647.

24. Hayes AH Jr. Triethylene dihydrochloride for treatment of penicillamine intolerant patients with Wilson's disease; invitation to submit new drug application. *Fed Reg* 1982; 47(186):42175–42176.

25. Patterson WP. Zinc induced copper deficiency Mega mineral sidero-blastic anemia. *Ann Intern Med* 1985; 103(3):385–386.

26. Brewer GJ. Oral zinc therapy for Wilson's disease. *Ann Intern Med* 1983; 99:314–320.

27. Sternlieb I. Wilson's disease. Indications for liver transplant. *Hepatology* 1984; 4(1):15S–17S

28. Travis J, Salvesen GS. Human plasma proteinase inhibitors. *Annu Rev Biochem* 1983; 52:655–709.

29. Alagille D. α_1 antitrypsin deficiency. *Hepatology* 1984; 4(1):11S–14S.

30. Sveger T. Liver disease in alpha$_1$ antitrypsin deficiency detected by screening of 200,000 infants. *N Engl J Med* 1976; 294:1316–1321.

31. Sveger T. Alpha$_1$ antitrypsin deficiency in early childhood. *Pediatrics* 1978; 62:22–25.

32. Sharp HL. Alpha$_1$ antitrypsin. An ignored protein in understanding liver disease. *Semin Liver Dis* 1982; 2(4):314–328.

33. Erikson S, et al. Risk of cirrhosis and primary liver cancer in alpha$_1$-anti-trypsin deficiency. *N Engl J Med* 1986; 314(12):736–739.

34. Gadek JE, Crystal RG. Experience with replacement therapy in the destructive lung disease associated with severe α_1 anti-trypsin deficiency. *Am Rev Respir Dis* 1983; 127(Suppl 2):545–546.

35. Rosenberg S, et al. Synthesis in yeast of a functional oxidation-resistant mutant of human α_1 anti-trypsin. *Nature* 1984; 312:77–80.

36. Hood JM, et al. Liver transplantation for advanced liver disease with alpha$_1$ anti-trypsin deficiency. *N Engl J Med* 1980; 302:272–275.

37. Brady RO, Barranger JA. Glucosylceramide lipidosis: Gaucher's disease. In: *Metabolic Basis of Inherited disease*, 5th ed. New York: McGraw-Hill, 842–856.

38. James SP, et al. Liver abnormalities in patients with Gaucher's disease. *Gastroenterology* 1981; 80:126–133.

39. Sales JEL, Hunt AH. Gaucher's disease and portal hypertension. *Surg* 1970; 57:225.

40. Kozower M, Kaplan MM, Kanfer JN, et al. Esophageal varies in a 60 year old man with Gaucher's disease. *Dig Dis* 1974; 19:565.

41. Brady RO, et al. Replacement therapy for inherited enzyme deficiency. Use of purified glucocerebrosidase in Gaucher's disease. *N Engl J Med* 1974; 291:989.

42. Brady RO. Sphingomyelin lipidoses: Niemann Pick disease. In: *Metabolic Basis of Inherited Disease*, 5th ed. New York: McGraw-Hill, 1983, pp. 831–841.

43. Brady RO. The metabolism of sphingomyelin II. Evidence of an enzymatic defect in Niemann Pick disease. *Proc Natl Acad Sci USA* 1966; 55:366.

44. Kampine JP, et al. Diagnosis of Gaucher's disease and Niemann-Pick disease with small samples of venous blood. *Science* 1967; 15:86.

45. Schneider EL, et al. Prenatal Niemann-Pick disease. Biochemical and histological examination of a 19-gestational week fetus. *Pediatr Res* 1972; 6:720.

46. Cori GT, Cori CF. Glucose-6-phosphatase of the liver in glycogen storage disease. *J Biol Chem* 1952; 199:661–667.

47. *Metabolic Basis of Inherited Disease: Glycogen Storage Diseases*, 5th ed. New York: McGraw-Hill, 1983, pp. 141–166.

48. Howell RR. Hepatic adenomata in patients with type I glycogen storage disease. *JAMA* 1976; 236:1481–1484.

49. Greene HL. Glycogen storage disease. *Semin Liver Dis* 1982; 2(4):291–301.

50. Edelstein G, Hirshman CA. Hyperthermia and ketoacidosis during anaesthesia in a child with glycogen storage disease. *Anesthesiology* 1980; 52:90–92.

51. Greene HL, et al. Type I. Glycogen storage disease. A metabolic basis for advances in treatment. *Adv Pediatr* 1979; 26:63–92.

52. Bur IM, et al. Comparison of the effects of total parenteral nutrition, continuous intragastric feeding and portacaval shunt on a patient with Type I glycogen storage disease. *J Pediatr* 1974; 85:792–795.

Editorial Comment

Lest the surgeons be misled by the title, *Metabolic Liver Diseases*, into the belief that these disorders are esoteric entities of no importance or significance to them, it is well to emphasize certain facts relating to these disorders.

Hemochromatosis, once a cirrhotic process has developed, carries a risk of 20% of developing hepatocellular carcinoma that must be recognized early if there is to be any chance of resection for cure. Wilson's disease does not often present with the problems of portal hypertension common to other types of cirrhosis, but progressive liver failure in these young patients should raise the question of liver transplant.

Alpha$_1$ antitrypsin deficiency has been treated by Starzl initially with portacaval shunting and more recently by liver transplant that, as Starzl states in a following section, "provides a metabolic 'cure' and the protein phenotype of the recipient becomes that of the donor for the lifetime of the graft." The same applies to glycogen storage disease.

In Gaucher's disease, thrombocytopenia may provide an indication for splenectomy. Thus, this and the following chapter both serve to emphasize the need for the surgeon to become familiar with these previously abstruse disorders.

Chapter 6
Surgery for Metabolic Liver Disease

THOMAS E. STARZL

There is no aspect of intermediary metabolism in which the liver is not involved. Consequently, it is not surprising that inborn errors of metabolism can be influenced by operations on the liver. This chapter will describe how the course of liver-based inborn errors of metabolism can be changed by two kinds of hepatic operations, portacaval shunt and liver transplantation.

Portal Diversion

Mechanism of Effects

Venous blood from the splanchnic viscera has liver-supporting qualities not found to the same degree in other kinds of arterial or venous blood (1–6). The main splanchnic venous "hepatotrophic" factors are almost certainly endogenous hormones of which the single most important is insulin. Deprivation of the liver of the so-called "hepatotrophic effects" of portal blood has been noted under several experimental conditions (including portacaval shunt) to cause hepatocyte atrophy, deglycogenation, and fatty infiltration. With electron microscopic studies, relatively specific findings have been disruption and reduction of the rough endoplasmic reticulum (RER) and diminution of its lining polyribosomes (1,3–7). Since RER is the "factory" of the cell, a consequent reduction in many biosynthetic processes would be expected. Numerous studies have verified this hypothesis.

For example, the effect of portal diversion on hepatic lipid metabolism has been unusually well studied. Reductions of more than 80% in hepatic cholesterol and/or triglyceride or lipoprotein synthesis have been demonstrated in rats, dogs, swine, and baboons (1,3). Reductions in hepatic lipid synthesis also have been documented in

patients treated by us with portacaval shunt for familial hypercholesterolemia (FH) (8–10), and it has been shown that total body cholesterol is greatly reduced (10). Thus, lipid homeostasis is altered to an extraordinary degree by portacaval shunt, with the reduction in hepatic lipid synthesis being the greatest change.

Bile acid synthesis also is greatly reduced by portacaval shunt (1,8,10). Another synthetic pathway that has been well studied after portal diversion is the hepatic urea (Krebs-Henseleit) cycle, which has been shown by Reichle et al. to be depressed by Eck's fistula in rats (11) and dogs (12). They also demonstrated a reduction in several of the enzymes involved in this metabolic pathway.

Many studies during the 1970s and mid-1980s, summarized elsewhere (1), have shown that portacaval shunt lowers the activity of the hepatic microsomal mixed-function enzyme system. Aside from illustrating the principle of a wide-ranging decline in hepatic metabolic functions after portacaval shunt, these observations are of potential specific importance because the microsomal mixed-function enzyme system, for which multiple cytochrome P450 and P448 species serve as terminal oxidases, metabolizes a variety of drugs and foreign chemicals, as well as endogenous compounds such as steroids and fatty acids. The depression of this broad-ranging enzyme system would relate to many of the metabolic effects of portal diversion.

Clinical Applications of Portal Diversion

Portacaval shunt has been used to palliate hepatic-based inborn errors of carbohydrate, lipid, and protein metabolism. Although these were great advances at the time, such surgical therapy has

Table 6.1. Patients with GSD Treated by Portal Diversion[a]

Patient No.	Age (yr)	GSD Type	Date of Operation	Preoperative Symptoms			Persistent Hypoglycemia Postoperatively	Survival After Shunt
				Hypogly-cemia	Acidosis	Growth Retard-ation		
1	8	III	October 15, 1963	Yes	Yes	Yes	No	Alive 22½ years
2	7	I	June 26, 1968	Yes	Yes	Yes	—	Died 2 days
3	7	I	May 2, 1972	Yes	Yes	Yes	Yes[b]	Alive 14 years
4	11	I	May 17, 1972	Yes	Yes	Yes	No	Died 4¾ years
5	10	VI	August 2, 1972	—	—	Yes	—	Alive 13⅔ years
6	5	III	November 7, 1972	Yes	Yes	Yes	No	Alive 13½ years
7	3	III	November 8, 1972	Yes	Yes	Yes	Yes[b]	Alive 13½ years
8	8	I	August 13, 1973	Yes	Yes	Yes	Yes[c]	Alive 12⅔ years
9	12	I	December 14, 1973	Yes	Yes	Yes	Yes[b]	Alive 12½ years
10	1	I	October 2, 1976	Yes	Yes	Yes	Yes[b]	Alive 9½ years

[a] Patients 1 and 2 had portacaval transposition; all others had portacaval shunt.
[b] Overnight feeding via nasogastric tube starting 2½–4 years after portacaval shunt.
[c] Underwent orthotopic liver transplantation February 12, 1982, and is alive 4 years later (see text).

been rendered obsolete by the even more effective procedure of liver transplantation. Nevertheless, the information obtained has been important in understanding hepatic physiology in humans, and will be briefly described here.

GLYCOGEN STORAGE DISEASE

Portal diversion was first performed for glycogen storage disease more than 20 years ago (13) with a rationale that is naive in retrospect. It was hoped that by short-circuiting splanchnic venous blood around the liver, glucose would be made more readily available to peripheral tissues with relief of the hypoglycemia caused by glycogen storage disease (GSD), and that the liver would be coincidentally deglycogenated. The animal experiments cited in Mechanism of Effects, above, suggest that the consequences of portacaval shunt are far more subtle and wide-ranging than this simple view.

That first patient had type III GSD. She is still alive more than 20 years after portacaval transposition. The bypassed portal venous blood was replaced with blood returning from the inferior vena cava, an operation which was first described in animals by Child et al. (14). The transposition was used in order to avoid the potential hazards of Eck's fistula. It was appreciated then, and amply confirmed since (1,7), that most animals, including subhuman primates, develop wasting and encephalopathy after portal diversion, but it was not appreciated that humans would be an exception to this generalization.

Two more portacaval transpositions were per-

formed, one by Riddell et al. (15). In Riddell's patient, the cavoportal anastomosis clotted (16). The other attempt cost the life of our second patient; the liver was unable to transmit the rerouted vena caval flow, causing hepatic swelling and uncontrollable acidosis (17).

Subsequently, the simpler procedure of portacaval shunt has been used (16). To our knowledge, end-to-side portacaval shunt was used in all later patients. By the spring of 1973 (16), our own series of patients had reached seven, and six more had been formally reported in the literature from other centers. Subsequently, our patients increased in number to 10. Type I disease (glucose-6-phosphatase deficiency) was the indication for treatment in six patients, type III disease (amylo-1, 6-glucosidase deficiency) in three, and type 6 disease (phosphorylase deficiency) in one (Table 6.1).

Metabolic Effects
Most of the children who had pre-existing hypoglycemia did not obtain relief from this problem after portal diversion, or the relief was not complete. Thus, night feedings usually had to be continued. Studies of plasma insulin and glucagon in several of these patients showed marked elevations of the insulin response to a glucose meal, and smaller increases in the glucagon curve. However, the glucose tolerance curves were very little different before and after operation (1).

Liver glycogen concentrations in all those patients who were later biopsied were not changed. In spite of this, in several of our patients and in those reported by others, the liver underwent an

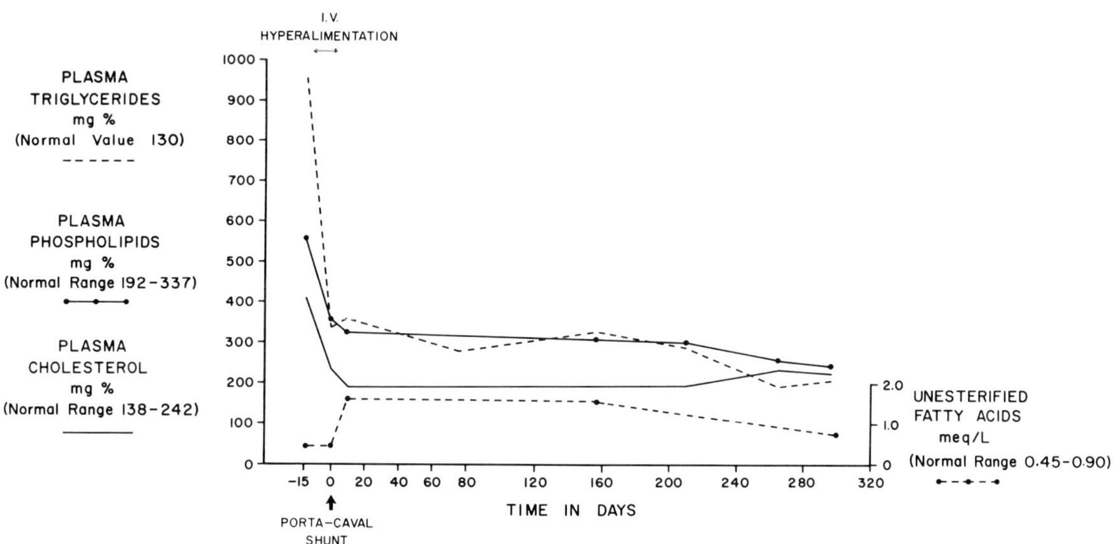

Figure 6.1. Effect of parenteral hyperalimentation and end-to-side portacaval shunt on the plasma lipids of a patient whose diagnosis was type I glycogen storage disease. Note the rapid and relatively complete reversal of all abnormalities. (Reproduced by permission from Starzl TE, Putnam CW, Porter Ka, et al. Portal diversion for the treatment of glycogen storage disease in humans. *Ann Surg* 1973; 178:525–539.)

obvious reduction in size as measured with liver scan planimetry. Even if obvious shrinkage did not occur, postoperative biopsies always showed a diminution in individual hepatocyte size similar to that produced in animals by portacaval shunt (16).

In contrast to the incomplete relief of hypoglycemia, there was profound and permanent relief of all components of the hyperlipidemia that is a characteristic of type I disease (Fig. 6.1). Correction of other metabolic defects was observed, including abnormal bleeding, uric acid elevation, and abnormal calcium metabolism (16). These observations have been confirmed by others (18–20).

Growth
All 10 of our patients had growth retardation before portacaval shunt. Increases in height, which in most cases had virtually ceased, occurred postoperatively at rates in the first year of approximately 0.5 centimeters per month. Quantitative measures of growth were obtained with radiographic techniques (16). An example of the results is shown in Figure 6.2. Comparison of the wrist and hands in this 7-year-old stunted child before and 11½ months after operation showed the phenomenal effects of bone-age doubling. In addition to the size change, mineralization occurred, as did the appearance of new wrist bones. Circulating

somatotrophin in these patients was normal. The growth spurts may have been at least partially attributable to the increased insulin distribution to the periphery mentioned earlier, since insulin has been recognized to be a major growth hormone, comparable in potency to somatotrophin. The simpler possibility that better nutrition was responsible must also be considered.

Encephalopathy and Other Risks
One patient exhibited hepatic encephalopathy 8 years after end-to-side portacaval shunt for type I glycogen storage disease, and also developed multiple filling defects in her enlarged liver. The diseased liver was replaced at transplantation. The metabolic abnormalities of type I GSD that had not been normalized by the portacaval shunt were completely relieved (21).

One other child developed a blood ammonia concentration of 85 micrograms per 100 milliliters (normal less than 60 μg/100 ml for that laboratory), but there were no symptoms of encephalopathy. This patient died almost 5 years after portacaval shunt during an attempt at transcaval radiographic visualization of the portacaval anastomosis. Except for the slightly elevated blood ammonia concentration, her standard liver functions were normal. At autopsy, the liver had macroadenomatosis, very

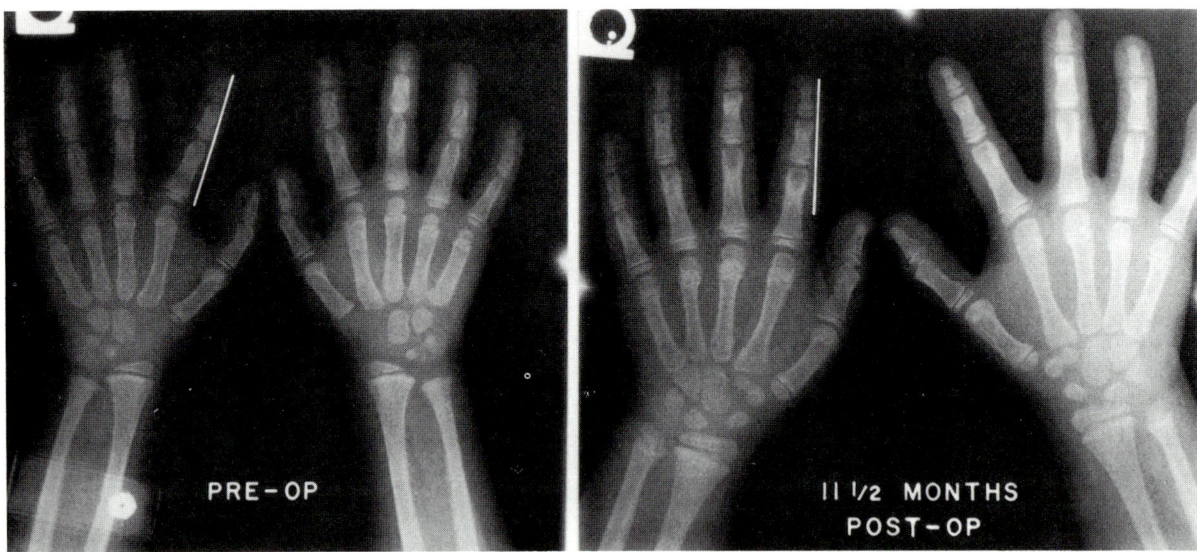

Figure 6.2. The dramatic wrist and hand bone growth and mineralization in a patient with type I GSD during the first $11\frac{1}{2}$ postoperative months. The bracket on the left index finger is 5 cm in length. (Reproduced by permission from Starzl TE, Putnam CW, Porter KA, et al. Portal diversion for the treatment of glycogen storage disease in humans. *Am Surg* 1973; 178:525–539.)

similar to that in the child who underwent transplantation. An autopsy finding that had not been suspected in life was advanced right ventricular hypertrophy and dilatation. The smaller pulmonary arteries and arterioles had medial muscle hypertrophy, medial and intimal fibrosis, scattered fibrinoid necrosis, and numerous plexiform lesions. Such cardiopulmonary complications have been documented in other patients with type I GSD and other liver diseases (22).

The macroadenomatosis seen in both of the foregoing patients is common in patients with type I GSD, and was reported in seven of eight non-shunted patients aged 3 to 28 years (23).

Present Status of Portal Diversion
Portacaval shunt in the treatment of GSD has been supplanted by the continuous night feeding schedule advocated by Greene et al. (24) and Crigler and Folkman (25). Failures of this more conservative approach should be considered for liver transplantation (see Liver Transplantation, Mechanism of Effect, below).

FAMILIAL HYPERCHOLESTEROLEMIA

In March 1973, a 12-year-old girl with homozygous FH was treated with an end-to-side portacaval shunt; her serum cholesterol concentration fell markedly (26) (Fig. 6.3). By March 1982, we had treated 12 patients with FH in this way (27), eight children and four adults.

In patients with this disease, there is an absence or deficiency of cell membrane lipoprotein receptors (28,29) and thus, a switch-off mechanism to control lipid (especially cholesterol) synthesis is not present. All but two patients were homozygous for the FH abnormality as judged by measure of low-density lipoprotein (LDL) receptors on cultured fibroblasts obtained from all patients (28,29). The other two patients had heterozygous disease.

Effect on Serum Lipids
Total serum cholesterol concentrations fell significantly in every patient after portacaval shunt (27). The total cholesterol declines ranged from 20% to 55.4% (average 33.8%) and were maintained throughout the period of study. With the fall in cholesterol concentration, tendinocutaneous xanthomas regressed or disappeared in every patient (Fig. 6.4). An anticholesterolemia response after portal diversion has been confirmed by numerous other authors [summarized in Starzl et al. (27)], at the time tendinocutaneous xanthomas have regressed. Hoeg et al. (30) have reported a postoperative increase in hepatic lipoprotein receptors in

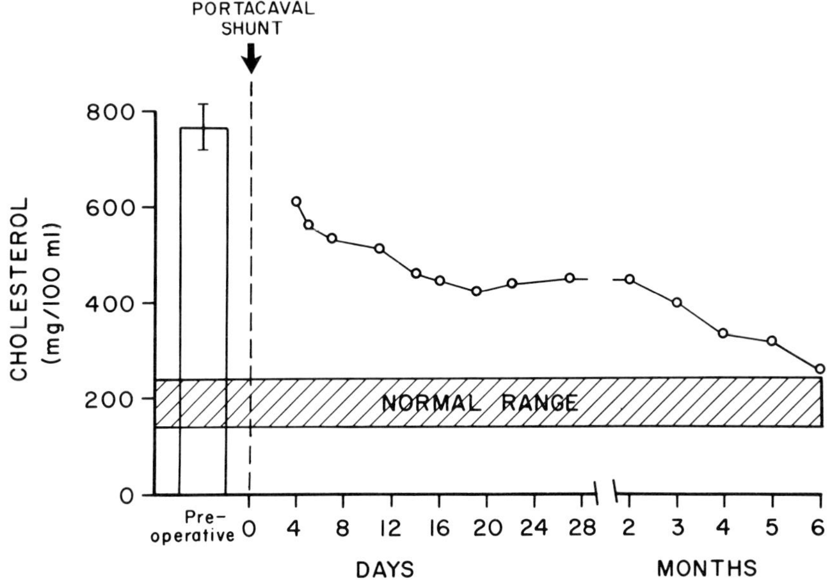

Figure 6.3. Serum cholesterol concentration after portacaval shunt in a patient of our FH series. (Reproduced by permission from Starzl TE, Chase HP, Putnam CW, Porter KA. Portacaval shunt in hyperlipoproteinemia. *Lancet* 1973; 2:940–944.)

one of our patients. Although an increase of receptors could have contributed to an antilipidemic effect of portal diversion, the principal effect probably was caused by reduced cholesterol and lipoprotein synthesis (1,3,8,10–12).

Morbidity
The invariable and long-lasting lipid lowering in our 12 patients was achieved without surgical morbidity. The physical development of those children who were normal before operation has pro-

ceeded, and the growth of those who were stunted before has moved toward normal. Emotional or intellectual deterioration secondary to the portal diversion has not occurred, although one child had an acute episode of encephalopathy, which was managed with diet (27).

Effect on Cardiovascular Disease
Reversal of aortic stenosis was seen in two of our patients, but regression of atheromas in the coronary arteries and aorta was not regularly accom-

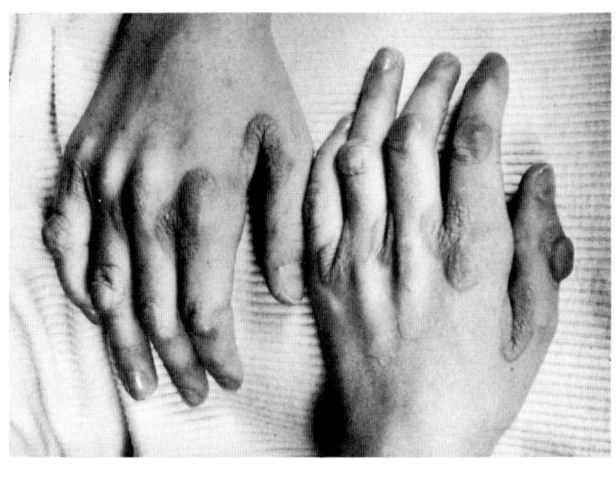

A

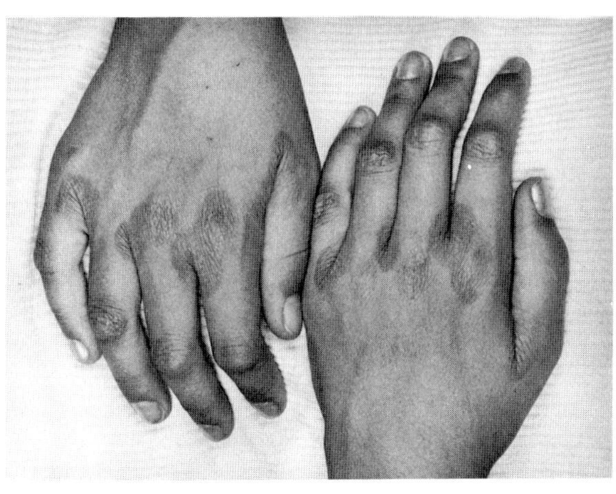

B

Figure 6.4. The hands of patient 1 of the hyperlipidemia series (A) 2 weeks before and (B) 16 months after portacaval shunt.

plished (27). Small and Shipley (31) have examined the factors that could preclude the reversal of atherosclerosis; some of these, including secondary fibrosis, would not be corrected completely by the resorption of intravascular xanthomas.

Present Status of Portal Diversion
The palliation is incomplete, since restoration of normal serum cholesterol values has not been achieved in any patient with homozygous disease. In contrast, the metabolic abnormalities of FH can be completely corrected by the ultimate step of liver transplantation, which will become the preferred method of treatment in the near future (see Clinical Applications of Liver Transplantation, below) in medically refractory cases.

ALPHA$_1$-ANTITRYPSIN DEFICIENCY

Patients with this disorder have a low level plasma alpha$_1$-antitrypsin (an alpha-globulin), a high incidence of pulmonary complications, and an increased incidence of liver disease. The basis for the liver injury may be the hepatic production of an abnormal alpha$_1$-antitrypsin, which cannot be effectively transported out of the liver cells and which consequently becomes sequestered within the hepatocytes near the RER (32). Irritation by the entrapped glycoprotein has been the postulated cause of the hepatic cirrhosis, portal hypertension, and hepatic failure that follow.

We have performed end-to-side portacaval shunt in three children with the cirrhotic liver disease of alpha$_1$-antitrypsin deficiency (33). Follow-up reports are available at $6\frac{1}{2}$, 8, and nearly 10 years. Standard liver function tests have not changed greatly since the portacaval shunt, although the plasma ammonia levels have been elevated in all three patients. Patient 2 has had mental slowness, which may be a symptom of encephalopathy.

The most objective evidence that the natural history of the disease was favorably altered came from the histopathologic studies of operative and postoperative biopsies in patients 2 and 3 (33). In patient 2, a biopsy 9 months after the portal diversion showed that the number of hepatocytes that contained alpha$_1$-antitrypsin globules was diminished to 28.5%, compared with 38.2% at the time of the original operation. The hepatocytes were 22% smaller and the amount of RER in their cytoplasm was greatly reduced.

In patient 3, the percentage of hepatocytes containing alpha$_1$-antitrypsin globules was 44.5% at the time of operation, and 48.2 and 38.7% at 7 and 13 months, respectively, after portacaval shunt. The hepatocytes were 15% and 20% smaller at these postoperative periods. The percentage of hepatocytes containing alpha$_1$-antitrypsin globules was reduced to 20.4% in the biopsy taken at 2 years, 11 months. The hepatocytes remained 20% smaller than in the preoperative biopsy, and the amount of both RER and smooth endoplasmic reticulum in their cytoplasm was reduced. The severity of the macronodular cirrhosis was unaltered.

We believe that the portacaval shunt diminished the synthesis of the abnormal alpha$_1$-antitrypsin, presumably by altering the function of the RER and its ribosomes (see Portal Diversion, Mechanism of Effects, above) without commensurately reducing the transport of this glycoprotein. With a better equilibrium between the production and transport of the alphaglobulin, it is possible that its intracellular accumulation has been slowed or probably even reversed (33).

No further portacaval shunts have been carried out in patients with alpha$_1$-antitrypsin deficiency for more than 6 years. It has been established that liver transplantation provides a metabolic "cure" and that the protein phenotype of the recipient becomes that of the donor for the lifetime of the graft (see Liver Transplantation, Mechanism of Effect, below).

Liver Transplantation

Mechanism of Effect

The use of portal diversion to treat liver-based inborn errors of metabolism requires the creation of an abnormal physiologic state for the liver in order to achieve countervailing metabolic objectives. A more direct and satisfactory approach is to provide a phenotypically normal liver. Studies of haptoglobin (34–36), group-specific component (36,37), and numerous other products of hepatic synthesis (21,32,38–40) have shown that liver homografts permanently retain their original metabolic specificity after transplantation. Consequently, liver transplantation has been recognized for a number of years (37,41) as a potentially decisive way to treat those inborn errors of metab-

Table 6.2. Inborn Errors of Metabolism Corrected by Liver Transplantation—Cases from Personal Series

Disease	Cases	Enzyme Defect	Metabolic Cure	Longest Survival (yr)
Alpha$_1$-antitrypsin deficiency	38	Unknown	Yes	10
Wilson's disease	14	Unknown	Yes	15½
Tyrosinemia	6	Fumarylacetoacetate hydrolase	Yes	4½
Type IV GSD	4	Amylo-1,4 transglucosidase (branching enzyme)	Yes	1½
Hemophilia-A	3	Unknown	Yes	1
Crigler-Najjar syndrome	2	Glucuronyl-transferase	Yes	4[a]
Familial hypercholesterolemia	2	None: deficient lipoprotein receptors	Yes	2
Type I GSD	1	Glucose-6-phosphatase	Yes	4
Niemann-Pick disease	1	Sphingomyelinase	Possibly	1½[b]
Sea-blue histiocyte syndrome	1	Unknown	No	4
Cystic fibrosis	1	Unknown	Not studied	1½
Hemochromatosis	1	Unknown	Yes	2
Type I oxalosis	1	Thiamin-pyrophosphate–dependent carboligase	Probably	Unknown[c]

[a] Longest survivor reported by Professor H. Wolff, Berlin, East Germany.
[b] Patient treated by Dr. Pierre Daloze, Notre Dame Hospital, Montreal; died of neurologic complications.
[c] Patient of Professor Roy Calne, Cambridge, England.

olism that result partly or completely from defects in hepatic function.

In many of the diseases for which liver transplantation has been carried out, a specific enzyme is missing as exemplified by the GSDs. With other disorders (e.g., Wilson's disease), the pathogenesis is not well understood even today (Table 6.2). In some of these conditions, the exact role of liver was not known until a study of patients after transplantation proved that the defect was hepatic. In two of these diseases, familial hypercholesterolemia and hemophilia, the transplantation itself became the most powerful of research tools while at the same time benefiting the patient.

Clinical Applications of Liver Transplantation

The inborn errors of metabolism for which liver transplantation has been carried out are shown in Table 6.2. In the majority of such patients, the inborn error has itself been responsible for damage to the liver, in which case the conventional indication of liver failure prompted the liver replacement. However, a small but particularly interesting minority of transplantations have been carried out solely for the purpose of correcting the inborn error itself, and in these cases, a morphologically normal liver has been removed and replaced with a homograft. Examples include familial hypercholesterolemia, congenital oxalosis, and Crigler-Najjar syndrome. In the following descriptions, emphasis is on those inborn errors that were once treated with portal diversion, but for which the most desirable treatment today probably is liver replacement.

GLYCOGEN STORAGE DISEASE

An 8-year-old girl with type I GSD underwent an end-to-side portacaval shunt in 1973. Although she had reasonable palliation from her multiple symptoms, she eventually developed hepatic encephalopathy, and in addition, her liver developed masses that were suspected of being hepatomas. In January 1982, her diseased liver was removed, the portacaval shunt was taken down, and a phenotypically normal liver was implanted. Her recovery was relatively uncomplicated, and all of the metabolic stigmata of type I GSD (mentioned in Glycogen Storage Disease, Metabolic Effects, above) were corrected (21). Prior to operation, she required frequent night feedings, and if she fasted for more than a few hours, her blood sugars dropped to below 10 mg%. Afterward, she could fast indefinitely. Some months postoperatively, her portal vein thrombosed, but she developed extensive collaterals to the hepatic graft and she has had no evidence of encephalopathy or liver failure during her 4 postoperative years.

Four patients with type IV GSD (see Table 6.2) have had their cirrhotic livers removed and replaced. Two of these children died perioperatively.

The other two have normal function 3 and 18 months postoperatively. A 1-year biopsy of the child with the longest survival has shown no evidence of recurrent disease.

FAMILIAL HYPERCHOLESTEROLEMIA

A 6-year-old girl with severe hypercholesterolemia and atherosclerosis had two defective genes at the LDL receptor locus, as determined by biochemical studies of cultured fibroblasts. One gene, inherited from the mother, produced no LDL receptors; the other gene, inherited from the father, produced a receptor precursor that was not transported to the cell surface and was unable to bind LDL. The patient degraded intravenously administered ^{125}I-LDL at an extremely low rate, indicating that her high plasma LDL-cholesterol level was caused by defective receptor-mediated removal of LDL from plasma. After transplantation of a liver and a heart from a normal donor, the patient's plasma LDL-cholesterol level declined by 81%, from 988 to 184 mg%. The fractional catabolic rate for intravenously administered ^{125}I-LDL, a measure of functional LDL receptors in vivo, increased by 2.5-fold. Thus, the transplanted liver, with its normal complement of LDL receptors, was able to remove LDL cholesterol from plasma at a nearly normal rate. We concluded from these observations that a genetically determined deficiency of LDL receptors could be largely reversed by liver transplantation. These data have underscored the importance of hepatic LDL receptors in controlling the plasma level of LDL cholesterol in human beings (42).

The foregoing hypothesis that the disease was caused by deficient LDL receptors has not excluded the further possibility that the hepatocytes of the metabolically abnormal liver overproduce cholesterol. A second patient, an 11-year-old boy, underwent liver transplantation on December 6, 1985. His serum cholesterol also fell to essentially normal levels. Presently, he is on a medical ward at the National Institutes of Health undergoing extensive postoperative metabolic studies. Although his heart had been gravely damaged by the high cholesterol of his disease, heart transplantation was not required. A residual high-grade stenosis of one of the coronary arteries has been treated by an internal mammary artery–coronary artery bypass.

It has become clear that liver transplantation "cures" familial hypercholesterolemia. Furthermore, the performance of the liver replacement has permitted the most decisive studies on the pathogenesis of the disease that have ever been possible.

ALPHA$_1$-ANTITRYPSIN DEFICIENCY

Serum alpha$_1$-antitrypsin levels, which normally are 200 to 300 mg%, usually are about one-tenth of this value in patients who develop alpha$_1$-antitrypsin-associated liver disease. Patients at risk can be identified by Pi (protease inhibitor) phenotypes, the ZZ marker usually being associated with the liver disease. More than a decade ago, it was demonstrated that the serum alpha$_1$-antitrypsin levels were brought to normal, and that the new Pi type of liver recipient permanently became that of the donor (32,41). Alpha$_1$-antitrypsin deficiency has been the inborn error of metabolism most commonly treated by liver transplantation (see Table 6.2). Realization of the effectiveness of liver replacement has prompted us to discontinue efforts at portal diversion, particularly since portacaval shunts can jeopardize candidacy for the definitive procedure of transplantation.

OTHER INBORN ERRORS

Among the first 500 liver transplantations carried out by us under cyclosporine-steroid therapy, there were almost a dozen inborn errors (see Table 6.2). One of the most significant observations (in 1985) has been that classical hemophilia is completely corrected by liver replacement (43). The explanation of hemophilia has been unknown, but the predominance of opinion has been that the liver was not central to the pathogenesis. With the simple expedient of liver transplantation, this doctrine was overthrown, and subsequent gene probe studies have verified the hepatocyte as the location of factor VIII production.

Summary

Complete portal diversion can palliate at least three inborn errors of metabolism, GSD, FH, and alpha$_1$-antitrypsin deficiency. However, these three liver-based inborn errors of metabolism, as well as numerous other inborn errors, can be metabolically cured by the transplantation of phenotypically normal livers.

References

1. Starzl TE, Porter KA, Francavilla A. The Eck fistula in animals and humans. *Curr Probl Surg* 1983; 20(11):688–752.
2. Starzl TE, Francavilla A, Halgrimson CG, Francavilla FR, et al. The origin, hormonal nature, and action of hepatotrophic substances in portal venous blood. *Surg Gynecol Obstet* 1973; 137:179–199.
3. Starzl TE, Lee I-Y, Porter KA, Putnam CW. The influence of portal blood upon lipid metabolism in normal and diabetic dogs and baboons. *Surg Gynecol Obstet* 1975; 140: 381–396.
4. Starzl TE, Porter KA, Kashiwagi N, Lee IY, et al. The effect of diabetes mellitus on portal blood hepatotrophic factors in dogs. *Surg Gynecol Obstet* 1975; 140:549–562.
5. Starzl TE, Porter KA, Kashiwagi N, Putnam CW. Portal hepatotrophic factors, diabetes mellitus and acute liver atrophy, hypertrophy and regeneration. *Surg Gynecol Obstet* 1975; 141:843–858.
6. Starzl TE, Porter KA, Watanabe K, Putnam CW. The effects of insulin, glucagon and insulin/glucagon infusions upon liver morphology and cell division after complete portacaval shunt in dogs. *Lancet* 1976; 1:821–825.
7. Putnam CW, Porter KA, Starzl TE. Hepatic encephalopathy and light and electron micrographic changes of the baboon liver after portal diversion. *Ann Surg* 1976; 184: 155–161.
8. Bilheimer DW, Goldstein JL, Grundy SM, Brown MS. Reduction in cholesterol and low density lipoprotein synthesis after portacaval shunt surgery in a patient with homozygous familial hypercholesterolemia. *J Clin Invest* 1975; 56:1420–1430.
9. Ginsberg H, Davidson N, Le N-A, Gibson J, et al. Marked overproduction of low density lipoprotein apoprotein-B in a subject with heterozygous familial hypercholesterolemia: Effect of portacaval shunting. *Biochim Biophys Acta* 1983; 712:250–259.
10. McNamara DJ, Ahrens EH Jr, Kolb R, Parker TS, et al. Cholesterol homeostasis in two familial hypercholesterolemic patients with a portacaval anastomosis. *Circulation* 1982; 66(Suppl 11):159.
11. Reichle FA, Bernstein MR, Hower RD, et al. Urea cycle enzyme activity in human hepatic cirrhosis and after experimental portacaval shunt. *Surg Forum* 1973, 24.246–248.
12. Reichle FA, Rao NS, Reichle RM, Chang KHY. The mechanism of postshunt liver failure. *Surgery* 1977; 82:738–749.
13. Starzl TE, Marchioro TL, Sexton AW, Illingworth B, et al. The effect of portacaval transposition upon carbohydrate metabolism: Experimental and clinical observations. *Surgery* 1965; 57:687–697.
14. Child CG, Barr D, Holswade GR, Harrison CS. Liver regeneration following portacaval transposition in dogs. *Ann Surg* 1953; 138:600–608.
15. Riddell AG, Davies RP, Clark AD. Portacaval transposition in the treatment of glycogen storage disease. *Lancet* 1966; 2:1146–1148.
16. Starzl TE, Putnam CW, Porter KA, Halgrimson CG, et al. Portal diversion for the treatment of glycogen storage disease in humans. *Ann Surg* 1973; 178:525–539.
17. Starzl TE, Brown BI, Blanchard H, Brettschneider L. Portal diversion in glycogen storage disease. *Surgery* 1969; 65: 504–506.
18. Corbeel L, Hue L, Lederer B, DeBarsy T, et al. Clinical and biochemical findings before and after portacaval shunt in a girl with type Ib glycogen storage disease. *Pediatr Res* 1981; 15:58–61.
19. Folkman J, Philippart A, Tze W-J, Crigler J Jr. Portacaval shunt for glycogen storage disease: Value of prolonged intravenous hyperalimentation before surgery. *Surgery* 1972; 72:306–314.
20. Liebschutz D, Soper RT. Portacaval shunt in siblings for type I glycogenosis. *J Pediatr Surg* 1976; 11:557–561.
21. Malatack JJ, Finegold DN, Iwatsuki S, Shaw BW, et al. Liver transplantation for Type I glycogen storage disease. *Lancet* 1983; 1:1073–1076.
22. Levine OR, Harris RC, Blanc WA, Wellins RB. Progressive pulmonary hypertension in children with portal hypertension. *J Pediatr* 1973; 83:964–972.
23. Howell RR, Stevenson RE, Ben-Menachem Y, Phyliky RL, et al. Hepatic adenomata with type I glycogen storage disease. *JAMA* 1976; 236:1481–1484.
24. Greene HL, Slonim AE, O'Neill JA, Burr IM. Continuous nocturnal intragastric feedings for management of type I glycogen storage disease. *N Engl J Med* 1976; 294:1125–1129.
25. Crigler JF Jr, Folkman J. Glycogen storage disease. New approaches to therapy. In: Porter R, Whelen J, eds. *Hepatotrophic Factors*. Ciba Foundation Symposium No. 55. Amsterdam: Elsevier/Excerpta Medica, 1978, pp. 331–356.
26. Starzl TE, Chase HP, Putnam CW, Porter KA. Portacaval shunt in hyperlipoproteinemia. *Lancet* 1973; 2:940–944.
27. Starzl TE, Chase HP, Ahrens EH Jr, McNamara DJ, et al. Portacaval shunt in patients with familial hypercholesterolemia. *Ann Surg* 1983, 198:273–283.
28. Goldstein J, Brown MS. Binding and degradation of low density lipoproteins in cultured human fibroblasts: Comparison of cells from a normal subject and from a patient with homozygous familial hypercholesterolemia. *J Biol Chem* 1974; 249:5153–5162.
29. Goldstein JL, Dana SE, Brunschede GY, Brown MS. Genetic heterogeneity in familial hypercholesterolemia: Evidence for two different mutations affecting functions of low density lipoprotein receptor. *Proc Natl Acad Sci USA* 1975; 72:1092–1096.
30. Hoeg JM, Demosky SJ Jr, Schaefer EJ, Starzl TE, Brewer HB Jr. Characterization of hepatic low density lipoprotein binding and cholesterol metabolism in normal and homozygous familial hypercholesterolemic subjects. *J Clin Invest* 1984; 73:429–436.
31. Small DM, Shipley GG. Physical chemical basis of lipid deposition in atherosclerosis: The physical state of the lipids helps to explain lipid deposition and lesion reversal in atherosclerosis. *Science* 1974; 185:222–229.
32. Hood JM, Koep LJ, Peters RL, Schroter GPJ, et al. Liver transplantation for advanced liver disease with alpha$_1$-antitrypsin deficiency. *N Engl J Med* 1980; 302:272–275.
33. Starzl TE, Porter KA, Francavilla A, Iwatsuki S. Reversal of hepatic alpha$_1$-antitrypsin deposition after portacaval shunt. *Lancet* 1983; 2:724–726.
34. Starzl TE, Marchioro TL, Rowlands DT Jr, Kirkpatrick CH, et al. Immunosuppression after experimental and clinical homotransplantation of the liver. *Ann Surg* 1964; 160:411–439.
35. Merrill DA, Kirkpatrick CH, Wilson WEC, Riley CM. Change in serum haptoglobin type following human liver transplantation. *Proc Soc Exp Biol Med* 1964; 116:748–751.
36. Kashiwagi N, Groth CG, Starzl TE. Changes in serum haptoglobin and group specific component after orthotopic liver homotransplantation in humans. *Proc Soc Exp Biol Med* 1968; 128:247–250.
37. Kashiwagi N. Special immunochemical studies. In: Starzl TE, ed. *Experience in Hepatic Transplantation*. Philadelphia: WB Saunders, 1969, pp. 394–407.

38. Alper CA, Johnson AM, Birtch AG, Moore FD. Human C'3: Evidence for the liver as the primary site of synthesis. *Science* 1969; 163:286–288.
39. Alper CA, Raum D, Awdeh Z, Petersen BH, Taylor PD, Starzl TE. Studies of hepatic synthesis *in vivo* of plasma proteins, including orosomucoid, transferrin, alpha$_1$-antitrypsin, C8, and Factor B. *Clin Immunol Immunopathol* 1980; 16:84–89.
40. Raum D, Marcus D, Alper CA, Levey R, Taylor PD, Starzl TE. Synthesis of human plasminogen by the liver. *Science* 1980; 208:1036–1037.
41. Starzl TE, Iwatsuki S, Van Thiel DH, Gartner JL, et al. Evolution of liver transplantation. *Hepatology* 1982; 2:614–636.
42. Bilheimer DW, Goldstein JL, Grundy SC, Starzl TE, Brown MS. Liver transplantation provides low density lipoprotein receptors and lowers plasma cholesterol in a child with homozygous familial hypercholesterolemia. *N Engl J Med* 1984; 311:1658–1664.
43. Lewis JH, Bontempo FA, Spero JA, Ragni WV, Starzl TE. Liver transplantation in a hemophiliac. (Letter to the Editor) *N Engl J Med* 1985; 312:1189.

Editorial Comment

The chapters that are concerned with inborn errors of metabolism relating directly or indirectly to the liver, are a well-orchestrated combined effort of two leaders in that field, Marshall Kaplan in medicine and Thomas Starzl in surgery.

Dr. Kaplan has presented a wide-ranging dissertation on a number of different familial disorders, and has then deferred in terms of surgical treatment to the section specifically related to this therapeutic approach.

Dr. Starzl has covered the main inborn errors of metabolism (specifically relating to surgical procedures). These include glycogen storage disease, familial hypercholesterolemia, alpha$_1$-antitrypsin deficiency, isolated examples of rare entities such as congenital oxalosis, and the Crigler-Najjar syndrome. The earlier imaginative approaches to some of these metabolic defects by portal diversion have contributed over the years, not only to a therapeutic program for these children, but also toward a better understanding of the abnormal metabolic defects.

Starzl's pioneer work in liver transplantation has made this somewhat formidable procedure a more acceptable and effective type of therapy. Orthotopic liver transplantation carried out for a number of inborn errors in metabolism, as Dr. Starzl points out, has replaced portal diversion as the surgical therapy in this area. In many of these instances, the metabolic defect results in the liver damage, which, in turn, proved to be the surgical indication for transplantation, but in a number of other instances the defect itself was the rationale for treatment by liver replacement. It is in this group in particular that liver transplantation has not only proved to be therapeutically effective, but also has contributed enormously to an increasing understanding of some of the puzzling enzymatic and other defects that are reflected in these inborn errors of metabolism. Observations are still emerging and may have widespread applications, for example, the suggested evidence that the hepatocyte is the site of the defect that results in classical hemophilia.

This review provides a succinct but hardly cursory review of a fascinating segment of human disease.

Chapter 7
Hepatitis and the Blood Bank

WALTER H. DZIK

Surgery of the liver may frequently involve extensive blood support. In recent years the issues surrounding safe blood transfusion have become more complex. This chapter reviews the use of blood products in patients with liver disease, the management of patients undergoing massive transfusion, and the risk of transmission of disease by blood transfusion to patients or by needlestick injury to health care workers.

National Blood Supply

In the United States three organizations—the American Association of Blood Banks, the American Red Cross Blood Services, and the Council of Community Blood Centers—are responsible for collection of the majority of blood donated for transfusion. In these organizations only volunteer blood donors are used as a source of whole blood or blood components: packed red cells, fresh frozen plasma (FFP), platelet concentrates, and cryoprecipitate. In contrast, certain blood derivatives, for example, factor VIII concentrate, are produced in part by commercial for-profit suppliers who continue to use paid plasma donors.

Although the virtual elimination of paid blood donors that occurred in the 1970s improved the safety of the blood supply, transfusions still transmit disease. The importance of transfusion-transmitted diseases has resulted in more complex screening of blood donors. All donors are questioned regarding prior exposure to or symptoms of hepatitis and acquired immune deficiency syndrome (AIDS). All donors must be afebrile. Donors are tested for hepatitis B surface antigen (HB_sAg), exposure to syphilis, and for antibody to the human immunodeficiency virus (HIV)/human T-cell lymphotropic virus-III (HTLV-III) virus. Some centers may do additional testing such as antibody to

cytomegalovirus (CMV). Testing donors for exposure to human T-cell lymphotropic virus-I (HTLV-I) may become a requirement in the near future. Because the most important transfusion-transmitted disease remains non-A, non-B hepatitis, the three national blood organizations recommended that their members establish before June 1987 the testing of all donors for the presence of an elevated serum alanine aminotransferase (ALT) level or a positive antibody to hepatitis B core antigen (anti-HB_c). These two tests were implemented as surrogate markers for the carrier state of non-A, non-B hepatitis. Earlier studies had suggested that donors with abnormalities of either the ALT or anti-HBc had a higher likelihood of transmitting non-A, non-B hepatitis through transfusion (1,2). Although each test is nonspecific, estimates suggest that 30% to 40% of transfusion-transmitted non-A, non-B cases may be averted by ALT and anti-HB_c testing of all donors. However, since these two tests have limited sensitivity, transfusion-transmitted non-A, non-B hepatitis continues to occur. Therefore, all multiply transfused patients should be considered as potentially exposed to non-A, non-B hepatitis. (See Transfusion-Transmitted Diseases: Risk to the Patient and Surgeon, below.) Health care workers treating the patient who has received multiple transfusions should not only wear gloves, but also should take precautions to avoid inadvertent puncture wounds from needlestick accidents. Detailed guidelines for health care workers are periodically issued from the Centers for Disease Control.

Increasing recognition of the importance of limiting donor exposures in patients facing uncomplicated elective surgery has renewed interest in autologous predeposit of blood. Most patients are able to donate one or more units of their own blood prior to elective surgery. Though autologous predeposit is not suitable for seriously ill individuals with advanced liver disease who require complicated surgery, the procedure should be seriously considered for all elective surgery patients who are capable of donating and who are not expected to require support with multiple blood products. Recombinant erythropoietin, when available, will increase the ability of patients to supply their own blood needs and should reduce exposure to homologous blood products. A second means of reducing exposure of the patient to transfusion-transmitted diseases is through the use of intraoperative blood salvage (see Massive Transfusion in Hepatic Surgery, below).

Blood Support for the Patient with Liver Disease

Patients with serious liver disease are likely to require support with a broad range of blood components. Although whole blood was for many years the most commonly transfused product, there is an increasing tendency to manage patients with specific components. The demand for blood and the shortage of blood donors provide additional pressure to produce components so that each donation may serve several recipients. Whole blood, although now in short supply, remains a reasonable product to manage the acutely bleeding patient. The more readily available packed red cells plus saline, albumin, or FFP is more frequently used to manage acute bleeding. Prior to the development of platelet concentrates, fresh blood served as a source of platelets. Fresh blood is no longer a reasonable request and carries a higher risk of transfusion-transmitted CMV infection compared with packed cells.

Packed Red Blood Cells

Packed red blood cells are the most common blood component transfused. Using current anticoagulant-preservative solutions, packed cells may be stored for at least 1 month following donation. The observation that the concentration of ammonia and amino acids in the plasma of stored blood is elevated following several weeks of storage raised concern over the effect of red cell transfusions on recipients prone to encephalopathy in the setting of hepatic failure (3). However, there is no evidence that patients with advanced liver disease are

more likely to develop hepatic encephalopathy when transfused with packed cells stored for 4 weeks compared with packed cells stored for shorter periods of time or compared with washed red cells. When ordering blood, hepatic surgeons should take advantage of "type and screen" policies, which have been introduced in transfusion services nationwide (4). For hospitalized patients at risk for sudden unexpected bleeding, a routine "type and screen" order allows the transfusion service to determine the ABO and Rh type of the patient, "screen" the patient's serum in advance for the presence of non-ABO red cell antibodies, and keep residual serum in the laboratory. Should transfusion be necessary, an immediate-spin (5-minute) cross-match to verify ABO compatibility is generally all that is required to release blood for transfusion to those patients whose antibody "screen" showed no antibodies outside the ABO system. Although the majority of transfused patients with liver disease do not make antibodies to blood group antigens, liver disease patients as a group produce such antibodies more frequently than other patient groups that require frequent transfusions. Such antibodies make it more difficult to identify blood suitable for transfusion. As there is no way to predict which patients make blood group antibodies and no way to prepare red cells so that they are not immunogenic, open communication between the hepatic surgeon and the blood bank is needed to manage patients with significant blood group antibodies.

Fresh Frozen Plasma

Patients with liver failure frequently require FFP to correct the coagulation deficiencies of liver disease. The exact indications for FFP are not established and a National Institutes of Health (NIH) Consensus Development Conference held in 1984 considered the product overused (5). FFP is plasma separated from whole blood within 6 hours of collection and stored frozen. It has essentially a normal concentration of blood electrolytes and plasma proteins. Each unit has a risk of transfusion-transmitted disease equivalent to that of packed cells. Once thawed it may not be refrozen and so should be ordered wisely. Patients with severe liver disease are frequently deficient in all coagulation factors except factor VIII, which is produced at extrahepatic sites. Therefore, FFP is commonly used to correct coagulation abnormalities in liver disease. However, before FFP is given, three simple questions should be answered.

1. *Is the patient deficient in vitamin K?* Patients may be malnourished, may be receiving antibiotics and have abnormal bowel function with bacterial overgrowth, or may have impaired enterohepatic bile circulation with decreased ability to absorb fat-soluble vitamins. Any of these factors can rapidly deplete vitamin K stores, thereby interfering with the terminal activation of clotting factors II, VII, IX, and X. Since factor VII has the shortest circulating half-life (approximately 7 hours), levels of factor VII decline most quickly when vitamin K deficiency develops. This results in a prolongation of the prothrombin time (PT), as this coagulation test is most sensitive to factor VII deficiency. FFP, by providing exogenous factor VII, will correct the PT only temporarily since the half-life of the transfused factor VII is also short. Vitamin K supplementation should be given parenterally since its gastrointestinal absorption is slow and unpredictable in seriously ill patients. The improvement in coagulation in response to parenteral vitamin K begins within 8 to 12 hours after its administration. Patients with significant liver disease usually do not completely correct their PT with vitamin K due to poor synthesis of coagulation factors.

2. *Is the patient bleeding primarily due to a lesion or a coagulopathy?* Most significant gastrointestinal bleeds in patients with liver disease are not due to the coagulopathy of liver disease but rather result from an anatomic lesion such as varices, gastritis, or ulcers. There is little or no evidence to suggest that patients with mild to moderate prolongation of the PT (14–16 seconds, with a normal time equal to 11–13 seconds) and a bleeding gastrointestinal lesion will profit from supplemental infusions of FFP.

3. *Should a measured coagulopathy in the nonbleeding patient be treated?* Mild to moderate deficiencies of factor VII will prolong the PT in vitro before the deficiency reaches a level of in vivo hemostatic significance. Experience with patients receiving vitamin K antagonists has shown that individuals frequently tolerate moderate to marked deficiencies of multiple clotting factors without spontaneous hemorrhage. Liver failure patients have a more serious and complicated derangement of coagulation than that seen with individuals on coumadin. Nevertheless experience with patients in fulminant hepatic failure awaiting transplantation has shown that nonbleeding patients do not require the large volumes of supplemental FFP that would have to be given in order to normalize laboratory coagulation values. Similarly, there is no evidence that prophylactic infusions of FFP given to nonbleeding patients prior to surgery are of benefit. In the nonbleeding patient a PT less than or equal to 1.5 times the upper limit of normal (20 seconds) may be a reasonable goal.

Platelet Concentrates

Platelet concentrates are prepared from individual units of donated blood. Six to eight units of platelets from the same number of different donors are pooled prior to transfusion. Pooled platelet concentrates, therefore, carry an increased risk of transfusion-transmitted diseases. Platelets may also be prepared from a single donor using automated apheresis machines that collect the equivalent of 6 to 8 U of platelets from one individual. The transfusion of 6 to 8 U of platelets should raise the average adult recipient's platelet count by approximately 70,000 platelets per microliter. A lower response occurs if the recipient has splenomegaly, sepsis, systemic viral infection, disseminated intravascular coagulation (DIC) or antibodies to human leukocyte antigens (HLAs), platelet antigens, or drug antigens. Multiply transfused patients with serious liver disease may have, therefore, several conditions that produce refractoriness to platelet support. A platelet count taken 1 hour post-transfusion is a simple and efficient way to screen for complications that interfere with platelet survival. A poor increment in the 1-hour count post-transfusion should initiate a diagnostic evaluation of the probable cause of platelet refractoriness and reassessment of the goal of platelet support. The template bleeding time is the single best test to evaluate platelet function. However, care should be taken in patients with liver disease when ordering this test. Skin edema and malnutrition with weight loss each may produce falsely elevated bleeding times.

Cryoprecipitate

Cryoprecipitate is cold-insoluble globulin that precipitates when previously frozen plasma is thawed in the cold. Cryoprecipitate is rich in factor VIII coagulant protein, von Willebrand's factor, fibrinogen, and factor XIII, as well as fibronectin. Since cryoprecipitate does not contain all the other coagulation factors, it cannot be considered a concentrated version of FFP and is not a suitable substitute for FFP in bleeding patients with severe liver disease and multiple coagulation deficiencies. In fact, cryoprecipitate is generally not indicated in liver failure patients who characteristically have well-preserved factor VIII levels and who usually have fibrinogen levels above 80 milligrams per deciliter. There is no solid current evidence to support its use in patients with liver disease as a source of exogenous fibronectin.

Cryoprecipitate may, however, improve platelet function, particularly in patients with uremia (6). Patients with hepatorenal syndrome or uremia from other causes may develop prolonged bleeding times and dysfunction of platelet-endothelial interaction. Von Willebrand's factor supplied by cryoprecipitate may improve platelet-endothelial adhesion and platelet plugging in uremia. A similar effect results from endogenous release of von Willebrand's factor by des-argenine d-amino vasopressin (DDAVP), an analogue of vasopressin. At least one study has suggested that DDAVP shortens the bleeding time in patients with cirrhosis. The beneficial effect of DDAVP likely results from its action on the endothelial cells of blood vessels. However, desperately ill patients with uremia and platelet dysfunction who are receiving pitressin or intravenous pressors probably derive little additional benefit from DDAVP.

Albumin

Hypoalbuminemia is nearly universal in patients with significant chronic liver failure. Despite the large numbers of such patients, the indications for the use of albumin are not established. Albumin is derived from plasma pooled from many donors. The albumin is extracted by a modification of the original Cohn cold-ethanol fractionation process developed during World War II. The extracted albumin is then heated to 60°C for 10 hours, which serves to inactivate virus contamination. Albumin does not transmit hepatitis, CMV, or HIV infection. It is, therefore, a safe source of colloid volume expansion. Albumin is packaged in two concentrations. Five percent albumin (5 grams per 100 milliliters) comes in 250-ml bottles (12.5 total g) and represents a physiologic concentration of protein in electrolytes. Twenty-five percent albumin is packaged in 50-ml vials (also 12.5 total g) and has an unphysiologic concentration of protein. Concentrated albumin is commonly referred to as "salt-poor"; however, the concentrated form has only 30 fewer milliequivalents of sodium per bottle than physiologic (5%) albumin. Physiologic albumin is indicated as a volume expander in patients with acute hypovolemia. It is also indicated for volume resuscitation in hypotensive patients following large-volume paracentesis (7).

The use of repeated albumin infusions in patient with chronic liver disease who have cirrhosis ascites and edema is less well established. Radiolabeled albumin studies have shown that transfused albumin quickly accumulates in the ascites and other extravascular sites (8). To raise the serum protein level in chronic liver disease, enteral or parenteral hyperalimentation is generally of greater benefit to the patient than repeated albumin infusions.

The indications for 25% albumin are even less well established. It is less suitable for immediate volume resuscitation than 5% albumin. Although of unproven benefit, concentrated albumin is used frequently to supplement parenteral hyperalimentation in catabolic patients with acute physiologic stress and serum albumin levels below 2 g/dl. Concentrated albumin infusions followed by diuretics have also been used in an attempt to stimulate diuresis in liver failure patients with total body salt and water overload but decreased effective intravascular volume. Such treatment is felt by some hepatic surgeons to risk precipitating variceal hemorrhage or acute pulmonary edema. Although a short-term increase in urine output frequently occurs, there is no conclusive evidence that a greater net volume reduction occurs in a shorter time than is achieved by a more traditional fluid management. One group studied an albumin-diuretic protocol in stable cirrhotics but was unable to show any benefit over conventional treatment (9). Albumin for diuresis, although of unproven benefit, is probably reasonable in the acutely ill patient in the intensive care unit (ICU) setting who is unresponsive to judicial fluid management and diuretics.

Massive Transfusion in Hepatic Surgery

Strictly defined, massive transfusion is the transfusion of greater than one blood volume in a 24-hour period. This corresponds to approximately 10 U in the average-sized adult. Patients with bleeding complications of severe liver disease and patients undergoing hepatic surgery or hepatic transplantation may frequently require even much greater volumes of blood support. Such patients require a skilled and coordinated approach to the management of the coagulopathy and metabolic complications that frequently arise in massive transfusion.

Logistics and Resources

Hepatic surgery and transplantation programs require sophisticated support by anaesthesia, ICU services, the laboratory, and transfusion services. The best care occurs when hepatic surgeons and transfusion service directors establish open and frequent communication regarding difficult patients, problems with blood supply, and management options. In addition to frequent informal meetings we have found preoperative consultation to the transfusion service a valuable way to insure smooth delivery of care to patients likely to require ultramassive transfusion.

The use of intraoperative blood salvage is a highly advantageous mechanism for increasing the blood resources available to the surgeon. A variety of devices are available that collect blood shed during surgery, process it, and return it to the patient intraoperatively. Using these devices, blood is drawn into a suction wand held by the surgeon and there mixed with some form of anticoagulant. Although heparin is used at many centers, we prefer to use exclusively citrate to avoid any concern over systemic anticoagulation. Because 250 ml of salvaged packed cells [hematocrit (Hct) = 55%] is routinely washed with 750 ml of saline, the concentration of plasma debris, vasoactive substances, activated clotting factors, fibrin(ogen) degradation products (FDPs), and hemolytic by-products are reduced to approximately 1/800 of their original concentration. The direct reinfusion of unwashed shed blood is less desirable since this results in reinfusion of activated clotting factors, activated fibrinolysins, and FDPs, all of which can promote continued coagulopathy. Moreover, direct reinfusion of large quantities of free hemoglobin can result in impaired renal function, particularly in patients with a reduced glomerular filtration rate. Following the wash step, the salvaged red blood cells can be pumped from the machine to a labeled sterile blood bag or returned directly to the recipient via a rapid transfusion device. Automated autotransfusion with washing is extremely safe for the patient and has numerous advantages over banked blood: it is faster, it introduces no additional risks of ABO clerical mishaps, and it limits donor exposures. The technique is also especially valuable in patients with alloantibodies who need antigen-negative blood that is in limited supply. Most importantly, intraoperative salvage decreases the drain on the blood supply that is imposed by massive transfusion cases. In our hospital it has been highly advantageous during hepatic resections and liver transplant surgery where an average of 47% of the patients' red cell needs are provided by salvaged blood (10). The relative proportions of the total red cell needs generated by intraoperative salvage increases with increasing total blood need.

Blood salvaged by intraoperative autotransfusion is returned to the patient as saline-suspended packed cells. It does not contain useful quantities of platelets or coagulation factors so that supplemental transfusions with these components need to continue during massive transfusion cases using intraoperative blood salvage. Intraoperative blood salvage is generally contraindicated when the operative field is bacterially contaminated or when the operative procedure is the resection of a nonmetastatic primary tumor.

Bleeding Complications

Excessive bleeding during major hepatic surgery is quite common. The most frequent source of such bleeding are surgical sites where hemorrhage is occurring locally. Systemic coagulopathy with generalized bleeding is not uncommon, and is more frequent in the setting of massive transfusion. Three factors contribute to the coagulopathy of massive transfusion during hepatic surgery: dilution; fibrinolysis and DIC; and impairment of the interaction between platelets, fibrin, and endothelial cells. Most patients have a combination of these three disorders, each of which is considered in turn below.

DILUTIONAL COAGULOPATHY

Dilutional coagulopathy is especially relevant in hepatic surgery since most patients enter the operating room with less than normal levels of coagulation proteins. In addition, patients with chronic liver disease may have significant thrombocytopenia due to the hypersplenism of portal hypertension. As blood loss at surgery is replaced by transfusions of packed cells lacking viable platelets or coagulation factors, the concentration of platelets and coagulation factors remaining in the circulation declines exponentially. Approximately 40% of initial levels are present after one blood volume exchange and 15% remain after two blood volumes (10 liters of volume in a 70-kilogram adult). Dilution of coagulation proteins also occurs and is the basis for surgical rules of thumb regarding the number of units of FFP that should be transfused for a given number of packed cells. When critically evaluated, however, such rules may be insufficient and even misleading in the management of hepatic surgery with massive transfusion. The most effective approach is to establish a mechanism for rapid monitoring during surgery of the platelet count, the coagulation proteins, and fibrinolysis. Some liver transplant programs rely on the intraoperative thromboelastogram and many others simply establish in-house STAT labs near the operating room that can measure the hematocrit, PT, activated partial thromboplastin time (aPTT), fibrinogen, and platelet count with rapid turnaround times. An operating room flow sheet charting the course of the patient's coagulation results and the amount of blood transfused is a simple but invaluable mechanism for selecting the proper mix of packed cells, platelet concentrates, and FFP. Dilutional coagulopathy is easily suspected when the patient has a prolonged PT or aPTT that corrects in vitro with an admixture of an equal volume of normal plasma.

Studies in massive transfusion have underscored the importance of thrombocytopenia in dilutional coagulopathy (11). Platelets not only serve as the first line of hemostasis, but also serve as the physical surface on which the formation of fibrin clot develops. Platelet plugging is therefore essential for normal clot formation. Since normal clotting can occur despite a reduction of coagulation proteins to 30% of normal, dilution during massive transfusion may result in significant

thrombocytopenia before a significant reduction in coagulation proteins develops. Thus transfusion of platelet concentrates may be more effective than FFP. In the absence of additional coagulation abnormalities a platelet count of 50,000 to 100,000/μl is probably adequate.

FIBRINOLYSIS AND DIC

A combination of fibrinolysis and DIC is present in patients with hepatic ischemia. The mechanism underlying the fibrinolysis and DIC of hepatic ischemia is outlined in Figure 7.1. Both processes can deplete circulating platelets and coagulation

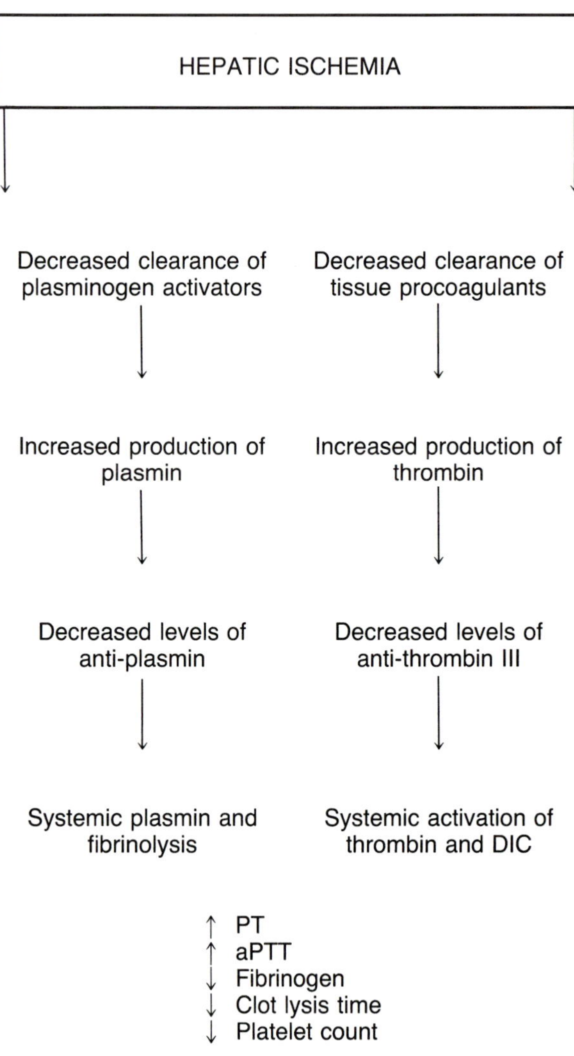

Figure 7.1. Mechanism of fibrinolysis and DIC in hepatic ischemia.

proteins, prolong the PT and aPTT, shorten the clot lysis time, and result in generalized bleeding. In patients with sepsis or with shunts that return ascites to the venous circulation, DIC is the predominant mechanism and dramatic elevation of FDPs, decreased fibrinogen, and thrombocytopenia often develop with concomitant generalized bleeding. More commonly the development of shock and tissue hypoperfusion promotes a deterioration in coagulation (12). Shock produces ischemia of all vascular beds especially those of the limbs and mesentery. Ischemic cells presumably release procoagulant material that activates the coagulation cascade and generates thrombin. Thrombin has multiple effects that lead to the depletion of circulating reserves of platelets and coagulation factors, as well as activation of protein C and secondary fibrinolysis. Once begun, the unregulated production of fibrin(ogen) degradation products can serve to further inhibit clot formation. Shock also may provoke a diffuse primary activation of the fibrinolytic system through release of tissue plasminogen activator (tPA) by vascular endothelial cells. Plasminogen activators such as tPA promote localized fibrinolysis by generating plasmin within the forming clot. Patients with cirrhosis have been shown to be deficient in natural inhibitors of fibrinolysis such as antiplasmin and plasminogen activator inhibitor. Liver disease and impaired hepatic blood flow as a result of shock amplify the pathophysiology of fibrinolysis, since tPA is normally cleared from the circulation by the liver. When such clearance is reduced, tPA may activate plasminogen to plasmin in the systemic circulation with resulting generalized fibrinolysis. Fibrinolysis and DIC may be life-threatening coagulopathies in hepatic surgery resulting in diffuse uncontrolled bleeding. The principal treatment is the correction of the underlying shock, acidosis, and sepsis (if present). Epsilon aminocaproic acid (EACA) is a potent inhibitor of the fibrinolytic system in humans. In patients with excessive bleeding due to fibrinolysis, EACA is indicated. The drug, however, should not be used as the sole agent in the treatment of patients with DIC. In DIC, EACA may prevent lysis of disseminated clotting in renal, cardiac, or central nervous system vascular beds with resultant thrombosis of vital organs. Careful patient assessment and monitoring by someone experienced in the complex coagulopathy of hepatic insufficiency is recommended when using systemic EACA.

PLATELET-ENDOTHELIAL INTERACTION

Platelet plugging begins when platelets bind to disrupted endothelium. This process, termed "platelet adhesion," depends on von Willebrand's factor. Adherent platelets undergo a release reaction to recruit additional platelets, which cluster in the process of aggregation. Platelet aggregation depends chiefly on platelet-platelet binding via fibrinogen. Fibrin clot forms on the surface of these aggregated platelets. In hepatic surgery with massive transfusion, platelet endothelial interaction may be deranged (13). Although transfusion of platelet concentrates promotes hemostasis, these platelets initially have subnormal aggregation due to the effects of storage. DIC, if present, decreases circulating platelets by consumption. Systemic fibrinolysis can also impair platelet function. Impaired platelet-endothelial binding is unusual as an isolated disorder in liver failure, but probably exists in a large proportion of hepatic surgery patients with massive transfusion. Therapy is supportive. The use of DDAVP or cryoprecipitate should be considered for patients with generalized bleeding or long template bleeding times who have adequate platelet numbers and adequate coagulation proteins. Cryoprecipitate is rich in factor VIII–von Willebrand multimers (platelet-adhesive proteins) as well as in fibrinogen (platelet aggregation protein). However, cryoprecipitate is not a source of the multiple coagulation proteins found in FFP.

DDAVP is an analogue of pitressin with little pressor or cardiovascular effect. DDAVP has been shown to promote hemostasis not only in the setting of uremia but also following cardiac surgery (14). DDAVP is felt to improve platelet-endothelial interaction through its ability to stimulate endogenous release of high-molecular-weight multimers of von Willebrand's factor. Although it would seem beneficial in the coagulopathy of massive transfusion during hepatic surgery, DDAVP is also known to stimulate release of activators of fibrinolysis. The role of DDAVP in patients with severe liver disease is uncertain. One report suggested a beneficial effect on the bleeding time in patients with cirrhosis (15).

Metabolic Complications

Massive transfusion in hepatic surgery threatens the patient with several serious metabolic complications. Most important are those that decrease left-ventricular performance and tissue perfusion. The adverse cardiovascular effects of the rapid infusion of large volumes of cold blood stored at 4°C was recognized in early studies of massive transfusion patients. The widespread availability of blood warmers has virtually eliminated this problem. Nevertheless in major hepatic operations such as transplants where the body cavity is open for extended periods of time, the core body temperature can fall significantly. Extremely rapid transfusion can exceed the capacity of standard blood warmers and contribute to hypothermia and poor cardiac performance.

ACIDOSIS

During storage, blood develops both a metabolic acidosis and a respiratory acidosis in vitro. During massive transfusion these administered acids must be buffered and excreted by the recipient. However, the degree of acidemia produced by blood products is relatively insignificant compared to that generated by the lactic acidosis that the patient produces in response to prolonged hypoperfusion, shock, and inadequate transfusion support. Following massive transfusion, especially that containing large volumes of FFP, a metabolic alkalosis is frequently seen (16). This results in part from metabolism of the citrate in stored blood to bicarbonate. Data from liver transplant patients in our institution suggest that the metabolism of excess citrate is slowed by alkalemia since in the immediate postoperative period, patients exhibit a metabolic alkalosis with an elevated anion gap and elevated plasma citrate levels (17).

Although emphasized in the past, the potassium load contributed by banked blood is relatively small. During liquid storage of red cell products, there is a progressive decline in the function of red cell ATP pumps and a progressive "leak" of intracellular potassium into the plasma. A plasma potassium in the range of 13 to 21 mEq/L has been repeatedly measured in plasma of 7- to 21-day-old citrate-phosphate-dextrose-(CPD)stored whole blood (3). In point of fact, however, the potassium load per unit of blood represents only 4 to 7 mEq since a unit of whole blood contains only 300 ml of plasma. Hyperkalemia when present in massive transfusion is usually due to an accompanying acidemia due to tissue hypoperfusion. Such a situation needs prompt recognition since both acidemia and hyperkalemia aggravate the cardiac effect of hypocalcemia caused by citrate infusion (see Citrate Toxicity, below). Severe hepatic ischemia (shock liver) will also result in hyperkalemia due to the massive release of intracellular potassium from ischemic hepatocytes.

Despite the measurement of high potassium in units of blood during storage, the serum potassium in patients undergoing massive transfusion generally declines following transfusion. In 21 patients receiving an average 33 U of blood, the potassium level fell from a pretransfusion value of 4.26 ± 0.48 to a post-transfusion value of 2.99 ± 0.49 mEq/L (16). Hypokalemia develops following massive transfusion principally because the transfused red cells that have "leaked" potassium during blood storage, metabolically revive following transfusion and act as "sponges" to take up potassium and restore intracellular potassium levels.

CITRATE TOXICITY

Citrate toxicity is particularly relevant during massive transfusion in hepatic surgery since the liver is the principal organ for metabolism of citrate. Trisodium citrate is universally used as the anticoagulant that prevents donor blood from clotting in the bag. Citrate is a potent chelator of calcium. Blood does not clot in the absence of free (ionized) calcium. If the recipient of massive transfusion cannot metabolize the administered citrate, he or she will continue to chelate calcium, resulting in a lowering of the level of ionized calcium with cardiovascular toxicity.

Guidelines exist for supplemental calcium administration during massive transfusion. Such rules, however, are generally inappropriate and frequently are incorrectly based on the number of units given. Moreover, these guidelines were developed during a time when whole blood rather than components was used. It should be emphasized that the citrate anticoagulant stays with the plasma. Thus a patient who receives 5 U of citrate-phosphate-dextrose-adenine-1 (CPDA-1) packed cells (Hct 80% and plasma volume approximately 50 ml/U) receives the same citrate load as is given in a single unit of FFP. Moreover FFP, due to its low viscosity, is frequently administered very rapidly. Citrate toxicity depends on the quantity of citrate per kilogram of body weight per minute (rate administered) versus the ability of the recipient to metabolize citrate and preserve the level of free calcium.

In the clinical setting of massive transfusion the cardiac toxicity of citrate is complex. Hypothermia, hyperkalemia, and acidemia all serve to augment the myocardial depression of hypocalcemia (18). These three metabolic derangements, which are frequently present in shock and tissue hypoperfusion, lower the threshold for poor left ventricular performance due to citrate, and increase the potential for a dangerous downward spiral during massive transfusion accompanied by shock. Therefore, avoidance of shock and tissue hypoperfusion remain of paramount importance in preventing toxicity to the cardiovascular system during massive transfusion.

Predicting citrate toxicity is difficult. The degree of such toxicity not only depends on the rate of administration; the rate of metabolism of citrate; the presence of hyperkalemia, hypothermia, and acidemia; and the duration of rapid citrate infusion, but also on the ability of the recipient to respond to citrate with sudden elaboration of parathyroid hormone, the recipient's ability to mobilize bony stores of calcium, the level of calcium binding proteins, and the recipient's individual end-organ susceptibility to citrate effects (18). The earlier work of Howland demonstrated that, although hypocalcemia was frequently accompanied by a prolonged Q-T interval on the electrocardiogram, the Q-T interval was often prolonged despite normal cardiac performance (19). Thus the Q-T interval is too nonspecific to be used as a guide to calcium supplementation. Such monitoring is best accomplished through the use of ion-selective probes capable of rapid clinically useful measurement of the blood ionized calcium level. A routine total blood calcium level is not useful in the management of massive transfusion because toxicity is dependent on the lowering of *ionized* calcium through chelation by citrate. Because the liver is the major organ for citrate metabolism, adults with severely impaired liver function or liver perfusion are more inclined to citrate toxicity. In our hospital the most pronounced degree of citrate toxicity has been seen in the setting of liver transplantation whenever rapid blood infusion occurs during the

period of time when the recipient's liver has been removed. Hypotension due to hypocalcemia secondary to citrate intoxication in this setting may be mistakenly attributed to hypovolemia, resulting in still more rapid blood administration and cardiac standstill.

The adverse cardiovascular effects of hypocalcemia secondary to citrate toxicity during liver transplantation have been reported (20). The literature provides no strict guidelines for calcium supplementation. In our own program we provide supplemental calcium during hepatic transplantation when the ionized calcium falls below 50% of the patient's preoperative baseline ionized calcium. Excessive calcium administration is to be avoided since, as the excess citrate is metabolized, free calcium is returned to the circulation. Severe iatrogenic hypercalcemia and death have been reported. Outside the setting of hepatic surgery with truly massive (rapid) blood transfusion, there are few instances of citrate toxicity requiring calcium supplementation. A complete review of citrate toxicity in massive transfusion has been published (21).

Transfusion-Transmitted Diseases: Risk to the Patient and Surgeon

The transmission of disease has remained the most common adverse consequence of blood transfusion. A variety of microorganisms can be transmitted by transfusion. Table 7.1 lists the more common pathogens seen in transfusion recipients in developed nations. The relative importance of each depends on the region of the world supplying the blood. In the Western world and the United States in particular, viruses are the most common

Table 7.1. Agents Transmitted by Transfusions

Parasites	Viruses
Plasmodium species	Non-A, non-B hepatitis
Babesia	CMV
Trypanasoma cruzii	Hepatitis B
	Delta-agent
	HIV/HTLV-III
Bacteria	HTLV-I
Staphylococcus epidermidis	EBV
Staphylococcus aureus	
Multiple species of	
gram-negative rods	
Treponema	

Abbreviations: EBV, Epstein-Barr virus; other abbreviations as in text.

pathogens. The viruses responsible for non-A, non-B hepatitis are the most important for patients receiving blood. CMV, hepatitis B virus, and HIV are of lesser risk. Since each of these viruses has also been transmitted by needlestick accidents, they represent an important occupational hazard to hepatic surgeons and other health care workers. However, not all parenteral blood exposures carry equal risk. At least four factors determine the risk of acquiring transfusion-transmitted disease: the kind of blood product, the volume of blood administered, the number of donor exposures, and the immune status of the recipient. Blood products such as albumin, which are heated to high temperatures for long durations during processing, carry no known risk of transfusion-transmitted viral disease. In contrast, unheated products prepared from multiple donors, for example, certain clotting factor concentrates, carry an extremely high risk of contamination. Commonly used volunteer donor products such as packed cells and FFP have essentially equal risk with regard to hepatitis. CMV, a virus trophic for leukocytes, is likely to be more often transmitted by fresh blood than stored blood since leukocytes deteriorate during blood storage. Transfusion-transmitted viruses have different infectivity for low-volume exposures such as occur in needlestick accidents. For example, studies suggest that hepatitis B virus may have a much higher transmission rate than HIV following needlestick exposure. Furthermore, the rate of seroconversion for recipients of an entire unit of HIV-infected blood appears to be significantly higher than the seroconversion rate following (low-volume) needlestick exposure to HIV-infected blood. For the patient receiving multiple blood transfusions, the number of donor exposures is the most important risk factor for transfusion-transmitted disease. Preoperative blood deposit (autologous blood), intraoperative blood salvage, limitation of postoperative blood tests, and scrutiny of the indications for blood transfusions are all important means to limit donor exposures. Finally, the immune status of the recipient is critical in assessing the risk of transfusion-transmitted disease. Antibodies to HB_sAg, whether obtained via previous infection or vaccination, are protective. Antibodies to HIV may not be. Whereas CMV infection can produce a serious systemic illness in immunocompromised hosts, CMV is generally of little consequence to the healthy recipient in the setting of accidental needlestick exposure. Each of these four viruses is considered below in turn.

Non-A, Non-B Hepatitis Agents

The inability to isolate the viruses responsible for non-A, non-B hepatitis has prevented the development of tests specific for these agents. The prevalence of infection with non-A, non-B hepatitis in patients or blood donor populations can therefore only be estimated. Non-A, non-B hepatitis is a diagnosis of exclusion. The prevalence of a carrier state in blood donors has been estimated through prospective studies of recipients of transfusion. In these studies serial liver function tests were monitored to identify possible cases of posttransfusion hepatitis. After excluding recipients considered to have transaminase elevations due to other causes and subtracting the background incidence of transaminase elevations in a control population of untransfused patients, the prevalence of non-A, non-B carriers in the volunteer donor pool could be estimated. Several independent studies concluded that the prevalence of active carriers of non-A, non-B agents ranged from 1% to 3% in the donor population (22,23). Since most patients receive more than 1 U of blood, approximately 10% of recipients become infected. The rate of infection increases dramatically in multiply transfused patients or in recipients of blood from nonvolunteer donor sources. With the introduction in 1987 of ALT and anti-HB_c testing of all volunteer blood donors, the rate of transmission of non-A, non-B hepatitis by transfusion is expected to decrease by 30% to 40%.

More than one virus is probably responsible for non-A, non-B hepatitis (24). Cross-inoculation studies in chimpanzees suggest that at least two different strains are capable of producing separate infections (25). The inability to serologically detect non-A, non-B viral agents may be due to efficient viral protein coat production with minimal circulating antigen.

The clinical course of non-A, non-B hepatitis is generally indolent. Acute fulminant hepatic failure can occur. The majority of cases, however, are without symptoms and go undetected. Following intravenous exposure the incubation time to transaminase elevation ranges from 2 to 12 weeks. Transaminases may elevate for a period of weeks and return to normal or may fluctuate over time with no specific pattern. Extrahepatic manifestations and serum sickness are generally not found. Although many patients recover completely, there is a high propensity for the development of a chronic carrier state and chronic liver disease among those patients who have chronic transaminase elevation. Chronically infected patients may develop cirrhosis. Studies of individuals with chronic transaminase elevations considered secondary to non-A, non-B hepatitis suggest that 20% to 50% of individuals develop chronic active hepatitis and 20% cirrhosis (26,27). Chronic active hepatitis secondary to non-A, non-B agents may be less aggressive than that due to hepatitis B. The indolent nature, chronicity, and propensity for inducing chronic active hepatitis and cirrhosis make non-A, non-B hepatitis of particular importance not only to those blood transfusion recipients expected to have a reasonable chance at 5-year survival, but also to health care workers exposed to patients' blood through needlestick injuries. Though commonly used in needlestick cases, there is no solid evidence that intramuscular gamma globulin is protective against non-A, non-B infection (28).

Cytomegalovirus

CMV is a member of the herpes family of viruses (29). It is a DNA virus capable of infecting nearly all human cells and spreading through the bloodstream as well as by contiguous cell-cell contact. Like other herpes viruses, latent CMV infection frequently occurs, and reactivation of previous infection occurs in immunosuppressed patients. The virus replicates in the nucleus of the host cell and acquires its viral coat from the cell's nuclear membrane. During viral infection, CMV produces perinuclear cytoplasmic inclusions representing intact and defective viral particles. In blood the virus can exist in free form in the plasma, but is more commonly cell-associated and found in leukocytes.

CMV is common in the human adult population. The presence of antibodies to CMV are used as a marker of previous infection. Since the virus remains latent for years, some antibody-positive individuals are capable of transmitting infection through transfusion. The prevalence of antibody-positive individuals in the general population is high. In Washington, D.C., greater than 80% of adults over age 35 were found to have comple-

ment-fixing antibodies to CMV (29). The proportion of antibody-positive individuals in the population increases with increasing age. Most antibody-positive blood donors are not viremic at the time of donation. Studies have suggested that the risk of infection post-transfusion is approximately 1% to 2%/U (29).

Transmission of CMV by blood transfusion was first noted in the setting of early cardiopulmonary bypass surgery and the "postperfusion" syndrome. Multiple studies have documented that seronegative recipients of blood from seropositive donors may seroconvert. The majority of such infections are asymptomatic. Approximately 3% of patients exposed to multiple donors develop symptomatic infection. The most common manifestation of CMV infection post-transfusion is a heterophile-negative mononucleosis syndrome with fever, lymphadenopathy, splenomegaly, atypical lymphocytes, and a mild hepatitis developing approximately 30 days after transfusion. Transaminase elevations may persist for weeks and the illness may be mistakenly attributed to non-A, non-B hepatitis, drug hepatitis, or other causes. Clinical manifestations may be subtle and may suggest other diagnoses.

In two clinical settings, CMV infection is particularly severe: neonates and immunosuppressed patients. In these two groups post-transfusion CMV may produce a constitutional illness with high fever, significant hepatitis, gastrointestinal bleeding, thrombocytopenia, and life-threatening pneumonia. Organ transplant patients are particularly susceptible to morbidity from CMV infections (29). Illness generally develops 1 to 4 months after transplant. Serious graft failure may occur following liver transplantation. A synergy between graft rejection and CMV infection may exist.

"CMV-negative blood" is collected from donors found to lack antibody to CMV. Given the high prevalence of CMV antibody in adults, CMV-negative blood is in short supply in many transplant centers. CMV-negative blood is indicated for premature infants born to CMV-negative mothers and in severely immunosuppressed individuals, for example, organ transplant recipients who are CMV antibody negative prior to transfusion and transplantation. CMV-negative blood is of no proven benefit for immunosuppressed CMV-positive patients. Studies published in 1986 suggested that passive transfer of CMV-antibody via transfusion of purified immunoglobulin preparations (CMV hyperimmune globulin) may be of clinical benefit in reducing the morbidity of CMV infection in transplant patients (30).

Hepatitis B

Hepatitis B virus is a DNA virus and a member of the Hepadna viridae of viruses. It is one of the best-characterized viruses and its 3200-base pair genome has been sequenced and cloned. The complete virion with surface antigen, DNA, and DNA polymerase is referred to as the *Dane particle*. During viral replication in humans many defective virus structures are made in addition to Dane particles, resulting in antigen (HB_sAg) detectable by various serologic means. The initial discovery of this antigen in the blood of an Australian aborigine with chronic active hepatitis led to the development and widespread application of diagnostic hepatitis serology.

The universal testing of blood donors for the presence of HB_sAg has led to the virtual elimination of post-transfusion hepatitis B. However, occasional cases of post-transfusion hepatitis B continue to occur since some donors who are chronic carriers have a level of HB_sAg below the level of detection of current screening tests (radioimmunoassay or enzyme-linked immunosorbant assay). The recent introduction of monoclonal antibodies directed against HB_sAg for use in HB_sAg detection in vitro may further improve the sensitivity of blood donor screening tests. Because paid-donor sources of blood have been shown to have a high prevalence of HB_sAg-positive individuals, reliance on volunteer blood donors remains a mainstay of preventing post-transfusion hepatitis B. Although testing of all donors for the presence of hepatitis B core antibody (anti-HB_c) was recently introduced as a surrogate test to detect carriers of non-A, non-B hepatitis, this additional serologic screen is expected to also identify some donors who are carriers of hepatitis B but test negative for HB_sAg. Despite current donor screening methods, pooled coagulation factor concentrates prepared from plasma batches of hundreds of donors continue to be occasionally contaminated with hepatitis B.

The clinical course of hepatitis B infection should be well known to hepatic surgeons, is covered in other chapters of this volume, and will not be considered here. Instead, the approach to the needlestick injury or injury to other mucous mem-

branes from a parenteral exposure to hepatitis B is reviewed. Following needlestick injury from a patient, the HB_sAg status to the patient should be determined. All HB_sAg-positive individuals should be considered infectious. Hepatitis B_c antigen (HB_cAg)-positive individuals are at even greater risk of transmitting infection. In certain endemic areas, consideration should be given to whether or not the patient may also have coinfection with delta-agent. Equally important, the antihepatitis B surface antibody (anti-HBs) status of the individual stuck with the needle (the recipient) should be determined. Anti-HBs positive individuals are protected from hepatitis B infection. If the recipient is anti-HB_s-positive, then no further action need be taken regarding the needlestick risk of hepatitis B. If the recipient is anti-HB_s negative and the patient is HB_sAg positive, then the recipient should be treated with hepatitis B hyperimmune globulin (HBIG) as soon as possible. This intramuscular preparation differs from gamma globulins since HBIG contains approximately 1000-fold higher titer of anti-HB_s. The injection of anti-HB_s provides immediate passive immunity. In addition to HBIG, hepatitis B vaccine should probably also be administered in order to provoke active immunity (28).

All hepatic surgeons should be vaccinated against hepatitis B if they do not already possess anti-HB_s as a result of previous infection (31). Several varieties of vaccine preparation exist including vaccine derived from HB_sAg-positive plasma that has been rendered noninfectious, as well as vaccine produced in vitro in yeast using techniques of molecular biology. Extensive testing of vaccine recipients has shown that both vaccines are safe and efficacious (32). Hepatitis B vaccine appears to have no risk of transmitting HIV infection. The duration of antibody response is not predictable. Therefore hepatic surgeons should have surveillance follow-up testing for anti-HB_s at approximately 3-year intervals to document active anti-HB_s activity. Booster injections may be required.

HIV

HIV, also referred to as HTLV-III and lymphadenopathy-associated virus (LAV), belongs to the family of retroviruses. Retroviruses are so named because these RNA viruses are capable of transcribing information from RNA to DNA, which is the reverse process of usual mammalian cell transcription. Although initially it was felt that HIV infection was restricted to T lymphocytes, subsequent work demonstrated that lymphocytes, macrophages, and brain cells were important reservoirs of infection. The transmission of HIV by blood transfusion and organ transplantation has been unequivocally demonstrated. Other human retroviruses include HTLV-I and HTLV-II, both of which are associated with chronic viral infection and lymphocyte abnormalities. It is very likely that transmission of such viruses may also occur via blood transfusion, although the prevalence of infection in donors and thus the potential for transmission in the U.S. population is exceedingly low. In areas of the world endemic for HTLV-I, however, seroconversion by transfusion has been documented. Widespread testing of blood donors in the U.S. for exposure to HTLV-1 may become required in the near future.

The recognition of transmission of HIV infection by blood transfusion resulted in the rapid deployment in the spring of 1985 of screening tests for the presence of antibody to HIV. At the time of writing a useful test for HIV antigen has been developed, but has not been implemented for screening blood donors. The elimination of blood products from donors found to test positive for antibody to HIV (anti-HIV) resulted in a definite decline in the incidence of transfusion-acquired HIV infection. Nevertheless, because of the long incubation period of viral infection with HIV virus, cases of symptomatic HIV infection resulting from transfusions given prior to donor testing are expected to occur for some time. In 1987 the Centers for Disease Control announced that some patients transfused before widespread donor screening was available be considered for anti-HIV testing.

There is now ample evidence to suggest that health care workers are not at high risk for acquiring HIV infection through contact with infected patients. In a study of nearly one thousand health care workers with parenteral exposure to HIV-infected patients, only two individuals developed a seroconversion (33). Thus the "attack rate" following needlestick injury of HIV virus is much lower than that following accidental inoculation with blood from a hepatitis B–positive patient. Nevertheless, well-documented cases of needlestick transmission of HIV infection have occurred. For surgeons and surgical teams operating on an ever-increasing number of HIV-infected persons, the issue of needlestick injuries remains a difficult one. Concern has also been expressed over the risk to patients from HIV-infected surgeons (34). Surgeons will need to keep informed on the complexities of testing patients for HIV infection. Although current evidence would suggest that the usual antibody response to HIV infection does not provide protection, the possibility of neutralizing (protective) antibodies remains. Should such protective antibodies exist, the possibility of an effective vaccine would represent a breakthrough in disease prevention. Until that time, HIV infection and AIDS are likely to represent an ever-increasing threat to both patients and health care workers.

References

1. Stevens CE, Aach RD, Hollinger FB, Mosley JW, et al. Hepatitis B virus antibody in blood donors and the occurrence of non-A, non-B hepatitis in transfusion recipients. *Ann Intern Med* 1984; 101:733–738.
2. Alter HJ, Purcell RH, Holland PV, Alling DW, Koziol DE. Donor transaminase and recipient hepatitis: Impact on blood transfusion services. *JAMA* 1981; 246:630–634.
3. Huestis DW, Bove JR, Busch S, eds. *Practical Blood Transfusion*, 2nd ed. Boston: Little, Brown, 1976.
4. *Standard for Blood Banks and Transfusion Series*, 12th ed. Arlington, Virginia: American Association of Blood Banks, 1987.
5. *Fresh Frozen Plasma: Indications and Risks*. National Institutes of Health Consensus Development Conference. Bethesda, Maryland: National Institutes of Health, 1984.
6. Carvalho ACA. Bleeding in uremia—a clinical challenge. *N Engl J Med* 1983; 308:38–39.
7. Tullis JL. Albumin: Background and use. *JAMA* 1977; 237:335, 460.
8. Sgouris JT, Rene A, eds. *Proceedings of the Workshop on Albumin*. Publication no. 76-925. Bethesda, Maryland: National Institutes of Health, 1976.
9. Wilkinson P, Sherlock S. The effect of repeated albumin infusions in patients with cirrhosis. *Lancet* 1962; 1:1125–1129.
10. Dzik WH, Jenkins R. Use of intraoperative blood salvage in liver transplantation. *Arch Surg* 1985; 120:946–948.
11. Counts RB, Haisch C, Simon TL, Maxwell NG, Heimbach DM, Carrico CJ. Hemostasis in massively transfused trauma patients. *Ann Surg* 1979; 190:91–99.
12. Harke H, Rahman S. Haemostatic disorders in massive transfusion. *Bibl Haematologica* 1980; 46:179–188.
13. Slichter SJ. Identification and management of defects in platelet hemostasis in massively transfused patients. In: *Massive Transfusion in Surgery and Trauma*. New York: Alan R. Liss, 1982.
14. Salzman EW, Weinstein MJ, Weintraub RM, et al. Treatment with desmopressin acetate to reduce blood loss after cardiac surgery. A double-blind randomized trial. *N Engl J Med* 1986; 314:1402–1406.
15. Burroughs AK, Matthews K, Qadiri M, Thomas N, Kernoff P, Tuddenham E, et al. Desmopressin and bleeding time in patients with cirrhosis. *Br Med J* 1985; 291:1377–1381.
16. Howland WS. Calcium, potassium, and pH changes during massive transfusion. In: Nusbacher J, ed. *Massive*

Transfusion 1978. Washington, D.C.: American Association of Blood Banks, 1978.

17. Driscoll DF, Bistrian BR, Jenkins RL, Randall S, et al. The development of metabolic alkalosis following massive transfusion during orthotropic liver transplantation. *Crit Care Med* (in press).

18. Collins JA. Massive blood transfusion. *Clin Haematol* 1976; 5:201–222.

19. Howland WS, Schweizer O, Carlon GC, Goldiner PL. The cardiovascular effects of low levels of ionized calcium during massive transfusion. *Surg Gynecol Obstet* 1977; 145: 581–586.

20. Kost GJ, Jammal MA, Ward RE, Sajwat AA. Monitoring of ionized calcium during human hepatic transplantation. *Am J Clin Path* 1986; 86:61–70.

21. Dzik WH, Kirkley SA. Citrate toxicity during massive blood transfusion. *Trans Med Rev* 1988 (in press).

22. Gitnick G. Non-A, non-B hepatitis. Etiology and clinical course. *Annu Rev Med* 1984; 35:265–278.

23. Wick MR, Moore S, Taswell HF. Non-A, non-B hepatitis associated with blood transfusion. *Transfusion* 1985; 25:93–101.

24. Bradley DW, Maynard JE. Etiology and natural history of post-transfusion and enterically-transmitted non-A, non-B hepatitis. *Semin Liver Dis* 1986; 6:56–66.

25. Hollinger FB, Mosley JW, Szmuness W, Aach RD, Peters RL, Stevens C. Transmission-transmitted virus study: Experimental evidence for two non-A, non-B hepatitis agents. *J Infect Dis* 1980; 142:400–407.

26. Koretz RL, Stone O, Gitnick G. The long-term course of non-A, non-B post-transfusion hepatitis. *Gastroenterology* 1980; 79:893–898.

27. Alter HJ, Hoofnagle JH. Non-A, non-B: Observations on the first decade. In: Vyas GN, Dienstag JL, Hoofnagle JH, eds. *Viral Hepatitis and Liver Disease*. Orlando, Florida: Grune & Stratton, 1984, pp. 345–354.

28. Seeff LB, Hoofnagle JH. Immunoprophylaxis of viral hepatitis. *Gastroenterology* 1979; 77:161–186.

29. Ho M. Cytomegalovirus: Biology and infection. In: Greenough WB, Merigan TC, eds. *Current Topics in Infectious Disease*. New York: Plenum, 1982.

30. Tegtmeier GE. Cytomegalovirus infection as a complication of blood transfusion. *Semin Liver Dis* 1986; 6:82–95.

31. Centers for Disease Control: Recommendations for protection against viral hepatitis. *MMWR* 1985; 34:313–335.

32. Stevens CE, Taylor PE, Tong MJ, Toy PT, Vyas GN. Hepatitis B vaccine: An overview. In: Vyas G, Dienstag JL, Hoofnagle JH, eds. *Viral Hepatitis and Liver Disease*, New York: Grune & Stratton, 1984.

33. McCray E, Cooperative Needlestick Surveillance Group. Occupational risk of the acquired immunodeficiency syndrome among health care workers. *N Engl J Med* 1986; 314: 1127–1132.

34. Sacks JJ. AIDS in a surgeon. *N Engl J Med* 1985; 313:1017–1018.

Editorial Comment

If there is any area of general surgery that is dependent upon availability of rapid and adequate blood replacement, it is in surgery of the liver, where advances in transplantation and hepatic resection as well as the successful management of variceal hemorrhage have been possible only because of this factor.

Thus, it seemed important to devote a chapter to this problem and Dr. Dzik has given us a global picture of the national and local problems concerned with procurement, distribution, and administration of blood and blood products. In the latter category, we have an expert's view on fresh frozen plasma, platelet concentrates, cryoprecipitate and albumin with the composition, indications for usage and administration, and the relative value under varying circumstances.

Intraoperative blood salvage has been a major asset to our Department of Surgery and to our Blood Bank, and the subject is well covered.

Complications attributable to hepatic surgery such as dilutional coagulopathy, fibrinolysis and disseminated intravenous coagulopathy, platelet endothelial reactions, citrate toxicity, and other metabolic disorders have been covered thoroughly, but in a way calculated to educate rather than confuse an attending surgeon or gastroenterologist.

The section on transfusion-transmitted disease has, since the advent of HIV, assumed particular importance to hospital personnel as well as to patients, so the surgeon or internist in charge must have a sound working knowledge of this area.

For anyone who is not fortunate enough to have someone like Dr. Dzik immediately available, this chapter is absolutely essential and for the rest of us, it is certainly both interesting and informative.

Chapter 8
Cirrhosis

DANIEL K. PODOLSKY
KURT J. ISSELBACHER

Cirrhosis represents the final common pathway of liver injury. Although etiologically discrete hepatic disorders usually demonstrate distinguishable pathologic and clinical features initially, as liver injury progresses to a state of irreversible chronic scarring, distinguishing characteristics are increasingly less prominent and the nonspecific features of cirrhosis predominate. Although uniformity of morphologic and clinical features is not complete, the fundamental processes of hepatocyte necrosis, collapse of supporting reticulin network, and subsequent connective tissue deposition with distortion of the vascular bed that lead to cirrhosis are independent of the nature of the initial disease process. Hepatic response to continued injury includes the extensive fibrosis and nodular regeneration, which are the essential features of cirrhosis. The clinical manifestations of cirrhosis follow directly from the pathologic findings. Hepatocyte necrosis and loss of functioning hepatocellular mass lead to jaundice, edema, coagulopathy, and a variety of metabolic abnormalities. Fibrosis and distorted vasculature lead to portal hypertension and its sequelae, including gastroesophageal varices and splenomegaly. Ascites and hepatic encephalopathy result from both hepatocellular insufficiency and portal hypertension.

Classification of the various types of cirrhosis based solely on etiology or morphology is unsatisfactory. A single pathologic pattern may result from a variety of insults, while the same insult may produce several morphologic patterns. Nevertheless, most types of cirrhosis may be usefully classified by a mixture of etiologically and morphologically defined entities. In the United States and other developed countries, alcoholic, postnecrotic, and biliary cirrhosis are most commonly encountered. Less frequently cirrhosis may be related to cardiac disease, a reflection of metabolic and/or inherited disorders or the consequence of drug therapy.

Alcoholic Liver Disease and Cirrhosis

Alcoholic cirrhosis, historically referred to as Laennec's cirrhosis, is the most common type of cirrhosis encountered in North America and many parts of Western Europe and South America. It is usually characterized by diffuse fine scarring, fairly uniform loss of liver cells, and small regenerative nodules; therefore, it is sometimes referred to as micronodular cirrhosis. However, micronodular cirrhosis may also result from other types of liver injury (e.g., following jejunoileal bypass), and thus alcoholic cirrhosis and micronodular cirrhosis are not necessarily synonymous. Conversely, alcoholic cirrhosis may progress to macronodular cirrhosis.

Alcoholic cirrhosis is only one of many consequences resulting from chronic alcohol ingestion and it often accompanies other forms of alcohol-induced liver injury. There are three principal alcohol-induced hepatic lesions: (1) alcoholic fatty liver, (2) alcoholic hepatitis, and (3) alcoholic cirrhosis. These morphologic categories are rarely found in a pure form, and features of each may be present to varying degrees in an individual patient.

Although chronic alcoholism is clearly the major cause of alcoholic cirrhosis, the quantity and duration of drinking necessary to cause cirrhosis remain unclear. The typical alcoholic patient with cirrhosis has had a daily consumption of a pint or more of whiskey, several quarts of wine, or an equivalent amount of beer for at least 10 years. The amount and duration of ethanol ingestion, rather than the type of alcoholic beverage or the pattern of ingestion, appear to be the important determinants of liver injury. In general, the latent period preceding the development of cirrhosis is inversely related to the level of daily alcohol intake. Although rates of ethanol metabolism are under genetic control, no metabolic defect has been identified in cirrhotic patients or their families to suggest a unique "susceptibility" to ethanol or its toxic effects. Although malnutrition per se does not appear to lead to cirrhosis, nutritional factors may augment the detrimental effects of chronic alcohol ingestion on the liver. The finding that only 10% to 15% of alcoholics develop cirrhosis suggests that other factors may affect the impact of alcohol on the liver. Significantly, women appear to be more susceptible to alcohol-induced liver injury, suggesting that hormonal factors may also play a role.

Alcoholic fatty liver occurs in most heavy drinkers but is reversible on cessation of alcohol consumption and is not thought to be an inevitable precursor of alcoholic hepatitis or cirrhosis. In contrast, alcoholic hepatitis, an inflammatory lesion characterized by infiltration of the liver with leukocytes, liver cell necrosis, and alcoholic hyalin, is thought to be the major precursor of cirrhosis. Subsequent healing accompanied by fibrosis distorts the normal lobular architecture. Indeed, deposition of collagen in perivenular spaces may be the earliest manifestation of the process that leads to centrilobular perivenous fibrosis and ultimately cirrhosis.

In alcoholic fatty liver, the liver is enlarged, yellow, greasy, and firm. Hepatocytes are distended by large cytoplasmic fat vacuoles that push the hepatocyte nucleus against the cell membrane. Accumulation of fat in the liver of the alcoholic results from the combination of impaired fatty acid oxidation, increased uptake and esterification of fatty acids to form triglycerides, and diminished lipoprotein biosynthesis and secretion.

In alcoholic hepatitis the morphologic features include hepatocyte degeneration and necrosis, often with ballooned cells, and an infiltrate of polymorphonuclear leukocytes and lymphocytes. The polymorphonuclear cells may encircle damaged hepatocytes that contain Mallory's bodies or alcoholic hyalin. These are clumps of perinuclear, deeply eosinophilic material believed to represent aggregated intermediate filaments. Mallory's bodies are highly suggestive of, but not specific, for alcoholic hepatitis, since morphologically similar material has been seen in association with morbid obesity, jejunoileal bypass surgery, poorly controlled diabetes mellitus, and a variety of other disorders. Deposition of collagen around the central vein and in perisinusoidal areas, often termed central hyaline sclerosis, may be associated with an increased likelihood of progression to cirrhosis. With continued alcohol intake and destruction of hepatocytes, fibroblasts (including myofibroblasts with contractile properties) appear at the sites of injury and stimulate collagen formation, which ultimately results in alcoholic cirrhosis. Weblike septa of connective tissue appear in periportal and pericentral zones and connect portal triads and central veins. This fine connective tissue network surrounds small masses of remaining liver cells that regenerate and form nodules. Although regeneration occurs within the small remnants of parenchyma, cell loss generally exceeds replacement. With continuing hepatocyte destruction and collagen deposition, the liver shrinks in size, acquires a nodular appearance, and becomes hard as cirrhosis develops. Although alcoholic cirrhosis is usually a progressive disease, appropriate therapy and strict avoidance of alcohol may arrest the disease at most stages and permit functional improvement.

Clinical manifestations of alcoholic fatty liver are often minimal or entirely absent, and the disorder may not be recognized unless another illness (frequently alcohol-related) brings the patient to medical attention. Hepatomegaly, at times accompanied by tenderness, may be the only finding. Jaundice, ascites, and edema are only seen with more serious liver injury.

The clinical severity of alcoholic hepatitis varies enormously, ranging from an asymptomatic or mild illness to fatal hepatic insufficiency. Typically, the clinical features of alcoholic hepatitis resemble those of viral or toxic liver injury. Patients often experience anorexia, nausea and vomiting, malaise, weight loss, abdominal distress, and jaundice. Fever as high as 103°F may be seen in about one-half of patients. On physical examination, tender hepatomegaly is common and splenomegaly is found in about one-third of patients. The patient may have cutaneous arterial "spider" angiomata and jaundice. More severe cases may be complicated by ascites, edema, bleeding, and encephalopathy. Continued alcohol excess and poor dietary habits usually lead to repeated acute episodes of hepatic decompensation. Some patients die during these acute exacerbations, but most recover after several weeks or months. After complete abstinence, clinical recovery may be protracted and histologic abnormalities can persist up to 6 months or longer.

Alcoholic cirrhosis may also be clinically silent; in fact 10% of cases are discovered incidentally at laparotomy or autopsy. In many patients, symptoms are insidious in onset, occurring usually after 10 or more years of excessive alcohol use and progressing slowly over subsequent weeks and months. Anorexia and malnutrition lead to weight loss and a reduction in skeletal muscle mass. The patient may experience easy bruising, increasing weakness, and fatigue. Eventually the clinical manifestations of hepatocellular dysfunction and portal hypertension ensue, including progressive jaundice, bleeding from gastroesophageal varices, ascites, and encephalopathy. The abrupt onset of one of these complications may be the first event prompting the patient to seek medical attention. In other cases, cirrhosis first becomes evident when the patient requires treatment of symptoms related to acute alcoholic hepatitis.

A firm, nodular liver may be an early sign of disease; the liver may be either enlarged, normal, or decreased in size. Other frequent findings include jaundice, palmar erythema, spider angiomas, parotid and lacrimal gland enlargement, clubbing of fingers, splenomegaly, muscle wasting, and ascites with or without peripheral edema. Men may have decreased body hair and/or gynecomastia as well as testicular atrophy which, like the cutaneous findings, result from disturbances in hormonal metabolism including increased peripheral formation of estrogen due to diminished hepatic clearance of the precursor androstendione. Testicular atrophy may reflect hormonal abnormalities or the toxic effect of alcohol on the testes. In women, signs of virilization or menstrual irregularities may occasionally be encountered. Dupuytren's contractures reflecting fibrosis of palmar fascia with resulting flexion contracture of the digits are associated with alcoholism but are not specifically related to cirrhosis.

Over a period of 3 to 5 years, the cirrhotic patient typically becomes emaciated, weak, and chronically jaundiced. Ascites and other signs of portal hypertension become increasingly prominent.

Most patients with advanced cirrhosis die in hepatic coma, commonly precipitated by hemorrhage from esophageal varices or intercurrent infection, especially spontaneous bacterial peritonitis. Progressive renal dysfunction often complicates the terminal phase of the illness.

In more advanced alcoholic liver disease, abnormalities of laboratory tests are common. Anemia may result from acute and chronic gastrointestinal blood loss, coexistent nutritional deficiency, hypersplenism, and a direct suppressive effect of alcohol on the bone marrow. Hemolytic anemia, presumably due to effects of hypercholesterolemia on erythrocyte membranes resulting in unusual spurlike projections (acanthocytosis), has been described in some alcoholics with cirrhosis. Leukocytosis is often present in severe alcoholic hepatitis; however, some patients with this disorder may have leukopenia and thrombocytopenia due to hypersplenism or an inhibitory effect of alcohol on the bone marrow. Mild or pronounced hyperbilirubinemia may be found, usually in association with varying elevations of serum alkaline phosphatase levels. The serum alanine aminotransferase (ALT) [serum glutamic pyruvic transaminase (SGPT)] is frequently elevated, but levels greater than 300 units are unusual and should prompt one to look for other coincident or complicating factors. In contrast to viral hepatitis, the serum aspartate aminotransferase (AST) is usually disproportionately elevated relative to ALT (AST/ALT ratio > 2). This discrepancy may result from the proportionally greater inhibition of ALT synthesis by ethanol, which may be partially reversed by pyridoxal phosphate.

The serum prothrombin time is frequently prolonged, reflecting reduced synthesis of clotting proteins, most notably the vitamin K–dependent factors (see coagulopathy, below). The serum albumin level is usually depressed, while serum globulins are increased.

Hypoalbuminemia reflects in part overall impairment in hepatic protein synthesis, while hyperglobulinemia is thought to result from nonspecific stimulation of the reticuloendothelial system. Elevated blood ammonia levels in patients with hepatic encephalopathy reflect diminished hepatic clearance because of impaired liver function and shunting of portal venous blood around the cirrhotic liver into the systemic circulation (see Chapter 12B).

A variety of metabolic disturbances may be detected including hypomagnesemia, hypophosphatemia, hypokalemia, and hyponatremia. Glucose intolerance due to endogenous insulin resistance may be present; however, clinical diabetes is uncommon. Central hyperventilation may lead to respiratory alkalosis in patients with cirrhosis. Dietary deficiency and increased urinary losses lead to hypomagnesemia and hypophosphatemia.

Alcoholic cirrhosis should be strongly suspected in patients with a history of prolonged or excessive alcohol intake and physical signs of chronic liver disease. The clinical features and laboratory findings are usually sufficient to provide a reasonable indication of the presence and extent of hepatic injury. Although a percutaneous needle biopsy of the liver is not usually necessary to confirm the typical findings of alcoholic hepatitis or cirrhosis, it may be helpful in distinguishing patients with less advanced liver disease from those with cirrhosis, and in excluding other forms of liver injury such as viral hepatitis. Biopsy may also be helpful as a diagnostic tool in evaluating patients with clinical findings suggestive of alcoholic liver disease who deny alcohol intake. In patients with features of cholestasis, ultrasonography may be appropriate to exclude the presence of extrahepatic biliary obstruction. When the clinical status of an otherwise stable cirrhotic patient deteriorates without an obvious explanation, complicating conditions, such as infection, portal vein thrombosis, and hepatocellular carcinoma, should be sought. Abstinence from alcohol as well as early and appropriate medical care can decrease long-term morbidity and mortality, and delay or prevent the appearance of further complications. Patients who have had a major complication of cirrhosis and who continue to drink have a 5-year survival of less than 50%. However, those patients who remain abstinent have a substantially better prognosis. In general, overall outlook in patients with advanced chronic liver disease remains poor; most of these patients eventually die as a result of massive variceal hemorrhage and/or profound hepatic encephalopathy.

Therapy is largely supportive. Specific treatment is directed at particular complications such as variceal bleeding, ascites, etc. Some studies suggest that administration of prednisone or prednisolone in moderately large doses may be helpful in patients with severe alcoholic hepatitis and encephalopathy. However, the use of corticosteroids in acute alcoholic hepatitis remains controversial and is not recommended. More recently, chronic treatment with low doses of propylthiouracil (300 mg/d) has been reported to improve survival in patients with alcoholic liver disease, including those with features suggesting a poor prognosis.

In the absence of signs of impending hepatic coma, the patient should be placed on a diet containing at least 1 gram protein per kilogram of body weight and 2000 to 3000 calories per day. Use of diets enriched in branched-chain amino acids has been advocated in patients predisposed to hepatic encephalopathy but the value of these diets in patients with compensated cirrhosis is unproven. Daily multivitamin supplements should be prescribed, with the addition of large parenteral doses of thiamine in patients with Wernicke-Korsakoff disease. The patient should be made to realize that there is no medication that will protect the liver against the effects of further alcohol ingestion. Therefore, alcohol should be absolutely forbidden and the patient encouraged to participate in an appropriate alcohol counseling program.

All medicines must be administered with caution in the patient with cirrhosis, especially those eliminated or modified through hepatic metabolism or biliary pathways. In particular, care must be taken to avoid overzealous use of drugs that may directly or indirectly precipitate complications of cirrhosis. For example, vigorous treatment of ascites with diuretics may result in electrolyte abnormalities or hypovolemia, which can precipitate or lead to coma. Similarly, even modest doses of sedative can lead to deepening encephalopathy.

Postnecrotic Cirrhosis

Postnecrotic cirrhosis represents the final common pathway of many types of advanced liver injury. *Coarsely nodular, posthepatitic,* and *multilobular cirrhosis* are terms synonymous with postnecrotic cirrhosis. The term "cryptogenic cirrhosis" has been used interchangeably with postnecrotic cirrhosis, but this designation should be reserved for those cases in which the etiology of cirrhosis is unknown (approximately 10% of all patients with cirrhosis).

Epidemiologic and serologic evidence suggests that viral hepatitis (hepatitis B or non-A, non-B) may be an antecedent factor in at least one-fourth of cases of apparently cryptogenic postnecrotic cirrhosis.

Postnecrotic cirrhosis is characterized morphologically by extensive confluent loss of liver cells, stromal collapse and fibrosis resulting in broad bands of connective tissue containing the remains of many portal triads, and irregular nodules of regenerating hepatocytes, varying in size from microscopic to several centimeters in diameter. A broad spectrum of disorders and toxins may cause postnecrotic cirrhosis, including drugs. In some instances, advanced alcoholic liver disease and primary biliary cirrhosis may lead to postnecrotic cirrhosis.

The postnecrotic liver is typically shrunken in size, distorted in shape, and composed of nodules of liver cells separated by dense and broad bands of fibrosis. In patients with cirrhosis of known etiology in whom there is progression to a postnecrotic stage, the clinical manifestations are an extension of those resulting from the initial disease process. Usually clinical symptoms are related to portal hypertension and its sequelae such as ascites, splenomegaly, hypersplenism, encephalopathy, and bleeding esophageal varices. The hematologic and liver function abnormalities resemble those seen with other types of cirrhosis. In a few patients with postnecrotic cirrhosis the diagnosis may be made incidentally at operation, at postmortem, or by a needle biopsy of the liver performed to investigate asymptomatic hepatosplenomegaly.

Postnecrotic cirrhosis should be suspected in patients with signs and symptoms of cirrhosis or portal hypertension. Needle or operative liver biopsies confirm the diagnosis, although nonuniformity of the pathologic process may result in sampling errors. The diagnosis of cryptogenic cirrhosis is reserved for those patients in whom no known etiology can be demonstrated. About 75% of patients have progressive disease despite supportive therapy and die within 1 to 5 years from complications including exsanguinating variceal hemorrhage, hepatic encephalopathy, or superimposed hepatocellular carcinoma.

Management is usually limited to treatment of the complications of portal hypertension, including control of ascites; avoidance of drugs or excessive protein intake that may induce hepatic coma; and prompt treatment of infections. In patients with asymptomatic cirrhosis, expectant management alone is appropriate. In patients in whom postnecrotic cirrhosis has developed as a result of a treatable condition (e.g., Wilson's disease, hemochromatosis), therapy directed at the primary disorder may limit further progression.

Biliary Cirrhosis

Biliary cirrhosis results from injury to or prolonged obstruction of either the intrahepatic or extrahepatic biliary system. It is associated with impaired biliary excretion, destruction of hepatic parenchyma, and progressive fibrosis. Primary biliary cirrhosis is characterized by chronic inflammation and fibrous obliteration of intrahepatic bile ductules. Secondary biliary cirrhosis is the result of long-standing obstruction of the larger extrahepatic ducts. Although primary and secondary biliary cirrhosis are separate pathophysiologic entities with respect to the initial insult, many clinical features are similar.

Primary Biliary Cirrhosis

The cause of primary biliary cirrhosis remains unknown. Several observations suggest that a disordered immune response may be involved. Most importantly, a circulating IgG antimitochondrial antibody is detected in more than 95% of patients with primary biliary cirrhosis and only rarely in other forms of liver disease. Elevated serum levels of IgM and cryoproteins consisting of immune complexes capable of activating the alternate complement pathway are also found in 80% to 90% of patients. In addition, lymphocytes are prominent in the portal regions and surround damaged bile ducts.

Primary biliary cirrhosis is often divided into four stages based on morphologic findings. The earliest recognizable lesion (stage 1), termed *chronic nonsuppurative destructive cholangitis*, is a necrotizing inflammatory process of the portal triads. It is characterized by destruction of medium and small bile ducts, a dense infiltrate of acute and chronic inflammatory cells, mild fibrosis, and occasionally bile stasis. At times, periductal granulomata and lymph follicles are found adjacent to affected bile ducts. Subsequently, the inflammatory infiltrate becomes less prominent, the number of bile ducts is reduced, and smaller bile ductules proliferate (stage 2). Progression over a period of months to years leads to a decrease in interlobular ducts, loss of liver cells, and expansion of periportal fibrosis into a network of connective tissue scars (stage 3). Ultimately, cirrhosis, which may be micronodular or macronodular, develops (stage 4).

Many patients with primary biliary cirrhosis are asymptomatic, and the disease is initially detected on the basis of elevated serum alkaline phosphatase levels (two- to fivefold) during routine screening. Serum 5'-nucleotidase activity is also elevated while serum bilirubin aminotransferase levels are usually normal. The diagnosis is supported by a positive antimitochondrial antibody test (titer > 1:40). The majority of such patients remain asymptomatic and do not develop progressive liver injury.

Among patients with symptomatic disease, 90% are women aged 35 to 60 years. The earliest symptom is usually pruritus, which may be either generalized or limited initially to the palms and soles. After several months or years, jaundice and gradual darkening of the exposed areas of the skin (melanosis) may ensue. Other clinical manifestations of primary biliary cirrhosis reflect impaired bile excretion. These include steatorrhea and the malabsorption of lipid-soluble vitamins, often resulting in easy bruising (vitamin K deficiency), bone pain due to osteomalacia (vitamin D deficiency), occasionally night blindness (vitamin A deficiency), and dermatitis (possibly vitamin E and/or essential fatty acid deficiency). Protracted elevation of serum lipids, especially cholesterol, leads to subcutaneous lipid deposition around the eyes (xanthelasmas) and over joints and tendons (xanthomas). Over a period of months to years, the itching, jaundice, and hyperpigmentation slowly worsen. Eventually signs of hepatocellular failure and portal hypertension develop and ascites appear. Death due to hepatic insufficiency usually occurs within 5 to 10 years after the first signs of the illness and is often precipitated by uncontrolled variceal hemorrhage or infection.

Physical examination may be entirely normal in the early phase of the disease, when patients are asymptomatic or pruritus is the sole complaint. Later there may be jaundice of varying intensity, hyperpigmentation of the exposed skin areas, xanthelasmas and tendinous and planar xanthomas, moderate to striking hepatomegaly, splenomegaly, and clubbing of the fingers. Bone tenderness,

signs of vertebral compression, ecchymoses, glossitis, and dermatitis may all be noted. Clinical evidence of the sicca syndrome can be found in as many as 75% of patients and serologic evidence of autoimmune thyroid disease in 25%. Other conditions encountered with increased frequency include rheumatoid arthritis; calcinosis cutis, Raynaud's phenomenon, sclerodactyly, and telangiectasia (CRST) syndrome; scleroderma; pernicious anemia; and renal tubular acidosis.

As the disease evolves, the serum bilirubin level rises progressively and may reach 30 mg/dL or more in the final stages. Serum aminotransferase values rarely exceed 150 to 200 U.

Hyperlipidemia is common, and a striking increase of the serum unesterified cholesterol is often noted. An abnormal serum lipoprotein (lipoprotein X) may be present in primary biliary cirrhosis but is not specific and appears in other cholestatic conditions. Similarly, the finding of elevated liver copper levels in patients with primary biliary cirrhosis is not specific and is found in all disorders in which there is prolonged cholestasis.

The diagnosis of primary biliary cirrhosis should be considered in middle-aged women with unexplained pruritus or an elevated serum alkaline phosphatase and in whom there may be other clinical or laboratory features of protracted impairment in biliary excretion. Although a positive serum antimitochondrial antibody determination provides important diagnostic evidence, false-positive results do occur and therefore liver biopsy should be performed to confirm the diagnosis. In most patients the biliary tract should be evaluated to exclude remediable extrahepatic biliary tract obstruction, especially in view of the frequent presence of coexisting cholelithiasis.

There is no specific therapy for primary biliary cirrhosis. Corticosteroids are ineffective and may actually worsen the bone disease. D-penicillamine has been tried because of its ability to chelate copper and because of its possible antifibrotic and immunomodulating activities. However, the drug appears to be ineffective and has a high incidence of unacceptable side effects. Some have suggested that azathioprine may be helpful in slowing the progression of disease.

Treatment is generally directed toward the relief of symptoms. Although the mechanism of the protracted pruritus is not entirely clear, cholestyramine, an oral bile salt–sequestering resin, may be helpful in doses of 8 to 12 g/day to decrease both the pruritus and the hypercholesterolemia. Steatorrhea can be reduced by a low-fat diet and substituting medium-chain triglycerides for dietary long-chain triglycerides. Fat-soluble vitamins A, D, and K should be given by parenteral injection at regular intervals. Osteomalacia may be ameliorated by dietary calcium supplements in conjunction with oral vitamin D. In advanced disease, 25 or 125 hydroxl D_3 may be preferred to vitamin D since poor hepatic function may limit conversion of vitamin D to the active metabolites. The management of ascites, variceal hemorrhage, and encephalopathy is described in chapters 13, 17 and 18. The role of hepatic transplantation for patients with primary biliary cirrhosis is under study; this may offer the best, and only, hope for survival in patients with end-stage disease.

Secondary Biliary Cirrhosis

Secondary biliary cirrhosis results from prolonged partial or total obstruction of the common bile duct or its major branches. In adults, obstruction is most frequently caused by postoperative strictures or gallstones, usually with superimposed infectious cholangitis. Chronic pancreatitis may lead to biliary stricture and secondary cirrhosis. Secondary biliary cirrhosis may also develop in patients with pericholangitis or idiopathic sclerosing cholangitis. Patients with malignant tumors of the common bile duct or pancreas rarely survive long enough to develop secondary biliary cirrhosis. In children, congenital biliary atresia and cystic fibrosis are common causes of secondary biliary cirrhosis.

The pathogenesis of secondary biliary cirrhosis appears clear. Unrelieved obstruction of the extrahepatic bile ducts leads to bile stasis and focal areas of centrilobular necrosis followed by periportal necrosis, proliferation, and dilatation of the portal bile ducts and ductules, sterile or infected cholangitis with accumulation of polymorphonuclear infiltrates around bile ducts, and progressive expansion of portal tracts by edema and fibrosis. Extravasation of bile from ruptured interlobular bile ducts into areas of periportal necrosis leads to the formation of "bile lakes" surrounded by cholesterol-rich pseudoxanthomatous cells. In general, at least 3 to 12 months is required for biliary obstruction to result in cirrhosis. Relief of the obstruction is frequently accompanied by biochemical and morphologic improvement.

Secondary biliary cirrhosis should be considered in any patient with clinical and laboratory evidence of prolonged obstruction to bile flow, especially when there is a history of previous biliary tract surgery or gallstones, bouts of ascending cholangitis, or right upper quadrant pain. Cholangiography (either percutaneous or endoscopic) usually demonstrates the underlying pathologic process.

The signs and symptoms of secondary biliary cirrhosis are similar to those of primary biliary cirrhosis. Jaundice and pruritus are usually the most prominent features. In addition, fever and/or right upper quadrant pain, reflecting bouts of cholangitis or biliary colic, are typical. The manifestations of portal hypertension are found only in advanced cases.

Elevation in serum alkaline phosphatase and conjugated hyperbilirubinemia are nearly always present. There is a moderate increase in serum aminotransferases. When the disease is complicated by cholangitis, elevations in aminotransferase levels and leukocytosis are more pronounced. As in primary biliary cirrhosis, there are abnormalities in serum lipids (including the presence of lipoprotein X) and laboratory findings consistent with steatorrhea. However, the antimitochondrial antibody test is usually negative.

Relief of obstruction to bile flow, by either surgical or endoscopic means, is the most important step in the prevention and therapy of secondary biliary cirrhosis. Effective decompression of the biliary tract results in a significant improvement in both symptoms and survival, even in patients with established cirrhosis. When obstruction cannot be relieved, as in sclerosing cholangitis, antibiotics may be helpful acutely in controlling superimposed infection or, when administered on a chronic basis, as prophylactic therapy in suppressing recurring episodes of ascending cholangitis.

Miscellaneous Types of Cirrhosis

Cardiac Cirrhosis

Prolonged severe right-sided congestive heart failure may lead to chronic liver injury and cardiac cirrhosis, which may be distinguished from both reversible passive congestion of the liver due to

Table 8.1 Cirrhosis and/or Liver Disease Associated with Metabolic, Hereditary, Infectious, Drug-related, and Other Types of Disorders

Inherited and Metabolic Disorders
  Alpha-1-antitrypsin deficiency
  Fanconi's syndrome
  Galactosemia
  Gaucher's disease
  Glycogen storage disease
  Hemochromatosis
  Hereditary fructose intolerance
  Hereditary tyrosinemia
  Wilson's disease
Infectious diseases
  Brucellosis
  Ecchinococcus
  Schistosomiasis[a]
  Toxoplasmosis
  Viral hepatitis (hepatitis B; non-A, non-B hepatitis;
    hepatitis D; cytomegalovirus)
Drugs and toxins
  Arsenicals
  Isoniazid
  Methotrexate
  Methyldopa
  Oral contraceptives (Budd-Chiari syndrome)
  Oxyphenasitin
  Perhexilene maleate
  Pyrrolidizine alkaloids (venocclusive disease)
Other or Unproven Causes
  Chronic inflammatory bowel disease
  Cystic fibrosis
  Diabetes mellitus
  Graft-versus-host disease
  Jejunoileal bypass
  Sarcoidosis

[a] The clinical manifestations in such cases are largely secondary to portal hypertension.

acute heart failure and acute hepatocellular necrosis ("ischemic hepatitis" or "shock liver") resulting from systemic hypotension and hypoperfusion of the liver. With prolonged passive congestion and ischemia from poor perfusion secondary to reduced cardiac output, necrosis of centrilobular hepatocytes ensues and leads to fibrosis in these central areas. Ultimately centrilobular fibrosis develops with collagen extending outward in a characteristic stellate pattern from the central vein. Gross examination of the liver shows alternating red (congested) and pale (fibrotic) areas, a pattern often referred to as "nutmeg liver." Improvement in management of cardiac disorders, particularly advances in surgical treatment, has reduced the frequency of cardiac cirrhosis.

Metabolic, Hereditary, and Drug-related Types of Cirrhosis

Cirrhosis or hepatitis may result from a wide variety of other processes encompassing the spectrum of etiologic factors listed in Table 8.1. Although some of these disorders have distinctive clinical or morphologic features, the manifestations of cirrhosis are largely independent of the underlying pathogenic mechanism.

References

1.　Beswick DR, Klatskin G, Boyer JC. Asymptomatic primary biliary cirrhosis. A progress report on long-term follow-up and natural history. *Gastroenterology* 1985; 89:267–271.

2.　Borowsky SA, Strome S, Lott E. Continued heavy drinking and survival in alcoholic cirrhotics. *Gastroenterology* 1981; 80:1405–1409.

3.　Christensen E, Crowe J, Doniach D., Popper H, Ranek L, Rodés J, et al. Clinical pattern and course of disease in primary cirrhosis based on an analysis of 236 patients. *Gastroenterology* 1980; 78:236–246.

4.　Long RG, Scheuer PJ, Sherlock S. Presentation and course of asymptomatic primary biliary cirrhosis. *Gastroenterology* 1977; 72:1204–1207.

5.　James O. Primary biliary cirrhosis—a revised clinical spectrum. *Lancet* 1981; 1:1278–1281.

6.　Neuberger J, Christensen E, Portmann B, Caballeria J, Rodes J, Ranek L, et al. Double blind controlled trial of d-penicillamine in patients with primary biliary cirrhosis. *Gut* 1985; 26:114–119.

7.　Maddrey WC, Boitnott JK, Bedine MS, Weber FL, Mezey E, White RI. Corticosteroid therapy of alcoholic hepatitis. *Gastroenterology* 1978; 75:193–199.

8.　Mendenhall CL, Anderson S, Garcia-Pont P, Goldberg S, Kiernan T, Sieff LB, et al. Short-term and long-term survival in patients with alcoholic hepatitis treated with oxandrolone and prednisone. *N Engl J Med* 1984; 311:1464–1470.

9.　Matloff DS, Selinger MJ, Kaplan MM. Hepatic transaminase activity in alcoholic liver disease. *Gastroenterology* 1980; 78:1389–1392.

10.　Orrego H, Blake JE, Blendis LM, Compton KV, Israel Y. Long term treatment of alcoholic liver disease with propylthiouracil. *N Engl J Med* 1987; 317:1421–1427.

11.　Powell WJ, Klatskin G. Duration of survival in patients with Laennec's cirrhosis. *Am J Med* 1968; 44:406–420.

12.　Sorensen TIA, Orholm M, Bentsen KD, Hoybye G, Eghoje K, Christoffersen P. Prospective evaluation of alcohol abuse and alcoholic liver injury in men as predictors of development of cirrhosis. *Lancet* 1984; 2:241–244.

13.　Theodossi A, Eddleston ALWF, Williams R. Controlled trail of methylprednisolone therapy in severe acute alcoholic hepatitis. *Gut* 1982; 23:75–79.

14.　Van Thiel DH, Lipsitz HD, Porter LE, Schade RR, Gottlieb GR, Graham TO. Gastrointestinal and hepatic manifestations of chronic alcoholism. *Gastroenterology* 1981; 81:594–615.

15.　Zetterman RK, Sorrell MF. Immunologic aspects of alcoholic liver disease. *Gastroenterology* 1981; 81:616–624.

Editorial Comment

Dr. Isselbacher and Dr. Podolsky have emphasized in this excellent chapter on the cirrhotic liver the difficulties that exist in terminology and classification. For example, one can classify changes in the liver from the point of view of etiology and refer to either alcoholic hepatitis or to alcoholic cirrhosis. On the other hand, one can categorize the pathologic description and refer to a liver as reflecting micronodular or macronodular cirrhosis. There is so much overlap in utilizing either type of terminology that the classification the authors have presented, and described so well in the subsections of the chapter, is probably the most useful approach.

There is purposely little in this chapter on pathophysiology and hemodynamics. The problems concerned with the concomitant destruction and fibrosis, which can occur simultaneously in the liver from a variety of insults, result in varying degrees of pre- or postsinusoidal block. Obviously, extrahepatic occlusion of the portal vein represents a presinusoidal block, whereas obstruction to the outflow from the liver either in the vena cava or hepatic veins produces an effective postsinusoidal block. The cirrhotic process, however, leads to tremendous variations in the end result and may effectively result in either pre- or postsinusoidal block, in the intrahepatic portion of the inflow and outflow vascular channels. This subject is very well covered in Chapter 12B that relates to the hemodynamics of the portal circulation, the development of ascites, the utilization of various types of shunts in decompressing an obstructed portal or sinusoidal bed, and in many other chapters throughout this volume. Thus, it is appropriate that this material is not repeated in any great detail in this particular chapter.

It is obvious that no mention has been made of the incidence of malignant disease in certain types of cirrhosis. While the development of primary hepatocellular carcinoma is not as common in micronodular cirrhosis as it is in hemochromatosis or macronodular disease, nonetheless the preponderance of micronodular or alcoholic cirrhosis in total number of cases is such that most of the malignant hepatomas arise in the alcoholic liver. In other parts of the world, the epidemiology is totally different; it is true that the sequelae of hepatitis B infestation include a high incidence of malignant change and the resulting tumors are a common cause of death in the Orient and Africa.

No more than passing reference is made in this chapter to one of the major problems of cirrhosis—the development of portal-azygous collateral channels, commonly referred to as esophageal varices. These dilated, thin-walled veins under high pressure are the source of repeated and often fatal massive hemorrhages. They have been the object of much surgical and medical effort; however, thus far no final and conclusive answer to this problem has been found.

Orthotopic transplantation of the liver is covered in chapter 23, which deals with all aspects of this relatively new therapeutic approach to liver disease. Obviously, various types of cirrhosis in its terminal phase can provide a major source of patients for this dramatic but highly effective form of therapy. In this context, we might call attention to the fact that the antimitochondrial antibodies referred to by the authors in the section on biliary cirrhosis have been found to persist in all patients who have had total hepatectomies so that, while serving as an excellent diagnostic marker for the disease of biliary cirrhosis, these are not purely a locally generated phenomenon and persist even in individuals with a new and completely healthy organ.

PART III
Assessment and Diagnosis

Chapter 9
Clinical Laboratory Evaluation of the Liver

BENJAMIN GERSON

Organization of the Liver

The liver classically is viewed functionally and microscopically as being organized at the level of lobules. Each approximately hexagonal lobule is 1 to 2 millimeters in diameter, oriented around a central vein. The central vein of the lobule is a branch of the hepatic vein. Peripheral to each of the lobules and forming the boundaries of each lobule, are the portal tracts, or portal triads. Each portal tract is made up of connective tissue containing a branch of the hepatic artery, a biliary tract branch, and a branch of the portal vein. The blood supply to the liver parenchyma (the hepatocytes) is approximately 30% to 40% from the hepatic artery, with the remainder coming from the portal vein (1). An alternative view of the organization of the liver at the functional and microscopic level is that the portal triad is the central unit and that the central veins mark the periphery of what may be termed portal lobules. A functional unit called the acinus is centered around the portal vein and hepatic artery branches, which leave the portal tracts at intervals and run along the sides of the hexagonal lobules. The functional unit in this model then consists of pie-shaped segments of contiguous lobules (1,2).

Regardless of the functional organization model, histologically the hepatocytes are organized in rows of pairs making sheets or plates, which variously are described as cribiform, branching, or anastomosing. The classically described lobule has pairs of uniform appearing hepatocytes arranged in cords that are radially distributed around the central vein, some terminating at the portal triads. The hepatocytes of the adult are characterized by their monotonous appearance. Mitoses and binucleation are unusual. Some variation appears in later adult life as there is a normal loss of individ-

ual cells with compensatory hypertrophy and regeneration (1).

Vascular spaces called sinusoids are between the rows of hepatocytes. The blood flowing within the sinusoids is a mix of hepatic arterial and portal venous blood from the portal triad, draining into the central vein. The sinusoids are lined by fenestrated endothelial cells and scattered reticuloendothial system cells referred to as Kupffer cells. The Kupffer cells are phagocytic macrophages that may ingest bacteria or other foreign matter from the blood as it flows through the sinusoids (3). The narrow Disse's space lies between the sinusoid and the hepatocytes. Microvilli of the hepatocytes protrude into the Disse's space. An additional cell, Ito's cell, which is a fat-containing lipocyte, is found in this space as well (1).

The biliary system originates in the center of the classical lobule. Bile canaliculi are between the adjacent hepatocytes of the plates. They merge as they approach the lobule periphery, draining into intermediate canals of Hering, which become the interlobular bile ducts within the portal triads. The canaliculi between individual hepatocytes have a diameter of 1 to 2 micrometers, being formed by grooves along adjacent cells. The channel walls are the external surfaces, that is, the plasma membranes of the hepatocytes. Microvilli protrude into these canaliculi. Bile duct epithelium first appears at the level of Hering's canals.

Clinical Laboratory Procedures

Clinical laboratory results that are indicators of hepatic disease are very useful in patient care. No individual procedure, however, is sufficient for most clinical situations. Therefore, selected groups of clinical laboratory procedures may be employed to pursue a particular aspect of hepatic status.

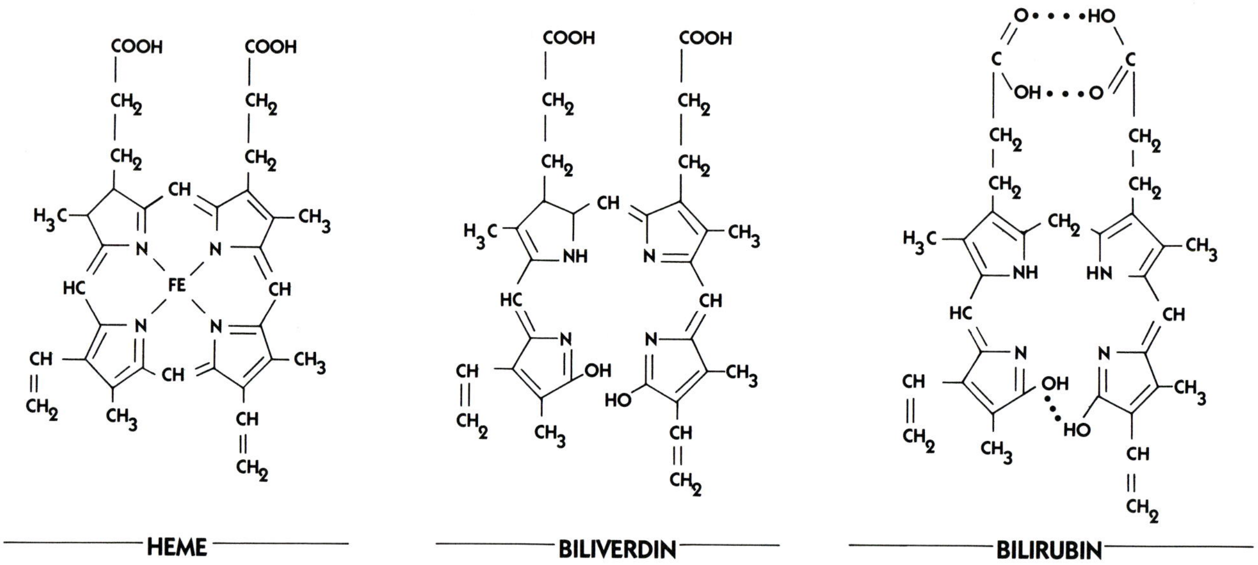

Figure 9.1. Structures of heme, biliverdin, and bilirubin.

Only the more common clinical laboratory tests related to the liver will be reviewed.

Clinical Laboratory Tests Based on Excretory Function

The excretions of endogenously produced bilirubin and of bile acids are the most frequently employed modern clinical laboratory techniques for assessing liver function based on excretory function. Not to be discussed due to diminishing use are tests based on the excretion of exogenously administered dyes, such as indocyanine green.

Bilirubin

Quantification of bilirubin is a common clinical laboratory procedure, and one that is very useful in classifying hepatic (as well as nonhepatic) diseases. Bilirubin is the principal pigment of bile, consisting of four pyrrole rings (Fig. 9.1) (4). There are three sources of bilirubin. Mostly it is a product of the biotransformation (catabolism) of hemoglobin in the reticuloendothelial system cells (Fig. 9.2). Approximately 80% to 85% of bilirubin in serum is derived from the senesence of mature red blood cells (3–6). Most of the rest results from the degradation of heme containing enzymes of the liver and elsewhere (myoglobin, cytochromes, catalase), with an additional small contribution from

the destruction of immature erythrocytes in the bone marrow (ineffective erythropoiesis) (4). The phagocytosis of hemoglobin by the reticuloendothelial cells takes place primarily in the liver, spleen, and bone marrow. The protoporphyrin is separated from the iron and globin portions of the molecule. The protein portion of hemoglobin, globin, is reused by the body. The iron likewise enters the body's stores for reuse. The heme porphyrin (protoporphyrin IX) ring is oxidatively opened at the alpha-methene bridge, mediated by the enzyme heme oxygenase, resulting in the formation of biliverdin with the release of carbon monoxide (3,5,6,7). Reduction (hydrogenation) of biliverdin by the action of the enzyme biliverdin reductase results in bilirubin. Carbon monoxide is produced as well.

Bilirubin present in the systemic circulation is being transported to the liver. Within the systemic circulation, bilirubin is bound to protein, mainly albumin (see Fig. 9.2). Bilirubin is found bound to gamma globulins, lipoproteins, and erythrocyte membranes as well when present in high concentrations (8). There are two types of bilirubin-albumin complexes. The first is a strong association of two molecules of bilirubin with two molecules of albumin (see delta-bilirubin, below). The second is a weaker bond (4). Once within the sinusoids, bilirubin becomes dissociated from the albumin in order to be translocated to the inner surface of the

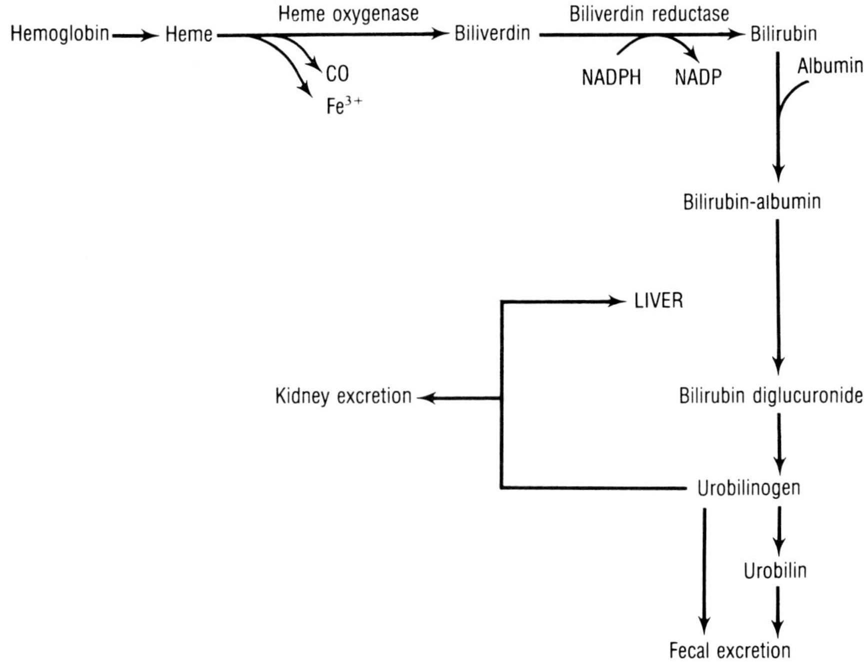

Figure 9.2. Production of bilirubin from hemoglobin, and subsequent biotransformation. One mole each of carbon monoxide (CO), bilirubin, and ferric iron (Fe^{3+}) are produced.

hepatocyte plasma membrane. The translocation process probably involves binding to proteins located within the membrane. This is an active transport (most likely) or facilitated diffusion saturable process and is subject to competitive inhibition (4,5,6,8). Bilirubin within the hepatocyte is reversibly bound to soluble proteins. The two which account for most of the intracellular binding are Z protein and ligandin (6).

When a cell is homogenized in vitro, the smooth endoplasmic reticulum fragments re-form into vessicles called microsomes. For this reason, the enzymes associated with the smooth endoplasmic reticulum frequently are referred to as the microsomal enzymes (the enzymes of the rough endoplasmic reticulum are involved in protein synthesis). Conjugation (esterification) of bilirubin, mainly with glucuronate, is a "synthetic" reaction that takes place in the endoplasmic reticulum of the hepatocyte resulting in the formation of bilirubin mono- and diglucuronide. Synthetic reactions sometimes are referred to as phase II reactions to distinguish them from phase I reactions, which are actual modifications of chemical structure (9). The conjugate product is more polar and so is more water-soluble, a property that enhances excretion.

The first step in this process actually is esterification of one propionyl group by way of the microsomal (endoplasmic reticulum) enzyme uridine diphosphate-glucuronyl transferase (UDPG-T). Synthetic reactions require an energy source, which generally is ATP. These reactions are characterized by the formation of an active nucleotide as an intermediate and a transferring enzyme that catalyzes the final conjugation step. Mercapturic acid formation is an exception (Fig. 9.3) (9).

The formation of glucuronic acid (a glucose derivative) derivatives is the most prominent of the several hepatic synthetic pathways. The chemical groups that undergo conjugation with glucuronic acid are aliphatic and aromatic alcohols (hydroxyl groups), some carboxyl groups, sulfhydryl groups, mercapto groups, dithiocarboxyl groups, and primary and secondary aromatic and aliphatic amines. The enzyme uridine diphosphate glucuronyl transferase and the coenzyme uridine-5'-diphospho-alpha-D-glucuronic acid (UDPGA) carry out this reaction. Glucuronic acid from UDPGA is transferred to the aglycone by the enzyme. The product is either an ether or ester glucuronide. Glucuronyl transferase, which has more than one form, is found predominantly in hepatic endoplas-

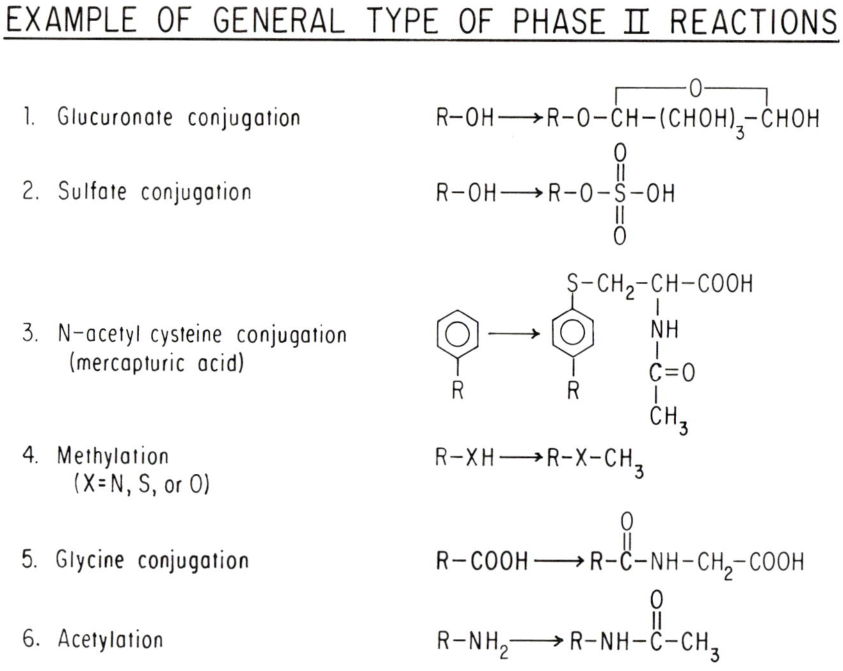

EXAMPLE OF GENERAL TYPE OF PHASE II REACTIONS

1. Glucuronate conjugation $R{-}OH \longrightarrow R{-}O{-}CH{-}(CHOH)_3{-}CHOH$ (ring O)

2. Sulfate conjugation $R{-}OH \longrightarrow R{-}O{-}\overset{O}{\underset{O}{S}}{-}OH$

3. N-acetyl cysteine conjugation (mercapturic acid)

4. Methylation (X = N, S, or O) $R{-}XH \longrightarrow R{-}X{-}CH_3$

5. Glycine conjugation $R{-}COOH \longrightarrow R{-}\overset{O}{C}{-}NH{-}CH_2{-}COOH$

6. Acetylation $R{-}NH_2 \longrightarrow R{-}NH{-}\overset{O}{C}{-}CH_3$

Figure 9.3. Synthesis (phase II) reactions. (Reprinted by permission from Gerson B. *Essentials of Therapeutic Drug Monitoring*. New York: Igaku-Shoin, 1983.)

mic reticulum (it is a microsomal enzyme). This enzyme activity is present also in kidney, intestine, skin, brain, and spleen. Conjugation may occur at OH, NH, S, or ester sites. The glucuronide derivatives of various substances may be excreted either in urine or bile, depending on their polarity and molecular weight. Molecular weights greater than 300 and low water solubility (relatively low polarity) favor biliary excretion. Glucuronides are secreted by the active transport mechanism for anions. Those eliminated via the biliary route may subsequently become substrate for intestinal beta-glucuronidase, which hydrolyzes the glucuronide and liberates substrate that may (or may not) be reabsorbed.

Sulfuric acid esters or ethereal sulfates may be formed by the reaction of phenolic and aliphatic hydroxyl groups and of certain amino groups with activated sulfate. The responsible enzymes are found in the soluble fraction (cytoplasm) of the liver cells. The final step is catalyzed by a sulfotransferase of which there are several with various specificities. Sulfation occurs either at an O or NH site.

Age affects biotransformation. Glucuronidation is not fully developed in preterm infants. Sulfate conjugation, however, is approximately at adult levels. Both premature and full-term neonates ex-

hibit especially deficient hepatic metabolic capacity for the first 15 days of life. This is in part due to differences in hemodynamics relative to adults as well as to reduced activity and number of enzymes. Immaturity of the glucuronyl transferase system is responsible for a relative reduction in conjugation activities. Early development of sulfate conjugation activity in some cases compensates for the lack of glucuronyl transferase activity.

The major form of bilirubin within the hepatocyte is the monoglucuronide. The major form in the bile, however, is the diglucuronide. The principal source of bilirubin diglucuronide is a transesterification catalyzed by a canalicular membrane-associated enzyme. Two molecules of the monoglucuronide are dismutated into one molecule of bilirubin diglucuronide, and one molecule of unconjugated bilirubin. Additionally, some monoglucuronide acts as substrate for UDPG-T and may be converted to the diglucuronide (8). However, it is not clear whether the conversion of the monoglucuronide to the diglucuronide is catalyzed by the same canalicular membrane enzyme or another enzyme (UDPG-T) (6). Alternatively, a sulfate group may be added by the action of the enzyme sulfotransferase (4). It is the glucuronide esters (mono- and di-) and/or the sulfate ester that is referred to as conjugated bilirubin, and that is secreted by active transport into the bile canaliculi, eventually ending up in the intestines as part of the bile. Of the glucuronides in bile, the diglucuronide accounts for approximately 90%, and the monoglucuronide for approximately 10% (4–6).

Approximately 200 to 300 milligrams of bilirubin is produced daily by a healthy adult (3,6). To be excreted, the bilirubin must be in a water-soluble form, that is, conjugated as the glucuronide or sulfate form. Almost all of the bilirubin formed is eliminated in the feces. Urine normally contains very little bilirubin. Bilirubin in serum classically is referred to as direct and indirect. This terminology is rooted in the historical observation that normal serum bilirubin would react with diazotized sulfanilic acid (Ehrlich diazo reagent) only after the addition of alcohol (4,5,10). Bile pigment, it was noted in contrast, would react without the addition of alcohol. This led to the terminology "direct" for bilirubin that would react rapidly without the addition of alcohol (or some other promoter with contemporary methods) and "indirect" for that which would react rapidly only with the addition of alcohol (11). It was clear to early investigators that some change occurs to bilirubin within the liver. Clinical laboratory methods for quantification of bilirubin based on the diazo reaction are still in wide use in modern clinical laboratories, perhaps being the most commonly employed at this time.

The indirect bilirubin is unconjugated albumin bound in transit to the liver. Unconjugated bilirubin is not water soluble, and so will not react with the diazo reagent without the addition of alcohol, in which both are soluble. Being bound to albumin, unconjugated bilirubin generally does not appear in urine except in trace quantities; it should normally not be filtered by the glomerulus or be secreted by the renal tubules. Direct bilirubin reacts rapidly with the diazo reagent without the requirement that alcohol be added. Direct bilirubin is 75% to 95% diglucuronide, the rest consisting of other slightly less water-soluble compounds, including bilirubin sulfates and monoglucuronides (4,6,12). It is both protein-bound and free (not protein-bound) so that it may be filtered by the glomerulus and be excreted into the urine in situations in which it appears in excess in the serum.

The classification of direct and indirect bilirubin has persisted even with modern clinical laboratory methods. Although the above classic description persists in the practice of medicine, five species of bilirubin have been identified in human serum: unconjugated, monoglucuronide, diglucuronide, sulfates, and delta-bilirubin (13,14). Classical direct bilirubin consists of monoglucuronide, diglucuronide, sulfates, and delta-bilirubin (8,14). Delta-bilirubin is the fraction of serum bilirubin that is covalently bound to albumin, but reacts directly with the diazo reagents of modern bilirubin quantification techniques employing such reagents (8,11). Delta-bilirubin comprises only less than 20% of total serum bilirubin in adults with no hepatobiliary disorders, or with disorders characterized by disorders associated with increases primarily of the unconjugated fraction (8,11). Delta-bilirubin may, however, comprise more than 50% of total serum bilirubin in conditions associated with elevations of conjugated bilirubin. The clinical role of quantification of delta-bilirubin is not established at the time of this writing, although work toward that end is in progress (8,11,14).

Total serum bilirubin fluctuates with gender and with age (4,13,15). With the understanding that there are variations among methods in use in clinical laboratories, normal total bilirubin in serum is 1.0 milligram/decaliter or less, almost exclusively unconjugated (3–5,13). Enough of this unconjugated bilirubin may behave in laboratory methods like conjugated bilirubin to result in an apparent "normal" direct bilirubin of approximately 0.2 to 0.4 mg/dl. It should be noted that discussions of bilirubin variously refer to either serum or plasma concentrations. Serum and plasma concentrations are interchangeable for total bilirubin (4,16). The normal variation of total serum bilirubin is important to keep in mind when interpreting clinical laboratory results. Normal within-day variation may be 14%, and day-to-day variation may be 22% for an individual patient (4,12). Individual-to-individual variation is great also, being reported as high as 47% (4,13,17). A frequently overlooked cause of intraindividual variation of serum bilirubin is fasting, although it was described in 1906. Fasting elevates bilirubin in well and ill individuals, possibly causing normal levels to go into the abnormal ranges (18).

There are potential interferences with the various methods used to quantify bilirubin. The physician should check with the laboratory to see which apply to the particular method in use. Hemolysis may lead to an artificially elevated "bilirubin" due to hemoglobin undergoing the same diazo reaction as does bilirubin. This is particularly likely to be encountered when collecting specimens from neonates, or when using any capillary blood samples. Hyperuricemia, the presence of caffeine, the presence of any of several drugs (phenazopyridine, rifapicin, theophylline, l-dopa, alpha-methyldopa), and the presence of biologic substances (histidine, tyrosine, vitamin A, xanthophylline) may cause apparent increases of bilirubin (4,13). Lipemia, as well, is a recognized potential interference with bilirubin quantification methods (4).

When bilirubin's concentration in the serum rises, the pigment begins to be deposited in the sclera of the eyes and in the skin. This visible yellow color is referred to as jaundice, alternatively as icterus (3,19). Visible jaundice relates to total serum bilirubin levels of approximately 2.5 mg/dl (5,6). There are many classifications of jaundice to be found in the literature. One of the more frequently employed is based on the presumed site of the physiologic or anatomic abnormality. Using this scheme, jaundice is classified as prehepatic, hepatic, or posthepatic. Jaundice may be due to increases of either unconjugated and/or conjugated bilirubin. This is the basis of an alternative classification of jaundice, using the classical indirect and direct nomenclature. An unconjugated jaundice is one in which greater than 80% of the total serum bilirubin is indirect. A classification incorporating aspects of both classifications is presented in Table 9.1.

Excess bilirubin being presented to the liver is the etiology of prehepatic, unconjugated hyperbilirubinemia (Fig. 9.4). Hemolysis is the most common cause of this type of jaundice. In the adult this usually results from the premature breakdown of erythrocytes and/or ineffective erythropoiesis. Total serum bilirubin generally does not exceed 4 mg/dl. The reason that indirect, unconjugated bilirubin is predominant is that the production of bilirubin exceeds the bilirubin biotransformation capacity of the liver. Physiologic jaundice of the newborn is a not uncommon unconjugated hyperbilirubinemia. Newborns typically have serum unconjugated bilirubin concentrations that are greater than those of healthy adults. About half of newborns may become clinically jaundiced during the first 5 days of life (6). Idiopathic, physiologic neonatal hyperbilirubinemia may result from he-

Table 9.1. Classification of Hyperbilirubinemia

Unconjugated (indirect bilirubin)
  Prehepatic
    Overproduction of erythrocytes
      Hereditary spherocytosis
      Neonates
    Defective globin synthesis (hemoglobinopathy, thalassemia)
    Feto-maternal incompatibility
    Hemolysis
    Ineffective erythropoiesis
    Physiologic neonatal jaundice[a]
  Hepatic
      (hepatocellular)
    drugs (some)
    Crigler-Najjar syndrome
    Gilbert's syndrome
    Physiologic neonatal jaundice[a]

Conjugated (direct)
  Hepatic
    Drugs, some
    Hepatocellular diseases (including viral, toxic, alcoholic hepatitis)
    Dubin-Johnson syndrome
    Rotor's syndrome
  Posthepatic: extrahepatic obstruction

[a] This appears in prehepatic and hepatic hyperbilirubinemia because of the heterogeneous causes. See text.

molysis, ineffective erthyropoiesis, or increased heme hepatic catabolism (4,20). Bilirubin toxicity in the neonate results from the conversion of unconjugated bilirubin to an insoluble acid derivative that forms a complex with membrane-associated phospholipids, particularly those of nerve cell mitochondria (4,21). Concentrations of unconjugated bilirubin in serum exceeding 15 mg/dl are encountered in approximately 5% of neonates (6). The risk of kernicterus in this setting appears when serum concentrations reach the 18 to 20 mg/dl range (4). The risk may be present at lower concentrations if albumin's binding capacity for bilirubin is diminished for any reason (competition by drugs, etc.) (4,22).

The problem in hepatic jaundice caused by unconjugated bilirubin is either removal from the blood, or conjugation within the liver. Gilbert's syndrome (nonhemolytic unconjugated hyperbilirubinemia) is characterized by impaired uptake of bilirubin by hepatocytes due to a reduction of binding sites (4). There is also a reduction of clearance of bilirubin by hepatocytes and decreased UDPG-T activity. The prevalence of Gilbert's syndrome is approximately 4% to 5% (23). It may be the most common cause of isolated hyper-

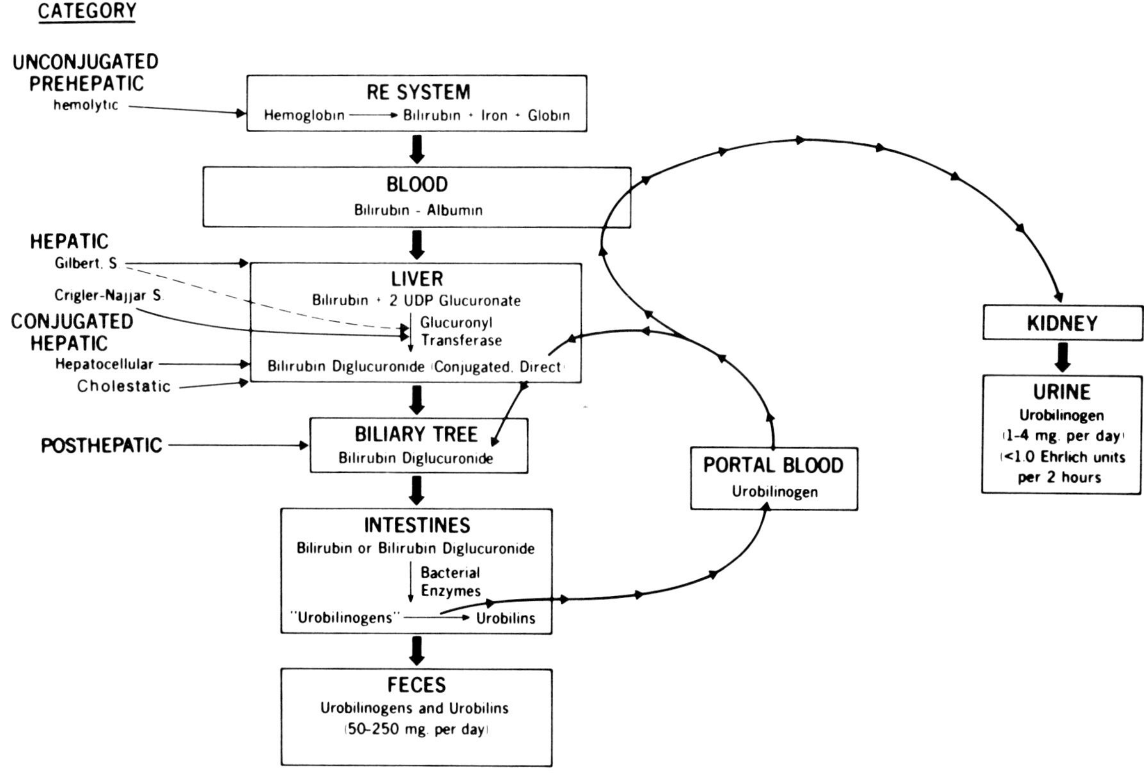

Figure 9.4. Schematic representation of bilirubin metabolism. The classification of jaundice is shown on the left, the arrows pointing to the site of the physiologic defect responsible for the respective category of jaundice. (Reprinted by permission from Zimmerman H. Function and integrity of the liver. In: Henry JB, ed. *Clinical Diagnosis and Management by Laboratory Methods*, 17th ed. Philadelphia: WB Saunders, 1984.)

bilirubinemia (24). Affected patients have mild icterus but are relatively asymptomatic. A useful guideline is that total serum bilirubin usually is less than 3 mg/dl in this entity, although it may be as high as 10 mg/dl (4,6). There are two types of Gilbert's syndrome. Type I is inherited as an autosomal-recessive trait. There are no glucuronide derivatives in the bile, and there is no response to a phenobarbital challenge. The more common type II Gilbert's syndrome is transmitted as an autosomal dominant. In this entity, the total bilirubin concentration in serum is lower. There are glucuronide derivatives in the bile and there is a response to phenobarbital resulting in normalization of the bilirubin concentration (4). A more serious abnormality is Crigler-Najjar syndrome, which results from a deficiency of the enzyme UDPG-T. There are two subtypes of the syndrome. Complete absence of the enzyme, type I, is rare. Bile is colorless as no conjugated bilirubin is

formed. Total serum bilirubin concentrations of 20 to 50 mg/dl are expected (6). This disease is uniformly fatal, with patients typically dying in infancy due to the development of kernicterus. A less severe deficiency, type II, is characterized by the formation of some conjugated bilirubin. The total serum bilirubin concentration typically is less than 20 mg/dl. Some drugs may also cause this type of jaundice (Table 9.2).

Conjugated jaundice may be subdivided into hepatic and posthepatic types. The hepatic type includes several inherited and acquired defects, as well as being the result of some drugs. Dubin-Johnson syndrome and Rotor's syndrome are two hereditary disorders of defective excretion of bilirubin by the hepatocyte, resulting in elevations of conjugated bilirubin in serum. Dubin-Johnson syndrome is caused by a defect in the transport of bilirubin glucuronides from the endoplasmic reticulum to the bile canaliculi of the hepatocyte

Table 9.2. Drugs Associated with Hepatotoxicity

Cholestasis		
Aminosalicylic acid	Erythromycin estolate	Oral contraceptives
Androgens	Estrogens	Penicillin
Azathioprine	Gold sodium thiomalate	Phenothiazines
Benzodiazepines	Imipramine	Progestins
Carbamazepine	Meprobamate	Propoxyphene
Carbarsone	Methimazole	Sulfonamides
Chlorpropamide	Nicotinic acid	Sulfones
Hepatocellular injury		
Acetaminophen	Ethionamide	Penicillin
Allopurinol	Halothane	Phenazpyridine
Aminosalicylic acid	Ibuprofen	Phenobarbital
Amitriptyline	Indomethacin	Phenylbutazone
Androgens	Iron salts	Phenytoin
Asparaginase	Isoniazid	Probenecid
Aspirin	MAO inhibitors	Procainamide
Azathioprine	Mercaptopurine	Propylthiouracil
Carbamazepine	Methotrexate	Pyrazinamide
Chlorambucil	Methoxyflurane	Quinidine
Chloramphenicol	Methyldopa	Sulfonamides
(occasional)	Mithramycin	Tetracyclines
Chlorpropamide	Nicotinic acid	Trimethadione
Dantrolene	Nitrofurantoin	Valproic acid
Disulfiram	Oral contraceptives	Warfarin (rare)
Estrogens	Papaverine	
Ethanol (excess)	Paramethadione	

Abbreviations: MAO, monoamine oxidase.

(8,25). More common causes of jaundice of this type are the various forms of hepatitis (viral, toxic, alcoholic) and other hepatocellular diseases.

Posthepatic jaundice refers to extrahepatic mechanical obstruction of the flow of bile into the intestines. Examples of causes of this type of conjugated hyperbilirubinemia include choledocholithiasis, various tumors (carcinomas of the head of the pancreas, common bile duct, ampulla of Vater, and others), fibrosis of the head of the pancreas, and common bile duct strictures (6). Conjugated bilirubin in serum rises and there is a loss of normal fecal color (becoming so-called "clay colored") when bile ceases to flow into the intestines. As would be expected, conjugated bilirubin appears in the urine, and urine urobilinogen concentrations decrease (see below) (3,19,26).

The detection of bilirubin in the urine is useful. If present, it indicates an excess of conjugated bilirubin in the serum of a jaundiced patient. The etiology may still be hepatic or posthepatic. There are situations in which bilirubin may be present in the urine of a patient who is not jaundiced. These include early anicteric hepatitis, metastatic carcinoma, and early obstruction of the biliary tree (4).

Keep in mind that the detection of bilirubin in the urine is not quantitative, and that there are different sensitivities among the various methods in use in clinical laboratories.

Urobilinogen

Bilirubin glucuronides are hydrolyzed (become unconjugated) by the action of beta-glucuronidase after entering the intestinal tract. The sources of the enzyme are hepatocytes, intestinal epithelium, and bacteria. The unconjugated bilirubin is subsequently reduced, resulting in a group of pigments collectively referred to as the urobilinogens: stercobilinogen, mesobilinogen, and urobilinogen. Subsequent oxidation converts the colorless urobilinogens to red-brown stercobilin, mesobilin, and urobilins (see Fig. 4.2) (3,4,6). Some of the urobilinogens, usually less than 10% but sometimes up to 20%, are reabsorbed into the portal circulation to be reexcreted by the liver into the bile (6). A small portion remains in the blood and is excreted in the urine after being filtered by the kidney. The formation of urobilinogen is decreased in all conditions in which liver secretion or the biliary drain-

Table 9.3. Urobilinogen in Urine

Decreased
Complete biliary obstruction
Increased
Cholangitis
Hemolysis, hemolytic anemias
Hemorrhage into tissues
Hepatic parenchymal (hepatocellular) damage

age of bilirubin is impaired (6). Conditions characterized by decreased load of urobilinogen returning to the liver, as in biliary obstruction, would be expected to show a decrease of urine urobilinogen; conversely, nonobstructive causes ordinarily would be expected to show increased urine urobilinogen (see Fig. 9.4) (6). Fecal urobilinogen, as quantified in the usual clinical laboratory procedures, is the total of urobilinogen and urobilin (4). Fecal urobilinogen likewise is diminished with biliary obstruction. Approximately half of the secreted conjugated bilirubin is biotransformed to substances other than the urobilinogens (6). Although urobilinogen may be quantified in the urine or in the feces, the value of this in patient care is of questionable value (6). It appears that the result of this clinical laboratory test adds no information to that obtainable by alternative means. Concentrations in urine are decreased in posthepatic (obstructive) jaundice, and in some situations involving hepatic jaundice (Table 9.3). Elevated levels may be seen in nonjaundiced patients in cases involving cirrhosis of the liver, metastatic carcinoma, and congestive heart failure. Marked fecal urobilinogen decreases (less than 5 milligrams per 24 hours) characterize posthepatic (obstructive) jaundice, but moderate decreases may be seen also with hepatocellular disease. Hemolysis may lead to marked elevation (greater than 250 mg/24 hr) of fecal urobilinogen.

Bile Acids

Bile has several constituents: bile pigments, primarily bilirubin esters; bile acids or salts; cholesterol; and various other substances derived from the blood (3). Although up to 3 L of bile may be produced per day, only approximately 1 liter is excreted. About 500 to 600 milliliters of bile enters the duodenum each day. Some of the constituents of bile have an important role in the digestion and absorption of lipids.

Cholesterol is synthesized continually by all tissues, but primarily by the liver and the small intestine (6). The cholesterol undergoes a variety of biotransformations with a portion resulting in the endogenous anions known as bile acids. Production of bile acids, along with the ability of the bile acids to solubilize additional cholesterol, are the major mechanisms of cholesterol elimination from the body (6). The bile acids contain one, two, or three hydroxy groups at positions 3, 7, and 12 and a carboxyl group at the end of the side chain. The primary bile acids, cholic (3, 7, 12 hydroxy) and chenodeoxycholic acids (3, 7 hydroxy), are derived from cholesterol in the liver. They are conjugated subsequently at the carboxylic acid carbon with the amino acids glycine or taurine. The bile acid conjugates are referred to as the bile salts. The primary bile acids, then, are found in four forms: cholyltaurine, cholylglycine, chendeoxycholyltaurine, and chenodeoxycholylglycine. The conjugates of the primary bile acids are more polar (water soluble) than are the unconjugated forms. The glycine conjugates predominate by 3:1 or 4:1 in healthy individuals. Unconjugated bile acids are not present in bile (6). The secretion of bile acids generates osmotic water flow and is a major factor regulating bile formation and flow (6). The excretion of the bile salts is by active transport into the canaliculi. Bile acids are stored in the gallbladder where they become concentrated by up to 10-fold between meals or during fasting (3). Up to 95% of the total body bile acid pool is contained within the gallbladder under conditions of fasting, at which point serum bile acid concentrations are at their lowest (6). Bacterial enzyme (7-alpha-dehydroxylase) action within the terminal ileum and colon results (by dehydration) in the formation of the secondary bile acids, and deoxycholic and lithocolic acids (Figs. 9.5, 9.6).

The bile acids undergo enterohepatic recirculation (see Fig. 9.6). Two mechanisms are involved. The predominant mechanism is active transport of all of the conjugated bile acids, and occurs in the distal ileum (6). The second mechanism is passive (nonionic) diffusion in the jejunum and colon. As such, the relative abilities of each of the bile acids to be reabsorbed is dependent on their relative pKa's, which determine their degree of ionization at any given pH within the jejunum. It is the unconjugated bile acids plus the glycine conju-

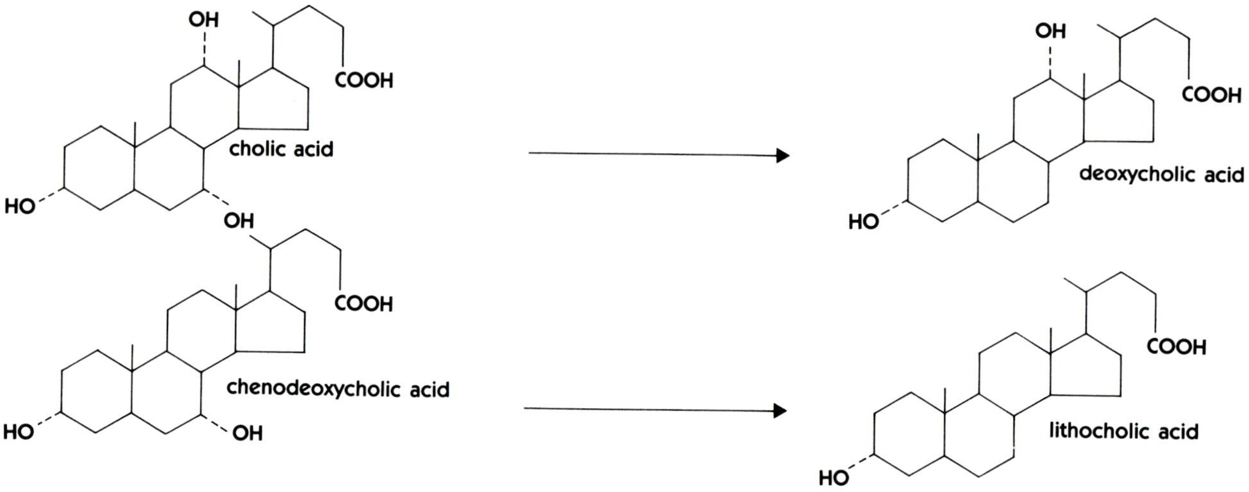

Figure 9.5. Primary and secondary bile acids. The secondary bile acids are derived from the primary bile acids due to the enzymatic (7-alpha-dehydroxylation) action by the normal flora of the gastrointestinal tract.

gates of the dihydroxy bile acids (-cholic and -chenodeoxycholic) that will be nonionized and therefore be reabsorbed by passive diffusion under these conditions (6). Passive reabsorption of the secondary bile acids takes place in the colon. Passive reabsorption of the chenodeoxycholic acid conjugate takes place in the jejunum (5). This enterohepatic recirculation (see Fig. 9.6) takes place from two to five times daily (19,27). The approximate proportions of the bile acids in normal bile of an adult are 38% cholate conjugates, 34% chenodeoxycholate conjugates, 28% deoxycholate conjugates, and 1% to 2% lithocholate conjugates (6).

Once in the portal vein, the bile acids are tightly bound to protein. Although the portal vein concentration of bile acids is very high, the systemic circulation concentrations normally are very low due to the liver's ability to extract them. Approximately 80% of cholic acid and 60% of chenodeoxycholic acid are removed from blood in one pass through the liver. Systemic circulation bile acid concentration may rise after a meal. The relative proportions of the bile acids in the systemic circulation change from fasting to postprandial conditions due to differences in the relative reabsorption of the bile acids by the passive diffusion mechanism described above (6).

Monitoring of bile acids in serum is a sensitive but not specific indicator of liver status. Occult liver disease may cause serum bile acid concentra-

tions to be abnormal even when other "liver function tests" are within their reference (normal) ranges. Bile acids in the systemic circulation, however, reflect the status of not only the liver, but that of the gallbladder and intestines as well since they are part of the enterohepatic recirculation. It is the lack of specificity of derangement of serum bile acid concentrations that has limited the interest in this clinical laboratory procedure. The physician should check with the individual laboratory concerning the particular reference ranges in use at the individual laboratory. Representative reference ranges for serum are: cholic—0.12 to 0.61 microgram per milliliter; cholylglycine—0.12 to 0.14 μg/ml; chenodeoxycholic—0.16 to 0.98 μg/ml; and deoxycholylglycine—0.02 to 0.04 μg/ml.

There have been four approaches to incorporating the monitoring of serum bile acids into patient care: two involve quantification of total bile acids, one involves removal from the sample of a bile acid previously administered to the patient, and the last involves fractionation into the di- and trihydroxy bile acids (5). *Total bile acids* have been quantified in fasting and postprandial serum specimens. Fasting serum concentrations are always elevated in patients with hepatitis (acute and chronic viral, and alcoholic), cirrhosis, posthepatic (obstructive) jaundice, and intrahepatic cholestasis (see Fig. 9.4). It is obvious that although this clinical laboratory finding is sensitive, it is not specific. The fast serum bile and test is useful for

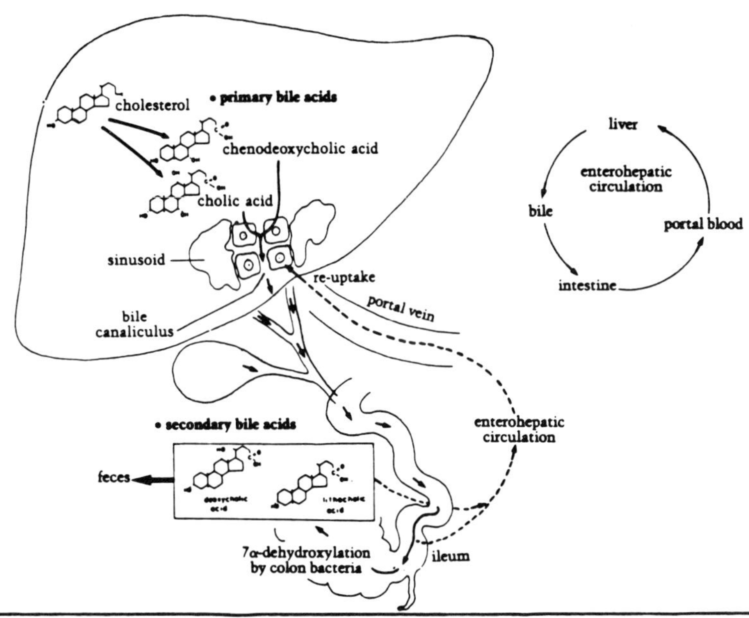

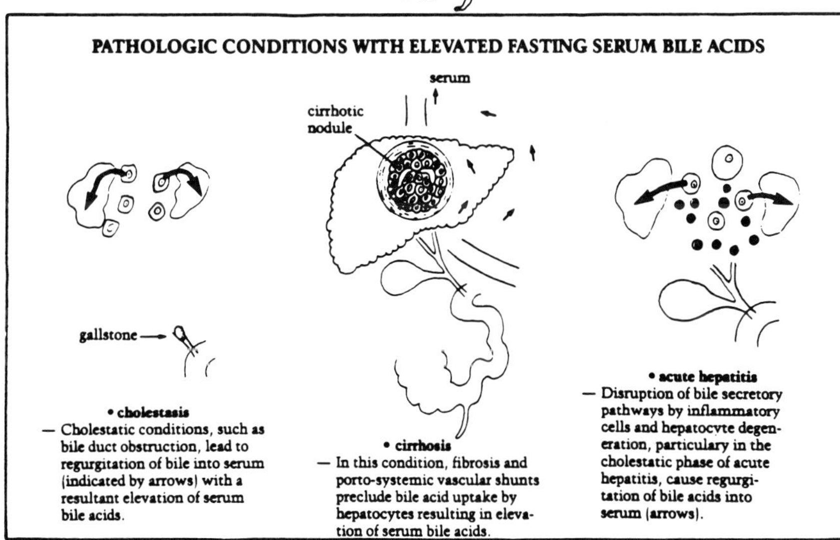

Figure 9.6. Summary of bile acids. (Reprinted by permission from *Lab Report for Physicians*.)

detecting occult portal cirrhosis. The *postprandial test* involves quantifying the bile acids after a meal, and as such may be viewed as an endogenous loading test. This procedure is based on the postprandial contraction of the gallbladder and the fact that the bile acids are concentrated in the bile as described above. All forms of hepatobiliary disease cause an increase of the postprandial rise of serum bile acids. Postprandial testing may be sensitive to hepatobiliary disease, but is of limited value in

differential diagnosis. The *bile acid tolerance test* involves the intravenous administration of exogenous bile acid, either unlabeled cholylglycine or some radiolabeled bile acid. Either the fractional disappearance or a retention at some predetermined time (10 minutes) may be monitored. This is a sensitive technique, the clinical role of which remains to be established. Finally, the *ratio of the dihydroxy to trihydroxy bile acids* may be monitored in serum. The theory behind this approach is attractive. A patient with posthepatic jaundice (obstruction) or intrahepatic cholestasis would be expected to be characterized by elevated total serum bile acid concentrations secondary to the blockage of excretion, and to have a high proportion of the trihydroxy bile acids since hepatocellular function is preserved. This latter is due to the fact that the primary bile acids do not reach the gut to be subject to bacterial action. Conversely, with hepatocellular disease, a decrease of trihydroxy bile acids in the serum would be anticipated. The relative ratios would then be of help in differential diagnosis. For instance, the ratio of cholylglycine (trihydroxy, see Fig. 9.5) to chenodeoxycholylglycine (dihydroxy, see Fig. 9.5) is less than 1 in approximately 80% of patients with hepatocellular disease, and greater than 1 in approximately 80% of pateints with cholestatic disease. As a practical matter, however, technical problems in the quantification of bile acids have precluded wide application of this approach.

Clinical Laboratory Tests Based on Serum Enzymes

Living cells produce enzymes that are biocatalysts and that increase the rate of chemical reactions. The same reactions would occur in tissues, but at a slower rate. Enzymes do not induce reactions that cannot occur. Virtually all important biochemical reactions in the body are enzyme mediated (28).

Enzymes are classified into six groups according to an international classification.

1. Oxidoreductases catalyze a variety of oxidation-reduction reactions, frequently using coenzymes. Included here are enzymes that are referred to as dehydrogenase, oxidase, peroxidase, and reductase.
2. Transferases catalyze various group transfers, such as amino, carboxyl, and acyl. These enzymes are referred to as aminotransferase (alternatively transaminase), acyltransferase, and transcarboxylase.
3. Hydrolases catalyze the cleavage of bonds between carbon and another atom or carbon by the addition of water. These enzymes are referred to as amylase, esterase, peptidase, phosphatase, and urease.
4. Lysases catalyze the cleavage of carbon-carbon, carbon-sulfur, and certain carbon-nitrogen (excluding peptide) bonds. These enzymes are referred to as decarboxylase, lysase, and dehydratase.
5. Isomerases catalyze racemization of optical or geometric isomers and certain intramolecular oxidation-reduction reactions. These enzymes are referred to as epimerase, racemase, and mutase.
6. Ligases catalyze the formation of bonds between carbon and oxygen, sulfur, nitrogen, or other atoms. These enzymes are referred to as synthetase and carboxylase.

For each enzyme, there are two names. The systematic name consists of two parts. The first gives the name of the substrate(s). The second indicates the type of reaction catalyzed by the group of enzymes. If two substrates are involved, both names are used, separated by a colon. The working or practical name is one that is suitable and convenient for daily use. It may or may not be identical to the systematic name or be a modification thereof. It should be noted that the familiar uppercase abbreviations are not recognized or encouraged nomenclature according to the above rules (25,29,30). The practice, however, is well established and widely accepted. The systematic name is associated with a numerical code designation preceded by the letters "EC" standing for Enzyme Commission. The numerical designation of each enzyme consists of four numbers, each separated by periods. The first number defines the class of the enzyme. The next two numbers indicate the subclass and sub-subclass to which the enzyme is assigned. The last number is the specific serial number given to each enzyme in its subsubclass. For alkaline phosphatase (ALP) the designation is EC 3.1.3.1., orthophosphoric acid monoester phosphorylase (Table 9.4).

Some enzymes are widely distributed among tissues. These ubiquitous enzymes include lactate dehydrogenase (LD), aldolase (ALS), phosphohexoisomerase (PHI), and malate dehydrogenase (MD). Other enzymes are characteristic of a limited number of tissues. Ornithine carbamoyl transferase (OCT) and iditol dehydrogenase (ID) are considered to be "liver" enzymes. Creatine kinase (CK) is found in muscle and brain. An increase in the serum activity of a ubiquitous enzyme has less clinical specificity than does an increase of an enzyme with a limited tissue distribution.

Table 9.4. Enzymes of Clinical Interest

Trivial, Common Name	Practical Name	Standard Abbreviation	Systematic Name	EC Code
Aldolase	Aldolase	ALS	D-Fructose-1,6-diphosphate D-glyceraldehyde-3-phosphate lyase	4.2.13
Alkaline phosphatase	Alkaline phosphatase	ALP	Orthophosphoric monoester phosphohydrolase	3.1.3.1
Amylase	Amylase	AMS	α_1,4-Glucan 4-glucanohydrolase	3.2.1.1
Creatine phosphokinase	Creatine kinase	CK	Adenosine triphosphate: creatine phosphotransferase	2.7.3.2
Glutamate oxalacetate transaminase	Aspartate transaminase	AST	L-Aspartate: 2-oxoglutarate aminotransferase	2.6.1.1
Isocitrate dehydrogenase	Isocitrate dehydrogenase	ICD	L-Isocitrate: NADP oxidoreductase (decarboxylating)	1.1.1.42
Lactate dehydrogenase	Lactate dehydrogenase	LD	L-Lactate: NAD oxidoreductase	1.1.1.27
Lipase	Lipase Triacylglycerol lipase	LPS	Triacylglycerol acyl-hydrolase	3.1.1.3
Pseudocholinesterase	Cholinesterase	CHS	Acylcholine acyl-hydrolase	3.1.1.8

Abbreviations: NAD, nicotinamide-adenine dinucleotide; NADP, nicotinamide-adenine dinucleotide phosphate.

The enzymes found in the systemic circulation of patients are derived from the various tissues of the body (see Table 9.4). They gain access from intact as well as from injured or disrupted cells. The release of enzymes into the circulation does not require coincident tissue necrosis. Increase of permeability of cell membranes, considered to be reversible, without identifiable damage, is widely accepted as the explanation for this phenomenon. An example of this phenomenon occurring under "normal" circumstances is the changes in skeletal muscle permeability under the conditions of contraction and relaxation. Irreversible permeability of cell membranes, however, characterizes cell death.

Enzymes normally are present in serum in such small quantities that the enzyme activity rather than the amount is measured. The activity generally is measured by the rate at which a reaction involving a particular substrate is catalyzed. Various inhibitors and/or activators may be important as well.

The activity in serum of any specific enzyme or isoenzyme may be increased or decreased relative to a reference (normal) range. Increases may be due to (1) an increase in release from tissue(s), (2) an increase in the intracellular concentration available for release, (3) an increase in the tissue mass producing the enzyme, (4) a decrease in the normal elimination (degradation and/or excretion) processes. Decreases result from (1) a decrease in enzyme production, either as a primary or acquired deficiency; (2) the presence of inhibitors; (3) a lack of necessary cofactors.

The fate of enzymes released into serum is not completely understood. A trivial amount may be retaken up for reuse. Excretion accounts for a small amount of the clearance from serum of enzymes. Some other mechanism, such as phagocytosis by macrophages, accounts for the majority of such clearance.

Enzymes that are quantified by their activity in human serum may be segregated into four groups as they relate to liver function (5). Group I is comprised of those enzymes that tend to be characterized by higher serum activities (levels) with obstructive jaundice than with acute hepatitis. The members of this group that are commonly available for quantification by clinical laboratories are ALP and gamma-glutamyl transpeptidase (GGT). Other members of this group are 5'-nucleotidase (5'-NT) and leucine aminopeptidase (LAP). Group II is comprised of those enzymes that tend to be characterized by higher serum activities with acute hepatitis than with obstruction. The commonly available members of this group are aspartate aminotransferase (AST), formerly referred to as serum glutamate oxaloacetic transaminase (SGOT); and alanine aminotransferase (ALT), formerly referred to as serum glutamate pyruvic transaminase (SGPT). Other members of this group include OCT, isocitric dehydrogenase (ICD), aldolase (ALS), iditol (sorbitol) dehydrogenase (ID), and others. Group III is comprised of those enzymes that tend to be characterized by only slightly elevated or normal serum activities with both acute hepatitis and obstruction. The commonly available

Table 9.5. Examples of Reference Ranges of Total ALP Activity

Method	Substrate	Reference Range (U)	Equivalent IU[a]	SI Units (nkat/L)
Bodansky's	B-Glycerophosphate	1.5–4.0/dl	8–22 mIU/ml	135–370
Shinowara's	B-Glycerophosphate	2.2–6.5/dl	15–35 mIU/ml	250–585
King-Armstrong	Phenylphosphate	3.7–13.0/dl	25–72 mIU/ml	420–1540
Bessey's	p-Nitrophenylphosphate	0.8–2.9/1000 ml	13–38 mIU/ml	220–635

[a] Approximations.

members of this group include lactate dehydrogenase (LD), creatine phosphokinase (CK), and lipase. Group IV is comprised of those enzymes that tend to be characterized by decreased serum activity with acute hepatitis and normal or slightly decreased activity with obstruction. The only common available member of this group is cholinesterase.

As a practical matter, the enzymes that usually are regarded as being most useful for the evaluation of the liver are ALT and AST, alkaline phosphatase, and GGT. These enzymes may be divided into three groups: (1) membrane-bound, (2) cytosolic, and (3) mitochondrial. ALP and GGT are membrane-bound glycoprotein enzymes.

Alkaline Phosphatase

ALP was among the first of the enzymes in which there was interest in quantification in serum as indicators of clinical status. It was noted more than 50 years ago that total serum ALP activity would fluctuate with osseous as well as hepatobiliary disease (31,32). ALP is found most richly in the sinusoids and the endothelium of the central vein and periportal veins, with smaller concentrations being found in the biliary canaliculi (33).

The phosphatases are relatively nonspecific hydrolytic enzymes (they belong to the hydrolase group of the international classification) that catalyze the cleavage of phosphoryl (phosphate) bonds. It should be appreciated that the phosphatases are not one enzyme but a group of related enzymes. Three types of phosphatases are commonly recognized: ALK with optimal activity at approximately pH 8.6 to 10.3, acid phosphatase with optimal activity at pH 4.9 to 5.0, and red cell phosphatase with optimal pH at 5.5 to 6.0 (29).

More than one ALP form is present in almost every serum of normal healthy individuals. Liver and bone type of ALP almost always are present in

sera from normal individuals, although the bone ALP activity may be low in some adults' sera. The relative serum activities of each vary with age (34).

The reference (normal) range for total ALP activity in serum depends on the quantification procedure that is performed (Table 9.5). The physician should check with the individual laboratory to determine the particular range in use. The range of total ALP activities in serum observed among normal individuals is wide. Distribution is such that a change of approximately 41 units per liter for men and 50 U/L for women [para-nitrophenylphosphate (PNPP) as substrate, 37 degrees C] must be observed to qualify as a reference change; a reference change for this purpose for healthy individuals is a difference between two successive values that would be statistically significant, $p \le$ 0.05, in 95% of such persons (36–42). The intraindividual within-day biologic variation is about 4%, while day-to-day variation is as high as 8% to 10% (39–44).

Age, sex, and sex-related factors (i.e., puberty, menopause) are well recognized as being very influential on total serum ALP activity (see Table 9.6). Total ALP as well as bone ALP activities in serum are greater in children than in adults. The relative proportion of bone-derived ALP in serum is greater when normal bone growth is occurring, and so is greater in children's and adolescents' than in normal adults' sera. This is due to ossifi-

Table 9.6. Examples of Reference Values for ALP[a]

Source	Patient's Age				
	2–13 yr (%)	2–15 yr (%)	13–17 yr (%)	18–30 yr (%)	Adult (%)
Intestinal	12	1.7–12	1.5	8.5	8
Liver	9	8–9	11.5	33.5	25
Bone	77	80–89	87	58	67

[a] The data in this table are presented as examples of typical results encountered.

from chondroblasts and osteoblasts (45). The higher total serum ALP activity of children relative to adults reflects not only bone growth but that of connective tissue in general (45). This activity is relatively stable up to approximately age 10 years. Total serum ALP activity peaks in boys at approximately age 15 years, decreasing to adult levels by approximately age 20 years. For girls, the peak is reached at approximately age 12 years, decreasing to adult levels by approximately age 18 years (40,45). From a quantitative point of view the activities of the intestinal and liver fractions are independent of age. Changes in total serum ALP activity with age are due mainly to fluctuations of bone ALP (40,46). The liver component of normal total serum ALP activity increases with age, with a late increase of bone activity noted in the elderly (47). The liver form of ALP found in the sera of normal individuals is derived from hepatic endothelial cells (48). Total ALP activity in serum is linked to sexual maturity; moreover, only the bone isoenzyme activity is altered with the change in hormonal state of the individual, at least for girls. Bone-derived ALP is correlated with height and weight in young people (40). Height and weight do not influence adult total ALP levels, except in cases of obesity in women. Bone, though not liver, ALP activity in serum is lower in girls who have not achieved menarche than in their age-matched counterparts who have (40). There is a slight increase of liver isoenzyme with age, plus a difference of bone-derived ALP activity between men and women (40,46). Statistically significant but clinically unimportant differences in total ALP serum concentrations between the sexes exist at certain ages, but not at others (47,49). In individuals greater than age 20 years, men are characterized by higher total and bone ALP activity in serum. After menopause, this difference is lost, sometimes even reversed. It is most important to realize that the above data are derived from studies of large populations. Application to the individual patient may be inappropriate. The best approach is to have method specific age-adjusted reference ranges for total serum ALP as well as each ALP form.

The mechanisms that primarily account for increases of total serum ALP activity are (1) an increase in the tissue source as well as tissue concentration, as in Paget's disease of bone, osteogenic sarcoma, fracture healing, and rickets; and

(2) decreased elimination, as in obstructive hepatobiliary disease. Patients of blood groups B and O have higher total serum ALP activities than do patients who are group A, while group AB patients are intermediate (Table 9.7). Secretor status is important as well, especially for the intestinal isoenzyme (3,40,47,52,53). It has been demonstrated that a postprandial rise of total serum ALP may be noted in almost all patients. However, the greatest increase from fasting levels is noted in patients who are blood group B or O and who are secretors of ABH blood group substances (52). Nonsecretors of any ABO blood group show little or no change (52). Decreased serum ALP activity due to decreased enzyme production is recognized in the genetically transmitted disease hypophosphatasia (54).

Hypophosphatasia is an inherited condition resembling rickets; it was first described in 1943 (55). It is the major cause of a decreased serum ALP in infants and children. The activities of liver, bone, and kidney ALP are all depressed (56). About 15 to 20 cases of hypophosphatasia in adults have been reported (54). The clinical constellation consists usually of low total serum ALP activity, low leukocyte ALP activity, and elevated serum and urinary phosphoethanolamine concentrations (54). Some patients have manifestations of immunodeficiency. The increased incidence of infections is related to the leukocyte ALP deficiency. Affected patients excrete above-normal amounts of ethanolamine phosphate and inorganic phosphate, consistent with the view that ethanolamine phosphate may be a natural substrate of ALP. The clinical entity of hypophosphatasia may not be homogeneous, as not all patients display all of the expected deficiencies (53). Other changes that may be seen include growth retardation, pseudofractures, deformities due to defective epiphyseal calcification, chondrocalcinosis, and premature loss of deciduous teeth. In its most severe form, there may be no supporting bone for the cranial and thoracic cavities. What ALP activity there is in serum appears to be derived from intestine. Affected patients may display a postprandial rise in serum ALP activity (53). Other causes of decreased serum ALP activity (see Table 9.5) are deficiencies of Mg^{2+} or An^{2+}, pernicious anemia (returning to normal after vitamin B_{12} administration), hypothyroidism, cachexia, and high serum inorganic phosphate. Thyroid hormone and vitamin B_{12} are re-

Table 9.7. Total Serum Alkaline Phosphatase Activity

Increased	Decreased
Biliary tract disease	Deficiencies
Obstruction	Mg^{2+}, Zn^{2+}, O
Primary biliary cirrhosis	Vitamin C
Blood group: higher in individuals of blood	Vitamin B_{12}
groups B, O	Drugs
Bone disease	Antilepileptic
Neoplastic (cancer)	Steroids
Primary neoplasm-osteogenic sarcoma	Birth control
Metastatic tumor-osteoblastic lesions	Estrogen-progesterone
Non-neoplastic	Hereditary hypophosphatasia
Acromegaly	Hyperalimentation possibly due to deficiency
Osteitis deoformans (Paget's disease of bone)	Lead
Osteomalacia	Malnutrition-protein deficiency
Fracture healing	Milk-alkali syndrome
Rickets	Myxedema
Drugs	Pernicious anemia
Gastrointestinal diseases	Scurvy
Ulcers, infarction	Thyroid—hypothyroidism
Malabsorption—decreased calcium	Transfusions—whole blood
absorption	Uropathy, obstructive
Ulcerative colitis	Vitamin D excess
Hepatic diseases	Wilson's disease (sometimes)
Focal—space-occupying	
Generalized—hepatitis, fatty liver, mononucleosis	
Hyperphosphatasia	
Intravenous albumin (sometimes)	
Myocardial infarction, failure	
Pancreatitis	
Parathyroid	
Hyperparathyroidism, pseudohyperparathyroidism	
Primary, secondary	
Pseudohyperparathyroidism	
Pregnancy	
Pulmonary infarction	
Renal infarction	
Splenic infarction	
Thyroid	
Hyperthyroidism	
Thyrotoxicosis	

quired for normal osteoblastic function. Attention must always be directed to the possibility of an in vitro interference as discussed previously.

The causes of elevation of total serum ALP are many, making it relatively nonspecific (see Table 4.7) (57–59). The magnitude of the elevation may be useful, keeping in mind that there is a wide range of "normal" among individuals. Total ALP activity in serum tends to be greater in biliary tract disease than in space-occupying lesions of the liver. The variety of hepatobiliary diseases that may elevate total serum ALP activity includes hepatitis (of any etiology), cirrhosis, fatty liver, drug reactions, hepatobiliary obstruction (of any etiology), primary biliary cirrhosis, and space-occupying lesions (including malignant and nonmalignant entities). Injury to the hepatocyte results in an increase of ALP production. ALP of hepatic origin, however, may be from the hepatocytes or from the endothelial cells lining the sinusoids. Elevation in serum of hepatic ALP is a sensitive indicator of cholestasis, but will not differentiate intrahepatic from extrahepatic causes (Table 9.8; see Table 9.7) (60). There are, however, limitations to the sensitivity and therefore the clinical value of total ALP activity determinations (61). Enzyme activity along hepatic sinusoids increases in diseases such as acute and chronic hepatitis and acute extrahepatic biliary obstruction, while activity in canaliculi is unchanged. ALP activity of the canaliculi does increase in association with various malignant tumors, autoimmune (collagen vascular) diseases, centrilobular necrosis, chronic extrahepatic obstruction, and several weeks of moder-

Table 9.8. Guidelines for Magnitude of Total Serum ALP Activity Increases

×2	Hepatitis—acute viral, toxic, alcoholic cirrhosis
	Fatty liver, acute
×5	Infectious mononucleosis
	Postnecrotic cirrhosis
×10	Drug cholestasis
	Biliary obstruction—choledocholithiasis Carcinoma, head of pancreas
×15–20	Primary biliary cirrhosis
	Carcinoma, metastatic or primary to liver
×30–40	Paget's disease of bone

Table 9.9. Gamma-Glutamyl Transferase—Causes of Elevations of Serum Activity[a]

| Liver metastasis |
| Liver tumors |
| Acute pancreatitis |
| Cholestasis |
| Drug-related hepatitis |
| Alcoholic cirrhosis |
| Viral hepatitis |
| Secondary liver injuries |
| Myocardial infarction |
| Hyperlipoproteinemia, type IV |
| Diabetes mellitus |
| Rheumatic diseases |
| Infectious mononucleosis |
| Chronic persistent hepatitis |
| Fatty liver |

[a] These are listed in approximate order of the relative increase that characterizes each (66).

hepatic obstruction, and several weeks of moderate alcohol consumption in normal volunteers (48,62). Although an increase in the synthesis of ALP precedes an increase in total ALP activity in serum, there is some additional factor that determines by how much or even if the serum total ALP will increase (63). Total parenteral nutrition (hyperalimentation) is associated with an increase of synthesis of liver ALP and subsequent increase in serum activity levels (60). A similar rise will be seen in approximately half of patients with uncontrolled diabetes. Interestingly, ALP has been reported to not be elevated in post–liver transplant (pediatric) patients (64).

Gamma-Glutamyltransferase

GGT concentration is greatest in bile canaliculi and the bile duct epithelium of the periportal region. This enzyme may be found in the lipocytes of Disse's space. It is found in other tissues with secretory or absorptive capacity as well: proximal renal tubules and Henle's loop, pancreatic acinar tissue, pancreatic ductules, and intestinal brush borders (65). Liver, spleen, and lungs contain the enzyme as well. Though the exact nature of its physiologic role is unclear, GGT appears to be involved in (1) protein synthesis, (2) glutamine activity, (3) mercapturic acid synthesis, (4) transmembrane transfer of amino acids and peptides, and (5) glutathione hydrolysis.

GGT is very sensitive to impairment of the liver's excretory capacity (Table 9.9). Frequently it is the first abnormal liver function test demonstrated in the serum of heavy drinkers (3). The highest levels are seen in biliary obstruction. The exquisite sensitivity of this marker, however, contributes to a relative lack of specificity. Most hepatobiliary diseases and some nonhepatobiliary disorders can lead to an increase of GGT activity in serum. Nonhepatobiliary causes of elevations include myocardial infarction, acute and chronic pancreatitis, carcinoma of the pancreas, diabetes mellitus, renal insufficiencies, and many others (66). Countless drugs may cause elevations of GGT activity in serum. Social drinkers and patients with minimal liver disease (even biopsy normal) may have elevations of GGT (65). Elevations in the absence of jaundice are considered to be indicative of hepatic neoplasm. Elevations in concert with elevated alkaline phosphatase confirm hepatic disease (67). GGT may be elevated in post–hepatic transplant (pediatric) patients (68). Efforts to improve specificity have generated interest in GGT isoenzymes. There is at this time no clear relationship between the isoenzyme patterns and diagnostic entities (65).

Serum and (heparinized) plasma GGT values are identical. Hemolysis generally does not alter GGT activity in patient specimens when hemoglobin is below 300 mg/dl (66). GGT levels are high in newborns, decreasing quickly by age 2 months, reaching their lowest levels by age 3 years after which they start to increase. However, there is a distinct decrease of activity in men after age 55 years, and in women after age 65 years (66). There is a small difference in the reference (normal) range for men and women. A representative range for men is 8.0 to 35.0 U/L, and for women 5.0 to 25.0 U/L (66). Many clinical laboratories will have only one range that is applied to all adults. The physician should check with the individual laboratory to determine the particular reference range in use.

Aminotransferases

AST and ALT together are referred to as the aminotransferases. AST catalyzes the synthesis and degradation of aspartic acid, resulting in the formation of oxaloacetic acid and 2-oxoglutaric acid. The 2 oxacids thus transformed enter the tricarboxylic acid cycle and are involved indirectly in gluconeogenesis (69). AST is found in almost all tissues, but most richly (in decreasing order) in heart, liver, skeletal muscle, kidney, and brain. Elevations of serum AST in both cardiac and hepatic necrosis have been recognized for a long time (Table 9.10) (5). Striking elevations of AST activity (10–200 times) are seen in the serum of patients with acute hepatic necrosis (viral hepatitis, carbon tetrachloride poisoning, drug-induced injury), while posthepatic jaundice and intrahepatic cholestasis result in less dramatic (10 times) elevations (Fig. 9.7) (5). Of patients with alcoholic cirrhosis, 60% to 70% are characterized by elevations of serum AST (less than 10 times) (5). Chronic active hepatitis may be characterized by serum AST activities that are very low or very high, but in any case indicating the severity of the disease. Metastatic (to the liver) tumors also may or may not be associated with elevations of serum AST activity levels. Lymphoma, leukemia, and infectious mononucleosis (80% of patients with the last) may be associated with elevations of AST. AST may be elevated transiently within a few days of hepatic transplantation, although it may not be a sensitive indicator or predictor of graft function as levels

Table 9.10. Aspartate Aminotransferase—Causes of Elevations of Serum Activity[a]

Hepatitis, acute viral
Hepatitis, toxic
Myopathy
Myocardial infarction, acute
Pulmonary infarction
Hepatitis, chronic active
Hepatitis, alcoholic
Obstructive jaundice
Cirrhosis
Tumors of the liver, primary and metastatic
Secondary hepatic failure
   Hemolytic syndromes
   Leukemia
   Parasitic infections
   Brucellosis

[a] These are listed in approximate order of the relative increase that characterizes each (69).

may remain low in spite of clinical evidence of deterioration (70). AST activity in serum will be below the reference (normal) range in vitamin B_6 deficiency associated with pregnancy or renal dialysis, and in the terminal stage of hepatic diseases. The reference range used by an individual laboratory varies depending on the particular method of quantification employed. Some age and sex variation is to be expected for AST. Representative reference ranges are men, 14 to 35 U/L; women, 13 to 28 U/L. A particular laboratory may employ only one range for all adults.

ALT is involved in the synthesis of and degradation of amino acids (transaminations), and therefore has a role in the metabolism of proteins. Pyruvate is a product of these reactions. The pyruvate can be used in carbohydrate metabolism (via the Embden-Meyerhof pathway) and/or in lipid metabolism. Vitamin B_6, pyridoxal phosphate, is required as a cofactor for ALT (71). ALT is found mostly in liver, but also in kidney and skeletal muscle. ALT generally is considered to be relatively more "liver-specific" (3). It is always higher than AST in acute liver injury uncomplicated by muscle injury or alcoholism (see Fig. 9.7). It may be elevated, however, in nonhepatic clinical entities such as rhabdomyolysis, polymyositis, dermatomyositis, infectious mononucleosis, parasitosis, yellow fever, brucellosis, and primary as well as metastatic hepatic tumors, leukemias, and renal infarction (Table 9.11) (69). Furthermore, ALT activity may fail to rise in the serum of patients with alcohol-related liver disease (72). In contrast, AST is almost always elevated in these latter patients. An AST/ALT ratio of greater than 2 is typical of alcoholic cirrhosis or alcoholic hepatitis.

ALT activity in serum will be elevated (see Table 9.9) in patients with acute viral hepatitis and other causes of hepatic necrosis. ALT is the first enzyme whose activity is increased in serum in acute hepatitis. This increase is seen during the 2 weeks immediately following the clinical onset of the disease, decreasing steadily until the sixth week (71). Posthepatic jaundice and intrahepatic cholestasis result in mild (10–200 times) elevations of serum ALT activity. Less dramatic elevations (less than 10 times) characterize metastatic (to the liver) carcinoma, alcoholic and primary biliary cirrhosis, and alcoholic hepatitis. ALT values are as high or higher than are AST values in acute viral hepatitis,

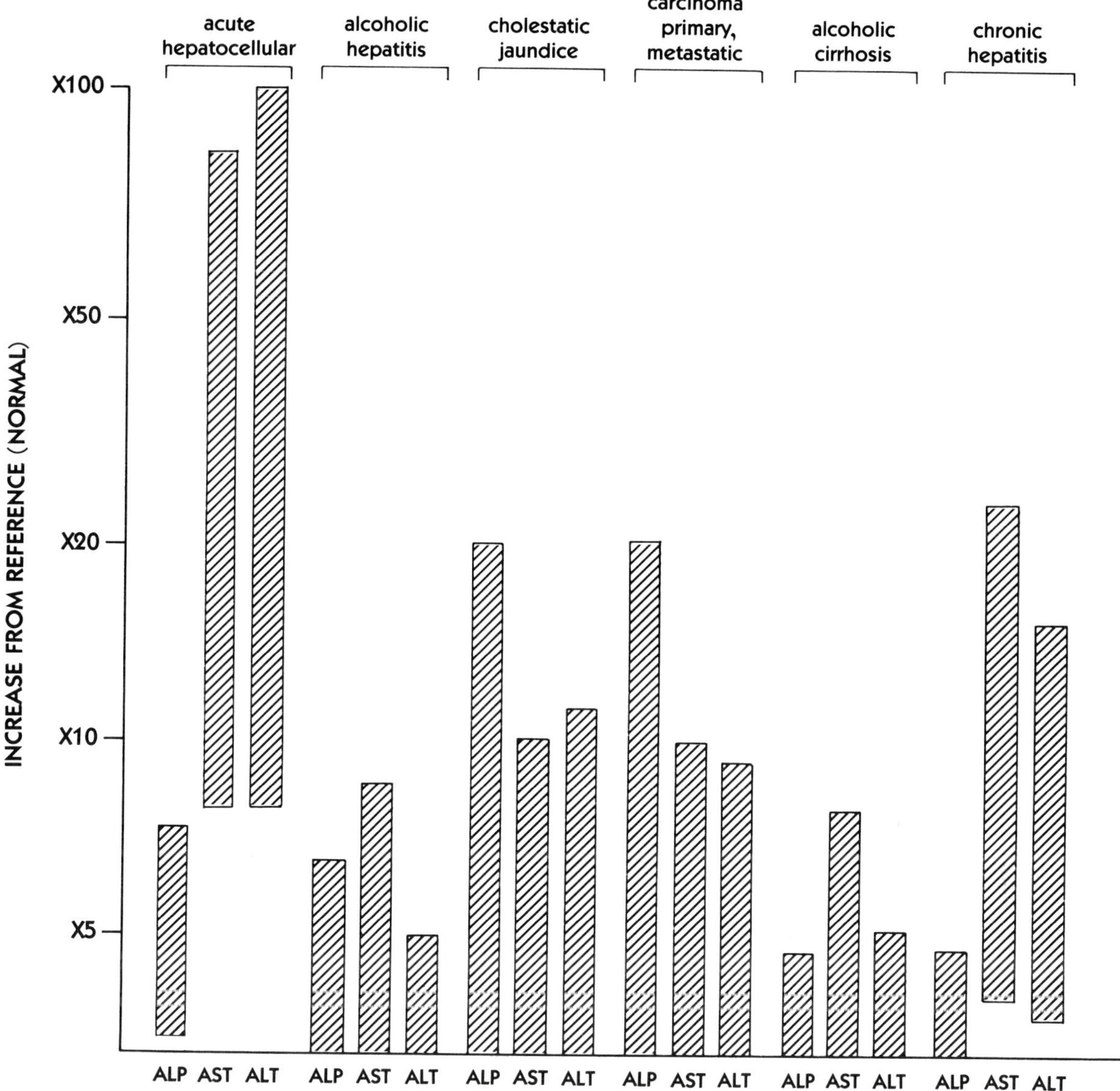

Figure 9.7. ALP, AST, and ALT. The relative ranges of elevation of each of these enzymes in various clinical entities are shown. Note that the baseline is the upper end of the reference (normal) range.

posthepatic jaundice, or intrahepatic cholestasis. They are lower than AST values in cirrhosis, alcoholic hepatitis, and metastatic carcinoma. ALT increases with chronic hepatitis are not as great as those seen with acute hepatitis. In chronic active hepatitis and cirrhosis, ALT activity may display periodic elevations. In cirrhosis, the ALT activity in serum reflects the degree of hepatocellular damage (71). No elevations are seen immediately after myocardial infarction, in contrast to AST. Below reference range (normal) activities in serum may be seen in vitamin B_6 deficiency (associated with pregnancy) and in the terminal stages of hepatic diseases (71). ALT activity in serum varies with age. It is stable in boys from ages 4 to 18, increasing steadily in men to age 45, and decreasing after age 65 years. In women, ALT activity decreases from age 4 to 18 years, increasing to age 65, then

Table 9.11. Alanine Aminotransferase—Causes of Elevations of Serum Activity[a]

Hepatitis, acute viral
Hepatitis, toxic
Hepatic failure by hypoxia
Obstructive jaundice
Hepatitis, chronic alcoholic
Cirrhosis
Tumors of the liver, primary and metastatic
Secondary hepatic failure
Leukemia
Parasitic infections
Infectious mononucleosis
Brucellosis
Myocardial infarction

[a] These are listed in approximate order of the relative increase that characterizes each (71).

decreasing. Overall, ALT levels in women tend to be lower than those in men (71). Interindividual variation in ALT activity is great. The particular reference (normal) range used by a clinical laboratory depends on the particular method employed for quantification. Representative ranges are: men, 14 to 45 U/L; women, 11.5 to 40 U/L (71). A par-ticular laboratory may employ only one range for all adults.

Frequently the aminotransferases are monitored simultaneously. Some generalizations are helpful. Monitoring of aminotransferases is of use in helping to differentiate hepatocellular from posthepatic disease (see Fig. 9.7). Aminotransferase elevations in the absence of acute necrosis or ischemia of another organ suggest hepatocellular damage. Biliary obstruction is associated with minimal or no increases. Mild elevations may be encountered with mild chronic or focal liver diseases such as subclinical or anicteric viral hepatitis, alcoholic cirrhosis, granulomatous diseases, and tumor invasion (3). The most dramatic elevations of AST and ALT are seen with acute viral and then other causes of hepatitis. Elevations greater than 10 times the upper limit of normal are unusual in posthepatic jaundice. Intrahepatic cholestatic diseases are characterized by AST and ALT activity levels similar to those of posthepatic obstruction. Hepatic cirrhosis, even when accompanied by deep jaundice, is characterized by moderate elevation of AST and even less dramatic elevations of ALT. Keep in mind that both of these enzymes, in particular AST, may be elevated on the basis of nonhepatobiliary disease(s) (5).

Clinical Laboratory Tests Based on Hepatic Synthetic Ability

Coagulation

The liver plays a well-recognized central role in the maintenance of hemostasis. Coagulation abnormalities in liver disease sometimes are complex as the liver has more than one role in the production and control of the coagulation and fibrinolytic systems. Most coagulation factors, which are proteins, are synthesized in the liver. Additionally, the activity of some is dependent on vitamin K (Table 9.12). Decreases of the vitamin K–dependent factors (II, VII, IX, X) are the earliest changes seen in liver diseases. Fibrinogen levels may be increased (it may behave as an acute phase reactant, as in acute viral hepatitis, for example) or decreased, depending on the type of liver disease. Vitamin K is required for post-translational carboxylation of the vitamin K factors within hepatocytes (6). The various coagulation factors interact in a modified cascade fashion (Fig. 9.8). Additional proteins important in hemostasis are synthesized in the liver as well: plasminogen, alpha$_2$-antiplasmin, antithrombin III. Severe clotting abnormalities are seen when there is widespread hepatic parenchymal cellular damage. More localized disease involving bile ducts and or malignancy may be characterized by large areas of preserved parenchymal tissue still able to produce coagulation factors in sufficient quantity to maintain hemostasis.

Table 9.12. Coagulation Factors—Those Which Are "Vitamin K–Sensitive" and Those Synthesized in the Liver Are Indicated

Name	No.	Vitamin K–Sensitive	Synthesized in Liver
Fibrinogen	I		+
Prothrombin	II	+	+
Tissue factor	III		
Calcium	IV		
Proaccelerin	V		+
Proconvertin	VII	+	+
Antihemolytic factor	VIII		
Christmas factor	IX	+	+
Stuart-Power factor	X	+	+
Plasma thromboplastin antecedent	XI		+
Hageman's factor	XII		+
Fibrin-stabilizing factor	XIII		+
Prekallikrein factor	PK		+
High-molecular-weight kininogen	HMWK		+

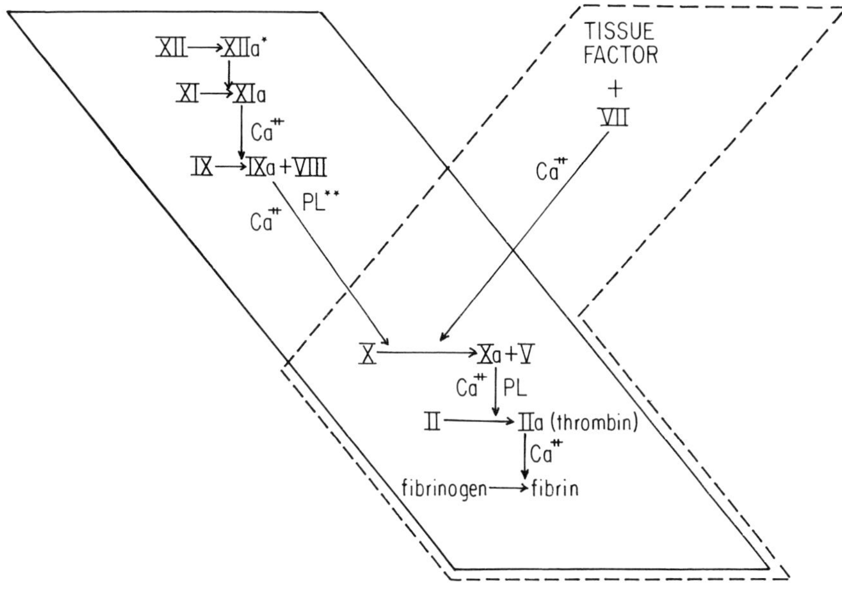

Figure 9.8. Simplified scheme of the coagulation pathways. a*, activated enzymatic factor; PL**, phospholipid. The intrinsic system is outlined by solid lines, the extrinsic system by broken lines. The region common to both is the "final common pathway." (Reprinted by permission from Gerson B. *Essentials of Therapeutic Drug Monitoring*. New York: Igaku-Shoin, 1983.)

The liver also has a role in clearing activated coagulation factors. This influences the fibrinolytic system. The enzyme plasmin is derived from plasminogen via several sources including activated factor XII (XIIa). Liver-related coagulation problems then may be viewed as an imbalance of either not enough synthesis, or not enough clearance (increased fibrinolysis). Plasmin sequentially cleaves bonds in fibrin molecules, releasing fibrin degradation products (FDP), producing clot lysis. FDP may be monitored in patient specimens.

Vitamin K has a well-recognized role in coagulation; it acts in the final steps of hepatic synthesis of coagulation factors II, VII, IX, and X by attaching gamma-carboxyglutamic acid residues at several sites on the respective molecules (see Table 9.12). These residues allow the fixation of Ca^{2+} to a reaction surface in the steps of the coagulation pathway that require formation of complexes on the surface of platelets. In the absence of vitamin K, the factor proteins are still synthesized and enter the circulation with their gamma-carboxyglutamic acid sites missing. These abnormal proteins are called protein-induced vitamin K absence (PIVKA) and possess anticoagulant activity, presumably because they competitively inhibit the remaining normal vitamin K factors. Despite the presence of PIVKA, absence of vitamin K primarily results in a factor deficiency state, that is, decreased concentrations of functional factors II, VII,

IX, and X, rather than a condition produced by a circulating anticoagulant.

In inadequate vitamin K levels, the order of disappearance of factors from the blood is correlated with their half-lives. Factors VII, IX, X, and II have half-lives of 6, 20, 40, and 60 hours, respectively, and disappear in that order. Inadequate diet, biliary obstruction, intestinal malabsorption, and gut sterilization by antibiotics may contribute to clinical vitamin K deficiency. Coumarin anticoagulant effects are similar to vitamin K deficiency, and are detectable after 24 hours due to factor VII deficiency, but are not physiologically maximal until several days have passed and factors IX and X are sufficiently depleted. On vitamin K replacement, the depleted factors return in the same order as their disappearance. Parenteral administration of vitamin K reverses the abnormalities when they are the result of obstruction because the vitamin K, being fat soluble, depends on the presence of bile salts for absorption. Diffuse hepatocellular disease is not responsive to vitamin K administration because of decreased synthetic capacity.

The two most commonly utilized clinical laboratory procedures for the assessment of coagulation are the prothrombin time (PT) and the activated partial thromboplastin time (aPTT), which measure the extrinsic and intrinsic pathways of the coagulation scheme, respectively (Fig. 9.8). There are additional tests of hemostasis that may be of help in special situations. The PT may be abnormal in liver-associated coagulopathy since the test is sensitive to several factors synthesized in the liver (6). The reduction of the vitamin K–dependent factors results in a prolonged PT and, to a lesser extent, a prolonged aPTT. The PT may be prolonged in acute viral hepatitis (or it may be normal), acute liver failure, cirrhosis, Wilson's disease, hemochromatosis, obstructive jaundice, biliary cirrhosis, and hepatoma. The aPTT may be prolonged or normal in acute viral hepatitis and obstructive jaundice. It may be prolonged, shortened, or normal in cirrhosis, Wilson's disease, and hemochromatosis.

The PT is measured simply by adding a source of tissue factor and Ca^{2+} to citrated platelet-poor plasma at 37°C and measuring the time until clot formation. This test measures the "intactness" of the extrinsic coagulation system (see Fig. 9.8), which is dependent on the presence of factors II, VII, and X, three of the four vitamin K factors, as well as factor V and fibrinogen. In respect to monitoring coumarin, it is usually assumed that the two other factors in the extrinsic system, factor V and fibrinogen, are present in adequate concentrations; however, some PT reagents are specifically designed to monitor coumadin therapy and already contain these two factors.

The response to vitamin K as a test useful in the differential diagnosis of jaundice is based on the above. The effect of vitamin K administration on PT helps to distinguish between vitamin K deficiency and hepatocyte synthetic deficiency (5). Administration of vitamin K usually returns a prolonged PT to normal in a patient with deep posthepatic (obstructive) jaundice. Failure of a standard dose of vitamin K to return the PT to normal suggests the presence of intrinsic hepatocellular disease.

The aPTT is performed on citrated plasma by first adding a contact activating agent activating the contact factors (e.g., kaolin, ellagic acid, celite) and a standardized phospholipid preparation as a platelet substitute incubating and then adding a source of Ca^{2+}. The time for clot formation is then measured. The aPTT is prolonged in defects involving the intrinsic pathway (including factors XII, XI, IX, VIII, X, V, II, and fibrinogen) or by inhibitors.

A common approach is to assess the PT, and if prolonged in a deeply jaundiced patient, to administer 10 mg of vitamin K intramuscularly daily for 1 to 3 days. Normalization, if it is to occur, generally is seen by 24 hours, but may take up to 72 hours. There are certain limitations to this approach. Problems of hemostasis will not always be a complication of hepatobiliary disease due to the functional reserve of the liver (6). The PT may be only minimally prolonged in patients with posthepatic jaundice. Furthermore, any "response" to vitamin K administration may be too small to make one comfortable with the response as being conclusive. Another limitation is that intrahepatic disease (intrahepatic cholestasis) may mimic posthepatic disease in that minimal hepatocellar disease may give a response similar to that of posthepatic jaundice. Finally, any cause of malabsorption or the administration of oral antimicrobial agents that affect the bacterial flora may potentiate cause vitamin K deficiency and hypoprothrombinemia. While this approach is still in use, it properly should be considered archaic. Alternative nonclinical laboratory techniques better suited to helping to distinguish intrahepatic from posthepatic disease are available. Testing of a defect of coagulation clearly should not be considered to be a screening procedure. It may be of use in following the progress of disease or of assessing the risk of bleeding before undertaking a traumatic procedure (6). The degree of prolongation of the PT in a patient known to have hepatocellular (intrahepatic) disease is useful as a monitor of the severity of the disease. Dramatic prolongation with acute viral hepatitis is an ominous sign. Similarly, such a change in a patient known to have alcoholic cirrhosis indicates substantial compromise of hepatocellar function.

Clinical Laboratory Tests Based on Metabolic Function

Ammonia, Amino Acids, and Hepatic Coma

The gastrointestinal tract is the main source for ammonia in the systemic circulation (Fig. 9.9) (6). Bacterial (particularly those of the cecum) proteases, ureases, and amine oxidases work on the nitrogen-containing foods and other constituents that are part of the colonic contents, resulting in ammonia. The hydrolysis of glutamine in both the large and small intestines results in ammonia as well. This ammonia, as well as ammonia ingested as ammonium salts, is absorbed into the portal vein (5). The concentration of ammonia in the portal vein is in the range of 5 to 10 times greater than that of the systemic circulation. It is the Krebs-Henseleit urea cycle within the hepatocytes that biotransforms the portal vein derived ammonia. Little ammonia normally escapes the liver into the hepatic vein to get into the systemic circulation (5). Excess ammonia exerts toxic effects on the central nervous system.

Hyperammonemia may be on the basis of any one of several defects. Deficiencies of urea cycle enzymes are the most common cause of hyperammonemia in infants. Other inherited disorders of metabolism involve the biotransformation of dibasic amino acids and the biotransformation of organic acids such as propionic acid, methylmalonic acid, isovaleric acid, and others. The acquired causes of hyperammonemia are hepatic disease (hepatocellular failure as in toxic or fulminant viral hepatitis and Reye's syndrome), or shunting of blood by passing the liver (as in cirrhosis), dramatic gastrointestinal bleeding (enhanced bacterial biotransformation of blood proteins), excess dietary protein, constipation infections, certain drugs, and acid-base imbalance (6).

Special mention should be made of the considerations involving the proper collection of samples for the quantification of ammonia. Ammonia concentration in collected blood rises rapidly due to the enzymatic deamination of labile amides such as glutamine. This artifact can be minimized by taking some precautions (74–76). Venous blood should be drawn into chilled, heparinized collection devices, which are placed into ice water for transport to the laboratory. The patient should be nonsmoking and at rest. Fist clenching and any other activity that might disturb acid base balance should be avoided. Muscular activity can increase venous blood ammonia concentration. The specimen on ice should be delivered to the laboratory within 10 minutes. The reference (normal) range for serum ammonia varies from laboratory to laboratory. Representative values are: mean 42.0 grams per deciliter with a range of 12.0 to 76.5 g/dl (74).

Hepatic coma is an entity associated with hyperammonemia. Its cause, however, is complex. Although blood ammonia and cerebrospinal fluid (CSF) ammonia concentrations are elevated in hepatic encephalopathy, no single blood or CSF constituent that may be quantified by the clinical laboratory correlates well with the degree of mental impairment. There are two prominent theories at this time with regard to the pathogenesis of hepatic coma. One relates to the toxic effects of ammonia, mercaptans, and fatty acids. The second relates to changes in the neurotransmitters of the central nervous system, which are derived from

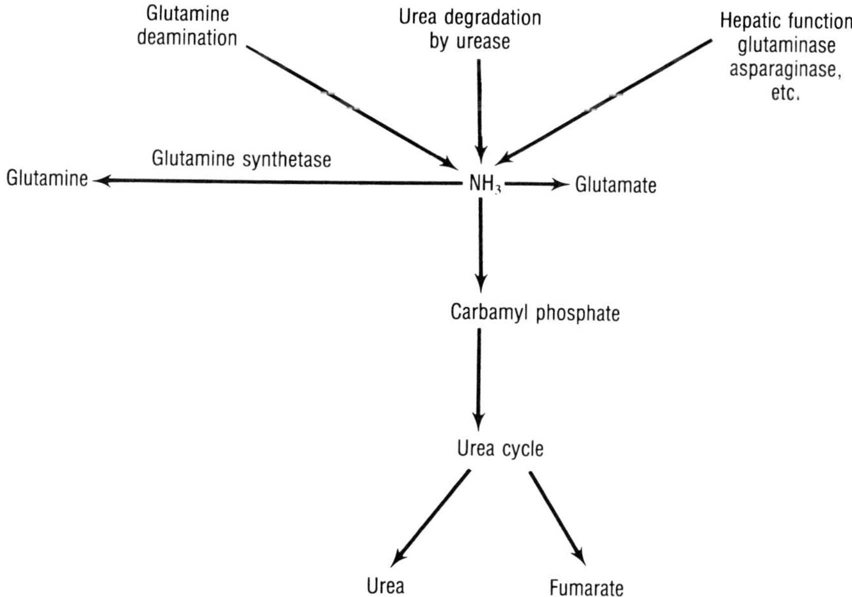

Figure 9.9.   Simplified representation of the various aspects of ammonia (NH$_3$) biotransformation.

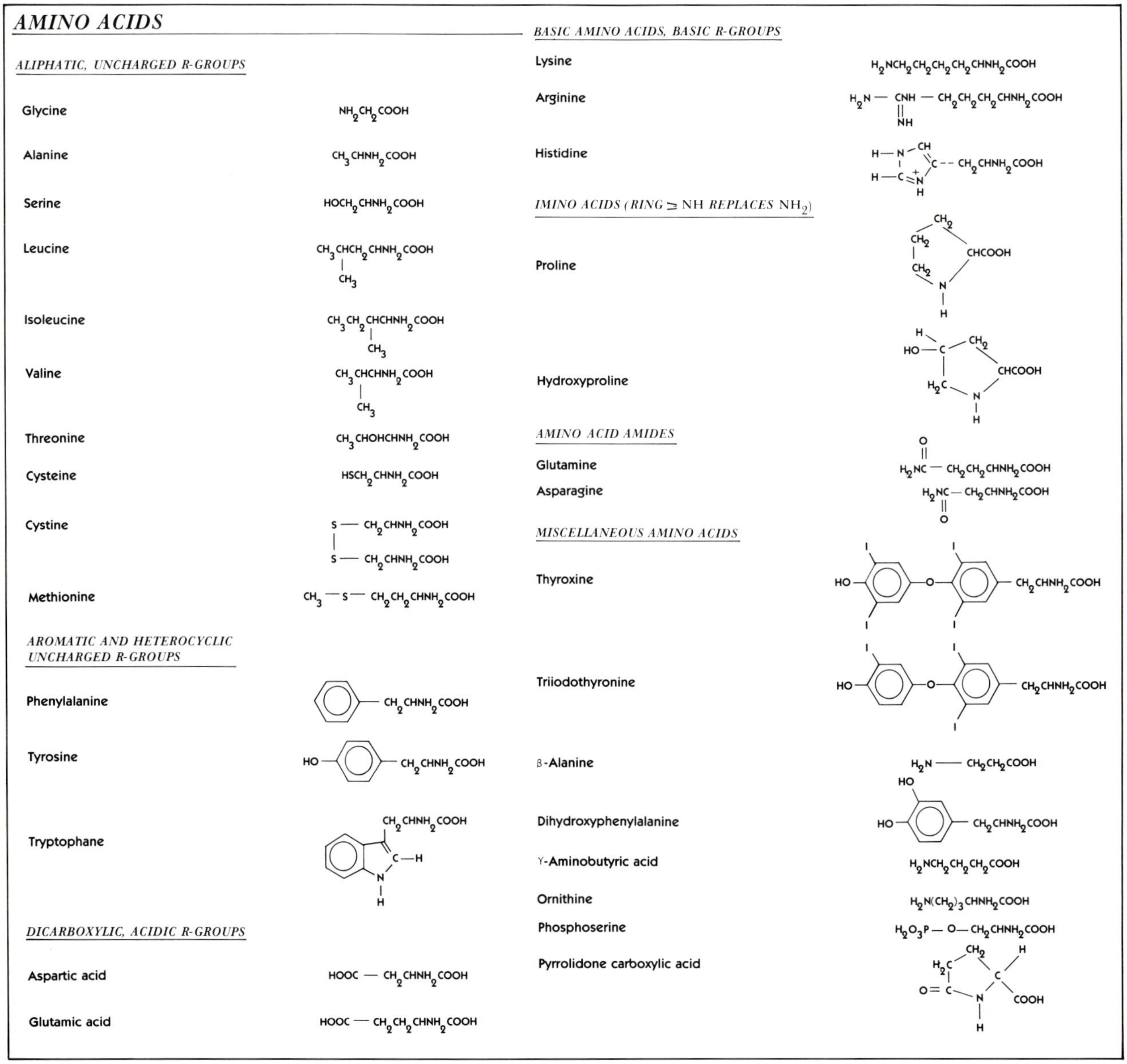

AMINO ACIDS

ALIPHATIC, UNCHARGED R-GROUPS

Glycine — NH_2CH_2COOH

Alanine — CH_3CHNH_2COOH

Serine — $HOCH_2CHNH_2COOH$

Leucine — $CH_3CHCH_2CHNH_2COOH$ (CH_3)

Isoleucine — $CH_3CH_2CHCHNH_2COOH$ (CH_3)

Valine — $CH_3CHCHNH_2COOH$ (CH_3)

Threonine — $CH_3CHOHCHNH_2COOH$

Cysteine — $HSCH_2CHNH_2COOH$

Cystine — $S-CH_2CHNH_2COOH$ / $S-CH_2CHNH_2COOH$

Methionine — $CH_3-S-CH_2CH_2CHNH_2COOH$

AROMATIC AND HETEROCYCLIC UNCHARGED R-GROUPS

Phenylalanine

Tyrosine

Tryptophane

DICARBOXYLIC, ACIDIC R-GROUPS

Aspartic acid — $HOOC-CH_2CHNH_2COOH$

Glutamic acid — $HOOC-CH_2CH_2CHNH_2COOH$

BASIC AMINO ACIDS, BASIC R-GROUPS

Lysine — $H_2NCH_2CH_2CH_2CH_2CHNH_2COOH$

Arginine — $H_2N-CNH-CH_2CH_2CH_2CHNH_2COOH$ (NH)

Histidine

IMINO ACIDS (RING $\supseteq$ NH REPLACES NH_2)

Proline

Hydroxyproline

AMINO ACID AMIDES

Glutamine — $H_2NC-CH_2CH_2CHNH_2COOH$ (O)

Asparagine — $H_2NC-CH_2CHNH_2COOH$ (O)

MISCELLANEOUS AMINO ACIDS

Thyroxine

Triiodothyronine

ß-Alanine — $H_2N-CH_2CH_2COOH$

Dihydroxyphenylalanine

γ-Aminobutyric acid — $H_2NCH_2CH_2CH_2COOH$

Ornithine — $H_2N(CH_2)_3CHNH_2COOH$

Phosphoserine — $H_2O_3P-O-CH_2CHNH_2COOH$

Pyrrolidone carboxylic acid

Figure 9.10. The amino acids.

amino acids. Aromatic amino acids (Fig. 9.10) are precursors of several neurotransmitters. In the CSF of patients suffering from hepatic encephalopathy, there are elevations of the concentrations of the amino acids phenylalanine, tyrosine, tryptophan, threonine, serine, and glutamine. Glutamine, an amino acid amide, is synthesized in the central nervous system (CNS) from ammonia and glutamic acid. Increases in ammonia result in increases of glutamine in the CSF (5). Glutamine, an amino acid amide (see Fig. 9.10), concentration in CSF correlates the best of any available clinical laboratory test with the severity of coma. Other amino acid concentrations (including phenylalanine, tyrosine, and methonine) do not correlate with the overall clinical course of a patient (70,77). The upper limit of normal for CSF glutamine is 20 mg/dl (5).

There are potential alternative applications of amino acid quantification to patient care that are the subject of clinical investigations. There are patterns of amino acid abnormalities that characterize patients with advanced hepatic disease. In chronic liver failure, it is reported that the levels of phenylalanine, tyrosine, tryptophan, and methionine are elevated; and that the levels of isoleucine, leucine, and valine are depressed (70,78,79). Elevated levels of aromatic amino acids and generally reduced levels of branched-chain amino acids are typical of patients with end-stage liver disease (80). Generalized hyperaminoacidemia characterizes acute hepatic failure, with the exception that the branched amino acids typically are within the reference (normal) range or may be minimally elevated (70,81). The branched-chain to aromatic amino acid (BC/AA) molar ratio normally is 3.0 to 3.5, but may be lower, typically below 2.0, in hepatic failure (70). Successful medical treatment of the underlying severe chronic liver disease is reflected by elevation of abnormally low ratios. Patients who fail to improve clinically or who suffer relapses tend to be characterized by ratios that remain abnormally low (70,82). It has been reported, furthermore, that the BC/AA ratio correlates with the clinical status of patients after liver transplantation (68,70). Plasma levels of aromatic amino acids decline and levels of branched-chain amino acids rise. This change occurs within several days, and its failure to occur, or to occur transiently, may be evidence of failure of the transplanted liver (70).

Serum Proteins

Many proteins are manufactured in the liver. These include albumin, various globulins, and coagulation factors. The coagulation factors have been dealt with in a separate section of this chapter. Monitoring changes in the concentrations of various proteins in serum forms the basis of several clinical laboratory procedures for assessing liver status. Essentially these procedures are in three groups: (1) quantification of specific individual proteins, of which albumin is the most pertinent; (2) electrophoresis; (3) turbidometric (flocculation) tests. The last of these are not in wide use any longer, and will not be discussed.

Albumin comprises about two-thirds of the total protein in the systemic circulation. It is synthesized by the hepatocytes. Its half-life is about 20 days. The maintenance of oncotic pressure is mostly (80%) due to albumin. Normal albumin fluctuates with sex and age. A representative reference range, however, is 3.7 to 4.8 g/dl, although particular ranges in individual laboratories may be slightly different. Edema begins when the serum albumin falls below the 2 to 3 g/dl range. Albumin has a secondary, but important role in the transport of endogenous (bilirubin, for instance) and exogenous (drugs, for instance) substances (9).

Albumin is easily quantified in a rapid, accurate, and precise manner in almost all clinical laboratories. It is both an index of severity and of prognosis in patients with chronic hepatic disease (5). Impaired synthesis of albumin is seen in both hepatitis and cirrhosis. In patients with cirrhosis, there is a direct correlation between the degree of hypoalbuminemia and the severity of ascites. Albumin concentrations in the serum of patients with acute liver disease (viral or toxic hepatitis) tend to remain within the reference (normal) range or be slightly depressed at most.

Serum protein electrophoresis is a qualitative and semiquantitative screening technique that may be useful in the setting of suspected hepatobiliary disorders. Immunoglobulins (which comprise a large portion of the "gamma" globulins, and a portion of the "beta"-globulins) may be increased in active macronodular cirrhosis and chronic active hepatitis. Biliary cirrhosis classically may result in a pattern of elevations of the alpha$_2$- and beta-globulins, often accompanied by an increase in the gamma-globulins (usually IgM). The alpha$_2$- and beta-globulins may be elevated in the serum of patients with posthepatic jaundice. Alcoholic cirrhosis may be characterized by an increase of the gamma globulins (IgG in this case) or of the proteins between beta and gamma (so-called beta-gamma bridging, usually due to a polyclonal increase of IgA). Caution must be exercised when interpreting the results of serum protein electrophoresis. The classical five-band pattern (albumin, alpha$_1$, alpha$_2$, beta, gamma) is being replaced in modern clinical laboratories by high-resolution electrophoretic techniques. Their resolution of eight or greater bands makes the traditional pattern associations archaic. The individual members of a band are now identifiable, making specific protein information available. The increased gamma globulin concentrations that may characterize chronic active hepatitis, cryptogenic cirrhosis and "subacute" viral hepatitis consists mainly

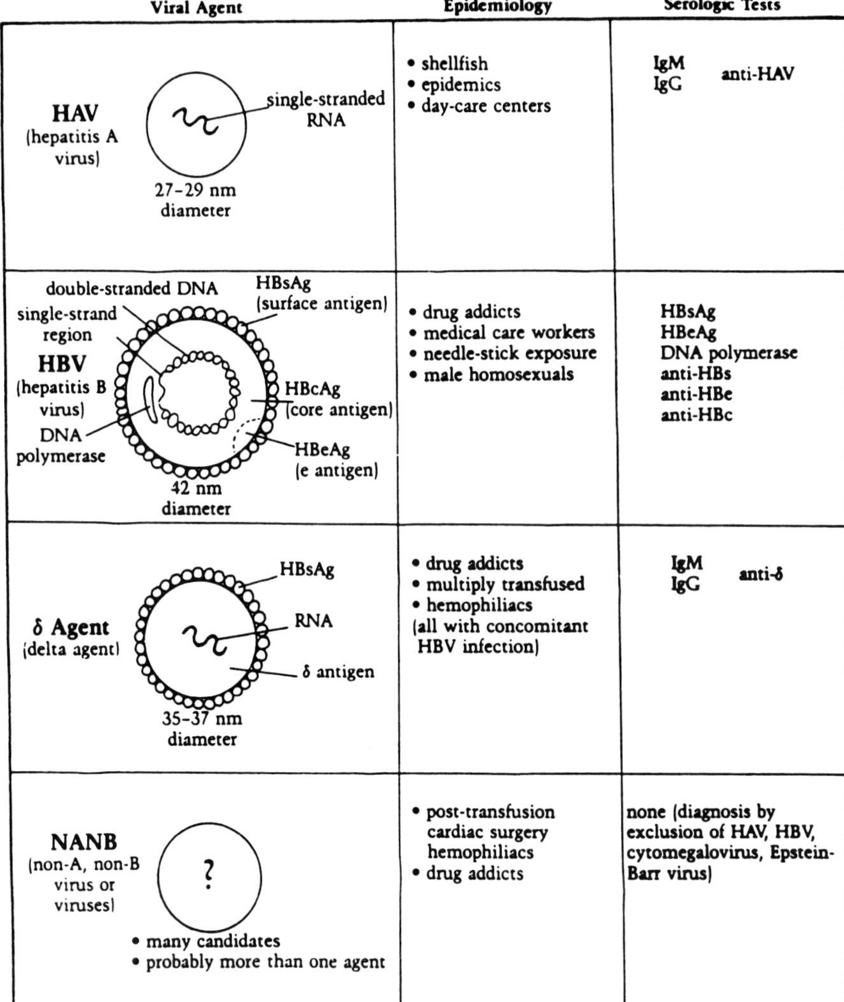

Figure 9.11. The hepatitis viruses. Although acute hepatitis may be caused by a number of viral agents, including cytomegalovirus, Epstein-Barr virus, and herpes virus, the specific hepatotropic viruses called the "hepatitis viruses" now comprise a number of varying agents. Certain of these agents, particularly hepatitis B virus, non-A, non-B virus(es) and delta-agent, may also lead to chronic hepatitis and cirrhosis. These agents are shown.

of IgG. It is IgA usually, only sometimes IgG or IgM, that is elevated in alcoholic cirrhosis. IgM is the cause of the gamma globulin increase that may accompany primary biliary cirrhosis, with minor contributions by IgA and IgG. It is strongly recommended that specific protein quantification be used rather than relying on protein electrophoresis.

Markers of Viral Hepatitis

There are several clinical laboratory procedures that are helpful in establishing the diagnosis of viral hepatitis, and in differentiating among the various types. Several of these procedures have been mentioned in the previous sections of this chapter. The clinical laboratory procedures used with respect to viral hepatitis form a natural group of tests. It is beyond the scope of this chapter to discuss individual clinical entities, including hepatitis. Specifics of each type of viral hepatitis will not be dealt with, except for some comments on delta hepatitis, as this subject is not widely dealt with in currently available textbooks.

Viral hepatitis is recognized at the time of this writing to be of four varieties: (1) type A, alternatively referred to as infectious hepatitis; (2) type B, alternatively referred to as serum hepatitis; (3) delta hepatitis; (4) so-called "non-A, non-B" (NANB) hepatitis. The viruses that cause types A and B are well described (Fig. 9.11). Clinical laboratory tests for antigens and antibodies associated with these are widely available. Delta virus (sometimes referred to as delta-agent) has been de-

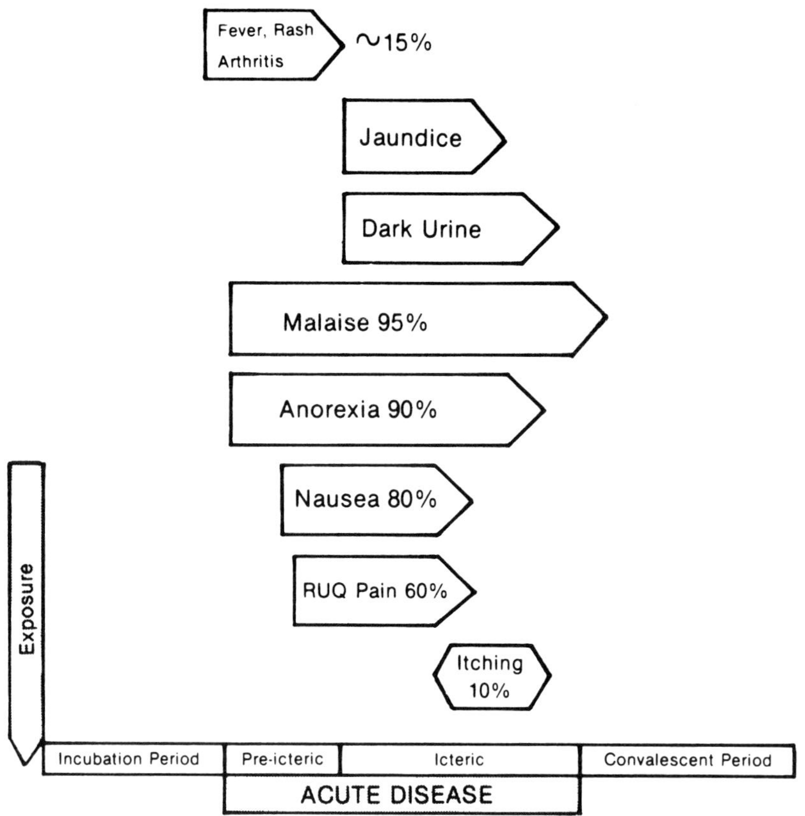

Figure 9.12. The course of symptoms in typical acute viral hepatitis. The timing and incidence of the major symptoms during the four clinical periods of this disease are shown. (Reprinted by permission from Hoofnagle JH. Type A and type B hepatitis. *Lab Med* 1983; 14: 705–716.

scribed recently (83,84). Serologic tests associated with delta virus should be widely available shortly. NANB is the least well defined at this time. The diagnosis of NANB viral hepatitis is made by default at this time, when type A and type B have been ruled out by the absence of their markers (see below). No satisfactory immunologic markers for NANB hepatitis for routine clinical laboratory use are available at this time.

The variable clinical course of acute viral hepatitis ranges from asymptomatic to fatal. A useful classification based on outcome is (1) typical, acute icteric hepatitis; (2) subclinical and anicteric hepatitis; (3) fulminant hepatitis; (4) chronic hepatitis (85). The clinical presentation and clinical laboratory findings typical of acute viral hepatitis are presented in Figures 9.12 and 9.13. The usual course of the serologic markers of type A hepatitis are summarized in Figure 9.13. Chronic hepatitis, hepatic inflammation, and necrosis lasting for at least 6 months occur in about 10% of patients with type B hepatitis and 10% to 60% of those with NANB hepatitis. It tends not to occur in type A hepatitis (see Fig. 9.14) (85). In dealing with

chronic hepatitis, it is important to eliminate entities such as Wilson's disease and alpha$_1$-antitrypsin deficiency. After eliminating these, there are three major groups: (1) autoimmune; (2) type B chronic hepatitis, with or without delta hepatitis (see below); (3) NANB chronic hepatitis. The autoimmune group may be subdivided into a milder chronic persistent hepatitis, and a more severe chronic active hepatitis on histologic grounds. The course of serologic markers for acute type B and chronic type B hepatitis are summarized in Figures 9.15 and 9.16, respectively. Note that the persistence of HB$_s$Ag in a patient's serum for more than approximately 3 months suggests either chronic hepatitis or the presence of a carrier state (5).

With respect to type B hepatitis, the detection of antibodies in a patient's serum to hepatitis B core antigen (anti-HB$_c$Ag) may be of help (Table 9.13). There is a period of time at which hepatitis B surface antigen (HB$_s$Ag) has disappeared, but antibody to surface antigen (anti-HB$_s$) has not yet appeared. This is referred to as the "core" window. It is possible to distinguish between IgM class and IgG class anti-HB$_c$Ag. This in turn allows

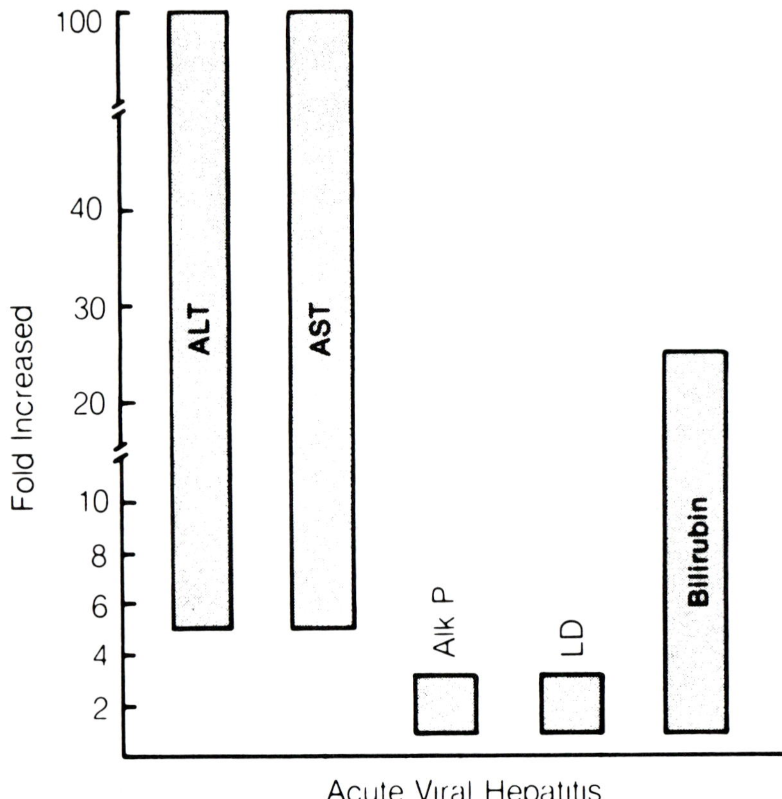

Figure 9.13. The typical range of results of biochemical laboratory tests in acute viral hepatitis. Most characteristic is the marked and simultaneous increase in levels of ALT and aspartate aminotransferase (AST) with minimal elevations in levels of Alk and LD. (Reprinted by permission from Hoofnagle JH. Type A and type B hepatitis. *Lab Med* 1983; 14:705–716.

one to distinguish between current acute type B hepatitis and remote or chronic infection (86). The IgM class of antibody is characteristic of primary immunologic responses. IgM class of anti-HB$_c$Ag persists at high titer for about 6 months. IgG class antibodies are characteristic of secondary immunologic responses. IgG class of anti-HB$_c$Ag appears subsequent to the IgM class, indicative of a conva-

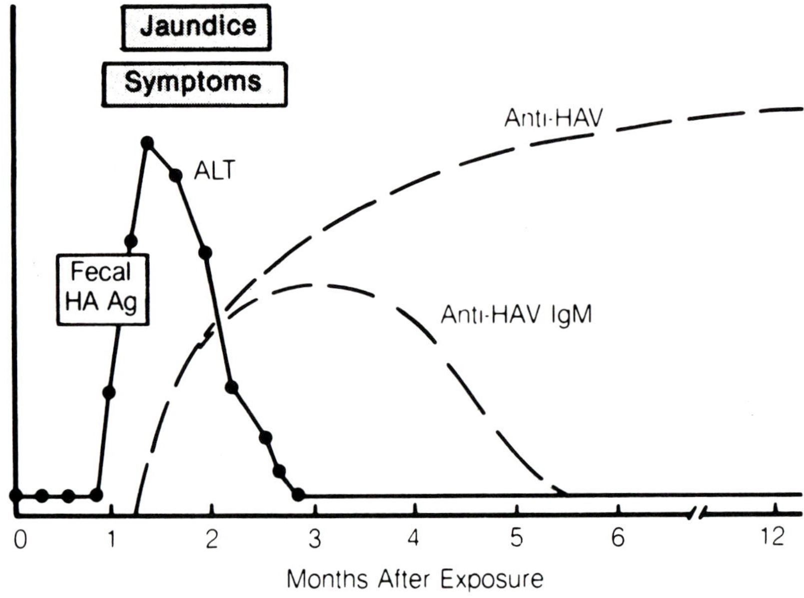

Figure 9.14. The clinical, serologic, and biochemical course of typical type A hepatitis. ALT, alanine aminotransferase; anti-HAV, antibody to hepatitis A virus; HA Ag, hepatitis A antigen. (Reprinted by permission from Hoofnagle JH. Type A and type B hepatitis. *Lab Med* 1983; 14:705–716.)

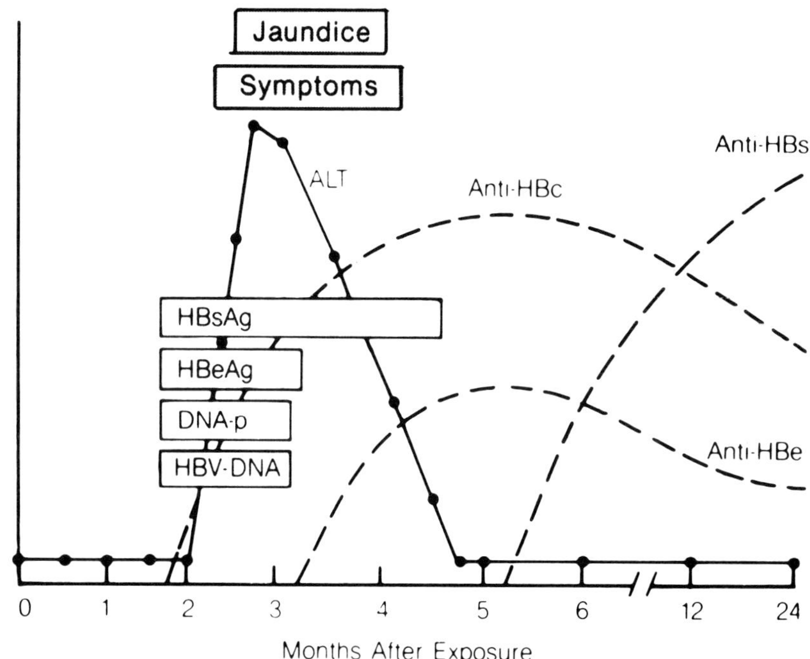

Figure 9.15. The clinical, serologic, and biochemical course of typical acute type B hepatitis. ALT, alanine aminotransferase; anti-HB$_c$, antibody to hepatitis B core antigen; anti-HB$_e$, antibody to hepatitis Be antigen, anti-HB$_s$Ag, antibody to hepatitis B surface antigen; DNA-p, serum hepatitis B virus DNA polymerase activity; HBV-DNA, serum hepatitis B virus DNA. (Reprinted by permission from Hoofnagle JH. Type A and type B hepatitis. *Lab Med* 1983; 14: 705–716.)

lescent stage. By comparing the IgM anti-HB$_c$Ag titer to the total HB$_c$Ag (the test quantifies IgM plus IgG antibody), one may estimate the relative amounts of IgM and IgG antibody. The simultaneous presence of HB$_s$Ag and relatively high titers of IgG class anti-HB$_c$Ag may indicate a chronic type B viral hepatitis (Figs. 9.17, 9.18).

The detection of the hepatitis B antigen (HB$_e$Ag) and antibody to it (anti-HB$_e$Ag) is of use in dealing with type B viral hepatitis as well. HB$_e$Ag is found in the serum of some patients who are HB$_s$Ag positive. It rarely occurs in the absence of HB$_s$Ag in the serum. When present, HB$_e$Ag is taken to be indicative of a high virus load and a high degree of

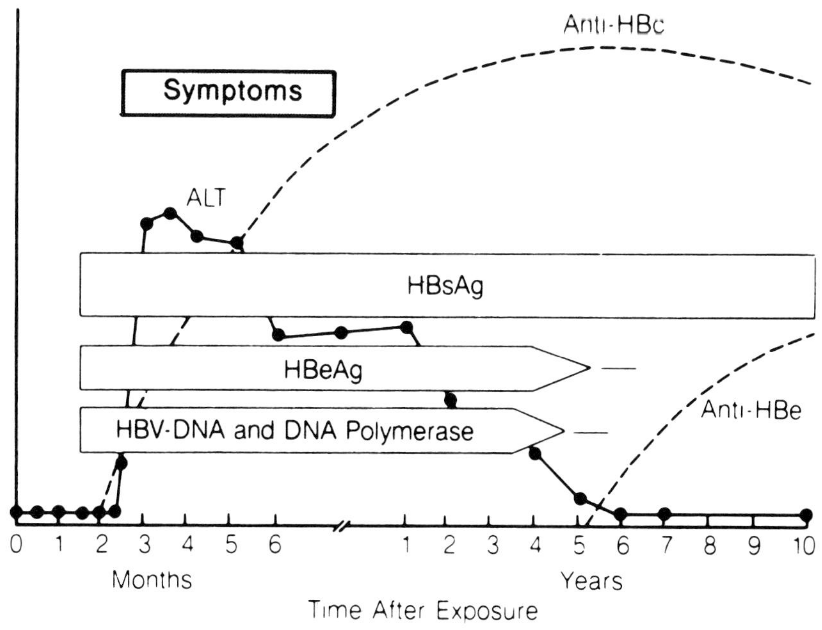

Figure 9.16. Clinical, serologic, and biochemical course of chronic type B hepatitis infection. (Reproduced by permission from Hoofnagle JH. Type A and B hepatitis. *Lab Med* 1983; 14:705–716.

Table 9.13. Hepatitis Type B—Serologic Tests

Disease Stage	HB_sAg	Anti-HB_s	Anti-HB_c	HB_eAg	anti-HB_e
Acute					
Early	+	−	+	±	−
Convalesence	−	−	+	−	−
Recovery	−	+	+	−	±
Chronic	+	−	+	±	−
Carrier state	+	−	+	±	±

Abbreviations: anti-HB_c, antibody to hepatitis B core; anti-HB_e, antibody to hepatitis Be antigen; anti-HB_s, antibody to hepatitis B surface antigen; other abbreviations as in text.

infectivity. Recovery is characterized by the disappearance of HB_eAg and the appearance of anti-HB_e (see Fig. 9.16). The persistence of HB_eAg in a patient who has also the persistence of HB_sAg

increases the likelihood that the carrier is actively infected (5).

Testing for DNA polymerase in serum gives information similar to that derived from testing for HB_eAg (see Figs. 9.15, 9.16) (85). That is, its presence in detectable quantities in a patient's serum is associated with high levels of hepatitis type B virus. Clinical laboratory methods for testing for DNA polymerase are tedious and complicated at this time. As this testing appears not to add information not available by alternative means, it is not recommended. The same is applicable to testing for the virus itself in serum.

Hepatitis D virus, sometimes referred to as delta-agent, is a small RNA virus consisting of a

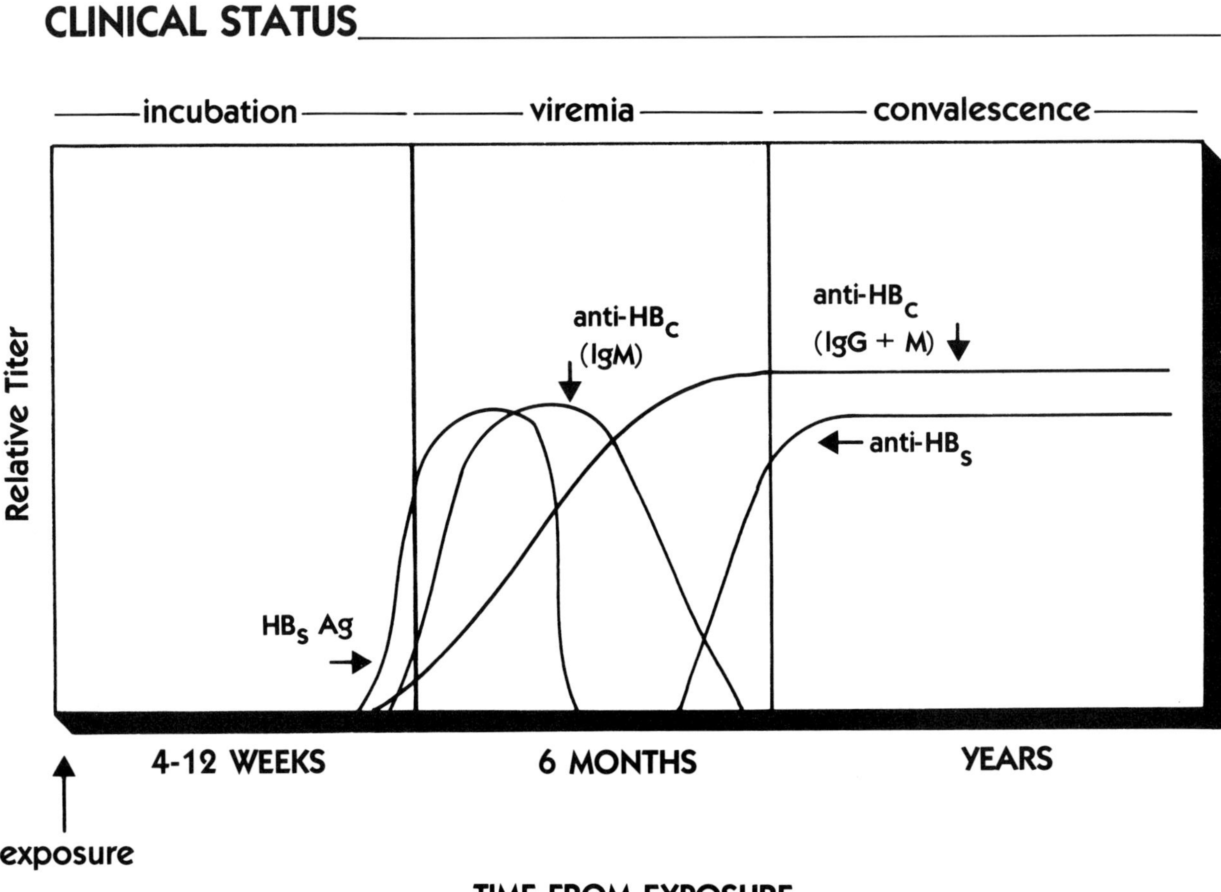

Figure 9.17. IgM class anti-HB_c is usually detected 1–3 weeks after HB_sAg becomes detectable in type B acute hepatitis. It is no longer detectable 6 months after the initial onset of symptoms. A period of time exists between the disappearance of HB_sAg and the apppearance of anti-HB_s (core window), during which anti-HB_c may be the only marker of viral hepatitis present. Anti-HB_c (IgG + IgM), IgG and IgM antibodies to hepatitis B core antigen; anti-HB_c (IgM), IgM antibody to hepatitis B core antigen; anti-HB_s (IgG + IgM), IgG and IgM antibodies to hepatitis B surface antigen; HB_sAg, hepatitis B surface antigen.

CLINICAL STATUS

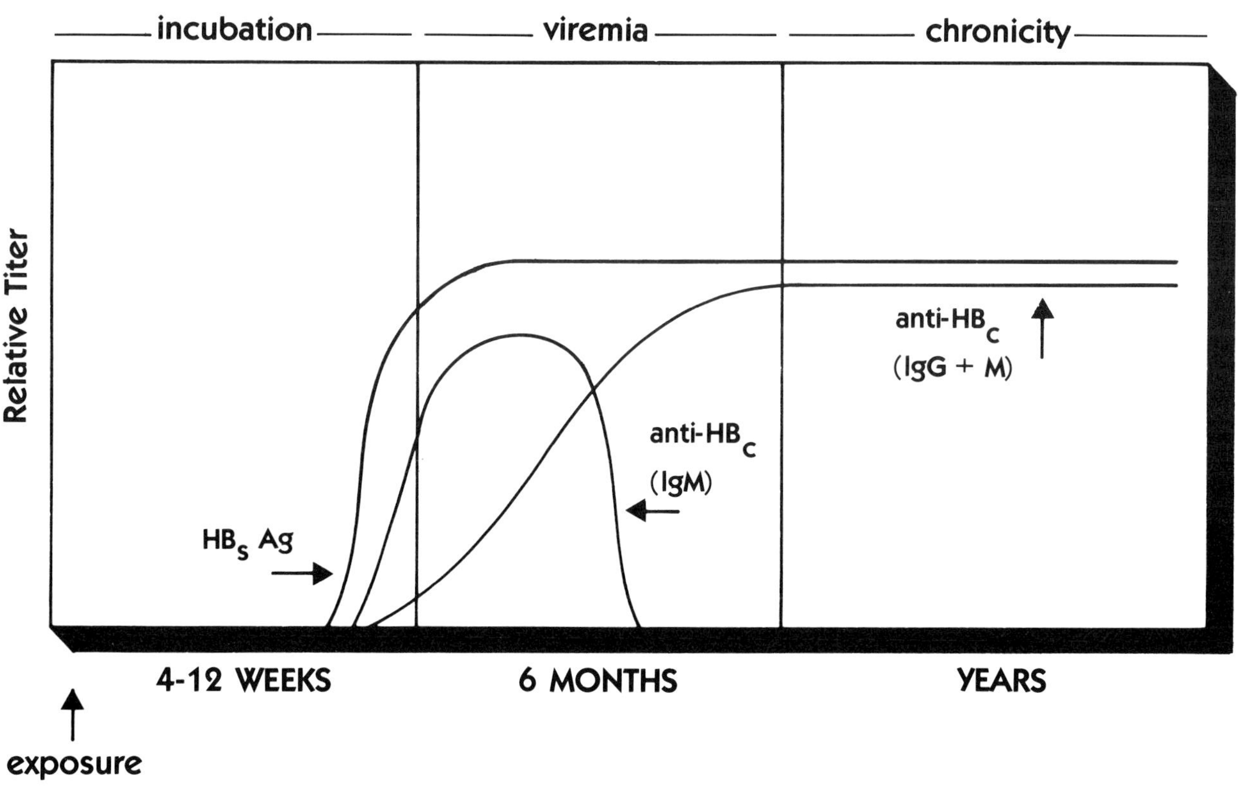

Figure 9.18. IgM class anti-HB$_c$ is usually detected 1–3 weeks after HB$_s$Ag becomes detectable in chronic type B hepatitis. It is no longer detectable 6 months after the initial onset of symptoms, even though HB$_s$Ag may remain indefinitely. For explanations of abbreviations, see Figure 9.16.

delta-antigen core and an outer coat of HB$_s$Ag. Delta hepatitis occurs only in individuals who have had hepatitis type B infection. The delta-agent is delta-RNA, encapsulated by type B hepatitis surface antigen (see Fig. 9.11). There are two situations, then, in which to consider delta-hepatitis: (1) simultaneous hepatitis B and delta-hepatitis as an acute event and (2) subsequent delta-

hepatitis in a persistent HB$_s$Ag-positive patient (superinfection of a hepatitis type B "carrier"). Delta-hepatitis, therefore, may be a cause of either an acute or a chronic hepatitis. This entity, therefore, enters into the differential diagnosis when dealing with fulminant hepatitis, severe chronic active hepatitis, and cirrhosis.

In one study conducted in the United States,

Table 9.14. Delta Hepatitis—Clinical Laboratory

	Acute	Chronic
Serum		
Delta-antigen	Rare, ominous sign	Absent
Anti-delta-antigen, IgM class	Transient	Present, high titers
Anti-delta-antigen, IgG class	May not develop	Present, high titers
Liver tissue		
Delta-antigen in nuclei	Present	Present

approximately 5% of HB$_s$Ag-positive patients from a group consisting of drug addicts, hemophiliacs, transfusion recipients, homosexuals, and US-relocated Vietnamese were positive for antibodies to delta-hepatitis virus (87). Among drug addicts and hemophiliacs in a different study, the rate was more than 50% positive in patients with chronic hepatitis B (88).

There are clinical laboratory procedures that will assist the clinician in making the diagnosis of delta hepatitis (see Table 9.14). The delta-antigen may be identified in the nuclei of liver cells in tissue obtained by biopsy. Alternatively, serum may be examined for antigen and antibodies. Delta-antigenemia is unusual, in contrast to type B hepatitis; when present, it is associated with extensive necrosis, as in fulminant hepatitis. IgM class antibody to delta-virus may be seen in acute delta-hepatitis. Past delta-hepatitis infection is associated with IgG antibody to delta-virus, whereas IgM class antibody is present in low titer or may be absent (Table 9.14). Persisting high titers of IgM and IgG antibodies to delta-virus indicate ongoing infection. Another finding in some patients is that there may be a transient decrease of the HB$_s$Ag titer, indicating persistent delta-hepatitis virus replication (89). The reason for this is that, as a so-called "defective interfering virus," delta-virus takes over the hepatocellular synthetic machinery for its own replication, at the expense of the type B hepatitis virus replication.

References

1. Robbins SL, Cotran RS, Kumar V. *Pathologic basis of disease*, 3rd ed. Philadelphia: WB Saunders, 1984, pp. 884–942.
2. Rapaport AM. The structural and functional units of the human liver (liver acinus). *Microvasc Res* 1973; 6:212.
3. Johns DF, Fody EP. Liver function. In: Bishop ML, Duben-Von Laufen JL, Fody EP, eds. *Clinical Chemistry*. Philadelphia: JB Lippincott, 1985, pp. 437–451.
4. Notter D. Bilirubin. In: Siest G, Henny J, Schiele F, Young DS, eds. *Interpretation of Clinical Laboratory Tests*. Foster City, California: Biomedical Publications, 1985, pp. 146–163.
5. Zimmerman H. Function and integrity of the liver. In: Henry JB, ed. *Clinical Diagnosis and Management by Laboratory Methods*, 17th ed. Philadelphia: WB Saunders, 1984, pp. 217–250.
6. Balisteri WF, Shaw LM. Liver function. In: Tietz NW, ed. *Textbook of Clinical Chemistry*. Philadelphia: WB Saunders, 1986, pp. 1373–1433.
7. Schmid R. Bilirubin metabolism—state of the art. *Gastroenterology* 1978; 76:1307–1312.
8. Singh J, Bowers LD. Serum bilirubin species: Analysis and clinical utility. *Lab Med* 1985; 16:597–601.
9. Gerson B. *Essentials of Therapeutic Drug Monitoring*. New York: Igaku-Shoin, 1983, pp. 1–54.
10. Van den Bergh AAH, Snapper J. Die Farbstoffe des Blutserums. *Deutsches Arch Klin Med* 1913; 110:540–561.
11. Kubasik NP, Mayer TK, Bhaskar AG, Sine HE, D'Souza JP. The measurement of fractionated bilirubin by Ektachem film slides. *Am J Clin Pathol* 1985; 84:518–523.
12. Statland BE, Winkel P. Problems of precision and accuracy related to specimen collection and handling. *Clin Chem* 1976; 24:60–73.
13. Doumas BT, Kwok-Cheung PP, Perry BW, Jendrezejczak B, McComb RB, Schaffer R, et al. Candidate reference method for determination of total bilirubin in serum: Development and validation. *Clin Chem* 1985; 31:1779–1789.
14. Lo DH, Wu TW. Assessment of the fundamental accuracy of the Jendrassik-Grof total and direct bilirubin assays. *Clin Chem* 1983; 29:31–36.
15. Muraca M, Blanckaert N. Liquid-chromatographic assay and identification of mono- and diester conjugates of bilirubin in normal serum. *Clin Chem* 1983; 29:1767–1771.
16. Lum G, Gambino SR. A comparison of serum versus heparinized plasma for routine chemistry tests. *Am J Clin Pathol* 1974; 61:108–113.
17. Harris EK, Brow SS. Temporal changes in the concentrations of serum constituents in healthy men. Distribution of within-person variances and their relevance to the interpretation of differences between successive measurements. *Ann Clin Biochem* 1979; 16:169–176.
18. Barrett PVD. Hyperbilirubinemia of fasting. *JAMA* 1971; 217:1344–1353.
19. Gornall AG. *Applied Biochemistry of Clinical Disorders*. Philadelphia: Harper and Row, 1980.
20. Bartoletti AL, Stevenson DK, Ostrander CR, Johnson JD. Pulmonary excretion of carbon monoxide in the human infant as an index of bilirubin production. *J Pediatr* 1979; 94:952–955.
21. Brosden R. Bilirubin transport in the newborn infant, reviewed with relation to kernicterus. *J Pediatr* 1980; 96: 349–356.
22. Gerson B. *Essentials of Therapeutic Drug Monitoring*. New York: Igaku-Shoin, 1983.
23. Owens D, Evans J. Population studies on Gilbert's syndrome. *J Med Genet* 1975; 12:152–156.
24. Chan K, Scott MG, Wu T, Clouse RE, Calvin DR, Koenig J, et al. Inaccurate values for direct bilirubin with some commonly used direct bilirubin procedures. *Clin Chem* 1985; 31:1560–1563.
25. Dubin IN, Johnson FB. Chronic idiopathic jaundice with unidentified pigment in liver cells: A new clinicopathologic entity with a report of 12 cases. *Medicine* 1954; 33:155–197.
26. Sherlock S. *Diseases of the Liver and Biliary System*, 6th ed. Oxford: Blackwell Scientific Publications, 1981.
27. Pennington CR, Ross PE, Bouchier I. Serum bile acids in the diagnosis of hepatobiliary disease. *Gut* 1977; 18:903–908.
28. Montgomery R, Dryer RL, Conway TW, Spector AA. *Biochemistry, a Case Oriented Approach*. St. Louis: CV Mosby, 1980, pp. 92–149.
29. Kachmar JF, Moss DW. Enzymes. In: Tietz NW, ed. *Fundamentals of Clinical Chemistry*, 2nd ed. Philadelphia: WB Saunders, 1976, pp. 565–698.
30. *Report of the Commission on Enzymes of the International Union of Biochemistry*. New York: Pergamon Press, 1961.
31. Roberts WM. Variations in the phosphatase activity of the blood in disease. *Br J Exp Pathol* 1930; 11:90–95.

32. Robinson R. *The significance of Phosphoric Esters in Metabolism*. New York: New York University Press, 1982.

33. Davis TE, Kahan L, Tormey DC, et al. Clinical studies of a fast homoarginine sensitive alkaline phosphatase in patients with cancer. *Cancer* 1981; 41:1110–1114.

34. Stinson RA, Seargeant LE. Comparative studies of pure alkaline phosphatases from five human tissues. *Clin Chim Acta* 1981; 110:261–272.

35. Harris EK. Some theory of reference values. II. Comparison of some statistical models of intraindividual variation in blood constituents. *Clin Chem* 1976; 22:1343–1350.

36. Harris EK. Step by step algorithm for computing critical range of next observation based on previous time series. *Clin Chem* 1977; 23:2179–2180.

37. Harris EK, Cooil BK, Shakarji G, Williams GZ. On the use of statistical models of within person variation in long term studies of healthy individuals. *Clin Chem* 1980; 26:383–391.

38. Hill PG, Sammonds HG. An interpretation of the elevation of serum alkaline phosphatase in disease. *J Clin Pathol* 1967; 20:654–659.

39. Pickup JF, Harris EK, Kearns M, Brown SS. Intra-individual variation of some serum constituents and its relevance to population-based reference ranges. *Clin Chem* 1977; 23:842–850.

40. Schiele F, Henny J, Hitz J, Petitclerc C, Gueguen R, Siest G. Total bone and liver alkaline phosphatase in plasma: Biological variations and reference limits. *Clin Chem* 1983; 29:634–641.

41. Statland BE, Winkel P, Killingsworth LM. Factors contributing to intra-individual variation of serum constituents: 6. Physiological day to day variation in concentrations of 10 specific proteins in sera of healthy subjects. *Clin Chem* 1976; 22:1635–1638.

42. Williams GZ, Widdowson GM, Penton J. Individual character of variation in time-series studies of healthy people 11: Differences in values for clinical chemical analyses in serum among demographic groups, by age and sex. *Clin Chem* 1978; 24:313–320.

43. Harris EK, Yasaka T, Horton MR, Shakarji G. Comparing multivariate and univariate subject-specific reference regions for blood constituents in healthy persons. *Clin Chem* 1982; 28:422–426.

44. Winkel P, Statland BE, Bokelund H, Johnson EA. Correlation of selected serum constituents: I. Interindividual variation and analytical error. *Clin Chem* 1975; 21:1592–1600.

45. Morton BD III, Statland BE. Serum enzyme alterations in polymyositis. Possible pitfalls in diagnosis. *Am J Clin Pathol* 1980; 73:556–557.

46. Statland BE, Nishi HH, Young DS. Serum alkaline phosphatase: Total activity and isoenzyme determinations made by centrifugal fast analyzer. *Clin Chem* 1972; 18:1468–1474.

47. Moss DW. Alkaline phosphatase isoenzymes. *Clin Chem* 1982; 28:2007–2016.

48. Hagerstrand I. Distribution of alkaline phosphatase activity in healthy and diseased human liver tissue. *Acta Pathol Microbiol Scand Sect A* 1975; 83:519–526.

49. Fleisher GA, Eickelber ES, Elveback LR. Alkaline phosphatase activity in the plasma of children and adolescents. *Clin Chem* 1977; 23:469–472.

50. Horne M, Cornish CJ, Posen S. Use of urea denaturation in the identification of human alkaline phosphatases. *J Lab Clin Med* 1968; 72:905–915.

51. Warnes TW, Hine P, Kay P. Polyacrylamide gel disc electrophoresis of alkaline phosphatase isoenzymes in bone and liver disease. *J Clin Pathol* 1976; 29:782–787.

52. Langman MJS, Leuthold E, Robson EB, Harris J, Luffman JE, Harris H. Influence of diet on the "intestinal" component of serum alkaline phosphatase in people of different ABO blood groups and secretor status. *Nature* 1966; 212:41–43.

53. Warshaw JB, Littlefield JW, Fishman WH, Inglis NR, Stolbach LL. Serum alkaline phosphatase in hypophosphatasia. *J Clin Invest* 1971; 50:2137–2142.

54. Pillans PI, Berman P, Saunders SJ. Cholestatic jaundice with a normal serum alkaline phosphatase level: Another case of hypophosphatasia in an adult? *Gastroenterology* 1983; 84:175–177.

55. Rathbun JC. Hypophosphatasia. A new developmental anomaly. *Am J Dis Child* 1948; 75:822–831.

56. McKenna MJ, Hamilton TA, Sussman HH. Comparison of human alkaline phosphatase isoenzymes. Structural evidence for three protein classes. *Biochem J* 1979; 181:67–73.

57. Lai CL, Lam KC, Wong KP, Wu PC, Todd D. Clinical features of hepatocellular carcinoma: Review of 211 patients in Hong Kong. *Cancer* 1981; 47:2746–2755.

58. Mettler FA, Christie JH, Crow NE, Garcia JF, Wicks JD, Bartow SA. Radionuclide bone scan, radiographic bone survey, and alkaline phosphatase. *Cancer* 1982; 50:1483–1485.

59. Spooner RJ, Smith DH, Bedford D, Beck PR. Serum gamma-glutamyl-transferase and alkaline phosphatase in rheumatoid arthritis. *J Clin Pathol* 1982; 35:638–641.

60. Wolf P. Clinical significance of an increased or decreased serum alkaline phosphatase level. *Arch Pathol Lab Med* 1980; 102:497–501.

61. Gerson B, Menduke H, Boitnott JK, et al. Lipoprotein X and alkaline phosphatase as indicators of cholestasis. *Johns Hopkins Med J* 1979; 144:41–44.

62. Hagerstrand I, Lindholm K, Lindroth Y. Endothelial and bile canalicular alkaline phosphatase in human liver and serum. *Scand J Clin Lab Invest* 1976; 36:131–135.

63. Schlaeger R, Haux P, Kattermann R. Studies on the mechanism of the increase in serum alkaline phosphatase activity in cholestasis: Significance of the hepatic bile acid concentration for the leakage of alkaline phosphatase from rat liver. *Enzyme* 1982; 28:3–13.

64. Simonsen R, Virji MA. Interpreting the profile of liver function tests in pediatric liver transplants. *Clin Chem* 1984; 30:1607–1610.

65. Nemesanszky E, Lott JA. Gamma-glutamyltransferase and its isoenzymes: Progress and problems. *Clin Chem* 1985; 31:797–803.

66. Siest G, Schiele F, Artur Y. Gamma-glutamyltransferase. In: Siest G, Henny J, Schiele F, Young DS, eds. *Interpretation of Clinical Laboratory Tests*. Foster City, California: Biomedical Publications, 1985, pp. 235–252.

67. Bayer PM, Hotschek H, Knoth E. Intestinal alkaline phosphatase and the ABO blood group system—a new aspect. *Clin Chim Acta* 1980; 108:81–87.

68. Fath JJ, Ascher NL, Konstantinides FN, Bloomer J, Sharp H, Najarian JS, et al. Metabolism during hepatic transplantation: Indicators of allograft function. *Surgery* 1984; 96:664–674.

69. Vincint-Viry M, Galteau MM, Schiele F. Aspartate aminotransferase. In: Siest G, Henny J, Schiele E, Young DS, eds. *Interpretation of Clinical Laboratory Tests*. Foster City, California: Biomedical Publications, 1985, pp. 130–145.

70. Reilly JJ, Halow GM, Gerhardt AL, Ritter PS, Gavaler JS, Van Thiel D. Plasma amino acids in liver transplantation:

Correlation with clinical outcome. *Surgery* 1985; 97:263–270.

71. Vincent-Viry M, Schiele F, Galteau MM. Alanine aminotransferase. In: Siest G, Henny J, Schiele F, Young DS, eds. *Interpretation of Clinical Laboratory Tests.* Foster City, California: Biomedical Publications, 1985, pp. 69–83.

72. Matloff DS, Selinger MJ, Kaplan MM. Hepatic transaminase activity in alcoholic liver disease. *Gastroenterology* 1980; 78:1389–1392.

73. Arkin CF. Anticoagulant Agents. In: Gerson B, ed. *Essentials of Therapeutic Drug Monitoring.* New York: Igaku-Shoin, 1983, pp. 263–284.

74. Svensson G, Anfalt T. Rapid determination of ammonia in whole blood and plasma using flow injection analysis. *Clin Chim Acta* 1982; 119:7–14.

75. Glasgow AM. Clinical application of blood ammonia determinations. *Lab Med* 1981; 12:151–157.

76. Colombo JP, Peheim E, Kretschmer R, Dauwalder H, Sidiropoulos D. Plasma ammonia concentrations in newborns and children. *Clin Chim Acta* 1984; 138:283–291.

77. Rossle M, Luft M, Herz R, Klein B, Lehmann M, Gerok W. Amino acid, ammonia and neurotransmitter concentrations in hepatic encephalopathy: Serial analysis in plasma and cerebrospinal fluid during treatment with an adapted amino acid solution. *Klin Wochenschr* 1984; 62:867–875.

78. Milsom J, Morgan M, Sherlock S. Factors affecting plasma amino acid concentrations in control subjects. *Metabolism* 1979; 28:313–319.

79. Fischer J, Rosen HM, Ebeid AM. The effect of normalization of plasma amino acids on hepatic encephalopathy in man. *Surgery* 1976; 80:77–91.

80. Cerra FB, Caprioli J, Siegel J, McMenamy R, Border J. Proline metabolism in sepsis, cirrhosis, and general surgery. *Ann Surg* 1979; 190:577–586.

81. Rosen HM, Yoshimura N, Hodgman JM. Plasma amino acid patterns hepatic encephalopathy of differing etiology. *Gastroenterology* 1977; 72:483–487.

82. McCullough AJ, Czaja AJ, Jones JD, Go V. The nature and prognostic significance of serial amino acid determinations in severe chronic active liver disease. *Gastroenterology* 1981; 81:645–652.

83. Rizetto M, Verme G. Delta hepatitis—present status. *J Hepatol* 1985; 1:187–193.

84. Rizetto M. The delta agent. *Hepatology* 1983; 3:729–737.

85. Hoofnagle JH. Type A and type B hepatitis. *Lab Med* 1983; 14:705–716.

86. Taswell HR, Czaja AJ, Nelson CA. Viral hepatitis: Diagnostic test using anti-HB$_c$ (IgM). *Mayo Clin Proc* 1985; 60:488–489.

87. Shields MT, Czaja AJ, Taswell HF. Frequency and significance of delta antibody in acute and chronic hepatitis B. A United States experience. *Gastroenterology* 1985; 89:1230–1234.

88. Rizetto M, Shih JW-K, Gocke DJ, Purcell RH, Verme G, Geri JL. Incidence and significance of antibodies to delta antigen in hepatitis B virus infection. *Lancet* 1979; 2:986–990.

89. Govindarajan S, Valinluck B. Serum hepatitis B virus-DNA in chronic hepatitis B and delta infection. *Arch Pathol Lab Med* 1985; 109:398–399.

Editorial Comment

"Clinical Laboratory Evaluation of the Liver" by Dr. Gerson may belie, in the simplicity of the title, the sophistication of his description of the various studies available for evaluation of the liver in almost every possible phase of disorder and disease. Certainly, the larger portion of the material that Dr. Gerson is presenting is of extreme importance to any surgeon undertaking procedures involving this complex organ. In addition, however, there is sufficient depth in the chapter to interest almost any scholar who has developed direct or peripheral interest in the extraordinary complexity of the biochemical and metabolic functions of the body subserved by the hepatocellular function.

The clinical surgeon can refer to this chapter selectively for specific problems, although the possibility of unexpected encounters should lead him to develop, through a mechanism such as this, a reasonably intimate knowledge of the pathophysiology of this organ.

As a brief adjunct to this chapter, the editor would suggest an essay by Helzberg and Spiro (1), which emphasizes the pitfalls of interpreting LFTs (liver function tests) in following patients with a malignancy that may metastasize to the liver.

References

1. Helzberg JH and Spiro HM. 'LFT's' test more than the liver. *JAMA*, 1986; 256:3006–3007.

Chapter 10
Diagnostic Imaging of the Liver

ROBERT A. KANE

Diagnostic imaging of the liver has undergone revolutionary changes in the past decade, primarily as a result of the development of ultrasonography and computed tomography (CT). Although there is still important information to be gained from plain films, radionuclide scans, and angiographic examination, CT and ultrasound have become the principal and often the sole means of diagnostic imaging of the liver because of their excellent anatomic resolution and definition of a variety of pathologic states. Radionuclide scanning has become less important as an anatomic imaging modality but more important for functional imaging, which can be achieved with various biliary agents. Intraoperative ultrasonography has added yet another dimension, offering even better anatomic resolution than can be achieved by standard ultrasound or CT. Finally, the development of magnetic resonance imaging (MRI) promises to have a significant impact on liver imaging, with some investigators claiming that MRI may be the imaging method of choice for a variety of liver diseases.

Many of the liver imaging tests offer complementary information to one another, and it may be clinically helpful to use more than one modality. At other times, tests may be redundant. This chapter discusses the findings in each of the modalities in a variety of disease processes affecting the liver and biliary tree and attempts to provide guidelines for rational and efficient use of the various imaging modalities.

Anatomy

The anatomy of the liver can be analyzed in several different ways. Lobar and segmental topographic anatomy of the liver is best demonstrated by ultrasound and CT. In this anatomic division of the liver, there are four main divisions, the right lobe, the medial and lateral segments of the left lobe, and the caudate lobe (1,2).

The right lobe consists of all of the liver substance to the right of an imaginary plane running from the sulcus for the inferior vena cava posteriorly, to the gallbladder fossa anteriorly. In most persons, the right lobe constitutes the major portion of the liver. The right lobe is further subdivided into anterior and posterior segments, which can be identified by visualizing the bifurcation of the right portal vein into anterior and posterior divisions (Fig. 10.1), as well as by visualization of the right hepatic vein, which courses between the anterior and posterior divisions of the right lobe.

The right lobe of the liver is contiguous with the medial segment of the left lobe (also known as the quadrate lobe) and also communicates posteriorly with the caudate lobe of the liver via a parenchymal bridge known as the caudate process of the right lobe. The boundary between the medial segment of the left lobe and the right lobe is identified by the course of the middle hepatic vein, which runs in the relatively avascular plane between the right and left lobes (Fig. 10.2). An incomplete fissure, known as the chief fissure of the liver, forms another landmark for the boundary between the right and left lobes. On ultrasound examination this is seen as an echogenic linear structure coursing from the right portal vein to the neck of the gallbladder (Fig. 10.3). The medial segment of the left lobe extends from the anterior surface of the liver posteriorly to the porta hepatis. The lateral segment of the left lobe is separated from the medial segment by the undivided left portal vein (umbilical segment). More caudally, the ligamentum teres (3) forms the boundary between medial and lateral segments of the left lobe (Fig. 10.4), and the left hepatic vein forms another

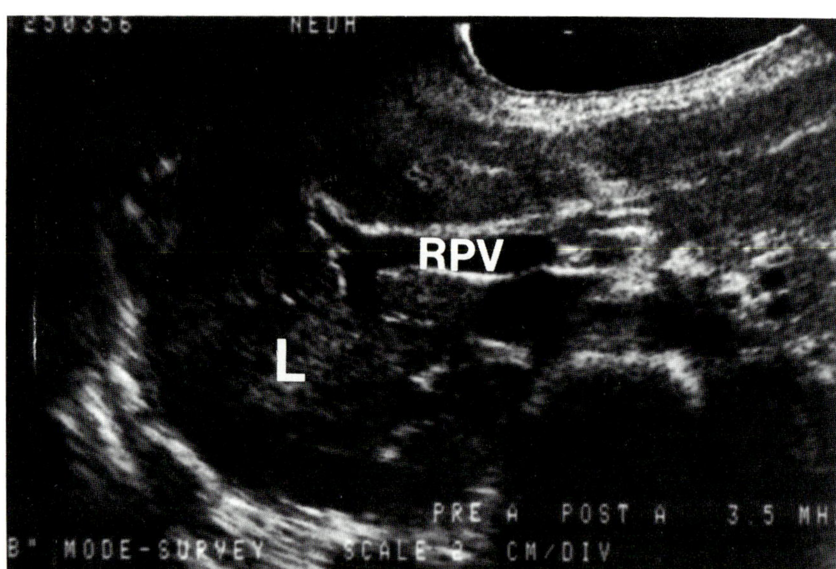

Figure 10.1. Transverse ultrasound showing the bifurcation of the right portal vein (RPV) into anterior and posterior divisions. L, liver.

boundary vessel between these two segments. The left lateral segment is also an anterior structure, with its posterior margin being defined by the porta hepatis and caudate lobe of the liver.

The caudate lobe is a deep or posterior lobe of the liver and extends from the porta hepatis leftward toward or across the spine (4). The anterior surface of the caudate lobe is defined by the fissure for the ligamentum venosum (5), a remnant of the sinus venosus seen in embryonic life (Fig. 10.5).

The caudate lobe is unique in that it derives its arterial, portal venous, and biliary supply from both the right and left common trunks; the left and right lobes of the liver receive their vascular and biliary supply exclusively from the left or right portal venous, hepatic arterial, and biliary trunks. The left and caudate lobes of the liver are quite variable in size but are most often significantly smaller in volume than the right lobe.

In the normal liver, 60% to 80% of the incoming blood flow is via the portal vein, which is formed

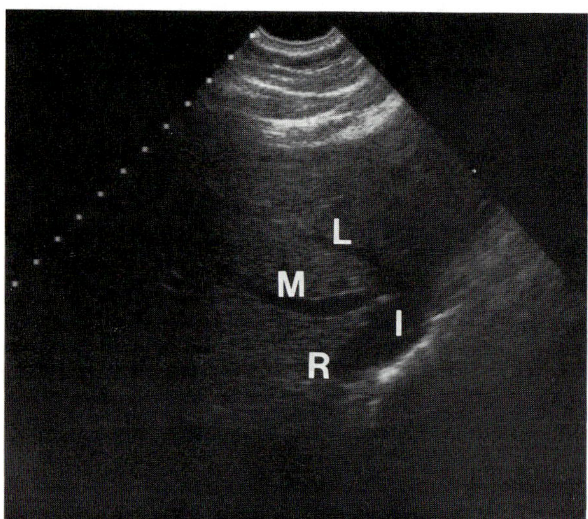

Figure 10.2. Confluence of left (L), middle (M), and right (R) hepatic veins with the inferior vena cava (I).

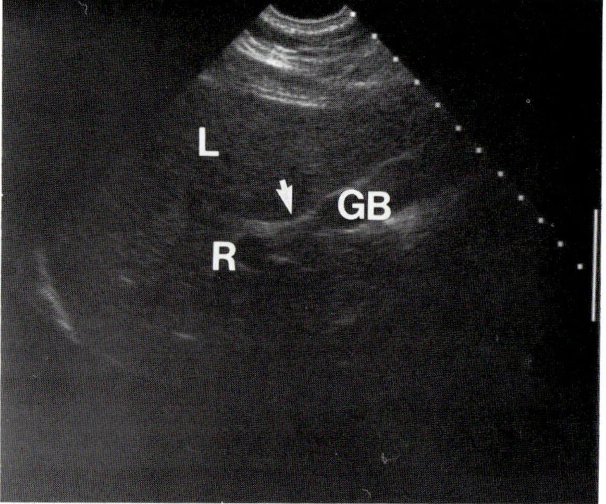

Figure 10.3. The chief fissure (*arrow*) of the liver (L) extending from the neck of the gallbladder (GB) to the right portal vein (R).

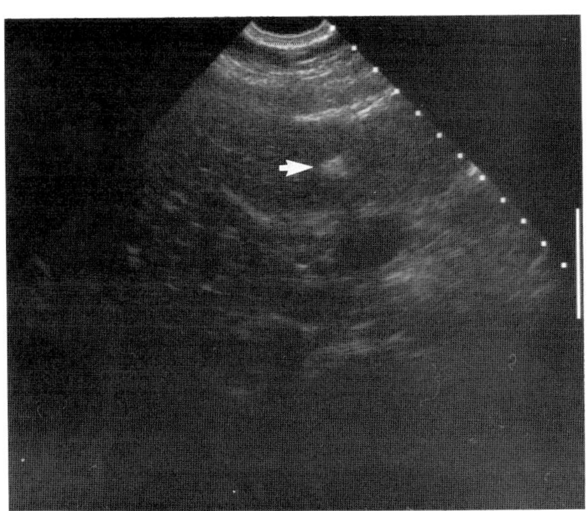

A

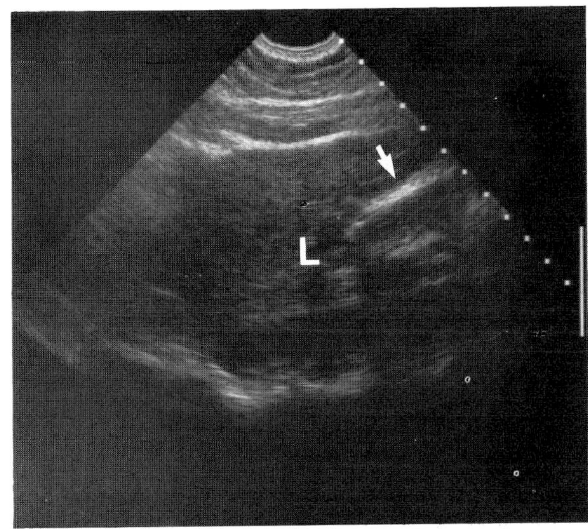

B

Figure 10.4. Ligamentum teres. (*A*) Appears as a rounded echogenic structure (*arrow*) on transverse view. (*B*) Appears linear on sagittal views arising from the left portal vein (L) and extending caudally to the free edge of the liver.

by the confluence of the splenic vein and the superior mesenteric vein in the region of the head of the pancreas. The portal vein then courses anterolaterally through the hepatoduodenal ligament to the porta hepatis (Fig. 10.6), where it bifurcates into main right and left trunks as well as supplying small penetrating branches to the cau-

date lobe (6). The hepatic arterial supply to the liver is quite variable (7). Typically the hepatic artery arises as one of the three major branches of the celiac artery and courses to the right side to the porta hepatis, where it branches into three main trunks, the right, middle, and left hepatic arteries, as well as again supplying small twigs to the caudate lobe. The middle hepatic artery supplies

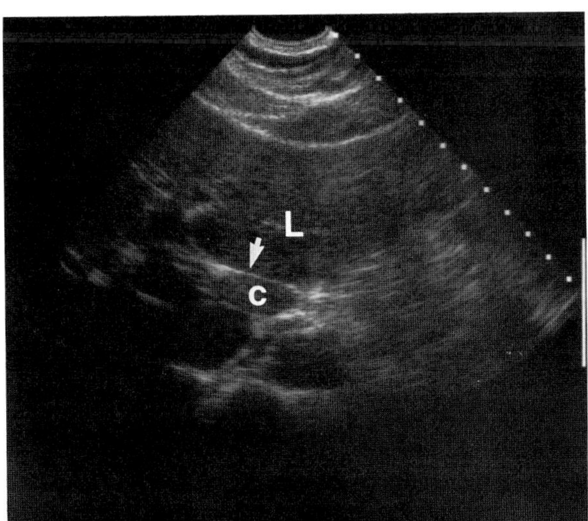

Figure 10.5. Fissure for the ligamentum venosum (*arrow*) dividing the left lateral segment (L) from the caudate lobe (C).

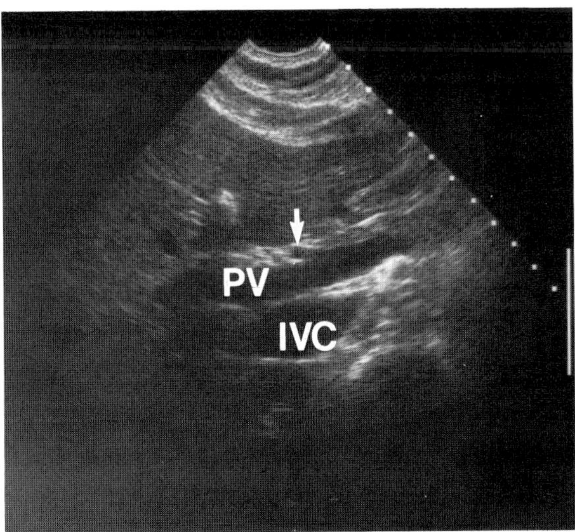

Figure 10.6. The main portal vein (PV) and hepatic artery (*arrow*) anteriorly. IVC, inferior vena cava.

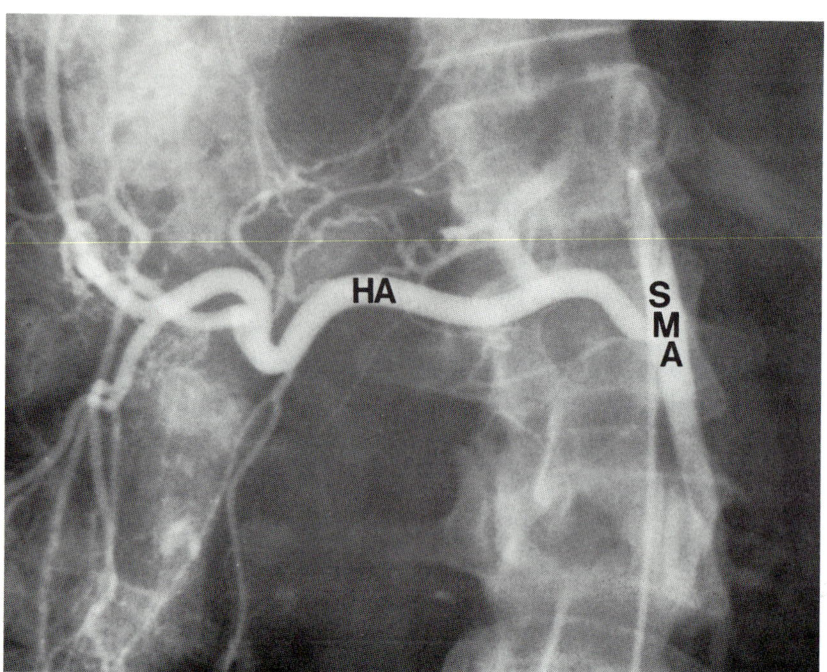

Figure 10.7. Selective arteriogram showing the hepatic artery (HA) arising aberrantly from the superior mesenteric artery (SMA).

basically the medial segment of the left lobe, whereas the left hepatic artery supplies the lateral segment (8). There is considerable variability in the arterial supply to the liver, however (9). In 25% of patients, there is either partial or complete relocation of the right hepatic artery to the superior mesenteric artery (Fig. 10.7). A replaced right hepatic artery is frequently seen in angiography and can indeed be recognized on ultrasound and CT examinations, where it is seen usually to course posterior to the portal vein into the porta hepatis (Fig. 10.8). Similarly, an accessory or replaced left hepatic artery can be seen in approximately 12% of patients, usually arising from the left gastric artery. Occasionally the entire hepatic artery may arise aberrantly either from a common celiac/mesenteric trunk, or directly from the aorta. Because of the considerable variability of the arterial supply to the liver, many surgeons find preoperative angiography indispensable for planning hepatic resections.

The intrahepatic biliary anatomy is discussed later in the chapter. The lymphatic vessels draining the liver are not visualized on CT or ultrasound examinations, but can be seen with some frequency during transhepatic cholangiography (10), when either the percutaneous skinny needle enters directly into a lymphatic or contrast material is forced through the hepatic parenchyma into draining lymphatic vessels (Fig. 10.9). The lymphatics arise in the perisinusoidal Disse's space, then drain into small lymphatics that tend to converge

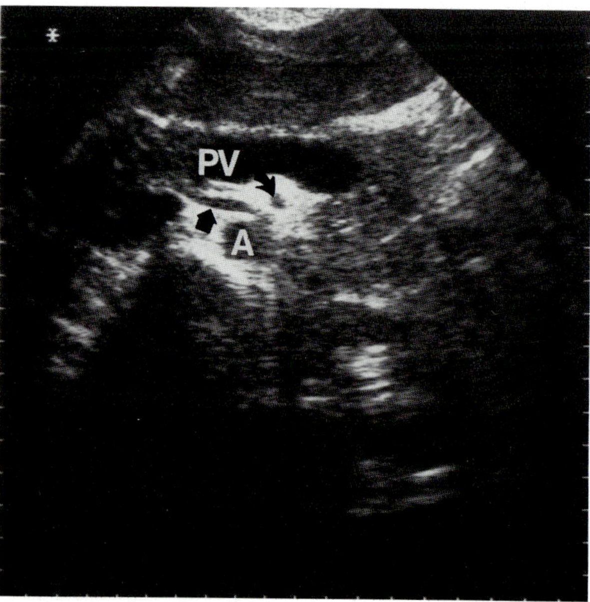

Figure 10.8. Accessory right hepatic artery (*arrow*) arising from the superior mesenteric artery (*curved arrow*) and coursing posterior to the portal vein (PV). A, aorta.

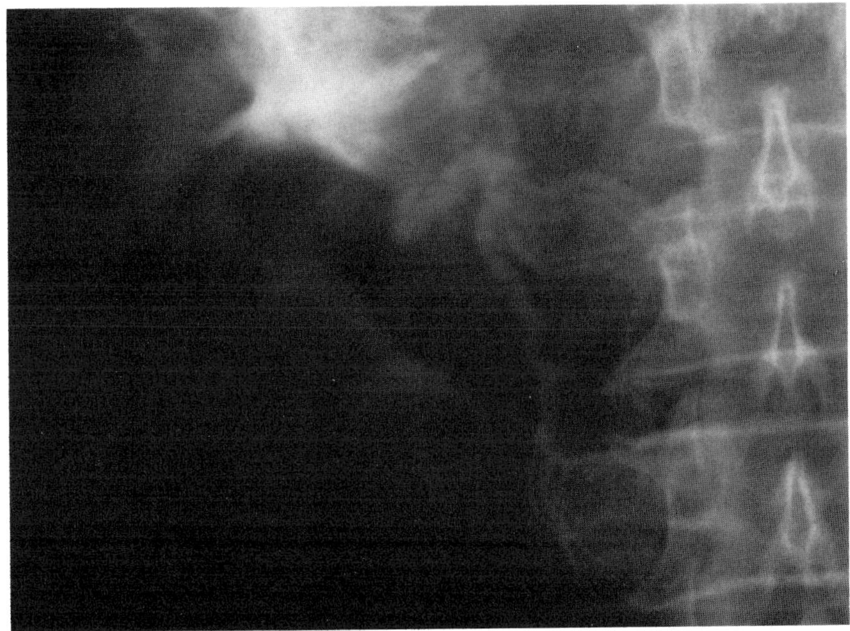

Figure 10.9. Transhepatic cholangiogram resulting in opacification of hepatic lymphatic channels in the porta hepatis and hepatoduodenal ligament.

into larger draining channels in the porta hepatis, exiting the liver along the hepatoduodenal ligament and draining into periportal and celiac lymph nodes. Although no diagnostic conclusions can be drawn from observation of the hepatic lymphatics, it is important to recognize their appearance and course in order to avoid confusing these channels with other biliary or vascular structures.

Diffuse Parenchymal Diseases

Cirrhosis

Hepatic cirrhosis may present with a variety of appearances, depending upon the stage of the disease. With acute alcoholic hepatitis, there may be generalized hepatomegaly, which can be recognized in images of kidneys, ureters, and bladder (KUB) as a soft tissue density filling the right upper quadrant and displacing the hepatic flexure of the colon inferiorly and at times displacing the duodenum toward the left. These changes, as well as posterior displacement and sometimes flattening of the right kidney, can also be visualized by CT. Hepatomegaly is somewhat more difficult to visualize on real-time ultrasonography, in which only a small portion of the liver is seen in any one section, but the contours of the liver are typically rounded or bulging as opposed to the usual tapered contour

(11). In addition, the volume of the right lobe can be judged relative to the right kidney. In a sagittal section through the liver and kidney, normally the area of liver is approximately twice that of the kidney, whereas with marked hepatomegaly the ratio may be 3:1 or 4:1, and flattening of the right kidney can also be seen (Fig. 10.10). Hepatomegaly can be well assessed by radionuclide technetium sulfur colloid scanning, in which the cephalocaudal dimension of the liver can be judged relative to a centimeter marker, the normal dimensions being less than 12 to 15 centimeters (Fig. 10.11).

With progressive damage to the liver, the right lobe becomes scarred and shrunken, while the left lobe and caudate lobe often undergo compensatory hypertrophy. The small right lobe may be recognized on plain films by high position of the hepatic flexure, but this is more readily visualized by ultrasonography, CT, and radionuclide scanning. In fact, a ratio of the size of the caudate lobe to the size of the right lobe has been proposed as a diagnostic criterion of cirrhosis by ultrasonography and CT (12), although this will only define cirrhosis in the later stages (Fig. 10.12). At ultrasonography the texture of the cirrhotic liver appears changed from the normal liver's usual homogeneous pattern and fine echo texture, to a coarse, inhomogeneous pattern with increased echogenicity and increased attenuation of the sound beam

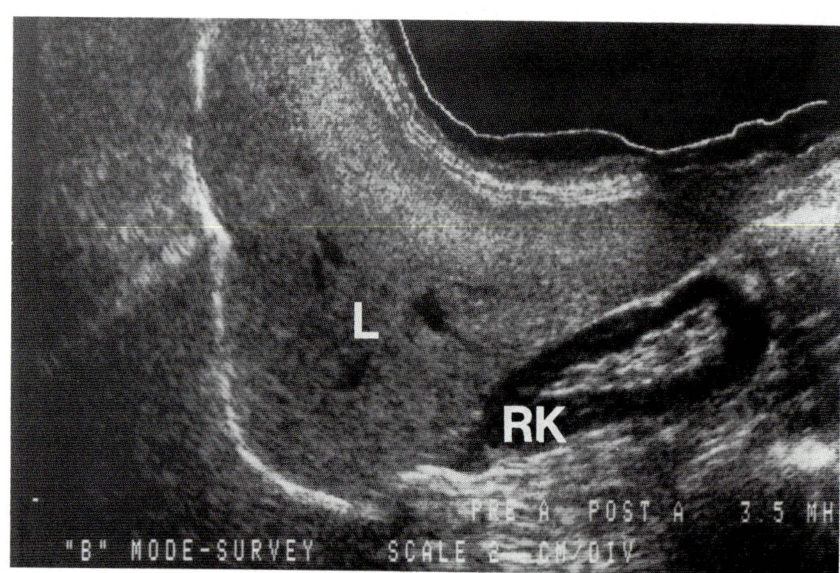

Figure 10.10. Sagittal ultrasound showing enlargement of the liver (L) with flattening of the right kidney (RK).

(13) (Fig. 10.13). Similar changes can be seen in fatty infiltration of the liver (14,15), however, and the ability to distinguish between these two entities is limited. The density and homogeneity of the liver as determined by CT do not change significantly with cirrhosis, but the distribution of radioactivity on technetium sulfur colloid is disrupted (16), with a typical nonhomogeneous uptake of isotopes, often accompanied by a shift of activity to the spleen and bone marrow with more severe

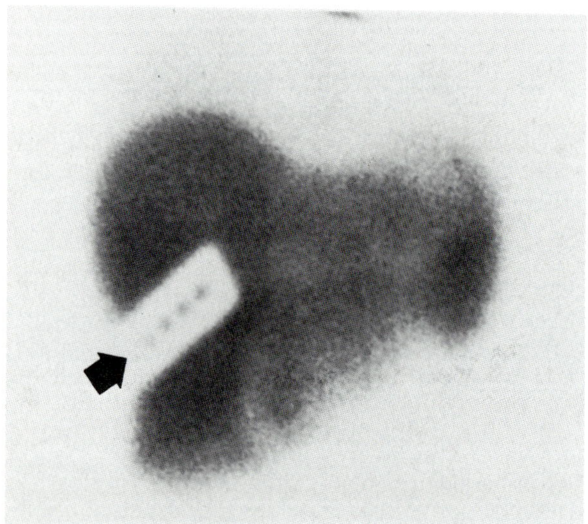

Figure 10.11. Technetium sulfur colloid liver scan demonstrating hepatomegaly. The photopenic marker (*arrow*) is 10 cm long.

stages of cirrhosis (Fig. 10.14). The inhomogeneous uptake can also be seen with fatty infiltration, but the splenomegaly and shift of the radiocolloid to the spleen and bone marrow are generally seen only with cirrhosis.

With arteriography, there are several findings seen in cirrhosis including enlargement of the common hepatic artery, reflecting increased arterial flow to the liver to accommodate the diminished portal flow (17). As the liver shrinks, the peripheral arterial branches become tortuous and redundant, giving a "corkscrew" appearance (Fig. 10.15). The capillary phase of a hepatic arteriogram may show mottled parenchymal opacification, and with very severe cirrhosis there may occasionally be arterioportal shunting, although the presence of shunting should raise strong suspicion of a possible hepatoma.

As the liver attempts to repair itself from the damage of cirrhosis, regenerative nodules develop. Typically these are very small (less than 5 millimeters). They are usually not visualized as discrete nodules by any of the imaging modalities but are rather lost in the generalized inhomogeneous background. Occasionally nodularity along the surface of the liver can be perceived by CT or ultrasound if the regenerative nodules are sufficiently large. Rarely giant regenerative macronodules can occur that may simulate the presence of neoplasm complicating the cirrhosis (Fig. 10.16), such as a hepatoma (18). Radionuclide evaluation

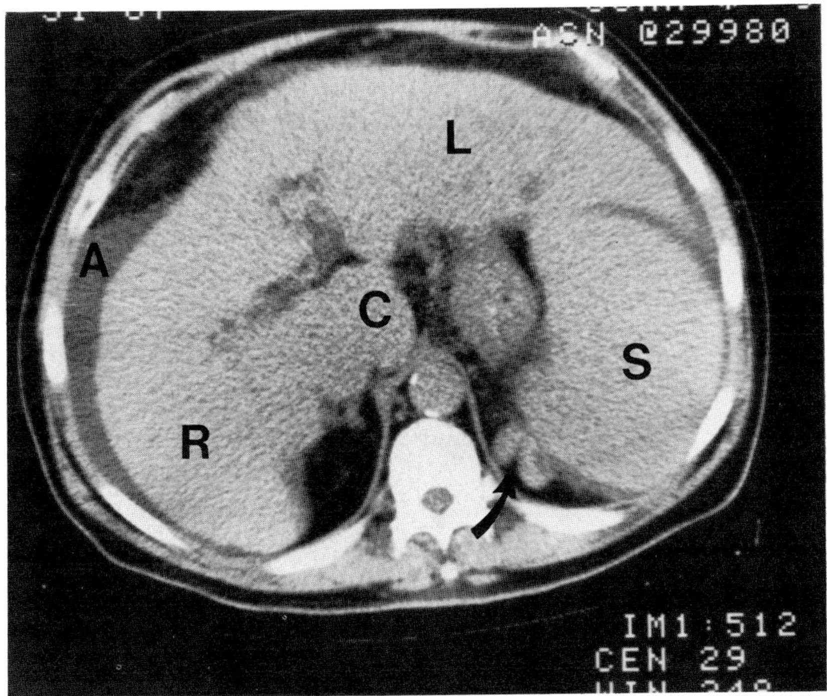

Figure 10.12. Hepatic cirrhosis with shrinkage of the right lobe (R) and hypertrophy of the left lateral segment (L) and caudate lobe (C). Note the perisplenic varices (*arrow*). S, spleen; A, ascites.

of these giant regenerative nodules is helpful since most of these will take up technetium sulfur colloid because of the presence of reticuloendothelial cells (19), whereas the hepatoma should be consistently cold on sulfur colloid scan.

Ascites frequently are present with cirrhosis, and if massive they can be detected by plain film of the abdomen. One of the earlier signs of ascites is loss of the fat pad that surrounds the posteroinferior margin of the right lobe of the liver. This is a deep space within the abdomen where ascites frequently collects, displacing the liver away from the adjacent retroperitoneal fat, and thereby obliterating the liver angle (Fig. 10.17). With more massive

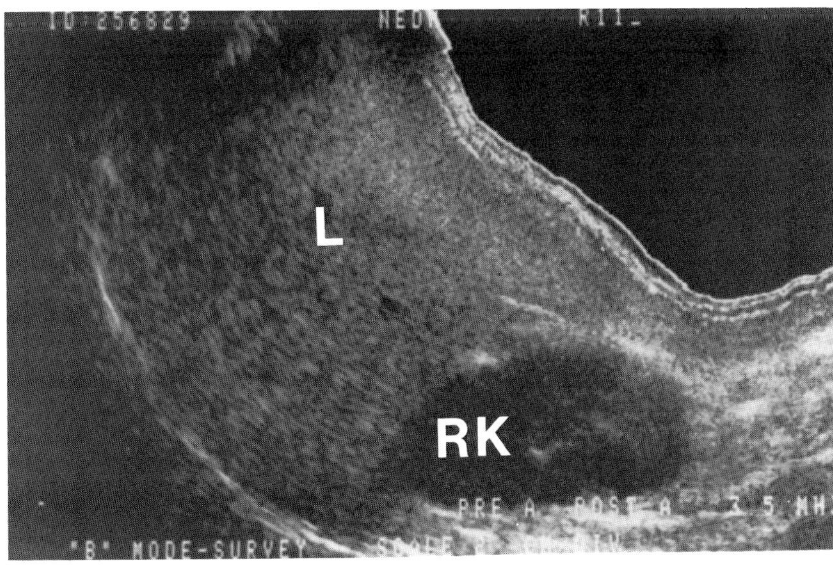

Figure 10.13. Highly echogenic liver (L) making the right kidney (RK) appear much more hypoechoic than normal. This pattern is seen in cirrhosis and fatty infiltration of the liver.

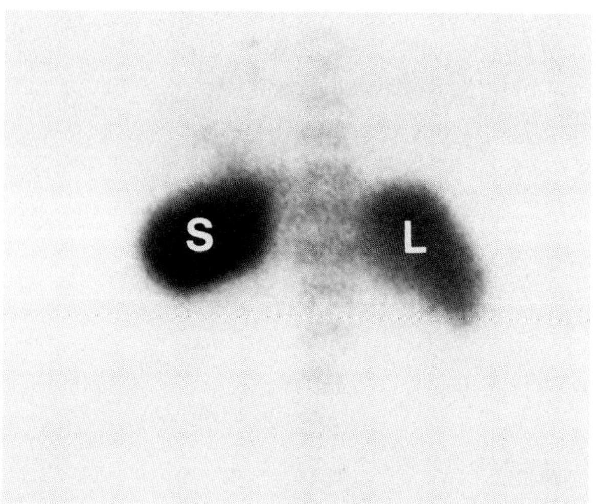

Figure 10.14.   Posterior view of technetium sulfur colloid liver scan showing a shift of activity from the liver (L) to the spleen (S) and to the bone marrow in the vertebral column, a finding typically seen with advanced cirrhosis.

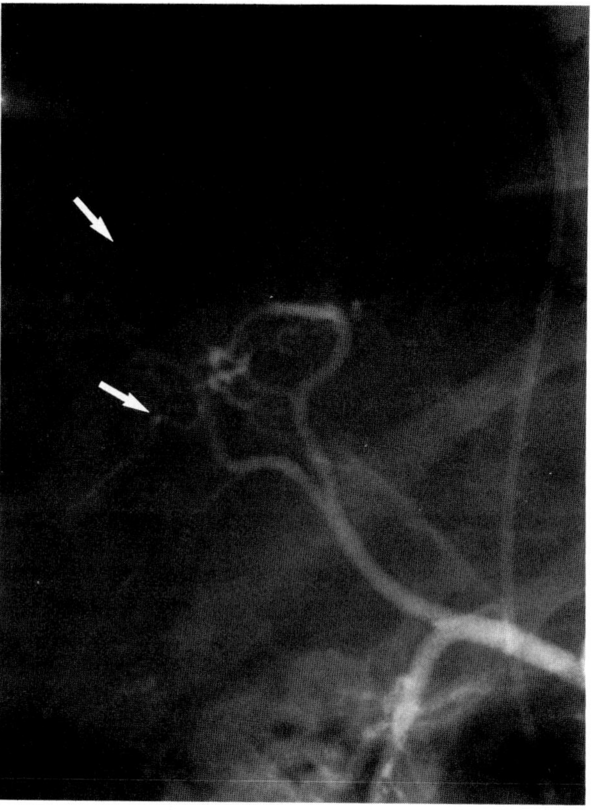

Figure 10.15.   Hepatic arteriogram demonstrating a corkscrew appearance to several of the right hepatic arteries (*arrows*) due to the loss of volume from cirrhosis. The catheter shown is in the right hepatic vein for wedge-pressure measurement.

ascites, fluid can be seen accumulating in the pelvis, obscuring the usual pelvic fat seen superior and lateral to the urinary bladder. Apparent displacement of the ascending and descending colon from the adjacent properitoneal fat can also be recognized because of the bulging flanks, and finally the gas-filled small bowel and transverse colon can be seen to float centrally within the abdomen when the patient is supine.

CT and ultrasound are much more sensitive in detecting minimal ascites, which is typically first seen around the lateral margin of the liver or spleen and in Morrison's pouch (the posterior subhepatic space), as well as in the pelvis. This is seen as a homogeneous low density on CT (Fig. 10.18), intermediate between the soft tissues and the fat in the retroperitoneum. Ascites is anechoic by ultrasonography unless complicated by bleeding, infection, or other inflammation, at which point the fluid may contain some more echogenic material (Fig. 10.19).

As portal hypertension develops, there are no specific plain film findings seen but the development of esophagogastric varices can be fairly well demonstrated by barium swallow and upper gastrointestinal tract series. Esophageal varices are seen as curvilinear serpiginous filling defects in the barium-filled esophagus (Fig. 10.20). Small varices are often obscured by a fully distended esophagus

but can be sometimes visualized as the esophagus is relaxed and partially collapsed. Similarly, serpiginous or nodular filling defects may be seen in the stomach, especially in the cardia and fundus and less frequently in the antrum and duodenum.

Varices can also be recognized quite readily by ultrasonography and CT. Barium is probably more sensitive in detecting the esophageal varices, but varices along the lesser and greater curvature of the stomach may be better shown by ultrasound and CT. At ultrasonography, varices appear as extremely tortuous tubular or serpiginous anechoic structures (20), typically seen posterior to the left lobe of the liver along the lesser curvature of the stomach, or medial to the spleen along the greater curvature of the stomach (Fig. 10.21). The appearance is quite characteristic and diagnostic. Lesser curvature varices can be traced back to a dilated coronary vein, which can be seen to arise

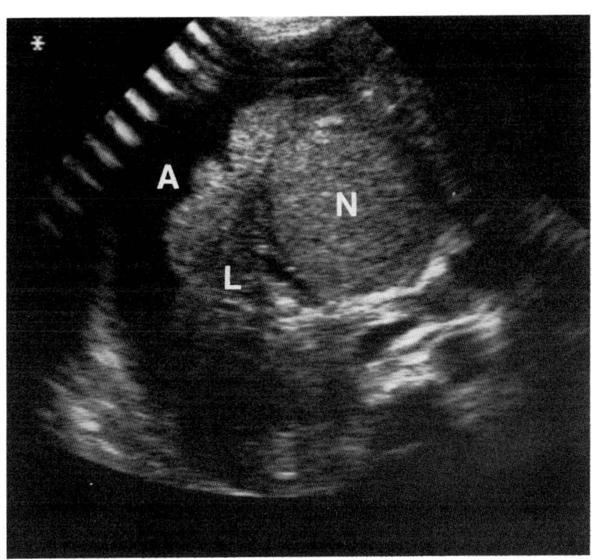

Figure 10.16. Giant regenerative macronodule (N) surrounded by a scarred cirrhotic liver (L). A, ascites.

from the confluence of the splenic and portal veins with advanced portal hypertension. The coronary vein is never seen in a normal setting. On CT scanning without contrast, varices may be visualized but can be confused with lymphadenopathy because of their rounded nodular appearance. However, a bolus injection of intravenous contrast material and subsequent dynamic scanning over these areas will show intense opacification (Fig. 10.22), thereby conclusively demonstrating their vascular nature (21).

With severe portal hypertension, spontaneous portosystemic shunts occur with some frequency. The most common shunt that can be recognized sonographically is the splenorenal shunt (20), with collaterals extending from the splenic vein into the region of the left adrenal gland and subsequently draining via the inferior adrenal vein into the left renal vein and inferior vena cava (Fig. 10.23). Alternatively, collaterals may extend around the lateral and inferior margins of the left kidney via capsular veins, which subsequently drain directly

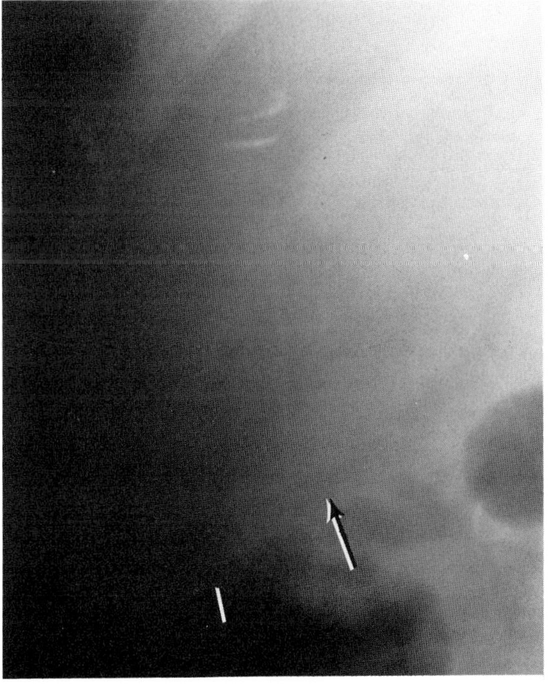

A

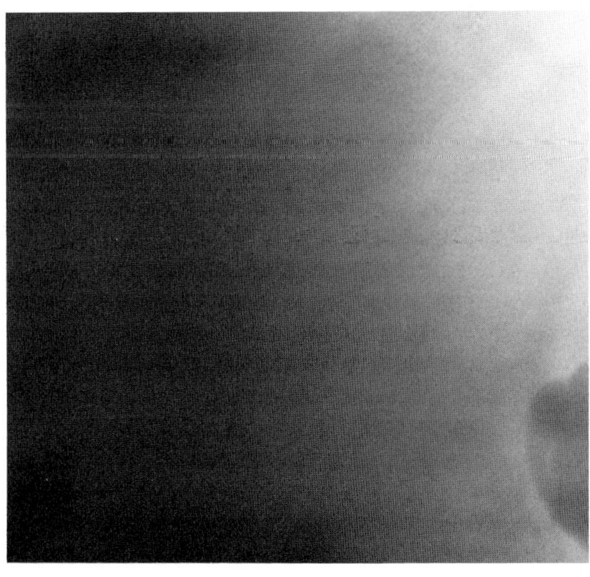

B

Figure 10.17. (*A*) Plain film of the abdomen demonstrating the normal radiolucent fat (*arrows*) surrounding the tip of the right lobe of the liver. (*B*) The same view of the same patient after development of ascites resulting in obliteration of the fat surrounding the liver angle.

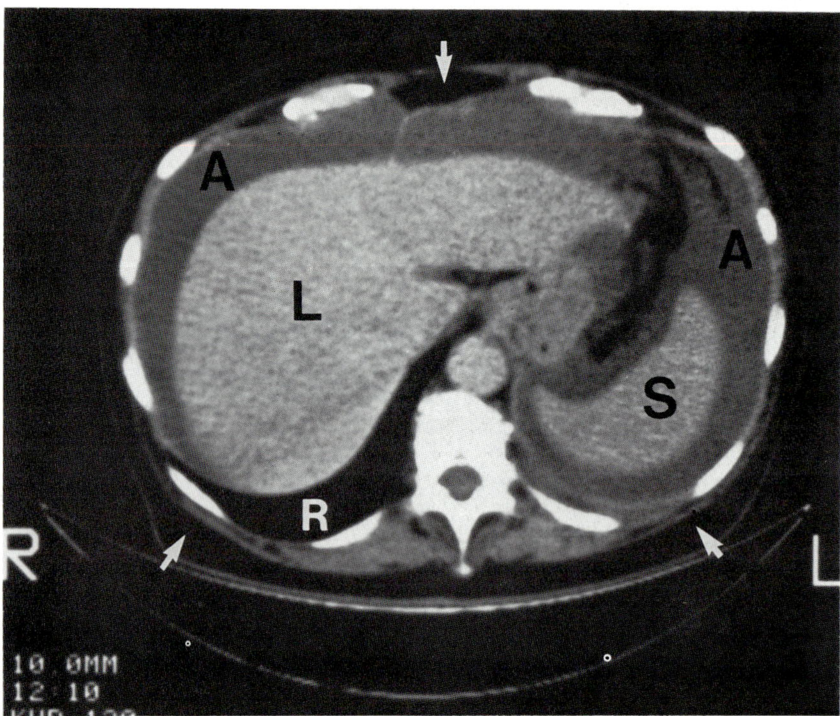

Figure 10.18. The CT density of ascites (A) is less than that of the liver (L) and spleen (S) but greater than the density of subcutaneous fat (*arrows*) and air in the right lung base (R).

into the left renal vein. Much less commonly other shunts may be identified including a mesocaval shunt with collaterals extending from branches of the superior mesenteric vein around the duodenal C-loop and head of the pancreas, into the right renal vein and inferior vena cava (Fig. 10.24). Collaterals may also be seen in the retroperitoneum, as well as in the pelvis, when hemorrhoidal veins or gonadal veins are used for the portosystemic connection.

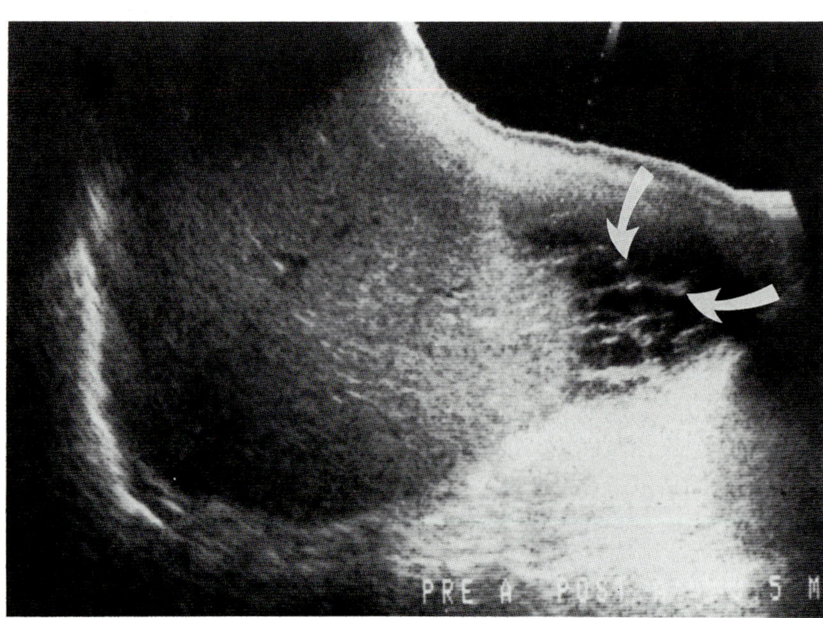

Figure 10.19. The presence of strands or echogenic material within ascites (*arrows*) indicates either blood, purulent material, or inflammation. Uncomplicated ascites are echo-free.

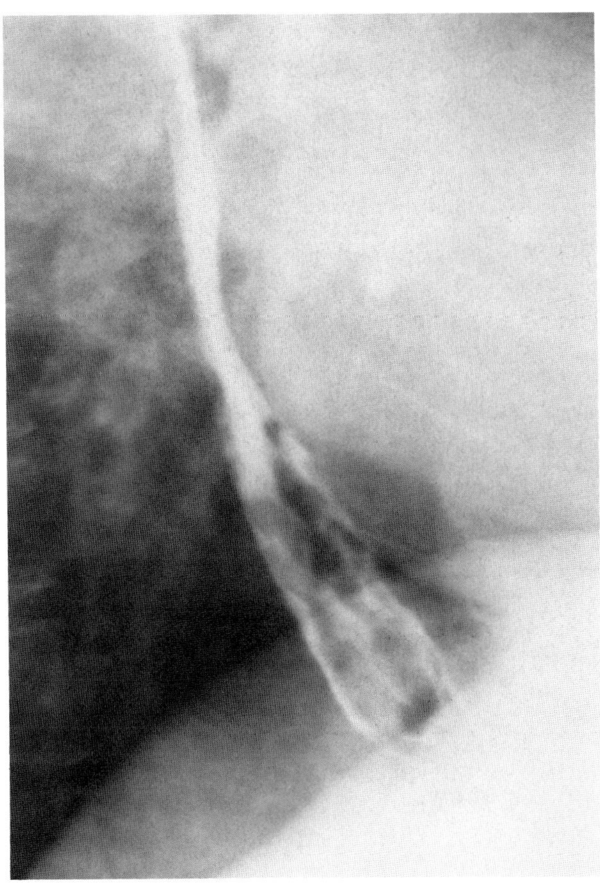

Figure 10.20. Barium swallow showing displacement of the barium by multiple serpiginous filling defects caused by lower esophageal varices.

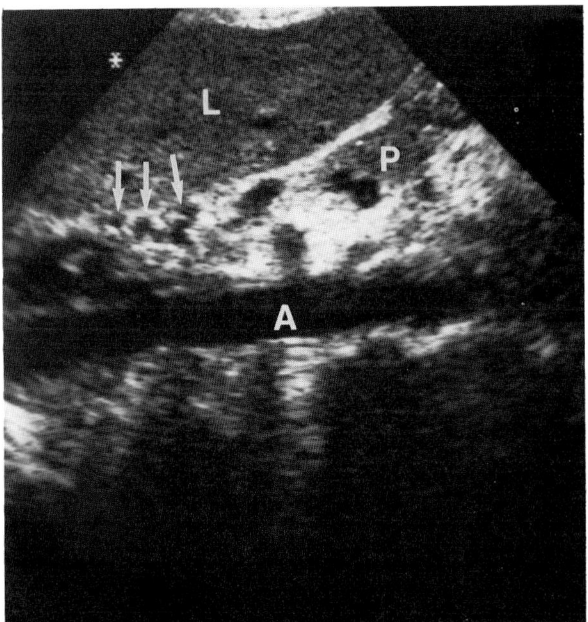

Figure 10.21. Sagittal ultrasound just to the left of midline, demonstrating multiple, tortuous, tubular, hypoechoic varices (*arrows*) posterior to the left lobe of the liver (L). A, aorta; P, body of pancreas.

Recanalization of the umbilical vein is felt to be a specific sonographic sign of portal hypertension (22). This vein is normally obliterated immediately after birth, but collaterals can develop with portal hypertension. The appearance is that of a fluid-filled (Fig. 10.25), anechoic, tubular structure located centrally within the ligamentum teres, which is normally homogeneous and hyperechoic in consistency. When large, the patent umbilical vein can be traced through the liver to the anterior peritoneal surface and followed down to the periumbilical region, where there is collateralization to branches of the inferior epigastric veins that drain into the iliac veins. This collateral pathway is typically seen in conjunction with the caput medusa on the surface of the abdomen.

Occlusion of the main portal vein, whether in conjunction with hepatic cirrhosis or occurring separately as a result of pylephlebitis, is often accompanied by development of portal-to-portal collaterals, the so-called cavernous transformation of the portal vein (23). This is readily recognized by ultrasound and CT as a nest of nodular or serpiginous vascular channels in the porta hepatis (Fig. 10.26). Collateral vessels may often be seen in the wall of the gallbladder also in the presence of portal vein occlusion. Cavernous transformation may occur as an unsuspected coincidental finding on routine CT or ultrasound scans when the patient is completely asymptomatic and there is no clinical evidence of portal hypertension elsewhere.

Angiography is, of course, the most effective means for evaluating portal hypertension. Arterial portography can be performed by injecting contrast material into the splenic and superior mesenteric arteries and filming delayed images as the contrast material passes into the splenic and superior mesenteric veins and subsequently into the portal vein (17). Esophagogastric varices are particularly well shown by this technique, and large patent umbilical veins may also be demonstrated, but frequently smaller varices are not seen as a result of respiratory motion. A more complete demonstration of all portosystemic collaterals can

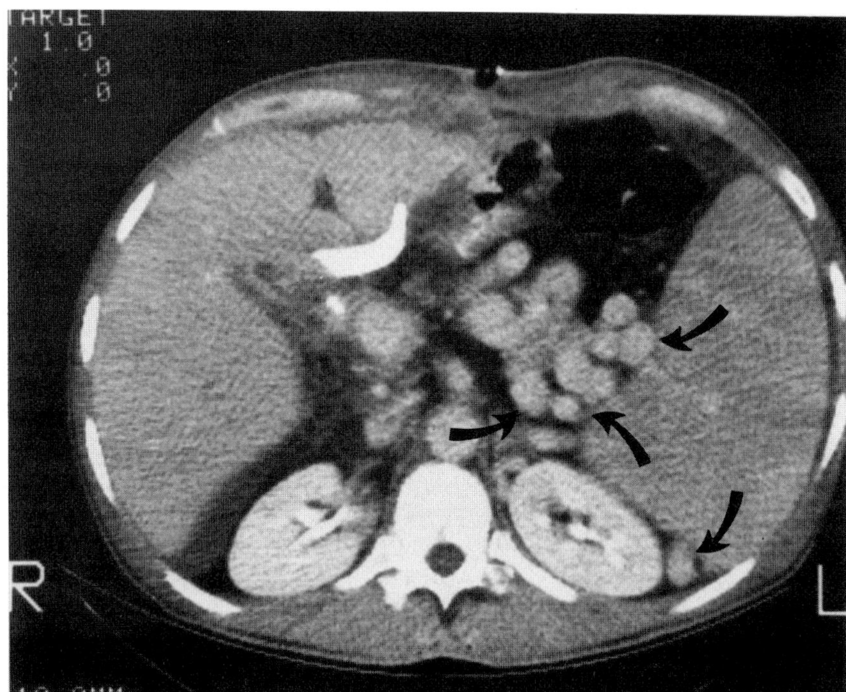

Figure 10.22. Multiple retroperitoneal varices (*arrows*) show enhancement on CT scanning after intravenous contrast administration.

be obtained by percutaneous transhepatic portography, in which a catheter is placed into the liver parenchyma and injections are made into a portal venous radicle with retrograde filling of the entire portal system. This is a time-consuming study, however, and is not used widely because the major collateral pathways can be demonstrated by arterial portography. Transhepatic portography has been used in an attempt to treat variceal bleeding by introducing sclerosing agents selectively into the coronary vein or branches feeding the bleeding varices. Hepatic venous catheterization can also be performed via the femoral vein and inferior vena cava. Pressures can be obtained by wedging the catheter distally in a hepatic vein; this reflects the sinusoidal pressure. A free hepatic vein pressure can also be obtained, and by subtracting the free hepatic vein pressure from the wedged pressure, a corrected sinusoidal pressure can be obtained that indicates the severity of the

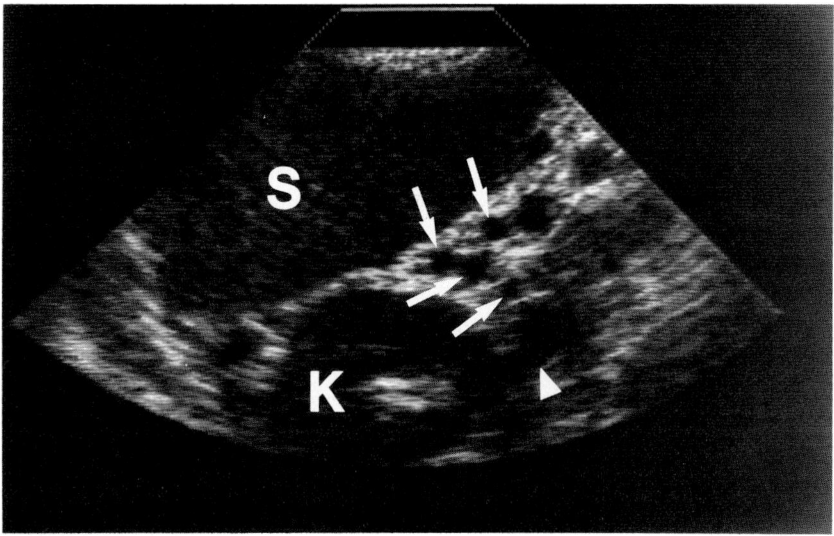

Figure 10.23. Spontaneous splenorenal shunt. The small perisplenic varices (*arrows*) could be traced in real time to the left renal vein (*arrowhead*). S, spleen; K, left kidney.

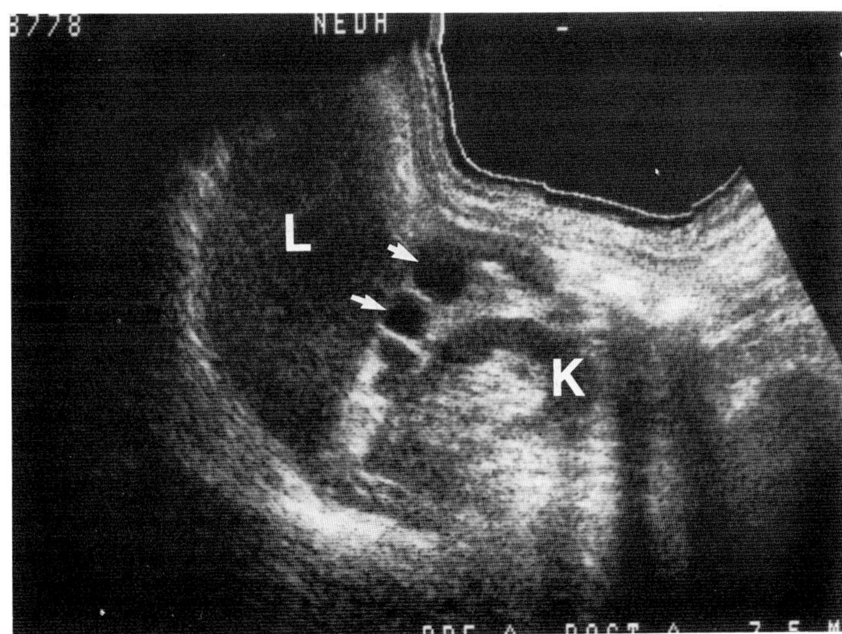

Figure 10.24. Right upper quadrant varices (*arrows*) between the liver (L) and the right kidney (K) as part of a spontaneous mesocaval shunt.

portal hypertension. The normal corrected wedge pressure is approximately 5 to 10 millimeters of mercury, and is considerably higher than this in advanced cirrhosis. Hepatic venography can also be performed to assess patency of the hepatic veins and to exclude hepatic venous occlusive diseases as a cause of portal hypertension (25). With cirrhosis the hepatic venous radicles are diminished in number and irregular in contour.

Both arterial and transhepatic portography may also demonstrate occlusion or thrombosis within the portal venous system, which may occur spontaneously as a result of slow flow. The presence of thrombus within the portal venous system is of great significance, especially if a portal venous shunt or hepatic transplantation is planned, because the presence of significant thrombus may make these surgical procedures impossible. By angiography, thrombus appears as a filling defect within the contrast-filled portal venous system (Fig. 10.27).

Thrombus can also be recognized as a filling defect on dynamic CT scanning with contrast enhancement of the portal vein (Fig. 10.28) (26). At ultrasonography, thrombus is readily seen as echogenic material filling the normally anechoic lumen of the portal vein or its radicles (Fig. 10.29) (27). The presence of portal vein thrombus should always alert one to the possibility of a hepatocellular carcinoma, which frequently will invade the portal venous system and grow within the lumen as tumor thrombus (28). Chronic portal vein thrombus often calcifies. This can be recognized by CT and ultrasound and is occasionally seen on plain films of the abdomen (Fig. 10.30).

Fatty Infiltration

Fatty infiltration of the liver may occur in a variety of conditions including diabetes, morbid obesity, following prolonged hyperalimentation, as a result of chemotherapy, and in association with cirrhosis and alcoholic hepatitis. The liver is frequently enlarged and has a lower density on CT scanning than normal (Fig. 10.31). Normally the density of the liver and spleen are quite similar, 40 to 60 Houndsfield units (HU), whereas with fatty infiltration the density of the liver will be significantly lower than that of the spleen (15). This is best appreciated in non-contrast-enhanced scans, as the iodine content of contrast material will increase overall liver density and may mask the changes of fatty infiltration. Ultrasonographically the liver will show increased echogenicity with an inhomogeneous pattern and enlarged blotchy echo pattern (14). There is also increased attenuation of the soundwaves as transmitted through the liver (Fig. 10.32). There has been a great deal of work attempting to distinguish the morphologic changes of cirrhosis from fatty infiltration by analyzing

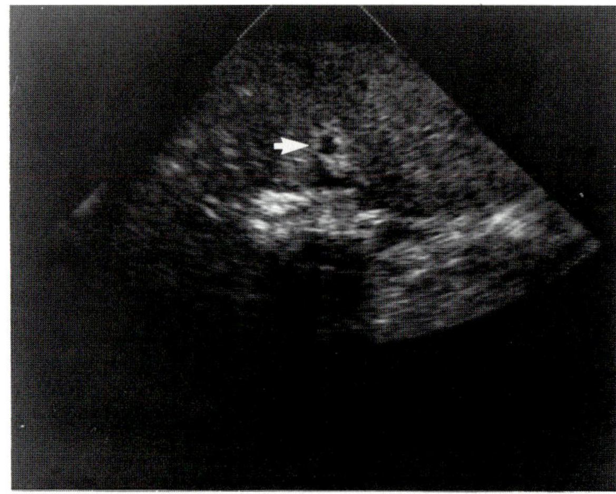

A

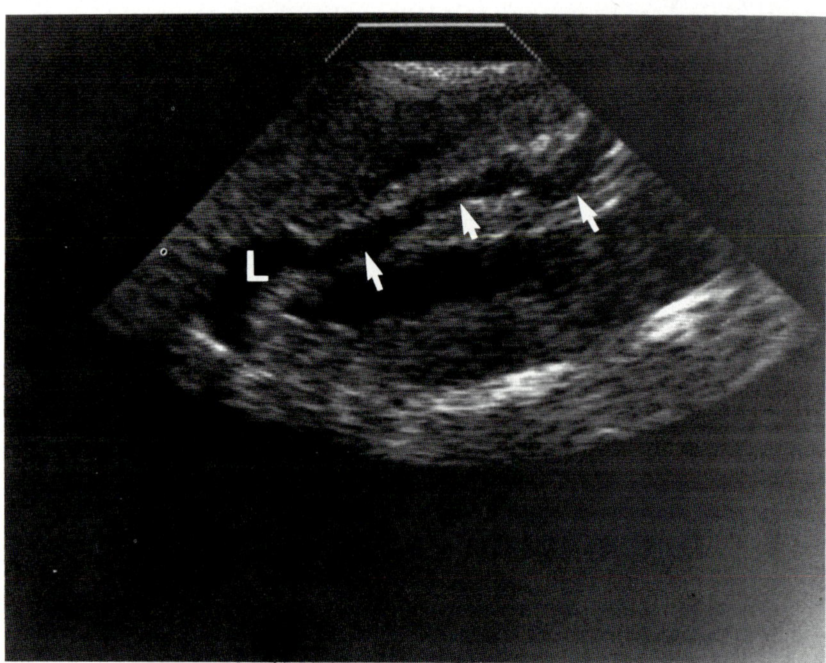

Figure 10.25. (*A*) Patent umbilical vein. Transverse ultrasound shows a bull's-eye appearance to the ligamentum teres (*arrow*) due to the recanalized umbilical vein within the ligament. (*B*) Sagittal scan shows the patent umbilical vein (*arrows*) as a tubular echolucent structure surrounded by the hyperechoic ligamentum teres. L, left portal vein.

B

histograms of echo amplitude through sections of the liver, but in general the two conditions are indistinguishable; indeed the increased echogenicity of cirrhosis may in part be due to the presence of increased fat in the liver. On MRI, the liver appears brighter when there is diffuse fatty infiltration, with shortened T_1 and prolonged T_2 relaxation times (29).

Usually, fatty infiltration is a diffuse process involving all of the liver, but it may occasionally be more patchy or even focal in nature. This may lead to the appearance of a pseudomass on CT or ultrasound, which is discussed in a later section.

Storage Diseases

Increased iron storage within the liver as a result of hemochromatosis can be detected by CT as a result of the overall increase in density of the liver parenchyma secondary to the iron deposition.

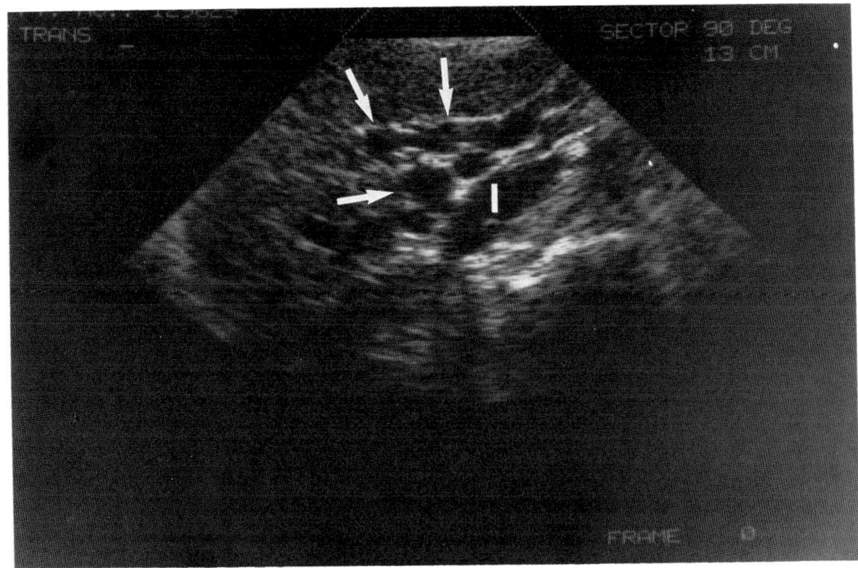

A

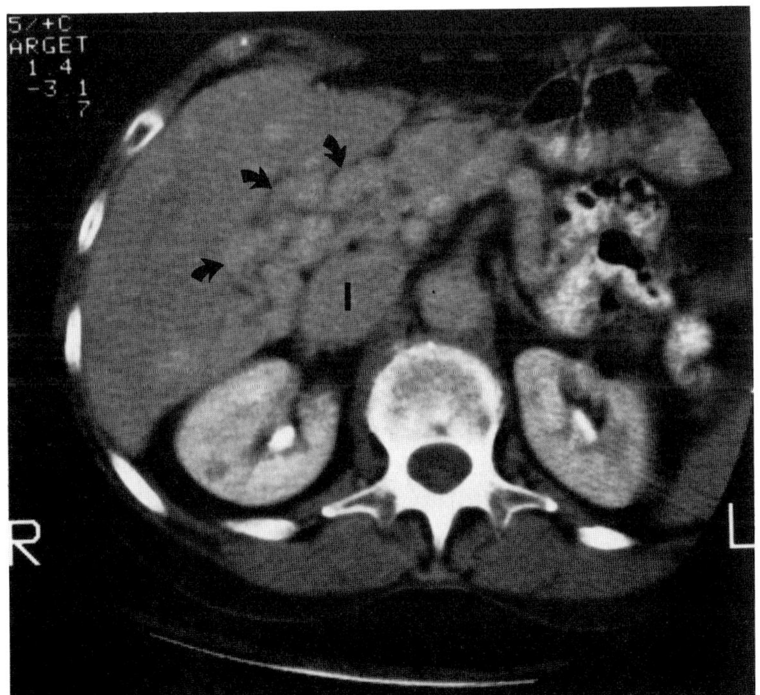

B

Figure 10.26. Cavernous transformation of the portal vein. (*A*) Multiple, hypoechoic tubular channels in the porta hepatis (*arrows*) replacing the occluded portal vein. (*B*) The collateral vessels (*arrows*) show increased density on CT after bolus injection of contrast material, thereby establishing their vascular nature. I, inferior vena cava.

Thus the liver, with a density of 100 HU or more, is often twice or more as dense as the spleen (Fig. 10.33) (30,31). Despite the readily recognizable changes on CT, there are usually no detectable sonographic changes in hemochromatosis, except for changes as a result of the development of hepatic cirrhosis. Magnetic resonance imaging shows diagnostic changes with hemochromatosis.

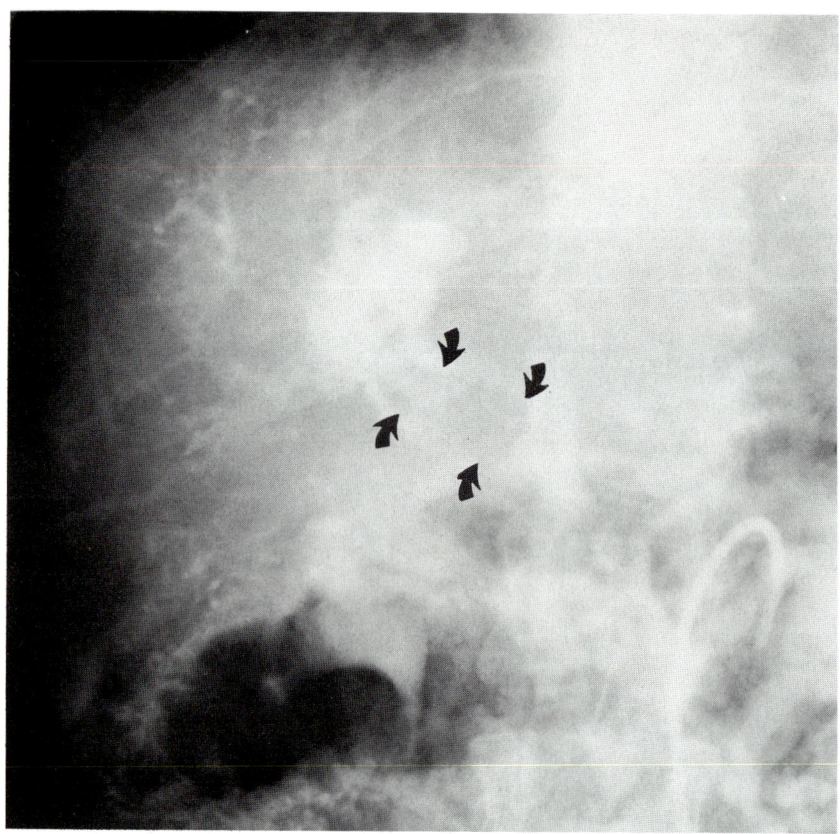

Figure 10.27. Portal vein thrombus as seen on the venous phase of a superior mesenteric arteriogram as a filling defect (*arrows*) within the opacified portal vein.

The increased iron content results in shortening of the T_1 and T_2 relaxation times (Fig. 10.34), giving the liver a low signal on both T_1- and T_2-weighted scans (32).

There is a marked increase in the incidence of hepatocellular carcinoma in patients with hemochromatosis. These carcinomas can be either focal masses or infiltrating neoplasms and can be recognized as such on the various imaging modalities (see "Malignant Tumors," page 210).

Glycogen storage disease (von Gierke's disease) results in hepatic enlargement and increased echogenicity at ultrasonography as well as increased attenuation of sound throughout the infiltrated liver (33). The density of the liver is also increased on CT. There is an increased incidence of hepatic adenomas in this condition, sometimes with malignant degeneration and development of hepatocellular carcinoma. The adenomas described in this condition appeared as hyperechoic solid masses, with some heterogeneity in larger lesions due to necrosis or hemorrhage (34). Notable was the apparent enhanced sound transmission deep to the solid tumors (35).

Thorium oxide (Thorotrast) was used in the 1930s and 1940s as an angiographic contrast material. Although unknown at the time, this is a long-lived radioactive contrast material emitting alpha radiation, and its use resulted in development of numerous neoplastic lesions in the liver including cholangiocarcinoma, hepatocellular carcinoma, and angiosarcomas (36). Thorotrast accumulated in the reticuloendothelial cells of the liver, spleen, and lymph nodes. These structures all show markedly increased radiodensity on plain films and CT, and both the liver and spleen are usually small and shrunken in size as well. If the typical pattern is recognized on plain films, CT should be performed to assess for development of neoplastic degeneration (Fig. 10.35).

Wilson's disease, the accumulation of copper within the liver, leads to hepatic cirrhosis and portal hypertension. These changes can be readily recognized by ultrasonography, although there are no specific changes in the hepatic parenchyma from the copper deposition per se. Similarly, amyloid infiltration of the liver may be recognized as diffuse hepatic enlargement without morphologic

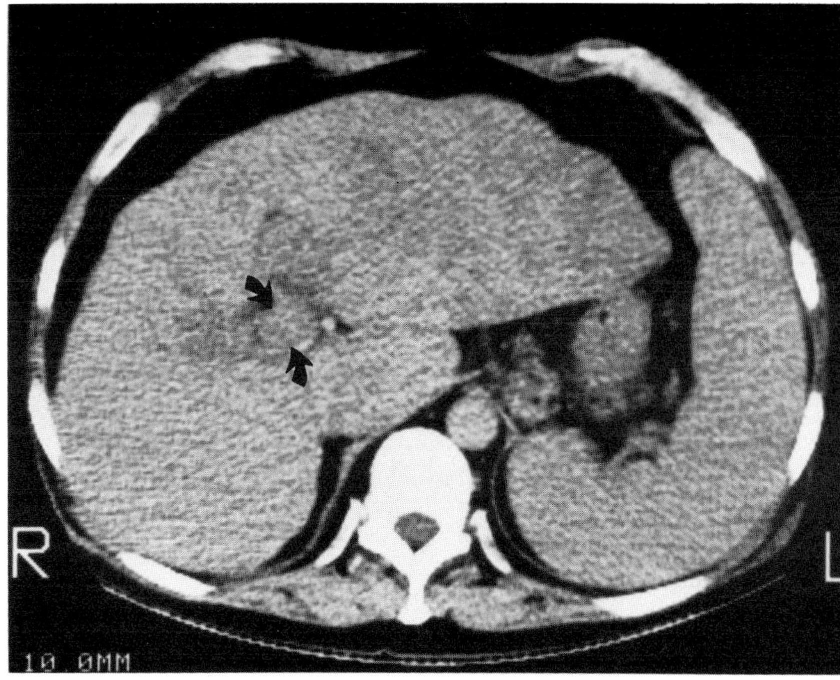

Figure 10.28. Tumor thrombus in the portal vein appears as an isodense filling defect (*arrows*) on contrast-enhanced CT scan.

change, although increased echogenicity of the kidneys has been described in amyloid infiltration. Large, discrete deposits of amyloid in the liver appear as focally low density areas on CT without significant enhancement following contrast injection (37). These focal deposits also show decreased activity on technetium sulfur colloid scan. The appearance may simulate neoplasm or focal fatty infiltration.

Hepatitis

Most patients with acute hepatitis have no need for liver imaging, and indeed there are few if any

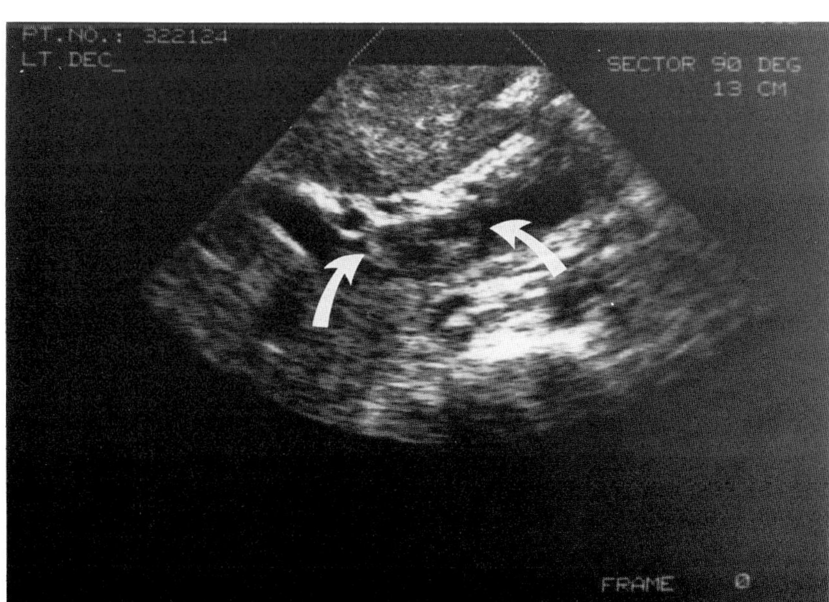

Figure 10.29. Echogenic thrombus (*arrows*) partially filling the lumen of the portal vein.

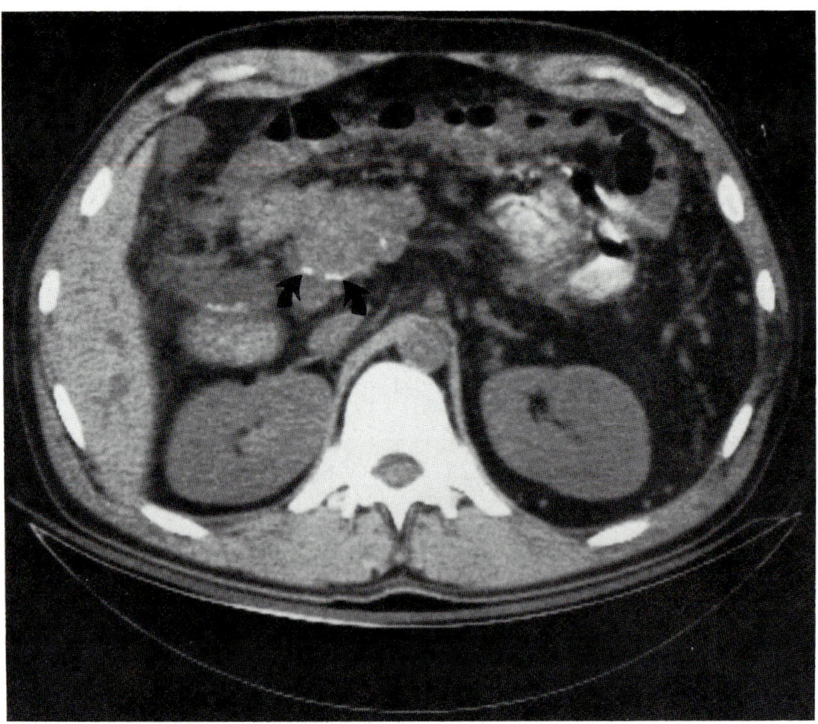

A

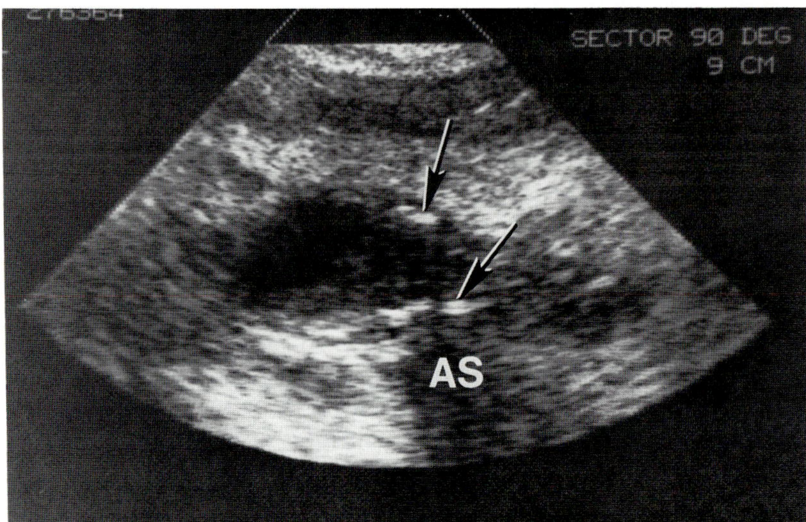

B

Figure 10.30. Chronic portal vein thrombus with calcification. (*A*) Rimlike calcification is seen in the superior mesenteric vein on CT (*arrows*). (*B*) Echogenic calcified thrombus (*arrows*) with acoustic shadowing (AS).

diagnostic patterns. Most often the ultrasound architectural pattern is normal, although a diminished parenchymal echogenicity with resultant accentuation or increased brightness of the periportal collagen has been described (38). In our experience this is infrequently seen, however. Radionuclide liver scan may show some inhomogeneity but there are generally no CT changes of note. Consistent changes on MRI have been noted with acute hepatitis, with increased signal inten-

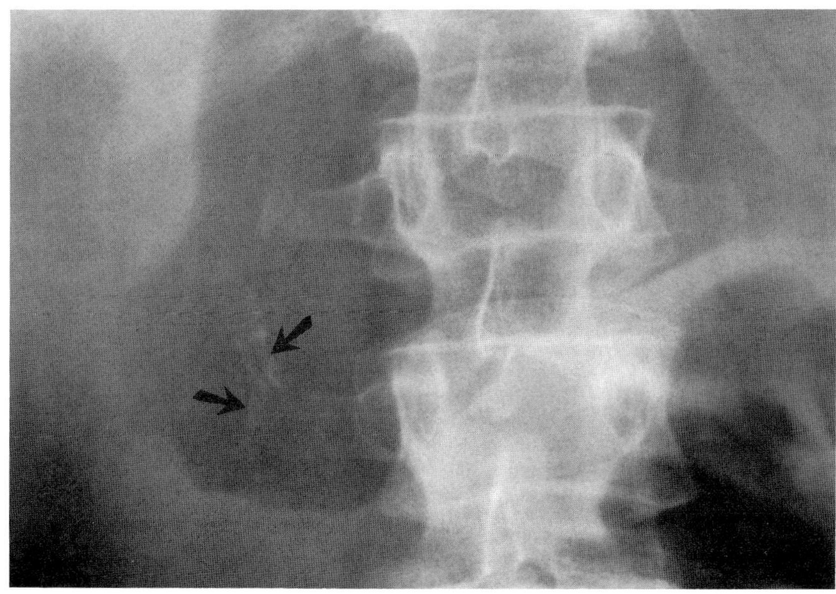

C

Figure 10.30 (continued). (C) Plain film visualization of calcified portal vein thrombus (*arrows*).

sity as a result of prolongation of T_1 and T_2 relaxation times, presumably due to increased water (edema) within the liver (29).

With chronic hepatitis, many changes can be seen with various imaging modalities, most of which are a result of fibrosis and subsequent cirrhotic changes. Perhaps the most useful role for imaging in patients with suspected hepatitis is to exclude biliary obstruction as a cause for the clinical findings.

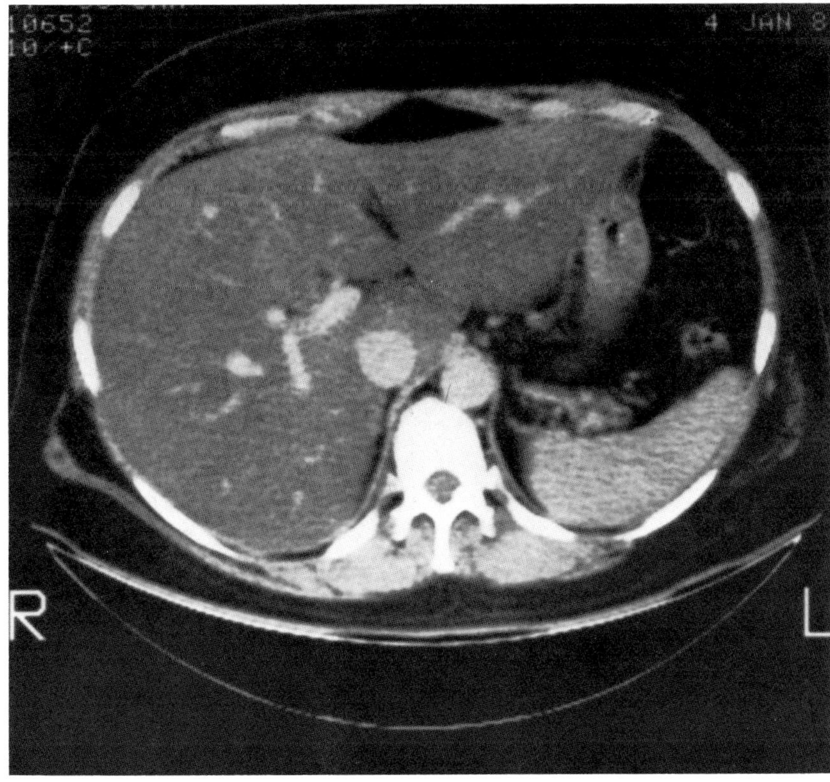

Figure 10.31. Diffuse fatty liver. The CT density is much lower (−13 HU) than that of the spleen, making the portal and hepatic veins stand out against the much lower density hepatic parenchyma.

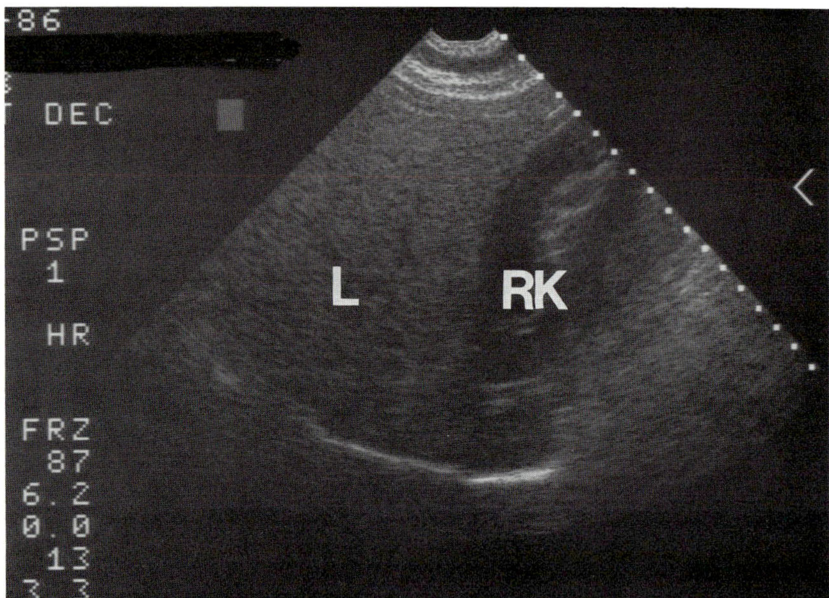

Figure 10.32. Diffuse fatty liver. On ultrasonography shows increased echogenicity, making the renal cortex appear more hypoechoic than usual. RK, right kidney; L, liver.

Focal Disease Processes

Infection

Pyogenic liver abscesses are most often secondary to Gram-negative rods such as *Escherichia coli*, anaerobic streptococci, *Bacteroides* species, and *Clostridium* species. The most common source of these abscesses is biliary tract infection, which may be a complication of stones and biliary tract obstruction or pancreatitis. Other common sources

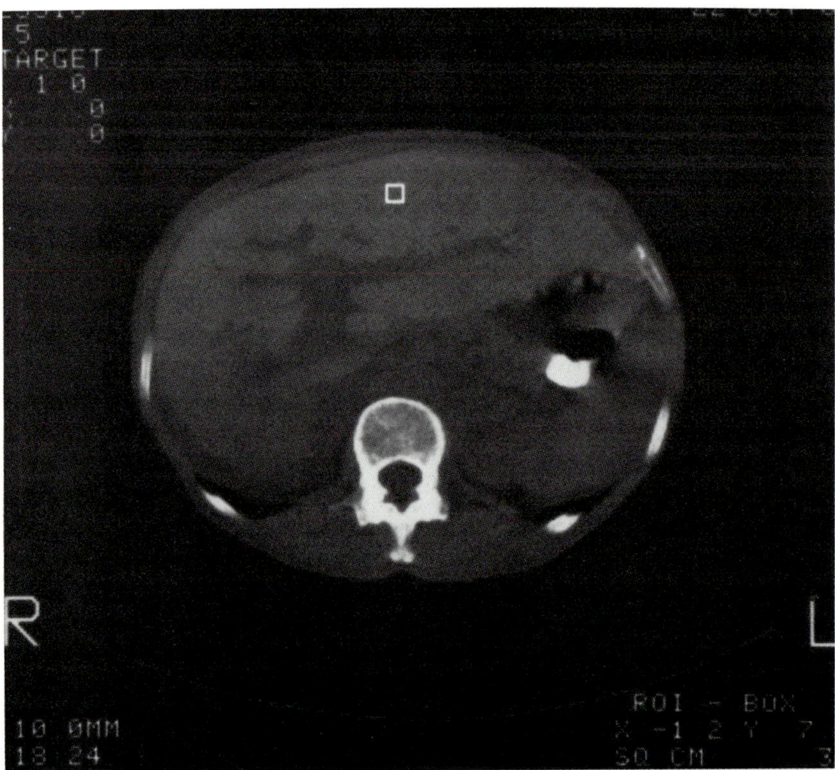

Figure 10.33. Hemochromatosis. The liver CT density is markedly increased (95 HU) relative to the spleen, making the portal vasculature stand out in negative contrast to the liver parenchyma.

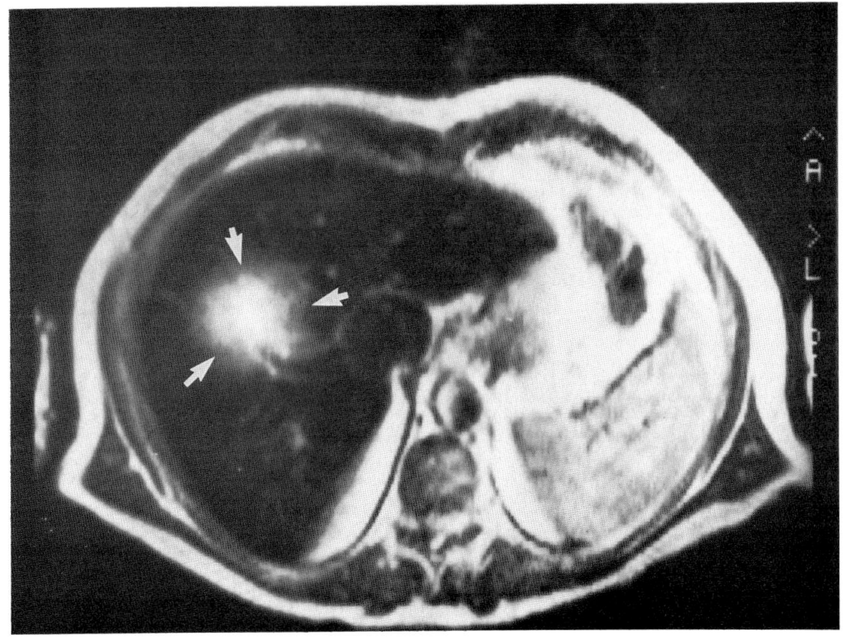

Figure 10.34. Hemochromatosis with hepatoma, MRI. The paramagnetic effects of iron in the liver result in extremely low signal intensity. The higher intensity mass centrally (*arrows*) is caused by a hepatocellular carcinoma.

include peridiverticular abscesses, inflammatory bowel disease, and appendicitis. If these abscesses are undrained, there is an extremely high mortality rate; consequently, early diagnosis and either percutaneous or surgical drainage are essential.

Plain films of the abdomen show no findings with the usual hepatic abscess unless there is gas contained within the lesion. In this setting, a mottled or bubbly gas collection may be seen projected over the liver and air-fluid levels may be seen on decubitus or upright films. Care must be taken not to mistake colonic gas for an abscess when the hepatic flexure is high in position, as can be seen with Chiliaditi's syndrome, where the hepatic flexure extends anterior to the liver up to the diaphragm. Similarly, if there has been previous hepatic resection, the colon may ride higher than usual.

Because of its nonspecificity, radionuclide scanning has little role in assessment for hepatic abscesses, but a sufficiently large abscess would appear as a focal cold area. Lesions smaller than 2 to 3 cm may not be visualized, however. Gallium-67 citrate scanning is useful in detecting inflammatory and infectious foci, which will show increased uptake relative to the normal liver parenchyma (Fig. 10.36) (39). However, this is also not specific, as hepatomas and some lymphomas may also show gallium positivity.

Ultrasound is a rapid and accurate means of assessing for hepatic abscesses, most of which are hypoechoic relative to the surrounding liver parenchyma with well-defined back walls and posterior acoustic enhancement as a result of their fluid content (40). The internal texture depends on the composition of the abscess and may vary from almost anechoic to a mixed pattern, and occasionally one may encounter hyperechoic abscesses (Fig. 10.37). This is more common in early stages before extensive liquefaction has occurred. If extremely high amplitude echoes are seen within an abscess, this is an indication of gas formation (41), and one may see associated acoustic shadowing or reverberation artifacts from the foci of gas (Fig. 10.38). Lesions as small as 1 to 2 cm can be regularly identified, and frequently multiple abscesses are encountered. The walls are often somewhat irregular in contour, and two abscesses within the same patient may have different appearances depending upon the age, degree of inflammation, and amount of liquefaction. The most diagnostic feature is increased sound transmission through the fluid medium, resulting in posterior acoustic enhancement. This is not always seen, however, especially in early infectious lesions, which are more cellular in nature. Differential diagnosis would include necrotic neoplastic lesions and hematomas.

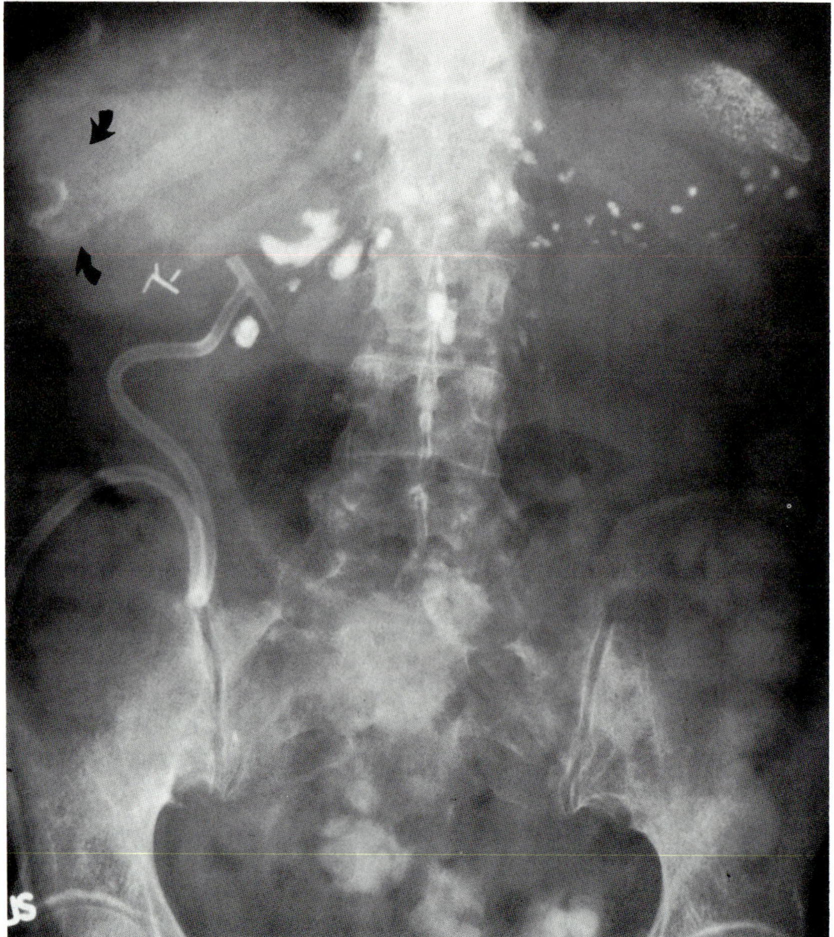

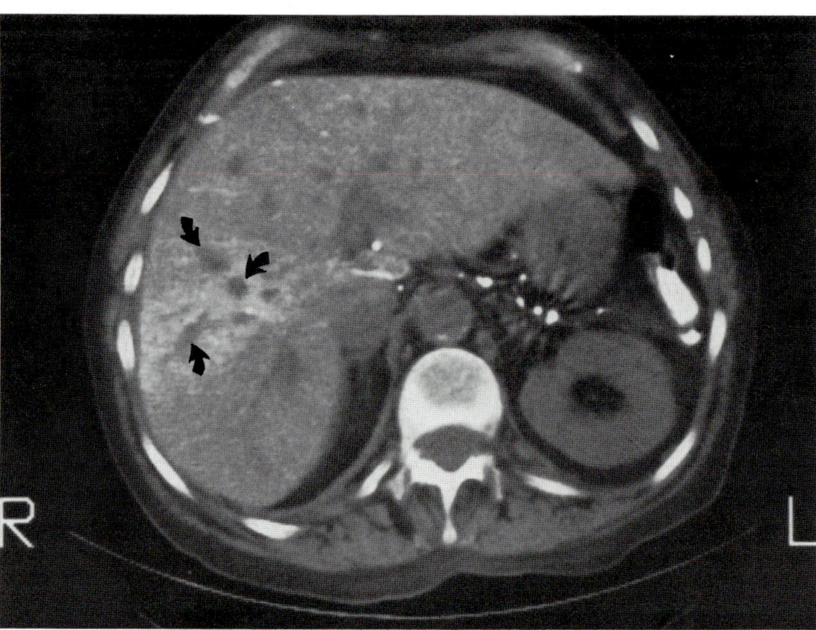

Figure 10.35. Thorotrast toxicity. (*A*) KUB shows a small hyperdense spleen, multiple dense celiac periportal and peripancreatic lymph nodes, and some less well defined, increased density in the liver (*arrows*) due to retained thorium oxide. (*B*) CT shows increased density in the lymph nodes and liver, as well as low-density dilated bile ducts (*arrows*) caused by a Thorotrast-induced cholangiocarcinoma.

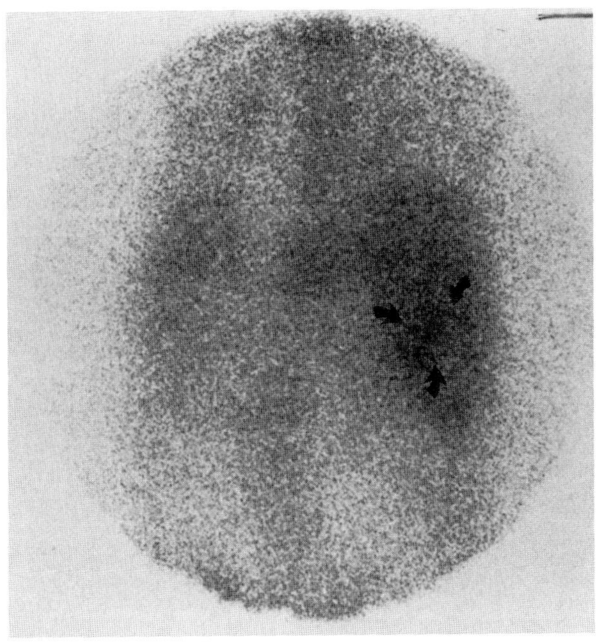

Figure 10.36. Hepatic abscess. Posterior view of a gallium scan showing slightly increased accumulation in the inferior right lobe (*arrows*) at the site of a pyogenic liver abscess.

CT scanning is equally accurate in the diagnosis of liver abscesses, most of which show uniform low density, with CT numbers ranging from 10 to 30 HU (42). The margins between the abscess and the surrounding liver are usually fairly sharp (Fig. 10.39), and there is no enhancement following intravenous injection of contrast material, although the interface between the abscess and liver parenchyma may show some enhancement (43). More aggressive or acute abscesses may have poor wall definition (Fig. 10.40). Gas formation within an abscess is readily detected either as bubbles or as air-fluid levels. As with ultrasound, on CT hematomas and necrotic liver tumors may appear similar to liver abscesses. Acute hematomas will have a higher density but chronic hematomas may be in the same range as abscesses. In addition, hepatic cysts can potentially be confused with abscesses on CT, although the values for cysts are generally closer to 0 HU.

Both CT and ultrasound are also excellent in assessing infectious collections around the liver in the subhepatic and subphrenic spaces (Fig. 10.41). Both modalities are also useful in guiding catheter placement for percutaneous drainage of liver abscesses (42,44,45), a highly successful technique that usually obviates the necessity for open surgi-

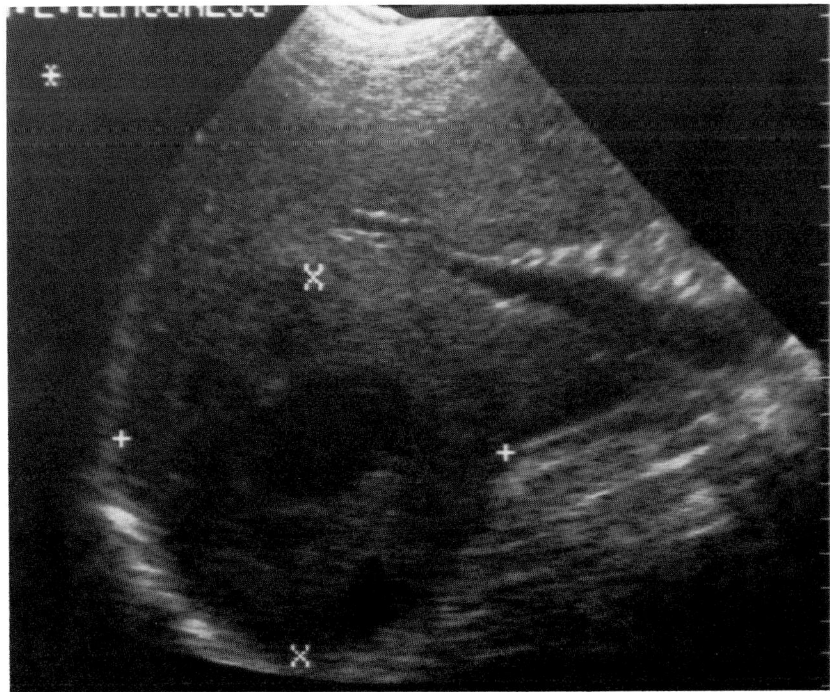

Figure 10.37. Liver abscess. Note the mixed echogenicity of this large abscess (*between calipers*) with both isoechoic and hypoechoic liquified areas seen.

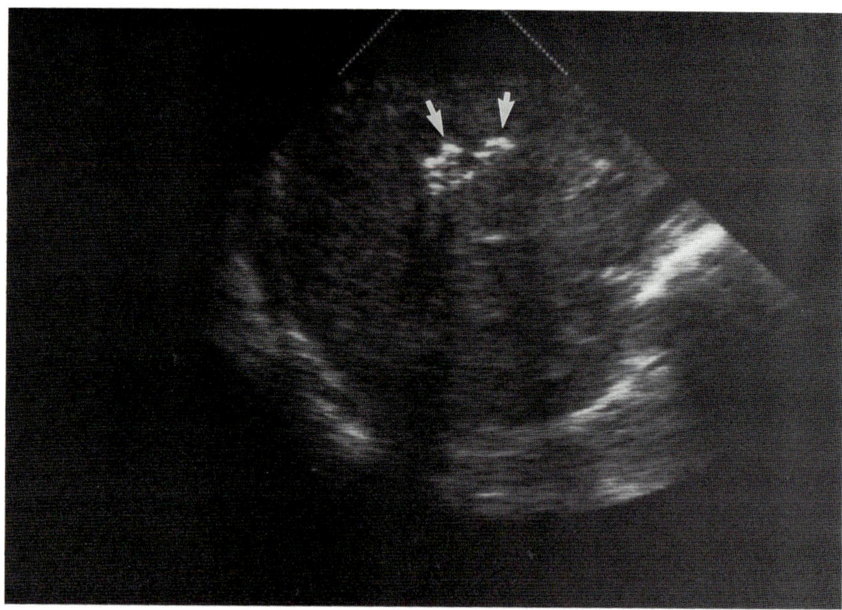

Figure 10.38. Gas-containing hepatic abscess. The gas-containing areas are markedly hyperechoic (*arrows*) and are associated with posterior acoustic shadowing.

cal drainage. Finally, both CT and ultrasound are also useful in following the healing of intrahepatic abscesses (46). In very obese patients or patients who are postoperative with large abdominal incisions, CT is probably preferable to ultrasound, which may be limited in these situations. Otherwise, because of the lack of ionizing radiation, ultrasound is the best initial imaging modality to assess for liver abscesses.

Amebic liver abscesses are perhaps the most common liver infections worldwide and are seen frequently in southwestern sections of the United States. The infection is usually in the right colon and invades the liver via the portal venous route.

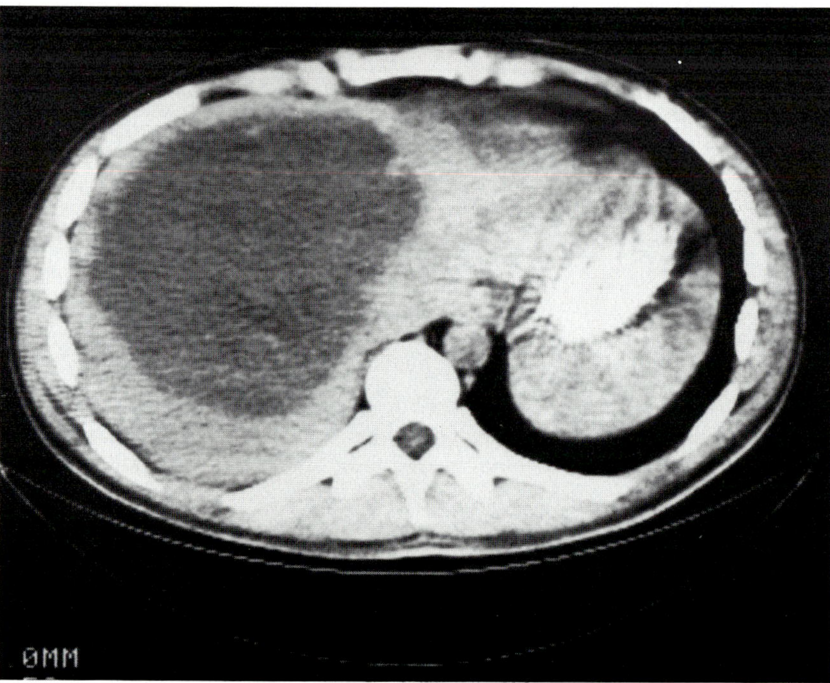

Figure 10.39. Large, low-density liver abscess in the dome of the liver. Note the sharp margins and lack of contrast enhancement.

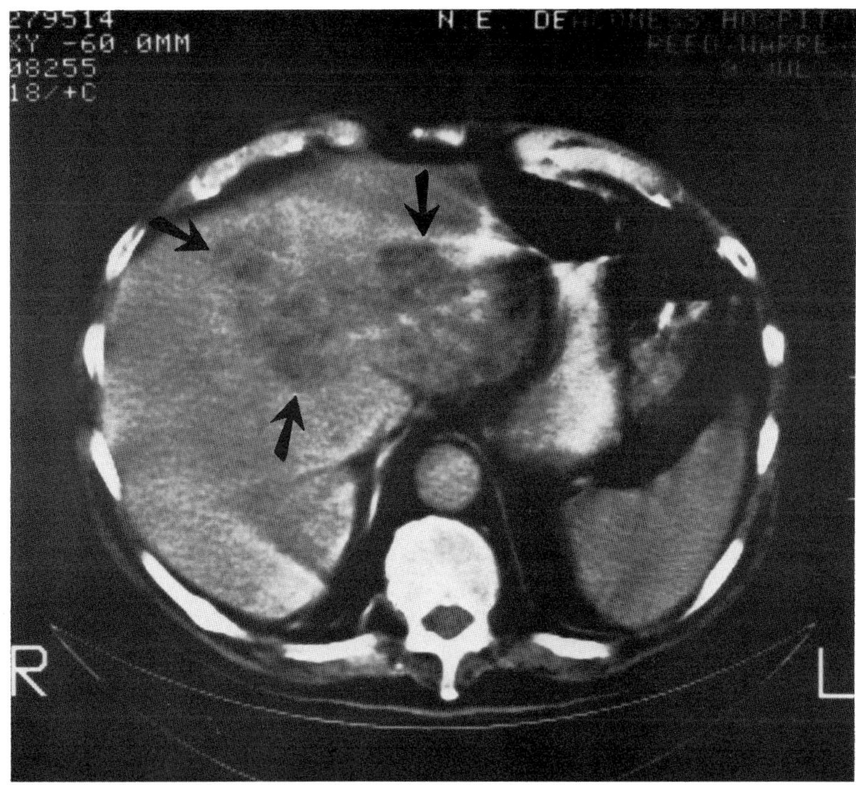

Figure 10.40. Phlegmonous liver abscess. This acute abscess shows less well-defined margins and a mottled consistency (*arrows*) indicating its partially solid, partially cystic nature. Over time the abscess will become more completely liquified.

Sonographically, most amebic abscesses are hypoechoic and homogeneous in texture with poorly defined walls (47). The homogeneity and lack of well-defined walls are features that help distinguish amebic abscesses from pyogenic abscesses, but the most characteristic feature of amebic abscesses is their peripheral subcapsular location, in contrast to the more central position of most pyo-

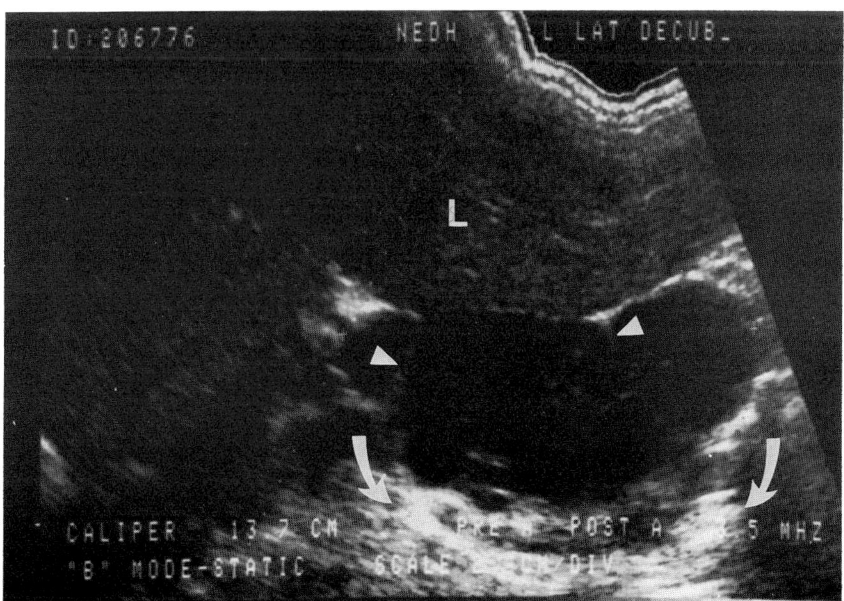

Figure 10.41. Subhepatic abscess. Large hypoechoic fluid collection beneath the liver (L). Note the bright posterior border (*arrow*) indicating its fluid composition. Note also the septations (*arrowheads*) and the speckled internal echoes due to purulent debris.

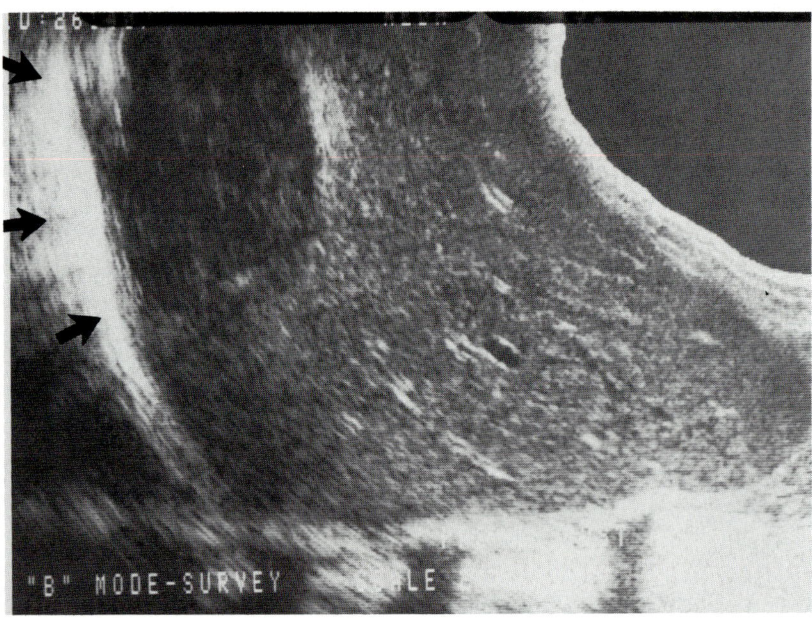

A

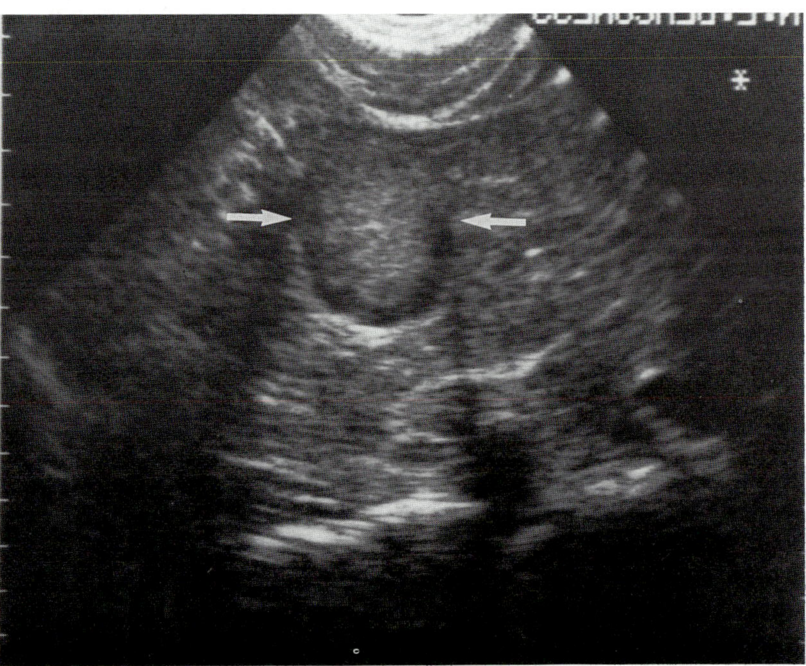

B

Figure 10.42. Amebic liver abscesses. (*A*) This lesion is basically hypoechoic with rather poorly defined margins and marked posterior acoustic enhancement (*arrows*) indicating fluid content. Note the peripheral subcapsular location, typical for amebic abscess. (*B*) Partially treated amebic abscess (*arrows*) with resultant increased echogenicity, iso-echoic to the surrounding liver.

genic abscesses. The margins of amebic abscesses are usually fairly sharp and smooth, even though the walls are not well defined. Posterior acoustic enhancement is typically noted (Fig. 10.42). In one large series approximately 10% of amebic abscesses were reported to be hyperechoic, and with treatment echogenicity will frequently increase in lesions that were echo-poor prior to therapy (48).

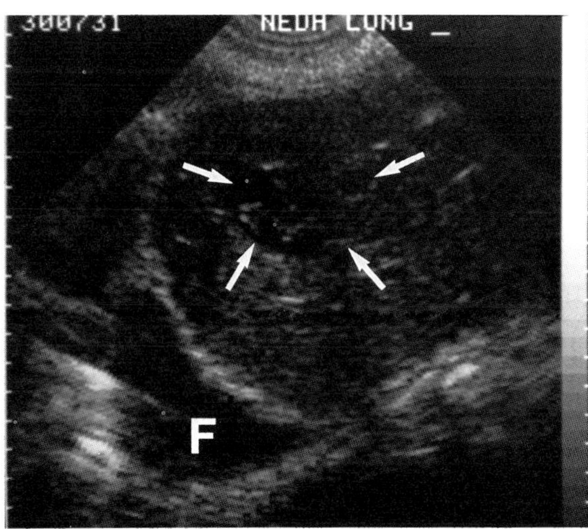

Figure 10.43. Echinococcal cyst. Hypoechoic cystic lesion (*arrows*) centrally within the right lobe of the liver. Note the internal septations forming small daughter cysts. F, right pleural effusion.

Most amebic liver abscesses can be successfully treated medically without internal drainage. Persistent echogenic or cystic abnormalities may remain long after clinical improvement, even up to 12 months or more (49).

Echinococcal cysts of the liver, secondary to hydatid infestation, most often present as multilocular cystic masses, although unilocular cysts may also be seen. The demonstration of smaller daughter cysts around the periphery of a larger cyst is a diagnostic finding but is not seen frequently (Fig. 10.43). Multiple thin and even thick septations throughout a cystic mass may simulate the appearance of a biliary cystadenoma (Fig. 10.44). Sonographically the cysts are typically anechoic and the walls are well defined, with acoustic enhancement posterior to the cyst (50). On CT scanning the cysts are typically low in density, similar to the density of water (0 HU). Inactive lesions may show cyst wall calcification. Occasionally a more solid echogenic appearance can be seen in an active echinococcal lesion (51). This may be a result of extremely small daughter cysts that are rapidly proliferating, or it may be an indication of superinfection of the echinococcal lesion with a bacterial infection. CT density will also increase in the presence of superinfection. Percutaneous aspiration or drainage of echinococcal lesions is not generally recommended. The diagnosis may be made serologically, and severe anaphylaxis may occur if the cyst contents and scolices are spilled into the peritoneal cavity.

Hepatic schistosomiasis, although infrequent in this country, is a major worldwide health hazard, resulting in extensive periportal fibrosis and pres-

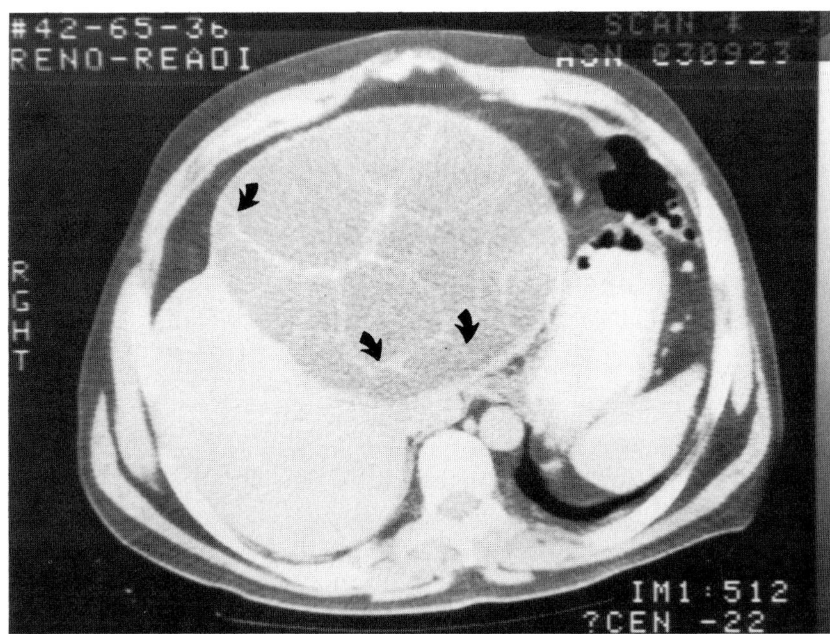

Figure 10.44. Biliary cystadenoma. The large septated cystic mass could be confused with an echinococcal cyst because of the small peripheral septations (*arrows*) suggesting the formation of daughter cysts.

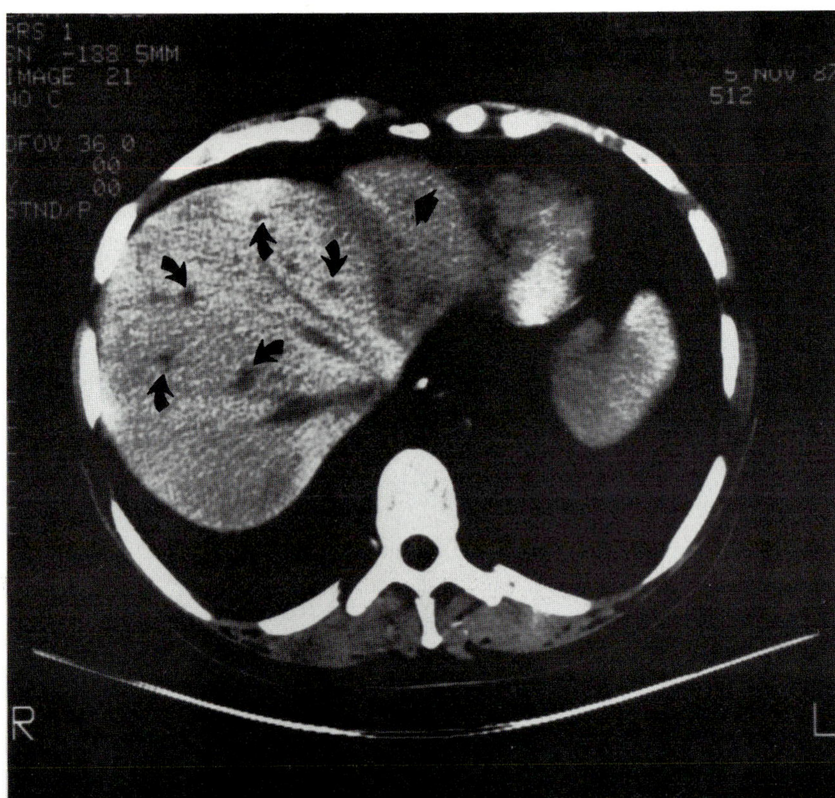

Figure 10.45. Hepatic candidiasis. Multiple, hypodense lesions of less than 1 cm (*arrows*) representing *Candida* microabscesses. Note the high-density center in one of the lesions (*arrowhead*) caused by conglomeration of fungal mycelia.

inusoidal portal hypertension. This results in a characteristic sonographic appearance consisting of dense, hyperechoic bands of tissue extending along the branches of the intrahepatic portal vein radicles (52). These are much thicker and more echogenic than the usual periportal collagen and can be seen extending all the way to the peripheral liver margin. Frequently a radiolucent tubular structure can be seen within the echogenic bands representing the encased portal veins. On CT, the periportal fibrosis appears as low-density periportal bands extending into the periphery of the liver. On nonenhanced scans this appearance might suggest dilated biliary radicles, but with intravenous contrast material the hypodense areas show marked contrast enhancement (53), serving to distinguish this entity from biliary ductal dilatation.

Fungal infection of the liver occurs almost exclusively in immunocompromised patients, especially patients undergoing bone marrow suppression therapy for leukemia, patients with acquired immune deficiency syndrome, and patients who are immunosuppressed following transplantation pro-

cedures. The most common infecting organism is *Candida* and the infection is usually diffuse or multifocal. Since this is a blood-borne infection, frequently other solid organs such as the spleen are also involved. The lesions are generally multiple and quite small, often no more than 1 cm in diameter (Fig. 10.45). Sonographically a typical target appearance has been described consisting of an anechoic cystic lesion with a central hyperechoic focus. This is thought to be due to a nidus of fungal mycelia within an otherwise necrotic and pus-filled lesion (54). On CT the lesions are low in density; occasionally high-density centers can also be seen on CT, again giving a target appearance. The target appearance is fairly specific and the diagnosis can be confirmed by needle biopsy.

While the liver may be involved with granulomatous disease in patients with tuberculosis, there are few if any diagnostic imaging findings. Involvement of the liver occurs in miliary tuberculosis, but the lesions are too small to be resolved, although hepatomegaly is usually present and there is a report of overall increase in echogenicity in the hepatic parenchyma secondary to miliary

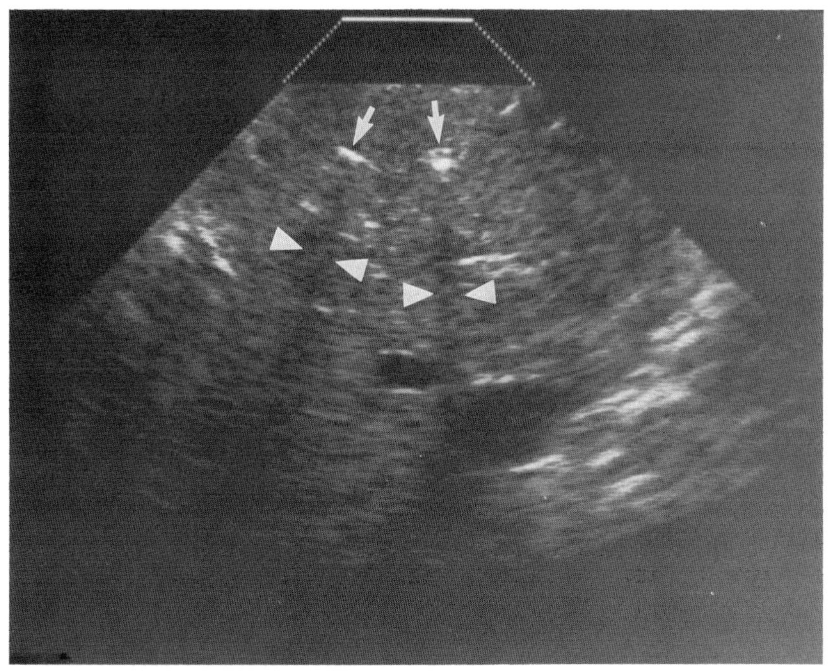

Figure 10.46. Air within intrahepatic bile ducts. The gas is highly reflective, causing very bright echoes (*arrows*) and posterior acoustic shadowing (*arrowheads*).

tuberculosis (55). However, this pattern was deemed indistinguishable from that of cirrhosis and other entities causing increased hepatic echogenicity. Similarly, sarcoidosis frequently involves the liver but is not detectable by current imaging methods. Chronic granulomatous disease of childhood, which is an x-linked recessive defect in leukocyte function, has an effect on the liver by virtue of the increased incidence of recurrent pyogenic infections. Consequently, single or multiple hepatic abscesses may be visualized in children with this disorder (56).

Finally, air may be seen within the liver parenchyma within either the bile ducts or the portal vein radicles (57). Biliary air is usually central within the liver while portal venous air tends to be in the periphery. Although linear, low-density air collections can be seen on plain films, the sensitivity of detection of air in the liver is much greater on CT (linear, low-density streaks) and ultrasonography, where air appears as very bright echogenic lines that often seem to scintillate or shimmer during real-time examination (Fig. 10.46). Air within the bile ducts is most often the result of previous biliary surgery, of endoscopic sphincteroplasty, or occasionally of rupture of a stone from the gallbladder or common duct into the gastrointestinal tract. The presence of air does not necessarily connote cholangitis. Air within the portal venous system, however, is usually an ominous sign often associated with necrotizing enterocolitis in infants or diffuse ischemic bowel disease in adults.

Benign Tumors

Cysts

The common benign focal hepatic lesion is the simple cyst, which may be solitary or multiple and occurs in approximately 5% of the population. Typically the cysts are unilocular, thin-walled, and smooth in contour. Although septations can be seen occasionally on sonography, a cyst is anechoic with sharp, smooth margins and enhanced transmission of sound through the lesion (58). On CT, cysts are also sharp and smooth-walled with homogeneous low density ranging from 0 to 15 HU, consistent with water density (Fig. 10.47). Cysts may be complicated by hemorrhage and infection, and infected cysts appear similar to hepatic abscesses, as described previously. Hemorrhage into a cyst will produce echogenic cyst fluid, and occasionally a fluid-fluid layer may be seen. Acute hemorrhage into a cyst may be recognized on CT by the high density of the blood, but

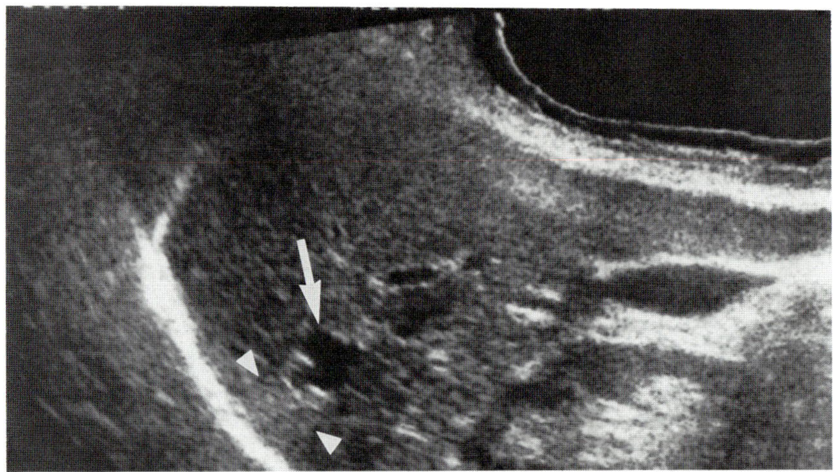

A

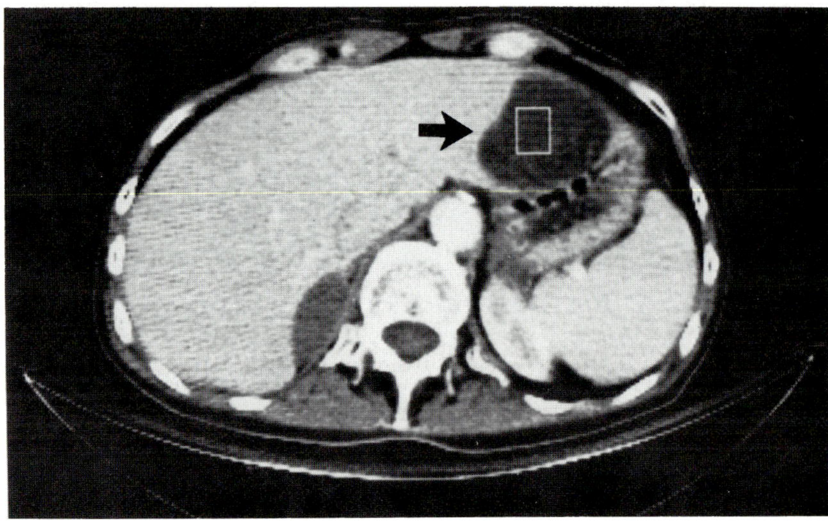

B

Figure 10.47. (*A*) Small septated cyst (*arrow*). Note the anechoic appearance, the sharp margins, and the acoustic enhancement posteriorly (*arrowheads*). (*B*) Left lobe cyst (*arrow*) with smooth, sharp margins and CT density measuring 0 HU.

old or chronic hemorrhage lacks this characteristic feature. Calcification of a cyst wall may occur following old trauma or infection and typically shows a thin, rimlike, high-density appearance on CT and increased echogenicity with acoustic shadowing on ultrasound. On MRI, hepatic cysts have prolonged T_1 and T_2 values (59) and hence appear of low intensity on T_1-weighted scans and of high intensity on T_2-weighted scans (Fig. 10.48). This appearance may be mimicked by cavernous hemangioma of the liver. Adult polycystic renal disease may also affect the liver in a certain percentage of patients, who usually present with multiple small

hepatic cysts that cause no impairment of liver function (60). Cysts may also be seen in the spleen and pancreas in this entity.

Hemangioma

Apart from cysts, the most common benign tumor of the liver is the cavernous hemangioma, which may be seen in up to 7% of the general population, as determined by autopsy series. These lesions may also be single or multiple and have a characteristic sonographic appearance consisting of a hyperechoic, homogeneous, and sharply margin-

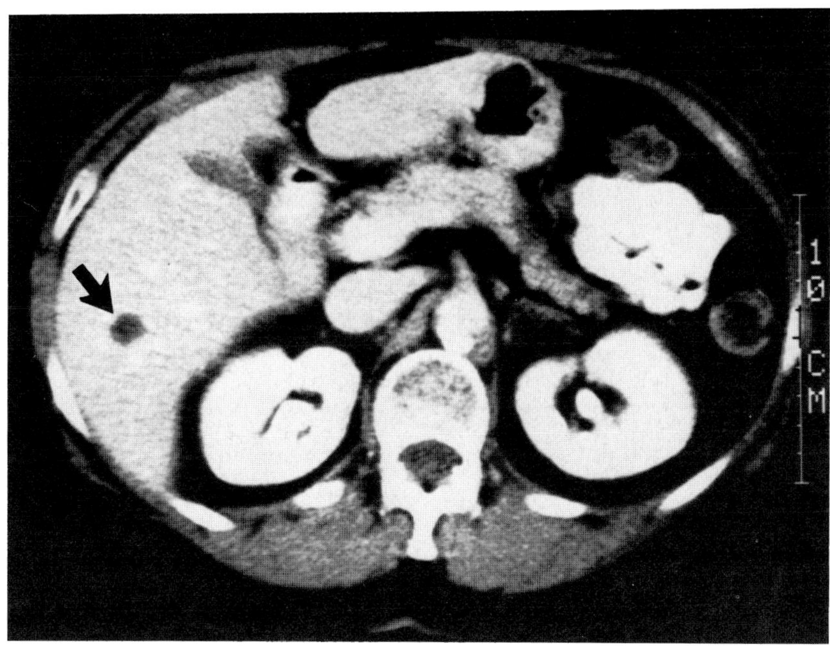

A

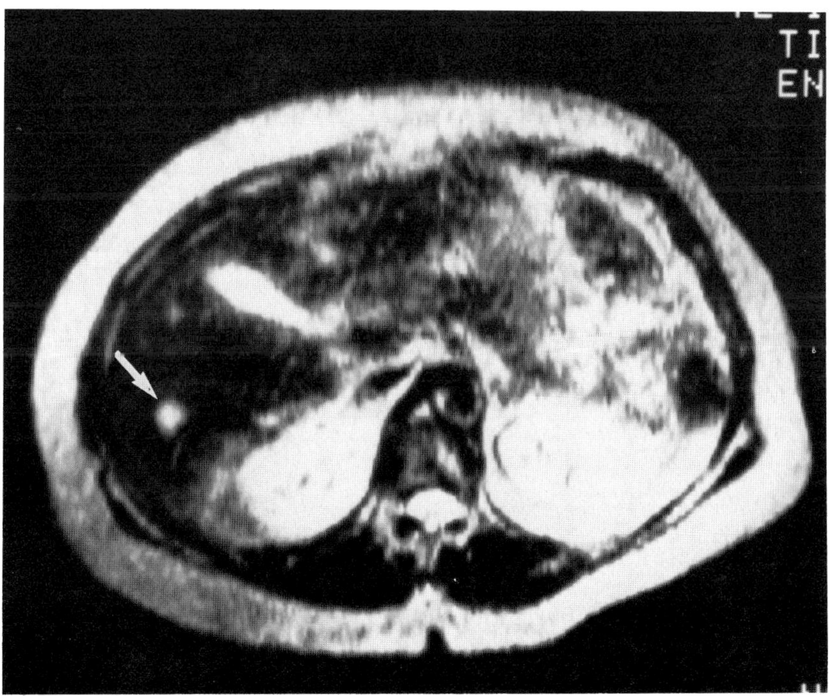

B

Figure 10.48. Hepatic cyst. (*A*) CT scan demonstrating small hypodense cyst (*arrow*). (*B*) Corresponding, heavily T_2-weighted MRI slice demonstrating characteristic high-intensity signal within the cyst (*arrow*).

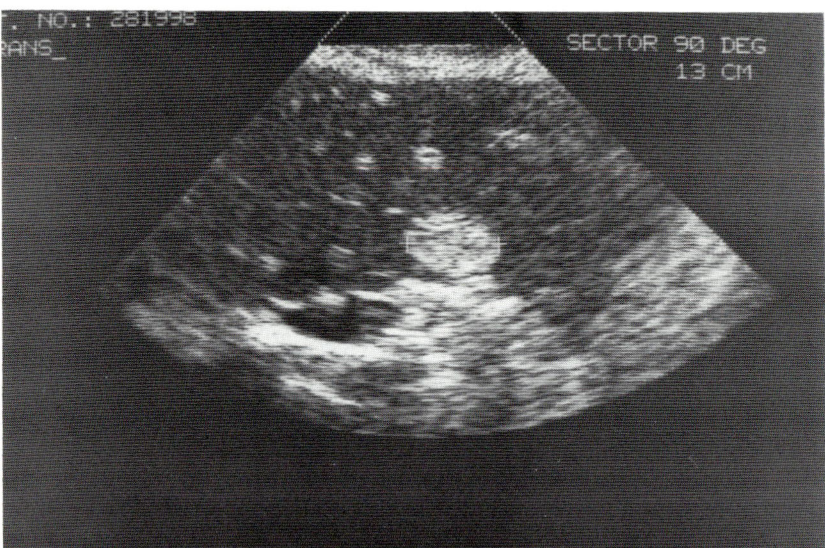

Figure 10.49. Liver hemangioma (*between cursors*). Note the hyperechoic homogeneous consistency and the sharp margins.

ated mass within the liver (61,62). Frequently acoustic enhancement may be seen posterior to the lesion as a result of its intensely vascular composition (Fig. 10.49) (63). Once the hemangioma is larger than 3 to 4 cm, echo-poor spaces can be seen within the lesion, corresponding to dilated vascular sinuses or lakes (Fig. 10.50). While most hemangiomas are located in the right lobe and are subcapsular in location, the lesions may be found in any portion of the liver. The ultrasonographic appearance is characteristic but not pathognomonic, as many other lesions may show a similar appearance, including both primary and metastatic hepatic tumors (64). Consequently, other modalities are utilized to attempt to reach a more specific diagnosis.

On CT scanning, the typical cavernous hemangioma has a low density without contrast enhancement. Rapid-sequence scanning following bolus injection of intravenous contrast material shows a characteristic enhancement pattern (65,66) consisting of fronds or fingers of enhancing tissue extending from the periphery toward the center of the lesion. Over time the lesion becomes more

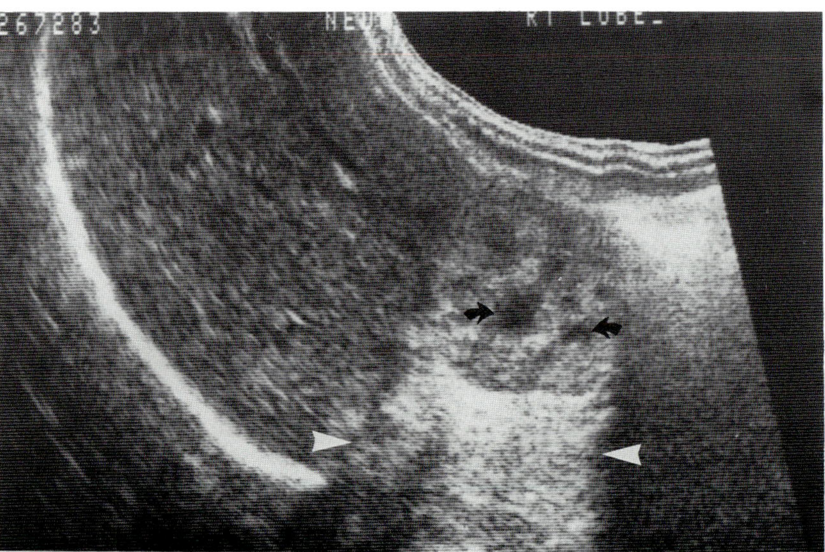

Figure 10.50. Large cavernous hemangioma demonstrating hypoechoic vascular lakes (*arrows*) within the hemangioma, as well as marked acoustic enhancement (*arrowheads*).

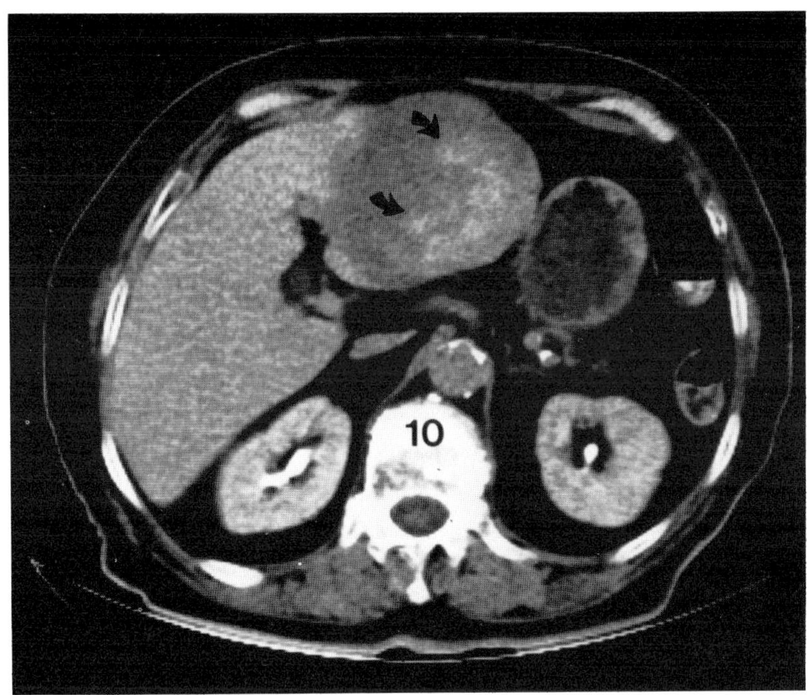

A

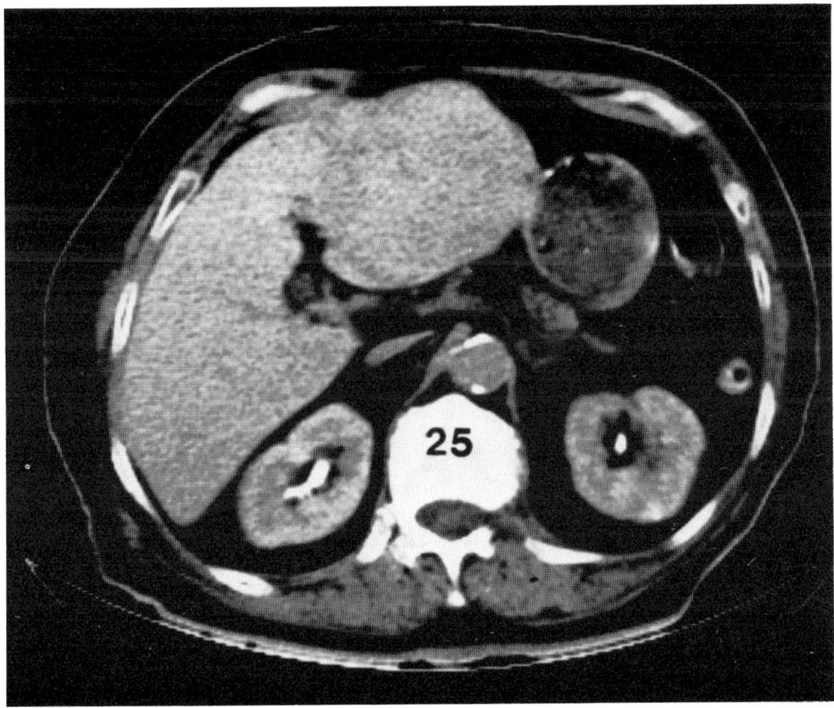

B

Figure 10.51. Cavernous hemangioma. (*A*) Dynamic contrast-enhanced CT 10 minutes after injection, demonstrating characteristic fingerlike enhancement of portions of the hemangioma (*arrows*). (*B*) Twenty-five minutes after injection, there is virtually homogeneous enhancement of the lesion.

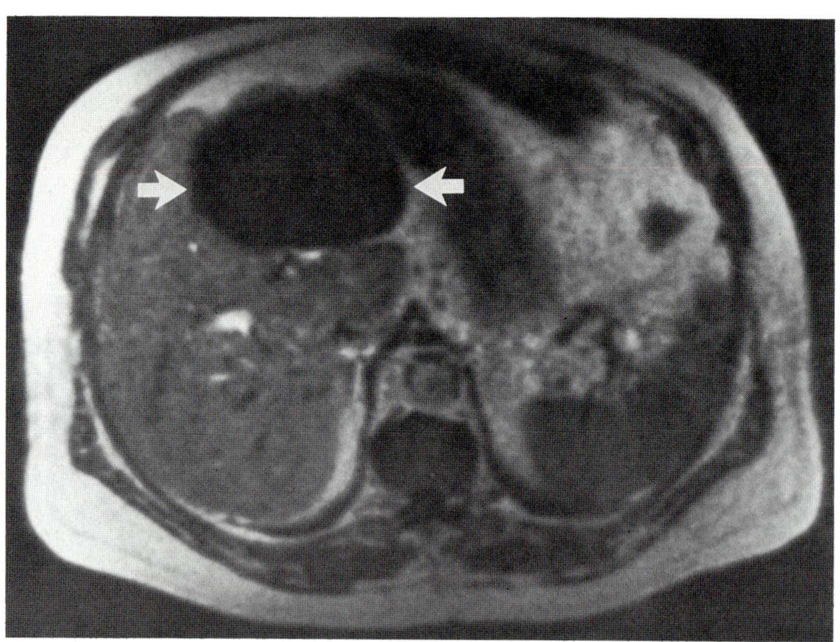

A

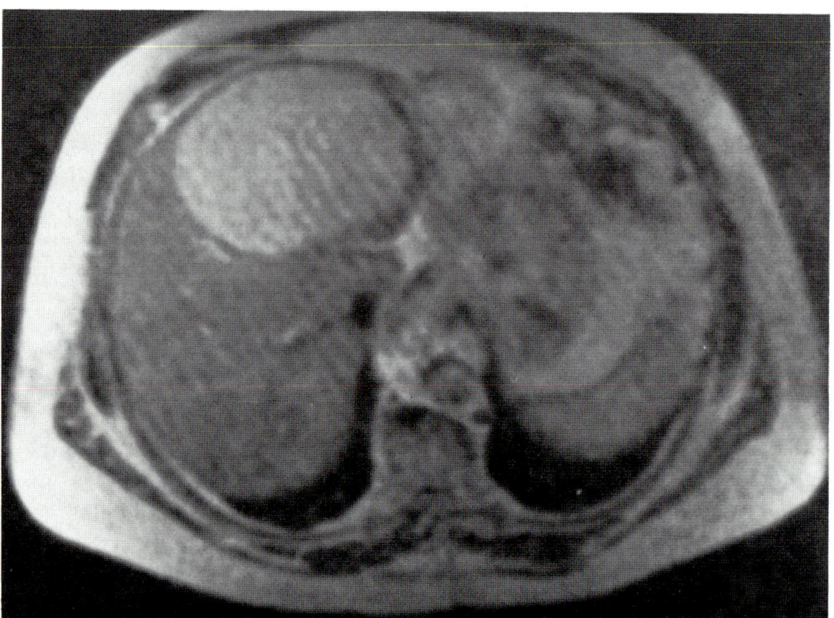

Figure 10.52. MRI of cavernous hemangioma. (*A*) T$_1$-weighted scan shows a large, low-intensity lesion (*arrows*) in the left lobe of the liver. (*B*) T$_2$-weighted sequence shows characteristic high signal intensity within the lesion.

B

completely enhanced, and on delayed scans it is homogeneously enhanced to an equal or greater degree than the surrounding liver parenchyma (Fig. 10.51). This is a diagnostic pattern for cavernous hemangioma but is only reliably seen in le-sions larger than 3 to 4 cm, approximately 80% of which will show this pattern. Radionuclide scanning of the liver with radiolabeled red blood cells is also a diagnostic imaging test for cavernous hemangioma. The hemangiomas show lack of activity

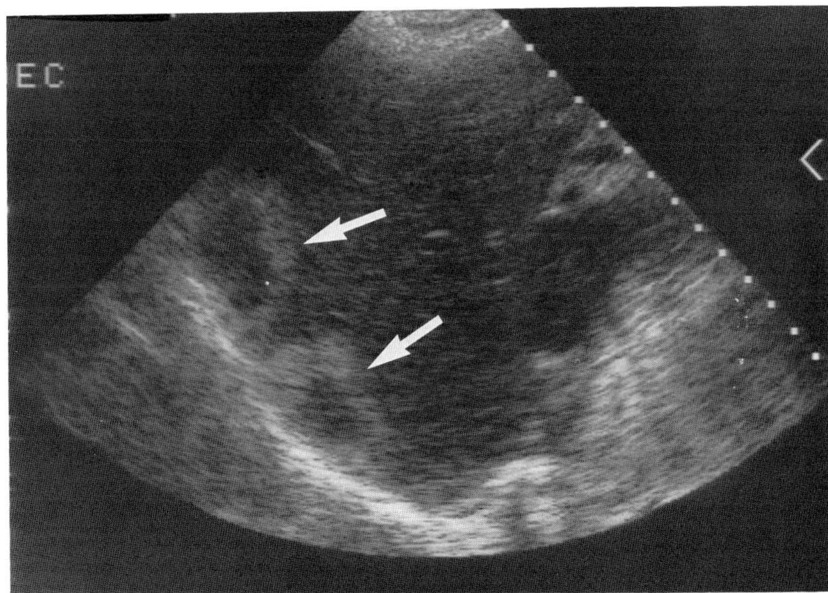

Figure 10.53. Fibrosed hemangiomas. Two large right lobe lesions (*arrows*) that are hyperechoic and sharply marginated but have central scarring that appears hypoechoic.

in the early flow phase but show increased activity on delayed scans, the activity persisting much longer than activity in the surrounding liver parenchyma (67). This is said to be more consistently diagnostic in small cavernous hemangioma than CT scanning. Magnetic resonance imaging also shows a diagnostic pattern for hemangiomas (68,69) consisting of long T_1 and long T_2 relaxations, resulting in a low-intensity appearance on T_1-weighted images and a high-intensity appearance on T_2-weighted scans (Fig. 10.52). This result is similar to that seen with hepatic cysts.

A small percentage of cavernous hemangiomas will undergo central scar formation, possibly due to ischemia and infarction (Fig. 10.53). This will result in an altered appearance on ultrasonography, with a central hypoechoic area surrounded by the more typical hyperechoic tissue. On CT, particularly after contrast enhancement, the central scar will remain as a sharply circumscribed low-density area, frequently linear or rectangular in appearance, surrounded by enhanced high-density tissue. The central scar may also have a differing signal intensity on MRI, with lower intensity signal within the scar on T_2 weighting.

With the variety of noninvasive techniques available, angiography is seldom required for the diagnosis of hemangioma. Nevertheless, there is a characteristic angiographic appearance consisting of intense and prolonged vascular staining, filling lakes or pools of contrast material, which may persist for 30 seconds or longer (Fig. 10.54). Usually the feeding hepatic artery is normal, or possibly slightly increased, in size while hypervascular malignant tumors such as hepatomas tend to have more dilated feeding vessels and less prolonged opacification. Finally, some investigators believe

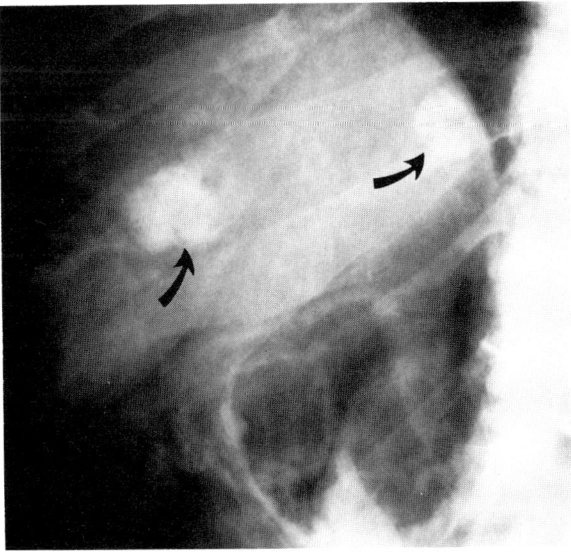

Figure 10.54. Two cavernous hemangiomas (*arrows*) exhibiting dense vascular blushes on hepatic arteriography. The staining persists well after contrast has washed out of the normal liver parenchyma.

that a guided needle biopsy may be diagnostic in confusing cases, either by aspiration of only blood without malignant cells or by demonstration of endothelial cells on cytologic smear (70). Fine 22-gauge needle biopsy is said to be safe, but serious, life-threatening hemorrhage has been reported with larger gauge needle biopsy of hemangiomas.

Hepatic Adenoma

Hepatic adenoma is an uncommon hepatic tumor, but its frequency has increased substantially due to the fact that long-term use of oral contraceptives is associated with an increased incidence of this tumor (71). Hepatic adenomas are also seen with increased incidence in patients with glycogen storage disease (von Gierke's disease) (35). The tumors are benign and well circumscribed, ranging from 2 to 10 cm or greater in size. The lesions are usually solitary, but multiple adenomas have been reported, particularly in glycogen storage disease. The lesions are frequently peripheral along the edge of the liver and may be exophytic. Hemorrhage into the lesion is not infrequent and spontaneous rupture with massive hemoperitoneum may occur (72). Consequently, surgery is recommended for this tumor.

Since the adenomas consist of hepatocytes and vascular tissue but lack bile ducts and reticuloendothelial cells, the lesions are cold on technetium sulfur colloid liver scanning (73). Sonographically the appearance is variable, with a relatively iso-echoic appearance frequently seen, but hypoechoic and hyperechoic adenomas may be encountered. In von Gierke's disease the adenomas have been described as hyperechoic with some acoustic enhancement (35). CT appearance of hepatic adenomas also shows variable density and variable contrast enhancement, with no single predictable diagnostic feature. Angiographically a characteristic hypervascularity is noted with normal-sized feeding vessels, draping of arteries over the lesion, and a dense parenchymal blush (Fig. 10.55). These features may also be seen with other benign and malignant liver tumors and there is no completely diagnostic feature to allow the preoperative diagnosis of hepatic adenoma to be made with certainty.

Focal Nodular Hyperplasia

This is another benign hepatic tumor most often seen in young females, although it is probably not directly associated with the use of oral contraceptives. This tumor is also well circumscribed and contains hepatic cells as well as bile ducts and Kupffer's cells in variable degree. Consequently, approximately one-half of the focal nodular hyperplasia (FNH) lesions will show uptake of technetium sulfur colloid to be either isointense or hyperintense compared with the surrounding normal parenchyma (75). This is a diagnostic feature of FNH since no other hepatic tumor has reticuloendothelial cells contained within it. Once again, on ultrasonography the lesion may be of greater, lesser, or equal echogenicity to the normal liver. CT density is also variable, although usually the lesions are somewhat less dense than normal liver (Fig. 10.56).

A central cleft or scar (Fig. 10.57) is characteristic of FNH and may be seen on CT, sonography (76), and MRI (77), as well as angiographically. The central scar is not completely diagnostic, however, as it also has been described in other lesions including hemangiomas, lymphoma, and fibrolamellar hepatoma (18). The angiographic appearance of FNH is similar to hepatic adenoma, although a typical spokewheel configuration of feeding vessels is described as a classic appearance (75), again relating to the deformity resultant from the central scar.

Lipomas

These are rare, benign liver tumors consisting of lipid-laden cells, resulting in a uniformly hyperechoic appearance on ultrasonography, similar to a hemangioma. When large, a lipoma may exhibit attenuation of sound with acoustic shadowing, in contrast to the posterior enhancement seen typically with a hemangioma. The CT appearance is diagnostic with low attenuation throughout the lipoma in the fat range of -30 to -100 HU (Fig. 10.58).

Cystadenoma

Biliary cystadenomas are again often seen in young females and frequently present as very bulky, large masses, seldom causing symptoms except for the large size. These tumors may be unilocular but are most frequently multilocular with thin septa and occasionally thicker septations and mural nodules (78). Rimlike calcification may also be encountered. Sonographically the appearance is that of any cystic lesion, with anechoic fluid

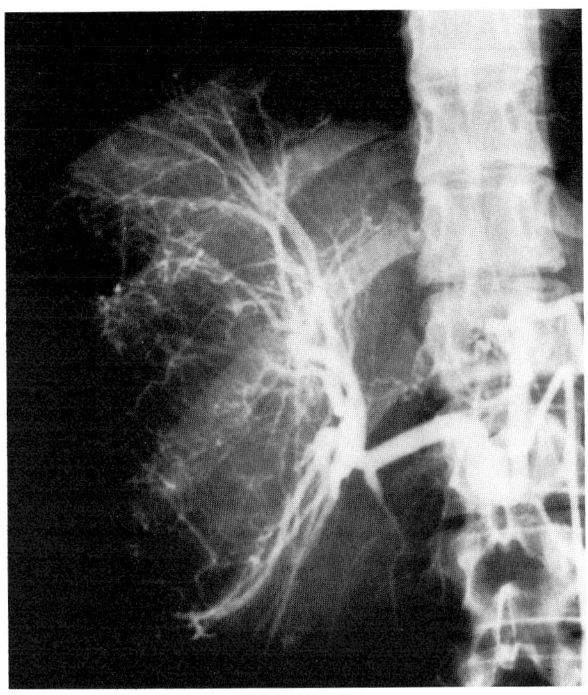

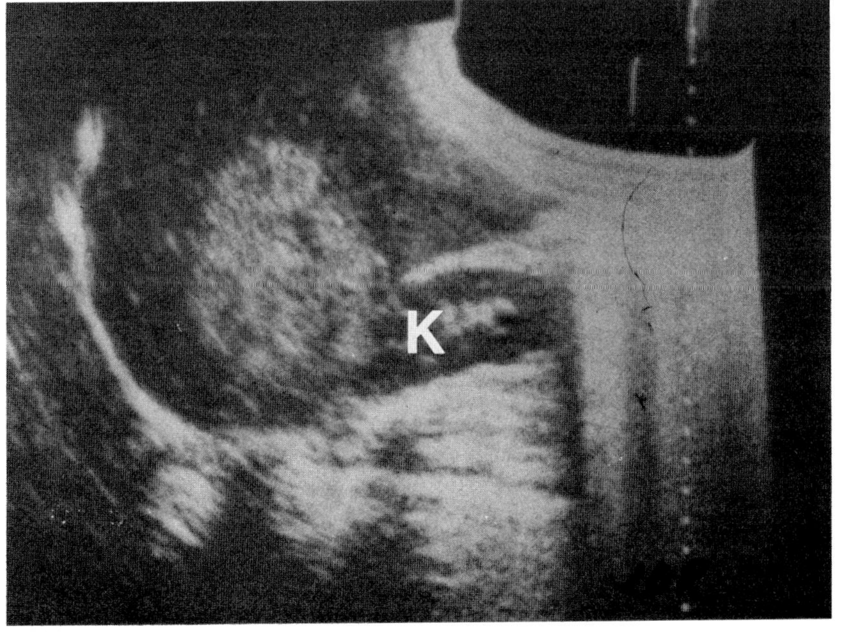

Figure 10.55. Hepatic adenoma. (*A*) Large right lobe mass demonstrating hypervascularity on arteriography but a normal-caliber hepatic artery. (*B*) The mass is markedly hyperechoic, somewhat similar to a hemangioma, but there is no acoustic enhancement. K, right kidney.

and sharp margins with acoustic enhancement. On CT, the fluid is usually low density but may occasionally be higher density if mucinous or crystalline fluid is present. This type of fluid may also cause fine echogenicity on sonographic study. The multiple septations within the lesion are frequently better seen sonographically than on CT (Fig. 10.59). The lesions are hypovascular on

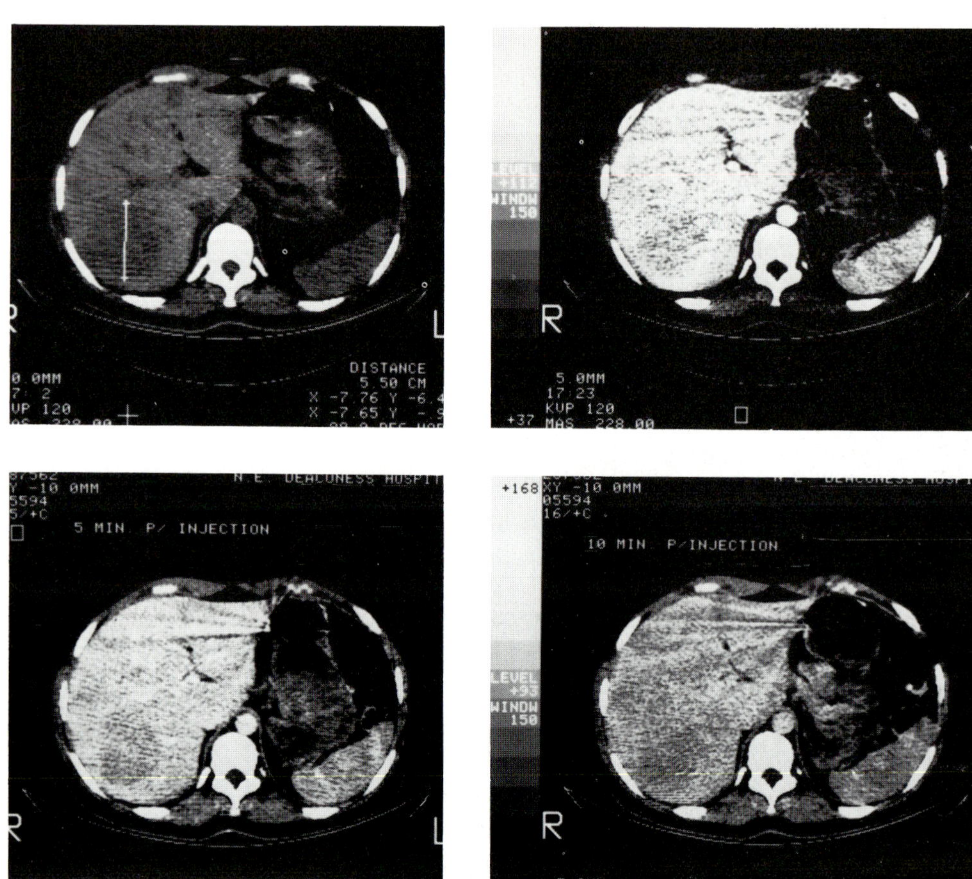

Figure 10.56. Focal nodular hyperplasia. (*A*) On CT the lesion, as marked by the cursors, is hypodense both before and after intravenous administration of contrast material. (*B*) The same lesion is hyperechoic on ultrasonography, as marked by the cursors.

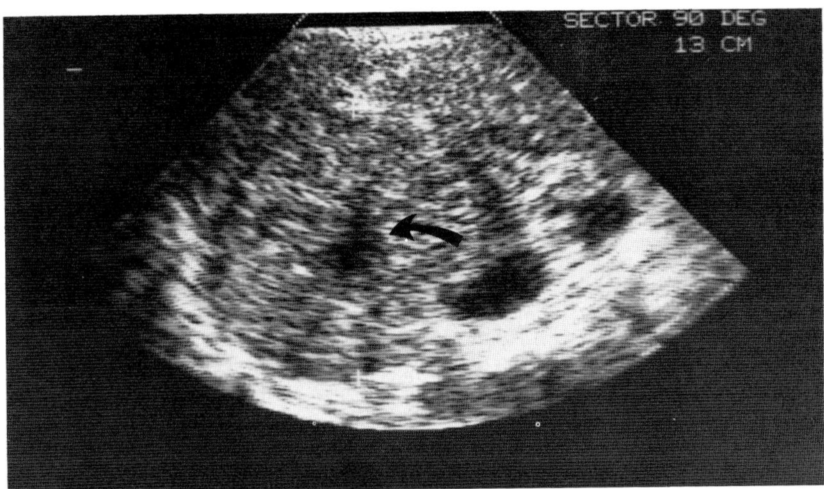

A

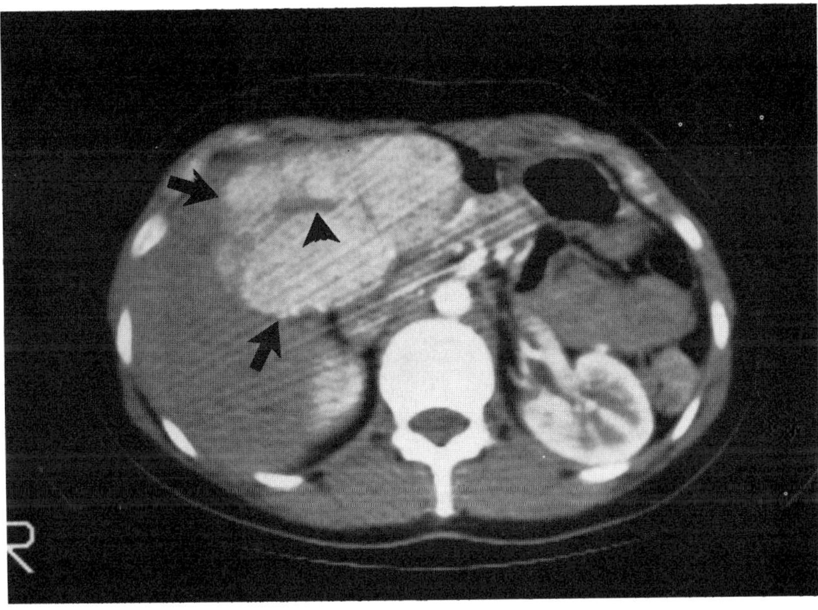

B

Figure 10.57. Focal nodular hyperplasia with central scar. (*A*) Slightly hyperechoic right lobe lesion (*between cursors*) with a linear hypoechoic central scar (*arrow*). (*B*) Left lobe lesion showing intense contrast enhancement (*arrows*) except for the hypodense central scar (*arrowhead*).

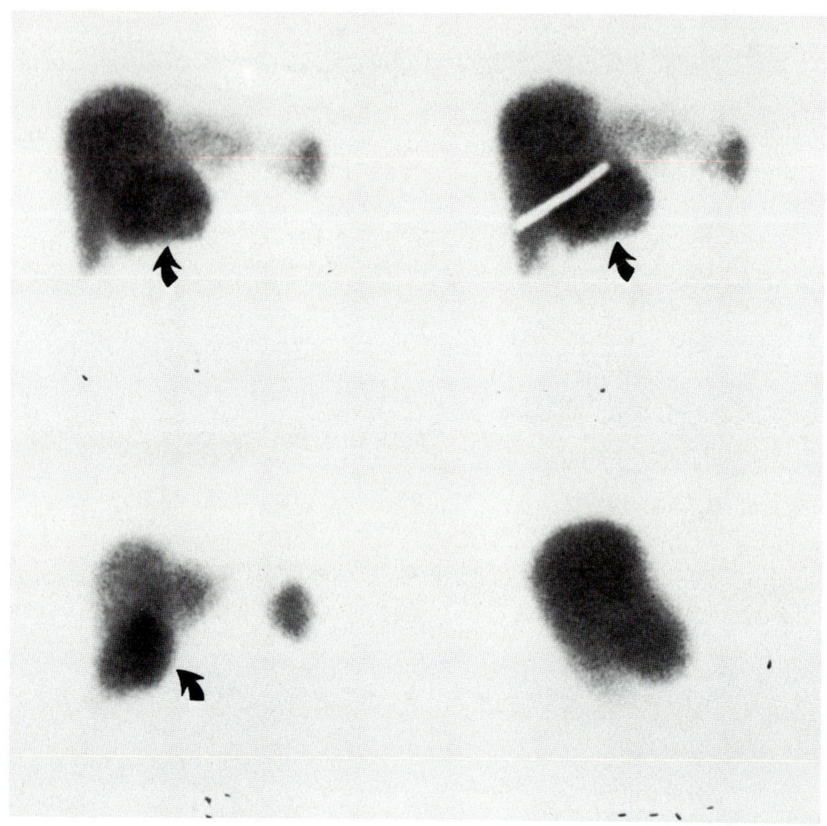

Figure 10.57 (continued). (C) Technetium sulfur colloid scan demonstrating activity within the FNH lesion (*arrows*). This is the same lesion as shown on the CT scan in part *B*.

C

angiographic examination. The vast majority of biliary cystadenomas are benign and there are no specific features to indicate carcinomatous degeneration. Rarely the cyst within the tumor may communicate with the bile ducts. Biliary cystadenomas may simulate the appearance of echinococcal cysts or less frequently cystic metastatic neoplasms, abscesses, or hematomas.

Malignant Tumors

Primary Tumors

Hepatocellular carcinoma is the most common primary hepatic tumor. In the United States this tumor is usually associated with underlying cirrhosis of the liver, whereas worldwide the tumor is more frequently associated with chronic B-positive hepatitis as well as with dietary carcinogens such as aflatoxin in Africa. The tumor has a protean appearance, ranging from a solitary discrete mass, to multifocal smaller nodules, to an infiltrative diffuse pattern (Fig. 10.60). The sonographic appearance may range from discrete hyperechoic masses simulating hemangiomas to isoechoic and hypoechoic lesions, as well as a diffuse disruption of underlying normal architecture of the infiltrating variety (79). Ultrasonography in a Japanese report was shown to be the most sensitive noninvasive means of detecting small hepatocellular carcinomas (80). On CT scanning, again there is no characteristic pattern, with low-density masses most typically seen, but isodense lesions and hyperdense lesions with calcifications are also described (81).

A characteristic of hepatocellular carcinoma is the tendency to invade either the portal venous or hepatic venous system (82,83). The presence of tumor thrombus growing within these veins can be readily demonstrated sonographically or on CT

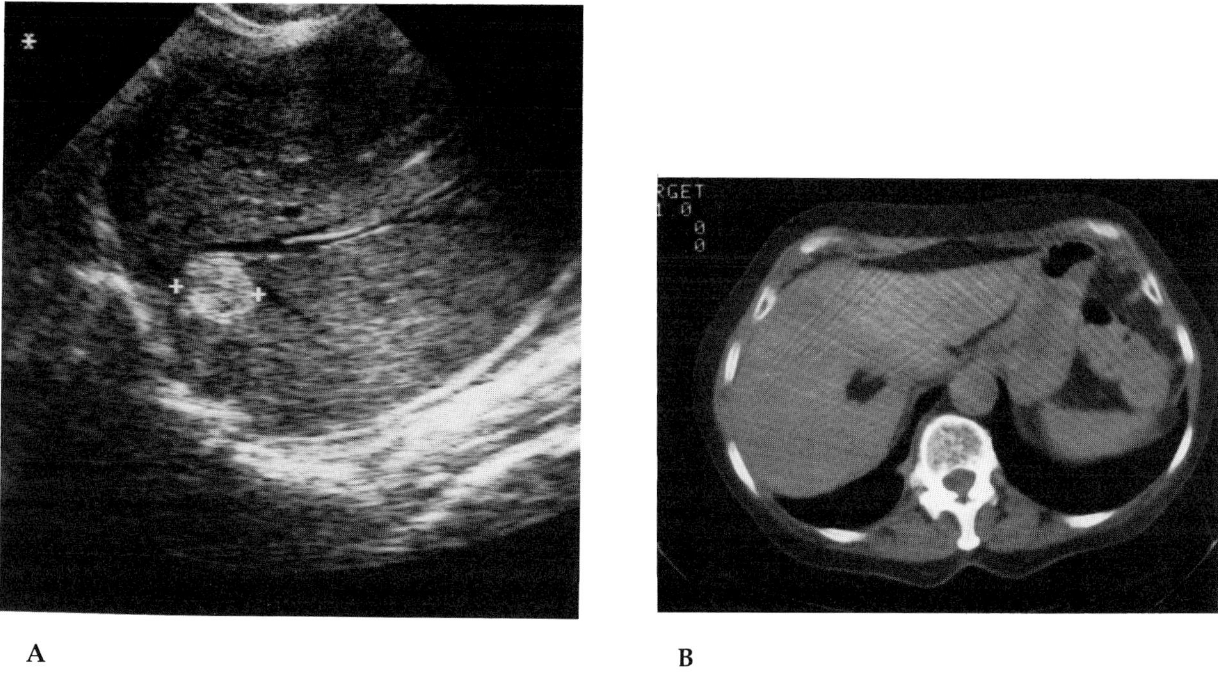

Figure 10.58.   Hepatic lipoma. (*A*) The lesion (*cursors*) is hyperechoic and homogeneous by ultrasonography, indistinguishable from a small hemangioma. (*B*) The CT density measured −84 HU, indicating a fatty lesion. Note the similar density to the subcutaneous fat.

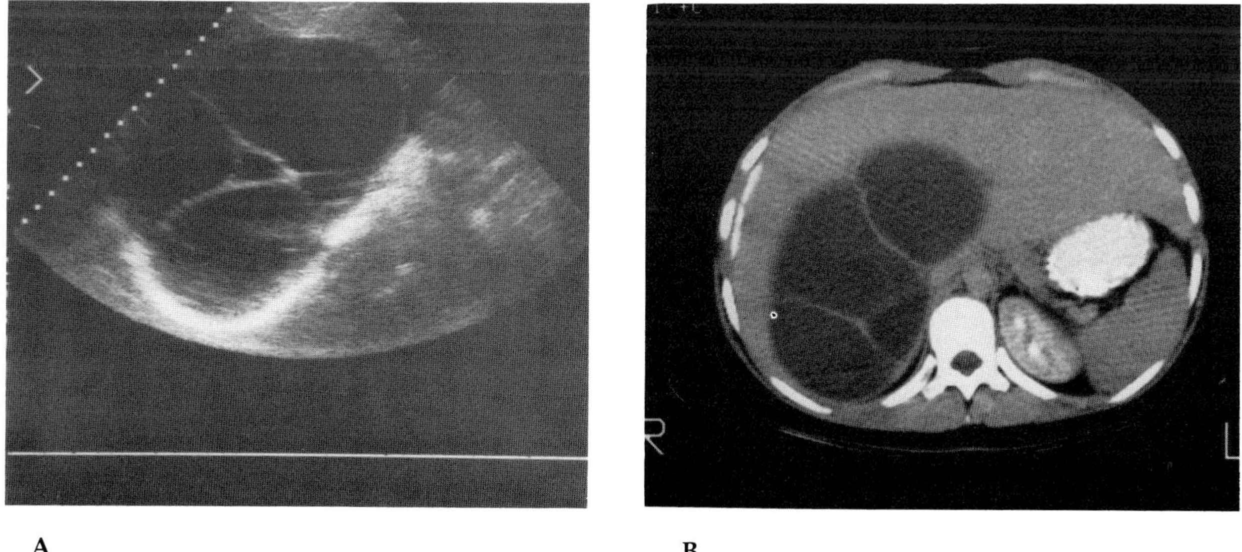

Figure 10.59.   Biliary cystadenoma. (*A*) Large, sharply marginated, hypoechoic mass with internal septations and acoustic enhancement, indicating its cystic nature. (*B*) Multiseptated hypodense mass on CT with CT density values similar to water density.

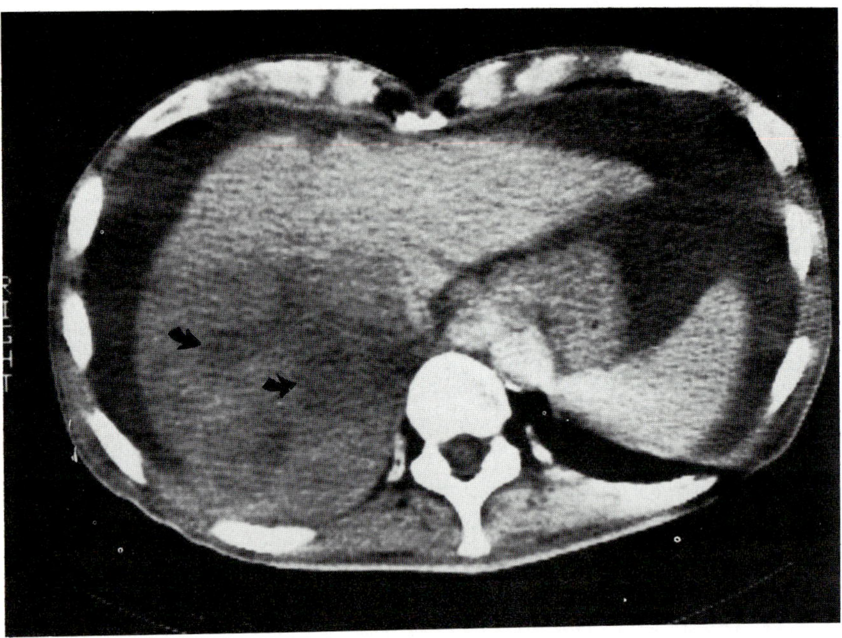

A

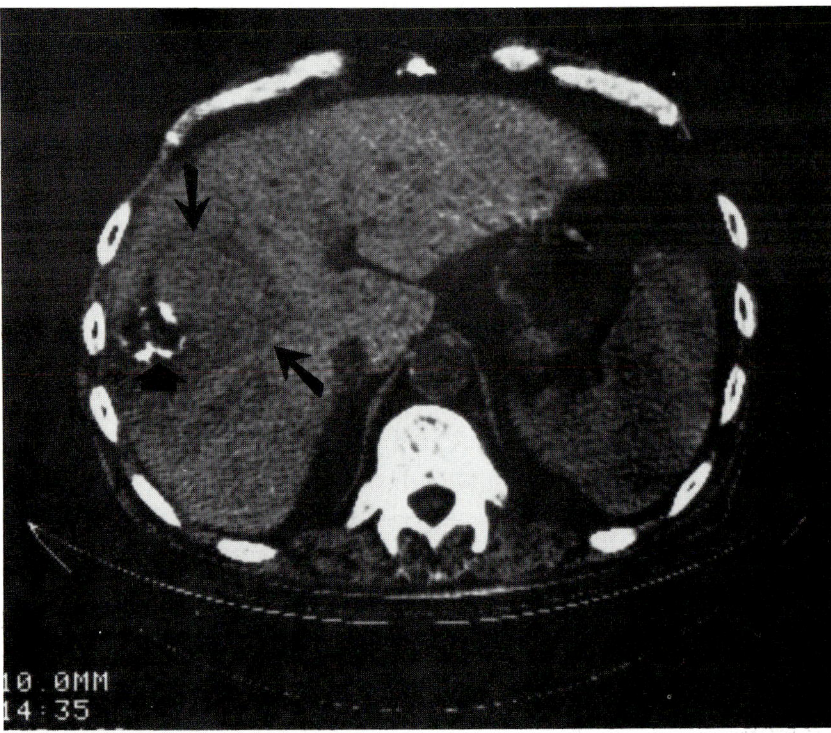

B

Figure 10.60. Hepatocellular carcinoma. (*A*) Contrast-enhanced CT showing large hypodense mass filling the right lobe of the liver. The areas of lowest density (*arrows*) correspond to tumor necrosis. (*B*) Nonenhanced CT showing a relatively isodense tumor (*arrows*) with high-density central calcification (*arrowhead*).

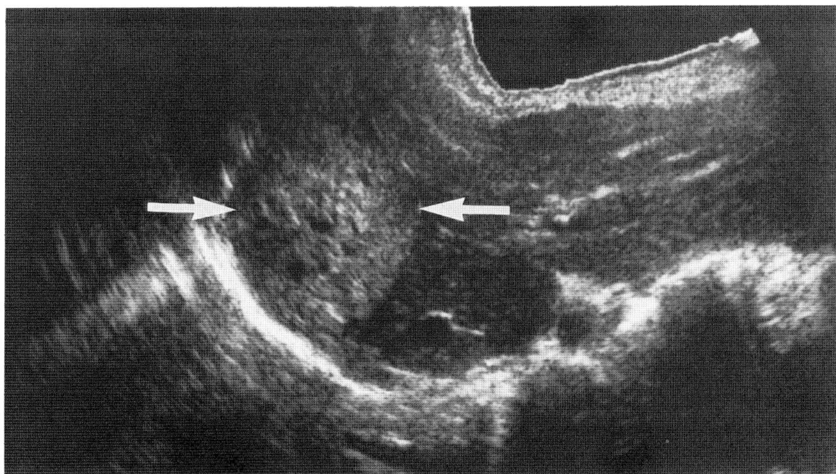

C

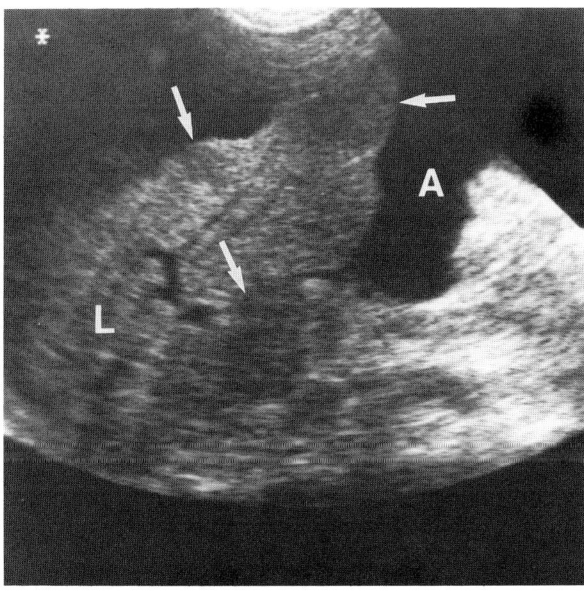

D

Figure 10.60 (continued). (C) Hyperechoic hepatoma (*arrows*) with an ultrasound appearance similar to a cavernous hemangioma. (D) Multifocal hypoechoic hepatomas (*arrows*) in a severely cirrhotic liver. L, liver; A, ascites.

scanning (Fig. 10.61). MRI may also be useful in demonstrating intravascular tumor growth.

Angiographically the typical hepatoma is fed by a dilated and tortuous hepatic artery, a feature that is seldom seen in other hepatic neoplasms. Irregular pooling of contrast material may be seen as well as malignant-type vasculature within the tumor, and arteriovenous shunting into the portal or hepatic veins is frequently seen (84), which is uncommon in other tumors. Opacification of the portal and hepatic veins will frequently demonstrate intravascular tumor thrombus (Fig. 10.62).

On radionuclide scanning, hepatomas are cold on technetium sulfur colloid, as are most other neoplasms apart from FNH, but hepatomas have an avidity for gallium-67 citrate (85), with reports of up to 90% positive gallium scans in some series (Fig. 10.63). Gallium positivity is, however, also seen with lymphoma as well as in inflammatory or infectious lesions.

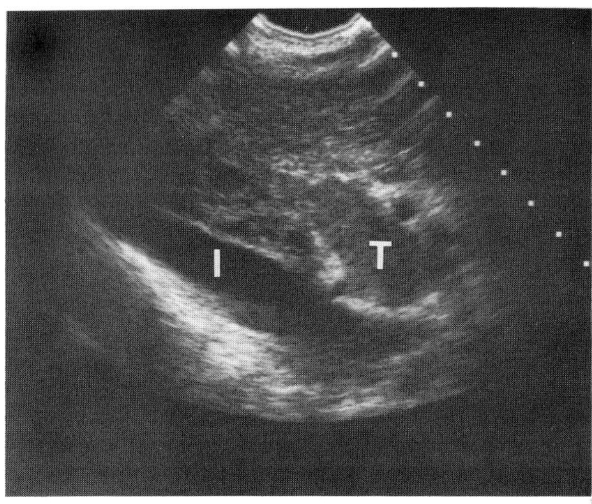
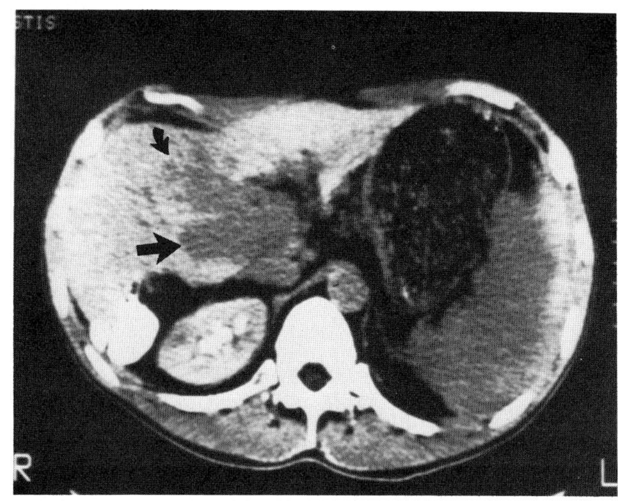

Figure 10.61. Tumor thrombus. (*A*) Sagittal ultrasound demonstrating echogenic tumor thrombus (T) filling the main portal vein. I, inferior vena cava. (*B*) Contrast-enhanced CT showing the hypodense tumor (*curved arrow*) and hypodense tumor thrombus growing in the portal vein (*straight arrow*).

Cholangiocarcinoma may affect the extrahepatic biliary tree, but a frequent site for this tumor is at the bifurcation of the common hepatic duct, the so-called Klatskin tumor. Central intrahepatic ductal dilatation is first seen, followed by more peripheral intrahepatic dilatation in the presence of a normal or small extrahepatic biliary system including the gallbladder (86). This serves to indicate the level of the obstruction at the porta hepatis, although frequently the tumor itself cannot be visualized by CT or ultrasound because of its infiltrating, nonmasslike behavior. Occasionally small or large hypoechoic hepatic masses can be seen secondary to cholangiocarcinoma (87), and low density, nonenhancing masslike areas may be seen on CT (Fig. 10.64). Angiographically the tumors are usually hypovascular, although peripheral cholangiocarcinomas may be hypervascular (88). On endoscopic retrograde cholangiopancreatography (ERCP) or PTC, the typical Klatskin tumor shows attenuation and obstruction of the main right and left hepatic ducts, with peripheral dilatation and a normal-caliber common duct (89).

Although central biliary obstruction defines the Klatskin tumor, other neoplasms may cause a similar effect, either via parenchymal metastatic disease invading the bifurcation or by nodal metastases to the lymph nodes in the porta hepatis from a variety of carcinomas and even lymphoma.

Other primary hepatic tumors such as angiosarcoma and hepatoblastoma are rare. The former tumor is a markedly hypervascular neoplasm that has been seen in association with thorium oxide (Thorotrast) toxicity. Hepatoblastoma is a tumor seen in the first year or two of life. The tumor may be calcified and has been described as either hyperechoic or cystic (90).

Metastatic Disease

Metastatic disease to the liver can take a focal or a diffuse infiltrating form. Focal hepatic metastases most often arise from the gastrointestinal tract, especially the colon, as well as from primary carcinomas of the lung, kidney, and nasopharynx, and from endocrine tumors. Focal metastases may also be seen with carcinoma of the breast and melanoma. The infiltrating metastatic pattern is most commonly seen with breast and lung carcinoma. Lymphoma may also be focal or diffuse while leukemic spread to the liver is nearly always a diffuse infiltrating pattern.

In the United States, metastatic disease is the most common neoplasm in the liver, although worldwide, hepatocellular carcinoma is more common. As with other tumors, there is no characteristic sonographic or CT appearance (Fig. 10.65). Lesions may be solid or cystic. Sonographically a

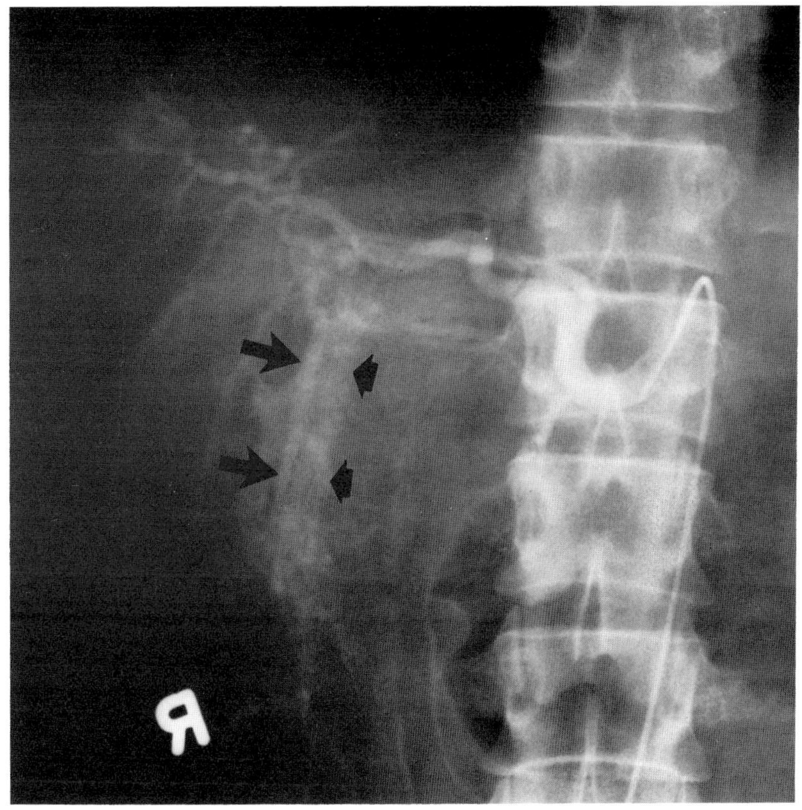

A

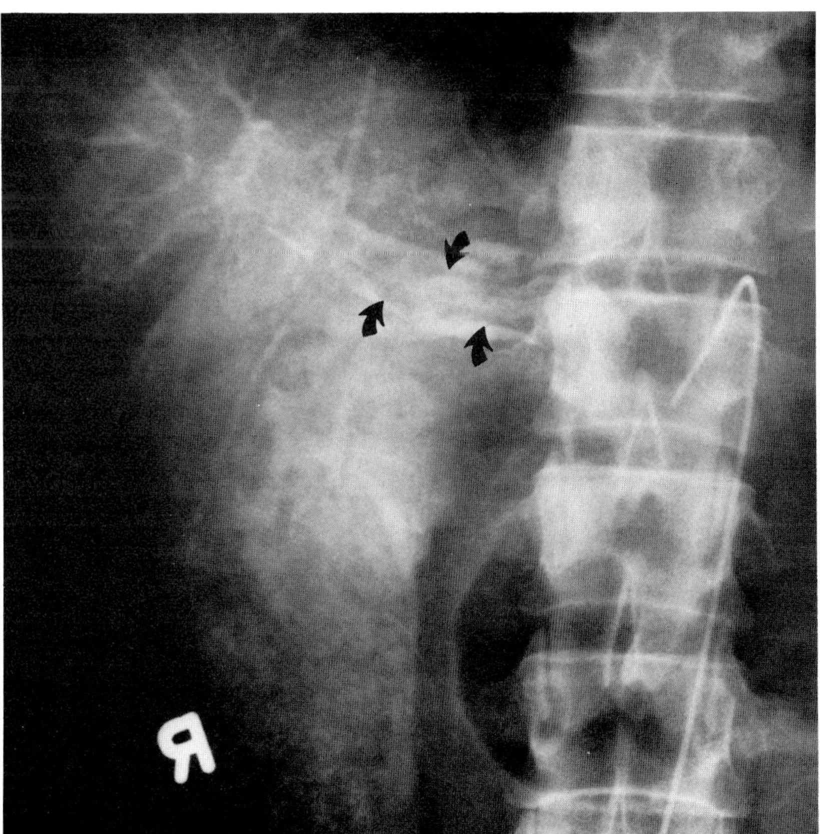

B

Figure 10.62. (*A*) Rapid arteriovenous shunting in hepatoma. The contrast in a right hepatic artery (*arrows*) is paralleled by immediate opacification of adjacent portal veins (*arrowheads*). (*B*) Subsequent opacification of the portal vein shows a filling defect (*arrows*) due to tumor thrombus.

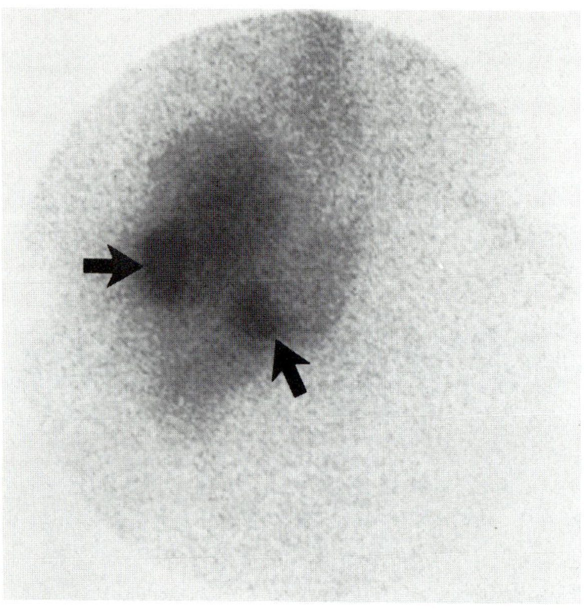

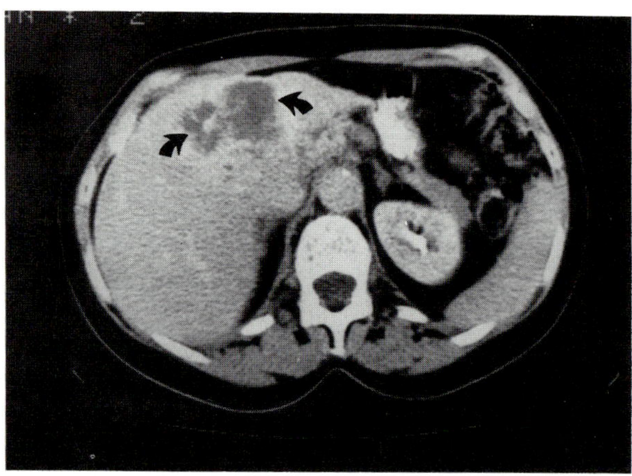

Figure 10.64.   Irregular hypodense mass on contrast-enhanced CT (*arrows*) secondary to cholangiocarcinoma.

Figure 10.63.   Gallium-67 citrate radionuclide scan demonstrating increased activity at two sites in the liver (*arrows*) corresponding to a multifocal hepatoma.

bull's-eye pattern with central increase in echogenicity is frequently seen with gastrointestinal tract tumors (91). Calcification within a metastatic nodule is also typically seen with mucin-producing adenocarcinomas of the gastrointestinal tract as well as in colon metastases (92). Liquefaction necrosis may be frequently seen in leiomyosarcomas as well as in aggressive lung metastases. Endocrine tumors and renal cell carcinoma may often be hyperechoic when small because of the intensely hypervascular nature of these tumors (93). Focal lymphoma within the liver is characteristically hypoechoic (94). Cystic metastases on the surface of the liver are frequently seen in ovarian carcinoma (95) and usually some wall thickening or mural nodularity can be appreciated.

The CT appearance of metastatic disease is also highly variable (Fig. 10.66), with increased or decreased density, cystic change, and calcification frequently seen (96). The technique of CT scanning may affect the appearance of the lesions. Some metastatic lesions will show an enhanced rim on dynamic CT angiography. Routine infusion of contrast material may make some lesions more visible but other lesions may become isodense and be missed with contrast enhancement (97). Some investigators advocate delayed CT scannings 6 hours

after infusion of contrast material (98). At this time, iodine is being excreted by the hepatocytes, which supposedly makes CT more sensitive in detecting focal lesions than scans obtained dynamically or with routine infusion techniques.

The excellent resolution achieved by CT and ultrasound has made radionuclide liver scanning relatively obsolete in assessment for metastatic disease, since the minimum size detectable on sulfur colloid scanning is 2 to 3 cm, whereas ultrasound and CT may detect lesions as small as 1 cm. Similarly, angiography is not utilized as a screening technique for metastatic disease both because of its invasive nature and because of its inability to detect small lesions. The exception to this is when hypervascular metastases are present, such as with renal cell carcinoma, and endocrine or carcinoid tumors. The intense hypervascularity of these lesions may make angiography the single most sensitive method for lesion detection.

Recent work in MRI has been controversial. Some investigators claim that fast T_1-weighted scanning sequences are more sensitive in lesion detection than CT scanning; other investigators find CT superior. The issue of which modality to choose for imaging the liver remains unsettled. As a practical matter, if high-quality ultrasonography is available, this should probably be the screening tool, because it is less expensive, but in many institutions the level of expertise or the type of equipment would dictate CT as a screening tool. The expense and limited availability of MRI at this time would suggest that it be reserved for assessment of complicated lesions or for screening high-risk patients in whom ultrasound or CT scans fail to show any lesions.

Finally, a word about intraoperative ultrasonography, which is probably the most sensitive technique in lesion detection. Although this is clearly not a screening tool, it is capable of picking up many lesions that are neither detected preoperatively nor detectable by the surgeon either visually or by palpation. This is particularly true of lesions smaller than 1 cm and especially those that are situated centrally within the left or right lobes of the liver (Fig. 10.67). Several studies (including our own) have documented the increased ability of intraoperative ultrasonography in lesion detection (99), and we feel that if aggressive hepatic resections are being performed for primary or metastatic hepatic malignancy, these patients should be routinely screened with intraoperative ultrasonography prior to resection. Lesions as small as 3 to 5 mm have been readily demonstrated.

Pseudomasses

Focal fatty infiltration of the liver and regenerative nodules both may present as focal masses in the liver that may simulate neoplasm. Regenerative nodules are seen in a setting of diffuse liver damage such as with chronic hepatitis and cirrhosis. These are usually very small, less than 5 mm, and often are not imaged. In the presence of ascites, a micronodular surface of the liver may be recognized sonographically or on CT scanning. Occasionally large regenerating macronodules may be encountered that can simulate hepatic neoplasm (100), notably a hepatoma arising in a cirrhotic liver. Sonographically the macronodules may be of variable echogenicity but are usually homogeneous. CT density and enhancement is also variable. We have seen a regenerative macronodule that has caused biliary obstruction, again simulating a hepatoma (Fig. 10.68). Most helpful in defining these regenerative macronodules is the radionuclide sulfur colloid scan, which should show relatively normal or increased activity within these nodules as a result of the phagocytic activity of the reticuloendothelial cells that engulf the colloid particles.

Focal fatty infiltration of the liver occurs frequently in patients with diabetes and in patients on intravenous hyperalimentation, as well as in patients with liver damage from hepatitis or cirrhosis, or from chemotherapy. Sonographically, focal fat deposits appear as hyperechoic lesions similar to that of hemangioma. However, the lesions are frequently flat or geographic in contour as opposed to the spherical nature of hemangiomas (101). In larger fatty deposits, portal or hepatic veins can be seen coursing through the fatty deposits without alteration (Fig. 10.69), a finding that rules out a solid space-occupying lesion. One frequent location for focal fatty infiltration is in the porta hepatis just anterior to the right portal vein and near the gallbladder bed (Fig. 10.70). The reason for this favored site is not well understood.

CT scanning is usually diagnostic of focal fatty infiltration by virtue of the lower CT density within the accumulations of fat (15). Similarly, vascular channels coursing through the areas of fatty infiltration can be seen on CT, especially with contrast enhancement. Care should be taken to perform the initial CT scans without intravenous contrast since subtle areas of lower density may be obscured by the overall enhancement of the liver following intravenous injection of contrast material (Fig. 10.71).

Occasionally there may be more diffuse fatty infiltration of the liver with focal sparing of small islands of uninvolved hepatic parenchyma. Sonographically these will appear as hypoechoic nodules surrounded by diffusely hyperechoic hepatic parenchyma. The reverse is seen on CT, with the islands of spared parenchyma appearing of higher density than the surrounding low-density fatty infiltration (Fig. 10.72). Unfortunately, it is not readily possible to distinguish small islands of hepatic parenchyma from nodular metastatic disease in the diffusely fatty liver, and frequently guided biopsy is necessary to make this distinction. Once again, the area around the porta hepatis is a favored site for focal sparing in the presence of diffuse fatty infiltration.

Trauma

Penetrating trauma to the liver, such as by stab wound or bullet wound, generally results in an acute surgical emergency due to hemorrhage and shock; consequently, the role of imaging in this setting is minimal because most patients immediately undergo surgery. With blunt abdominal trauma, however, diagnostic imaging frequently

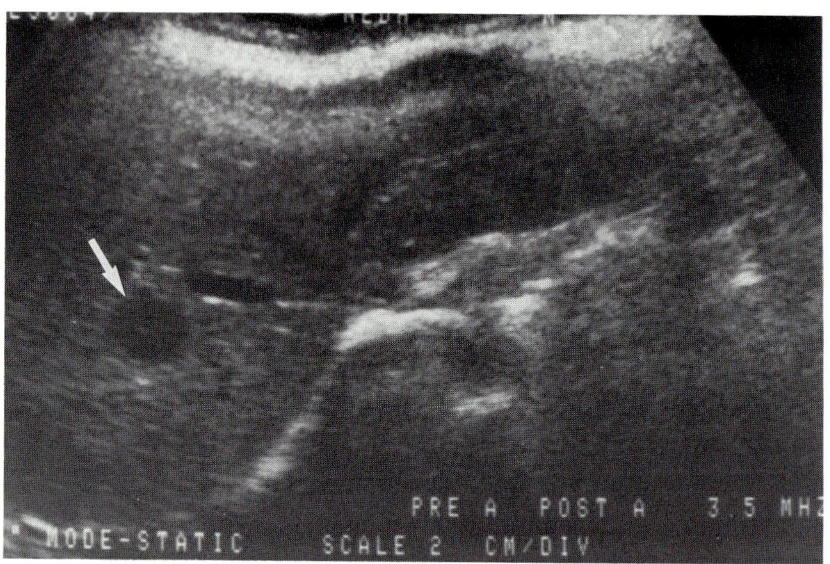

A

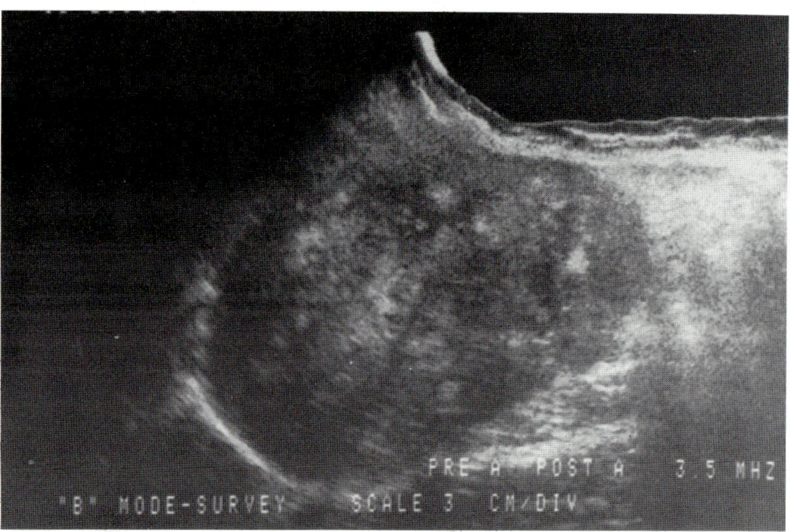

B

Figure 10.65. Metastatic disease—ultrasonography. (*A*) Hypoechoic nodule (*arrow*) secondary to metastatic oat cell carcinoma. (*B*) Multiple confluent hyperechoic metastases from duodenal carcinoma.

plays an important role in the evaluation of the patient. Plain film of the abdomen may show indications of an expanding liver mass by caudal and medial displacement of the hepatic flexure. This is a nonspecific finding that could be seen in an expanding intrahepatic hematoma or as a result of hemorrhage into the subhepatic space. A hematoma in the left lobe of the liver may show caudal and lateral displacement of the lesser curvature of the stomach. Fractures of the lower right ribs may

be observed, alerting one to the possibility of underlying hepatic trauma.

While radionuclide liver scanning formerly had a role in evaluation of liver trauma (102), it has largely been supplanted by CT scanning and ultrasonography, both of which can reveal with good anatomic detail the presence of intrahepatic or subcapsular hematomas. Sonographically the acute hepatic hematomas (103) are frequently echogenic due to organization of thrombus and

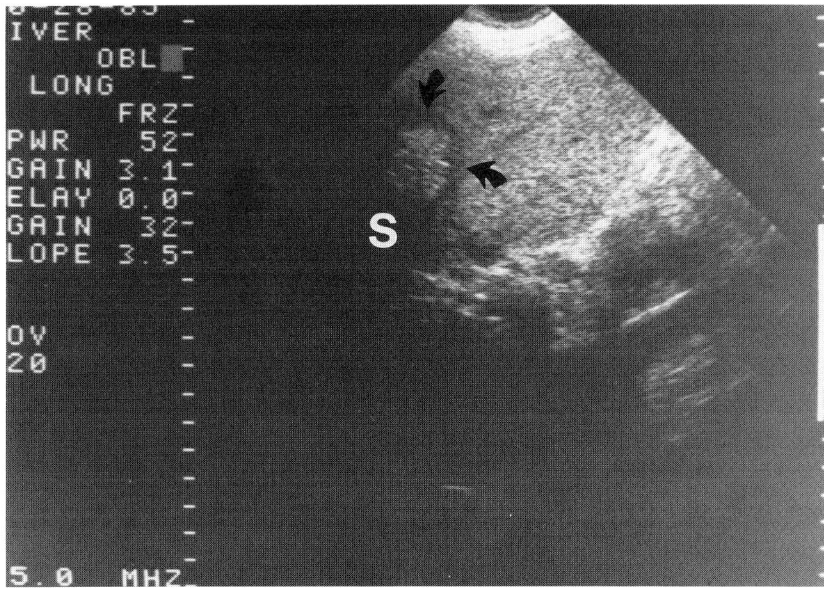

C

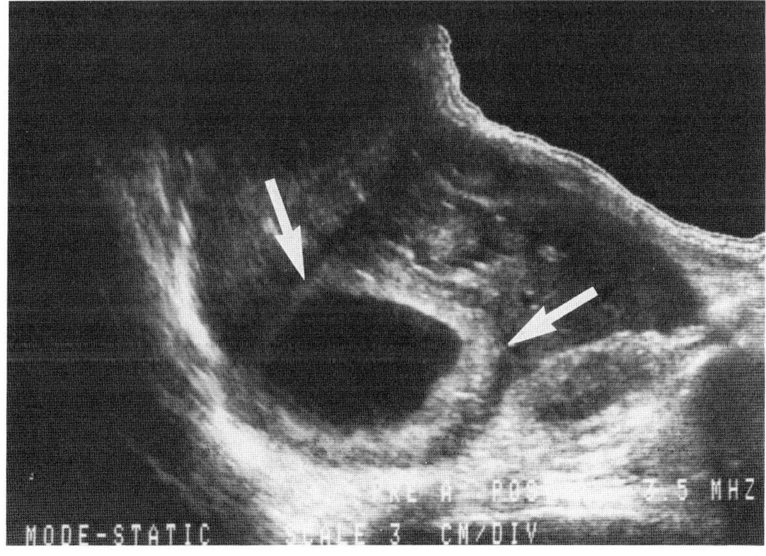

D

Figure 10.65 (continued). (C) "Bull's-eye" pattern of colon metastasis with hypoechoic rim (*arrows*) and hyperechoic center due to tumor calcification. Note the acoustic shadow (S). (D) Metastatic leiomyosarcoma. The largest lesion (*arrows*) has a cystic center due to liquefaction necrosis.

fibrin deposition. Over time, with clot retraction and reabsorption, large anechoic areas will be seen containing irregular echogenic material within. Occasionally fluid-fluid levels may be seen with anechoic serum superiorly and more echogenic cellular material in the dependent position.

Because ultrasound data can be obtained quickly and noninvasively, ultrasonography is frequently the first choice in evaluating hepatic trauma, but CT scanning is the preferable route of evaluation since it not only can indicate trauma to the liver but also can be used to assess fully the remaining intraperitoneal organs, as well as the retroperitoneum, for further involvement (104). Acute hemorrhage in the liver on CT is frequently manifested as a disruption in normal liver architecture with a

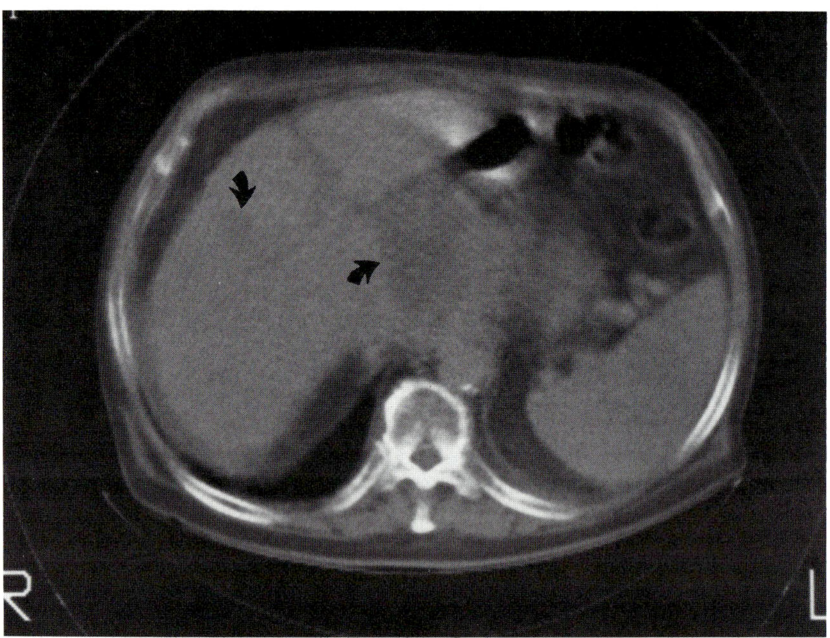

A

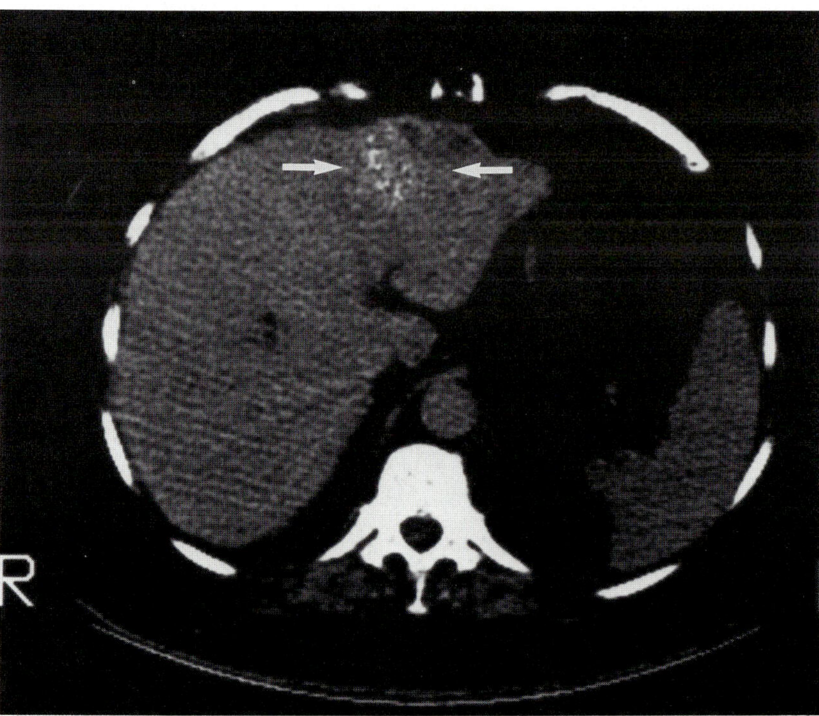

B

Figure 10.66. Metastatic adenocarcinoma on CT. (*A*) Two hypodense metastases (*arrows*). (*B*) Calcification in a left lobe metastasis manifested by multiple punctate high-density areas within the mass (*arrows*).

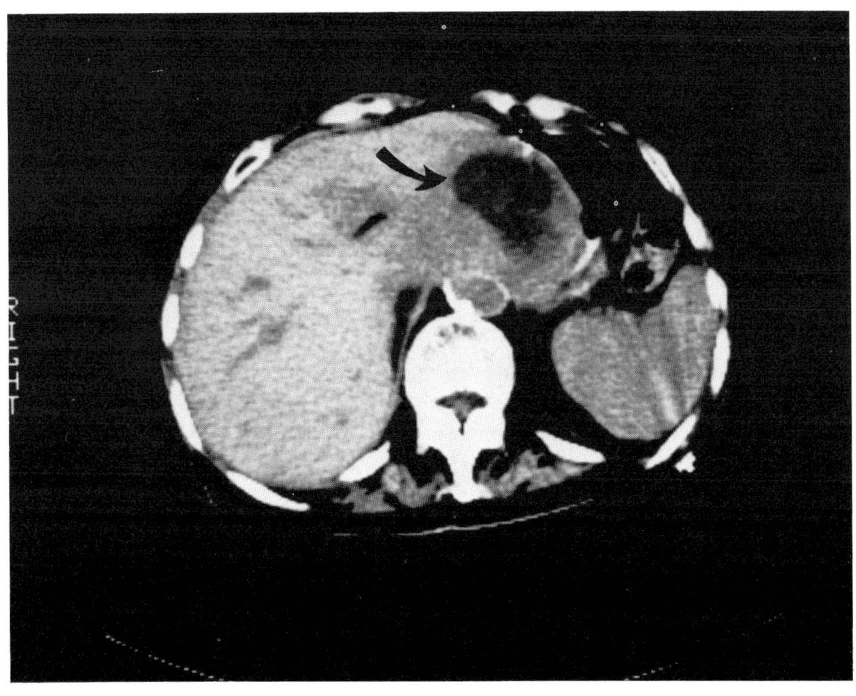

C

Figure 10.66 (continued). (*C*) Hypodense lesion (*arrow*) due to liquefaction necrosis.

slightly lower or slightly greater density than the surrounding liver parenchyma. Later the hematoma appears as a low-density lesion, usually fairly sharply marginated (Fig. 10.73). The appearance of high-density material within a low-density hematoma suggests fresh hemorrhage. Contrast enhancement may show active bleeding into acute hematomas and chronic hematomas may show rim enhancement.

Arteriography may be used in acute hepatic

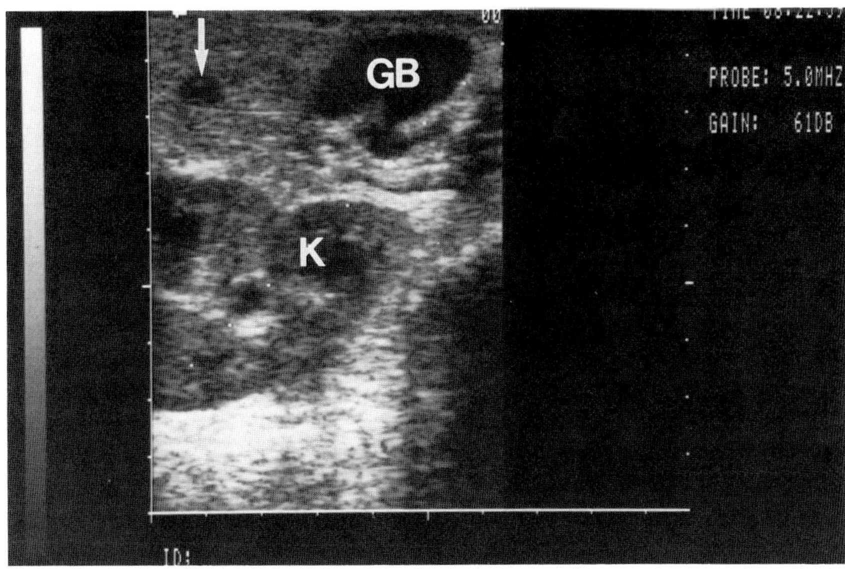

Figure 10.67. Proven liver metastasis of 5 mm (*arrow*) seen only on intraoperative ultrasonography. GB, gallbladder; K, right kidney.

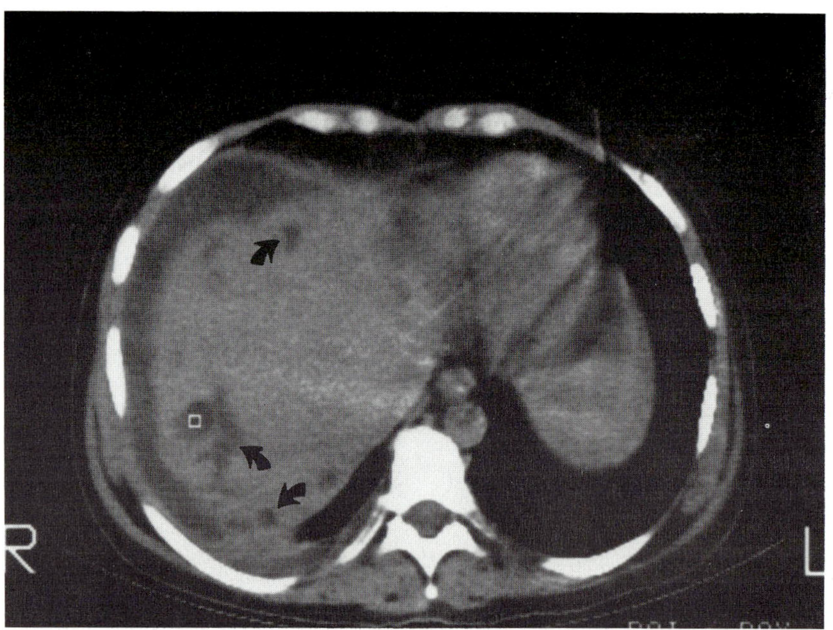

A

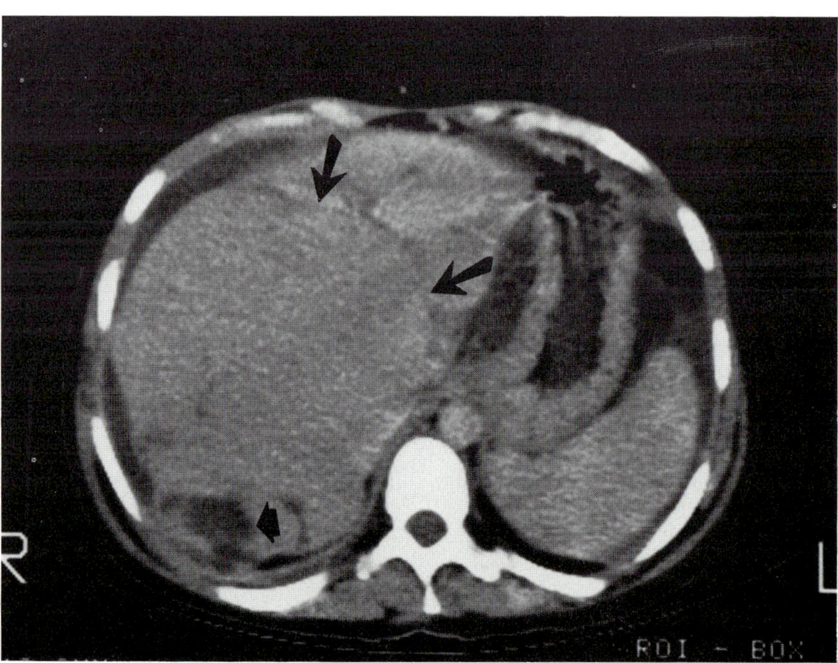

Figure 10.68. Regenerative macronodule. (*A*) CT scan through the high right lobe demonstrates dilated bile ducts (*arrows*). (*B*) The cause of the obstruction is a large isodense mass (*arrows*), a macronodule of regenerating liver tissue in a severely damaged liver. Hypodense area posteriorly (*arrowhead*) is another dilated bile duct.

B

trauma, primarily to evaluate for patency or disruption of the vascular supply to the liver. Therapeutic intervention via embolization of bleeding vessels can also be performed in the acute phase (105). Hematomas appear as masses displacing and stretching intrahepatic arteries and appearing as hypodense masses on the capillary-parenchymal phase of the arteriogram (Fig. 10.74). He-

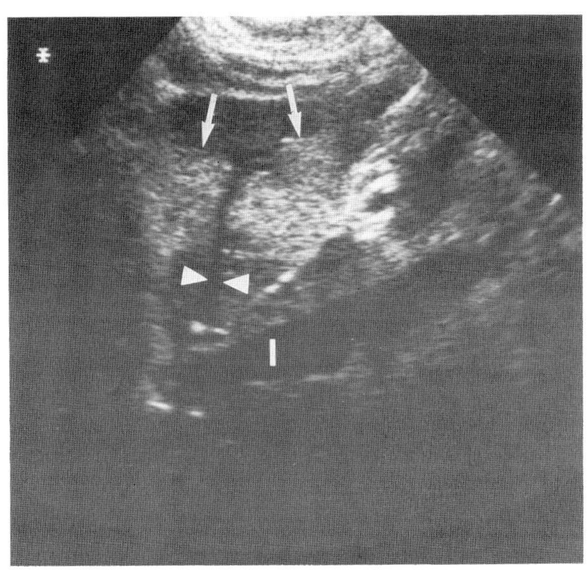

Figure 10.69. Focal fatty infiltration of the left lobe of the liver appears as a geographic, hyperechoic area (*arrows*). Note the hepatic vein (*arrowheads*) coursing through the "mass" without alteration or compression. I, inferior vena cava.

patic arteriography is also useful in the acute phase for identifying any anomalous arterial supply to the liver prior to potential surgical resections. Arteriography has a role in the post-acute phase in evaluation for the presence of pseudoaneurysms

and arteriovenous fistulas. Again, in the chronic phase, arteriography may demonstrate bleeding into the biliary tract as a result of fistulization from penetrating trauma. Hemobilia may also be recognized by sonography and CT, with clot visualized in the common bile duct and/or gallbladder (Fig. 10.75). It should be noted that complications of pseudoaneurysm, arteriovenous fistula, and hemobilia may also occur following iatrogenic trauma, for instance, following liver biopsy. One further complication of chronic liver trauma is infection, most often occurring as a result of disruption of the biliary tract or infection in a pre-existing hematoma. These post-traumatic infections appear similar to other forms of liver abscess, as described earlier in the chapter.

Intrahepatic Biliary Tract Disease

Many of the disorders of the biliary tract affect the common bile duct and gallbladder and are outside the scope of this chapter. However, when assessing the liver one frequently encounters changes intrahepatically that reflect disease of the extrahepatic biliary tract. In addition, there are some biliary-related diseases that express themselves primarily by their effect on the intrahepatic ducts. Consequently, a limited review of these disease entities is presented here.

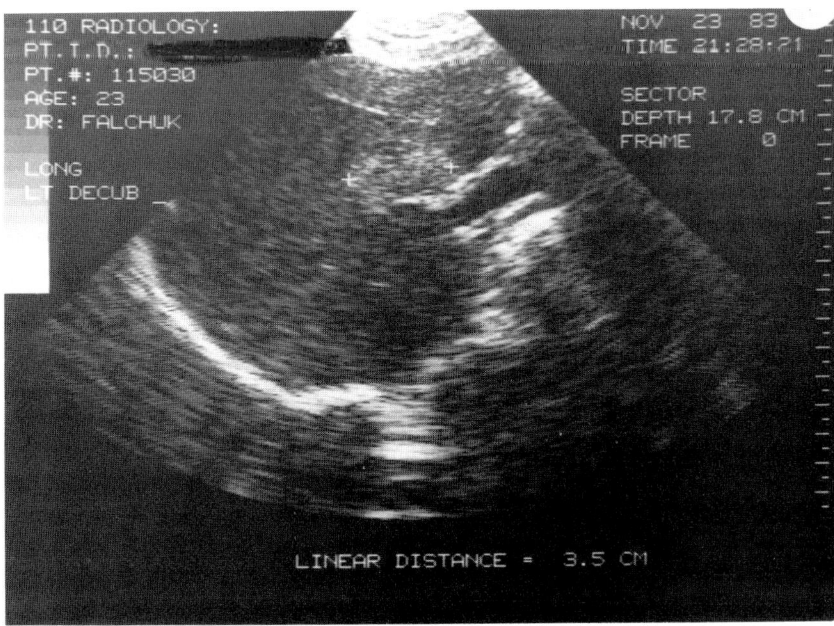

Figure 10.70. Focal fatty liver (*between cursors*) in the typical location immediately anterior to the right portal vein and porta hepatis.

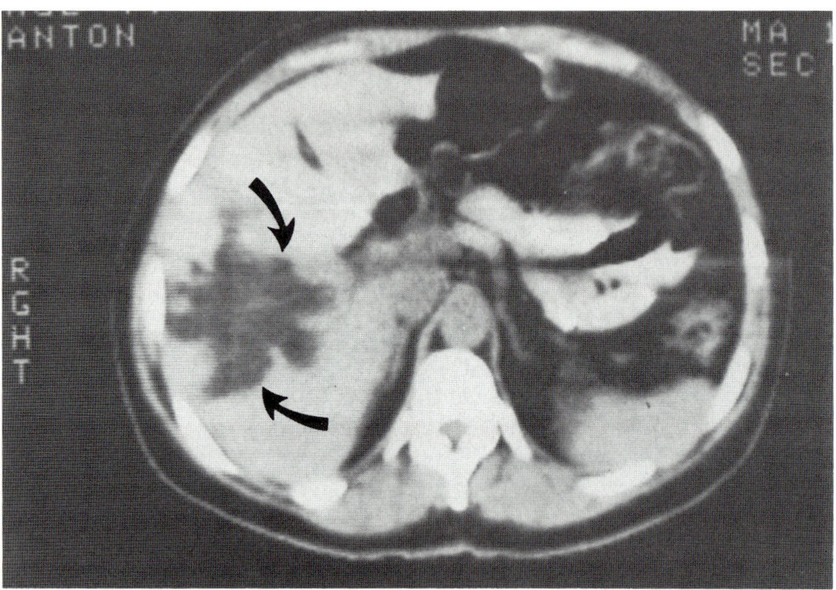

Figure 10.71. Focal fatty liver on CT with an unusual frondlike appearance (*arrows*). The negative CT density, however, indicates its fatty consistency.

Normal Anatomy

The common hepatic duct is formed by the confluence of the main left and right bile duct branches, which join together in the porta hepatis just anterior to the bifurcation of the portal vein. The common hepatic duct is best seen by ultrasound in the parasagittal oblique scans, where it appears as an anechoic tubular structure situated immediately anterior to the right hepatic artery and right main portal vein. Normally it measures no more than 5 to 6 mm in diameter. Occasionally the normal common hepatic duct can be imaged on CT scanning, with contrast enhancement, as a circular hypodense structure just anterior to the portal bifurcation. The central right and left bile ducts can occasionally be imaged for a few millimeters by ultrasound. These structures are situated immediately anterior to the main right portal vein and to the main left portal vein as it bifurcates into medial and lateral branches. These normal ducts are much smaller than the adjacent portal vein branches and frequently are too small to be visualized sonographically. Normal left and right ducts are seldom, if ever, seen on CT. Peripheral second order and more distal bile ducts are never normally visualized by CT or ultrasonography (106).

Direct visualization of the biliary tree and the liver is best obtained by transhepatic cholangiography, where a small needle is inserted into the liver substance and contrast material is infused directly into a peripheral bile duct, thereby filling out the intrahepatic and extrahepatic biliary tree (Fig. 10.76). Retrograde studies via ERCP can also demonstrate the intrahepatic ducts, although complete filling is much less often obtained than with transhepatic cholangiography. On either contrast study the normal bile ducts show a smooth tapering and regular branching pattern.

Biliary Obstruction

Ultrasonography is the imaging method of choice to assess for biliary obstruction. Dilatation of the common hepatic duct to a diameter greater than 6 mm is usually the first sign of biliary obstruction, followed by dilatation of the central and peripheral bile ducts. It should be noted that the common bile duct may increase slightly in diameter with age, and the normal value of 5 to 6 mm may be slightly greater in the elderly. Some authors allow 1 cm per decade of age, such that a patient in the 70s may have a 7 mm common bile duct and still be within normal range. A small percentage of patients may also show some enlargement of the common duct following cholecystectomy, up to 10 mm in diameter, although this is thought to occur infrequently in the absence of biliary obstruction (107). Also, if a patient has had a previous episode of bile duct obstruction and dilatation, the common duct may never return to a normal diameter even after relief of the obstruction.

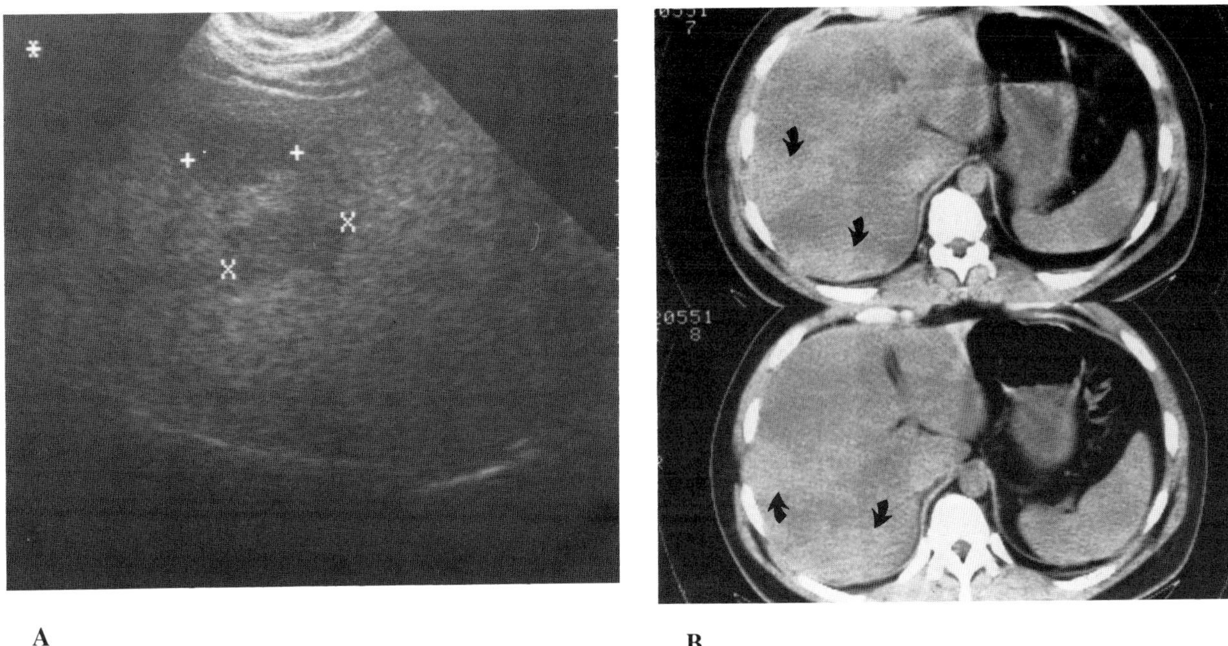

A   **B**

Figure 10.72.   Diffuse fatty infiltration with focal sparing. (*A*) Two geographic lesions (*between cursors*) appear hypoechoic but are really of normal echogenicity surrounded by hyperechoic fatty liver. (*B*) On CT, the overall liver is slightly hypodense, while the focally spared regions (*arrows*) are of more normal density, similar to that of the spleen.

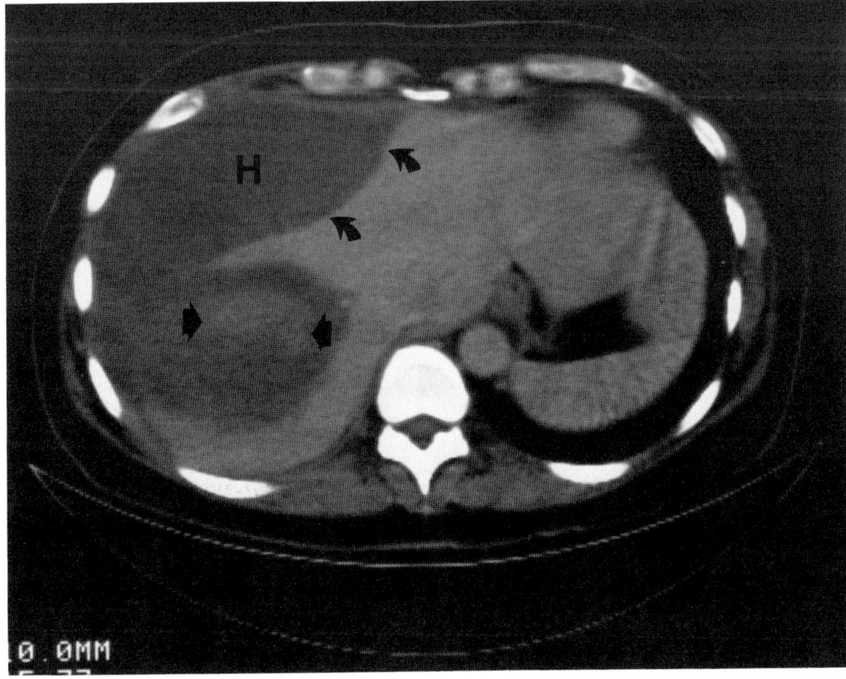

Figure 10.73.   Subcapsular and intrahepatic hematoma. The liver is compressed anteriorly (*arrows*) by a low-density fluid collection representing a chronic subcapsular hematoma (H). Fresh intrahepatic hemorrhage is represented by the higher density (*arrowheads*) centrally within the intrahepatic hematoma.

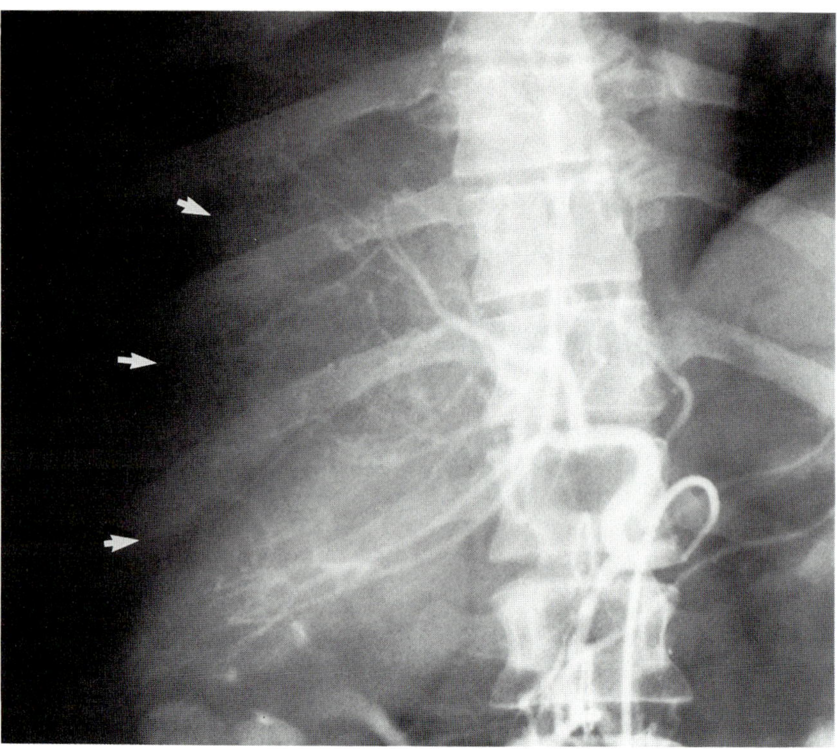

Figure 10.74. Hepatic arteriogram demonstrating a large subcapsular hematoma displacing the liver edge (*arrows*) well away from the costal margin and diaphragm.

These exceptions aside, the measurement of a common hepatic duct over 6 mm is a very strong indication of biliary tract disease. A useful means of assessing equivocal dilatation of the common hepatic duct is to challenge the patient with a fatty meal or intravenous cholecystokinin (108). Either of these approaches results in contraction of the gallbladder if present, relaxation of Oddi's sphincter, and increased bile flow from the hepatic parenchyma. A normal duct will remain the same or decrease in size following this stimulation. Any increase in diameter of the duct following this challenge is an indication of either an anatomic obstruction or a functional disorder such as spasm of Oddi's sphincter (Fig. 10.77).

The central right and left ducts, when dilated, are readily visualized and can be seen to approach 50% or more of the diameter of the corresponding portal vein segment. These ducts are also seen over a longer distance than when nondilated and frequently have undulating margins. The recognition of centrally dilated intrahepatic ducts has been termed the "shotgun" sign or "parallel channel" sign (Fig. 10.78) (109). Dilatation of the peripheral intrahepatic ducts has several findings at sonogra-

phy, including an increased number of tubular structures seen in the periphery of the liver, an increased branching pattern of the dilated ducts giving a stellate confluence (Fig. 10.79), irregularity of the bile duct walls, and occasionally acoustic enhancement posterior to the dilated ducts (110). On CT scanning, dilatation of the central and intrahepatic ducts is best recognized following contrast enhancement, in which the vessels and parenchyma will increase in density, bringing out the nonenhanced bile ducts, which will appear in tandem or parallel with the portal vein branches both centrally and peripherally in the liver (Fig. 10.80). The two direct methods of cholangiography (PTC and ERCP) show increased diameter of the common duct with obstruction distally to a diameter greater than 12 mm, and the intrahepatic dilatation is also readily demonstrated, as well as the tortuosity often associated with obstruction (Fig. 10.81).

One should be aware that with very acute obstruction of the common duct, as seen with an impacted stone, there may be no bile duct dilatation initially and this could contribute to false-negative results in noninvasive studies (111). The

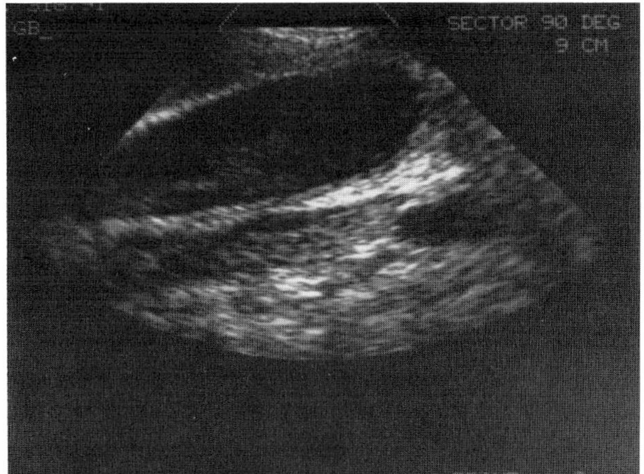

A

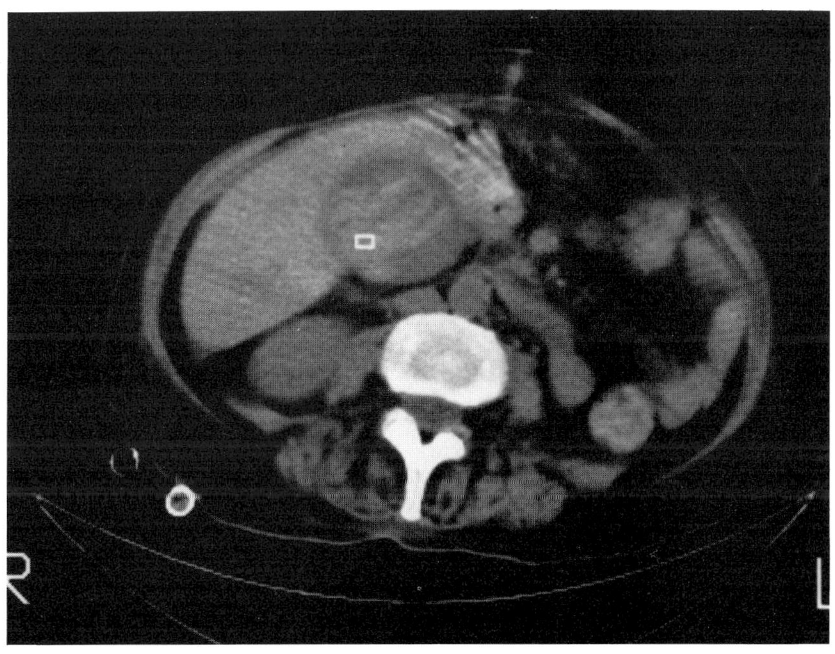

B

Figure 10.75. (*A*) Ultrasound image of the gallbladder showing echogenic thrombus in the lumen secondary to hemobilia from a septic pseudoaneurysm. (*B*) CT demonstrating high-density active hemorrhage within the gallbladder lumen.

vast majority of these patients, however, have classic physical symptoms of biliary colic as well as elevation of alkaline phosphatase, which should provide a high enough clinical suspicion to warrant further direct cholangiographic studies in the presence of negative noninvasive tests. In some series acute biliary obstruction due to stones with nondilated ducts occurs in up to 30% of patients (112).

Conversely, biliary dilatation may be detected by CT or ultrasound prior to the development of clinical jaundice and occasionally even before elevation of bilirubin. Again, the alkaline phosphatase level is nearly always elevated in this group of patients, but the lack of other clinical and laboratory findings should not lead one to dismiss the CT or ultrasound findings of bile duct obstruction.

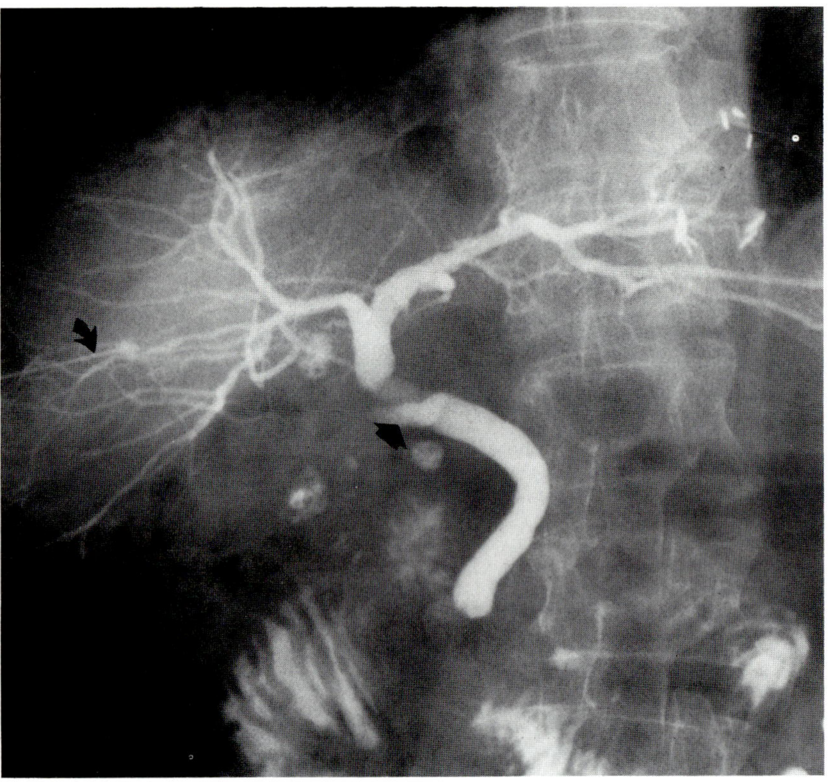

Figure 10.76. Normal transhepatic cholangiogram obtained by injecting contrast into a small biliary radicle in the right lobe via a fine needle (*arrow*). Note the fine tapering and normal branching pattern of the intrahepatic ducts. The cystic duct remnant is indicated (*arrowhead*).

Inflammatory or Infectious Diseases

In sclerosing cholangitis, the scirrhous nature of the periductal inflammation and fibrosis is so intense that frequently patients with jaundice and obstruction will not show any bile duct dilatation whatsoever. This may therefore result in false-negative results in CT and ultrasound studies. Occasionally one may see segmental or subsegmental dilatation of one or more groups of intrahepatic ducts where the sclerosing obstruction affects only the proximal bile duct. The same appearance may be seen with focal biliary obstruction from parenchymal hepatic tumors such as hepatoma, cholangiocarcinoma, and occasionally metastatic disease. Most commonly there is no bile duct dilatation whatsoever with sclerosing cholangitis. If the extrahepatic common duct is affected, thickening of the wall of the common bile duct can be appreciated at times by sonography (Fig. 10.82) (113).

The classic diagnostic pattern of sclerosing cholangitis is best seen on transhepatic cholangiography. The intrahepatic ducts are narrowed, are fewer ·in number, and frequently show a beaded appearance or alternating areas of stricture and mild dilatation (114). The strictures are multiple, diffuse, and variable in length (Fig. 10.83). The degree of dilatation is usually minimal as opposed to the dilatation typically seen with obstructions secondary to neoplasm. When the extrahepatic bile duct is involved it typically shows a beaded thickening of the wall, with multiple irregular strictures.

While the cholangiographic pattern is diagnostic, a similar pattern can often be seen with the development of cholangiocarcinoma. This tumor is often infiltrative and scirrhous, and may resemble sclerosing cholangitis. It is frequently impossible to distinguish one disease process from the other unless malignant vasculature associated with cholangiocarcinoma can be demonstrated angiographically, or a parenchymal liver mass is seen by CT or ultrasound in association with the bile duct obstruction.

Primary biliary cirrhosis generally has no diagnostic manifestations on any imaging modality,

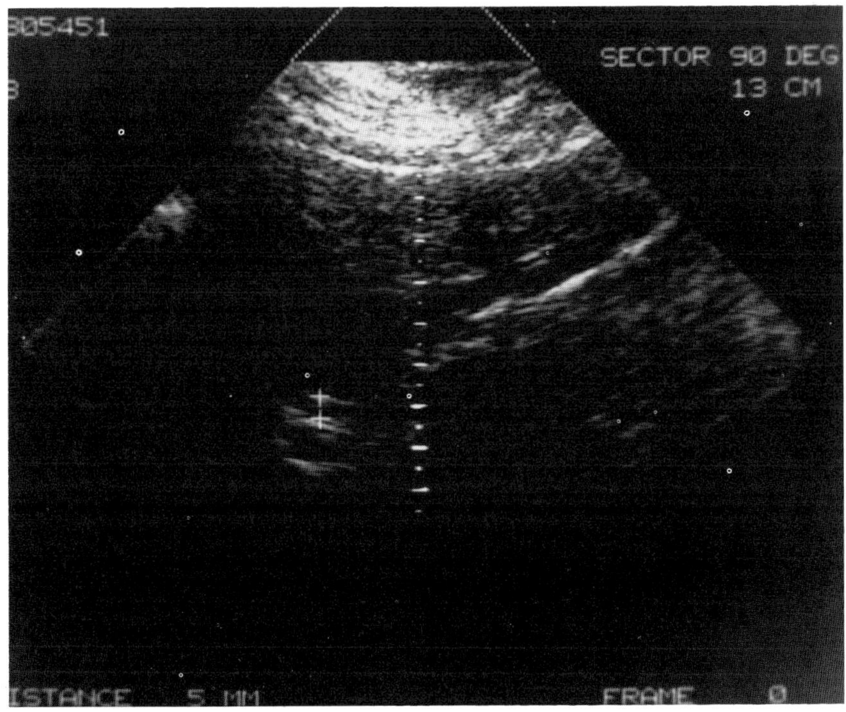

A

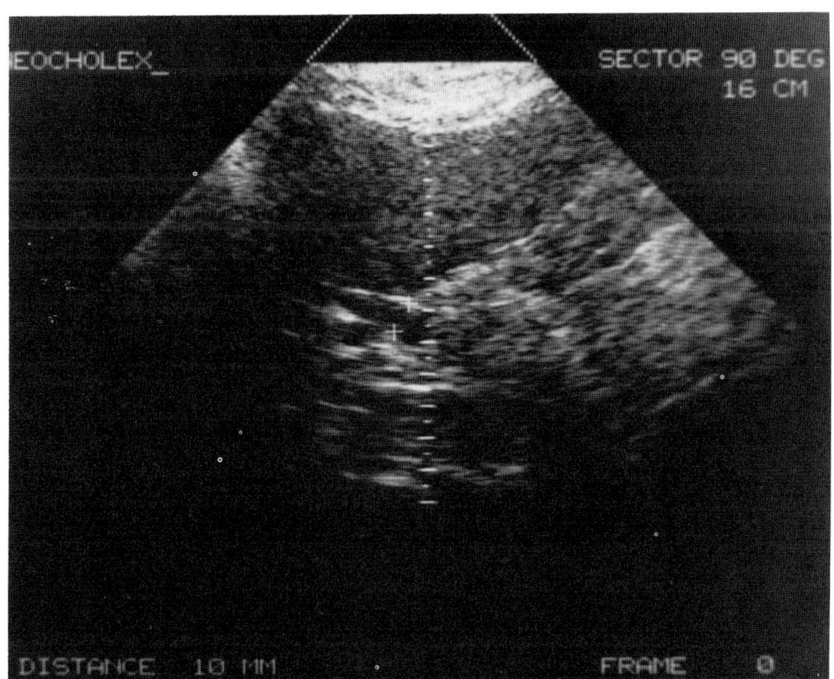

B

Figure 10.77. (*A*) Common hepatic duct measuring 5 mm in the fasting state. (*B*) Following a fatty meal, 30 minutes after *A* was obtained, the common hepatic duct is doubled in size to 10 mm, indicating either a mechanical obstruction or a functional sphincter abnormality distally.

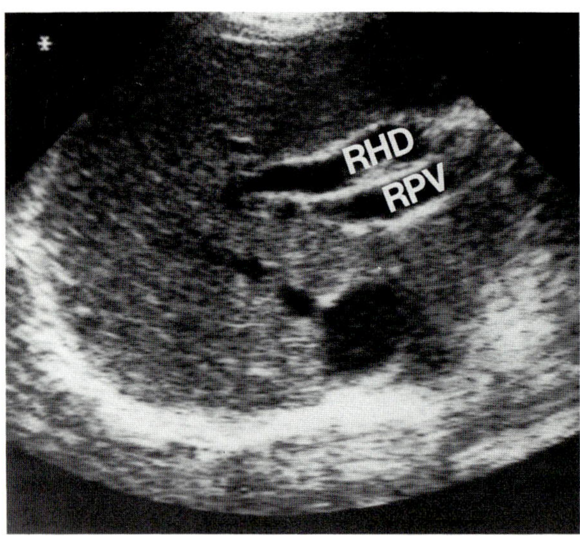

Figure 10.78. Positive "parallel channel" sign indicating dilatation of the central right hepatic duct (RHD) that is equal in diameter to the adjacent right portal vein (RPV).

other than the typical changes found with any other form of cirrhosis. Cholangiography may show some beading of the intrahepatic ducts, but this is probably merely the result of shrinkage of the overall liver volume as a result of the cirrhosis, and in fact this beading can be seen in other forms of cirrhosis as well.

Stones can occur in the intrahepatic biliary tree, particularly in the presence of long-standing obstruction. These are readily recognized sonographically as echogenic structures with posterior acoustic shadowing (Fig. 10.84). This appearance is seen regardless of the composition of the stones, whereas on CT scanning only calcified stones are readily recognized. The most reliable means for detection of intrahepatic biliary calculi is the use of direct transhepatic cholangiography to look for filling defects in the opacified ducts. ERCP is somewhat less effective due to the frequent incomplete filling of the intrahepatic ducts.

Ascending cholangitis may accompany the stones in the biliary tract, resulting in pain, fever, and frequently jaundice. If obstruction and superinfection occur, this can result in sepsis and the formation of multiple hepatic abscesses that can be readily revealed by CT and sonography. Ascending cholangitis without superimposed suppuration shows no diagnostic findings on CT or ultrasound.

Oriental cholangiohepatitis is a common disease in the Far East and Southeast Asia and may be seen in immigrants from these areas in the United States. These patients have recurrent episodes of cholangitis and sepsis with biliary colic, jaundice, and fever. Most of these patients have bacterial superinfection with *E. coli* and many of these patients also have infestation with the liver fluke,

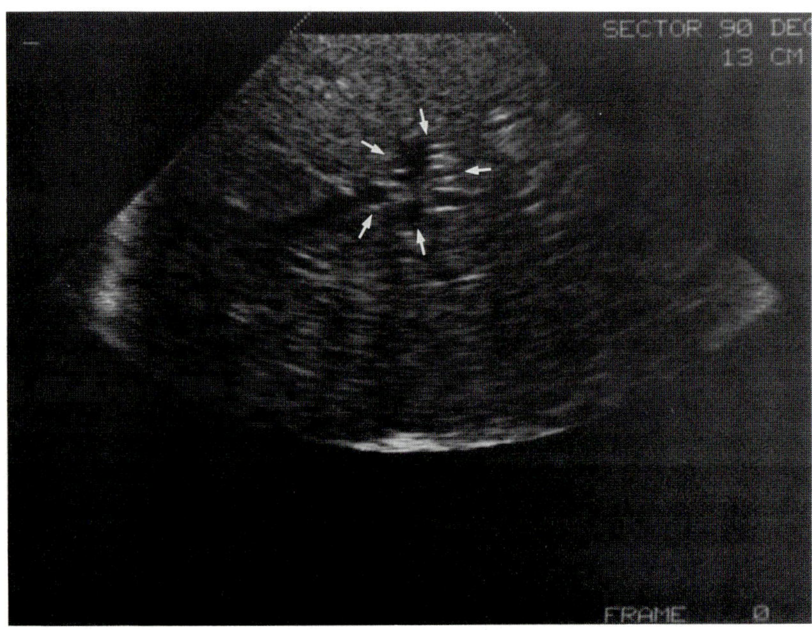

Figure 10.79. Peripheral intrahepatic ductal dilatation as manifested by increase in the number of tubular structures representing the dilated peripheral ducts (*arrows*), which converge in a stellate branching pattern.

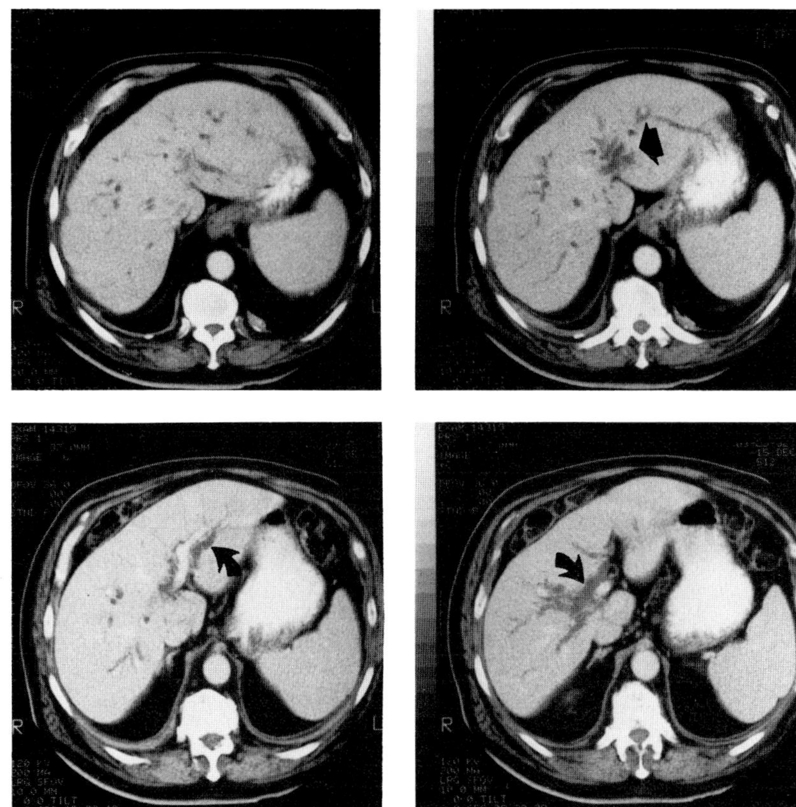

Figure 10.80. Following intravenous contrast, dilated ducts on CT are visualized as nonenhancing branching tubular structures that run in tandem with the portal venous branches (*arrows*). Note the stellate confluence of ducts in the left lobe (*arrowhead*).

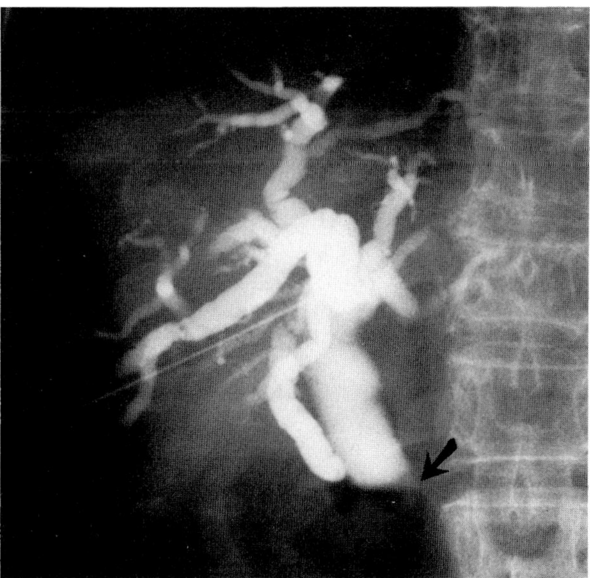

Figure 10.81. Transhepatic cholangiogram showing peripheral, central, and extrahepatic biliary dilatation due to complete obstruction of the common duct (*arrow*) by invading pancreatic carcinoma. Note the tortuosity of the intrahepatic ducts, a condition frequently seen in long-standing obstruction.

Clonorchis sinensis. Sonographically, the patients exhibit dilatation of the intrahepatic ducts and variably of the common duct as well (Fig. 10.85). Intrahepatic duct stones are frequently seen, although sometimes these stones are very soft and sludgelike, having an echogenicity similar to that of the surrounding liver, making them difficult to recognize. Frank hepatic abscesses and gas within the biliary tract are not uncommon in the presence of infection (115,116). CT findings also show ductal dilatation, abscesses, and intrahepatic gas. The stones may not be as well visualized on CT unless cholangiographic contrast material is administered, since the majority are nonradiopaque. On cholangiography, again ductal dilatation is seen, with areas of stricture, filling defects due to stones and sludge, and occasional direct communication into abscess cavities (Fig. 10.86). The branching pattern is abnormal with a decreased number of biliary radicles. Transhepatic drainage and stone retrieval from the intrahepatic ducts has been performed occasionally on these patients, with some success in temporarily relieving obstruction

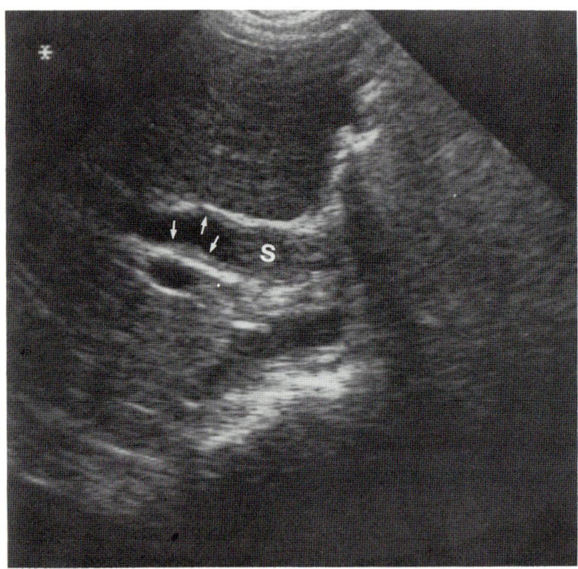

Figure 10.82. Sclerosing cholangitis. Thickening of the wall of the common hepatic duct can be seen (*arrows*) as well as thick bile or sludge (S) in the lumen more distally.

and clearing infection. The underlying disease process remains unaltered, however, and recurrent obstruction, stone formation, and infection will inevitably occur. There is also an increased incidence of cholangiocarcinoma developing in patients with Oriental cholangiohepatitis.

Other parasitic infestations of the biliary tract can be recognized. Ascariasis is common throughout the world and is seen in some endemic areas of the southeastern United States. The worms can be seen as filling defects in the common duct or gallbladder on cholangiographic studies (Fig. 10.87). The worms can be visualized as echogenic tubular or rounded structures sonographically, and parasitic or superimposed bacterial liver abscesses may result from obstruction secondary to the worms (117). Both amebiasis and echinococcal infestations of the liver may occasionally manifest changes in the biliary tract due either to pressure and narrowing or occasionally to direct communication with a bile duct.

Air may be recognized within the biliary tree sonographically (see Fig. 10.46), even when the ducts are not dilated, presenting as linear, highly echogenic foci with a shimmering or scintillating

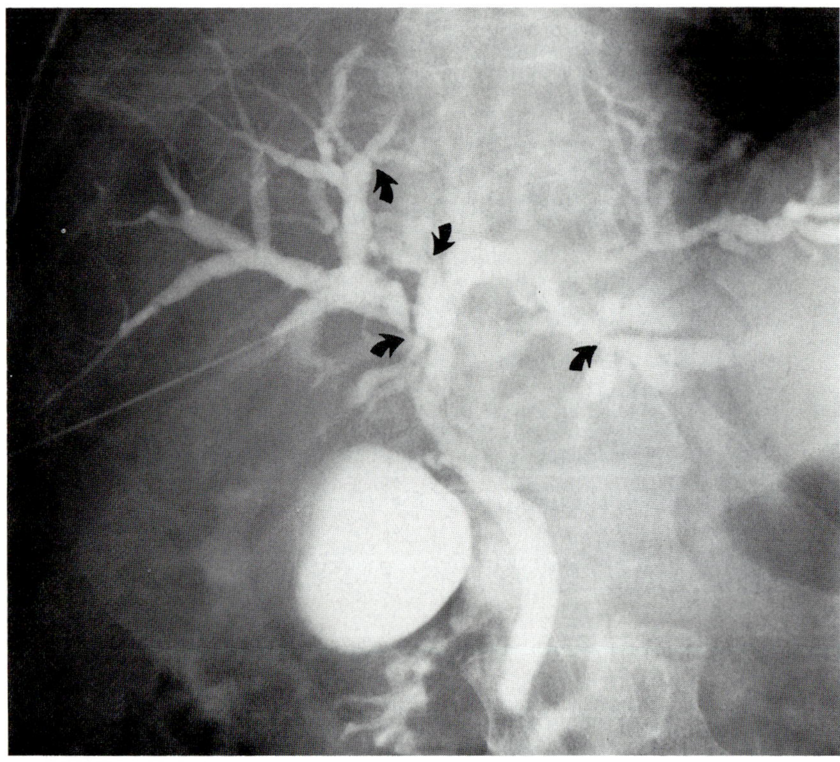

Figure 10.83. Sclerosing cholangitis. Transhepatic cholangiography shows the typical appearance with multiple strictures (*arrows*) and beading of the obstructed ducts. Note the rather minimal dilatation despite the multiple sites of obstruction.

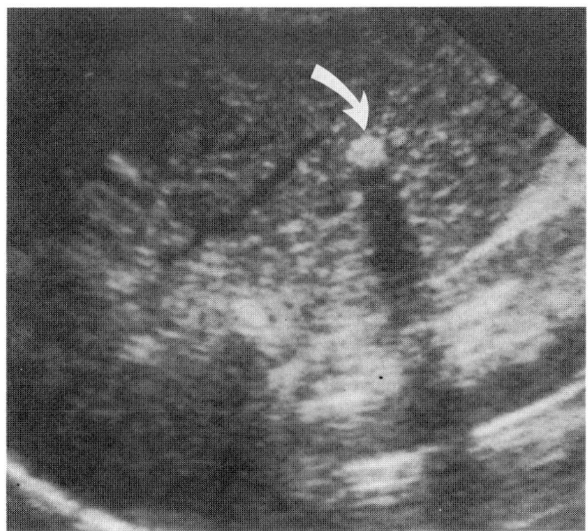

Figure 10.84. Ultrasound demonstration of intrahepatic biliary stones, which appear as bright echogenic structures (*arrow*) with posterior acoustic shadowing.

appearance on real-time examination as well as some acoustic shadowing. On CT, air in bile ducts appears as linear, low-density areas with density less than retroperitoneal fat. Biliary air tends to remain fairly central within the liver, as opposed to air in the portal venous system, which tends to lie in the periphery of the liver. Although air in the bile ducts may indicate suppurative cholangitis, it

may be seen in a variety of other noninfected conditions including recent passage of an impacted stone through the ampulla, choledochoduodenal, or choledochocolic fistula (which will also show air in the gallbladder bed), and any surgical or endoscopic procedures involving Oddi's sphincter. Rarely biliary air has been described in cases of encasement of the distal common duct and ampulla by carcinoma of the pancreas.

Congenital Diseases

Caroli's disease is a congenital autosomal-recessive disorder manifested by segmental saccular dilatation of the intrahepatic bile ducts, with variable involvement of the common duct, although most often the common duct is normal in caliber. This cystlike dilatation of the intrahepatic ducts results in a "lollipop" appearance on cholangiography (118). Both CT and sonography show multiple cystic areas as well as dilated intrahepatic ducts, and frequently stones can be recognized within the ducts or the cysts (Fig. 10.88). The superinfection may result in pyogenic material seen within the ducts or frank liver abscesses. Some investigators speculate a relationship of Caroli's disease with congenital hepatic fibrosis, a disease that is also congenital and usually lethal in childhood. In this entity there is bile duct proliferation and multiple

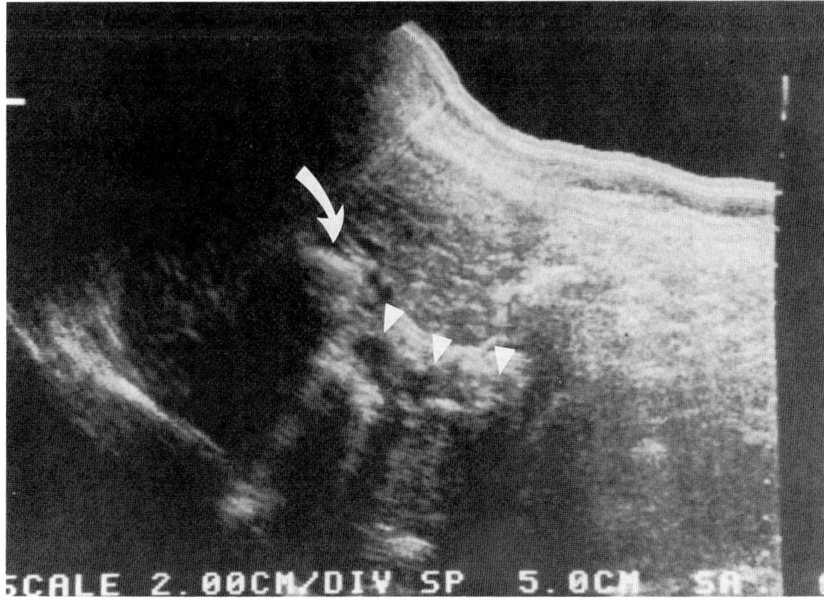

Figure 10.85. Oriental cholangiohepatitis. Ultrasound demonstrates intrahepatic stones (*arrow*) as well as dilatation of the common duct, which contains both sludge and stones (*arrowheads*).

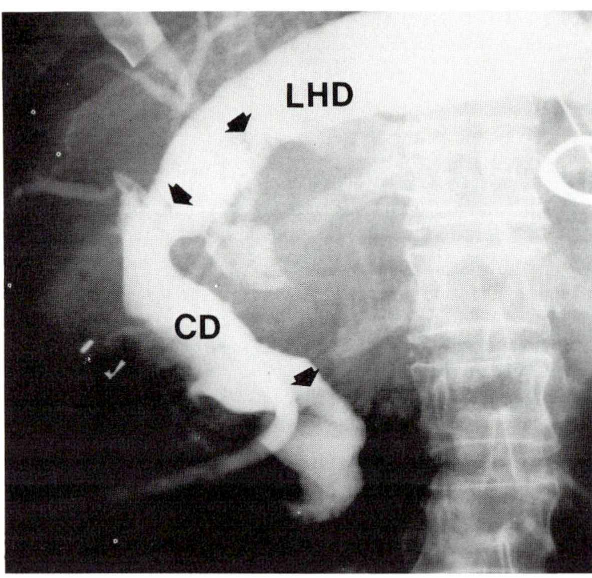

Figure 10.86. Oriental cholangiohepatitis. Intraoperative cholangiogram demonstrating gross dilatation of the common duct (CD) and left hepatic duct (LHD) with filling defects due to stones and sludge (*arrowheads*). Note the relatively normal caliber of right hepatic ducts.

strictures with proximal dilatation, but the dilatation is much less than in Caroli's disease and the predominant feature of this disease is the fibrosis and the resultant cirrhosis and portal hypertension.

Biliary atresia is a disease of the newborn due to congenital agenesis of all or portions of the biliary tract. This can present a difficult problem sonographically since nondeveloped ducts will of course not be visualized but normal intrahepatic ducts are usually not visualized either. The same problem pertains to CT scanning, and in this setting radionuclide biliary scanning is the best noninvasive means of evaluation (119). This is a functional test, and if it demonstrates normal passage of radioactivity into the gut, it is a conclusive demonstration of normal biliary tract function. The lack of excretion is more difficult to interpret since other entities such as neonatal hepatitis may cause parenchymal dysfunction, but an abnormal biliary scan is probably an indication to consider direct cholangiographic evaluation.

Choledochal cyst is another congenital abnor-

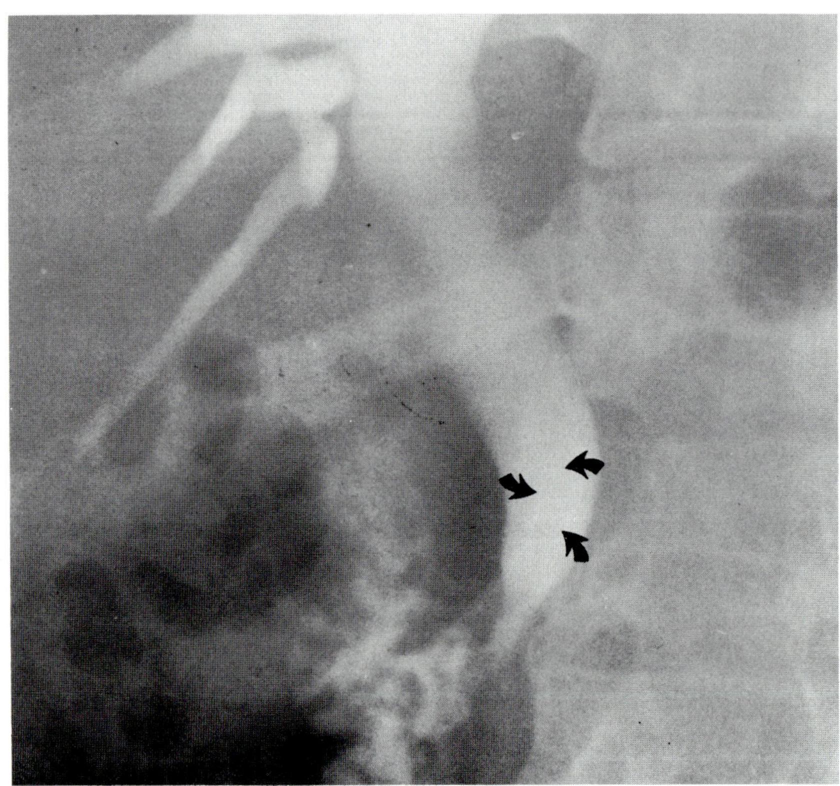

Figure 10.87. Ascariasis. Transhepatic cholangiogram demonstrating central and extrahepatic biliary dilatation. Faintly seen in the distal common duct is a tubular filling defect (*arrows*) caused by the parasite.

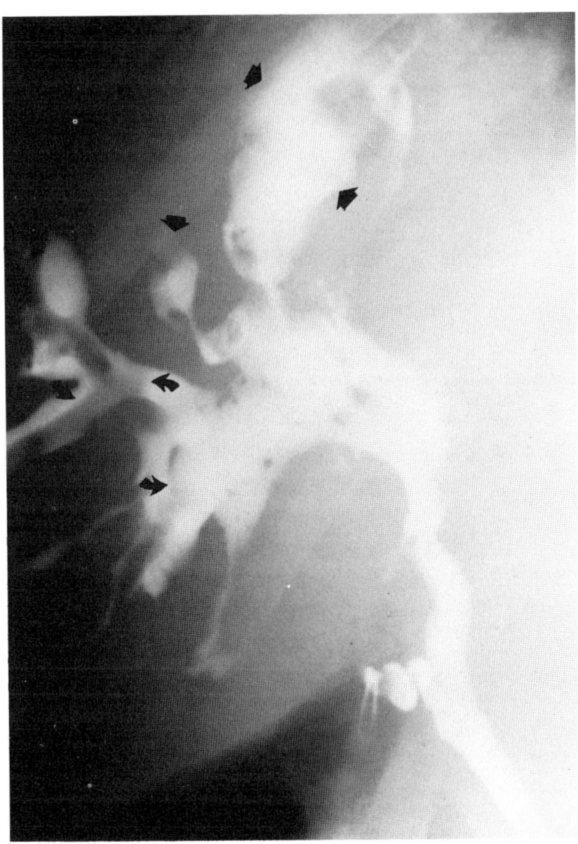

A

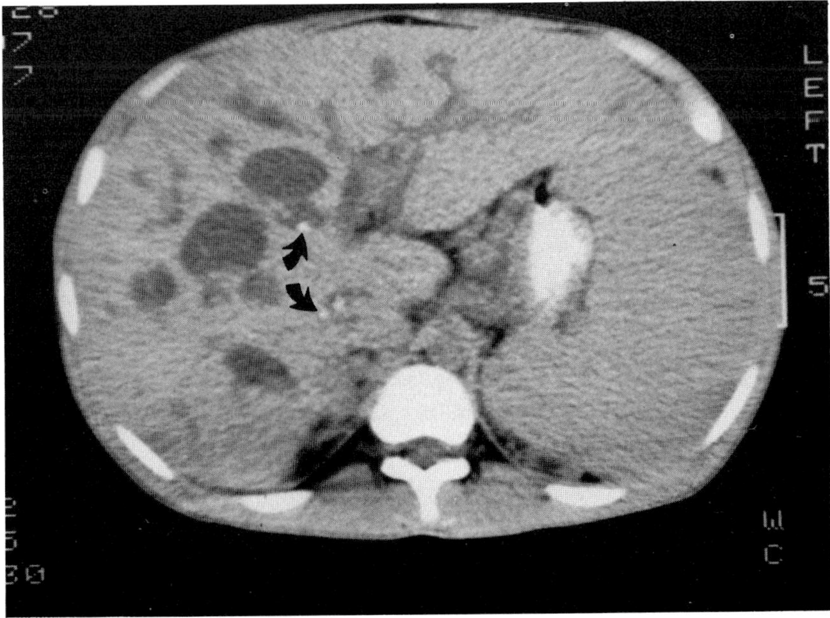

B

Figure 10.88. Caroli's disease. (*A*) ERCP demonstrating gross deformity and dilatation of the intrahepatic ductal system with multiple tubular filling defects (*arrows*) secondary to stones, sludge, and infectious material. Note the periductal extravasation (*arrowheads*) into infected cystic spaces. Also note the relatively normal appearance of the extrahepatic common duct. (*B*) CT on the same patient, demonstrating ductal dilatation and periductal cystic spaces, several of which are seen to contain stones (*arrows*).

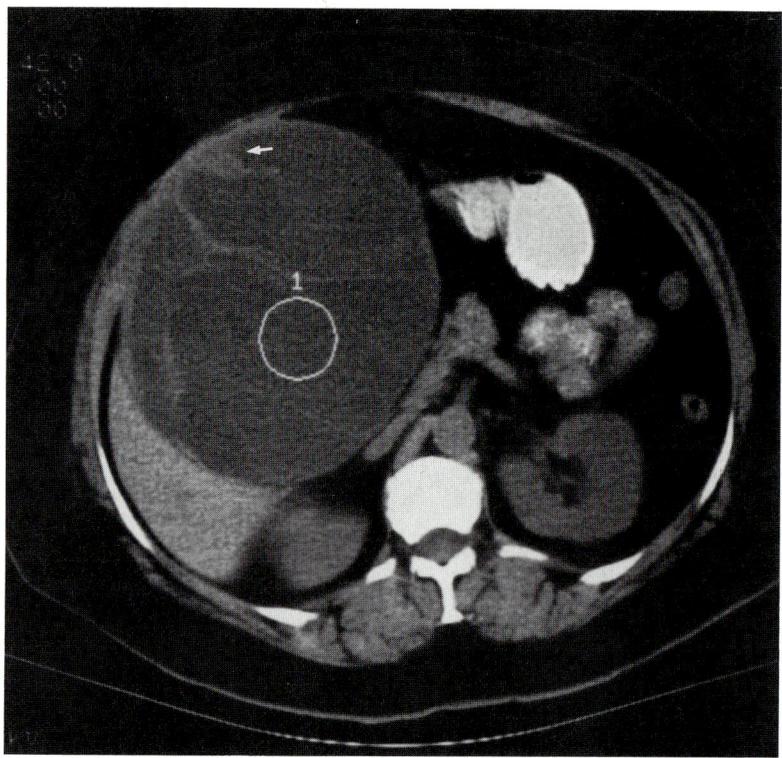

Figure 10.89. Biliary cystadenoma appearing as a sharply circumscribed, low-density cystic lesion on CT with fine internal septations. The CT density measures 10 HU. Note the small area of nodular wall thickening (*arrow*), which is frequently seen and does not necessarily indicate malignancy.

mality often seen in children or young adults who present with jaundice and pain. This entity represents massive dilatation of the common bile duct and common hepatic duct, but the intrahepatic ducts are frequently normal in caliber or at best only minimally dilated centrally (120). The disproportion between the extrahepatic ductal dilatation and the caliber of the intrahepatic ducts is a tip-off to the underlying diagnosis. It is felt this lesion results from an abnormal insertion of the distal common duct into the pancreatic duct, resulting in continual reflux of pancreatic enzymes into the common duct, causing irritation and stricture. Sepsis due to stones and cholangitis is frequently seen in patients with this condition, and there is also an increased incidence of cholangiocarcinoma, even after surgical correction of this entity.

Neoplastic Disease

The only benign intrahepatic biliary neoplasm likely to be encountered is the biliary cystadenoma. This is a cystic neoplasm seen most often in young women. The cysts may be unilocular but are more frequently multilocular (78). The walls and septations are usually thin but may in some cases be thickened and even nodular. Occasionally rim-like calcification may occur in the walls.

These lesions are seen easily by both CT (Fig. 10.89) and ultrasound, although the internal septations and architecture are better demonstrated by ultrasonography. The cyst fluid is usually clear sonographically but may have some echogenicity if there is crystalline material or blood contained within. Similarly, the CT density, although usually that of water, may be higher in the presence of mucin, cholesterol, hemosiderin, or infectious material. The lesions are hypovascular on angiography. Occasional cystadenocarcinomas are encountered; however, the vast majority of these lesions are benign and there are no distinct imaging criteria to predict malignancy unless frank neovascularity is seen angiographically. Because of their benign nature the lesions may occasionally grow extremely large before presentation. The vast majority of these lesions are isolated from the ducts, although arising from bile duct epithelium, but

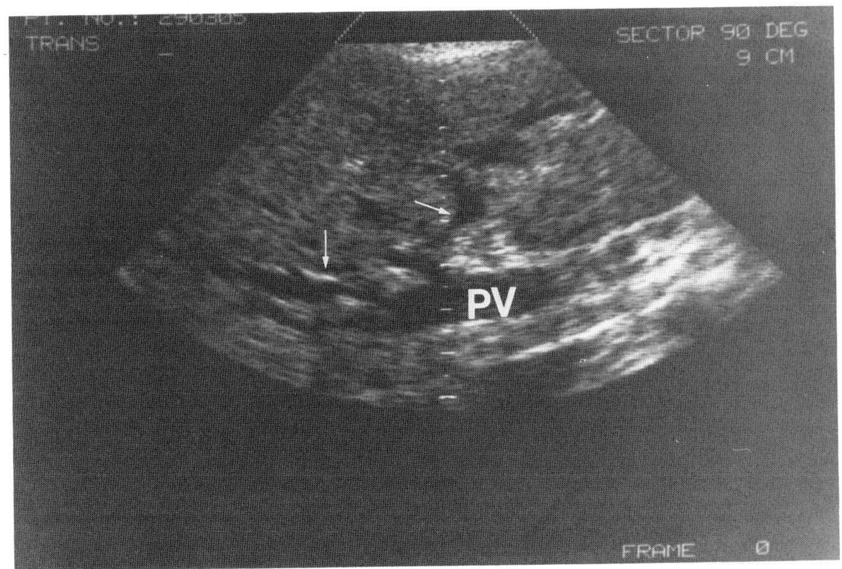

Figure 10.90. Cholangiocarcinoma. Centrally dilated left and right hepatic ducts (*arrows*) converge to the point of obstruction at the bifurcation in the porta hepatis. No mass could be visualized in this Klatskin tumor. PV, portal vein.

rarely these may communicate with the adjacent bile ducts.

Cholangiocarcinoma may arise in any portion of the biliary tree including the main bifurcation (the so-called Klatskin tumor), as well as the more peripheral intrahepatic ducts. The appearance of this tumor is protean. The majority of cases in our experience fail to show evidence of a discrete parenchymal hepatic mass on ultrasound or CT and merely show the effects of the bile duct obstruction (Fig. 10.90). In this group of patients angiography seldom shows evidence of tumor neovasculature. A lesser percentage of cases will show either small or large discrete masses in the

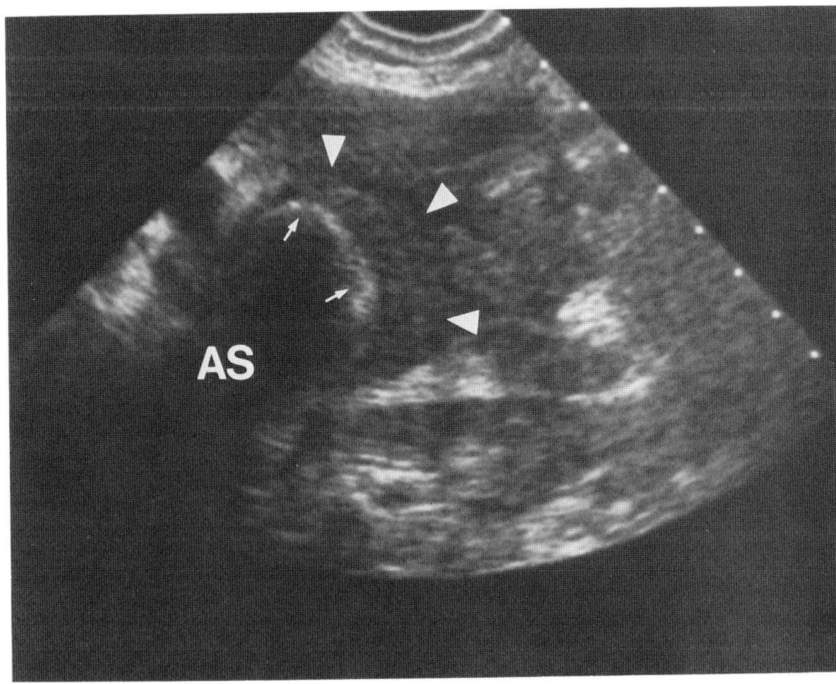

Figure 10.91. Gallbladder carcinoma. Ultrasound demonstrates a large gallstone (*arrows*) with acoustic shadowing (AS), surrounded by a soft tissue mass (*arrowheads*) representing the gallbladder carcinoma.

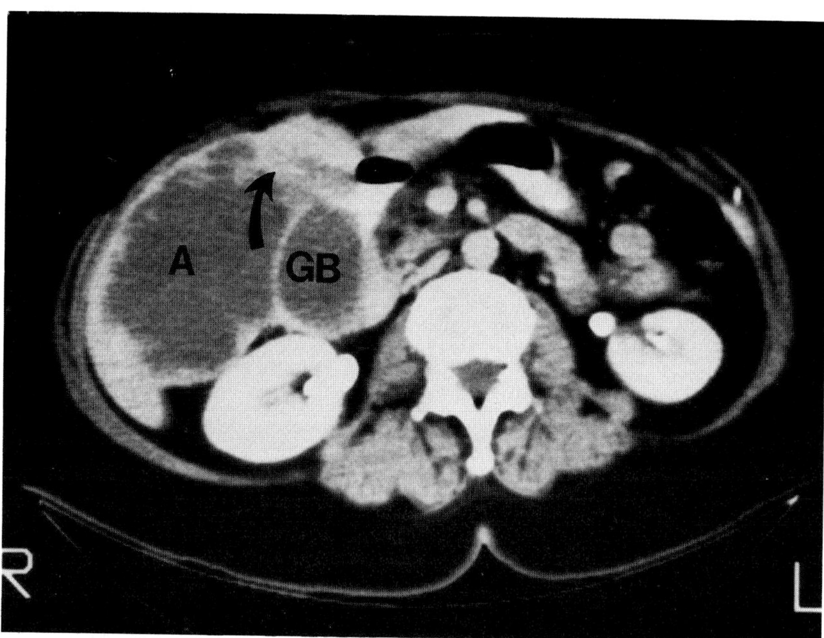

Figure 10.92. Gallbladder carcinoma with intrahepatic perforation. On this CT slice, the gallbladder (GB) appears to be intact with an anterior mass (*arrow*) adjacent to a large intrahepatic abscess (A). On lower cuts, the wall of the gallbladder was destroyed, resulting in communication between the abscess and the gallbladder lumen.

liver substance, which are usually hypoechoic and hypodense (see Fig. 10.64) (87). In this type, angiography may show tumor vasculature and occasionally a hypervascular tumor blush. Much less frequently, a discrete intraluminal mass can be seen growing within the lumen of the biliary ducts. Periportal lymph node metastases are also frequently visualized. The reason for the difficulty in visualizing most cholangiocarcinomas is their tendency to infiltrate submucosally along the course of the ducts. This type of tumor is difficult for the surgeon to palpate and is often even difficult for the pathologist to demonstrate because of the intense scirrhous reaction.

In contrast to cholangiocarcinoma, gallbladder carcinoma generally presents as a large intrahepatic mass obliterating the gallbladder itself. Frequently stones can be seen surrounded by neoplastic tissue (Fig. 10.91) (121). This, plus the lack of an identifiable normal gallbladder, provides the only clue to the diagnosis, since the parenchymal hepatic mass is indistinguishable from either primary or metastatic adenocarcinoma to the liver. Occasionally the tumor may perforate into the liver, resulting in a bizarre, complex appearance of neoplastic tissue and cystic areas of sterile or infected bile (Fig. 10.92).

Intrahepatic bile duct dilatation is of course seen secondary to a variety of other tumors causing biliary obstruction. If the common duct is also dilated, the obstruction is generally caused by tumors of the pancreas or Vater's ampulla or the duodenum. If the obstruction is at or just below the bifurcation, this is usually caused by metastatic lymphadenopathy from adenocarcinomas of the gastrointestinal tract, metastatic breast carcinoma, or occasionally lymphoma. If there is only segmental intrahepatic obstruction, this is usually due to parenchymal hepatic tumor, either primary hepatoma or metastatic lesions compressing or occasionally invading the ducts.

Conclusions

It is apparent that there are many complementary and supplementary types of diagnostic imaging of the liver. Although it is not possible to specify the optimal sequencing of tests for each clinical question, since equipment and expertise in imaging will vary from one institution to another, a few general guidelines may be of use. If high-quality ultrasound is available, this is recommended as the initial screening device for liver disease because it is noninvasive, fairly inexpensive, and capable of providing good information in a short period of time. In other settings, CT would be the preferable screening modality, since consistently good CT scans can be obtained without specific technical expertise. Frequently these two imaging modalities provide complementary information and further definition of disease, although often one or the other will suffice. Radionuclide evaluation of the liver has diminished in significance and is no longer considered to be the screening method of choice, although there are some very specific uses such as gallium scanning for hepatoma, hepatobiliary scanning for biliary obstruction, and tagged red cell scanning for hemangioma. The invasive imaging tests of the liver, including angiography, transhepatic cholangiography, and ERCP, should be reserved for those cases in which the noninvasive tests have not provided sufficient data for a comprehensive preoperative evaluation. The role of magnetic resonance imaging is yet to be fully determined in diagnostic evaluation of the liver, although there is promising work suggesting it may be very accurate in focal liver lesion detection (122). Finally, the use of intraoperative ultrasonography of the liver is to be encouraged because it appears to be capable of demonstrating many lesions that are neither imaged preoperatively nor seen or felt by the surgeon intraoperatively.

One final point to emphasize is that the quality of image interpretation is related to the skill and experience of the interpreter but is also dependent on adequate clinical information about the patient, since many disease processes have overlapping patterns of expression. The more fully informed the radiologist is regarding clinical data, the better the quality of interpretation should be.

References

1. Kane RA. Sonographic anatomy of the liver. *Seminars in Ultrasound* 1981; 2:190.
2. Sexton CC, Zeman RK. Correlation of computed tomography, sonography and gross anatomy of liver. *AJR* 1983; 141:711.
3. Sones PJ, Torres WE. Normal ultrasonic appearance of the ligamentum teres and falciform ligament. *J Clin Ultrasound* 1978; 6:392.
4. Brown BM, Filly RA, Callen PW. Ultrasonographic anatomy of the caudate lobe. *J Ultrasound Med* 1982; 1:89.
5. Parulekar SG. Ligaments and fissures of the liver: Sonographic anatomy. *Radiology* 1977; 130:409.
6. Carlsen EN, Filly RA. Newer ultrasonographic anatomy in the upper abdomen: I. The portal and hepatic venous anatomy. *J Clin Ultrasound* 1976; 4:85–90.
7. Ralls PW, Quinn MF, Rogers W, Halls J. Sonographic anatomy of hepatic artery. *AJR* 1981; 136:1059.
8. Nebesar RA, Kornblith PL, Pollard JJ, et al. Celiac and superior mesenteric arteries: A correlation of angiograms and dissections. Boston: Little, Brown, 1969.
9. Michels, NA. Blood supply to the upper abdominal organs with a descriptive atlas. Philadelphia: JB Lippincott, 1955.
10. Goldberg HI, Dodds WJ, Lawson TL, et al. Hepatic lymphatics demonstrated by percutaneous transhepatic cholangiography. *Am J Roentgenol* 1975; 123:415–419.
11. Gosink BB, Leymaster CE. Ultrasonic determination of hepatomegaly. *J Clin Ultrasound* 1981; 9:37.
12. Harbin WP, Robert NJ, Ferrucci JT. Diagnosis of cirrhosis based on regional changes in hepatic morphology. *Radiology* 1980; 135:273.
13. Taylor KJW, Gorelick FS, Rosenfield AT, Riely CA. Ultrasonography of alcoholic liver disease with histological correlation. *Radiology* 1981; 141:157.
14. Foster KJ, Dewbury KC, Griffin AH, Wright R. The accuracy of ultrasound in the detection of fatty infiltration of the liver. *Br J Radiol* 1980; 53:440.
15. Scatarige JC, Scott WW, Donovan PJ, et al. Fatty infiltration of the liver: Ultrasonographic and computed tomographic correlation. *J Ultrasound Med* 1984; 3:9.
16. Geslin GE, Pinsky SM, Poth RK, et al. The sensitivity and specificity of ^{99m}Tc-sulfur colloid liver imaging in diffuse hepatocellular disease. *Radiology* 1976; 118:115–119.
17. Reuter SR, Redman HC. *Gastrointestinal Angiography*, 2nd ed., chapters 4 and 5. Philadelphia: WB Saunders, 1977.
18. Kane RA, Curatolo P, Khettry U. "Scar sign" on computed tomography and sonography in fibrolamellar hepatocellular carcinoma. *J Comput Tomogr* 1987; 11:27–30.
19. Laing F, Brooke J, Federle M, Cello J. Noninvasive imaging of unusual regenerating nodules in the cirrhotic liver. *Gastrointest Radiol* 1982; 7:245–249.
20. Kane RA, Katz SG. The spectrum of sonographic findings in portal hypertension: A subject review and new observations. *Radiology* 1982; 142:453.
21. Ishikawa T, Tsukune Y, Ohyama Y, et al. Venous abnormalities in portal hypertension demonstrated by CT. *AJR* 1980; 134:271.
22. Funston MR, Goudie E, Richter IA, et al. Ultrasound diagnosis of the recanalized umbilical vein in portal hypertension. *J Clin Ultrasound* 1980; 8:244.
23. Marz M, Scheible W. Cavernous transformation of the portal vein. *J Ultrasound Med* 1982; 1:167.
24. Viamonte M, LePage J, Lunderquist A, et al. Selective catheterization of the portal vein and its tributaries. *Radiology* 1975; 114:457–460.
25. Maguire R, Doppman J. Angiographic abnormalities in partial Budd-Chiari syndrome. *Radiology* 1977; 122:629–635.
26. Pauls CH. Ultrasound and computed tomographic demonstration of portal vein thrombosis in hepatocellular carcinoma. *Gastrointest Radiol* 1981; 6:281.
27. Merritt CRB. Ultrasonographic demonstration of portal vein thrombosis. *Radiology* 1979; 133:425.
28. Subramanyam BR, Balthazar EJ, Hilton S, et al. Hepatocellular carcinoma with venous invasion: Sonographic-angiographic correlation. *Radiology* 1984; 150:793.
29. Stark DD, Bass NM, Moss AA, et al. Nuclear magnetic resonance imaging of experimentally induced liver disease. *Radiology* 1983; 148:743–751.
30. Chapman RWG, Williams G, Bydder G. Computed tomography for determining liver iron content in primary hemochromatosis. *Br Med J* 1980; 280:40.
31. Houang MTW, Skalicka A, Awzena X. Correlation between computed tomographic values and liver iron content in thalassemia major with iron overload. *Lancet* 1979; 8130:1322.
32. Stark DD, Moseley ME, Bacon BR, et al. Magnetic reso-

nance imaging and spectroscopy of hepatic iron overload. *Radiology* 1985; 154:137–142.

33. Grossman H, Ram PC, Coleman RA, et al. Hepatic ultrasonography in type I glycogen storage disease (von Gierke disease). *Radiology* 1981; 141:753.

34. Brunelle F, Tammam S, Odievre M, Chaumont P. Liver adenomas in glycogen storage disease of children: Ultrasound and angiographic study. *Pediatr Radiol* 1984; 14:94.

35. Bowerman RA, Samuels BI, Silver TM. Ultrasonographic features of hepatic adenomas in type I glycogen storage disease. *J Ultrasound Med* 1983; 2:51.

36. Janower ML, Sidel VW, Baker WH, et al. Late clinical and laboratory manifestations of Thorotrast administration in cerebral arteriography. *N Engl J Med* 1968; 279:186.

37. Suzuki S, Takizawa K, Nakajima Y, et al. CT findings in hepatic and splenic amyloidosis. *J Comput Assist Tomogr* 1986; 10:332–334.

38. Kurtz AB, Rubin CS, Cooper HS, et al. Ultrasound findings in hepatitis. *Radiology* 1980; 136:717.

39. Kuwar B, Alderson PO, Geisse G. The role of Ga-67 citrate imaging and diagnostic ultrasound in patients with suspected abdominal abscesses. *J Nucl Med* 1977; 18:534.

40. Kuligowska E, Conners SK, Shapiro JH. Liver abscess: Sonography in diagnosis and treatment. *AJR* 1982; 138:253.

41. Jones M, Kovac A, Geshner J. Acoustic shadowing by gas-producing abscesses. *South Med J* 1981; 74:247.

42. Haaga JR, Alfidi RJ, Havrilla TR, et al. CT detection and aspiration of abdominal abscesses. *Am J Roentgenol* 1977; 128:465–474.

43. Callen PW, Filly RA, Marcus FS. Ultrasonography and computed tomography in the evaluation of hepatic microabscesses in the immunosuppressed patient. *Radiology* 1980; 136:433–434.

44. Yaremchuk MJ, Kane R, Cady B. Ultrasound-guided catheter localization of intrahepatic abscesses: An aid in open surgical drainage. *Surgery* 1982; 91:482.

45. Kimura M, Tsuchiya Y, Ohto M, et al. Ultrasonically guided percutaneous drainage of solitary liver abscess: Successful treatment in four cases. *J Clin Gastroenterol* 1981; 3:61.

46. Weed TE, Merritt CRB, Bowen JC. Surgical management of multiple hepatic abscesses using ultrasonography for sequential evaluation. *South Med J* 1982; 75:1270.

47. Sukov RJ, Cohen LJ, Sample WF. Sonography of hepatic amebic abscesses. *AJR* 1980; 134:911.

48. Ralls PW, Quinn MF, Bowswell WD Jr., Colletti PM, et al. Patterns of resolution in successfully treated hepatic amebic abscess: Sonographic evaluation. *Radiology* 1983; 149:541.

49. Gooding GAW. Amebic abscess: Sonographic follow-up of persistent hepatic defects in two patients one year after successful treatment for amebiasis of the liver. *J Clin Ultrasound* 1981; 9:451.

50. Hadidi A. Sonography of hepatic echinococcal cysts. *Gastrointest Radiol* 1982; 7:349.

51. Barriga P, Cruz F, Lepe V, Lathrop R. An ultrasonographically solid tumor-like appearance of echinococcal cysts in the liver. *J Ultrasound Med* 1983; 2:123.

52. Fataar S, Bassiony H, Satyanath S. Characteristic sonographic features of schistosomal periportal fibrosis. *AJR* 1984; 143:69–71.

53. Fataar S, Bassiony H, Satyanath, et al. CT of hepatic *Schistosomiasis mansoni*. *AJR* 1985; 145:63–66.

54. Ho B, Cooperberg PL, Li DKB, et al. Ultrasonography and computed tomography of hepatic candidiasis in immunosuppressed patients. *J Ultrasound Med* 1982; 1:157.

55. Andrew WK, Thomas RG, Gollach BL. Miliary tuberculosis of the liver-another cause of the "bright liver" on ultrasound examination. *S Afr Med J* 1982; 62:808–809.

56. Garel L, Pariente DM, Nezelop C, et al. Liver involvement in chronic granulomatous disease: The role of ultrasound in diagnosis and treatment. *Radiology* 1984; 153:117.

57. Gosink BB. Intrahepatic gas: Differential diagnosis. *AJR* 1981; 137:763.

58. Taylor KJW, Viscomi GN. Ultrasound diagnosis of cystic disease of the liver. *J Clin Gastroenterol* 1980; 2:197.

59. Stark DD, Moss AA, Goldberg HI. Nuclear magnetic resonance of the liver, spleen, and pancreas. *Cardiovasc Intervent Radiol* 1986; 8:329–341.

60. Kuni CC, Johnson ML, Holmes JH. Polycystic liver disease. *J Clin Ultrasound* 1978; 6:332.

61. Onodera H, Ohta K, Oikawa M, et al. Correlation of the real-time ultrasonographic appearance of hepatic hemangiomas with angiography. *J Clin Ultrasound* 1983; 11:421.

62. Mirk P, Rubaltelli L, Bazzocchi M, et al. Ultrasonographic patterns in hepatic hemangiomas. *J Clin Ultrasound* 1982; 10:373.

63. Taboury J, Porcel A, Tubiana J-M, Monnier J-P. Cavernous hemangiomas of the liver studied by ultrasound: Enhancement posterior to a hyperechoic mass as a sign of hypervascularity. *Radiology* 1983; 149:781.

64. Bree RL, Schuab RE, Neiman HL. Solitary echogenic spot in the liver: Is it diagnostic of a hemangioma? *AJR* 1983; 140:41.

65. Freeny PC, Vimont TR, Barnett DC. Cavernous hemangioma of the liver: Ultrasonography, arteriography, and computed tomography. *Radiology* 1979; 132:143.

66. Itai Y, Ohtomo K, Araki T, et al. Computed tomography and sonography of cavernous hemangiomas of the liver. *AJR* 1983; 141:315.

67. Rabinowitz SA, McKusick KA, Strauss HW. ^{99m}Tc red blood cell scintigraphy in evaluating focal liver lesions. *AJR* 1984; 143:63–68.

68. Stark DD, Felder RC, Wittenberg J, et al. Magnetic resonance imaging of cavernous hemangioma of the liver: Tissue-specific characterization. *AJR* 1985; 145:213–222.

69. Itai Y, Ohtomo K, Furui S. Noninvasive diagnosis of small cavernous hemangioma of the liver: Advantage of MRI. *AJR* 1985; 145:1195–1199.

70. Solbiati L, Livraghi T, DePra L, et al. Fine needle biopsy of hepatic hemangiomas with sonographic guidance. *AJR* 1985; 144:471–474.

71. Baum JK, Holtz F, Bookstein JJ, et al. Possible association between benign hepatomas and oral contraceptives. *Lancet* 1973; 2:926–929.

72. Mays E, Christopherson WM, Mahr MM, et al. Hepatic changes in young women ingesting contraceptive steroids: Hepatic hemorrhage and primary hepatic tumors. *JAMA* 1976; 235:730–732.

73. Sandler MA, Petrocelli RD, Marks DS, Lopez R. Ultrasonic features and radionuclide correlation in liver cell adenoma and focal nodular hyperplasia. *Radiology* 1980; 135:393.

74. Casarella WJ, Knowles DM, Wolff M, et al. Focal nodular hyperplasia and liver cell adenoma: Radiologic and pathologic differentiation. *Am J Roentgenol* 1978; 131:393–402.

75. Rogers JV, Mack LA, Freeny PC, Johnson ML, Sones PJ.

Hepatic focal nodular hyperplasia: Angiography, CT, sonography and scintigraphy. *AJR* 1981; 137:983–990.

76. Scataridge JC, Fishman EK, Sanders RC. The sonographic "scar sign" in focal nodular hyperplasia of the liver. *J Ultrasound Med* 1982; 1:275.

77. Butch RJ, Stark DD, Malt RA. MR imaging of hepatic focal nodular hyperplasia (case report). *J Comput Assist Tomogr* 1986; 10:874–877.

78. Stanley J, Vujic I, Schabel SI, et al. Evaluation of biliary cystadenoma and cystadenocarcinoma. *GI Radiol* 1983; 8:245–248.

79. Kamin PD, Bernardino ME, Green G. Ultrasound manifestations of hepatocellular carcinoma. *Radiology* 1979; 131:459.

80. Cheu J-C, Sung J-L, Chen D-S, et al. Ultrasonography of small hepatic tumors using high resolution linear-array real-time instruments. *Radiology* 1984; 150:797.

81. Kuntslinger F, Federle MP, Moss AA, et al. Computed tomography of hepatocellular carcinoma. *AJR* 1980; 134: 431–437.

82. Vigo M, De Faweri D, Biondetti PR Jr, et al. CT demonstration of portal and superior mesenteric vein thrombosis in hepatocellular carcinoma. *J Comput Assist Tomogr* 1980; 4:627–629.

83. Harter LP, Gross BH, Hilaire JS, et al. CT and sonographic appearance of hepatic vein obstruction. *AJR* 1982; 139:176–178.

84. Okuda K, Obato H, Jinnonchi S, et al. Angiographic assessment of gross anatomy of hepatocellular carcinoma: Comparison of celiac angiograms and pathology in 100 cases. *Radiology* 1977; 123:21–29.

85. Brocerick TW, Gosink B, Menuck L, et al. Echographic and radionuclide detection of hepatoma. *Radiology* 1980; 135:149.

86. Machan L, Muller NL, Cooperberg PL. Sonographic diagnosis of Klatskin tumors. *AJR* 1986; 147:509–512.

87. Subramanyam BR, Raghavendra BN, Balthazar EJ, et al. Ultrasonic features of cholangiocarcinoma. *J Ultrasound Med* 1984; 3:405–408.

88. Walter JF, Bookstein JJ, Bouffard EV. Newer angiographic observations in cholangiocarcinoma. *Radiology* 1976; 118:19–23.

89. Legge DA, Carlson HC. Cholangiographic appearance of primary carcinoma of the bile ducts. *Radiology* 1972; 102: 259–266.

90. Miller JH. The ultrasonographic appearance of cystic hepatoblastoma. *Radiology* 1981; 138:141.

91. Green B, Bree RL, Goldstein HM, Stanley C. Gray scale ultrasound evaluation of hepatic neoplasms: Patterns and correlations. *Radiology* 1977; 124:203.

92. Bruneton JN, Ladree D, Caramella E, et al. Ultrasonographic study of calcified liver metastases. *Gastrointest Radiol* 1982; 7:61.

93. Rubaltelli L, Del Mashio A, Candiana F, Miotto D. The role of vascularization in the formation of echographic patterns of hepatic metastases: Microangiographic and echographic study. *Br J Radiol* 1980; 53:1166.

94. Ginaldi S, Bernardino ME, Jing BS, Green B. Ultrasonographic patterns of hepatic lymphoma. *Radiology* 1980; 136:427.

95. Federle MP, Filly RA, Moss AA. Cystic hepatic neoplasms: Complementary roles of CT and sonography. *AJR* 1981; 136:345.

96. Stephens DH, Sheedy PF II, Hattery RR, et al. Computed tomography of the liver. *Am J Roentgenol* 1977; 128:579–590.

97. Burgener FA, Hamlin DJ. Contrast enhancement of focal hepatic lesions on CT: Effect of size and histology. *AJR* 1983; 140:297–301.

98. Bernardino ME, Erwin BC, Steinberg HV, et al. Delayed hepatic CT scanning: Increased confidence and improved detection of hepatic metastases. *Radiology* 1986; 159:71.

99. Gozzetti G, Mazziotti A, Bolondi L, et al. Intraoperative ultrasonography in surgery for liver tumors. *Surgery* 1986; 99:523–530.

100. Laing F, Brooke J, Federle M, Cello J. Noninvasive imaging of unusual regenerating nodules in the cirrhotic liver. *Gastrointest Radiol* 1982; 7:245–249.

101. Scott WW, Sanders RC, Siegelman SS. Irregular fatty infiltration of the liver: Diagnostic dilemmas. *AJR* 1980; 135:67.

102. Gilday DL, Alderson PO. Scintigraphic evaluation of liver and spleen injury. *Semin Nucl Med* 1974; 4:357–370.

103. VanSonnenberg E, Simeone JF, Mueller PR, et al. Sonographic appearance of hematomas in the liver, spleen, and kidney; a clinical, pathologic, and animal study. *Radiology* 1983; 147:507.

104. Federle MP, Goldberg HI, Kaiser JA, et al. Evaluation of abdominal trauma by computed tomography. *Radiology* 1981; 138:637.

105. Ruben BE, Katzen BT. Selective hepatic artery embolization to control massive hepatic hemorrhage after trauma. *Am J Roentgenol* 1977; 129:253–256.

106. Kane RA. Ultrasonographic anatomy of the liver and biliary tree. *Semin Ultrasound* 1980; 1:87–95.

107. Mueller PR, Ferrucci JT Jr, Simeone JF, et al. Postcholecystectomy bile duct dilatation: Myth or reality? *AJR* 1981; 136:355–358.

108. Hopman WPM, Rosenbusch G, Jansen JBMJ, et al. Gallbladder contraction: Effects of fatty meals and cholecystokinin. *Radiology* 1985; 157:37–39.

109. Conrad MR, Landay MJ, Janes JO. Sonographic "parallel channel" sign of biliary tree enlargement in mild to moderate obstructive jaundice. *Am J Roentgenol* 1978; 130: 279–286.

110. Laing FC, London LA, Filly BA, Filly RA. Ultrasonographic identification of dilated intrahepatic bile ducts and their differentiation from portal venous structures. *JCU* 1978; 6:90–94.

111. Muhletaler CA, Gerlock AJ Jr, Fleischer AC, et al. Diagnosis of obstructive jaundice with nondilated bile ducts. *AJR* 1980; 134:1149–1152.

112. Cronan JJ, Mueller PR, Simeone JF, et al. Prospective diagnosis of choledocholithiasis. *Radiology* 1983; 146:467–469.

113. Carroll BA, Oppenheimer DA. Sclerosing cholangitis: Sonographic demonstration of bile duct wall thickening. *AJR* 1982; 139:1016–1018.

114. Geisse G, Melson GL, Tedesco FJ, et al. Stenosing lesions of the biliary tree: Evaluation with endoscopic retrograde cholangiography and percutaneous transhepatic cholangiography. *Am J Roentgenol* 1975; 123:378–385.

115. Ralls PW, Colletti PM, Quinn MF, et al. Sonography in recurrent Oriental pyogenic cholangitis. *AJR* 1981; 136: 1010–1012.

116. Federle MP, Cello JP, Laing FC, Jeffrey RB Jr. Recurrent pyogenic cholangitis in Asian immigrants. *Radiology* 1983; 146:753–754.

117. Cerri GC, Leite GJ, Simoes JB, et al. Ultrasonographic evaluation of ascaris in the biliary tract. *Radiology* 1983; 146:753–754.

118. Mittelstaedt CA, Volberg FM, Fischer GJ, et al. Caroli's disease: Sonographic findings. *AJR* 1980; 134:585.

119. Markle BM, Potter BM, Majd M. The jaundiced infant and child. *Semin Ultrasound* 1980; 1:123.
120. Kangarloo H, Sarti DA, Sample WF, et al. Ultrasonographic spectrum of choledochal cysts in children. *Pediatr Radiol* 1980; 9:15.
121. Yeh H-C. Ultrasonography and computed tomography of carcinoma of the gallbladder. *Radiology* 1979; 133:167.
122. Stark DD, Wittenberg J, Butch RJ, Ferrucci JT Jr. Hepatic metastases: Randomized, controlled comparison of detection with MR imaging and CT. *Radiology* 1987; 165:399.

Editorial Comment

This chapter covers an enormous amount of ground in terms of description and evaluation of the various techniques available to the radiologist for evaluation of liver disease. Although Dr. Kane's particular expertise among subspecialties of radiology lies in the field of ultrasound imaging, his interests have led him into close collaboration with the Department of Surgery in the preliminary evaluation of clinical problems, and in the operating room, where his use of intraoperative ultrasonic imaging has been invaluable to the surgeons.

Because of this interest in the liver, his review and assessment of the technology is of particular value to the surgeon. As more sophisticated technology has been brought to bear in the broad field referred to as radiology, it has been somewhat discouraging that very little has been replaced. Certainly, one rarely utilizes the Graham-Cole test any longer, but almost any other form of imaging of the liver and biliary tract still has a very specific utility and cannot be discarded as a possible adjunct evaluation.

Thus, the surgeon must develop his own expertise and experience in this particular technical field, and this review and assessment by Dr. Kane certainly provides an excellent mechanism for the education of all of us who are interested in surgery of the liver.

Chapter 11
Endoscopy and Laparoscopy in Liver Disease

HARRY ANASTOPOULOS
Z. MYRON FALCHUK

Endoscopy

Endoscopy plays a vital role in the evaluation of gastrointestinal tract diseases, as well as in the evaluation of potential complications of liver disease. The introduction of the flexible endoscopy by Hirschowitz et al. (1) allowed greater direct visualization of the intestinal tract than previously afforded by rigid endoscopes.

The utility of esophagogastroduodenoscopy is well established. This procedure is indispensable in the diagnosis of peptic esophagitis, peptic ulcerations, and upper tract malignancies, which can be missed or misinterpreted by radiologic contrast studies (2,3). In fact, endoscopy detects 95% of all lesions, in contrast to radiologic studies, which can miss up to 30% of lesions.

Endoscopy plays a helpful, if not essential role in the management of upper gastrointestinal (UGI) hemorrhage. Shallow lesions missed by routine contrast studies—such as erosive gastritis, Mallory-Weiss tears, or angiodysplasia—can be easily identified by direct endoscopic visualization. The endoscopic demonstration of a "visible vessel" in an ulcer crater is associated with a high risk of rebleeding. The use of techniques such as bipolar coagulation or Nd : Yag laser therapy allows those patients (greater than 85%) to be managed without surgical intervention.

Prompt recognition of a bleeding source in a patient with liver disease can be lifesaving. Studies done in the period 1976–1980 have shown that variceal hemorrhage accounts for only one-third to one-half of UGI hemorrhage in cirrhotic patients with varices. Gastritis and ulcer disease need to be strongly considered as potential sources (4–6). The treatment of varices is radically different from that of gastritis and ulcer disease. Prompt endoscopic

diagnosis confirming varices is mandatory so as to initiate appropriate therapy. The various medical modalities available to control variceal hemorrhage include vasopressin infusion, balloon tamponade, or emergency sclerotherapy.

Sclerotherapy techniques vary as to the type of sclerosant used (sodium morrhuate, thrombin, Keflin) and to the site of injection (paravariceal versus intravariceal), but the basic concept is the same. The injection of a sclerosant into or around a varix produces thrombosis and obliteration of the vessel, preventing or stopping bleeding. The long-term outcome of this approach is determined by the underlying liver disease.

ERCP

Endoscopic retrograde cholangiopancreatography is a unique diagnostic test that may also have therapeutic applications. The procedure has come a long way since Rabinov and Simon first cannulated the ampulla of Vater in 1965 (7).

The technique utilizes a lateral viewing endoscope through which numerous working accessories can be manipulated, for example, a cannulating catheter, papillotome, stone-retrieving basket, cytolology brush, nasobiliary catheter, and recently a peroral choledochoscope, allowing direct visualization of the biliary tree.

ERCP provides information leading to a vast diagnostic spectrum that combines details gained from routine endoscopy with subsequent evaluation of the biliary and pancreatic ductular systems. These include cytologic brushing, fluid sampling, and culture of pancreatic/biliary fluid. The procedure is an accepted diagnostic tool that helps distinguish intra- from extrahepatic cholestasis, especially in cases where choledocholithiasis, sclerosing cholangitis, ductular neoplasms, or extrahepatic neoplasms are suspected. The technique not only assists in the clinical diagnosis, but also delineates what surgical procedure should be performed in those instances where the problem requires an exploration. In a prospective study of 104 patients, the results of ERCP in jaundiced patients were compared with the final pathologic diagnosis established by surgery, liver biopsy, or autopsy. The overall sensitivity of ERCP was .99 and the specificity was .90, showing the reliability of this test (8).

The technique requires the use of routine endoscopic preparation, and the usual premedications such as meperidine and diazepam are used for sedation. 0.2 to 1 milligram of glucagon is administered intravenously to decrease duodenal activity, since a contracting duodenum makes cannulation of the ampulla of Vater very difficult. Once the ampulla is identified, the duodenoscope is positioned so that it lies approximately 90 degrees to the opening of the ampulla. After careful examination of the papilla, the radiopaque cannula is slowly advanced, either perpendicularly into the pancreatic duct or in the cephalad direction into the distal common bile duct. A 30% renografin solution is injected slowly by manual pressure. Fluoroscopy is used to demonstrate filling of the desired ducts and appropriate roentographic exposures are then made. In expert hands the procedure requires 15 to 30 minutes, and can be performed on an ambulatory basis (Figs. 11.1 to 11.4).

Successful cannulation occurs in 60% to 98% of the cases (9), and is directly related to the skill of the operator. A competent investigator can overcome such hazards as difficult catheter-duct alignment, the presence of separate ductular orifices, poorly controlled duodenal activity, and duodenal distortions secondary to previous surgery. One also needs to take into account the added difficulties in cases where duodenal diverticuli or pancreas divisum are present.

Complications include those inherent to endoscopy itself, that is, drug reactions, esophageal perforation, and those peculiar to ERCP. Asymptomatic amylase elevations have been documented in up to 70% of patients. Those values tend to return to normal in 3 to 5 days (10). Amylase levels of 2000 to 3000 IU/L are not uncommon and are probably the result of ampullary spasm or swelling after manipulation by the catheter. Clinically evi-

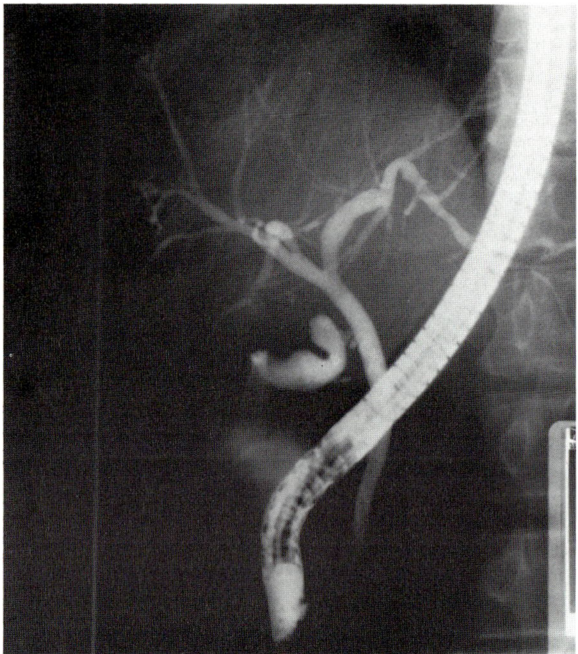

Figure 11.1. This diagnostic ERCP radiograph demonstrates normal anatomic findings. A smooth, 4- to 5-mm common bile duct leads into the typically spiral cystic duct and a partially filled gallbladder. The bifurcation is without irregularities and the intrahepatic ducts taper normally.

dent acute pancreatitis occurs in 1% to 7.4% of patients (11,12). The pathogenesis of the pancreatitis is not fully understood but appears to be related to the amount and rate of contrast injection. Care should be taken not to inject contrast with such pressure as to opacify the small intrapancreatic ductules, since this may result in damage to those structures and subsequent pancreatitis. Cholangitis is reported in less than 1% of patients and usually occurs in patients with an obstructed ductular system (13,14). This complication is minimized by pre- and postprocedure antibiotic administration, and if necessary, ductular decompression, either endoscopically (papillotomy, stent placement, nasobiliary catheter) or surgically (preferably within 24 to 36 hours).

Endoscopic Approach to Biliary Calculi

ERCP has its merits as more than just a diagnostic procedure. The introduction in 1974 of endoscopic papillotomy and common bile duct stone extraction has established a new standard for the management of isolated choledocholithiasis.

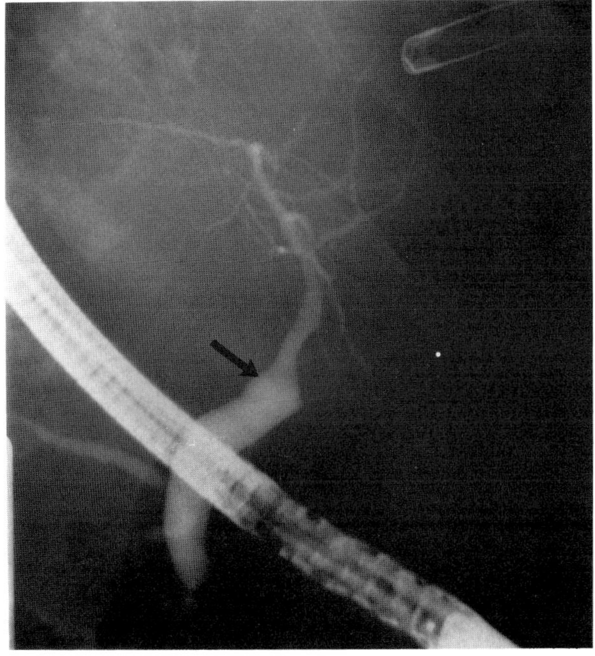

Figure 11.2. Fifty-two-year-old Hispanic woman with a past history of chronic active hepatitis complicated by cirrhosis, massive ascites, and recurrent variceal bleeds; the patient underwent a successful orthotopic liver transplant. In the subsequent 4 months after transplant, the patient's bilirubin slowly increased to 30 mg/dl. A diagnostic ERCP was performed to rule out obstruction. The ERCP radiograph shows a patent ductular system. The *arrow* points to the area of the anastomosis, with the patient's larger common bile duct being attached to the donor's slender duct. Serial liver biopsies showed the increased bilirubin to be secondary to chronic rejection.

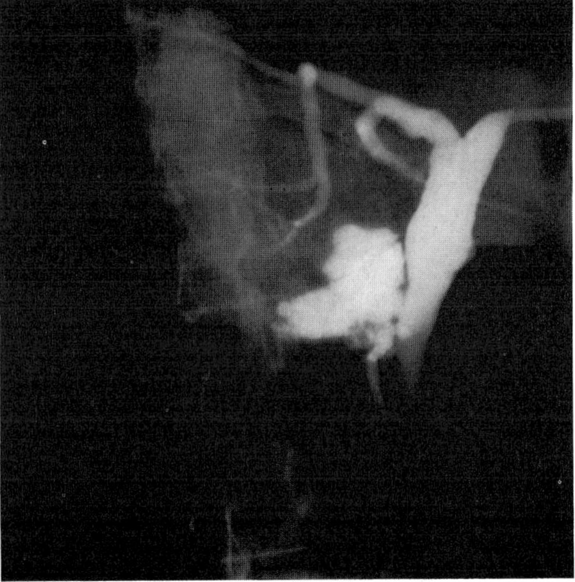

Figure 11.3. This ERCP radiograph, done in the evaluation of a 39-year-old man with a past history of ethanol abuse, demonstrates a normal common bile duct and communication of the pancreatic duct with a moderate-sized pseudocyst. The pseudocyst was followed by serial ultrasound examinations and regressed over a period of 7 weeks.

The technique requires the use of a papillotome, which is a catheter equipped with a specialized electric cauterizing/cutting tip. The technique accomplishes the mucosal transection of the sphincter of oddi and in effect creates a permanent biliary-enteric fistula that in theory (and usually in practice) allows free flow of bile and passage of any stones.

A papillotomy is difficult when the ampulla is located in a large duodenal diverticulum, is aberrant due to pancreas divisum, or is hard to access due to anatomic rearrangements after gastric surgery. These conditions are not contraindications, but do require experience and patience on the part of the operator to successfully accomplish the papillotomy.

Most stones less than 1 centimeter in diameter pass spontaneously within a day to weeks of the procedure (Figs. 11.5 and 11.6). Patients undergoing papillotomy should be hospitalized, since complications including bleeding and pancreatitis are more common than in ordinary ERCP procedures.

Active extraction of stones in the bile duct is accomplished by means of a balloon tip catheter, but more often a Dormier basket is needed. The balloon catheter is used on stones less than 1 cm in size. The catheter is inserted beyond the stone, inflated and then retracted—usually with the stone preceding it. The major drawback of balloon instruments is their fragility. This has prompted the development of devices (e.g., the Dormier basket) that under radiographic control are used to engage and (if necessary) fragment the stone in the common bile duct (Fig. 11.7). Active extraction becomes difficult in large, tortuous ducts, as well as in small ducts where the stone fills the lumen, and in cases of occlusive narrowing below the calculus. When stones are found to be embedded in the duct wall, attempts at fragmentation are warranted, but excessive manipulation is unwise since complications of infection, obstruction, and cholangitis are common in this setting.

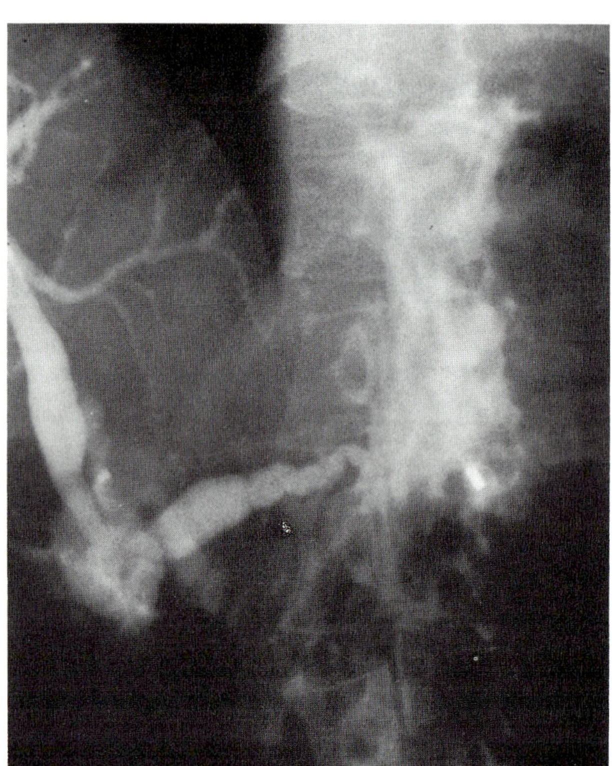

A

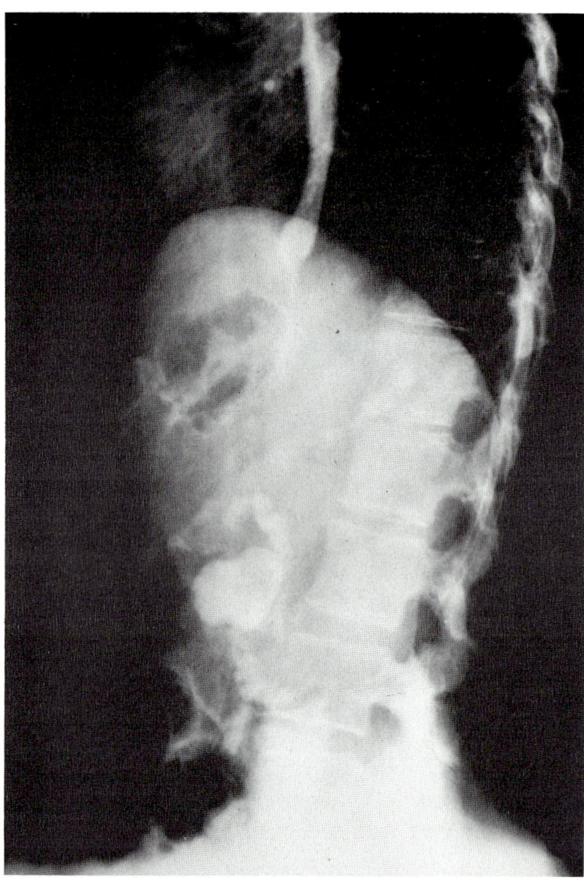

B

Figure 11.4.   This patient, a 59-year-old woman with a long history of ethanol abuse, was admitted with nausea, vomiting, epigastric pain, and a left pleural effusion. Serum amylase was 600 IU/L. Thoracentesis fluid produced an amylase of over 4000. The ERCP radiograph shows a dilated, irregular pancreatic duct consistent with chronic pancreatitis (A). There is extrasavation of contrast indicative of a pancreaticopleural fistula. This feature is well demonstrated on the lateral chest film (B). (Courtesy of Douglas Pleskow, MD.)

Indications for endoscopic papillotomy vary, but mainly this procedure is employed in the following:

1. Residual or recurrent common duct stones, especially in the elderly, regardless of their surgical risk
2. Common duct stones in high-surgical-risk patients who have an intact gallbladder

Calculi with a diameter of 2.5 cm or larger pose a technical problem, but extraction is not contraindicated. Attempts at removing large stones have a lower success rate, but are approachable using "crushing" baskets and catheter-directed dissolution techniques (Fig. 11.8). Chemodissolution using mono-octanoin is time-consuming and of limited effectiveness, but can be helpful in the management of intrahepatic stone disease (as in Caroli's disease).

Contact ultrasonic dissolution techniques require apposition of the stone and ultrasound tip to be effective. This relatively new modality is still undergoing clinical testing to see if it will have any major usefulness. Extracorporeal shock wave lithotripsy appears favorable in common duct stone management but sometimes requires papillotomy to allow large fragments of stones to pass. There-

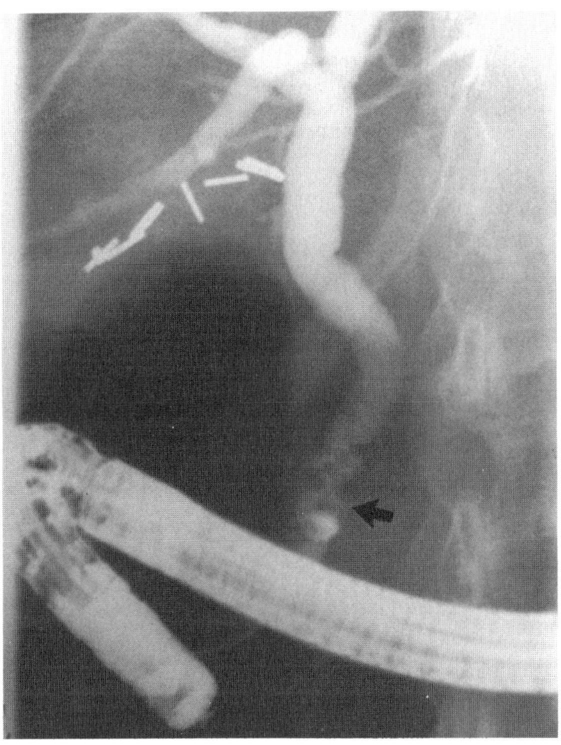

Figure 11.5. Thirty-four-year-old woman with recurrent abdominal pain. She had undergone a cholecystectomy 3 years earlier without complications. Evaluation with ultrasound showed a mildly diluted common duct without evidence of gallstones. The radiograph demonstrates multiple, faceted common duct calculi. The patient underwent an endoscopic sphincterotomy with passage of all common duct stones.

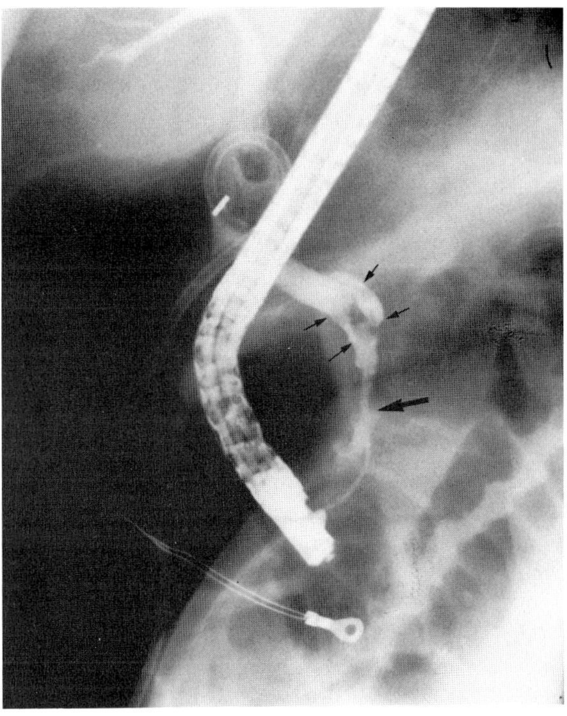

Figure 11.6. ERCP was performed in a 67-year-old man with fever and jaundice. The radiograph demonstrates several common duct stones (*small arrows*) impacted above a distal common duct stricture (*large arrow*). A papillotomy was performed, and subsequently balloon dilation of the stricture allowed passage of the calculi.

fore, lithotripsy is likely to be limited to situations of difficult stone extraction. Extensive trials of this technology are presently underway.

The contraindications to all the above stone removal techniques include a coagulopathy, a long stricture of the distal bile duct, and abnormalities of the proximal bile duct. It should also be recognized that unanticipated hemorrhage may follow papillotomy and require surgery to control the bleeding.

Success rates are relatively consistent in the literature—with papillotomy being achieved in approximately 95% of attempts and subsequent stone passage/retrieval in approximately 90% (15–21). The complication rates are as consistent. Early complications include hemorrhage, pancreatitis, cholangitis, and retroperitoneal perforation, and can occur in 8% to 10% of patients. Urgent surgery

is indicated in 1% to 2% of these, with a subsequent mortality of approximately 1% (15–22).

At this point there are few follow-up studies. A symptom recurrence rate of approximately 10% is reported. Two studies by Vallon and Cotton followed 148 patients after papillotomy and stone removal over a period of 1 to 7 years. Approximately 8% of their patients developed serious biliary problems (stenosis with and without recurrent calculi, or simply recurrent calculi alone) (22,23).

Neoptolemos studied 59 elderly patients (mean age 78) with intact gallbladders following successful papillotomy for common bile duct calculi. The patients were followed for 4 to 50 months (mean 17 months) and only 2 of the 53 patients who had undergone successful extraction required a subsequent cholecystectomy (24).

It is evident that an endoscopic approach to stone removal will play a vital role in the future—

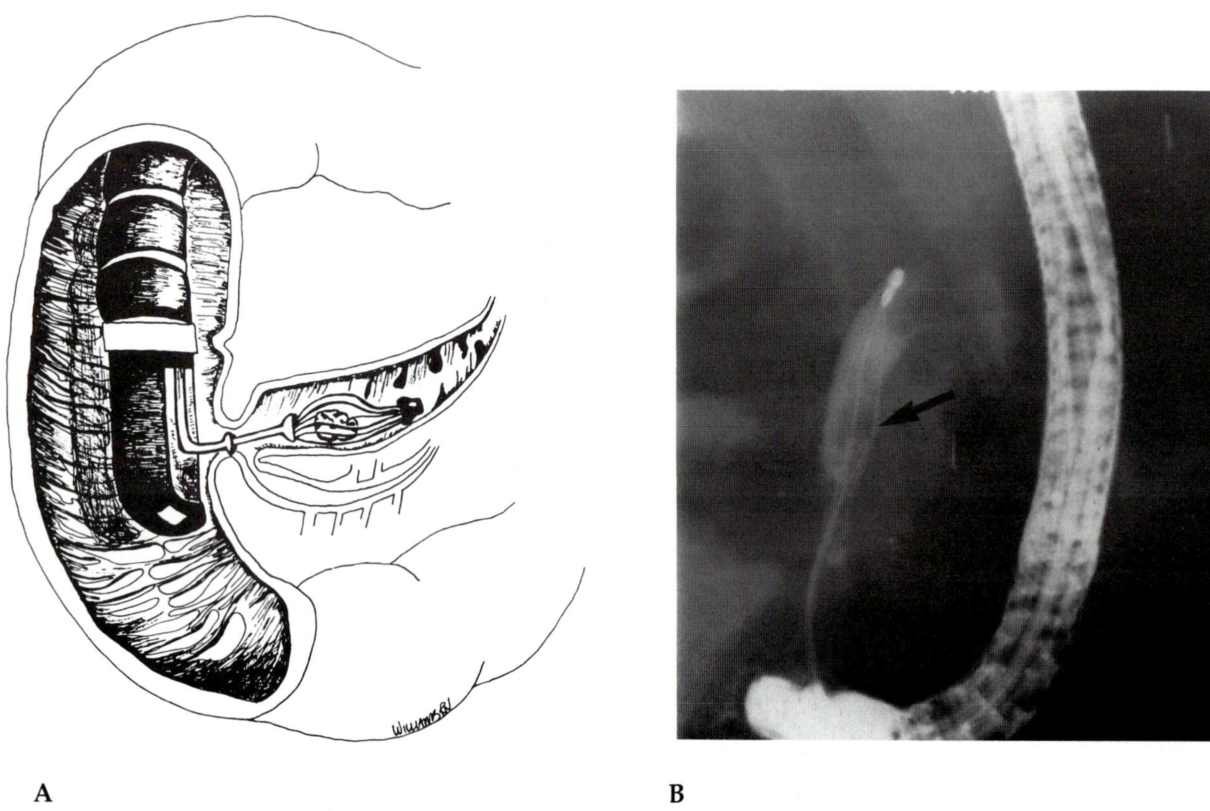

A   **B**

Figure 11.7.   Endoscopic extraction of a common duct stone with a Dormier basket (A). Prior to the extraction, a papillotomy is performed, producing a 6- to 9-mm incision through the inferior sphincter. The accompanying radiograph (B) illustrates cannulation of the duct postsphincterotomy with subsequent basket extraction of a 5-mm common duct stone (*arrow*).

especially in the aged patient with concurrent health problems that make surgery difficult or impossible. The role that the technique will play in relatively healthy, young patients remains to be fully defined, since surgical or other approaches to common duct stones or strictures are still major arms of the therapeutic armamentarium.

Prostheses

With the advent of ERCP and all the technologic advances in the instrumentation, the endoscopic insertion of a biliary prosthesis became possible. The singular indication for use of this device is to establish patency of the biliary tree to allow drainage of bile. In the majority of cases the procedure is mainly palliative, especially in the treatment of advanced pancreatic or ductular malignancy.

The devices—straight or mono/bipigtail catheters—are inserted using a large-channel, side-viewing endoscope. An initial ERCP is performed to define the biliary anatomy and to obtain appropriate brushing and biopsy specimens. There is disagreement whether an initial papillotomy is necessary, but it may facilitate the placement of larger-diameter stents and possibly prevent pancreatic duct occlusion secondary to the prosthetic stent.

Briefly, the technique requires an initial ERCP with subsequent guidance of a Teflon-coated wire across the stenotic area. A flexible catheter is then threaded over the wire past the obstruction, in order to obtain an accurate assessment of the structure. After removing the catheter, the appropriate prosthesis is fed down the guide wire by means of a "pushing" tube. The prosthetic stent is placed in the correct position under fluoroscopic guidance, with the duodenal end of the prosthesis projecting 1 to 2 cm intraluminally. The wire, "pushing" tube, and endoscope are then removed, allowing fluid to drain freely.

The procedure may be very difficult, even for an

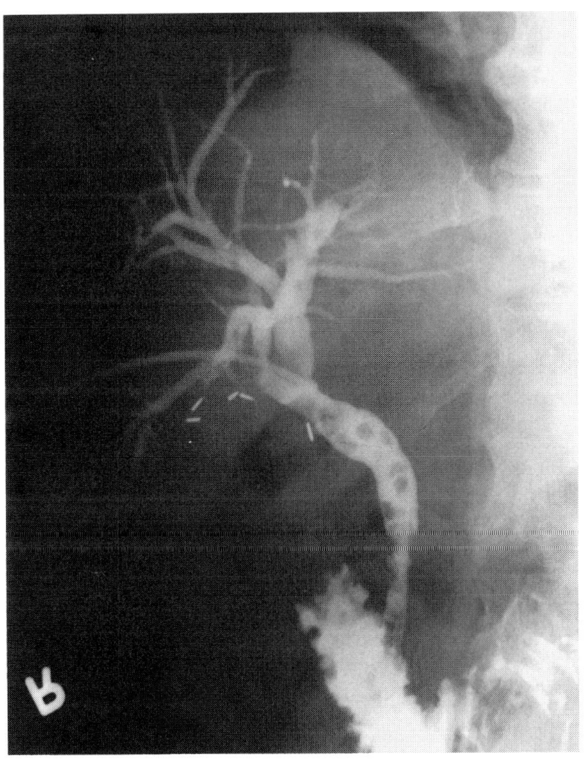

A

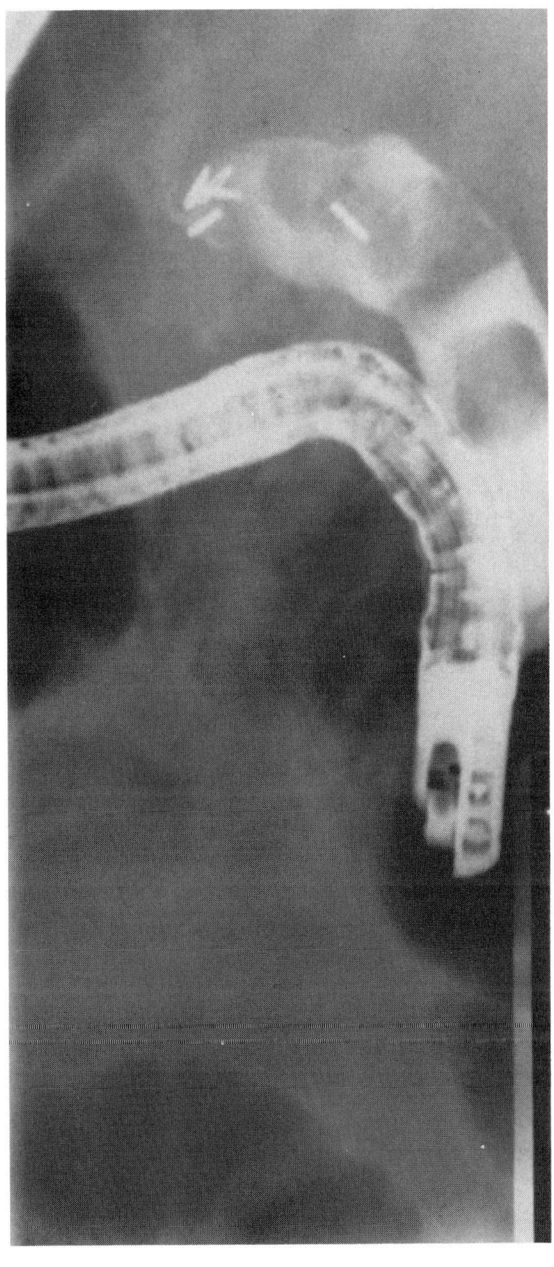

B

Figure 11.8. Seventy-eight-year-old man with jaundice and cholangitis. The patient had undergone cholecystectomy 10 years before. Radiograph (A) demonstrates a dilated common bile duct filled with stones up to 1.3 cm in diameter. A papillotomy was performed. Because the stones did not pass, a transhepatic catheter was placed and mono-octonoate was infused. Radiograph (B) demonstrates the transhepatic catheter in the common bile duct. The duct was cleared of calculi in 4 days.

experienced operator. Difficulties may arise from the initial papillotomy, or in the passage attempt of the prosthetic stent through a scirrhous malignancy. It is often necessary to dilate with a balloon-tipped catheter prior to stent placement. Certain lesions can be impossible to bypass, especially those that are tortuous or multiangulated, and thus may require a transhepatic or surgical drainage system. The special cases of duodenal diverticular disease and prior Billroth II surgery present additional technical problems in this situation as in ordinary ERCP.

To interpret results and outcomes, one needs to remember the nature of the disease being treated, usually obstructive/invasive pancreatic, gallbladder, or ductular carcinomas—diseases with survival rates usually less than 1 year.

Huibregtse has compiled a large series of over 1250 patients with ductular obstruction treated with endoscopic prostheses. In a consecutive series of 221 patients treated with endoscopic stenting, Huibregtse quoted an overall success rate of 90%, with the disappearance of jaundice in 80% (25). The mortality was 10% within 30 days, but two-thirds of these deaths were not directly related to complications of the procedure. Siegel reported similar success rates (89%) and no procedure-related deaths in his series of 227 patients (26).

Complications usually involve clogging of the prosthesis, either from clot or biliary sludge. In this event, there is a high incidence of cholangitis and recurrence of obstructive symptoms (up to 30% with small-caliber stents) (27).

Endoscopic stenting appears justified in certain clinical situations. It offers reasonable palliation with low morbidity and short hospital stays for selected patients with advanced obstructive and clearly demonstrated unresectable malignancies.

However, a relatively fit patient with a localized lesion should be treated surgically for a possible curative resection or longer-term palliation.

Laparoscopy

Laparoscopy is a technique that attempts to bridge the gap between clinical evaluation and open laparotomy. Its use in this country is not as broad as that in Europe or Japan, and has declined significantly with the advent of more sophisticated radiologic techniques, such as ultrasound or computed tomography (CT)-guided needle biopsy.

The procedure is relatively safe, and in experienced hands carries a diagnostic accuracy of over 84% (28). The indications for the procedure in liver disease are varied and include the following:

1. examination of the surface of the liver, and direct biopsy, if not contraindicated by bleeding problems
2. direct visualization of the gallbladder, especially in cases of suspected gallbladder neoplasm
3. peritoneal biopsy
4. differential diagnosis of ascites, whether secondary to the liver, peritoneum, female genitalia, or pancreas

The technique requires a direct cut down to the peritoneum through a locally anesthetized site, usually periumbilical. A limited examination can be performed under local anesthesia. However, for a more general examination of the peritoneal cavity, general anesthesia is necessary. An intra-abdominal dome of carbon dioxide is established using a Verres needle, to facilitate more room to maneuver and to provide better visualization. The Verres needle used for carbon dioxide insufflation has a blunt, spring-loaded tip, which protrudes beyond a sharp bevel. On entering the peritoneal space, the blunt end is advanced, preventing damage to adjacent viscera. Carbon dioxide is insufflated prior to advancing the laparoscope trocar. The scope is introduced and the examination can be performed with or without a secondarily placed manipulating probe.

Guided liver biopsies deserve special mention. Although CT-guided needle aspiration and biopsy have become the standard for most lesions, biopsy under direct visualization through the laparoscope is useful in assessing lesions not detected by CT scan (usually less than 1 cm). Many tumor metastases have similar densities as liver parenchyma and may not be visualized.

Laparoscopy is especially useful in the diagnosis of cirrhosis. A study by Pagliaro et al. (29) compared percutaneous biopsies to those obtained by laparoscopy, in patients with diffuse chronic liver disease. They found that percutaneous biopsy gave inconclusive results up to 20% of the time, while laparoscopic biopsies were 100% accurate in demonstrating the presence or absence of cirrhosis. Although they did not advocate the routine use of laparoscopic biopsies, they felt that in the evaluation of chronic liver disease without varices (varices have a high predictive value for portal hypertension and cirrhosis), laparoscopy should be the procedure of choice.

In the mid-1980s, laparoscopy has been used to stage gastric cancer. Possik et al. (30) employed laparoscopy to evaluate 360 patients with gastric cancer. They were able to discern serosal infiltration, lymph node metastases, peritoneal dissemination, and liver metastases, with a high confidence level equal to or better than that of ultrasonography or scintigraphy.

Laparoscopic evaluation is limited to direct visualization of the anteriormost portion of the abdominal viscera. Using a probe placed through a separate trocar stab wound, the omentum and bowel can be moved to allow better visualization. Palpation of the pancreas and liver is possible using the probe. Lysis of adhesions, directed tissue biopsies, and cauterization of bleeding sites can also be performed safely via the laparoscope.

References

1. Hirschowitz BI, Curtis IE, Peters CW, Pollard HM. Demonstration of a new gastroscope—the "fiberscope." *Gastroenterology* 1958; 35:50–53.
2. Keto P, Suoranta H, Ihamaki T, Melartin E. Double contrast examination of the stomach compared with endoscopy. *Acta Radiol Diagn* 1979; 5:762–768.
3. Thoeni RF, Cello JP. A critical look at the accuracy of endoscopy and double-contrast radiography of the upper gastrointestinal tract in patients with substantial UGI hemorrhage. *Radiology* 1980; 135:305–308.
4. Reynolds, TB. Interrelationships of portal pressure, variceal size, and upper gastrointestinal bleeding. *Gastroenterology* 1980; 79:1332–1333.
5. Pitcher J. Variceal hemorrhage among patients with varices and upper gastrointestinal hemorrhage. *Sout Med Journal* 1977; 70:1183–1185.
6. Novis BH, Days P, Barbezat GO, et al. Fiberoptic endoscopy and the use of Sengstaken tube in acute gastrointestinal hemorrhage in patients with portal hypertension and varices. *Gut* 1976; 17:258–263.
7. Rabinov KR, Simon M. Peroral cannulation of ampulla of Vater for direct cholangiography and pancreatography. *Radiology* 1965; 85:693–697.
8. Martzen P, Haubek A, Holst-Christensen J, Lejerstoffe J, et al. Accuracy of direct cholangiography by endoscopic or transhepatic route in jaundice—a prospective study. *Gastroenterology* 1981; 81:237–241.
9. Siegel JH. ERCP update: Diagnostic and therapeutic applications. *Gastroenterology* 1978; 3:311–318.
10. Blackwood WD, Vennes JA, Silvis SE. Post-endoscopy pancreatitis and hyperamylasemia. *Gastrointest Endosc* 1973; 20:56–58.
11. Nebel OT, Silvis SE, Rogers G, Sugawa C, et al. Complications associated with endoscopic retrograde cholangiopancreatography—results of the 1974 A.S.G.E. survey. *Gastrointest Endosc* 1975; 22:34–36.
12. Bilbao MK, Dotter CT, Lee TG, et al. Complications of endoscopic retrograde cholangiopancreatography—a study of 10,000 cases. *Gastroenterology* 1976; 70:314–320.
13. Martin TR, Greenen J, Raskin JB, Vennes JA, et al. The reduction of septic complications following endoscopic retrograde cholangiopancreatography in obstructed patients (abstr). *Gastrointest Endosc* 1979; 25:43.
14. Vennes JA. Infectious complications of gastrointestinal endoscopy. *Dig Dis Sci* 1981; 26:60–64.
15. Geenen JE, Vennes JA, Silvis SE. Résumé of a seminar on endoscopic retrograde sphincterotomy. *Gastrointest Endosc* 1981; 27:31–38.
16. Classen M. Endoscopic papillotomy—new indications, short- and long-term results. *Clin Gastroenterol* 1986; 15:457–469.
17. Safrany L, Cotton PB. Endoscopic management of choledocholithiasis. *Surg Clin North Am* 1982; 62:825–836.
18. Siegel JH. Endoscopic papillotomy in the treatment of biliary tract disease—258 procedures and results. *Dig Dis Sci* 1981; 26:1057–1064.
19. Safrany L. Endoscopic treatment of biliary tract disease. *Lancet* 1978; 2:983–985.
20. Cotton PB. Non-operative removal of bile duct stones by duodenoscopic sphincterotomy. *Br J Surg* 1980; 67:1–5.
21. Frakes JT. An evaluation of performance after informal training in endoscopic retrograde sphincterotomy. *Am J Gastroenterol* 1986; 81:92–105.
22. Cotton PB. Endoscopic management of bile duct stones (apples and oranges). *Gut* 1984; 25:587–597.
23. Vallon AG, Cotton PB. Clinical and endoscopic followup after *duodenoscopic sphincterotomy* (abstr). *Gut* 1982; 22:A889.
24. Neoptolemos JP, et al. The management of common bile duct calculi by endoscopic sphincterotomy in patients with gallbladders in situ. *Br J Surg* 1984; 71:69–71.
25. Huibregtse K, et al. Endoscopic palliative treatment in pancreatic cancer. *Gastrointest Endosc* 1986; 32:334–338.
26. Siegel JH, Snady H. The significance of endoscopically placed prostheses in the management of biliary obstruction due to carcinoma of the pancreas: Results of nonoperative decompression in 277 patients. *Am J Gastroenterol* 1986; 21:634–641.
27. Tytgat GNJ, et al. Endoscopic palliative therapy of gastrointestinal and biliary tumours with prostheses. *Clin Gastroenterol* 1986; 15:249–271.
28. Reynolds TB, Cowan RE. Peritoneoscopy. In: Wright R, Millward-Sadler GH, Alberti KGMM, Karran S, eds. *Liver and Biliary Disease*. Philadelphia: WB Saunders, 1985, pp. 633–646.
29. Pagliaro L, Rinaldi F, Craxi A, DiPiazza S, et al. Percutaneous blind biopsy versus laparoscopy with guided biopsy in the diagnosis of cirrhosis. *Dig Dis Sci* 1983; 28:39–43.
30. Possik RA, Franco EL, Pires DR, Wolthrath DR, et al. Sensitivity, specificity, and predictive value of laparoscopy for the staging of gastric cancer and for the detection of liver metastases. *Cancer* 1986; 58:1–6.

Editorial Comment

This chapter gives us a succinct but complete description of the utilization of endoscopic techniques in visualizing the gastrointestinal, biliary, and pancreatic ductal tract. Some of the descriptions extend to a point beyond the strict limitations of liver disease alone but for completeness and thoroughness, it would have been very difficult to eliminate some sections that relate only peripherally to disease of the liver itself.

The chapter also has an imposed limitation inasmuch as a previous chapter by Terblanche has gone into great detail on the use of sclerotherapy in the control of bleeding esophageal varices secondary to portal hypertension. In a way, one should read these chapters together. But one is concerned with endoscopy and laparoscopy primarily as a diagnostic modality, whereas the chapter on endoscopic sclerosing techniques is concerned directly with therapy and in that sense fits in closer to the pharmacological and surgical methods of controlling massive hemorrhage from varices.

Any comments by the editor on endoscopic techniques and treatment can be found at the close of Terblanche's chapter, 13B.

PART IV
Surgical Disorders and Techniques

Chapter 12
Portal Hypertension

Chapter 12A
Portal Hypertension: Background and General Evaluation

ARTHUR J. DONOVAN

1877–1945—Eck to Whipple

The last quarter of the nineteenth century witnessed the introduction of general anesthesia and the establishment of the principles of aseptic surgery. These developments created an environment permissive for the performance of elective surgery. In the burgeoning of surgery that ensued, innovative surgeons devised surgical techniques that they applied in the treatment of the complications of portal hypertension. These complications were hematemesis and ascites, and the efforts to treat portal hypertension have been previously reviewed (1,2).

By the turn of the century a remarkable understanding of the pathophysiology of portal hypertension existed. Banti in 1894 had emphasized what he believed to be vascular congestion as the cause of congestive splenomegaly (3). Others recognized the role of cirrhosis and obstruction to portal flow as a factor in development of ascites and as a cause of variceal hemorrhage. Indeed, in 1900, Preble reviewed 60 reported cases of esophageal varices, and discussed portal venous obstruction, collateral flow, and the role of spontaneous portal venous to systemic venous shunting in decompression of the portal circulation (4). Pick in 1909 introduced the concept of "hepatopetale" and "hepatofugale" flow (5). The principal intent of surgical endeavors was to decompress the portal system. Concern was directed more toward control of ascites then to the prevention of recurrent hematemesis.

A consideration of the role of surgery in the treatment of portal hypertension must begin with the experimental work of Nicholas V. Eck, a Russian surgeon. In 1877, he reported that he had anastomosed the portal vein to the vena cava of eight dogs (6). The portal vein was ligated on the hepatic side of the anastomosis, completely diverting portal blood into the vena cava. Only one of the eight dogs survived for greater than 1 week; that dog ran away at the end of $2\frac{1}{2}$ months. Despite these meager results, Eck had proven that portal blood could be diverted into the systemic venous system with survival of the animal. He suggested that it might be possible to treat some cases of "mechanical ascites" by such a fistula. Pavlov utilized the fistula in numerous studies of hepatic physiology and identified the fact that an Eck's fistula could result in a syndrome of meat intoxication (7).

The first major surgical procedure developed for the treatment of portal hypertension was omentopexy. This operation was designed to increase collateral portasystemic flow and to decompress the portal venous system. In 1896, Drummond and Morrison, an internist and a surgeon, respectively, described this procedure for treatment of ascites (8). The abdomen was entered, the parietal peritoneum scarified, and the omentum sutured to the parietal peritoneum in an attempt to stimulate collateral flow. The operation had actually been performed in 1889 by Talma, a German surgeon, but was not reported until 1898 (9). Omentopexy was an indirect form of portal systemic shunting and became known as the Talma-Drummond-Morrison operation.

Interest soon evolved in the feasibility of the direct method for decompression of the portal system by an anastomosis between the portal and systemic venous system as reported by Eck. The techniques of vascular anastomosis that had been developed by Carrell were an additional impetus in this direction (10).

The first direct anastomosis of the portal vein to the inferior vena cava for the treatment of portal hypertension was undoubtedly that performed by Vidal of Perigueux in 1903 (11). His report is included in a paper on the surgical treatment of ascites. He possessed a remarkable understanding of the pathophysiology of portal hypertension. In his discussion of "hypertension" in the "portale" circulation, Vidal expressed confusion as to why portal hypertension led to ascites. He pointed out that sphlancnic capillaries were in the submucosa and not the subserosa; diarrhea should result from venous obstruction. Vidal divided the portal vein in dogs and perfused the sphlancnic end with saline at a pressure of 30 centimeters. Fluid leaked into the enteric lumen rather than from the serosa. Vidal's selection of a pressure of 30 cm certainly suggests knowledge of portal pressures. He was convinced that portal systemic shunting had far more efficacy in the treatment of hematemesis from ruptured esophageal varices than of ascites. Hematemesis was, in his opinion, the more serious manifestation of portal hypertension. His surgical goal was reduction of pressure in the portal venous system; the standard operation was omentopexy.

The first direct portacaval shunt was performed by Vidal in a woman with recurrent hemorrhage whom he had scheduled for an omentopexy. The omentum was not suitable for this procedure and he performed an end-to-side portacaval shunt. This was accomplished in 45 minutes using Carrell's technique of vascular anastomosis. The patient recovered and did not have recurrence of hemorrhage. When fed protein, she developed a syndrome that he described as characteristic of "intoxication" with "ammoniacal substances which are toxic for the organism when the liver is no longer there to guard against this danger and transform them into urea and other waste products." He discovered that restriction of intake of protein would control this syndrome. The patient died several weeks later of an "intoxication" that he believed was the consequence of total portal diversion. Thus, Vidal established the feasibility of direct portacaval shunt in the human, observed that hemorrhage did not recur and that a syndrome of protein intolerance ensued, controlled by protein restriction. This one case encompasses two

subsequent dominant themes concerning portacaval anastomosis for treatment of portal hypertension—therapeutic efficacy in control of bleeding and the provocation of hepatic dysfunction.

Cases of direct portacaval shunts were reported sporadically during the next 25 years (2). A side-to-side anastomosis of the portal vein to the vena cava was established by Rosenstein in 1913 (12). This was intended to assure continued portal perfusion of the liver, a laudable goal not attainable by this procedure.

These early efforts at direct and indirect portal diversion were performed without firm criteria for selection of cases, without clear understanding of the role of hepatic functional impairment in morbidity and mortality, and usually for ascites. The endeavors were not successful. The incidence of recurrent ascites was high after omentopexy (13). The collective mortality for direct portacaval shunt was at least 50% (2). By the 1930s treatment of portal hypertension by either direct or indirect means of portal systemic shunting had been largely abandoned.

Interest in either ligation of the varices or reduction of flow into the varices as a method of treatment of portal hypertension arose early. In a report on splenic surgery in 1910, Mayo discussed splenectomy in the treatment of complications of cirrhosis of the liver (14). Although considerable interest in this approach persisted at the Mayo Clinic, this enthusiasm was not widely shared. Rowntree from the Mayo Clinic, in 1929, reported ligation of the coronary vein for variceal hemorrhage (15) and McIndoe, in 1933, suggested direct injection of paraesophageal veins with sclerosing agents (16). Transesophageal sclerotherapy was first reported by Crafoord and Frenckner in 1939 (17). None of these techniques were widely adopted. By the early 1940s, efforts at surgical treatment of portal hypertension had largely ceased. All of the interventional techniques currently used in the treatment of portal hypertension had been introduced—direct portal systemic shunts, vascular ligations to reduce flow into the varices, and sclerotherapy.

Interest in the surgical treatment of portal hypertension was reawakened in 1945 by Dr. Allen O. Whipple of the Columbia University College of Physicians and Surgeons and Presbyterian Hospital in New York. His report was entitled "The problems of portal hypertension in relation to hepatosplenopathies" (18). The work represented the collaborative efforts of surgeons, internists, and pathologists in the Spleen Clinic at the Presbyterian Hospital. Dr. Whipple was disillusioned with splenectomy and with indirect attempts such as omentopexy to control bleeding due to portal hypertension. He reemphasized the importance of obstruction to portal flow as the cause of portal hypertension. Whipple and associates, including Dr. William Blakemore, resorted to direct portacaval shunt. Initially, a vitallium prosthesis developed by Dr. Blakemore was used to create the end-to-side anastomosis between the portal vein and vena cava (19). Other prominent surgeons had also become interested in the surgical treatment of portal hypertension. Dr. Alfred Blalock of the Johns Hopkins Hospital preferred a direct suture technique for end-to-side portacaval shunt (20). Dr. Robert Linton of the Massachusetts General Hospital in Boston chose to perform a central splenorenal shunt (21).

Dr. Whipple emphasized strongly the importance of hepatic function as a predictor of survival. In 1945, the same year as Dr. Whipple's report, Ratnoff and Patek had published their classic article on the natural history of cirrhosis of the liver (22). This report clearly identified the importance of levels of hepatic function, hemorrhage, and ascites on survival. Portacaval shunt was performed by Dr. Whipple following hemorrhage from varices. He recognized that some cases of ascites might not recur following a portacaval shunt. The fact that a patent portacaval shunt was remarkably effective in preventing recurrent variceal hemorrhage became immediately apparent.

These early efforts of Whipple, Blalock, and Linton immediately established that the portacaval shunt could be performed in selected cases with a low operative mortality. A patent shunt was essentially synonymous with prevention of recurrent variceal hemorrhage. The long-term consequences of the operation remained to be determined. World War II had just concluded. Surgeons of a new generation were embarking on careers in academic surgery. Several accepted the challenge of further elucidation of our understanding of portal hypertension and of the role of surgery in its treatment. Among these was Dr. Charles Gardner Child III (Fig. 12A.1). His endeavors in this field over the ensuing 25 years illustrate the types of laboratory studies that were conducted, the clinical

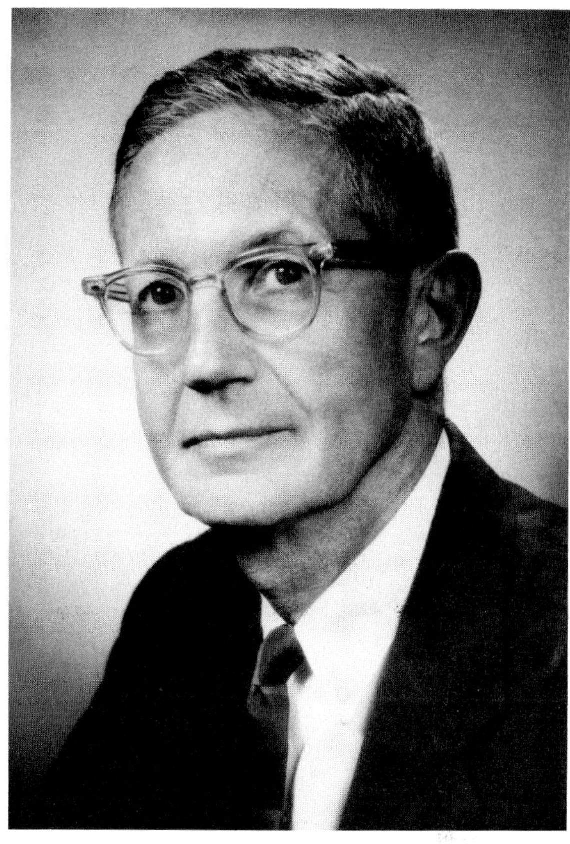

Figure 12A.1   Charles G. Child III, M.D., a member of the Faculty at Cornell University Medical College (1943–1953), Tufts University School of Medicine (1953–1958), the University of Michigan (1959–1978), and Emory University (1978–). Dr. Child was Professor and Chairman of the Department of Surgery at Tufts University and at the University of Michigan.

concerns that evolved, and some of the conclusions that were reached.

1945–1975—Charles G. Child III

Gardner Child graduated from Yale College in 1930 and from the Cornell University Medical College in 1934. He received his graduate education in surgery at the New York Hospital-Cornell Medical Center under Dr. George Heuer and completed the residency in 1942. Following service in the United States Navy, he joined the faculty at Cornell and embarked on a professional lifetime devoted to the study of the hepatic circulation, the liver, and portal hypertension. During the first 10 years, he was at Cornell and engaged in a series of laboratory and clinical investigations. These culminated in the publication in 1953 of a scholarly monograph, *The Hepatic Circulation and Portal Hypertension* (23).

Dr. Child recognized that the portal circulation of the dog differed markedly from that of the human, stating "I also felt that there might be some virtue in studying an animal with anatomical relationships more closely correlated with those of man than are those of the dog. I chose, therefore, as my experimental animal the Macaca Mulatta monkey" (23). Ligation of the portal vein in the dog was recognized to be invariably fatal. Hemorrhagic infarction of the gastrointestinal tract developed. Ligation of the hepatic artery led to death due to septic necrosis of the liver. The liver of the dog is teeming with virulent organisms; the liver of humans is sterile. The liver and portal circulation of the monkey more closely resembles in all respects those of man than the dog. Child demonstrated that either the portal vein or hepatic artery of the monkey could be ligated and that the animal would survive (23–25). The portal vein was ligated in a number of patients with carcinoma of the pancreas (25). The patients developed transient portal hypertension and survived.

Studies of the effect of blood flow on hepatic regeneration were conducted utilizing a technique for portacaval transposition. In this latter operation the portal vein and infrahepatic vena cava were divided. Portal blood was diverted into the cephalic end of the divided infrahepatic vena cava. Caval blood from the lower extremities was diverted into the hepatic end of the divided portal vein. End-to-end vascular anastomoses were performed. Child reported that regeneration of the liver following subsequent hepatic resection was dependent on volume of flow (26).

Subsequent experimental studies were conducted in Boston where Dr. Child was Professor and Chairman of the Department of Surgery at Tufts University from 1953 to 1958, and in Ann Arbor, Michigan, where he was Professor and Chairman of the Department of Surgery from 1958 to 1974. The hepatic circulation was reversed by a complex technique depicted in Figure 12A.2 (27). The vena cava was divided between the liver and the right atrium. A graft was placed between the side of the portal vein and the atrial end of the divided vena cava. The hepatic side of the suprahepatic cava was ligated. Thus, caval blood from below the diaphragm perfused the liver in a retro-grade fashion through the hepatic veins. The animals survived. Chronic ascites were produced by suprahepatic constriction of the vena cava and techniques for control of ascites such as ileoentrectopy (28), studied. These studies recognized the important role of hepatic venous outflow obstruction in the genesis of ascites. The effect of arterialization of the portal circulation on hepatic regeneration was investigated (29). The above are but some examples of the many areas of investigation into which Child's fertile imagination led him and his colleagues.

Dr. Child was a skilled clinician and a consummate technical surgeon. He had an intense interest in all of the clinical aspects of the treatment of portal hypertension. By the mid-1950s, he had recognized that portacaval shunt was effective in controlling variceal hemorrhage but that encephalopathy and deterioration of hepatic function occurred postoperatively in an unpredictable fashion (30). McDermott had, in 1954, refocused attention to the problem of the episodic stupor that might follow the portacaval shunt (31).

Surgery was usually performed electively after an episode of hemorrhage from varices and of subsequent evaluation of hepatic function. Thus, patients submitted to a shunt were self-selected. They had survived the hemorrhage and their physician believed that they had sufficient hepatic reserve to survive a major operation. Dr. Child emphasized that such selected patients should not be compared with a population that had bled but not been selected for operation. He became convinced that the alternatives of portacaval shunt and nonsurgical treatment should be compared in a randomized study of a group of patients, all of whom were equally suitable for a shunt (30).

Few institutions alone would accumulate sufficient clinical experience to answer this and other questions concerning the natural history and treatment of portal hypertension. Dr. Child, therefore, in 1957 organized the Boston Inter-Hospital Liver Group (BILGE). This group consisted of representatives from the Boston City Hospital, the Lemuel Shattuck Hospital, the Massachusetts General Hospital, the New England Medical Center, the Peter Bent Brigham Hospital, and the University Hospital (Boston University). All three medical schools in Boston were involved. The members, in addition to Dr. Child (Tufts), were Dr. Allan Callow (Tufts), Dr. Thomas Chalmers (Tufts), Dr.

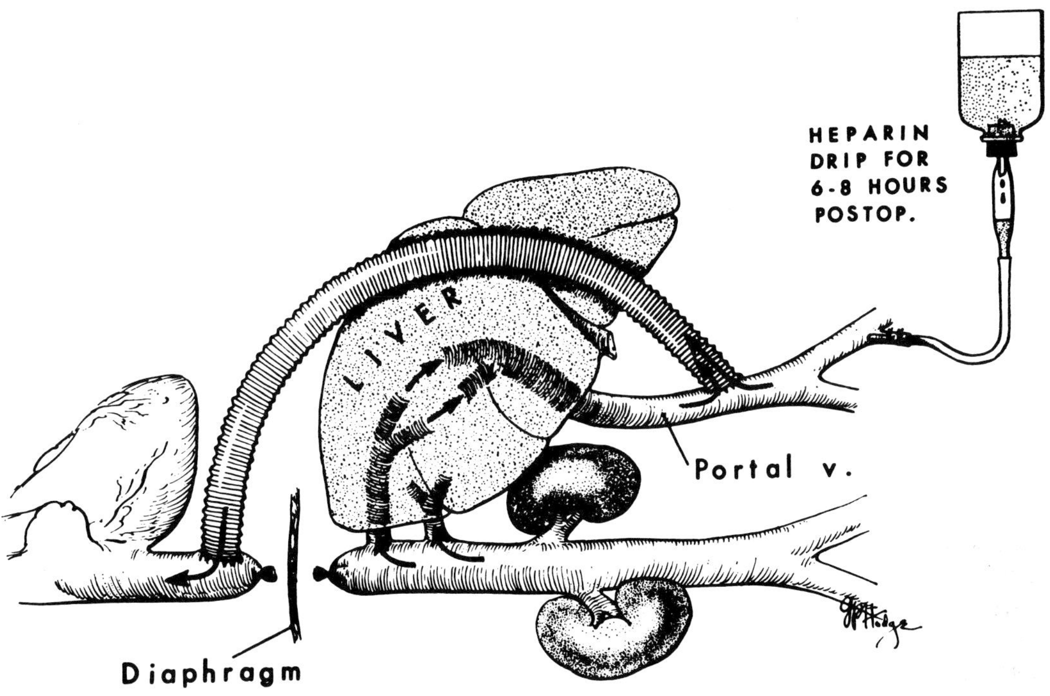

Figure 12A.2 Child's original technique of reversal of hepatic venous circulation in dogs, using crimped Teflon tubing: Animals survived up to 50 days. (Reproduced by permission from Child CG III, McDonough EF Jr., DesRochers GC. Reversal of hepatic venous circulation in dogs. *Ann Surg* 1959; 150:445–453.)

Chilton Crane (Harvard), Dr. Charles Davidson (Harvard), Dr. Franz Inglefinger (Boston University), and Dr. William McDermott (Harvard). The present author was Dr. Child's associate at Tufts and was the initial secretary of BILGE. There was immediate discussion of a randomized trial of therapeutic portacaval shunts. This was the era of infancy for randomized clinical trials. BILGE was in the forefront of those recognizing their importance in contrast to retrospective reviews with historical controls. The conviction of one institution as to the established therapeutic efficacy of the portacaval shunt precluded a study of the therapeutic portacaval shunt as the initial clinical trial. A clinical trial of the prophylactic portacaval shunt was conducted (32).

The study of the prophylactic shunt involved patients with a diagnosis of portal hypertension in whom varices were documented but in whom bleeding had not occurred. A therapeutic benefit for a prophylactic shunt was not established.

When Dr. Child moved to Michigan, BILGE continued its cooperative multi-institutional pro-

spective trials under the leadership of Dr. Thomas Chalmers. A classic study of the efficacy of the therapeutic portacaval shunt was ultimately performed (33). This revealed that although the shunt was highly effective in the prevention of variceal hemorrhage, survival was not altered. Patients who were shunted experienced an early mortality from perioperative complications and a later one from progressive hepatic decompensation that together were comparable to the mortality in control subjects who had not been subjected to a portacaval shunt. Their deaths were largely due to recurrents hemorrhage. Randomized studies by the Veterans Administration (34) and at the University of Southern California (35) arrived at essentially the same conclusion. If these studies are combined, there is a slight advantage for the surgical group. Some patients in the control group in all studies have been subjected to surgery because of recurrent episodes of hemorrhage from varices and have survived.

Child's interest in those factors that influenced mortality following portacaval shunt led him to

Table 12A.1. Clinical and Laboratory Classification of Patients with Cirrhosis in Terms of Hepatic Functional Reserve

Group Designation	"A" Minimal	"B" Moderate	"C" Advanced
Serum bilirubin[a] (mg%)	Below 2.0	2.0–3.0	Over 3.0
Serum albumin (g%)	Over 3.5	3.0–3.5	Under 3.0
Ascites	None	Easily controlled	Poorly controlled
Neurologic disorder	None	Minimal	Advanced, "coma"
Nutrition	Excellent	Good	Poor, "wasting"

[a] Equivocal in biliary cirrhosis.
Reproduced by permission from Child CG III: *The Liver and Portal Hypertension*, Vol. 1. Philadelphia: WB Saunders, 1964, p. 50.

focus increasingly on identification of criteria that might be applied in a prospective fashion to predict early operative survival. He adopted a scheme for classification of patients based on preoperative evaluation and which divided patients into A, B, and C categories. This is known as the Child's classification. Table 12A.1 is reproduced from his second monograph, entitled *The Liver and Portal Hypertension* (36), published in 1964. Child's classification considers the levels of serum bilirubin and serum albumin, the presence of ascites and its control, the presence or absence of neurologic symptoms, and the patient's nutrition. Mortality, as reported in his monograph, was directly correlated with this classification (Table 12A.2). Child's classification has been universally adopted. Reports of its validity as a predictor of postoperative mortality have been repeatedly published. Unfortunately, it does not accurately predict which patients will develop postshunt encephalopathy and slow deterioration of hepatic function, a still unresolved problem. Patients who are classified as Child's group A or B may in an apparently random fashion manifest deterioration of hepatic function following a shunt. Although the small contracted

Table 12A.2. Postoperative Mortality in Terms of Hepatic Function Among 128 Patients with Cirrhosis of the Liver Undergoing End-to-Side Portal Decompression

Group	No. Patients	Mortality
A (minimal impairment)	48	0.0%
B (moderate impairment)	46	9.0%
C (advanced impairment)	34	53.0%
	128	17.0%
A and B combined	94	4.3%

Reproduced by permission from Child CG III: *The Liver and Portal Hypertension*, Vol. 1. Philadelphia: WB Saunders, 1964, p. 51.

liver, alcoholic rather than postnecrotic cirrhosis, and hepatofugal rather than hepatopetal flow in the portal vein may be less favorable prognostic indicators, they are not, alone or in combination, of sufficient validity to be of firm assistance in predicting the course of the individual patient.

Two additional areas of intense discussion have been the treatment of the acute variceal hemorrhage and the selection of one or the other type of portacaval shunt. Dr. Child had an abiding interest in both subjects. He objected to the concept of an emergency shunt, preferring to consider the operation to be at the most urgent. Hemorrhage could almost always be controlled by pneumatic tamponade, the patient evaluated, and a decision made regarding surgery in the absence of the pressure associated with the acute event. Cases with significant hepatic dysfunction, often further compromised as a consequence of the episode of hemorrhage, were best served by a period of medical therapy and nutritional support prior to elective surgery. Child's category C could be converted to A or B. Acute alcoholic hepatitis with sclerosing hyaline necrosis could resolve (37). On rare occasions, pneumatic tamponade failed and recurrent hemorrhage from esophageal, or more likely from gastric, varices necessitated a true emergency shunt. The operative mortality of 42% reported by Orloff et al. for emergency shunt (38) supported Dr. Child's conservative policy. Dr. Child was not enthusiastic about direct transthoracic or transabdominal ligation of actively bleeding varices—an operation with inherent mortality that was likely to be followed by recurrent hemorrhage and the need for a portacaval shunt. He believed that the patient in whom pneumatic tamponade had failed and who was a candidate for an operation should have the definitive portacaval shunt and not a temporizing operation such as transesophageal ligation of varices.

Both in New York and Boston, Dr. Child performed the end-to-side portacaval shunt. The concept of continued portal perfusion after a side-to-side anastomosis does not withstand critical analysis, whether the anastomosis is of a direct side-to-side type or a functional side-to-side anastomosis such as the central splenorenal or mesocaval shunt. Portal blood will not perfuse the liver against a head of resistance if there is an adequate escape route through a fistula into the low-pressure caval system. Indeed, the hepatic end of the fistula in a side-to-side shunt is probably converted into an outflow tract from the liver (39). In a comparison of end-to-side and side-to-side portacaval shunt that was conducted in Michigan, Dr. Child found no benefit to the latter type of shunt in either mortality or in incidence of postoperative hepatic functional impairment (36).

Ascites as a manifestation of portal hypertension was treated by portacaval shunt in the 1950s and early 1960s. Child, as well as others, established that patients with hepatic function equivalent to a Child's A classification group, with the exception of ascites, manifested effective control of the refractory ascites after a portacaval shunt (30). Hepatic venous outflow obstruction is accepted as an important factor in the development of ascites and a side-to-side shunt to decompress both the hepatic and sphlancnic ends of the portal circulation in cases with ascites was recommended by many, including Orloff and Johansen (40). Eisenmenger and Nichols had reported (41) and Child confirmed that end-to-side portacaval shunt effectively controlled ascites in selected patients (30). By the mid 1960s the development of effective diuretics that promote sodium excretion had almost eliminated a role for surgery in the treatment of ascites.

Current Status

In the period 1975–1985, at least three interventional techniques have risen to prominence and considerable acceptance in the treatment of portal hypertension—the peritoneovenous shunt for treatment of refractory ascites, the selective distal splenorenal shunt, and sclerotherapy. Medical therapy has not been more notably successful than in the past (42).

Ruotte in 1907 utilized the saphenous vein as a conduit for ascitic fluid from the peritoneal cavity to the venous circulation (43). After establishing that the values in the saphenous vein were intact, he mobilized the proximal segment of the vein and passed it in retrograde fashion beneath the inguinal ligament and into the peritoneal cavity. A fish mouth incision was made into the cephalic end of the vein, which was then sutured to the peritoneum. The intact valves were supposed to prevent reflux of blood and to permit the passage of ascitic fluid into the venous circulation. The principle involved is identical to that of the pressure-activated valves that have now been developed for this purpose. Initially reported by Hyde and Eiseman in 1967 (44), these shunts have been further refined by LeVeen (45). A pressure-activated valve is placed subcutaneously. Connecting tubes lead into the peritoneal cavity and into the central venous system. Transfer of ascitic fluid through this shunt is almost invariably associated with a mild degree of hematologic abnormality consistent with subclinical disseminated intravascular coagulation; rarely does overt disseminated intravascular coagulation (DIC) develop. The peritoneal venous shunt is remarkably effective in control of chronic refractory ascites.

A type of portasystemic shunt that would prevent variceal hemorrhage without the risk of deterioration of hepatic function would be a major advance. W. Dean Warren of Atlanta and his associates developed the distal splenorenal shunt for this purpose (46). Patients initially selected for the operation were those with angiographically documented hepatopetale flow. The distal splenic vein is anastomosed to the side of the renal vein and the coronary vein is ligated. Varices thus drain in a retrograde fashion through the spleen, out the distal splenic vein, and into the renal vein. The operation is effective in control of variceal hemorrhage. Hemodynamic studies have documented continued perfusion of the portal system through the patent superior mesenteric vein. The effectiveness of this operation in the control of encephalopathy and in preservation of hepatic function has been independently reported by Langer and associates (47). Conn and colleagues conducted a randomized study of the distal splenorenal shunt and did not observe a benefit compared to the direct portacaval shunt (48). Further studies are necessary to establish the exact role of the distal spleno-renal shunt.

Generally, there has been disillusionment with the portacaval shunt for the treatment of portal hypertension and variceal hemorrhage. Despite control of hemorrhage, documentation of major impact on survival has not been established. Concurrently, there has been a recrudescence of interest in a direct approach to the varices, particularly by sclerotherapy. Initial efforts with splenectomy, coronary vein and other venous ligations, transesophageal ligation of varices, and sclerotherapy were abandoned because of the high incidence of recurrent hemorrhage. Sugiura in Japan has now reported an incidence of recurrent hemorrhage of less than 5% following splenectomy, periesophageal vascular ligations, and transesophageal ligation of varices (49). This experience has not been reproduced in this country, as recently emphasized by Johnson and his associates (50). Devascularization procedures in the United States are usually performed only in cases of thrombotic occlusion of the extrahepatic portal venous system, when a portasystemic shunt would not be possible and when hemorrhage is recurrent.

The renaissance of sclerotherapy owes its occurrence to the flexible fiberoptic endoscope, which has replaced the rigid esophagoscope. Repeated injections of varices with sclerosing solution can be carried out with ease and with minimal morbidity. The procedure can be performed during the acute episode of bleeding. The number of transfusions required and incidence of rebleeding are reported to be reduced in randomized studies with both acute and chronic sclerotherapy (51,52). Warren et al. have reported in 1986 a randomized trial comparing chronic sclerotherapy with the distal splenorenal shunt (53). Sclerotherapy was superior in survival, transfusion requirements, and incidence of hepatic failure. Approximately one-half of patients bleed following sclerotherapy. These patients can be subjected to a portacaval shunt. In 1985, enthusiasm for sclerotherapy is waxing and enthusiasm for the portacaval shunt is waning. Both Warren (53) and Telfer B. Reynolds (42), a distinguished hepatologist, have concluded that patients with cirrhosis who bleed from esophageal varices are best served by an initial trial of sclerotherapy, with a distal splenorenal shunt as the procedure of choice for those in whom sclerotherapy has failed, as manifested by recurrent hemorrhage.

The vast majority of patients with portal hypertension have cirrhosis of the liver. This process, once established, is not reversible by currently available therapeutic modalities. Hepatic transplantation does not yet carry an acceptably low morbidity and adequate donors are not available for its general use in the treatment of cirrhosis of the liver. An effective form of lathyrism that eliminates scar tissue has not been developed. Pharmacologic techniques that effectively reduce portal pressure have not evolved. Surgery is thus directed to the secondary effects of a grave disease for which there is not a satisfactory treatment. The physician must steer between the Scylla and Charybdis of the morbidity of complications of uncorrected portal hypertension on one side, and the deterioration of hepatic function that may occur consequent to surgical therapy on the other.

References

1. Donovan AJ, Covey PC. Early history of the portacaval shunt in humans. *Surg Gynecol Obstet* 1978; 147:423–430.
2. Donovan AJ. Surgical treatment of portal hypertension: An historical perspective. *World J Surg* 1984; 8:626–645.
3. Banti G. Splenomegaly with cirrhosis of the liver. *Sperimentale* 1894; 48:901–912.
4. Preble RB. Conclusions based on sixty cases of fatal gastrointestinal hemorrhage due to cirrhosis of the liver. *Am J Med Sci* 1900; 119:263–280.
5. Pick L. Uber totale hemangiomatose obliteration des pfortaderstammes und uber hepatopetale kolateralbahnen. *Virchows Arch Pathol Anat Physiol Klin Med* 1909; 197:490–530.
6. Eck NV. On the question of ligature of the portal vein. *Voen Med J* 1877; 130:1–2. (Translation in *Surg Gynecol Obstet* 1953; 96:375–376)
7. Hahn M, Massen M, Nencki M, Pavlov J. Die Eck'sche Fistel zwischen der unteren Hohlvene und der Pfortader und ihre Folgen fur den Organismus. *Arch Exper Pathol Pharmokol* 1893; 32:161–210.
8. Drummond D, Morison R. A case of ascites due to cirrhosis of the liver cured by operation. *Br Med J* 1896; 2: 728.
9. Talma S. Chirurgische Offnung neuer Seitenbahnen fur das Blut der Vena porta. *Berl Klin Wochenschr* 1898; 35:833–836.
10. Carrel A, Morel. Anastomose bout à bout de la jugulaire et de la carotide interne. *Lyon Med* 1902; 99:114.
11. Vidal M. Traitement chirurgical des ascites dans les cirrhoses du foie. *16th Cong Franç Chir* 1903; 16:294–304.
12. Rosenstein P. Uber die Behandlung der Lebercirrhose durch Anlegung einer Eck'schen Fistel. *Arch Klin Chir Berl* 1912; 98:1082–1092.
13. Cates HB. Surgical treatment for cirrhosis: Prognosis subsequent to omentopexy. *Arch Intern Med* 1943; 71:183–205.
14. Mayo WJ. Principles underlying surgery of the spleen with a report of ten splenectomies. *JAMA* 1910; 54:14–18.
15. Walters W, Rowntree LG, McIndoe AH. End result of the tying of the coronary vein for prevention of hemorrhage from esophageal varices. *Proc Staff Meet Mayo Clin* 1929; 4: 263–264.

16. Kegaries DL. The venous plexus of the esophagus: Its pathologic and clinical significance (Discussion by McIndoe). *Proc Staff Meet Mayo Clin* 1933; 8:160–165.

17. Crafoord C, Frenckner P. New surgical treatment of varicose veins of the esophagus. *Acta Otolaryngol* 1939; 27:422–429.

18. Whipple AO. The problem of portal hypertension in relation to hepatosplenopathies. *Ann Surg* 1945; 122:449–475.

19. Blakemore AH. Portacaval anastomosis: Report on fourteen cases. *Bull NY Acad Med* 1946; 22:254–263.

20. Blalock A. The use of shunt or by-pass operations in the treatment of certain circulatory disorders, including portal hypertension and pulmonic stenosis. *Ann Surg* 1947; 125:129–141.

21. Linton RR. Portacaval shunts in the treatment of portal hypertension with special reference to patients previously operated upon. *N Engl J Med* 1948; 238:723–727.

22. Ratnoff OD, Patek AJ Jr. The natural history of Laennec's cirrhosis of the liver. *Medicine* 1942; 21:207–268.

23. Child CG III. The Hepatic Circulation and Portal Hypertension. Philadelphia: WB Saunders, 1954.

24. Child CG III, McClure RD Jr, Hays DM. Studies on the hepatic circulation in the Macaca mulatta monkey and in man. *Surg Forum* 1951; 2:140–146.

25. Child CG III, Holswade GR, McClure RD Jr, Gore AL, O'Neill EA. Pancreaticoduodenectomy with resection of the portal vein in the Macaca mulatta monkey and in man. *Surg Gynecol Obstet* 1952; 94:31–45.

26. Child CG III, Barr D, Holswade GR, Harrison CS. Liver regeneration following portacaval transposition in dogs. *Ann Surg* 1953; 138:600–608.

27. Child CG III, McDonough EF Jr, DesRochers GC. Reversal of hepatic venous circulation in dogs. *Ann Surg* 1959; 150:445–453.

28. Wilson JT, Child CG III. Resorption of experimental ascites in the dog by ileoperitoneopexy. *Surg Forum* 1958; 9:554–557.

29. Zuidema GD, Gaisford WD, Abell MR, Brody TM, Neill SA, Child CG III. Segmental portal arterialization of canine liver. *Surgery* 1963; 53:689–698.

30. Child CG III, Donovan AJ. Current problems in management of patients with portal hypertension. *JAMA* 1957; 163:1219–1229.

31. McDermott WV Jr, Adams RD. Episodic stupor associated with an Eck fistula in the human with particular reference to the metabolism of ammonia. *J Clin Invest* 1954; 33:1–9.

32. Resnick RH, Chalmers TC, Ishihara AM, et al. A controlled study of the prophylactic portacaval shunt: A final report. *Ann Intern Med* 1969; 70:675–688.

33. Resnick RH, Iber FL, Ishihara AM, Chalmers TC, Zimmerman H, The Boston Interhospital Liver Group. A controlled study of the therapeutic portacaval shunt. *Gastroenterology* 1974; 67:843–857.

34. Jackson FC, Perrin EB, Felix WR, Smith AG. A clinical investigation of the portacaval shunt V. Survival analysis of the therapeutic operation. *Ann Surg* 1971; 174:672–701.

35. Reynolds TB, Donovan AJ, Mikkelsen WP, Redeker AG, Turrill FL, Weiner JM. Results of a 12-year randomized trial of portacaval shunt in patients with alcoholic liver disease and bleeding varices. *Gastroenterology* 1981; 80:1005–1011.

36. Child CG III. *The Liver and Portal Hypertension*. Philadelphia: WB Saunders, 1964.

37. Mikkelsen WP, Turrill FL, Kern WH. Acute hyaline necrosis of the liver: A surgical trap. *Am J Surg* 1968; 116:266–272.

38. Orloff MJ, Bell RH Jr, Hyde PV, Skivolocki WP. Long-term results of emergency portacaval shunt for bleeding esophageal varices in unselected patients with alcoholic cirrhosis. *Ann Surg* 1980; 192:325–340.

39. Britton RC, Shirey EK. Cineportography and dynamics of portal flow following shunt procedures. *Arch Surg* 1962; 84:25–33.

40. Orloff MJ, Johansen KH. Treatment of Budd-Chiari syndrome by side-to-side portacaval shunt: Experimental and clinical results. *Ann Surg* 1978; 188:494–512.

41. Eisenmenger WJ, Nickel WF. Relationship of portal hypertension to ascites in Laennec's cirrhosis. *Am J Med* 1956; 20:879–889.

42. Reynolds TB. What to do about esophageal varices (editorial). *N Engl J Med* 1983; 309:1575–1577.

43. Routte M. Abouchement de la veine saphene externe au pentouine pour resorber les epanchement siatiques. *Lyon Chir* 1907; 109:574–577.

44. Hyde GL, Eisemen B. Peritoneal atrial shunt for intractable ascites. *Arch Surg* 1967; 95:369–373.

45. LeVeen HH, Chriustoudias G, Ip M, Luft R, Falk G, Grosberg S. Peritoneovenous shunting for ascites. *Ann Surg* 1974; 180:580–591.

46. Warren WD, Zeppa R, Fomon JJ. Selective trans-splenic decompression of gastroesophageal varices distal splenorenal shunt. *Ann Surg* 1967; 166:437–455.

47. Langer B, Rotstein LE, Stone RM, et al. A prospective randomized trial of the selective distal splenorenal shunt. *Surg Gynecol Obstet* 1980; 150:45–48.

48. Conn HO, Resnick RH, Grace ND, et al. Distal splenorenal shunt vs. portal-systemic shunt: Current status of a controlled trial. *Hepatology* 1981; 1:151–160.

49. Sugiura M, Futagawa S. A new technique for treating esophageal varices. *J Thorac Cardiovasc Surg* 1973; 66:677–685.

50. Johnson G, Keagy BA. Should ablative operations be used for bleeding esophageal varices? *Ann Surg* 1986; 203:463–469.

51. Larsen AW, Cohen H, Zweiban B, et al. Acute esophageal variceal sclerotherapy: Results of a prospective randomized control trial. *JAMA* 1986; 255:497–500.

52. Korula J, Balart LA, Radvan G, et al. Perspective randomized controlled trial of chronic esophageal variceal sclerotherapy. *Hepatology* 1985; 5:584–589.

53. Warren WD, Henderson JM, Millikan WJ, Galambos JT, Brooks WS, Riepe SP. Preliminary report of a prospective randomized trial of distal splenorenal shunt versus endoscopic sclerotherapy for long-term management of variceal bleeding. *Ann Surg* 1986; 203:454–462.

Editorial Comment

Both Dr. Donovan and I were disappointed that illness prevented a major contribution to this book by Dr. Charles G. Child III, who had been a valued friend and colleague for so many years and who had made such major contributions to the field of portal hypertension.

It has been a particular pleasure for me to read this chapter and to see the prominent position that Dr. Donovan has given to his mentor and colleague. I am sure that this emphasis on the work of Dr. Child will be greeted with enthusiasm by surgeons of all ages involved in this complex and difficult area of surgical endeavor.

Chapter 12B
Hemodynamics of Portal Hypertension

JOSEF E. FISCHER

Normal Hepatic Blood Supply and Physiology

Normal Hepatic Blood Supply

Hepatic blood supply is noteworthy by its dual nature. The normal anatomic arrangement of the liver is that of single plates of hepatocytes opening directly on hepatic sinusoids and lined with Kupffer's cells—reticuloendotheliocytes. The relationship between hepatocytes and Kupffer's cells may be important in hepatic failure complicating sepsis (1).

Forty percent of the cardiac output is delivered by the hepatic artery and portal vein, entering at different levels of the hepatic sinusoid. The normal hepatic functioning unit is centered around the hepatic vein, the main effluent vessel. The portal triad—bile canaliculus, hepatic artery, and portal venule—is at the periphery. Hepatic artery blood more likely enters the sinusoid at the periphery of the hepatic lobule, giving a higher oxygen concentration at the periphery and the lowest at the central vein. Similarly, nutrient concentrations delivered by the portal venule are highest at the periphery and lowest at the central vein. Hepatocytes are in various degrees of activity, depending on blood supply and concentration of nutrients and oxygen. However, on an anatomic basis, the hepatic lobule centered around the portal triad with the central veins at the periphery is more correct. By this concept, central hepatocytes are in a higher functional state.

Portal Vein

A portal system is a venous system with two sets of capillaries separated by a vein. Only two portal systems are known: the neurohypophysis and the liver. In both, the first capillary system supplies a substance(s) useful for the function of the second structure. In the hepatic portal system, the gut supplies hormones and nutrients.

The liver, containing more than 600 enzymes, is both a synthetic and an excretory organ. Thus, in addition to clearing glucose and amino acids, and synthesizing and storing products for release following appropriate hormonal and nervous signals, the liver has degradative functions. Amines liberated by gut bacteria are degraded by liver monoamine oxidases. An example of what follows bypassing hepatic degradative function is the carcinoid syndrome in which kinins, substance P, serotonin, and perhaps prostaglandins are liberated by metastatic tumors within the liver. A controversial point in hepatic physiology is whether the liver *requires* these huge amounts of substrate to maintain normal function. Perhaps it does; chronic absence of portal flow, as in extrahepatic portal block in patients without liver disease, may result in deterioration of hepatic function and premature hepatic failure (2).

Hepatic Artery

Portal vein oxygen content is higher than other venous systems, but 50% of hepatic oxygen is supplied by the hepatic artery. Nutrients are in lower concentrations in the hepatic artery as compared with the portal vein. In classical hepatic physiology, portal vein blood is trophic: It contains nutrients and hormones from the gut or pancreas. Under some circumstances, however, increased hepatic artery flow may at least partially replace portal blood, as after end-to-side portacaval shunt, and may be associated with a better prognosis as reflected in longer survival and lower rates of severe encephalopathy (3). Similarly, inferior caval flow is better than no flow, as is seen following portacaval transposition in which caval blood perfuses the hepatic stump of the portal vein.

Portal Hypertension

Physiologic Basis of Portal Hypertension

Portal hypertension, a homeostatic mechanism, is an attempt by the liver (as it were) to maintain perfusion in the face of increased vascular resistance secondary to disordered architecture. This concept is critical when contemplating therapy of bleeding varices.

If portal hypertension is a homeostatic mechanism and the portal system does not have an intrinsic pump, the only mechanisms by which portal pressure can be increased are secondary to increased volume and/or cardiac output (increased flow), and/or abnormal connections(s) with the arterial circulation (higher pressure). Increased flow is secondary to increased plasma volume, due in turn to sodium and water retention. Whether true hepatic volume and aldosterone receptors exist is controversial, but it is universally agreed that there is decreased inactivation of antidiuretic hormone (ADH) and increased activity of the renin-angiotensin system, resulting in part in increased secretion of aldosterone. Whether decreased pulsatile perfusion contributes to the renin reflex is not clear. If present, it may be related to opening of peripheral shunts, perhaps secondary to decreased inactivation of estrogen and/or other vasodilatory substances such as substance P or vasoactive intestinal peptide, resulting in decreased pulsatile perfusion.

Shunting also results in secondary increase in cardiac output, again increasing portal perfusion. Another factor that may play a role in peripheral shunting is the loss of sympathetic tone, possibly secondary to the replacement of the normal neurotransmitter, norepinephrine, by octopamine and other false or less active neurotransmitters (4). Finally, abnormal arteriovenous connections in the splanchnic circulation expose the portal venous system to systemic arterial pressure. These shunts contribute to the "arterialization" of portal venous blood, with a higher perfusion pressure and increased oxygen content.

Regenerating Nodule—Single Blood Supply

The regenerating nodule is extremely vulnerable to hypotension and/or ischemia, because instead of the normal dual blood supply it is dependent largely on the hepatic artery. Regenerating nodules are formed by collapse of the reticulin framework following hepatocyte necrosis and increased scarring secondary to hyperplasia of collagen, surrounding each nodule by fibrous tissue. Normal perfusion anatomy is disrupted; only hepatic artery supplies the nodule. The hepatic artery is extraordinarily sensitive to sympathetic stimulation. This renders the resultant disordered hepatic architecture extremely vulnerable to hypotension or other noxious stimuli.

My clinical impression, although difficult to prove, is that a similar volume of blood loss from variceal bleeding is more damaging than that from gastritis or duodenal ulcer. This may be for two reasons:

1. The increased pressure of portal hypertension is a homeostatic mechanism for maintaining portal flow. Variceal bleeding opens a side-vent, as it were, in the portal system, decreasing portal pressure to a considerably greater extent than the corresponding decrease in intravascular volume.

2. The hepatic artery, as a splanchnic artery, is extremely sensitive to sympathetic stimulation, and responds to hypovolemia, with differentially greater vasoconstriction as compared with arteries to the brain or heart.

Thus, the patient with cirrhosis is extraordinarily vulnerable to bleeding, especially bleeding varices. Witness the mortality of 22% to 33% commonly reported for patients with variceal bleeding treated by sclerotherapy alone—a mortality merely the result of liver disease (5,6).

Types of Portal Hypertension

PRESINUSOIDAL BLOCK

Presinusoidal block is usually synonymous with "extrahepatic portal block," and also with portal vein thrombosis. In the United States, intrahepatic presinusoidal block is currently rare, but is likely to increase as people from countries afflicted with schistosomiasis immigrate. Portal vein thrombosis, usually idiopathic, may be secondary to splenectomy and/or pancreatitis. A history of omphalitis or the use of umbilical vein catheters in infancy may be obtained, but for the most part etiology is unknown.

In younger patients with bleeding esophageal varices secondary to extrahepatic portal block, hepatic function is usually well maintained, with occasional hepatic failure. However, as time goes on, "premature aging" of the liver occurs, ultimately resulting in a course indistinguishable from patients with cirrhosis. Ascites, encephalopathy, jaundice, the hepatorenal syndrome, and death occur at ages 40 or 50 (2). This is the best evidence I am aware of suggesting that the trophic nature of portal flow is necessary for maintenance of normal hepatic function.

In other countries, particularly Third World nations, portal hypertension of the intrahepatic presinusoidal block type is endemic secondary to schistosomiasis. Here again, hepatic function is well maintained so long as prograde portal flow is maintained. In the extensive literature concerning the treatment of variceal bleeding secondary to schistosomiasis, it is clear that any shunt operation for relief of portal hypertension is associated with higher late mortality from hepatic failure than other operations that maintain flow, such as devascularization.

POSTSINUSOIDAL BLOCK: STAGES OF
PORTAL HYPERTENSION

Postsinusoidal block secondary to deranged hepatic architecture is purportedly the most common type of portal hypertension in the United States, and is usually alcohol and/or hepatitis related. It is likely not purely postsinusoidal, but a mixed variety of presinusoidal and postsinusoidal scarring and deranged architectures leading to blockage at various levels of the portal bed. It is possible that pre- or postsinusoidal block dominates in different patients, and that this heterogeneity may be responsible for the difficulty in obtaining reproducible results in patient populations with portal hypertension.

Stages of portal hypertension include an early, hemodynamically insignificant phase where there may be piecemeal, perhaps bridging necrosis, collapse of the reticulum, and replacement by collagen. In most of the liver, however, normal architecture persists, with single plates of hepatic sinusoids in an orderly, lobular pattern. Retention of sodium, and either increased secretion or perhaps decreased inactivation of ADH may increase plasma volume. Corrected, wedged hepatic vein pressure does not exceed 10 centimeters of saline. Some abnormal collaterals are present, and small varices may or may not be present. The fraction of hepatic blood flow derived from the hepatic artery may be increased slightly from the normal range 20% to 35%, but not to the 50% level characteristic of patients with established cirrhosis of the liver. This suggests that portal system arteriovenous shunting is minimal.

Portal flow is prograde. If portal flow decreases suddenly, increased hepatic artery flow is capable of making up the difference, either because liver capacitance has not decreased to the extent where hepatic artery flow is fixed, or that the hepatic artery itself is capable of responding.

As cirrhosis progresses, flow becomes more "balanced" and, if at surgery a portal vein clamp is placed, pressure above the clamp ("liver side") and pressure below ("gut side") become more nearly equal. The portal vein tends to serve as an outflow tract, that is, the scarring and obstruction to outflow via the hepatic veins increase and the portal vein prograde flow diminishes. Finally, the postsinusoidal portal block becomes so severe that outflow through the central hepatic veins essentially ceases, and the portal vein is the outflow for the hepatic artery. This stage is the most advanced form of cirrhosis and represents a different physiologic state, creating an inherent bias against which some studies concerning shunts for portal hypertension must be measured. In some studies of distal splenorenal shunt, for example, patients with reverse portal flow have been excluded (7,8), thus effectively excluding the most advanced cirrhotics, a point that has escaped notice. Some other, usually total, shunt is chosen, a practice that results in a selective bias against other forms of shunt. Our own practice in doing a randomized, prospective trial comparing central and distal splenorenal shunts does not use direction of flow as a criterion for exclusion (9,10).

BUDD-CHIARI SYNDROME

When the hepatic veins, either smaller lobular veins or main hepatic veins, thrombose, the Budd-Chiari syndrome results, accompanied by pain, sudden massive ascites, fever, and toxicity. Clotting disorders, oral contraceptives, malignancy, and paroxysmal nocturnal hemoglobinuria are among causes. There are two Budd-Chiari syndromes, the first resulting from thrombosis of hepatic veins, and the second resulting from membranous valves in the inferior vena cava, the latter more common in Japan. Therapy depends on the extent of necrosis and degree of obstruction. In less severe cases, diuresis and anticoagulation may tide the patient over until recanalization.

If necrosis is substantial, some outflow must be provided, utilizing the portal vein as an outflow tract, by some form of side-to-side shunt—if the vena cava is not involved. If vena caval involvement is present, a long shunt from portal vein to right atrium is indicated. If caval membranes are present, angiographic dilatation may relieve the constriction, but may require several attempts.

Complications of Portal Hypertension

Ascites

Ascites is lymphatic fluid weeping from the surface of the liver. In ascites the degree of hepatic outflow block is very high; as a result, lymphatic drainage is increased up to 15 times normal as measured in the thoracic duct. When clearance of hepatic lymph is insufficiently rapid, lymphatics develop on the surface of the liver, which then leaks ascites, readily observed during operation on patients with tight ascites.

Ascites represent the most extreme case of fluid and water retention. Plasma volume is difficult to measure owing to the tremendous increase in extracellular fluid. It is likely near normal or possibly even increased in some patients, but in others (perhaps the majority), such as those with type I hepatorenal syndrome (see below), plasma volume seems decreased or, at least, that is how these patients react hemodynamically. Probably most of the physiologic hemodynamic behavior of patients with ascites is determined by the rapidity of the plasma volume achieving equilibrium with the ascites. In most patients, ascites is in delayed equilibrium with the plasma; it takes 24 hours for a substantial movement of fluid from the ascitic compartment to the plasma. This should be borne in mind when diuresing patients with tight ascites, as diuresis initially results in decreased plasma

volume, with decreased hepatic perfusion until the intravascular compartment refills.

Patients with stable tight, diuretic-resistant ascites are capable of prolonged survival, except for the inconvenience of tight ascites, and may respond to surgical procedures (11,12).

Variceal bleeding in a patient with tight ascites calls for a portal decompression procedure which decompresses the liver as well. While there have been occasional case reports of tight ascites being relieved by procedures that do not decompress the liver, such as end-to-side portacaval shunt (11), these are exceptions to the rule; some form of side-to-side shunt, such as a side-to-side or double-barreled portacaval, mesocaval, or central splenorenal shunt, is required. Decompressing the liver is also effective in that form of the "stable hepatorenal syndrome" (type I), which probably represents diuretic-resistant ascites in which diuretics have been pushed to the extent that plasma volume is progressively decreased and which thus results in incipient renal failure (11,12). In our current randomized, prospective trial comparing proximal and distal splenorenal shunts (9,10), patients with tight ascites have been difficult to manage following distal splenorenal shunt. Since the theoretical purpose of the distal splenorenal shunt is to compartmentalize the portal circulation into the right and left side of the portal circulation, and decompression of the liver is not achieved, it is apparent that distal splenorenal shunt is not the procedure of choice for the patient with tight ascites. Furthermore, in dissection of the renal vein it is often necessary to divide tissues that are in continuity with the cisterna chyli, at times resulting in chylous ascites (13,14).

Hepatorenal Syndrome

The true hepatorenal syndrome is usually a terminal event in hepatic failure. Throughout the years, confusion has arisen because patients with very tight postsinusoidal block have been suggested as having the hepatorenal syndrome; they usually respond to portal decompression provided the hepatic side of the portal vein is decompressed as well, thus providing outflow. Pathophysiologi-

Table 12B.1. Tentative Clinical Classification of Hepatorenal Syndrome

Characteristics	Type I	Type II
Cardiac index	Normal or decreased	Increased
Blood pressure	Normal or low	Decreased (by 5–30 mmHg)
Peripheral resistance	Normal or increased	Decreased
Intravascular volume	Low	Normal
Urinary Na	<10 mEq/L	<10 mEq/L
A-VO$_2$ difference	Normal	Decreased
Associated findings	Intractable ascites	Hepatic encephalopathy
	IVC-RA gradient	Acute hepatic insult
	High hepatic vein wedge pressure	
Pathophysiology	Effective hypovolemia	Maldistribution
	Portorenal reflex	
Diagnostic maneuver	Volume infusion	Tyramine-NE infusion
Therapy	Volume infusion	α-Adrenergic agents
	Ascites reinfusion	L-Dopa
	Peritoneoatrial shunt	
	Portal decompression	

Abbreviations: IVC-RA, inferior vena cava-right atrium; mEq/L, milliequivalents per liter; mmHg, millimeters of mercury; NE, norepinephrine; other abbreviations as in text.
Reproduced by permission from Fischer JE, Bower RH. Amino acids in liver disease. *In*: Epstein M, ed. *The Kidney in Liver Disease.* New York: Elsevier, 1982, p. 525.

cally, decreased renal perfusion is the result of hypovolemia and responds to volume. Hepatic function is stable. Cardiac index is normal or decreased, blood pressure normal or low, and peripheral vascular resistance is increased. The arteriovenous oxygen (A-VO$_2$) difference is normal. The clinical picture is hypovolemia rather than high-output vasodilation, as in hepatorenal syndrome complicating hepatic failure. In the latter situation, there is loss of sympathetic tone with shunting of blood through muscle, splanchnic bed and skin, a secondary rise in cardiac output, a low A-VO$_2$ difference, and frank hepatic failure (15). This latter type, type II, does not respond to portal decompression and/or LeVeen's shunt. If a Le-Veen's shunt is performed, disseminated intravascular clotting usually follows.

The pathophysiologic response of the kidney in type II hepatorenal syndrome is appropriate, in that there is differential vasoconstriction in response to effective hypovolemia and decreased pulsatile perfusion. The type I hepatorenal syndrome (Table 12B.1) usually responds to portal-hepatic decompression or peritoneal atrial shunt.

Bleeding Esophageal Varices

Bleeding esophageal varices is the most troublesome complication of portal hypertension. Although collaterals may form throughout the gastrointestinal tract, especially around the anus, and in various adhesions due to previous abdominal surgery, bleeding from other portal-systemic collaterals is rare compared with bleeding from gastric and esophageal varices, although why they bleed is not clear.

For 50 years controversy around portal decompression for bleeding esophageal varices has continued unabated. It is now accepted that depriving the liver of portal flow probably contributes to hepatic failure. One can frame the controversies in portal decompression as a balance between the need to decompress the elevated portal pressure to prevent further bleeding and the need to maintain hepatic-portal vein perfusion. This is the essence of the controversy.

It has been difficult to demonstrate improved outcome following therapeutic portacaval shunt; statistically significant improvement in long-term survival is only possible when one combines three major randomized series (16–19). The difficulty in demonstrating improved salvage following portacaval shunt explains the enthusiasm that welcomes new nonsurgical forms of therapy, whether their efficacy has been established or not. Witness the ready acceptance of propranolol for bleeding esophageal varices, despite difficulty in proving its efficacy and not a little suspicion that propranolol may contribute to deterioration of hepatic function.

Sclerotherapy, which once again has been resurrected (5), is the current beneficiary of enthusiasm on the part of nonshunt proponents. Although the number of late complications has not yet become fully apparent, large numbers of patients have been subjected to sclerotherapy, with some positive results. The difficulty is in those patients who either are not sufficiently responsible to attend their sclerotherapy sessions or in whom sclerotherapy proves ineffective because of large esophageal varices or bleeding from gastric varices. In this group it appears that the distal splenorenal shunt has become the gold standard against which other shunts must be compared (7,8). It is a difficult shunt and one not readily carried out by most surgeons, with significant operative mortality. The theoretical basis on which distal splenorenal shunt is based is sound: to separate the right and left sides of the portal circulation, decompress the esophageal varices via the left side and the spleen, and leave the right side intact to perfuse the liver.

There are several difficulties with this hypothesis as originally proposed:

1. Many patients in the original published series (7) were selected; a large percentage were nonalcoholics who, as proven by experience, have a better prognosis.
2. Patients with a retrograde portal flow were excluded. These patients have the most advanced form of cirrhosis; if they are excluded a more favorable group was subjected to distal splenorenal shunt.
3. It is impossible to permanently separate areas of high pressure and low pressure. Within 6 hours of a distal splenorenal shunt, collaterals reopen (20).

In six randomized prospective trials in which distal splenorenal shunt has been compared with other shunts, there was absolutely no difference in long-term survival (9,21–25). In three of the six studies, the incidence of encephalopathy has been lower (21–23), and in three of the studies (9,24,25), including one in Cincinnati in which distal splenorenal shunt was randomized against central splenorenal shunt (9), there was no difference in encephalopathy during more than 6 years of follow-up. Patients continue to accrue to this latter study.

In persistently bleeding varices, distal splenorenal shunt is probably at least as good as most other shunts, except with ascites or hypersplenism, in

which case a proximal splenorenal shunt should be performed. Given the complexities of alcoholics and cirrhotics, I am not convinced that for most patients it makes a great deal of difference. I believe that the ability to perform the operation without technical misadventures is an important part of portal hypertension surgery that has not been stressed sufficiently. Thus, each surgeon should carry out the operation with which he or she is most comfortable.

References

1. Keller GA, West MA, Cerra FB, Simmons RL. Multiple systems organ failure: Modulation of hepatocyte protein synthesis by endotoxin activated Kupffer cells. *Ann Surg* 1985; 201:87–95.
2. Thompson E, Williams R, Sherlock S. Liver function in extrahepatic portal hypertension. *Lancet* 1964; 2:1352–1356.
3. Panke WF, Rousselot LM, Burchell AR. A sixteen-year experience with end-to-side portacaval shunt for variceal hemorrhage: Analysis of data and comparison with other types of portasystemic anastomoses. *Ann Surg* 1968; 168: 957–965.
4. Fischer JE, Baldessarini RJ. False neurotransmitters and hepatic failure. *Lancet* 1971; 2:75–80.
5. Terblanche J, Yakoob HI, Bornman PC, Stiegmann GV, Bane R, Jonker M, et al. Acute bleeding varices. A five year prospective evaluation of tamponade and sclerotherapy. *Ann Surg* 1981; 194:521–530.
6. Palani CK, Abuabara S, Kraft AR, Jonasson O. Endoscopic sclerotherapy in acute variceal hemorrhage. *Am J Surg* 1981; 141:164–168.
7. Warren WD, Zeppa R, Fomon JJ. Selective trans-splenic decompression of gastroesophageal varices by distal spleno-renal shunt. *Ann Surg* 1967; 166:437–455.
8. Salam AA, Warren WD. Anatomic basis of the surgical treatment of portal hypertension. *Surg Clin North Am* 1974; 54:1247–1257.
9. Fischer JE, Bower RH, Atamian S, Welling R. Comparison of distal and proximal splenorenal shunts. A randomized prospective trial. *Ann Surg* 1981; 194:531–544.
10. Fischer JE, McKinley J. Comparative randomized study: proximal vs. distal splenorenal shunt. *Policlinico Sez Chir* 1985; 92:592–596.
11. Schroeder ET, Numann PJ, Chamberlain BE. Functional renal failure in cirrhosis: Recovery after portacaval shunt. *Ann Intern Med* 1970; 72:923–928.
12. Fischer JE, Foster GS. Survival from acute hepatorenal syndrome following splenorenal shunt. *Ann Surg* 1976; 184:22–25.
13. Freund H, Brewster D, Fischer JE. Letter: Total parenteral nutrition in post-Warren shunt chylous ascites. *Arch Surg* 1979; 114:345.
14. Maywood BT, Goldstein L, Busuttil RW. Chylous ascites after a Warren shunt. *Am J Surg* 1978; 135:700–702.
15. Fischer JE, Bower RH. Amino acids in liver disease. In: Epstein M, ed. *The Kidney in Liver Disease*. New York: Elsevier Biomedical, 1982, pp. 515–534.
16. Resnick RH, Iber FL, Ishihara AM, Chalmers C, Zimmerman H, the Boston Inter-Hospital Liver Group. A controlled study of the therapeutic portacaval shunt. *Gastroenterology* 1974; 67:843–857.

17. Mikkelsen WP. Therapeutic PC shunt. Preliminary data on controlled trial and morbid effect of acute hyaline necrosis. *Arch Surg* 1974; 108:302–305.
18. Jackson FC, Perrin EB, Felix RW, Smith AG. A clinical investigation of the portacaval shunt. Survival analysis of the therapeutic operation. *Ann Surg* 1971; 174:672–701.
19. Conn HO. Therapeutic portacaval anastomosis: To shunt to not to shunt. *Gastroenterology* 1974; 67:1065–1073.
20. Miallard JN, Falmant YM, Hay JM, Chandler JG: Selectivity of the distal splenorenal shunt. *Surgery* 1979; 86:663–671.
21. Reichle FA, Fahmy WF, Golsorkhi M. Prospective comparative clinical trial with distal splenorenal and mesocaval shunts. *Am J Surg* 1979; 137:13–21.
22. Rikkers LF, Rudman D, Galambos JT, et al. A randomized controlled trial of the distal splenorenal shunt. *Ann Surg* 1978; 3:271–282.
23. Langer B, Rotstein LE, Stone RM, Taylor BR, Patel SC, Blendis LM, et al. A prospective randomized trial of the selective distal splenorenal shunt. *Surg Gynecol Obstet* 1980; 150:45–48.
24. Villamil F, Redeker A, Reynolds T, Yellin A. A controlled trial of distal splenorenal and portacaval shunts (abstr). *Hepatology* 1981; 1:557.
25. Conn HO, Resnick RH, Grace CE, et al. Distal splenorenal shunt vs. portal-systemic shunt: Current status of a controlled trial. *Hepatology* 1981; 1:151–160.

Editorial Comment

Of all the topics included in this wide-ranging volume on surgery of the liver, it is perhaps most difficult to summarize the hemodynamics of portal hypertension in a clear, concise, and yet scientific way. Dr. Fischer has accomplished this admirably. As always, there are areas that overlap with other chapters. The anatomy included in this chapter is purposely sparse but certainly is complementary to the anatomic section earlier in the volume. Indeed, with such an excellent review of the hemodynamics associated with ascites in this chapter, one could ask, Why follow this with a separate chapter on ascites (See Chapter 18)?

In fact, the authors raised that question themselves and decided that the subject was so controversial and so clinically important that a chapter focusing on this facet of portal hypertension would be additive rather than repetitive. At any rate, the reader wishing to learn about hemodynamics of this peculiar vascular arrangement, and the inflow and outflow tracts of the liver, would do well to study the three major divisions of this chapter relating particularly to the anatomy, experimental hemodynamics, and clinical disease patterns associated with variations of blood flow.

Chapter 13
Acute Variceal Bleeding

Chapter 13A
Variceal Hemorrhage: Pharmacologic Approach

NORMAN D. GRACE

Hemorrhage from esophagogastric varices continues to be a major and potentially lethal complication of cirrhosis, with up to a 50% mortality with each bleeding episode. For years, standard therapy for control of hemorrhage has been balloon tamponade with variations of the Sengstaken-Blakemore tube for those patients failing conservative treatment. In experienced hands, initial control has been achieved in up to 94% of patients (1,2). However, use of the tube in less experienced hands is associated with a high complication rate (3). The rebleeding rate after initial control by balloon tamponade averages 25% to 30% and the mortality is up to 42%. For those who fail medical therapy, an emergency portasystemic shunt is associated with a 30% to 50% operative mortality (4).

As Graham et al. (5) have pointed out, 25% of all patients admitted with bleeding varices rebleed within the first 2 weeks; 31% rebleed within 6 weeks and this is associated with a 41% 6-week mortality. Therefore, therapy to prevent recurrent bleeding is vital in improving long-term prognosis. Although the portacaval shunt has been reasonably effective in preventing recurrent variceal hemorrhage, it has been associated with a high incidence of portasystemic encephalopathy and progressive hepatic failure (4). In addition, there is often a delay of several months between the initial bleeding episode and the shunt procedure while the patient's alcoholic hepatitis subsides and he or she becomes a "better" operative candidate. Thus, many of the studies of surgical therapy to prevent recurrent variceal hemorrhage have not included the high-risk patients who rebleed and succumb in the 6-week period following their index bleed. These observations have stimulated physicians to seek alternative approaches for the acute control of variceal hemorrhage and prevention of recurrent hemorrhage after initial stabilization.

Mechanism for Variceal Rupture

In the past 10 years, there has been a renewal of interest in the use of pharmacologic agents in the treatment of variceal hemorrhage. The rationale for their use is based on an understanding of the factors responsible for the development and rupture of esophageal varices. Two theories have received attention: (1) the erosion theory suggests that acid reflux leads to esophagitis and subsequent rupture of distal esophageal varices; (2) the explosion theory is based on the high pressure within the varix leading to rupture at a weak point in the wall, analogous to an over-inflated tire with a bubble.

There is abundant evidence that esophagitis plays little, if any, role in the initiation of variceal hemorrhage. Several investigators have demonstrated that patients with cirrhosis and portal hypertension have normal lower esophageal sphincter pressures and no increase in esophageal reflux when measured with a pH probe, compared to control populations (6–8). Esophageal specimens from patients undergoing esophageal resection and stapling for bleeding esophageal varices have failed to show histologic evidence of inflammation or erosion on histologic examination (9,10). In a prospective double-blind trial, MacDougall et al. (8) compared cimetidine, 1.6 grams per day, with a placebo for the prevention of recurrent variceal hemorrhage. The rebleeding rate in patients with cirrhosis was 62.5% for the cimetidine group and 75% for the placebo [not significant (NS)]. They concluded that gastric acid reflux does not initiate and cimetidine does not prevent recurrent esophageal variceal hemorrhage.

The occurrence of esophageal variceal hemorrhage has been related to both the size of varices and the degree of portal hypertension (11–17).

There is uniform agreement that large varices are at higher risk of bleeding than small varices. This is especially true if the varices are seen to have the red color sign at the time of endoscopy (18). There is less agreement about the role of portal hypertension in initiating bleeding. All investigations have found a threshold portal pressure gradient (measured either as the difference between hepatic wedged and free pressures or as the difference between portal venous pressure measured directly via the percutaneous transhepatic route and the inferior vena cava pressure) ranging from 10 to 12 millimeters of mercury, below which variceal bleeding does not occur (11–16). However, some investigators have found a higher hepatic venous pressure gradient in bleeders compared to non-bleeders (11–13) while others have found no difference (14–16). Even in the studies that found a difference, there is tremendous overlap between the groups so that the degree of elevation of portal pressure in a given patient is not predictive of the likelihood of variceal hemorrhage.

In addition to the size of varices and elevation of portal pressure as important risk factors for variceal hemorrhage, interest has centered on the concept of variceal wall tension as introduced by Groszmann (19,20). Using a modification of La-Place's law, wall tension (T) is a function of transmural pressure (TP) times the radius of the varix (r) over the wall thickness (w):

$$T = TP \times \frac{r}{w}$$

The transmural pressure is the difference between the pressure within the varix (reflecting portal pressure) and the intraluminal pressure within the esophagus. In general, the larger the varix, the greater is the radius of the varix and the thinner the wall. As the radius enlarges, the wall tension increases in an exponential fashion until the "rupture point" is reached. An in-depth explanation of this concept can be found in a 1986 review by Polio and Groszmann (20). Finally, there has been interest in the direct measurement of variceal pressure, obtained either by direct puncture techniques (21) or pressure-sensitive gauges (22–24) applied during endoscopy. Preliminary results suggest a good correlation between variceal pressure and variceal size but the relationship with portal pressure needs further clarification.

Pharmacology

Portal pressure is a function of portal blood flow and hepatic resistance. In patients with cirrhosis, there is a hyperdynamic circulation leading to an increase in portal blood flow (25,26). With a relatively fixed hepatic resistance and this increase in portal venous flow, the rate of increase in portal pressure relative to the increase in flow exceeds that in the normal liver.

In animal models and acute human experiments, vasopressin, a posterior pituitary hormone, has been shown to diminish mesenteric arterial blood flow, resulting in a decrease in portal venous flow and portal pressure (27,28). However, the reduction of portal flow is greater than the reduction of portal pressure, suggesting that there might be an increase in hepatic arterial flow to compensate partially for the decrease in portal venous flow. Unfortunately, vasopressin has significant systemic effects involving the cardiovascular and gastrointestinal systems, leading to a number of complications including hypertension, bradycardia, peripheral vasoconstriction, myocardial ischemia and infarction, cerebrovascular accidents, mesenteric angina, diarrhea, and hyponatremia with fluid retention (29). In addition, it causes release of plasminogen activator and factor VIII, although the clinical significance of their release is unclear (30). In an attempt to find an agent that will reduce portal pressure with minimal to absent side effects, a number of other agents have been explored. A group of drugs that act by causing splanchnic vasoconstriction leading to a reduction of gastroesophageal collateral blood flow and pressure include vasopressin analogues (terlipressin) (31), somatostatin (32,33), and β-adrenergic blockers (34–36). A greater reduction of portal pressure is achieved by nonselective β-adrenergic blockers (propranolol, nadalol) than by the β_1-selective blockers (atenolol, metoprolol). This occurs because of the former agents' ability to decrease splanchnic blood flow in addition to a reduction in cardiac output achieved by all of these agents (35). A second group of drugs, the vasodilators, have been shown to lower portal pressure, probably by a reflex splanchnic arterial vasoconstriction with a subsequent reduction in portal venous blood flow in response to venous pooling and vasodilatation in other parts of the circulatory system (20). In addition, they may decrease hepatic resistance by

Table 13A.1. Control of Acute Variceal Hemorrhage—Vasopressin Versus Conventional Therapy

Author (No.)	Therapy		Control of Hemorrhage		Rebleeding Rate (%)	Mortality
Merigan (50)	PPE	IV	16/29	$p < 0.01$	"Transient control"	12/15
	Plac		0/24			14/15
Conn (47)	VP—SMA		12/17	$p < 0.01$	45	9/17
	Conv		4/16		33	10/16
Mallory (48) [a]	VP—SMA		2/5	NS	N/A	2/5
	Conv		1/6			3/6
Fogel (49)	VP	IV	4/14	NS	N/A	7/14
	Plac		7/19			8/19
Total	VP		52%		25–45	59%
	Conv		18%		33–67	63%

Abbreviations: Conv, conventional therapy; Plac, placebo; PPE, posterior pituitary extract; SMA, superior mesenteric artery; VP, vasopressin.
[a] Estimate for patients with cirrhosis and bleeding varices.

causing a relaxation of myofibroblasts leading to an "opening up" of sinusoids (37). Nitroglycerin (28), isosorbide dinitrate (38,39), sodium nitroprusside (40), prazosin (41), clonidine (42,43), and verapamil (39,44,45) share some of these properties.

For clinicians, the value of these agents is dependent on their ability to control acute esophageal variceal hemorrhage, prevent its recurrence, and, hopefully, to improve survival of the patients. The remainder of this discussion will be directed to an analysis of a number of prospective controlled trials that have evaluated several of these agents.

Control of Acute Variceal Hemorrhage

Vasopressin

Since the mid-1970s, vasopressin has been widely employed for the control of acute variceal hemorrhage. Much of the early enthusiasm for vasopressin stemmed from the report of Baum and Nussbaum (46) that selective infusion of vasopressin via the superior mesenteric artery resulted in acute control of hemorrhage in 27 of 28 patients (96%). The failure of other investigators to duplicate these results has led to, at present, four controlled clinical trials comparing vasopressin to a placebo or conventional therapy (47–50) (Table 13A.1) and three comparing selective superior mesenteric artery infusion to systemic intravenous infusion of vasopressin (51–53) (Table 13A.2). The study designs and dose of vasopressin differed, and one study (50) used posterior pituitary extract. Employing a continuous infusion of vasopressin via the superior mesenteric artery, Conn et al. (47) found a significant benefit in the initial control of hemorrhage, with 12 of 17 patients (71%) responding in the vasopressin group, compared to 4 of 16 (25%) in the control group ($p < 0.001$). However, almost half the patients rebled after initial control, and there was no difference in survival. In a similarly designed study by Mallory et al. (48), two of five patients in whom the site of bleeding was esophageal varices were controlled with vasopressin compared to one of six patients receiving conventional therapy; however, the number of patients was too small for statistical analysis. Fogel et al. (49), comparing a continuous intravenous infusion of vasopressin to a placebo, found no difference in either the initial control of hemorrhage or survival. Using an intravenous infusion of posterior pituitary extract, Merigan et al. (50) were able to demonstrate transient control of initial hemorrhage in 55% of patients, compared to none in the placebo group ($p < 0.01$). If one takes some liberties and combines the data from these four

Table 13A.2. Control of Acute Variceal Hemorrhage by Vasopressin, IV Versus SMA Route

Author (No.)	Route	Control of Hemorrhage		Rebleeding Rate	Mortality
Johnson (51)	IV	7/11	NS	0/7	5/11
	SMA	7/14		3/10	4/14
Clanet (53)	IV	14/15	$p < 0.05$	N/A	12/18
	SMA	6/11			9/11
Chojkier (52)	IV	5/10	NS	2/5	7/10
	SMA	6/12		3/6	9/12
Total	IV	71%		17%	62%
	SMA	48%		38%	59%

studies, 52% of the vasopressin-treated population had initial control of hemorrhage, compared to 18% of the control population. None of the studies showed any improvement in survival.

Since selective catheterization of the superior mesenteric artery requires the presence of a radiologist and is associated with catheter complications, easier means of administering vasopressin were sought. In comparing a constant intravenous infusion of vasopressin with intra-arterial infusion, two studies (51,52) showed the routes were equally effective, while a third (53) usually showed an advantage with the intravenous route. The complications were similar in all these studies, negating the theoretical advantage of selective infusion. Since constant intravenous infusion of vasopressin was found to be at least as good as selective catheterization, it is the current route of choice, starting at a dose of 0.4 units per minute, with a maximum dose up to 0.8 U/min dependent on side effects of the drug.

There have been several major problems with the use of vasopressin. Almost half the patients do not exhibit initial response to the drug; there is a significant rebleeding rate after initial control; there are significant systemic complications associated with its use, as previously mentioned; and there is no improvement in survival associated with its use. Because of its relatively modest success in control of hemorrhage and the significant complication rate associated with its use, a search for better agents seemed warranted.

Terlipressin

Terlipressin (triglycyl-lysine vasopressin) is relatively inert but, with cleavage of the N-terminal glycyl residues, lysine vasopressin, the active component, is released. Because of the slow release of active drug, it can be given in bolus form, therefore avoiding the necessity for continuous infusion. However, this possible advantage would be negated if complications developed. In a prospective randomized trial, Freeman et al. (54) compared terlipressin (2 milligrams every 6 hours) with a continuous infusion of vasopressin (0.4 U/min) (Table 13A.3). They were successful in controlling hemorrhage in 7 of 10 patients (70%) receiving terlipressin, compared to 1 of 11 (9%) of patients randomized to the vasopressin group ($p < 0.02$). This is a surprisingly low success rate for vasopressin. A second study by Walker et al. (55) compared terlipressin (given as a 2-mg bolus followed by 1 mg every 4 hours) to a placebo. Interpretation of the results is complicated by the fact that both groups had concomitant use of the Sengstaken-Blakemore tube in about 80% of the patients. Successful control of hemorrhage was achieved in 20 of 25 patients (80%) on terlipressin, compared to 13 of 25 (52%) on the placebo ($p < 0.05$). Both studies showed a trend (not statistically significant) toward improved survival with terlipressin, and the systemic adverse effects were minimal. The number of patients evaluated is small, and further studies will be needed before its clinical usefulness can be established.

Table 13A.3. Control of Acute Variceal Hemorrhage by Terlipressin (Glypressin)

Author (No.)	Therapy	Maximum Dose	Control of Hemorrhage		Rebleeding Rate	Mortality
Freeman (54)	tGVP	2 mg q6hr	7/10	$p < 0.02$	0/7	1/10
	VP	0.4 U/min	1/11		0/1	4/11
Walker [a] (55)	tGVP	2-mg bolus 1 mg q4hr	20/25	$p < 0.05$	1/20	3/25
	Plac	—	13/25		3/13	8/25
Total	tGVP		77%		4%	11%

Abbreviations: tGVP,
[a] Both groups had Sengstaken-Blakemore tube used ~ 80% of time.

Nitroglycerin

In addition to producing a modest reduction in portal pressure, nitroglycerin has been shown to alleviate the systemic vasoconstrictive effects of vasopressin (28). In a prospective randomized trial, Gimson et al. (56) compared an intravenous infusion of vasopressin (initial bolus of 20 U followed by infusion of 0.4 U/min) to a similar infusion of vasopressin plus an intravenous infusion of nitroglycerin (median dose 300 micrograms per minute) (Table 13A.4). Evaluation following a 12-hour treatment period revealed control of hemorrhage in 68% of patients receiving the combination therapy compared to 44% receiving vasopressin alone ($p < 0.05$). There were fewer major complications with the combination therapy, but the transfusion requirements and early mortality were similar for both groups. A second randomized controlled trial by Tsai et al. (57) compared an intravenous infusion of vasopressin (initial dose 0.66 U/min) to a similar dose of vasopressin plus nitroglycerin given sublingually (0.6 mg every 30 minutes for 6 hours). There was no difference in the control of hemorrhage at 6 hours, but at 24 hours there was a definite trend in favor of the combination therapy (45% vs. 21%, NS). As in the previous study, there were fewer systemic adverse effects with the combination therapy but no differences in transfusion requirements or early mortality.

In the study by Gimson et al., half the patients had alcoholic liver disease and 61% were classified as Child's classification group C. Tsai et al. studied patients with hepatitis B surface antigen (HB_sAg)-positive posthepatitic cirrhosis including 38% with hepatomas. The higher mortality in the latter study (56% vs. 29%) may be a consequence of the type of liver disease. Despite differences in patient population, route of nitroglycerin administration (intravenous vs. sublingual), and duration of treatment, both studies show that the combination of

Table 13A.4. Control of Acute Variceal Hemorrhage by Nitroglycerin—VP Versus VP

Author (No.)	Therapy	Maximum Dose	Control of Hemorrhage		Rebleeding Rate	Mortality
Gimson (56)	VP	0.4 U/min	15/34	$p < 0.05$	NA	9/30
	VP NTG	0.4 U/min 400 μg/min	26/38		NA	9/32
Tsai (57)	VP	0.66 U/min	9/19	NS	NA	11/19
	VP NTG	0.66 U/min 0.6 mg/$\frac{1}{2}$ hr SL	11/20		NA	11/20
Total	VP		45%			41%
	VP/NTG		64%			38%

Abbreviations: NA, not available; NTG, nitroglycerin; SL, sublingual.

Table 13A.5. Control of Acute Variceal Hemorrhage—Somatostatin Versus Vasopressin

Author (No.)	Therapy	Maximum Dose	Control of Hemorrhage		Rebleeding Rate	Mortality
Kravetz (58)	SOM	500 μg/hr	26/30	NS	10/26	14/30
	VP	0.8 U/min	23/31		5/23	14/31
Jenkins (59)	SOM	250 μg/hr	10/10	$p < 0.01$	3/10	2/10
	VP	0.4 U/min	4/12		0/4	4/12
Total	SOM		90%		36%	40%
	VP		63%		19%	42%

Abbreviations: SOM, somatostatin.

vasopressin plus nitroglycerin markedly reduced the complications of vasopressin therapy and had superior control of variceal hemorrhage. However, neither study showed benefit in survival.

Somatostatin

Somatostatin lowers portal pressure by a vasoconstrictive effect on the splanchnic circulation, but, in contrast to vasopressin, it has very little effect on systemic blood flow (32). In a prospective randomized trial, Kravetz et al. (58) compared somatostatin, given as an initial bolus of 50 μg followed by a continuous infusion of 250 μg/hr, raised to 500 μg/hr if bleeding was not controlled, to a continuous intravenous infusion of vasopressin with a maximum dose of 0.9 U/min (Table 13A.5).

There was no significant difference in either control of hemorrhage (somatostatin 87% vs. vasopressin 74%) or early mortality (somatostatin 47% vs. vasopressin 45%). Somatostatin produced significantly fewer serious complications, leading the authors to conclude that it was the preferred treatment. However, the higher incidence of adverse effects with vasopressin may have been due to the unusually high dose employed in the study. Jenkins et al. (59) compared somatostatin (250-μg bolus followed by 250 μg/hr) to vasopressin (0.4 U/min) in a prospective randomized trial. Hemorrhage was controlled in 10 of 10 patients (100%) receiving somatostatin, compared to 4 of 12 patients (33%) on vasopressin ($p < 0.01$), but there were no differences in early mortality. Two patients receiving vasopressin had to be discontinued from the study due to serious adverse effects, compared to none in somatostatin. Although the number of study patients is small, somatostatin

appears to be at least as good as vasopressin in controlling variceal hemorrhage and is associated with fewer complications.

Summary

Although vasopressin is the only pharmacologic agent enjoying widespread use in this country for the initial control of variceal hemorrhage, it has definite limitations. There is no benefit in survival, a significant complication rate, and only a 50% success rate in the control of hemorrhage. Somatostatin and the combination therapy of vasopressin and nitroglycerin are clearly superior in the reduction of systemic side effects. Terlipressin may also be helpful in this regard. Early studies suggest that all of these agents are at least as good as and perhaps superior to vasopressin in controlling variceal hemorrhage, but none have been shown to enhance survival. However, survival may be influenced more by treatment to prevent recurrent hemorrhage than by therapy used for the initial control of bleeding. To date, there are no published controlled trials evaluating clonidine, prazosin, nitroprusside, verapamil, or prostaglandin inhibitors.

Prevention of Recurrent Variceal Hemorrhage

Despite initial control of variceal hemorrhage in patients with cirrhosis, there is a 25% risk of recurrent variceal hemorrhage within 2 weeks of the index bleed and 31% within 6 weeks (5). The efficacy of sclerotherapy and portasystemic shunts in the prevention of recurrent bleeding are discussed elsewhere. Of the pharmacologic agents

Table 13A.6. Propranolol for Prevention of Recurrent Variceal Hemorrhage–Results

| | Lebrec (60) | | Burroughs (61) | | Villeneuve (62) | |
	Prop	Plac	Prop	Plac	Prop	Plac
Recurrent bleeding						
1 yr	13%	58% ($p < 0.0001$)	46%	44%	71%	74%
2 yr	21%	68% ($p < 0.0001$)	72%	70%	78%	82%
Dropouts	8	4	4	0	8	2
Survival						
1 yr	94%	84% (NS)	85%	77%	61%	70%
2 yr	90%	57% ($p < 0.02$)			55%	62%
Adverse effects	Minor—10		Minor N/A		Minor N/A	
	Major—0		Major—6		Major—5	

Abbreviations: Prop, propranolol.

previously discussed that have the potential for lowering portal pressure, data from controlled clinical trials are available only for the β-adrenergic blockers.

Propranolol

Three major trials have compared propranolol to a placebo in the prevention of recurrent variceal hemorrhage (60–62). Lebrec et al. reported that propranolol, given in a dose adjusted to produce a reduction of 25% in the resting heart rate, was successful in preventing recurrent hemorrhage in patients bleeding from either esophageal varices or hemorrhagic gastritis (60). When only patients whose initial hemorrhage was from esophagogastric varices are considered, the rebleeding rate at 2 years was 14% for the propranolol group and 64% for the control group ($p < 0.001$) (Table 13A.6). Although the authors reported a survival benefit for propranolol, there are some valid questions

about the method used in constructing the survival curves. Patients who bled were dropped from the patient population at risk, leaving relatively few patients in a control group available for analysis in the second year of the study. In contrast, Burroughs et al. (61), using a similar method for determining the dose of propranolol, found no difference either in the control of hemorrhage or in survival. The latter study reported a higher complication rate associated with propranolol. Villeneuve et al. (62) also found no differences between patients treated with propranolol or placebo in either recurrence of hemorrhage from varices or in survival. Despite similarities in design, there are major differences between these studies that might explain the differing outcomes.

In the study by Lebrec et al., 88% of the patients had alcoholic liver disease; 72% were classified as Child's classification group A and had little to no ascites on admission to the study (Table 13A.7).

Table 13A.7. Propranolol for Prevention of Recurrent Variceal Hemorrhage—Study Characteristics

		Lebrec (60)[a]	Burroughs (61)	Villeneuve (62)
Patients				
Propranolol		38	26	42
Placebo		36	22	37
Alcoholic liver disease		88%	42%	72%
Child's	A	72%	60%	11%
classification	B	28%	30%	52%
	C	0	10%	37%
Ascites		Minimal to absent	34%	NA
Average dose (mg/day)		159 ± 83	198 ± 32	103 + 7
Interval between bleeding and start of treatment (days)		21 ± 12	11 ± 1	1

[a] 76%—site of bleeding—varices.

Table 13A.8. Prevention of Recurrent Variceal Hemorrhage—β-Blocker Versus Sclerotherapy

	O'Connor (64)	Alexandrino (65)	Fleig (66)	Dollet (67)	Westaby (68)
Patients					
Propranolol	28	34	34	20	48
SCT	25	31	36	24	52
Alcoholic	80%	NA	83%	NA	60%
Rebleeding rate					
β-Blocker	68%	44%	28%	15%	52%
	$p < 0.05$	$p < 0.05$	NS	NS	NS
SCT	36%	19%	29%	33%	42%
Survival					
β-Blocker	54%	NA	85%	80%	63%
SCT	60%		92%	75%	63%

Abbreviations: NA, not applicable; SCT, sclerotherapy.

The average dose of propranolol was slightly lower than that used by Burroughs et al. (61), possibly accounting for a lower incidence of significant side effects. In contrast, only 42% of the patients in the study by Burroughs et al. had alcoholic liver disease, 40% were classified as Child's group B or C, and one-third had ascites on admission to the study. Seventy-two percent of the patients studied by Villeneuve (62) had alcoholic liver disease and 89% were classified as Child's B or C. The average interval between the initial bleeding episode and the start of treatment was 21 days in the Lebrec study compared to 11 days in the Burroughs study and 1 to 2 days in the Villeneuve study, raising the possibility that some higher-risk patients may not have been included in the former study because of early recurrent hemorrhage.

Gatta et al. (63) recently compared nadolol, a nonselective β-blocker to placebo in the prevention of recurrent variceal hemorrhage. Nadolol has a theoretical advantage over propranolol in that it has a lower penetration of the blood–brain barrier, is not metabolized by the liver, and maintains renal blood flow. In a limited study with 12 patients in each group, the rebleeding rate was 18% in the nadolol group compared to 67% in the control group ($p < 0.01$; follow-up to 145 weeks). The survival rate was 92% for nadolol and 75% for placebo (NS).

A possible conclusion from these studies is that nonselective β-adrenergic blockers may have a role in the treatment of bleeding varices in alcoholic cirrhotics with mild liver disease but has a questionable place in the treatment of patients with nonalcoholic liver disease or more severe hepatic dysfunction. At this point, they should be restricted to investigational use.

β-blockers Versus Sclerotherapy

With the development of newer fiberoptic endoscopes, there has been a resurgence in the last decade of enthusiasm for sclerotherapy in the treatment of variceal hemorrhage. Preliminary reports of 4 prospective randomized studies have compared sclerotherapy with propranolol for the prevention of recurrent variceal hemorrhage (64–67) (Table 13A.8). All 4 groups dealt only with variceal bleeders but the type of liver disease and Child's classification group are available for just two groups. For all groups, propranolol dose was adjusted to yield a 25% decrease in the resting heart rate. The sclerotherapy technique varied with intra- and paravariceal injections, sessions twice per week to every 3 weeks, and a variety of agents. Two studies (64,65) found that sclerotherapy was preferable to propranolol in the prevention of recurrent variceal hemorrhage, while the other two found no difference (66,67). There were no survival differences for any of the studies. The complications were those usually associated with the two therapies.

Again we find a mixed review—half of the studies finding a preference for sclerotherapy over propranolol for the prevention of variceal hemorrhage and half finding no difference. However, Fleig et al. (66) note that control groups in other studies (60,61) had a higher rebleeding rate in one year than in their investigations and suggest that both sclerotherapy and propranolol are effective therapies. More importantly, none of the studies showed a survival advantage of either therapy. It is doubtful that an advantage will become apparent with more patients and longer follow-up, but it is possible that, when the full data are published,

Table 13A.9. β-Blockers for Prophylaxis Against Initial Variceal Hemorrhage

	Pascal (70)	*Pagliaro (71)*	*Lebrec (73)*	*Ideo (72)*
β-Blocker	Propranolol	Propranolol	Nadolol	Nadolol
Patients				
β-Blocker	118	85	53	30
Plac	112	89	53	27
Follow-up (mo)	14 ± 6	22 ± 9	12 ± ?	NA
Bleeding rate				
β-Blocker	17%[a] ⎫	~23% ⎫	10% ⎫	37% ⎫
	⎬ NS	⎬ NS	⎬ NS	⎬ $p < 0.05$
Plac	27% ⎭	~36% ⎭	18% ⎭	26% ⎭
Survival				
β-Blocker	72% ⎫	~60%	84%	85%
	⎬ $p < 0.05$			
Plac	51% ⎭	~72%	84%	80%

[a] Patients free of bleeding (cumulative - 2 yrs).
 Prop - 74%   Plac 39% (p < 0.05)

stratification of the subjects may reveal subgroups that may benefit.

Metoprolol, a $\beta1$ (cardioselective) blocking agent, has been compared with sclerotherapy in the prevention of recurrent variceal hemorrhage in a study by Westaby et al. (69). The choice of this agent preceded the publication of data showing nonselective agents were superior to $\beta1$ selective agents in reducing portal pressure (35). The patient population consisted of 15 patients randomized to metoprolol and 27 to sclerotherapy (Table 13A.8). They were predominantly nonalcoholic (59%) with 47% Child's classification A and 53% Child's classification B. The average dose of metoprolol was 300 mg/day, adjusted to yield a 25% decrease in resting heart rate. Sclerotherapy was significantly better than metoprolol in preventing recurrent bleeding (60% rebleeding for metoprolol vs. 35% for sclerotherapy). Data are not available for survival. Of interest, two of the patients who rebled on metoprolol had a 56% and 50% decrease in hepatic venous pressure gradient (HVPG), respectively, as determined 4 weeks after starting the drug. Prior to the time of recurrent hemorrhage, two patients had a decrease in HVPG to less than 10 millimeters of mercury, below the accepted "cutoff" for variceal hemorrhage.

Prophylactic Propranolol

Based on previous controlled trials, 25% of patients who have esophageal varices demonstrated by barium swallow or endoscopy, but have not yet bled, will have a significant bleed within a 3- to 4-year follow-up period. Although prophylactic portacaval shunts have successfully prevented bleeding, they have led to a higher mortality rate than a comparable control population, due to progressive hepatic failure with encephalopathy. In the mid-1980s there has been a renewal of interest in nonsurgical approaches to prophylaxis with the use of sclerotherapy or β-blockers. Four abstracts have compared β-blockers to a placebo (two propranolol, two nadolol) (70–73) (Table 13A.9). Pascal et al. (70) report data on 230 patients with endoscopically proven esophageal varices and Child's classification group A/B cirrhosis. Propranolol dosage was determined by a 25% decrease in resting heart rate. Their results (follow-up period of 436 ± 172 days) show a significant protective effect by propranolol for the prevention of bleeding when analyzed as the cumulative percentages of patients free of bleeding two years after inclusion in the study (propranolol 74% vs. placebo 39%). This difference was most dramatic for patients in poor condition. Unfortunately, only 29 of the 50 patients with upper gastrointestinal tract bleeding had endoscopic verification of the source of bleeding, a potential weakness in this study. However, only two of the 29 had a bleeding source other than varices. Two-year cumulative survival was significantly better in the propranolol group (propranolol 72% vs. placebo 51%, $p < 0.05$). The second study by Pagliaro et al. (70) compares 85 patients on an average dose of 84 mg propranolol/day, as determined by a 25% decrease in resting heart rate, with 89 patients on placebo. With a mean follow-up of 22 months on all patients entered, there has been no difference between the groups in either bleeding rate or survival. However, 25 patients were unable to continue taking propranolol because of adverse effects. This group of patients had a poorer outcome, both in terms of bleeding and survival. Comparing nadolol to placebo, Ideo et al. (71) found that nadolol was successful in preventing variceal hemorrhage while Lebrec et al. (72) showed a favorable trend that was not statistically significant. Neither study was able to demonstrate a difference in survival. These data are preliminary and it is too early to judge whether β-blockers will be useful prophylactic agents.

Conclusion

For initial control of esophageal variceal hemorrhage, both sclerotherapy and pharmacologic agents appear preferable to emergency portasystemic shunt surgery. Although the success rate for acute sclerotherapy is impressive, there are complications, and this treatment modality requires endoscopists skilled in the technique. It may be reasonable to initiate treatment with a pharmacologic agent, especially one that might avoid the systemic adverse effects of vasopressin. Sclerotherapy could then be used for patients failing the initial therapy.

Some controlled trials have shown sclerotherapy, portasystemic shunt surgery, and propranolol to have a beneficial effect in the prevention of recurrent variceal hemorrhage, and perhaps on survival, while others have failed to demonstrate efficacy. Currently, there are several studies in progress comparing two of these modalities and at least one comparing all three. At the present time, the data are insufficient to establish a treatment of choice. Currently there is no established therapy for prophylaxis against initial variceal hemorrhage.

References

1. Pitcher JL. Safety and effectiveness of the modified Sengstaken-Blakemore tube: A prospective study. *Gastroenterology* 1971; 61:291–298.
2. Hunt PS, Korman MG, Hansky J. An 8-year prospective experience with balloon tamponade in emergency control of bleeding esophageal varices. *Dig Dis Sci* 1982; 27:413–416.
3. Conn HO, Simpson JA. Excessive mortality associated with balloon tamponade of bleeding varices. *JAMA* 1967; 202:587–591.
4. Grace ND, Muench H, Chalmers TC. The present status of shunts for portal hypertension in cirrhosis. *Gastroenterology* 1966; 50:684–691.
5. Graham D, Smith JL. The course of patients after variceal hemorrhage. *Gastroenterology* 1981; 80:800–809.
6. Eckardt VF, Grace ND, Kantrowitz PA. Does lower esophageal sphincter incompetency contribute to esophageal variceal bleeding? *Gastroenterology* 1976; 71:185–189.
7. Eckhardt VF, Grace ND. Gastroesophageal reflux and bleeding esophageal varices. *Gastroenterology* 1979; 76:39–42.
8. MacDougall BRD, Williams R. Gastric acid reflux in the pathogenesis of variceal hemorrhage: A double blind trial of cimetidine treatment. *Hepatology* 1983; 3:69–73.
9. Ponce J, Froufe A, de la Morena E, et al. Morphometric study of the esophageal mucosa in cirrhotic patients with variceal bleeding. *Hepatology* 1981; 1:641–646.
10. Johnston GE. Oesophageal transection and devascularization procedures. In: Williams R, Westaby D, MacDougall BRD, eds. *Variceal Bleeding*. London: Royal Society of Medicine, 1982.
11. Viallet A, Marleau D, Huet M, et al. Hemodynamic evaluation of patients with intrahepatic portal hypertension. *Gastroenterology* 1975; 69:1297–1300.
12. Joly JG, Marleau D, Legare A, et al. Bleeding from esophageal varices in cirrhosis of the liver: Hemodynamic and radiologic criteria for the selection of potential bleeders through hepatic and umbilicoportal catheterization studies. *Can Med Assoc J* 1971; 104:576–580.
13. Garcia-Tsao G, Groszmann RJ, Fisher RL, et al. Portal pressure, presence of gastroesophageal varices and variceal bleeding. *Hepatology* 1985; 5:419–424.
14. Lebrec D, DeFleury P, Rueff B, et al. Portal hypertension, size of esophageal varices and risk of gastrointestinal bleeding in alcoholic cirrhosis. *Gastroenterology* 1980; 79:1139–1144.
15. Grace ND, Matloff DS, Bermann MM, et al. Is variceal hemorrhage related to variceal size or portal pressure? *Gastroenterology* 1986; 90:1729(A).
16. Vinel JP, Cassigneul J, Levade M, et al. Assessment of short term prognosis after variceal bleeding in patients with alcoholic cirrhosis by early measurement of portohepatic gradient. *Hepatology* 1986; 6:116–117.
17. Vinel JP, Cassigneul J, Louis A, et al. Clinical and prognostic significance of portohepatic gradient in patients with cirrhosis. *Surg Gynecol Obstet* 1982; 155:347–352.
18. Snady H, Feinman L. Prediction of variceal hemorrhage—a prospective study. *Gastroenterology* 1987; 92:1648(A).
19. Groszmann RJ. Reassessing portal venous pressure measurements. *Gastroenterology* 1984; 80:1611–1617.
20. Polio J, Groszmann RJ. Hemodynamic factors involved in the development and rupture of esophageal varices: A pathophysiologic approach to treatment. *Semin Liver Dis* 1986; 6:318–331.
21. Staritz M, Poralla T, Meyer Zum Buschenfelde KH. Intravascular oesoghageal variceal pressure (10 VP) assessed by endoscopic fine needle puncture under basal conditions, Valsalva's manoeuver and after glyceryl trinitrate application. *Gut* 1985; 26:525–530.
22. Gertsch PH, Bohnet J, Mosimann R. Endoscopic non-aggressive assessment of oesophageal variceal pressure compared with wedged hepatic venous pressure in alcoholic liver cirrhosis. *Endoscopy* 1983; 15:101–103.
23. Dawson J, Gertsch PH, Mosimann R, et al. Endoscopic variceal pressure measurements. Response to isosorbide dinitrate. *Gut* 1985; 26:843–847.
24. Leonard R, Polio J, Vogel G, et al. An improved pressure sensitive capsule for the endoscopic measurement of esophageal variceal pressure. *Gastroenterology* 1987; 92:1501(A).

25. Lebrec D, Bataille C, Bercoff E, et al. Hemodynamic changes in patients with portal venous obstruction. *Hepatology* 1983; 3:530–553.
26. Murray JF, Dawson AM, Sherlock S. Circulatory changes in chronic liver disease. *Am J Med* 1958; 24:358–367.
27. Barr JW, Lakin RC, Rosch J. Similarity of arterial and intravenous vasopressin on portal and systemic hemodynamics. *Gastroenterology* 1975; 69:13–19.
28. Groszmann RJ, Kravetz D, Bosch J, et al. Nitroglycerin improves the hemodynamic response to vasopressin in portal hypertension. *Hepatolgy* 1982; 2:757–762.
29. Rector WG. Drug therapy for portal hypertension. *Ann Intern Med* 1986; 105:96–107.
30. Cash JD, Gader AM, DaCosta J. The release of plasminogen activator and factor VIII to lysine vasopressin, arginine vasopressin, I-desamino-8-d-arginine vasopressin, angiotensin and oxytocin in man. *Br J Hematol* 1974; 27:363–364.
31. Blei AT, Groszmann RJ, Gusberg R, et al. Comparison of vasopressin and triglycyl-lysine vasopressin on splanchnic and systemic hemodynamics in dogs. *Dig Dis Sci* 1980; 25:688–694.
32. Bosch J, Kravetz D, Rodes J. Effects of somatostatin on hepatic and systemic hemodynamics in patients with cirrhosis of the liver: Comparison with vasopressin. *Gastroenterology* 1981; 80:518–525.
33. Barbare JC, Poupon R, Jaillen P, et al. The influence of vasoactive agents on metabolic activity of the liver in cirrhosis: A study of the effects of posterior pituitary extract, vasopressin, and somatostatin. *Hepatology* 1984; 4:59–62.
34. Lebrec D, Hillon P, Munoz C, et al. The effect of propranolol on portal hypertension in patients with cirrhosis: A hemodynamic study. *Hepatology* 1982; 5:523–527.
35. Hillon P, Lebrec D, Munoz C, et al. Comparison of the effects of a cardioselective and a nonselective β blocker on portal hypertension in patients with cirrhosis. *Hepatology* 1982; 2:528–531.
36. Garcia-Tsao G, Grace ND, Groszmann RJ, et al. Short-term effects of propranolol on portal venous pressure. *Hepatology* 1986; 6:101–106.
37. Bathal PS, Grossman HJ. Contractile fibroblasts in the pathogenesis of cirrhotic portal hypertension. *Hepatology* 1982; 2:155(A).
38. Blei AT, Gottstein J. Isosorbide dinitrate in experimental portal hypertension: A study of factors that modulate the hemodynamic response. *Hepatology* 1986; 6:107–111.
39. Freeman JG, Barton JR, Record CO. Effect of isosorbide dinitrate, verapamil, and labetalol on portal pressure in cirrhosis. *Br Med J* 1985; 291:561–562.
40. Gelman S, Ernst EA. Hepatic circulation during sodium nitroprusside infusion in the dog. *Anesthesiology* 1978; 49:182–187.
41. Mills PR, Rae AP, Farah DA, et al. Comparison of three adrenoreceptor blocking agents in patients with cirrhosis and portal hypertension. *Gut* 1984; 25:73–78.
42. Willett IR, Esler M, Jennings G, et al. Sympathetic tone modulates portal venous pressure in alcoholic cirrhosis. *Lancet* 1986; 2:939–943.
43. Moreau R, Lee SS, Nadengue A, et al. Hemodynamic effects of a clonidine-induced disease in sympathetic tone in patients with cirrhosis. *Hepatology* 1987; 7:149–154.
44. Reichen J, Hirlinger A, Ho HR, et al. Chronic verapamil administration lowers portal pressure and improves hepatic function in rats with liver cirrhosis. *J Hepatol* 1986; 3:49–58.
45. Kong CW, Lay CS, Tsai YT, et al. The hemodynamics effect of verapamil on portal hypertension in patients with postnecrotic cirrhosis. *Hepatology* 1986; 6:423–426.
46. Baum S, Nussbaum M. The control of gastrointestinal hemorrhage by selective mesenteric arterial infusion of vasopressin. *Radiology* 1971; 98:497–505.
47. Conn HO, Ramsby GR, Storer EM, et al. Intra-arterial vasopressin in the treatment of upper gastrointestinal hemorrhage: a prospective controlled trial. *Gastroenterology* 1975; 68:211–221.
48. Mallory A, Schaefer JW, Cohen JR, et al. Selective intra-arterial vasopressin infusion for upper gastrointestinal tract hemorrhage: A controlled trial. *Arch Surg* 1980; 115:30–32.
49. Fogel MR, Knauer CM, Andres LL, et al. Continuous intravenous vasopressin in active upper gastrointestinal bleeding: A placebo-controlled trial. *Ann Intern Med* 1982; 96:565–569.
50. Merigan TP, Plotkin GR, Davidson CS. Effect of intravenously administered posterior pituitary extract on hemorrhage from bleeding esophageal varices. *N Engl J Med* 1962; 266:134–135.
51. Johnson WC, Widrich WC, Ansell JE, et al. Control of bleeding varices by vasopressin: A prospective study. *Ann Surg* 1977; 186:369–376.
52. Chojkier M, Groszmann RJ, Atterbury CE, et al. A controlled comparison of continuous intra-arterial and intravenous infusions of vasopressin in hemorrhage from esophageal varices. *Gastroenterology* 1979; 77:540–546.
53. Clanet J, Tournet R, Fourtainier G, et al. Traitment par la pitressine des hemorrhagies par rupture de varices oesophagiennes chez le cirrhotique. Etude controles. *Acta Gastroenterol Belg* 1978; 41:539–543.
54. Freeman JG, Cobden I, Lishman AH, et al. Controlled trial of terlipressin (glypressin) versus vasopressin in the early treatment of oesophageal varices. *Lancet* 1982; 2:66–68.
55. Walker S, Stiehl A, Raedsch R, et al. Terlipressin in bleeding esophageal varices: A placebo-controlled, double-blind trial. *Hepatology* 1986; 6:112–115.
56. Gimson AE, Westaby D, Hegarty J, et al. A randomized trial of vasopressin and vasopressin plus nitroglycerin in the control of acute variceal hemorrhage. *Hepatology* 1986; 6:410–413.
57. Tsai YT, Lay CS, Lai KH, et al. Controlled trial of vasopressin plus nitroglycerin vs. vasopressin alone in the treatment of bleeding esophageal varices. *Hepatology* 1986; 6:406–409.
58. Kravetz D, Bosch J, Teres J, et al. Comparison of intravenous somatostatin and vasopressin infusions in treatment of acute variceal hemorrhage. *Hepatology* 1984; 4:442–446.
59. Jenkins SA, Baxter JN, Corbett W, et al. A prospective randomized controlled clinical trial comparing somatostatin and vasopressin in controlling acute variceal hemorrhage. *Br Med J* 1985; 290:275–278.
60. Lebrec D, Poynard T, Bernuau J, et al. A randomized controlled study of propranolol for prevention of recurrent gastrointestinal bleeding in patients with cirrhosis: A final report. *Hepatology* 1984; 4:355–358.
61. Burroughs AK, Jenkins WJ, Sherlock S, et al. Controlled trial of propranolol for the prevention of recurrent variceal hemorrhage in patients with cirrhosis. *N Engl J Med* 1983; 309:1539–1543.
62. Villeneuve JP, Layrargues GM, Infante-Riuard C, et al. Propranolol for the prevention of current variceal hemorrhage: A controlled trial. *Hepatology* 1986; 6:1239–1243.
63. Gatta A, Merkel C, Sacerdoti D, et al. Controlled trial of nadolol in the recurrence of variceal hemorrhage in patients with cirrhosis. *Hepatology* 1986; 6:788(A).

64. O'Connor KW, Lumeng L, Christiansen PA, et al. Propranolol therapy vs. two forms of sclerotherapy for variceal bleeding: 2nd report of a randomized prospective trial. *Gastrointest Endosc* 1985; 31:151(A).

65. Alexandrino P, Alves M, Correia JP. Controlled trial of propranolol and endoscopic sclerotherapy in the recurrence of variceal bleeding. *Hepatology* 1985; 5:990(A).

66. Fleig WE, Stange EF, Hunecke R, et al. Prevention of recurrent bleeding in cirrhotics with recent variceal hemorrhage: prospective, randomized comparison of propranolol and sclerotherapy. *Hepatology* 1987; 7:355–361.

67. Dollet JM, Champigneulle B, Evangelista M, et al. Sclerotherapy versus propranolol after first variceal hemorrhage in alcoholic cirrhosis. *Lancet* 1985; 2:97(LE).

68. Westaby D, Polson RJ, Gimson AFS, et al. Propranolol—A primary role for the prevention of recurrent variceal bleeding in compensated cirrhosis. *Hepatology,* 1987; 7:1030(A).

69. Westaby D, Melia WM, MacDougal BRD, et al. β1 selective adrenoceptor blockade for the long-term management of variceal bleeding. A prospective randomized trial to compare oral metoprolol with injection sclerotherapy in cirrhosis. *Gut* 1985; 26:421–425.

70. Pascal JP, Cales P, and a multicenter study group. Propranolol in the prevention of first upper gastrointestinal tract hemorrhage in patients with cirrhosis of the liver and esophageal varices. *N Engl J Med* 1987; 317:856–861.

71. Pagliaro L, Pasta L, D'Amico G, et al. A randomized clinical trial of propranolol for the prevention of initial bleeding in cirrhosis with portal hypertension. *N Engl J Med* 1986; 314:244–245(LE).

72. Ideo G, Grimoldi D, Fesce E, et al. Nadolol prevents the first variceal bleeding in cirrhotics. *Hepatology* 1986; 6:788(A).

73. Lebrec D, Poynard T, Capron JP, et al. A randomized trial of nadolol for prevention of gastrointestinal bleeding in patients with cirrhosis. Results at one year. *Hepatology* 1986; 6:788(A).

Editorial Comment

Although Chapter 13C of this volume emphasizes the use of emergency portacaval shunt in the treatment of variceal hemorrhage and has presented data that in the long-term follow-up are probably comparable in terms of mortality, rebleeding, and complication rate to other invasive and noninvasive approaches to this often disastrous problem of massive upper gastrointestinal hemorrhage secondary to portal hypertension, Dr. Grace has analyzed in some detail one of the alternative and noninvasive approaches to the control of hemorrhage.

In his analysis, Grace has emphasized particularly the utilization of vasopressin—a posterior pituitary hormone—which has been shown to diminish mesenteric arterial blood flow, thus decreasing the portal venous flow and pressure.

Despite the obvious appeal of a noninvasive pharmacologic approach, Dr. Grace's thoughtful analysis of the literature would certainly support the statement that none of the studies utilizing vasopressin alone showed any improvement in survival as compared with other therapeutic modalities. Dr. Grace has emphasized the major problems in the use of vasopressin, which emphasize the ineffectiveness of the response in almost half of the patients, a significant late rebleeding rate, significant systemic complications including those related to insufficiency of coronary flow, and, finally, the fact that no improvement in survival has been demonstrated. Other less widely known or utilized agents such as terlipressin, nitroglycerin, and somatostatin have also been analyzed, although many of the drugs that Dr. Grace referred to in passing have not been utilized in any randomized control fashion as yet.

Another important aspect of pharmacologic therapy of portal hypertension has been the interest that Lebrec's report on the prophylactic use of propranolol (reference 60 in Chapter 12C.1) has raised among those interested in this area. Again, this thoughtful analysis by Grace gives us a solid statistical base for maintaining some reservations about the effectiveness of this drug in long-term and prophylactic usage. Certainly, further investigation and studies are needed.

The final summary and conclusion of this chapter is excellent in terms of analysis and discouraging in terms of hope for improved therapy. At the time of writing, it is clear the data are insufficient to establish a solid choice for emergency treatment of variceal hemorrhage and as yet, there is no established therapy for prophylaxis against initial variceal hemorrhage.

Discouraging as this conclusion may be, it is certainly better to have a solid base that we can analyze for future introductions for therapy and modifications of existing methods.

Chapter 13B
Injection Sclerotherapy for Bleeding Esophageal Varices

JOHN TERBLANCHE

Sclerosis of varices was suggested by Walters of the Mayo Clinic in 1933 (1) and first used in a patient by Crafoord and Frenckner in 1936. This case report appeared in 1939 (2), and was soon followed by the pioneering work of Moersch (3) and Patterson and Rouse (4) in the United States in the early 1940s. The excellent results reported by Macbeth of Oxford in 1955 (5) tended to be overshadowed by the advent of portacaval shunting at that time. Renewed interest in sclerotherapy was stimulated by the report of Johnston and Rodgers from Belfast in 1973 (6). All of these workers used rigid endoscopes and intravariceal injections. Meanwhile, in Europe, Wodak, who was followed by Paquet, introduced a successful paravariceal or submucosal injection technique with a rigid endoscope (7,8). The preliminary results of the first controlled trial comparing sclerotherapy with medical management were published by the Cape Town group in 1979 (9). This, together with reports on the use of sclerotherapy for the management of acute variceal bleeding (10–15), led to a resurgence of interest in sclerotherapy in the early 1980s (16).

Several technical variants of sclerotherapy are available. The most common is a freehand intravariceal injection technique using a flexible endoscope without an anesthetic, injecting either ethanolamine oleate or sodium morrhuate. There is a considerable body of opinion in Europe that prefers a paravariceal (submucosal) injection technique using polidocanol. Studies in the 1980s have also evaluated combined intra- and paravariceal injection techniques with various sclerosants.

Sclerotherapy has become an established part of the management of acute variceal bleeding when hemorrhage does not respond to simple conservative measures. Sclerotherapy is also being widely evaluated as a form of therapy for the long-term management of patients after a variceal bleed. An ongoing controversy is whether sclerotherapy improves patient survival (17). In the 1980s interest has also focused on the use of sclerotherapy for prophylaxis in patients who had not yet bled from varices.

Technical Variants of Sclerotherapy

A variety of described techniques appear to be equally effective. Controlled trials are required to determine the best technique. Intending sclerotherapists are advised to learn one well-established technique and to apply it to their patients. This is best achieved by a period of observation and "hands-on" learning in a unit with an active and successful sclerotherapy program.

Rigid or Flexible Endoscope

Although the pioneers used rigid endoscopes (2–6,9,13) most groups have converted to the use of modern flexible fiberoptic endoscopes (11,12,14, 15). The members of the Cape Town group believe that the rigid endoscope still has a limited but important role in the management of some patients with acute variceal bleeding. This view is supported by other major groups (18–20).

The rigid endoscope technique requires special technical skill with the patient under general anesthesia. Despite these disadvantages there are specific advantages. The Cape Town group has used a modified wide-bore rigid 50-centimeter Negus's esophagoscope with a slot at the distal end (Fig. 13B.1). Once the endoscope has been passed

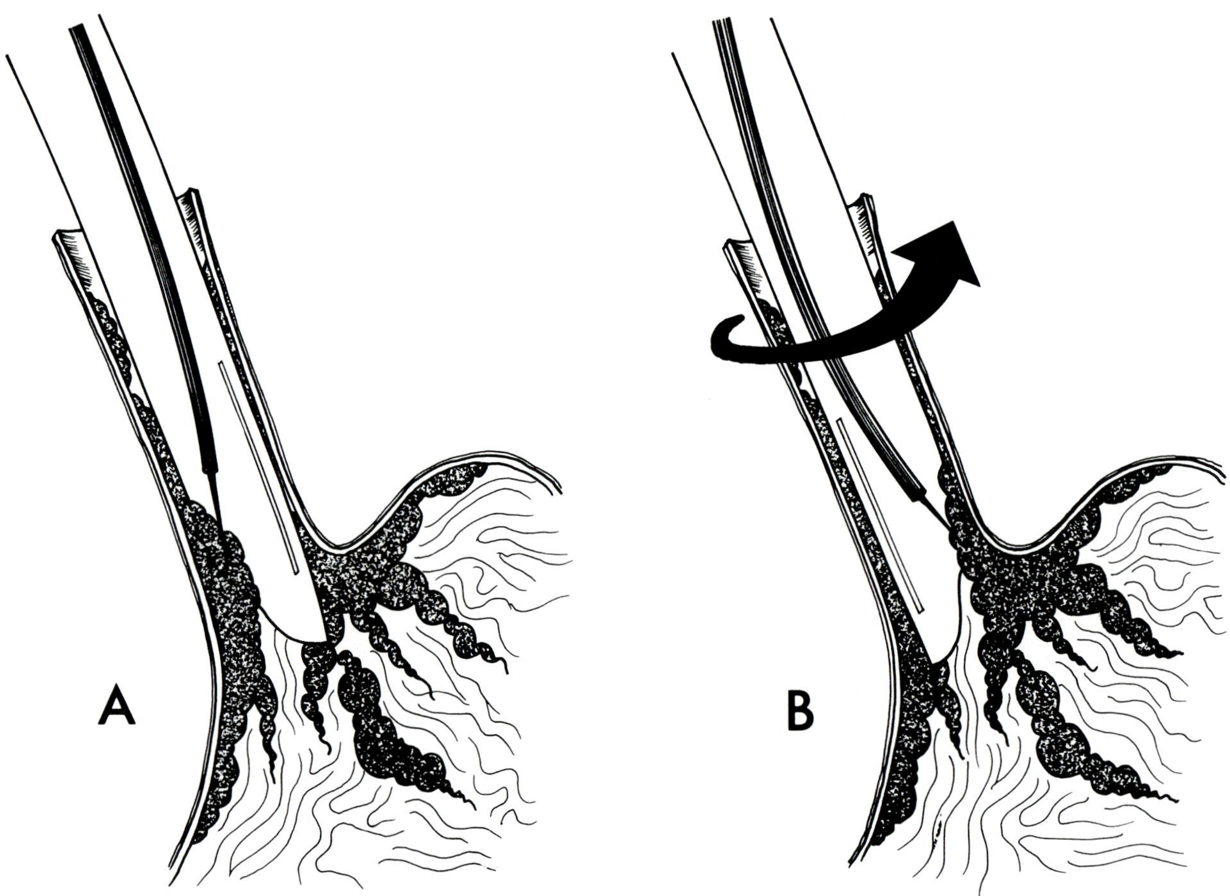

Figure 13B.1. Lower esophagus and upper stomach with the rigid Negus's esophagoscope (modified with a slot) in position in the lower esophagus. (*A*) Injection of the first varix. (*B*) Rotation of scope to compress the first varix while injecting next varix.

to the esophagogastric junction a single varix projects into the slot at the distal end facilitating injection, while the other varices are simultaneously compressed (Fig. 13B.1A). After injection, immediate rotation of the scope compresses the injected varix while the next varix presents in the slot ready for injection (Fig. 13B.1B). If bleeding recurs, it is easily controlled by compression and the scope's proximal fiber lighting does not become obscured. Suction is facilitated by the wide lumen of the endoscope (21). Several other rigid endoscopes are available and in use. The rigid Storz's scope with the excellent view produced by the Hopkins's optical system is favored by Paquet for paravariceal injection (19) and by Johnson of Sheffield for intravariceal injection (20).

The majority of sclerotherapists use the newer model, twin-channel flexible fiberoptic endoscopes, for freehand intravariceal injections (Fig. 13B.2). Modifications with proximal or distal balloons or combinations of balloons have been advocated but are seldom used today (12,14). The flexible outer sheath for use with a flexible scope (Fig. 13B.3), developed by the group at King's College Hospital, London, has been advocated and is said to provide some of the advantages of the rigid endoscope (11,15). A recent controlled trial concluded that the sheath was only marginally better than freehand injections in eradicating varices and preventing early rebleeds in long-term management (22). This together with the disadvantage of its discomfort if used with local anes-

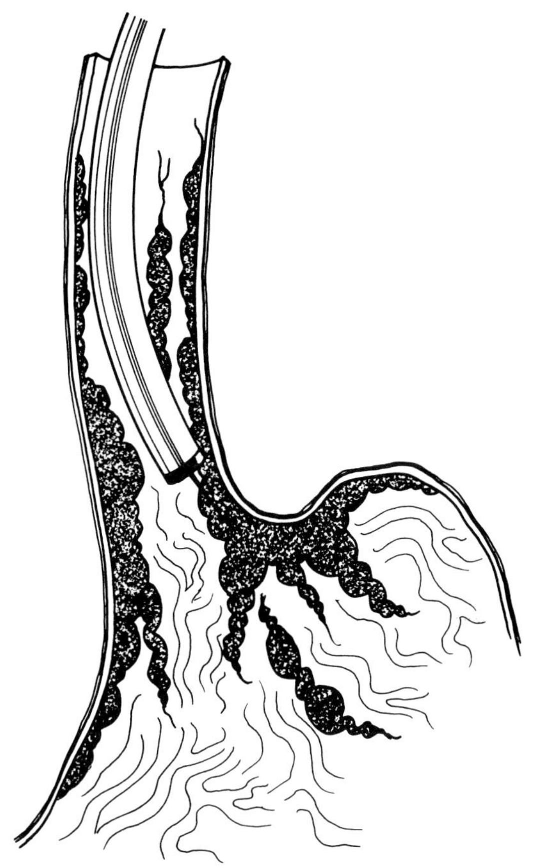

Figure 13B.2. Intravariceal injection with the flexible fiber-optic endoscope—freehand technique.

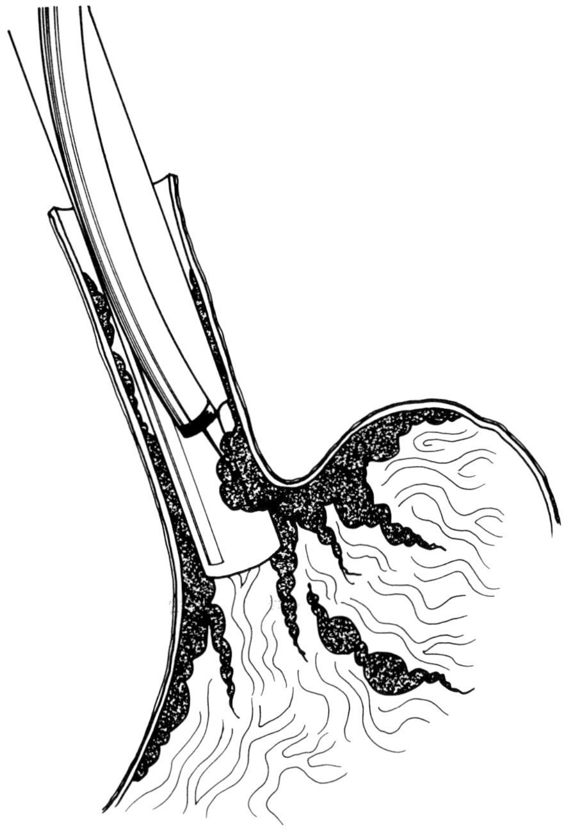

Figure 13B.3. Intravariceal injection with the flexible fiber-optic endoscope—oversheath technique (see ref. 11).

thetic or the need for a general anesthetic has prevented its widespread adoption.

Intravariceal or Paravariceal Injection

The original and most widely used technique is intravariceal injection (see Figs. 13B.1.–13B.3.). The aim is to thrombose the varices and thereby prevent further bleeding. In the paravariceal injection technique the sclerosant is injected submucosally adjacent to the varices (Fig. 13B.4)(19). Initially edema and swelling compress the variceal channels thereby controlling acute variceal bleeding. In the long term it produces thickening of the mucosa and submucosa preventing recurrent bleeds (19). Our group and others have described a third technique combining intravariceal and paravariceal injections (Fig. 13B.5) (23,24). The aim is to combine the advantages of both techniques. Recent work has questioned whether truly intravari-

ceal or truly paravariceal injections are always possible (25). The author's group currently favors an intravariceal technique but would combine this with paravariceal injections to control a local bleeding point.

Type, Volume, and Site of Injection of Sclerosant

The best sclerosant and optimal volume of each sclerosant to use is as yet unproven. Although sclerosants can be assessed in newly developed animal models (26,27), final assessment will have to be undertaken in controlled trials in humans.

The most widely used sclerosants for intravariceal injections have been ethanolamine oleate 5% and sodium morrhuate 5%. The author's group injects 6 to 8 milliliters of ethanolamine oleate into each varix as it presents in the slot in their rigid scope technique (see Fig. 13B.1) (21). Usually three

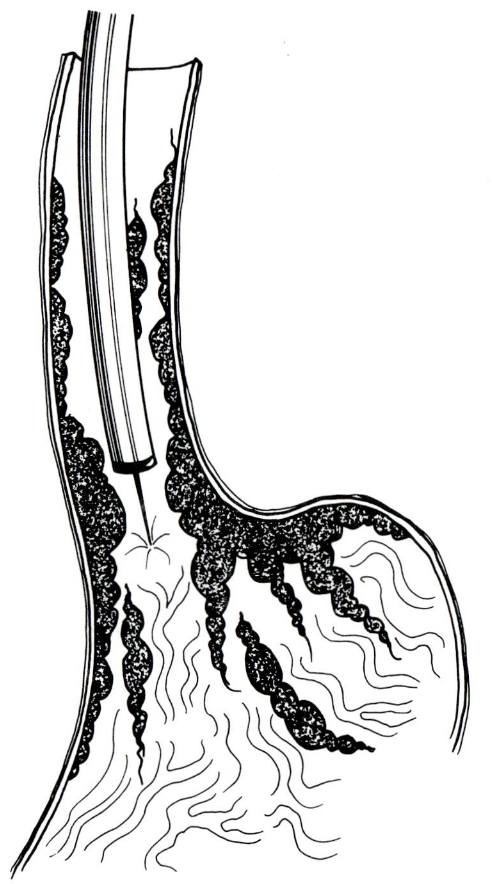

Figure 13B.4. Paravariceal injection with the flexible fiberoptic endoscope—freehand technique.

or four varices require injection, with a total of 18 to 24 ml being injected at the initial session. Lesser volumes are frequently required at subsequent injection sessions. Using the fiberoptic scope for freehand injections (see Fig. 13B.2), between 4 and 6 ml is injected per varix. With sodium morrhuate the amount should probably be limited to 4 to 6 ml per varix. Tetradecal (STD) may be too irritant if injected outside the varix and should not be used, although Rose and others have used it with success (25). Most authorities accept that intravariceal injections can be limited to the esophagogastric junction area only and need not be repeated up the length of the esophagus as was proposed originally.

The most commonly used solution for paravariceal injection (see Fig. 13B.4) is polidoconal. Paquet commences at the esophagogastric junction and injects 0.5 to 1.5 ml of 0.5% to 1% polidoconal

into each site between the varices. The procedure is repeated between 30 and 50 times while progressing proximally up the esophagus in a helical fashion, producing wheals at each injection site (19). Others have used a more concentrated solution of polidoconal but this has been associated with a high incidence of slough and stenosis (28).

In the combined intravariceal and paravariceal technique in Cape Town (see Fig. 13B.5) ethanolamine oleate has been used with injections limited to the esophagogastric junction only. One to 2 ml is injected into each submucosal site between the varices and 2 to 3 ml into each variceal channel (23). Today our group would use a greater volume injected into the varices. Soehendra and coworkers (24) have used 1% polidoconal for combined injections localized to the esophagogastric junction. They believe that initial perivascular injection compresses the varix, making subsequent intravariceal injection more effective in producing thrombosis of the compressed varix. They use a total of 60 ml of polidoconal at each session.

Injection Sclerotherapy for Acute Variceal Bleeding

Initial Management

Early management policy is discussed in Chapter 13A. The arguments for the policy used in Cape Town in the past have been presented in detail elsewhere (29,30). Patients with suspected variceal bleeding must be admitted to hospital and preferably managed in an intensive care unit. They are best treated in a unit with a special interest in liver disease. Standard resuscitation should include the use of fresh blood or blood components and fresh frozen plasma. Other supportive treatment is used as required. The cause of portal hypertension may be known from previous investigations. If not, detailed evaluation of etiology should be delayed until the initial hemorrhage has been controlled.

PHARMACOLOGIC MANAGEMENT

A continuous intravenous infusion of vasopressin with or without the addition of nitroglycerin has remained the mainstay of pharmacologic therapy to lower portal pressure. The hope is that this will control or reduce acute variceal bleeding. The only other pharmacologic agents shown to be of value in acute variceal bleeding to date are the synthetic vasopressin analogue, glypressin, and somatostatin, which are expensive and still under investigation.

EMERGENCY ENDOSCOPY AND SENGSTAKEN BALLOON TUBE TAMPONADE

Emergency fiberoptic endoscopy is essential in patients with massive upper gastrointestinal hemorrhage suspected to be due to varices. First, it will exclude those patients who do not have varices. Panendoscopy is required in patients who have varices to rule out another cause of bleeding in the stomach or duodenum. This is not always easy and is sometimes impossible when active bleeding or a large amount of blood clot is present in the stomach or esophagus. Despite these difficulties most patients with varices can be separated into one of three groups: those actively bleeding from varices, those with varices that have stopped bleeding, and those with varices who are bleeding from another lesion. In two prospective trials at our institution approximately one-third of patients fell into each of these three groups at the time of their index bleed (31,32). Patients with varices who are bleeding from another lesion, such as a peptic ulcer, are managed along the usual lines. When variceal bleeding is excessive at the time of emergency endoscopy, a Sengstaken balloon tube is inserted. The details of the use of the Sengstaken tube have been described elsewhere (21). We inflate the gastric balloon with 200 ml of air and hold this tightly in place against the esophagogastric junction by using a split tennis ball attached to the tube at the patient's mouth. In all uncooperative or stuperose patients, the airway should be protected by inserting an endotracheal tube prior to passing the Sengstaken tube.

Emergency Injection Sclerotherapy

This may be performed at the time of the emergency endoscopy or as a delayed urgent procedure the following day.

IMMEDIATE SCLEROTHERAPY

A major proponent of immediate sclerotherapy has been Lewis (33). Lewis emphasized that visualization at the time of the first endoscopy can be improved and the safety enhanced if the head of the bed is well raised and the stomach lavaged. Lewis injects sodium morrhuate intravariceally immediately proximal to the bleeding point at the commencement of the endoscopy. Once the bleeding has been controlled the diagnostic endoscopy is completed and all other variceal channels injected. The alternative paravariceal injection technique has also been successfully used at the time of the emergency endoscopy by Paquet in 81% of patients over a 4-year period (19). The present author recommends immediate sclerotherapy at the time of emergency endoscopy if the expertise is available and if it can be performed safely.

ALTERNATIVE OPTIONS

If the expertise for immediate sclerotherapy is not available and the patient has stopped bleeding, early sclerotherapy is advocated the following day. For those patients with active variceal bleeding, the Cape Town group has used a Sengstaken tube to control bleeding (21) while the patient is being resuscitated prior to urgent sclerotherapy (31). Successful control of variceal bleeding has been reported in over 90% of patients by a number of groups using different techniques (6,18,19,24,28, 31). Intravariceal, paravariceal, and combined injection techniques have all been used successfully.

CAPE TOWN RESULTS

All three techniques of sclerotherapy have been evaluated in Cape Town. The first study was a 5-year evaluation of combined balloon tube tamponade and sclerotherapy for patients with continued active variceal bleeding. Ethanolamine oleate was used for intravariceal injection via the rigid endoscope under general anesthesia. Sixty-six of 143 patients admitted during the 5-year trial period had balloon tube tamponade and were referred for injection sclerotherapy during at least one admission. They were admitted 93 times with episodes of continued active variceal hemorrhage and definitive control of variceal bleeding was achieved in 88 (95%) of the 93 admissions. A single injection was successful in 70% of patients while 22% required two or more injections. The mortality per hospital admission was 28% with no deaths directly attributable to uncontrolled continued variceal hemorrhage. Most deaths were due to end-stage liver failure, often contributed to by acute variceal bleeds (31). These results compare favorably with those of our previous prospective study of the use of the Sengstaken tube alone in patients with continued variceal bleeding. In this study the admission mortality was 60% and definitive control of variceal hemorrhage was only achieved in 40% of patients (32). We concluded that, although a correctly placed Sengstaken tube temporarily controls acute variceal bleeding, the addition of sclerotherapy is required to achieve definitive control of hemorrhage and improve survival (31).

Our second study has recently been completed (unpublished data). This prospective randomized controlled clinical trial was commenced in mid-1981 and designed to compare our previously used rigid endoscope intravariceal injection technique (see Fig. 13B.1) with a combined paravariceal and intravariceal technique using the flexible endoscope without an anesthetic (see Fig. 13B.5). In this combined technique 1 to 2 ml of ethanolamine oleate was injected into each submucosal site between the varices and 2 to 3 ml into each variceal channel in the lower esophagus immediately above the esophagogastric junction. A preliminary analysis of the index bleed admission, when 49 patients had been randomized, demonstrated over 90% control of variceal bleeding in both trial groups. Mortality was higher than in our previous study. This was probably related to a greater number of poor-risk Child's group C alcoholic cirrhotic patients being included in the new trial. We have concluded that in our hands both the rigid and the flexible endoscope techniques effectively control variceal bleeding in a population of poor-risk, predominantly alcoholic cirrhotic patients with continued variceal bleeding. In both groups sclerotherapy was performed after a period of Sengstaken tube intubation and resuscitation. The rigid scope appeared to have an advantage in the more difficult patients and in those who rebled during the injection procedure. Here the situation is easier to control with a rigid endoscope (unpublished data).

We have had a brief 6-month experience evaluating the paravariceal technique of Paquet using polidocanol as sclerosant in a nontrial situation. In our hands there was a relatively high incidence of mucosal ulceration and complications, and we have thus reverted to a predominantly intravari-

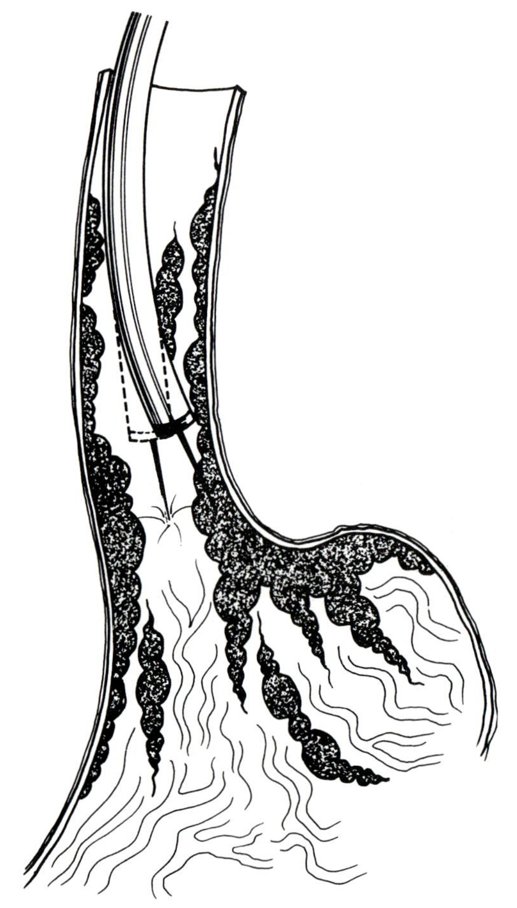

Figure 13B.5. Combined intravariceal and paravariceal injection with the flexible fiberoptic endoscope—the Cape Town technique with injections localized to the esophagogastric junction.

ceal technique using ethanolamine oleate and a flexible fiberoptic endoscope.

Current Cape Town Policy for Acute Variceal Bleeding

Patients with suspected variceal bleeding are admitted to hospital and resuscitated. A continuous intravenous infusion of pitressin, 0.4 units per minute, is commenced. Emergency endoscopy is performed on a 24-hour call basis, some 4 to 6 hours after the patient has been admitted to hospital. Where possible, sclerotherapy is performed at the time of the emergency endoscopy when variceal bleeding is diagnosed. If technical expertise is not available at that time, or if the patient is actively bleeding from varices, emergency sclerotherapy is delayed. A Sengstaken tube is only inserted in those patients who have active variceal bleeding and only these patients go on to have rigid endoscopic sclerotherapy under general anesthetic. All other patients are injected with the fiberoptic scope. Irrespective of whether a rigid or a fiberoptic scope technique is used, an intravariceal injection is currently preferred. Local paravariceal injection is added if there is bleeding at the time of endoscopy using the fiberoptic scope. Subsequent management after successful emergency sclerotherapy can either be repeated sclerotherapy or one of the surgical techniques detailed in Chapters 13C, 14, or 15.

Results from Other Major Centers

The Belfast group have published their 25-year experience using the rigid endoscope under general anesthesia (18). They achieved control of variceal bleeding in 91.4% of 396 hospital admissions in 264 patients with a low hospital mortality (14.9%). They conclude that sclerotherapy is valuable in the control of variceal hemorrhage where bleeding continues or recurs after vasopressin or tamponade.

Paquet of West Germany has achieved a 93% control rate in 386 patients using his paravariceal sclerotherapy technique with polidoconal injected with either a flexible or a rigid endoscope. Paquet's 22% patient mortality is surprisingly low considering that 68% of the patients had decompensated cirrhosis or liver coma (19).

Other major series include Soehendra's group, who use a combined intra- and paravariceal technique. They achieved successful control in 84% of 120 patients with an in-hospital mortality of 36.7% (24). Most groups use a flexible endoscope for emergency sclerotherapy. Inokuchi, who recently reported the massive Japanese experience of the surgical treatment of esophageal varices (34), has emphasized that sclerotherapy has taken over as the first line of management in Japan for acute variceal bleeding (35).

The only published controlled trial comparing sclerotherapy with emergency portacaval shunting included 52 Child's group C predominantly alcoholic cirrhotic patients. Although this failed to show a survival advantage for sclerotherapy, sclerotherapy was less costly than shunting (36). Another evaluation has concluded that injection

sclerotherapy was the most cost-effective management for acute bleeding varices (37).

In a controlled trial, Huizinga et al. concluded that emergency or urgent esophageal transection with an autosuture stapling device was better than sclerotherapy in high-risk patients (38), but their low control rate of variceal bleeding with sclerotherapy must lay their conclusion open to criticism.

Management of the Failures of Sclerotherapy

Sclerotherapy does fail in a small percentage of patients. The problem has been to identify these patients early and to determine the most appropriate therapy. A reanalysis of our 5-year study revealed that patients who required more than two emergency injection sessions had a mortality of 66%, which reached 89% if the good-risk Child's classification A patients were excluded (39). We have therefore recommended that a further bleed after a second injection session be immediately controlled by a Sengstaken tube and that one of the emergency surgical options be instituted after the patient has been resuscitated. These surgical options are discussed in Chapters 14a, 15. In our opinion either a devascularization and/or transection procedure or a standard end-to-side portacaval shunt should be performed in this small group of patients. We do not accept that these major surgical procedures are justified on a routine basis when the lesser procedure of sclerotherapy is so successful in the majority of patients.

Sclerotherapy in Long-Term Management

In 1985, the author has reviewed the role of sclerotherapy in long-term management (17) and concluded that repeated sclerotherapy offers a simple method for preventing recurrent variceal bleeds in patients who have bled from esophageal varices. Sclerotherapy reduces the incidence of life-threatening bleeds significantly, although there is still dispute whether the procedure improves survival (17). It is the therapy currently recommended for most patients in Cape Town. The most effective technique for sclerotherapy has still to be defined.

Repeated sclerotherapy has a number of advantages when compared with the more major surgical procedures presented in Chapters 13C, 14, 15.

It is the most direct and the simplest method of dealing with esophageal varices. Morbidity and mortality are low, which is important in poor-risk Child's classification C patients. In addition, it does not affect liver function or increase the incidence of encephalopathy. Both controlled (9,15,40–43) and uncontrolled studies (7,8,12–14,18,19,24,25,44,45) have clearly demonstrated that repeated sclerotherapy eradicates esophageal varices in most patients and, once varices have been eradicated, recurrent variceal bleeding is virtually eliminated if follow-up is adequate. When varices recur, which they usually do, frequently only one or two channels reappear and the recurrent varices are easy to re-eradicate (40).

There are also a number of problems associated with repeated sclerotherapy. The underlying portal hypertension remains unaltered and varices usually recur with the passage of time. Patients therefore require life-long follow-up and repeated injections to prevent recurrent variceal bleeds. The need for repeated injections also increases the chance of complications in any individual patient. An important problem is that prior to the varices being eradicated, which usually requires several courses of injections, patients continue to have variceal bleeds (9,15,19,22,40). The main unanswered question remains whether sclerotherapy improves long-term survival. This will be addressed below in considering the results of controlled studies.

Cape Town Studies

Intravariceal, paravariceal, and combined injection techniques as well as rigid and flexible endoscopes have been evaluated. Our initial study was the first randomized trial to compare sclerotherapy with conventional medical management and was conducted over a 5-year period commencing in 1975. Seventy-five patients with endoscopically proven variceal bleeding were prospectively randomized. The details of the trial have been published (9,40). Patients randomized for sclerotherapy were injected intravariceally with ethanolamine oleate via a rigid endoscope under general anesthesia with sclerotherapy being repeated at defined intervals. Eighty percent of the patients had cirrhosis and 70% were alcoholic cirrhotics. In the sclerotherapy group, varices were eradicated in 95% after a mean of 4.6 injections and remained eradicated for a

mean of almost 2 years. When varices recurred the re-eradication was easy. There were significantly fewer recurrent variceal bleeds in the sclerotherapy group than in the control patients and all recurrent bleeds occurred prior to eradication of varices, except in five patients. Thus recurrent variceal bleeds were virtually prevented with adequate follow-up after eradication of varices. The major disappointment in the trial was that no difference in survival was shown between the two groups (40). The major cause of mortality was the underlying liver disease and complications were not a major problem. At that time we concluded that repeated sclerotherapy was a viable alternative form of management for patients who had bled from esophageal varices (40).

The next Cape Town trial extended over 3 years from 1981 to 1984 (unpublished data). Intravariceal injections using the rigid Negus endoscope under general anesthesia were compared with a new combined intra- and paravariceal technique using ethanolamine oleate injected via a flexible endoscope without anesthetic. The trial included 71 randomized patients. Preliminary analysis revealed a larger percentage of poor-risk Child's classification C patients than in our previous trial. There was no difference in survival between the two groups. However, there were less complications in the fiberoptic group and more localized injection site leaks with the rigid scope. Eradication of varices was achieved equally in the two groups but the median number of injections required to achieve eradication was greater with the fiberoptic technique (seven vs. four injections). Nevertheless the time taken to achieve eradication was the same. Although there was no clear difference in the results with the rigid or the flexible scope, we are convinced that simple fiberoptic endoscopy is the preferred treatment for repeated chronic injections.

In a subsequent nonrandomized evaluation of paravariceal injections using polidoconal and Paquet's technique, we had more complications with slough and have subsequently adopted a mainly intravariceal sclerotherapy technique using ethanolamine oleate injected via a flexible endoscope.

In a separate group of 37 adult patients with extrahepatic portal vein obstruction, repeated sclerotherapy has been evaluated prospectively using our various techniques. Eradication required more injections over a longer period than in cirrhotic patients but control of major variceal hemorrhage was satisfactory with no deaths during a 9-year study period. We have concluded that injection sclerotherapy is a valuable form of treatment for adult patients with extrahepatic portal vein obstruction (unpublished data).

Other Major Studies

The two other controlled trials comparing repeated sclerotherapy with conventional medical management have similarly shown success in eradicating esophageal varices and preventing recurrent variceal bleeding. However, in both of these trials improvement in survival has been claimed in the sclerotherapy group (15,41), although in the Copenhagen trial *overall* survival was not significantly increased by sclerotherapy (41). The differences between these trials and the Cape Town trial require evaluation. Probably the most important difference was that sclerotherapy was used for life-threatening bleeds in the control patients in Cape Town, whereas it was not part of the regime in the other two trials. A significant number of the deaths were due to variceal bleeding in one trial (15) and the data are not readily apparent in the other trial (41). The London trial included 107 patients and used intravariceal injections of ethanolamine oleate via a flexible scope with an oversheath (see Fig. 13B.3) (15) whereas the Copenhagen trial, which included 187 patients, used paravariceal injections with polidocanol via a flexible scope (see Fig. 13B.4) (41). An important question asked by the Copenhagen group was to what extent the late benefits depended on the early commencement of sclerotherapy (41). We believe that a major factor accounting for the difference in survival in these studies was the successful use of sclerotherapy to treat acute variceal bleeds in the control patients in Cape Town. Smith and Graham have argued that to improve long-term survival it is necessary to improve survival for the early period after a variceal bleed and that early survival may be the best predictor of long-term survival (46,47). A preliminary report of a controlled trial from Los Angeles (48) as well as a detailed retrospective analysis of the experience at the Mayo Clinic (49) have failed to demonstrate improved survival in patients undergoing sclerotherapy. The question of improved survival in patients undergoing sclerotherapy therefore re-

mains an open one. Nevertheless excellent results have been published in a large number of uncontrolled studies using intravariceal sclerotherapy, mainly with the fiberoptic endoscope (12,14,20, 25,44,45). The long-term results of paravariceal sclerotherapy have also been excellent with Paquet reporting over 50% of 1123 patients surviving for 5 years or longer with 94% follow-up (19).

Conclusions

Workers in the field would concur that repeated injection sclerotherapy is the best treatment available today for poor-risk Child's classification C grade patients. Whether repeated sclerotherapy will prove to be the best therapy for good-risk Child's classification grade A and B patients, rather than the surgical options presented in Chapters 13, 14, 15, will have to await the results of future controlled trials. Sclerotherapy is nevertheless an acceptable alternative form of therapy for all patients who have bled from varices and should be considered in any individual patient as long as the necessary expertise is available. The role of medical therapy using β-blockade was dealt with in Chapter 13A but remains unproven in the author's opinion.

Prophylactic Sclerotherapy

If patients at high risk of bleeding from varices could be defined prior to the first variceal bleed, prophylactic therapy would be justified. Paquet (50) and Beppu (51) have claimed to have identified endoscopic findings that predict the likelihood of variceal bleeding. If confirmed, prophylactic therapy should once again be evaluated. In the past, prophylactic portacaval shunts failed to improve the survival in four controlled trials.

To date two encouraging randomized controlled clinical trials have been published in which prophylactic sclerotherapy was investigated. The first was Paquet's in 1982 (50). Paquet identified a high-risk group of patients with "black points" on their varices at endoscopy and prolonged prothrombin times. Sixty-five patients were randomized, 33 to conservative treatment and 32 to repeated sclerosis. Over a 2-year period 66% of control subjects compared with 6% of sclerosed patients bled from varices and 42% died compared with 6%. In a more recently published trial, Witzel et al. (52) of Berlin randomized 109 patients with cirrhosis and varices that had not bled. Over a 25-month period 57% of the control subjects and 9% of the sclerosed patients bled, with mortality rates of 55% and 23%, respectively. Like Paquet, Witzel et al. used paravariceal injection of polidocanol with a flexible endoscope for repeated sclerotherapy. The obvious conclusion from these studies is that prophylactic sclerotherapy should be undertaken in patients with large varices or those with endoscopic stigmata of likely bleeding.

However, the author shares the concern expressed by three major groups involved in sclerotherapy in letters to the *Lancet* (53–55) following the Berlin (52) report. Two of the letters (53,54) point out that the major fallacy of the study of Witzel et al. (52) is the exceedingly high variceal bleed rate in the control subject compared with other studies. Burroughs and Hamilton also emphasized that different therapy for acute bleeding episodes may explain the improved survival after sclerotherapy in both prophylactic studies, and that the conclusion that increased survival in treated patients was due to variceal prophylactic sclerotherapy requires reexamination (53).

Prophylactic nondecompression surgery is being evaluated in a major prospective study in Japan. Preliminary data have been published in 1984 by Inokuchi (56). The data have shown a reduction in the frequency of hemorrhage but no improvement in survival rate as yet. This trial differs from the sclerotherapy trials discussed above in that there was a very much lower frequency of hemorrhage in the Japanese control patients, who were virtually all nonalcoholic cirrhotics. The ultimate results may thus not be comparable with studies from elsewhere.

At this time prophylactic therapy is unjustified outside of controlled trials. This applies to sclerotherapy, major surgical procedures, or drug therapy with propranolol or other new agents. Prophylaxis remains one of the most exciting areas of clinical investigation in portal hypertension today. Several prospective randomized trials are being undertaken as of 1985 (57).

References

1. Walters W. In Kegaries DL. Discussion. The venous plexus of the esophagus: Its pathologic and clinical significance. *Proc Staff Meet Mayo Clin* 1933; 8:163–165.
2. Crafoord C, Frenckner P. New surgical treatment of varicose veins of the oesophagus. *Acta Otolaryngol* 1939; 27:422–429.
3. Moersch HJ. Treatment of esophageal varices by infection of a sclerosing solution. *JAMA* 1947; 135:754–756.
4. Patterson CO, Rouse MO. The injection treatment of esophageal varices. *JAMA* 1946; 130:384–386.
5. Macbeth R. Treatment of oesophageal varices in portal hypertension by means of sclerosing injections. *Br Med J* 1955; 2:877–880.
6. Johnston GW, Rodgers HW. A review of 15 years experience in the use of sclerotherapy in the control of acute haemorrhage from oesophageal varices. *Br J Surg* 1973; 60:797–800.
7. Wodak EE. Akute gastrointestinale blutung. Resultate der endokopischen sklerierung von osophagusvarizen. *Schweiz Med Wochenschr* 1979; 109:591–594.
8. Paquet K-J, Oberhammer E. Sclerotherapy of bleeding oesophageal varices by means of endoscopy. *Endoscopy* 1978; 10:7–12.
9. Terblanche J, Northover JMA, Bornman PC, et al. A prospective controlled trial of sclerotherapy in the long-term management of patients after esophageal variceal bleeding. *Surg Gynecol Obstet* 1979; 148:323–333.
10. Terblanche J, Northover JMA, Bornman PC, et al. A prospective evaluation of injection sclerotherapy in the treatment of acute bleeding from esophageal varices. *Surgery* 1979; 85:239–245.
11. Williams KGD, Dawson JL. Fibreoptic injection of oesophageal varices. *Br Med J* 1979; 2:766–767.
12. Lewis J, Chung RS, Allison J. Sclerotherapy of esophageal varices. *Arch Surg* 1980; 115:476–480.
13. Palani CK, Abuabara S, Kraft AR, Jonasson O. Endoscopic sclerotherapy in acute variceal hemorrhage. *Am J Surg* 1981; 141:164–168.
14. Takase Y, Ozaki A, Orii K, Nagoshi K, Okamura T, Iwasaki Y. Injection sclerotherapy of esophageal varices for patients undergoing emergency and elective surgery. *Surgery* 1982; 92:474–479.
15. Macdougall BRD, Westaby D, Theodossi A, Dawson JL, Williams R. Increased long-term survival in variceal haemorrhage using injection sclerotherapy. Results of a controlled trial. *Lancet* 1982; 1:124–127.
16. Conn HO. Endoscopic sclerotherapy: An analysis of variants. *Hepatology* 1983; 3:769–771.
17. Terblanche J. The long-term management of patients after an oesophageal variceal bleed: The role of sclerotherapy. *Br J Surg* 1985; 72:88–90.
18. Spence RAJ, Anderson JR, Johnston GW. Twenty-five years of injection sclerotherapy for bleeding varices. *Br J Surg* 1985; 72:195–198.
19. Paquet K-J. Endoscopic paravariceal injection sclerotherapy of the esophagus—indications, technique, complications: Results of a period of 14 years. *Gastrointest Endosc* 1983; 29:310–315.
20. Johnson AG, Simms JM, Stoddard CJ. Is there a role for injection sclerotherapy in the presence of active bleeding? In: Westaby D, Macdougall BRD, Williams R, eds. *Variceal Bleeding*. London, Pitman Medical, 1982:154–159.
21. Terblanche J. Treatment of esophageal varices by injection sclerotherapy. In: Maclean LD, ed. *Advances in Surgery*, Vol 15. Chicago: Year Book Medical, 1981, pp. 257–291.
22. Westaby D, Macdougall BRD, Melia W, Theodossi A, Williams R. A prospective randomized study of two sclerotherapy techniques for esophageal varices. *Hepatology* 1983; 3:681–684.
23. Terblanche J, Bornman PC, Jonker MAT, Kirsch RE,

Saunders SJ. Injection sclerotherapy of esophageal varices. *Semin Liver Dis* 1982; 2:233–241.

24. Soehendra N, de Heer K, Kempeneers I, Runge M. Sclerotherapy of esophageal varices: Acute arrest of gastrointestinal hemorrhage or long-term therapy? *Endoscopy* 1983; 15:136–140.

25. Rose JDR, Crane MD, Smith PM. Factors affecting successful endoscopic sclerotherapy for oesophageal varices. *Gut* 1983; 24:946–949.

26. Jensen DM. Sclerosants for injection of esophageal varices. *Gastrointest Endosc* 1983; 29:315–317.

27. Jensen DM, Machicado GA, Tapia JI, et al. A reproducible canine model of esophageal varices. *Gastroenterology* 1983; 84:315–317.

28. Sorensen T, Burcharth F, Pedersen ML, Findahl F. Oesophageal stricture and dysphagia after endoscopic sclerotherapy for bleeding varices. *Gut* 1984; 25:377–473.

29. Terblanche J, Bornman PC, Kirsch RE. Sclerotherapy for bleeding esophageal varices. *Annu Rev Med* 1984; 35:83–94.

30. Terblanche J. Sclerotherapy for emergency variceal bleeding. *World J Surg* 1984; 8:653–659.

31. Terblanche J, Yakoob HI, Bornman PC, et al. Acute bleeding varices. A five-year prospective evaluation of tamponade and sclerotherapy. *Ann Surg* 1981; 194:521–530.

32. Novis BH, Duys P, Barbezat GO, Clain J, Bank S, Terblanche J. Fibreoptic endoscopy and the use of the Sengstaken tube in acute gastrointestinal haemorrhage in patients with portal hypertension and varices. *Gut* 1976; 17:258–262.

33. Lewis JW. Survival and rebleed after acute and chronic injection sclerotherapy. In: Sivak MV, ed. *Endoscopic Sclerotherapy of Esophageal Varices*. New York: Praeger, 1984, pp. 89–97.

34. Inokuchi K. Present status of surgical treatment of esophageal varices in Japan: A nationwide survey of 3588 patients. *World J Surg* 1985; 9:171–180.

35. Inokuchi K. In Discussion. Portal hypertension. In: Kirsch RE, Kruskal JB, Csomos G, Terblanche J, eds. *Liver Update 2/1985*. London: Baillière Tindall, 1985, pp. 157–196.

36. Cello JP, Grendell JH, Crass RA, et al. Endoscopic sclerotherapy versus portacaval shunt in patients with severe cirrhosis and variceal hemorrhage. *N Engl J Med* 1984; 311:1589–1594.

37. Chung R, Lewis JW. Cost of treatment of bleeding esophageal varices. *Arch Surg* 1983; 118:482–485.

38. Huizinga WKJ, Angorn IB, Baker LW. Esophageal transection versus injection sclerotherapy in the management of bleeding esophageal varices in patients at high risk. *Surg Gynecol Obstet* 1985; 160:539–546.

39. Bornman PC, Terblanche J, Kahn D, Jonker MAT, Kirsch RE. Limitations of multiple injection sclerotherapy sessions for acute variceal bleeding. *S Afr Med J* 1986; 70:34–36.

40. Terblanche J, Bornman PC, Kahn D, et al. Failure of repeated injection sclerotherapy to improve long-term survival after oesophageal variceal bleeding. A five-year prospective controlled clinical trial. *Lancet* 1983; 2:1328–1332.

41. The Copenhagen esophageal varices and sclerotherapy project. Sclerotherapy after first variceal hemorrhage in cirrhosis. A randomized multicenter trial. *N Engl J Med* 1984; 311:1594–1600.

42. Yassin YM, Shrif SM. Randomized controlled trial of injection sclerotherapy for bleeding oesophageal varices—an interim report. *Br J Surg* 1983; 14:20–22.

43. Witzel L, Wolbergs E. Prospektive kontrollierte studie einer para—und intravariкösen verödungstherapie bei ösophagusvarizen. *Schweiz Med Wochenschr* 1984; 3:681–684.

44. Harris OD, Dickey JD, Stephenson PM. Simple endoscopic injection sclerotherapy of oesophageal varices. *Aust NZ J Med* 1982; 12:131–135.

45. Sivak MV, Stout DJ, Skipper G. Endoscopic injection sclerosis (EIS) of esophageal varices. *Gastrointest Endosc* 1981; 27:52–57.

46. Smith YL, Graham DY. Variceal hemorrhage. A critical evaluation of survival analysis. *Gastroenterology* 1982; 82:968–973.

47. Graham DY, Smith YL. The course of patients after variceal hemorrhage. *Gastroenterology* 1981; 80:800–809.

48. Balart LA, Larson AW, Radvan GA, Chapman DJ, Reynolds TB. A prospective controlled trial of endoscopic sclerotherapy in variceal bleeding: Progress report. *Hepatology* 1982; 2:732.

49. DiMagno EP, Zinmeister AR, Larson DE, et al. Influence of hepatic reserve and cause of esophageal varices on survival and rebleeding before and after the introduction of sclerotherapy: A retrospective analysis. *Mayo Clin Proc* 1985; 60:149–157.

50. Paquet K-J. Prophylactic endoscopic sclerosing treatment of the esophageal wall in varices—a prospective controlled trial. *Endoscopy* 1982; 14:4–5.

51. Beppu K, Inokuchi K, Koyanagi N, et al. Prediction of variceal hemorrhage by esophageal endoscopy. *Gastrointest Endosc* 1981; 27:213–218.

52. Witzel L, Wolbergs E, Merki H. Prophylactic endoscopic sclerotherapy of oesophageal varices. A prospective controlled study. *Lancet* 1985; 1:773–775.

53. Burroughs AK, Hamilton G. Prophylactic endoscopic sclerotherapy of oesophageal varices. *Lancet* 1985; 1:1105–1106.

54. Hayes PC, Westaby D, Williams R. Prophylactic endoscopic sclerotherapy of oesophageal varices. *Lancet* 1985; 1:1106.

55. Smith PM, Rose JDR. Prophylactic endoscopic sclerotherapy of oesophageal varices. *Lancet* 1985; 1:1106.

56. Inokuchi K. Prophylactic portal nondecompression surgery in patients with esophageal varices. *Ann Surg* 1984; 200:61–65.

57. Conn H. Portal hypertension. In: Kirsch RE, Kruskal JB, Csomos G, Terblanche J, eds. *Liver Update 2/1985*. London: Baillière Tindall, 1985, pp. 157–196.

Editorial Comment

Dr. Terblanche has presented an intensive series of studies beginning in 1975 and relating to the nonsurgical variceal sclerosis approach to bleeding esophageal varices.

The data presented would make it very difficult to refute the argument that immediate sclerotherapy in patients with significant bleeding from esophageal varices is the treatment of choice in the hands of Terblanche and his group, and probably in the hands of others as skilled and experienced with this technique as they are.

Comparing these results, both short- and long-term, with those described by Orloff, in Chapter

13C of this volume, who proposes immediate emergency portacaval shunt for all patients with bleeding esophageal varices, may leave the reader of this chapter in somewhat of a dilemma, since Dr. Orloff also marshalls some impressive arguments for emergency shunt as a direct and effective method of both emergency and long-term control of bleeding esophageal varices. Certainly, if one deals with a population who are unlikely to return for successive follow-up visits and treatment, there is considerable rationale for Orloff's position.

Terblanche points out the cost-effectiveness of variceal sclerosis as compared to emergency surgery, but does not present the total package costs if one includes the accepted necessity of repeated admissions for sclerosis over many, many weeks.

Despite the obvious success of the Cape Town method, Terblanche takes the usual balanced approach to the problem of bleeding esophageal varices and suggests that the ultimate effective program may include initial emergency variceal sclerosis followed by early surgery in patients who demonstrate early and massive recurrent bleeding.

Dr. Terblanche does not recommend, on the basis of present evidence, the use of sclerosis as a prophylactic measure, and this certainly agrees with previous studies negating the usefulness of prophylactic subsurgery. Terblanche does, however, state the reservation that further studies and information in this area are necessary before one can draw definitive conclusions in the general area of prophylactic treatment.

The superb results achieved by the Cape Town group in this extraordinarily difficult field testify to the skill and judgment of the operators. Whether or not similar results can be obtained by other less experienced and dedicated groups throughout the world remains to be seen. Nonetheless, the obvious success of this method in their hands warrants work toward obtaining a comfortable degree of experience and excellence in this approach to what has long been recognized as an extraordinarily difficult clinical problem.

Chapter 13C
Emergency Surgical Treatment of Bleeding Esophagogastric Varices in Cirrhosis

MARSHALL J. ORLOFF

The most frequent cause of death from upper gastrointestinal bleeding is rupture of an esophageal or gastric varix with hemorrhage. Until recently, approximately three of four cirrhotic patients who entered the hospital with their first episode of bleeding varices failed to leave the hospital alive. Table 13C.1, which shows the results of a number of studies conducted during the past 40 years, indicates that as of 1962 the immediate mortality rate of the first variceal hemorrhage averaged 73% (1–8). From these statistics, it is apparent that the emergency treatment of bleeding esophagogastric varices is the single most important aspect of the therapy of portal hypertension.

The precipitating cause of rupture of esophageal varices is uncertain. It has been proposed that erosion of the mucosa by reflux acid-peptic esophagitis is involved. However, in a gross and microscopic study of the distal esophagus in 20 patients at the time of bleeding we found esophagitis in only 1 patient (9). Moreover, bleeding from esophageal varices has been reported in patients with proven gastric achlorhydria. The evidence strongly suggests that increased hydrostatic pressure is responsible for "blowout" rupture of esophageal varices (9,10). It is important to point out that finding esophageal or gastric varices in a patient with cirrhosis does not mean that the patient will develop bleeding. In fact, only 25% to 35% of patients with proven varices ultimately bleed from the varices (11). However, once bleeding has occurred, the patient is almost certain to bleed again, usually within a year of the first bleeding episode. The prognosis and therapeutic implications of esophagogastric varices depend on whether or not bleeding has occurred.

Emergency Diagnosis

In most patients who enter the hospital with upper gastrointestinal hemorrhage, the diagnosis of bleeding esophagogastric varices depends on affirmative answers to three questions. Does the patient have cirrhosis? Does the patient have portal hypertension and esophagogastric varices? Are the varices the site of the bleeding, rather than some other lesions such as duodenal or gastric ulcer, gastritis, or hiatus hernia? Information sufficient to answer these questions almost always can be obtained within 4 to 5 hours of the patient's admission to the hospital by means of an organized diagnostic plan that includes some or all of the following steps:

1. *History and Physical Examination.* A history of chronic alcoholism, hepatitis, jaundice, previous bleeding episodes, melena, abdominal swelling, edema, and mental abnormalities, and the absence of symptoms of peptic ulcer suggest the diagnosis of cirrhosis. The most important physical findings are hepatosplenomegaly, spider angiomas, palmar erythema, collateral abdominal veins, muscle-wasting, jaundice, ascites, edema, and neurologic signs such as tremor and asterixis. In many patients, not all these classic signs are present. Confirmation of gastrointestinal bleeding by aspiration of the stomach through a nasogastric tube and by gross and chemical examination of the stool is an essential early measure and should really be considered part of the physical examination. A nasogastric tube should be inserted in all patients.

2. *Blood Studies.* Blood samples for typing and cross-matching and for studies are drawn immedi-

Table 13C.1. Mortality Rate of First Episode of Bleeding from Esophageal Varices in Patients with Cirrhosis

Author (No.)	Year Reported	Type of Hospital	No. Patients	Mortality (%)
Ratnoff and Patek (1)	1942	Five private-teaching	106	40
Higgins (2)	1947	City indigent	45	76
Atik and Simeone (3)	1954	City indigent	59	83
Nachlas et al. (4)	1955	City indigent	102	59
Cohn and Blaisdell (5)	1958	City indigent	456	74
Taylor and Jontz (6)	1959	Veterans	102	45
Merigan et al. (8)	1960	City indigent	74	76
Orloff (8)	1962	City indigent	87	84
			Total 1031	Mean 73

ately on hospital admission. Initial studies include a complete blood count, liver function tests [indocyanine green (ICG) excretion, prothrombin, bilirubin, alkaline phosphatase, albumin, globulin, glutamic oxalacetic transaminase, glutamic pyruvic transaminase], and determinations of urea nitrogen, electrolytes, pH, arterial blood gases, and blood alcohol. In our experience, the liver function test that is most consistently abnormal and of greatest value is ICG excretion, if performed in the absence of marked jaundice and after hypovolemic shock has been corrected. The prothrombin and serum bilirubin measurements also are often abnormal. It is not unusual for the other liver function tests to be normal in the presence of advanced cirrhosis.

3. *Esophagogastroduodenoscopy.* With the development of the flexible fiberoptic esophagogastroscope, endoscopy has become a well-tolerated, relatively simple procedure that can be performed rapidly at the bedside in the emergency room. It is the best diagnostic measure for demonstrating varices in the esophagus or stomach and for determining with certainty the presence or absence of gastritis and of the uncommon Mallory-Weiss syndrome. It makes possible the diagnosis of esophagogastric varices with a high degree of confidence (12).

4. *Upper Gastrointestinal Roentgenograms.* As soon as shock is corrected and the patient's condition stabilized, it has been our practice to perform a barium contrast upper gastrointestinal series. As experience with endoscopy has grown, many workers have discontinued the use of contrast x-ray studies, but we continue to obtain roentgenographic studies following endoscopy whenever there is the slightest doubt about the diagnosis of bleeding esophagogastric varices. Roentgeno-

graphic studies are directed at determining the presence or absence not only of esophageal or gastric varices, but also of other lesions such as a duodenal ulcer, gastric ulcer, or hiatus hernia. The literature contains many statements that suggest esophageal varices are demonstrated in only 50% to 60% of patients who have them. Our experience indicates that a skillful and interested radiologist can accurately demonstrate varices at the time of bleeding in more than 90% of cirrhotic patients (Fig. 13C.1).

5. *Hepatic Vein Catheterization.* This simple procedure, which has become a routine diagnostic measure in our institution, is used to determine wedged hepatic venous pressure (WHVP), free hepatic venous pressure, and inferior vena caval pressure. Hepatic vein catheterization is done whenever there is some doubt about the diagnosis, although it does not yield information that is as important as that obtained from the other studies. WHVP accurately reflects portal pressure in the common forms of cirrhosis and establishes the diagnosis of portal hypertension with certainty.

The emergency diagnosis of bleeding esophagogastric varices has been made accurately from information obtained in these first five steps in more than 99% of our patients (8,13). It has been regularly possible to complete these diagnostic measures within 4 to 5 hours of the patient's admission to the emergency room.

6. *Splenoportography and Splenic Manometry.* Visualization of the portal venous system is not usually required for emergency diagnosis of varix hemorrhage in patients with cirrhosis. In the few patients with normal liver function in whom extrahepatic portal obstruction is suspected, splenoportography provides crucial information about the site of obstruction and patency of the portal ve-

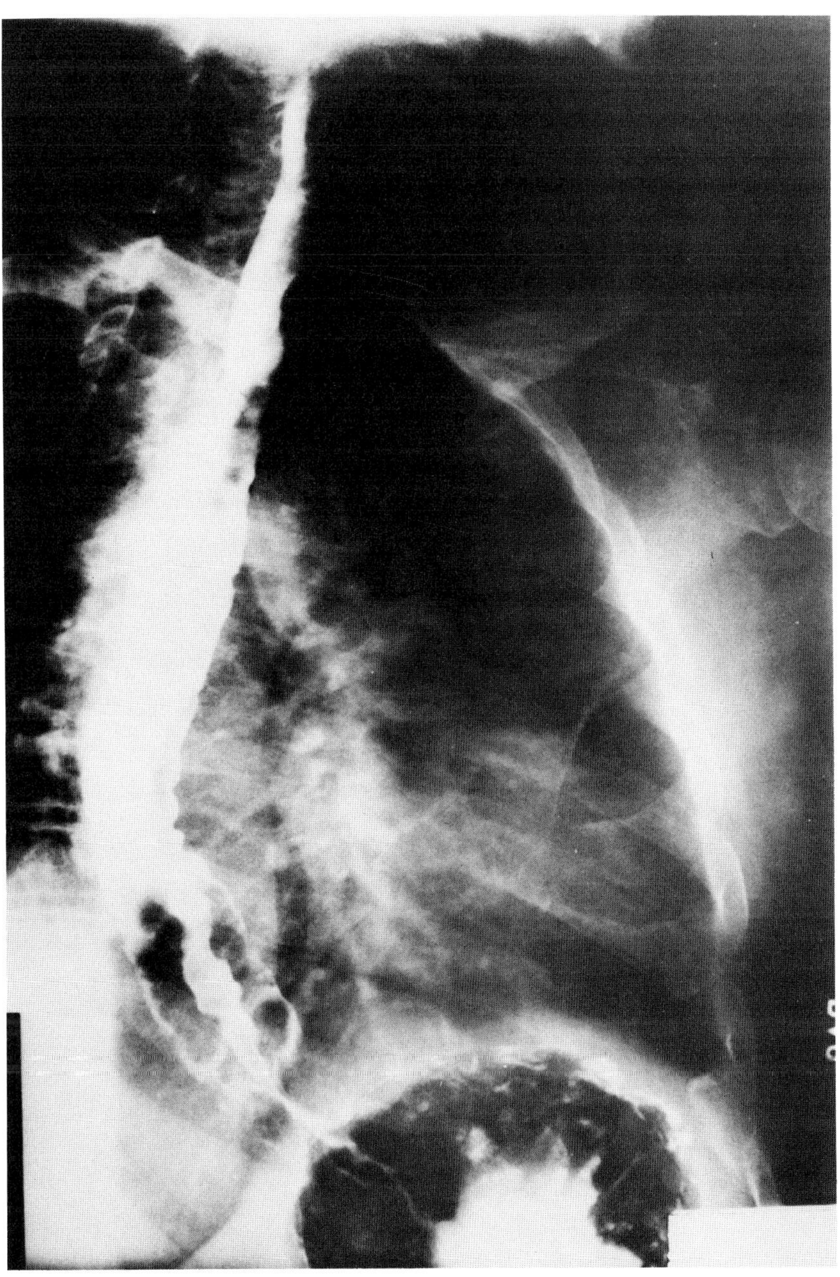

Figure 13C.1. Barium contrast upper gastrointestinal roentgenogram showing large esophageal varices. (Reproduced by permission from Orloff MJ. The liver. In: Sabiston DC, ed. *Davis-Christopher Textbook of Surgery.* Philadelphia: WB Saunders, 1981:1149–1207.)

nous system. Some years ago we regularly performed splenoportography as part of the emergency diagnostic workup in all patients. However, we discontinued use of the procedure in most patients with cirrhosis because it failed to yield information not provided by other, less invasive diagnostic tests. Splenic manometry is usually combined with splenoportography and offers an alternative to hepatic vein catheterization. If de-

sired, the splenic pulp pressure can be determined readily at the bedside by percutaneous puncture of the spleen under local anesthesia. Although this procedure does not determine the site of bleeding, it indicates the presence or absence of portal hypertension. Bleeding from esophageal varices infrequently occurs with a splenic pulp pressure below 250 millimeters of saline and rarely occurs with a pressure below 200 mm.

7. Splenic, Hepatic, Celiac, Left Gastric, and Superior Mesenteric Arteriography. Percutaneous selective catheterization and visualization of the splanchnic arteries provide interesting hemodynamic information about the status of the circulation in cirrhosis (14). With proper timing, injection of contrast media into the splenic artery or superior mesenteric artery provides delayed visualization of the portal vein and its collateral connections, a technique known as indirect portography. Arteriography and indirect portography have largely replaced splenoportography as the initial approach to visualization of the portal system because the risk and incidence of complications are somewhat lower. It is particularly useful in patients whose spleen has been removed previously. We have found that selective injection of the left gastric artery frequently produces excellent delayed visualization of esophageal varices. Selective arteriography is not an essential or routine emergency diagnostic procedure in cirrhotic patients with varix hemorrhage. After performing the procedure as a regular part of the emergency diagnostic workup in all patients over a period of seven years, we discontinued its routine use because it did not provide essential information.

Differential Diagnosis

The differential diagnosis of upper gastrointestinal bleeding in 99% of cirrhotic patients is confined to a consideration of six lesions in addition to ruptured varices. Three of these lesions, hemorrhagic gastric, duodenal ulcer, and gastric ulcer, are common. The other three lesions, gastric cancer, hiatus hernia, and the Mallory-Weiss syndrome, are infrequent causes of bleeding. Each of these conditions produces characteristic symptoms, and each can be ruled in or out by the combination of esophagogastroduodenoscopy and barium contrast upper gastrointestinal roentgenograms. Bleeding in cirrhotic patients originates from lesions other than esophagogastric varices in 20% to 25% of patients. While this statistic should serve to alert the clinician to a spectrum of etiologic considerations, it should not be interpreted as an indication that the diagnosis of varix hemorrhage is particularly complicated or cannot be made with accuracy. In point of fact, once esophagogastric varices are demonstrated, the chances that another lesion is responsible for the bleeding are not more than 10%. Furthermore, if instances of mild bleeding in cirrhotic patients with proven varices are eliminated, gastrointestinal hemorrhage will be found to arise from rupture of the varices in over 95% of patients. Thus, demonstration of esophagogastric varices in a cirrhotic patient with significant upper gastrointestinal bleeding provides overwhelming odds that the varices are the source of the hemorrhage.

General Measures of Emergency Treatment

Cirrhosis of the liver is a severe, debilitating disease with remote manifestations, only one of which is bleeding from esophagogastric varices. Death after varix rupture is frequently due to hepatic decompensation, renal failure, or infection, rather than to exsanguination. Although control of bleeding is of primary importance, the effectiveness of therapy of the underlying liver disease often determines the outcome. Therefore, there are certain general measures of treatment that apply to all patients, regardless of the specific forms of therapy used to stop the hemorrhage.

1. *Prompt Restoration of Blood Volume.* Vigorous replacement of blood loss with blood transfusions is essential. Large-bore intravenous catheters should be inserted in each arm at the start of therapy. Every effort is made to obtain fresh blood less than 12 hours old for administration because of the serious defects in coagulation associated with liver disease as well as those superimposed by multiple transfusions. Bleeding cirrhotic patients usually have thrombocytopenia in addition to abnormalities of the protein blood clotting factors. In addition, recent evidence indicates that the red blood cells of cirrhotic patients are deficient in 2,3-diphosphoglyceric acid, a substance that mediates the dissociation of oxygen from hemoglobin. The use of fresh blood has been recommended to correct the abnormality in oxygen transport. When fresh blood cannot be obtained, an acceptable alternative is the use of a combination of packed red blood cells, fresh frozen plasma, and platelet transfusions.

2. *Prevention of Hepatic Coma.* Although the nervous disorders associated with liver disease are diverse and poorly understood, the encephalopathy observed in patients with bleeding esophagogastric varices sometimes appears to be due to the absorption of large quantities of ammonia directly

into the systemic circulation through portal-systemic collateral veins. For this reason, measures directed at destroying ammonia-forming bacteria and eliminating all nitrogen from the gastrointestinal tract are initiated promptly. These include removal of blood from the stomach by lavage with iced saline through a nasogastric tube, instillation of cathartics (60 milliliters magnesium sulfate) and neomycin (4 grams) into the stomach, and thorough and repeated cleansing of the colon with enemas containing neomycin (4 grams per liter of water). The fear that insertion of a nasogastric tube will perforate the varices is unfounded, and such a tube should be placed at the start of the diagnostic workup. Although ammonia-binding agents, such as sodium glutamate and arginine, and ion exchange resins have been used, we have obtained no evidence that agents of this sort are of value.

3. *Support of the Failing Liver.* Parenterally administered hypertonic glucose solutions containing therapeutic doses of vitamins K, B, and C are included in the initial treatment regimen. Appropriate amounts of electrolytes are added to the parenteral fluids. In general, administration of sodium is avoided because patients with advanced cirrhosis usually have an increase in total body sodium and a tendency to retain salt and water.

4. *Frequent Monitoring of Vital Functions.* The usual techniques are used to determine the magnitude of bleeding and adequacy of blood volume replacement. These include measurements of vital signs, of urine output by way of an indwelling catheter, of central venous pressure by a polyethylene catheter threaded through an arm cutdown into the superior vena cava, of hematocrit, and of rate of blood loss by continuous suction through a nasogastric tube. Serial measurements of arterial blood pH and blood gases are facilitated by insertion of an indwelling catheter into the radial artery, which also makes possible continuous recordings of blood pressure. Because of the systemic circulatory abnormalities and hyperdynamic state that frequently exist in bleeding cirrhotic patients, we have added serial determinations of cardiac output by the dye dilution technique using ICG to our monitoring regimen, and occasionally we measure pulmonary artery wedge pressure by percutaneous insertion of a Swan-Ganz pulmonary artery catheter.

5. *Correction of Hypokalemia and Metabolic Alkalosis.* Most of the more than 1000 bleeding cirrhotic patients that we have studied have had significant hypokalemia and metabolic alkalosis preoperatively (15). The deleterious effects of hypokalemia are well known. In addition, alkalosis has a number of harmful consequences that include: (a) interference with the release of oxygen to the tissues by shifting the oxyhemoglobin dissociation curve to the left; (b) in combination with hypokalemia, precipitation of cardiac arrhythmias, particularly in patients taking digitalis; (c) potentiation of ammonia toxicity by elevating the tissue concentration of ammonia, and increasing the passage of ammonia across the blood-brain barrier; and (d) production of tetany by lowering the level of ionized calcium in extracellular fluid. Correction of hypokalemia and metabolic alkalosis is undertaken soon after admission to the hospital and consists of parenteral administration of large quantities of potassium chloride supplemented, occasionally, by infusion of an acidifying agent such as arginine hydrochloride or hydrochloric acid. Administration of potassium is usually required for several days in amounts occasionally as high as 500 millequivalents per day.

6. *Treatment of Hyperdynamic Cardiovascular State.* Many studies have shown that patients with cirrhosis and portal hypertension frequently have a hyperdynamic state that consists of a decrease in vascular tone and peripheral resistance, an increase in cardiac output, and an increase in venous oxygen saturation with widespread peripheral arteriovenous shunting and marked pulmonary arteriovenous admixture (16–18). These abnormalities are sometimes intensified by bleeding from esophagogastric varices or performance of a portacaval shunt, and high-output cardiac failure may develop, particularly in older patients and those with far-advanced liver disease. For this reason, we perform serial measurements of cardiac output in all patients both preoperatively and postoperatively. Patients with a hyperdynamic state and a cardiac output of 6 liters per minute or higher are digitalized over a 48-hour period, beginning preoperatively, before any signs of cardiac failure develop. Vigorous correction of hypovolemia is undertaken simultaneously. Once blood volume is restored, fluids are restricted to avoid circulatory overload, and diuretics are used if there are any signs of overhydration. Positive inotropic drugs are used when appropriate.

Specific Emergency Medical Therapy

Emergency medical treatment used specifically to stop varix bleeding includes esophageal balloon

Table 13C.2. Results of Esophageal Balloon Tamponade in Cirrhotic Patients with Bleeding Varices

Author (No.)	Year Reported	Type of Study	No. Patients	Initial Control (%)	Ultimate Control (%)	Mortality (%)
Ludington (19)	1958	Retrospective selective	58	75	43	—
Conn (20)	1958	Retrospective selective	50	70	—	82
Read et al. (21)	1960	Retrospective selective	38	84	24	74
Orloff et al. (22)	1962	Prospective unselective	45	56	20	82
Villanueva and Magnenat (23)	1964	Retrospective selective	64	64	—	69
Hermann and Traul (24)	1970	Retrospective selective	75	87	60	64
Pitcher (25)	1971	Prospective selective	50	92	82	36
Johansen and Baden (26)	1973	Retrospective selective	91	88	45	—
Novis et al. (27)	1976	Retrospective selective	42	85	46	60
Terés et al. (28)	1978	Prospective selective	79	86	38	26
Orloff et al. (29)	1986	Prospective unselective	22	52	36	64
			Total 614	Mean 76	Mean 37	Mean 59

tamponade, systemic intravenous administration of vasopressin (posterior pituitary extract), selective mesenteric intra-arterial administration of vasopressin, percutaneous transhepatic obliteration of varices, and endoscopic sclerotherapy (EST). Although each of these measures is capable of temporarily controlling bleeding varices, there is no solid evidence that they have significantly influenced the mortality rate of varix hemorrhage in cirrhotic patients. Emergency nonsurgical therapy is discussed in detail in other chapters, but I will comment briefly on the efficacy of these measures because we have conducted prospective studies of most of them.

Esophageal Balloon Tamponade

The most widely used nonoperative measure of therapy has been esophageal balloon tamponade. As shown in Table 13C.2, balloon tamponade undoubtedly stops varix bleeding initially in a large percentage of the patients in whom it is used (19–30). However, the results have been discouraging because many of the patients have resumed bleeding when the balloons were deflated. Moreover, we and others have observed frequent and sometimes lethal complications of balloon tamponade, which include perforation of the esophagus, asphyxiation from regurgitation of the balloon into the pharynx, and aspiration pneumonia (20,22,31). The ultimate mortality rate of cirrhotic patients treated by balloon tamponade is difficult to determine because most reports have failed to include such information; moreover, almost all reports have been based on retrospective reviews of the

medical records of highly selected patients. Nevertheless, no data indicate that balloon tamponade has measurably influenced the mortality rate of bleeding esophageal varices during a trial of 36 years. For these reasons, we have abandoned the use of balloon tamponade as a definitive form of treatment and use it only on infrequent occasions as a temporary measure to prepare patients for operation when massive bleeding cannot initially be controlled by other means.

Systemic Intravenous Vasopressin

In both experimental animals and humans, vasopressin (posterior pituitary extract) reduces portal pressure and blood flow by constricting the splanchnic arterioles. The response is directly related to the dose and rapidity of injection, and in the usual clinical dosage range has a duration of 1 hour or less. However, as shown in Table 13C.3, the transient reduction of portal pressure is sufficient to stop varix hemorrhage temporarily in a large percentage of patients (29,30,32,41). Unfortunately, most of the patients bleed again unless operation is performed within 8 hours of treatment, and subsequent administration of the drug is much less effective in stopping bleeding. Recently, continuous rather than bolus intravenous infusion of vasopressin in low doses has been tried in an attempt to lengthen the period of hemostasis. It is apparent, however, that vasopressin alone is not a definitive form of treatment but may be of considerable immediate value while other measures are being readied or the patient is being prepared for operation. Every patient with bleed-

Table 13C.3. Results of Systemic Intravenous Vasopressin Therapy in Cirrhotic Patients with Bleeding Varices

Author (No.)	Mode of Administration	No. Patients	No. Trials	Initial Control (%)	Ultimate Control (%)	Mortality (%)
Schwartz et al. (32)	Bolus	11	27	89	Infrequent	—
Merigan et al. (33)	Bolus	15	22	73	Infrequent	93
Shaldon and Sherlock (34)	Bolus	8	25	100	37	75
Johnson et al. (35)	Continuous infusion	11	11	64	64	45
Chojkier et al. (36)	Continuous infusion	10	10	50	30	70
Orloff et al. (37–40)	Bolus	180	180	95	Immediate operation	42
		84	84	95	Immediate operation	17
		32	32	91	Immediate operation	18
		38	38	87	18	—

ing esophageal varices is given vasopressin soon after admission to our institution. The agent is administered intravenously over a 15- to 20-minute period in a dose of 20 U of posterior pituitary extract (Pituitrin) diluted in 200 ml of solution. We have not observed any cardiac abnormalities from a single-dose bolus infusion of Pituitrin, but prolonged infusion may be hazardous in patients with coronary artery disease. Studies done in 1982 and 1984 have shown that adding nitroprusside (42) or nitroglycerin (43) to the administration of vasopressin reduces the deleterious cardiac effects of vasopressin while maintaining the beneficial reduction of portal pressure. Posterior pituitary extract (Pituitrin) is as effective in controlling bleeding as pure vasopressin. This measure of therapy has largely replaced esophageal balloon tamponade as our means of obtaining immediate control of hemorrhage.

Selective Mesenteric Intra-arterial Vasopressin

Continuous infusion of vasopressin into an indwelling catheter inserted in the superior mesenteric artery was introduced by Nusbaum et al. (44) in 1967 to control bleeding esophageal varices. Since that time, the technique has been widely used and rather uncritically accepted. The objective of the method is to obtain prolonged effects of vasopressin on the splanchnic circulation without systemic hemodynamic effects. However, a number of studies have shown that continuous selective mesenteric intra-arterial infusion of vasopressin often is accompanied by a decrease in cardiac output, a fall in femoral arterial Po_2, and a rise in arterial blood pressure, so that the systemic effects

of the drug clearly are not avoided (45,46). Moreover, portal venous Po_2 regularly falls during infusion, an undesirable side effect. Initial control of varix bleeding has been good, but it has not been superior to that obtained with much simpler and less invasive systemic intravenous administration of vasopressin (47–53). Most important, in the several prospective controlled clinical trials that have been performed recently, infusion of vasopressin into the superior mesenteric artery has been no more effective than systemic intravenous administration and has been associated with a higher incidence of complications (42,48). Moreover, it was found that mesenteric intra-arterial infusion of vasopressin failed to influence the mortality of varix hemorrhage when compared with conventional therapy. When the potential and actual complications of indwelling catheterization of the superior mesenteric artery are added to these recent findings, there is little to indicate that the selective intra-arterial technique is worthwhile.

Percutaneous Transhepatic Obliteration of Varices

From the mid-1970s to the early 1980s, some radiologists attempted to obliterate esophageal varices by percutaneous transhepatic catheterization of the portal vein and its branches and injection of blood clots, hemostatic polymers, or sclerosing solutions into the coronary vein and the varices (54–61). This method has been used in actively bleeding patients as emergency treatment, and in patients who have recovered from a bleeding episode as elective therapy. Substantial experience with the percutaneous transhepatic technique has accumulated, although many of the results reported in the literature are anecdotal. The incidence of rebleeding has been high, and there has been a substantial number of complications directly related to the procedure. Moreover, the procedure has failed to improve the survival rate of patients with varix hemorrhage. There is little question that the varices, if obliterated, will invariably recur; hence, the potential of this approach lies in the temporary control of active hemorrhage in the expectation of preparing the patient for definitive treatment. While opinion may differ on the likelihood that this technique will succeed, it is important to emphasize that it is an invasive and potentially dangerous measure that should not be widely attempted unless careful trials demonstrate its efficacy. The ultimate and essential test of any new therapeutic modality is its influence on the high mortality rate of the disease.

Endoscopic Sclerotherapy

Injection of sclerosing solutions into or around bleeding esophageal varices through an esophagoscope was first reported in 1939, but the technique was discarded in the 1950s in favor of portal-systemic shunting. In the early 1970s, however, there was a revival of EST, and currently there is widespread interest in this mode of treatment (62–75). Sclerotherapy has been used most often as emergency treatment for bleeding varices, but in the 1980s there has been increasing use of serial sclerotherapy as the sole form of long-term treatment (64,65,69,70–75).

Uncontrolled, predominantly retrospective evaluations of heterogeneous groups of selected patients indicate that emergency EST has controlled acute variceal hemorrhage in 71% to 96% of patients. Recurrent bleeding has been frequent, however, and hospital mortality rate has been substantial in patients with the types of liver disease common in the United States. Two randomized controlled trials in selected patients of long-term sclerotherapy aimed at obliterating all esophageal varices have shown a reduction in the frequency of subsequent bleeding episodes, but no improvement in survival compared to conventional medical treatment (64,68,72). To date, both the early and long-term results of EST are significantly inferior to our results of emergency portacaval shunt

Table 13C.4. Results of a 3-Year Study of Emergency and Long-term Endoscopic Sclerotherapy in 53 Unselected Patients with Cirrhosis and Bleeding Esophageal Varices— UCSD, 1983–1985

Rebleeding (%)	
After initial sclerotherapy	100
After final sclerotherapy	89
Mean emergency blood transfusions (U)	16.3
Death from rebleeding (%)	60
Portacaval shunt for rebleeding (%)	21
Follow-up as of 1986 (%)	98
Survived to leave hospital (%)	70
Currently alive (6–31 mo) (%)	33
Survivors who had portacaval shunt (%)	41
Actuarial 2-yr survival rate (%)	17

Abbreviations: UCSD, University of California, San Diego.

(EPCS) in patients with cirrhosis (see Emergency Portacaval Shunt, below).

In 1983, our division of gastroenterology undertook a study of emergency and long-term EST in unselected cirrhotic patients with bleeding esophageal varices (76). During the 3 years from 1983 through 1985, all of the patients admitted to our medical service with varix hemorrhage were treated by emergency EST, and then underwent serial EST for the long-term control of bleeding. A total of 53 patients had EST. Table 13C.4 shows the results.

All of the patients rebled from varices after emergency EST and 89% rebled after their final session of serial, long-term EST. The mean requirement of blood transfusions during the emergency period was 16.3 U. Although 70% of the patients survived to leave the hospital, 60% died from recurrent bleeding varices. Many of the survivors were alive only because a portacaval shunt was ultimately done to control the bleeding. As of 1986, only 33 percent of the group of 53 patients was alive, 6 to 31 months after the initial EST. The actuarial 2-year survival rate is only 17%, which is no different from the survival rate of 25% reported 45 years ago by Ratnoff and Patek (1), or the survival rate of 14% reported 24 years ago by the Boston Inter-Hospital Liver Group (11).

Specific Nonshunting Emergency Surgical Therapy

During the past 40 years, the widely accepted approach to the treatment of bleeding varices in patients with cirrhosis has involved the use of temporary nonsurgical emergency measures directed at stopping the hemorrhage so as to permit deliberate and methodical preparation of the patients for an elective portal-systemic shunt. This approach has been based on the belief that, on the one hand, it is often possible to stabilize and improve the underlying liver disease and, on the other hand, cirrhotic patients will not tolerate major operations performed under emergency circumstances in the face of hemorrhage. Considerable evidence indicates that this approach has not substantially influenced survival of the bleeding cirrhotic population, since two-thirds to three-fourths of the patients have died during the initial bleeding episode and only 15% to 20% have become eligible for elective therapy. Because of the failure of the "conventional" approach, there has been considerable recent interest in emergency surgical management. Experience is insufficient as yet to establish definite criteria for selection of patients for operation. Although it is clear that the risk of operation is great in patients with decompensated cirrhosis, it is also certain that such patients have little chance of surviving with nonoperative therapy. Currently, emergency operative treatment is largely confined to the use of three types of operations: (1) direct suture ligation of the bleeding varices, (2) esophagogastric devascularization procedures, and (3) emergency portal-systemic shunt. All three operations control varix bleeding initially in most patients. However, a major potential problem associated with all emergency operations is hepatic decompensation, which may result when a critically ill patient with a severely damaged liver is subjected to anesthesia and major trauma, in addition to hemorrhage.

Transesophageal Varix Ligation (Fig. 13C.2)

Although transesophageal ligation of esophageal varices was first described in 1949, reported experience with this procedure has not been large (77–80). The mortality rate has ranged from 15% to 86%. The largest reported series has involved 72 selected patients with an operative mortality rate of 50%. Because the value of this procedure was not clearly established, some years ago we undertook a prospective comparison of emergency transesophageal varix ligation and medical therapy (81). Every cirrhotic patient admitted to the hospital with varix bleeding was included in the study with no attempt at selection. The diagnostic workup

was completed within 6 hours and, in the surgical group, operation was performed within 8 hours of admission to the hospital. The study was conducted in comparable groups of chronic alcoholics with advanced cirrhosis and massive varix hemorrhage. Approximately half the patients in each group had jaundice and ascites, and one-fourth had hepatic encephalopathy. When feasible, the patients who survived emergency surgical or medical therapy were prepared for and underwent an elective portacaval shunt at a later date.

The results of this study are included in the summary presented in Table 13C.8. Emergency transesophageal varix ligation consistently controlled bleeding. The early survival rate was 54% following operative ligation compared with 14% in the medically treated patients. The 5-year survival rate was 21% in the surgical group and 3% in the medical group, and the 10-year survival rates were 11% and 0%, respectively. Our experience showed that varix ligation is not a definitive procedure, but rather must be considered the first of two stages in treatment, the second stage of which is an elective portacaval shunt. The refusal of some patients to undergo an elective shunt was invariably associated with rebleeding and played a major role in the declining survival rate. Moreover, in evaluating the long-term results of both varix ligation and medical therapy, the mortality rate of the subsequent elective portacaval shunt must be included.

A major reason for considering transesophageal varix ligation as emergency treatment for bleeding varices is the belief that it is an effective procedure of lesser magnitude than other emergency operations. Our experience has shown that such is not the case. The time required to perform the operation, the magnitude of the trauma, the metabolic response, and the effects on liver function are similar to those associated with EPCS. While varix ligation appears to have distinct advantages over medical therapy, it does not appear to be the best emergency surgical procedure available.

Esophagogastric Devascularization Procedures

Various esophagogastric devascularization procedures have been used as both emergency and elective treatment of bleeding esophageal varices (82–92). Included among these are (a) gastric or esophageal transection and reanastomosis, most recently done with the aid of a stapling gun, which

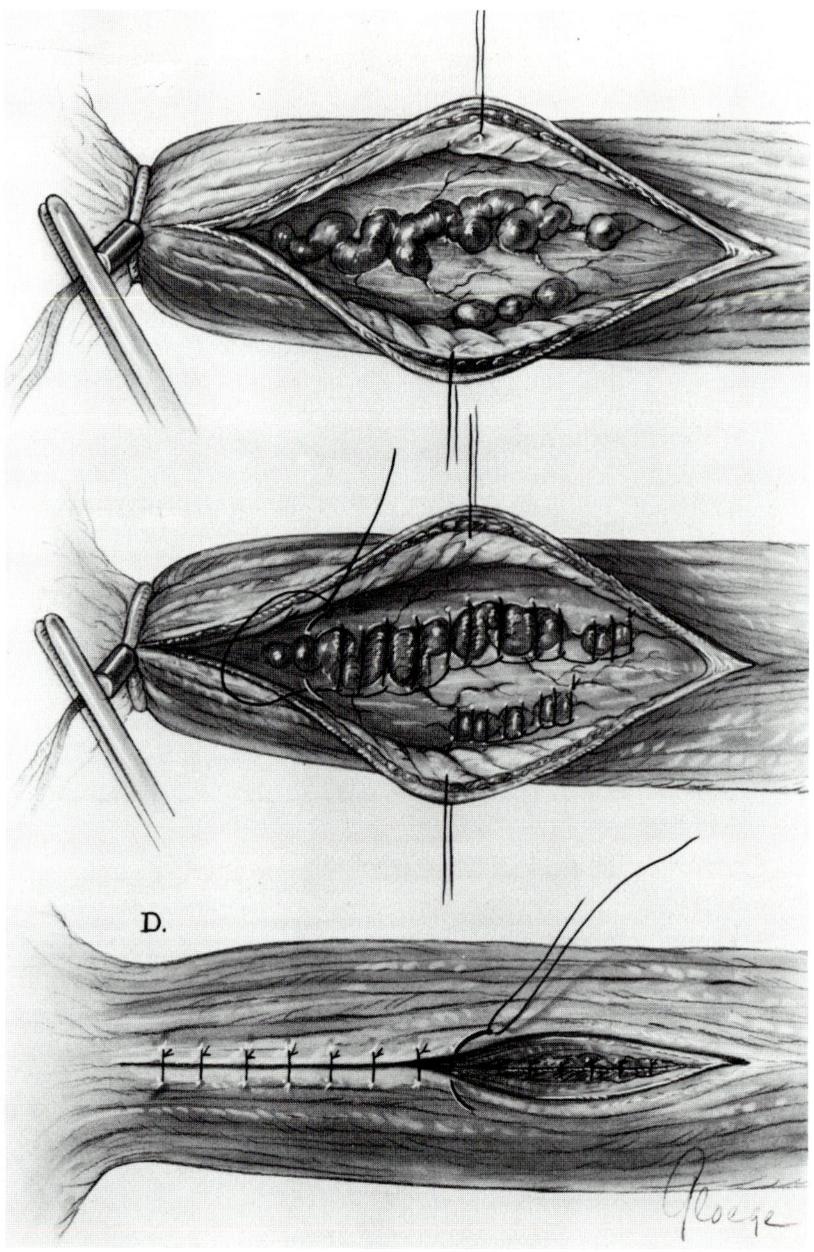

Figure 13C.2. Technique of transesophageal varix ligation. (Reproduced by permission from Orloff MJ. A comparative study of emergency transesophageal ligation and nonsurgical treatment of bleeding esophageal varices in unselected patients with cirrhosis. *Surgery* 1962; 52:103–116.)

is sometimes combined with splenectomy and extensive ligation of the veins around the distal esophagus and upper stomach; (b) esophagogastrectomy and pyloroplasty with or without interposition of a segment of colon or jejunum, and with or without ligation of collateral veins and splenectomy; (c) splenectomy alone or with coronary vein ligation; and (d) ligation of the hepatic, left gastric, and splenic arteries. By and large, these operations involve transection of the esophagus and/or resection of parts of the lower esophagus and upper stomach and/or extensive ligation of collateral veins that connect with the esophageal varices. The results of the various esophagogastric devascularization procedures are difficult to evaluate because most of the series are small, involve highly selected patients with many types of portal hypertension, and are retrospective in nature. By far, the greatest experience with these operations has been in Japan, where surgeons have largely abandoned portal-systemic shunting in favor of esophagogastric devascularization, which they have performed prophylactically, electively, and emergently (82,85,86,90). Japanese researchers have reported favorable results, but their reports do not lend themselves readily to analysis, and the results have not been verified in other countries. Moreover, in several reports the long-term survival rate of cirrhotic patients has been low. In the United States, esophagogastric devascularization procedures in cirrhotic patients have been associated with substantial mortality rates and a high incidence of recurrent varix bleeding.

Emergency Portacaval Shunt

Author's Prospective Study

Portal-systemic shunt is the only available definitive treatment for portal hypertension and esophagogastric varices. Numerous studies have shown that a technically satisfactory portacaval shunt permanently solves the problem of bleeding varices in the vast majority of patients. The obvious potential advantage of performing this procedure under emergency circumstances is that, unlike other forms of treatment, it can be expected to provide both immediate and prolonged control of varix hemorrhage. The question is, Can cirrhotic patients tolerate an operation of this magnitude when it is performed as an emergency in the face of bleeding? To answer this question, we have conducted a prospective study of EPCS, similar to our comparative evaluation of varix ligation and medical therapy (38,39,93–98). The study is distinguished from all other reported studies of emergency treatment in two respects: (a) it has involved *every* cirrhotic patient admitted with varix bleeding, regardless of his or her condition on admission; and (b) all of the patients have been operated on within 8 hours of admission to our emergency room or, in the occasional patient who started bleeding while in the hospital, within 8 hours of the onset of bleeding. Between 1963 and 1983, 264 consecutive, unselected patients underwent EPCS.

Follow-up study has been conducted in a special clinic, and the current status of 97% of the patients is known.

We have divided our 264 unselected patients into two groups: an Early Group of 180 patients operated on from 1963 up to 1978, and a Recent Group of 84 patients operated on from 1978 through 1983. The characteristics of the two groups were similar and are shown in Table 13C.5. Almost all of the patients were chronic alcoholics, and all had cirrhosis on liver biopsy. On admission, about half of the patients in each group had jaundice and ascites; 19% had frank encephalopathy or coma; 30% and 42%, respectively, had severe muscle wasting; and 82% and 90%, respectively, had a hyperdynamic state. Systemic intravenous Pituitrin temporarily controlled the varix bleeding in 95% of the patients and allowed sufficient time to complete the diagnostic workup. Emergency portacaval shunt promptly and perma-

Table 13C.5. Emergency Portacaval Shunt in Unselected Patients with Cirrhosis: Characteristics of Early Group (n = 180) and Recent Group (n = 84)

Pathologic Manifestations	Early Group (%)	Recent Group (%)
Hematemesis	98	94
Jaundice on admission	49	48
Ascites on admission	53	42
Encephalopathy on admission	19	18
Severe muscle-wasting	30	42
Hyperdynamic cardiovascular state	82	90
Liver dye retention ≥ 21%	95	92
Varices on endoscopy	98	100
Varices on roentgenography	95	97
Cirrhosis on liver biopsy	100	100
Portal hypertension by direct measurement	100	100

Treatment		
Temporary control by IV vasopressin	95	95
Permanent control by portacaval shunt	98	100
Blood transfusions		
<5000 ml	61	69
5000–7000 ml	16	21
>7000 ml	23	10
Type of shunt		
Side-to-side	83	74
End-to-side	15	26
Other	2	0
Skin-to-skin operating time		
<4 hr	45	57
4–5 hr	42	31
>5 hr	13	12
Gradient across shunt <50 mm	86	98

nently stopped the varix hemorrhage in 98% and 100% of the patients, respectively. The requirement for blood transfusion before and during operation for the two groups averaged 5.1 and 3.7 L, respectively. Side-to-side portacaval shunt was performed in 83% and 74% of the patients, respectively; end-to-side shunt in 15% and 26%; and another type of shunt in three patients in the Early Group. There was no difference in survival rate between patients with side-to-side anastomosis and those with end-to-side anastomosis. The "skin-to-skin" operating time, which included various measurements of splanchnic pressures and blood flows, averaged 4.1 hours, and was less than 5 hours in 87% and 88% of each group. All patients had portal hypertension with corrected free portal pressures, obtained by subtracting the inferior vena cava pressure, which averaged 267 mm saline. The portacaval anastomosis reduced the portal pressure to normal in all patients.

Table 13C.6 summarizes the long-term results of EPCS. In the Early Group, 58% of the 180 patients survived the operation, and the 5- and 12-year survival rates were 38% and 30%, respectively. In contrast, 83% of the Recent Group of 84 patients survived the shunt, and the 5-year survival rate was 72%. One-third of the patients in each group had a documented history of encephalopathy before the shunt (98). After the shunt, 31% of the Early Group and 16% of the Recent Group have had encephalopathy at one time or another. Severe

encephalopathy requiring chronic dietary protein restriction occurred in only 7% of the patients. At the time of discharge, 95% of patients in the Early Group, and 99% of patients in the Recent Group could tolerate a diet containing 80 g of protein per day. Long-term shunt patency has been demonstrated by *yearly* angiography in 99% of the early patients and 100% of the recent patients. The two thrombosed shunts in the Early Group were of the end-to-side type. Forty-eight percent of the survivors in the Early Group and 70% of the Recent Group have not consumed alcohol at any time during the follow-up period. The lower incidence in the Recent Group may be due to the fact that it has not been followed up for as many years as the Early Group. After 5 years, the general status of the survivors in the Early Group and Recent Group, respectively, is excellent or good in 62% and 69%, fair in 29% and 24%, and poor in 9% and 7%; all but one patient in the poor category have resumed heavy alcohol consumption. Sixty percent of the survivors have been gainfully employed or doing full-time housework during part or all of the follow-up period. Five years after the shunt operation, results of liver function tests showed an improvement over preoperative results in 44% of the Early Group and 52% of the Recent Group; no change in 33% and 35%, respectively; and worsening in 22% and 13%, respectively.

Beginning with the moment of admission and continuing through the lifelong follow-up visits, detailed data on every patient were recorded on standard forms and entered continuously into a computer analysis program. Since our study involved unselected patients, we carefully analyzed all factors present on admission that might have influenced survival, in the hope of identifying criteria for future selection of patients for operation. Table 13C.7 summarizes the preoperative findings obtained from the history, physical examination, and diagnostic workup that were associated with a statistically significant decrease in survival rate in the Early Group and, therefore, can be considered to be risk factors. Six such risk factors were identified: (a) presence of ascites on admission; (b) serum glutamic oxaloacetic transaminase (SGOT) level of 100 units per deciliter or higher; (c) bromsulphalein (BSP) retention greater than 50% in 45 minutes; (d) hypokalemic alkalosis with an arterial blood pH of 7.50 or greater and a serum potassium level below 3.5 mEq/L; (e) re-

Table 13C.6. Emergency Portacaval Shunt in Unselected Patients with Cirrhosis: Results of Long-Term Follow-up of Early Group (n = 180) and Recent Group (n = 84)

Results	Early Group (%)	Recent Group (%)
Operative survival (30 days or longer)	58	83
5-year survival	38	72
Actuarial 12-yr survival	30	—
Encephalopathy		
Before shunt	33	36
After shunt	31	16
Patency of shunt by yearly catheterization	99	100
Abstinence from alcohol	48	70
General status after 5 yr		
Excellent or good	62	69
Fair	29	24
Poor	9	7
Liver function after 5 yr		
Improved	44	52
Unchanged	33	35
Worse	22	13

Table 13C.7. Preoperative Risk Factors that Significantly Decreased Survival of the Early Group of 180 Unselected Cirrhotic Patients Treated by Emergency Portacaval Shunt

Risk Factors	Percent of Group	Survival (%)	Significance (p)
Ascites			
Present	53	46	<0.01
Absent	47	72	
SGOT			
≥100 U/dl	34	43	<0.01
<100 U/dl	66	70	
BSP retention			
>50%	21	36	<0.01
≤50%	79	66	
Hypokalemic alkalosis			
pH >7.5, K$^+$ <3.5	29	42	<0.05
pH ≤7.5, K$^+$ ≥3.5	71	67	
Blood transfusion			
≥5 L before and during operation	39	41	<0.001
<5 L before and during operation	61	70	
Last drank alcohol			
≤7 days before admission	71	53	<0.05
>7 days before admission	29	71	

quirement of 5 L or more of blood transfusion before and during operation; and (f) consumption of alcohol within 7 days prior to admission. Because the presence of these risk factors was associated with survival rates of from 36% to 53%, they cannot be considered contraindications to emergency shunt. Age, sex, jaundice, encephalopathy, severe muscle-wasting, a small liver, a large spleen, a history of delirium tremens, and the blood levels of bilirubin, albumin, and prothrom-

bin did not have a statistically significant influence on survival.

In 17 patients (9% of our series), jaundice, ascites, encephalopathy, and severe muscle-wasting were present concurrently on admission. All these patients had markedly disturbed liver function, and nine had an SGOT level above 100 U/dl. The operative survival rate of these patients with the most advanced stage of alcoholic cirrhosis was 47%, a rate similar to that of patients with ascites alone. However, 1 year after operation only 18% were still alive, and 5 years postoperatively, the survival rate was only 12%, so the outlook for these patients is grim under any circumstances. Nevertheless, without portacaval shunt, these pre-terminal cirrhotics rarely survive beyond 2 years.

Table 13C.8 compares the results of the three forms of emergency treatment of bleeding varices that we evaluated prospectively in unselected patients during the past 24 years, and Figure 13C.3 compares the cumulative survival curve of the Early Group of shunted patients with the survival curves resulting from the other two types of emergency therapy. Although these three groups of patients were not studied concurrently, they are similar from every standpoint. Early survival rates produced by the two forms of surgical therapy were substantially greater than that resulting from EMT. Five- and 12-year survival rates, both actual and actuarial, were significantly greater following emergency shunt than after either of the other two types of emergency therapy.

Figure 13C.4 compares the cumulative survival curve of the 84 patients in the Recent Group with

Table 13C.8. Comparison of Results of Emergency Portacaval Shunt, Transesophageal Varix Ligation, and Medical Treatment in Unselected Patients with Cirrhosis and Bleeding Varices

Clinical Factors and Survival Rates	Medical Treatment[a]	Varix Ligation[a]	Emergency Shunt	
			Early Group	Recent Group
No. patients	59	28	180	84
Jaundice on admission (%)	42	57	49	48
Ascites on admission (%)	41	50	53	42
Encephalopathy on admission (%)	25	25	19	18
Mean liver index on admission	2.8	2.8	2.4	2.6
Admission hemoglobin 11 g/dl or less (%)	70	71	71	74
Varices demonstrated (%)	95	100	100	100
Mean volume of blood transfused (L)	7.2	4.2	5.0	3.7
Early survival (30 days) (%)	17	54	58	83
5-yr survival (%)	3	21	38	72
12-yr survival (%)	0	11	30	—

[a] Followed by elective portacaval shunt when possible.

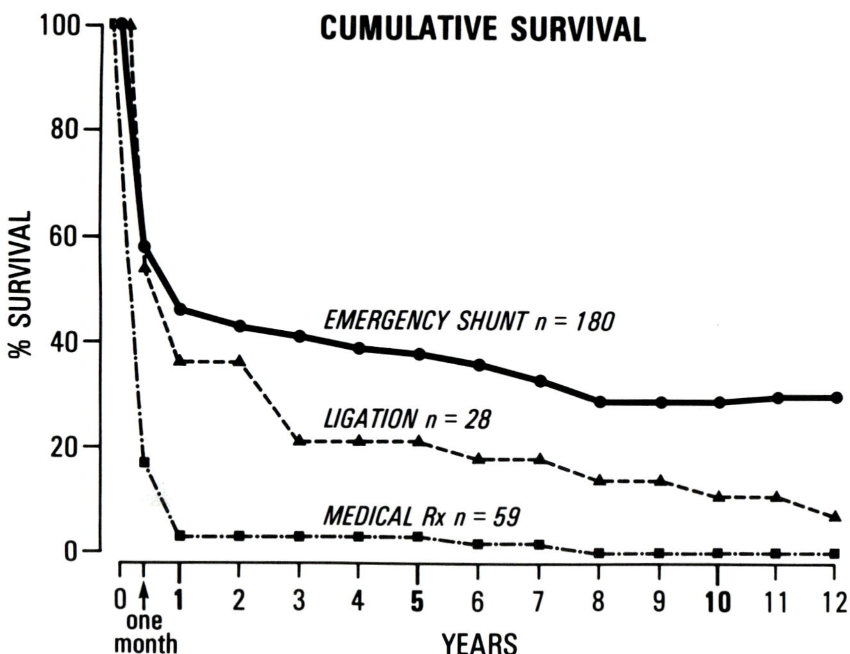

Figure 13C.3. Cumulative 5-year survival rates of patients with cirrhosis and varix hemorrhage following EPCS (Early Group), transesophageal varix ligation, and medical treatment.

that of the 180 patients in the Early Group. As our experience with EPCS has increased, there has been a striking improvement in results. In unselected patients, all comers included, operative survival rate has increased from 58% to 83%, and 5-year survival rate has almost doubled from 38% to 72%. It should be emphasized that *no* patient who came to us with bleeding varices was excluded from the emergency shunt program. Nonetheless, the 5-year survival rate of emergency shunt in *unselected* patients is now the same as or better than the 5-year survival rate of elective shunt in *highly selected* patients reported by others.

Many patients with alcoholic cirrhosis have not yet reached 50 years of age and, in the absence of liver disease, would have a life expectancy of more than 25 additional years. However, little information is available about survival beyond 5 years after treatment, and almost no information about the quality of life following any form of therapy. Of our 264 patients who underwent emergency portacaval shunt, 153 were operated on 10 or more years ago, and 45 survived for from 10 to 22 years. These 45 patients have undergone regular follow-up and the status of all of them is known (99).

Of the 45 long-term survivors, 20% were in Child's class A, 73% were in class B, and 7% were in class C at the time of operation. There was a substantial incidence of the six preoperative risk factors that we have found to adversely affect survival.

Table 13C.9 presents data on the quality of life in the patients who survived for 10 to 22 years. All of the patients were shown to have a patent portacaval anastomosis by yearly angiography, and no patient had gastrointestinal bleeding. Eight patients or 18% had portasystemic encephalopathy. Four of these patients had a single episode of encephalopathy early in their course, so that the incidence of significant, recurrent encephalopathy was 9%, and it was directly related to use of alcohol. Stated differently, encephalopathy played no role in the lives of 91% of the patients. It should be noted that 22% of the patients had encephalopathy before shunt.

Abstention from alcohol was total and continuous in 58% of the long-term survivors, and the abstainers had an excellent record of productive living and freedom from encephalopathy. Remarkably, 31% of the patients drank alcohol occasionally and 11% resumed regular use, yet they survived for many years. After 10 years, liver function had improved in 53%, was unchanged in 29%, and was worse in 18% compared to the function at the time of bleeding and operation. Excluding four patients who were 65 years or older at the time of operation and were classified as retired, 68% of the patients were gainfully em-

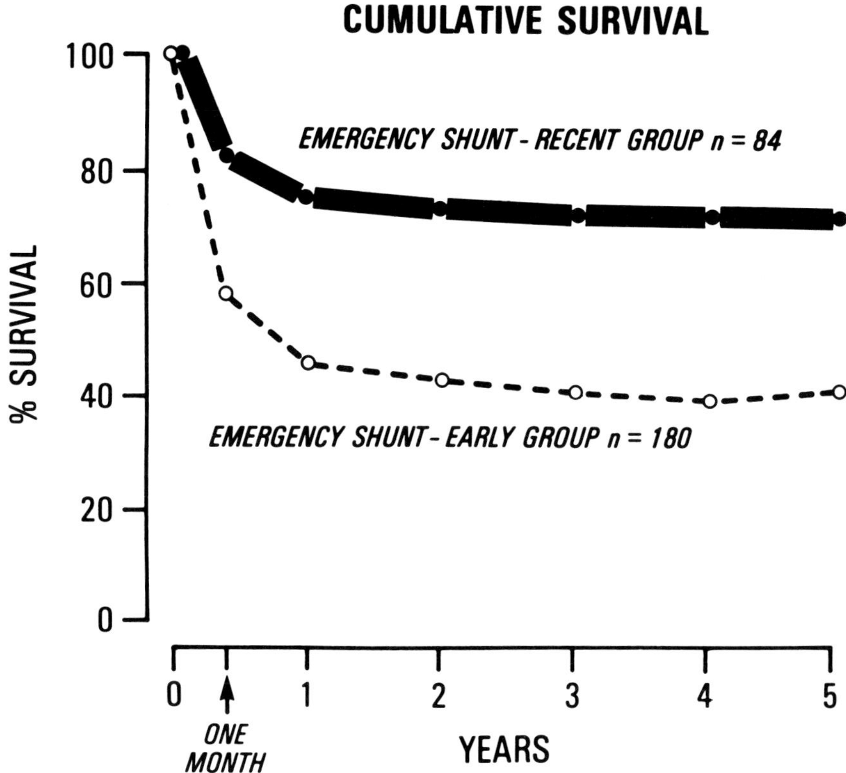

Figure 13C.4. Cumulative survival rate of 84 unselected patients with cirrhosis who underwent EPCS in the Recent Group, as compared with the cumulative survival rate of 180 patients in the Early Group.

ployed or doing full-time housework for part or all of the follow-up period. Ten years after emergency shunt, the general status of the patients was judged to be excellent or good in 73% and fair in 27%, almost all of whom had resumed use of alcohol. Not surprisingly, and in confirmation of our previous studies, the single factor that appeared to influence long-term survival was resumption of regular alcohol intake.

The results of our studies indicate that emergency portacaval shunt has improved both the immediate and long-term survival rates of cirrhotic patients with bleeding esophageal varices. As is true of survival statistics for cancer and other lethal disorders, the absolute survival rate is of limited meaning unless it is viewed in the context of the natural history of the disease. The 5- and 12-year survival rates in our experience to date are many times greater than those associated with EMT followed by elective portacaval shunt in the relatively small number of patients who survive. Undoubtedly, some patients with advanced cirrhosis

Table 13C.9. Quality of Life in 45 Unselected Cirrhotic Patients Who Survived for 10 to 22 Years After Emergency Portacaval Shunt

Criteria	Patients (%)
Shunt patency	100
Gastrointestinal bleeding	0
Encephalopathy at any time	18
Recurrent	9
Mild (single episode)	9
Existed before and after shunt	11
Alcohol intake	
None	58
Occasional	31
Regular	11
Liver function	
Improved	53
Worse	18
Unchanged	29
General health at 10 yr	
Excellent or good	73
Fair	27
Poor	0
Work status	
Working	68
Not working	32

will not survive with any form of therapy currently available. The problem is that criteria for identifying such patients are not yet known. The development of sound criteria for selecting patients for various forms of treatment unquestionably will improve the results of operative management. Until such guidelines are developed by well-controlled, prospective studies, or until alternative effective therapy is devised, emergency portacaval shunt appears to be the therapy of choice for most cirrhotic patients who bleed from esophageal varices.

Author's Recent Prospective Randomized Comparison of Emergency Portacaval Shunt and Emergency Medical Therapy

Although our studies showed that emergency portacaval shunt produced a much higher survival rate and much better quality of life than any other form of emergency therapy, a potential shortcoming in the comparisons described above is that they were not conducted concurrently in a randomized clinical trial. Therefore, in 1978 we initiated a prospective randomized trial comparing EPCS and EMT involving every patient, without selection, admitted to one of our hospitals with cirrhosis and bleeding esophagogastric varices (40,41). Survivors of EMT underwent an elective portacaval shunt within 9 to 30 days. All patients underwent exactly the same diagnostic workup described previously, and all patients received the same initial therapy. Randomization was done after the diagnosis of bleeding varices was made by drawing a card from an opaque, sealed envelope prepared by the biostatistician according to a randomization design. Randomization resulted in 21 patients receiving EPCS and 22 patients receiving EMT. EPCS was performed within 8 hours of initial contact, and EMT consisted of a continuation of initial therapy plus continuous systemic intravenous vasopressin and esophageal balloon tamponade. Randomization ended in 1983, and the follow-up rate to date has been 100%.

Table 13C.10 shows the characteristics of the two groups. The only significant difference between them was fewer Child's risk class A patients and more class C patients in the EPCS group. If anything, this difference would tend to favor EMT.

Table 13C.11 shows control of bleeding in the two groups of patients. As we have found consist-

Table 13C.10. Prospective Randomized Comparison of Emergency Portacaval Shunt and Emergency Medical Therapy Followed by Elective Shunt in Unselected Patients with Cirrhosis and Bleeding Varices: Characteristics of the EPCS Group (n = 21) and EMT Group (n = 22)

Pathologic Manifestations	EPCS (%)	EMT (%)
Drank alcohol ≤7 days before admission	62	59
Jaundice on admission	48	50
Ascites on admission	52	50
Encephalopathy on admission and/or past history	43	27
Severe muscle-wasting	81	59
Hyperdynamic cardiovascular state	90	91
Liver dye retention ≥50%	33	14
SGOT >100 U/dl	33	36
Varices on endoscopy	100	100
Elevated WHVP	100	100
Child's risk class		
A	10	45[a]
B	38	23
C	52	32

[a] $p < 0.01$.

ently in the past, 90% or more of patients responded initially to systemic intravenous vasopressin. However, after the initial response, the differences between the two groups were highly significant. Both early control and permanent control of bleeding were achieved in 100% of the shunted patients, but in only 45% and 36%, respectively, of the medically treated patients. Furthermore, the mean requirement for blood transfusions was three times greater in the EMT group than in the EPCS group, a very important difference in this day when every blood transfusion carries a substantial risk.

Table 13C.12 shows the survival rates in the two groups. Almost twice as many patients in the EPCS group survived to leave the hospital than in the EMT group. Actual survival after 1, 2, and 3 years was twofold or more than that in patients treated by EPCS than in patients treated by the combination of EMT and elective shunt. Five-year actuarial survival was almost three times greater after EPCS than after EMT-elective shunt. The difference in early survival rate between EPCS and EMT-elective shunt was particularly striking in Child's risk class B and C patients: 100% versus 20% in class B, and 64% versus 14% in class C.

When we compared the 21 patients assigned to the randomized EPCS group with the 84 unselected patients in our recent unrandomized series of EPCS, we found that the two groups were very

Table 13C.11. Prospective Randomized Comparison of Emergency Portacaval Shunt and Emergency Medical Therapy Followed by Elective Shunt in Unselected Patients with Cirrhosis and Bleeding Varices: Control of Bleeding

Control of Bleeding	EPCS (n = 21)	EMT (n = 22)	p
Initial response to IV vasopressin (%)	90	91	NS
Response to esophageal balloon tamponade (%)	—	50	—
Control during initial hospitalization (%)	100	45	<0.001
Permanent control (%)	100	36	<0.001
Blood transfusions during initial hospitalization—mean U	7.1 ± 1.1	21.4 ± 2.6	<0.001

similar from the standpoint of historical data, physical findings, laboratory data, operative data, portal pressure data, and requirement for blood transfusion. Furthermore, survival rates in the randomized series and the unrandomized series were quite similar. In addition, quality of life has been similar in the two groups of patients treated by EPCS. All patients have had permanent control of varix bleeding, more than two-thirds have abstained from alcohol, and the incidence of encephalopathy at any time (29% in the randomized group, 16% in the unrandomized group) has not been significantly different. Therefore, our results of EPCS over the past 9 years have been confirmed by our prospective randomized clinical trial.

Postoperative Care Following Emergency Portacaval Shunt

Patients with liver disease who bleed from esophageal varices are among the most seriously ill patients in any hospital, regardless of the specific therapy used to control the bleeding. In those who undergo emergency portacaval shunt, the expert-

Table 13C.12. Prospective Randomized Comparison of Emergency Portacaval Shunt and Emergency Medical Therapy Followed by Elective Shunt in Unselected Patients with Cirrhosis and Bleeding Varices: Survival Rates

Survival Rate	EPCS (n = 21) (%)	EMT (n = 22) (%)	p
Discharged from hospital alive	81	45	0.03
1 yr—actual	71	36	0.03
2 yr—actual	67	32	0.03
3 yr—actual	67	27	0.01
5 yr—actuarial	54	19	0.01
By Child's risk class—			
Discharged from hospital alive:			
A	100	80	NS
B	100	20	<0.01
C	64	14	<0.01

Abbreviations: NS, not significant.

ness of the postoperative care is a major factor in determining survival. All such patients should be admitted to an intensive care unit with equipment and personnel geared to managing the complicated problems associated with hepatic disease. A description of specific prophylactic and therapeutic aspects of postoperative care follows.

MONITORING

Careful monitoring of vital signs, central venous pressure, urine output, arterial pH, arterial and alveolar gases, fluid balance, body weight, and abdominal girth are essential. Serial electrocardiograms and determinations of cardiac output and peripheral resistance often are very helpful. Measurement of pulmonary artery wedge pressure with a Swan-Ganz catheter is indicated occasionally but not routinely. Serial measurements of liver function; of the formed elements in the blood, including platelets; of blood coagulation; of serum electrolytes; and of renal function must be done.

PARENTERAL FLUID THERAPY

Patients with cirrhosis are often waterlogged even before the onset of bleeding from varices, and they have a markedly impaired capacity to excrete water loads. The bleeding episode and the operation intensify renal sodium and water retention and exaggerate the already existing fluid intolerance. Parenteral fluid therapy should be calculated to maintain such patients on the dry side. Fluid losses are replaced by a solution of 10% dextrose in water containing vitamins B, C, and K. The total volume usually amounts to 1500 to 2000 ml/day, based on daily losses of 500 ml nasogastric aspirate, 500 to 1000 ml urine, 800 to 1000 ml insensible water, and a gain of 250 to 400 ml from endogenous water formation. Sodium is given only to replace nasogastric losses, which rarely exceed 30 to 40 mEq/day. Parenteral potassium therapy is started as soon as urine output is adequate, and is given in whatever amounts are necessary to maintain the serum potassium concentration between 4 and 5 mEq/L. Usually the requirement is 150 to 200 mEq/day, but doses as high as 500 mEq/day may be necessary. If metabolic alkalosis develops, as is often the case, it usually responds to repletion of potassium with large quantities of parenteral potassium chloride. In addition to crystalloid fluid therapy, it is often necessary to add colloid to replace continuing losses of blood and plasma. Transfusions of fresh blood are given for blood loss or a hematocrit below 30%. Type-specific, single-donor plasma, fresh frozen plasma, or salt-poor concentrated albumin is given for losses of fluid into the operation site and peritoneal cavity (acute ascites), as determined by the combined measurements of abdominal girth, central venous pressure, urine output, body weight, and hematocrit showing hemoconcentration.

PULMONARY THERAPY

Pulmonary complications, particularly infection and wet lung, are a major cause of morbidity and mortality in patients with cirrhosis and bleeding varices. In about 2% of our patients, it has been necessary to maintain the patient on a respirator for several days postoperatively. In such cases, mechanical ventilatory support usually can be provided through an endotracheal tube that may be left indwelling for 48 to 72 hours. Occasionally, it is necessary to perform a tracheostomy for ventilation and tracheobronchial toilet, but it should be recognized that complications of tracheostomy, particularly bleeding, are more frequent in cirrhotic patients than in others. Portable chest roentgenograms are obtained daily in patients on respirators or those having pulmonary problems. The decision to taper off and then discontinue mechanical ventilatory support is based on measurements of arterial blood and alveolar gases, ventilatory volumes, chest roentgenograms, and physical findings.

All patients not on a respirator are given continuous oxygen therapy by nasal catheter, nasal prongs, or mask for 5 to 7 days postoperatively because of the frequent cardiovascular abnormalities and arteriovenous shunting that exist in cirrhosis. From the start, all patients receive intensive respiratory therapy that consists of intermittent tracheobronchial aspiration, postural drainage, chest physiotherapy, intermittent positive-pressure respiration, frequent turning, encouragement to cough and breathe deeply, and the use of blow bottles and a humidifier. Diuretics may be of value in the treatment of pulmonary edema due to left heart failure or infection.

HYPERDYNAMIC CARDIOVASCULAR STATE

As mentioned previously, cirrhotic patients regularly have a hyperdynamic cardiovascular state and sometimes develop high output cardiac failure. In fact, 82% of our Early Group of patients who underwent emergency portacaval shunt, and 90% of our Recent Group had a cardiac output of 6 L/min or higher before and/or after operation. All such patients are digitalized over a period of 48 hours, parenteral fluid therapy is restricted to avoid circulatory overload, and inotropic drugs are given if myocardial performance is not satisfactory.

DELIRIUM TREMENS

Alcoholic cirrhotic patients frequently have delirium tremens following hemorrhage alone or in combination with a portacaval shunt or other operation. Delirium tremens by itself, in the absence of bleeding or an operation, is associated with a substantial mortality rate (100,101). When added to the stress of hemorrhage or a major operation, the mortality rate is even higher. Initial treatment consists of administration of a central nervous system depressant. We prefer intramuscular magnesium sulfate in doses of 2 g every 2 to 4 hours. If magnesium sulfate therapy is not rapidly effective, chlordiazepoxide hydrochloride (Librium) is added in a dose of 25 to 50 mg intramuscularly every 4 hours. Supportive treatment in the form of adequate parenteral fluids containing concentrated glucose and vitamins, antipyretic agents, and pulmonary therapy are important. This hyperactive, hypermetabolic disorder must not be confused with hepatic encephalopathy because a central nervous system depressant may be lethal in patients with hepatic encephalopathy. Intravenous alcohol is a severe hepatotoxin, and no basis exists for its use in cirrhotic patients with postoperative delirium tremens. Parenteral paraldehyde has no advantages over other hypnotic drugs and, in the author's opinion, should not be used because of the frequent soft tissue abscesses and noxious odor it produces.

HEPATIC FAILURE

The majority of patients appears to be in surprisingly good condition immediately following an emergency portacaval shunt. However, by the second or third postoperative day, some deterioration of liver function is noted in almost all patients. In many patients, the liver dysfunction stabilizes and then improves, but in some it progresses to hepatic coma and the full syndrome of hepatic failure, with jaundice, severe abnormalities of blood coagulation, ascites, and renal insufficiency. Liver failure is the most frequent cause of death in cirrhotic patients who bleed from esophageal varices, whether or not they have had a portacaval shunt. The hepatic coma that occurs during the immediate postoperative period is due to liver cell failure, and is not related to ammonia intoxication or systemic shunting of nitrogenous substances absorbed from the intestines (102–104). Unfortunately, there is no specific therapy for hepatic failure, and all that can be done is to provide parenteral nutritional support and symptomatic therapy of the individual abnormalities that arise. There is no evidence that exchange transfusion, hemodialysis, or extracorporeal perfusion of the blood through a pig, baboon, or human liver are of value in this situation. Spontaneous recovery sometimes occurs.

Because it is rarely possible to remove all of the blood from the gastrointestinal tract preoperatively, neomycin therapy (1 g every 6 hours by nasogastric tube), cathartics (60 ml magnesium sulfate per day by nasogastric tube), and a daily neomycin enema (4 g in 1 quart of water) are continued for 3 days postoperatively. If continued beyond three days, troublesome diarrhea usually follows. With this regimen, significantly elevated blood ammonia levels or signs of nitrogen-related encephalopathy rarely occur within the first postoperative week.

GASTRIC ACID HYPERSECRETION

Inconclusive evidence suggests that, following portacaval shunt, gastric acid hypersecretion develops and is associated with an increased incidence of peptic ulcer disease (105,106). To protect against this potential complication, nasogastric suction is continued for 3 or 4 days postoperatively and cimetidine or ranitidine is given throughout the stay. As soon as the nasogastric tube is removed, the patient is given hourly antacid therapy until his or her oral dietary intake is satisfactory, and then the antacid schedule is changed to between meals and at bedtime. An antacid that does not contain sodium is used. Antacid and cimetidine or ranitidine therapy are discontinued 3 months postoperatively.

RENAL FAILURE

Two common forms of renal dysfunction follow varix hemorrhage and portacaval shunt. The first is acute tubular necrosis, which results from a period of hypotension and consequent renal ischemia. It is manifested by oliguria, azotemia, hyperkalemia, a low fixed urine specific gravity and osmolality, substantial quantities of sodium in the urine, and a urine sediment containing casts and red blood cells. Treatment consists of stringent fluid restriction, measures to reduce serum potassium, and, if necessary, hemodialysis. The second renal disorder is spontaneous renal failure associated with hepatic decompensation, the so-called hepatorenal syndrome (107–109). It is more insidious in onset than acute tubular necrosis and is manifested initially by progressive azotemia without striking oliguria. In contrast to acute tubular necrosis, the urine specific gravity in the hepatorenal syndrome is variable and ranges up to 1.020, there is almost no sodium in the urine, the osmolality of the urine is high, and the urine sediment is normal. There is no specific treatment for spontaneous renal failure, and therapy is directed at reversing the hepatic decompensation, minimizing dilutional hyponatremia, and correcting problems as they appear. There is no indication for the use of diuretics and, in fact, they may intensify the renal abnormality. Numerous vasoactive agents have been used for the purpose of improving renal blood flow, but none has influenced the outcome. Hemodialysis has created more problems than it has solved. The mortality rate of the combined syndrome of hepatic and renal decompensation is very high.

INFECTION

Substantial evidence indicates that patients with cirrhosis have a high incidence of infection, perhaps because of their debilitated general condition. Surprisingly, wound and intraperitoneal infections following emergency portacaval shunt have been uncommon in our experience, occurring in only 3% of our patients. However, pulmonary infections have been common and urinary tract infections not infrequent. The value of prophylactic antibiotic therapy in this condition is uncertain. Appropriate antibiotics are given for proven infections, always on the basis of bacterial cultures and antibiotic sensitivity tests. We routinely obtain cultures of tracheal aspirates and urine during the early postoperative period to avoid delays in therapy should infection develop.

NUTRITION

Nutritional therapy is very important in liver disease (110). Oral diet is started as soon as the patient tolerates removal of the nasogastric tube for 24 hours, usually on the fifth or sixth postoperative day. Initially, a 500-mg sodium, 4000-calorie, high-carbohydrate, regular fat, 20-g protein, bland diet is introduced. There is no basis for restricting fat, and doing so only makes the diet unpalatable. The protein content of the diet is increased in 20-g increments every 3 days up to 80 g, and the patient is carefully observed and tested each day for signs of encephalopathy. If the patient tolerates 80 g protein per day, he or she is discharged on a 60-g protein diet after having received a diet list and specific instructions from a dietitian. Rigorous sodium restriction is continued for several months and, even after a year has elapsed, sodium intake is not allowed to advance above 2.5 g/day. Daily therapeutic doses of vitamins B and C are added to the diet.

ALCOHOLISM

A factor that influences long-term survival following portacaval shunt is abstinence or failure to abstain from alcohol. It is vitally important that a frank discussion be held with the patient regarding the serious dangers of further ingestion of alcohol. The help of psychiatrists and social workers should be obtained while the patient is in the hospital and continued after discharge. It is incumbent upon the surgeon to exploit his or her special relationship with the patient in a long-term effort to cure the underlying cause of the patient's liver disease.

FOLLOW-UP

A lifelong program of follow-up evaluation and treatment is a crucial part of the care of cirrhotic patients who have undergone portacaval shunt. The liver disease cannot be cured, but it can be stabilized to the point of permitting a long and productive life in reasonable comfort. After discharge from the hospital, outpatient visits are scheduled weekly for the first 8 weeks, monthly for the remainder of the first postoperative year, and every 3 months thereafter for the remainder of the patient's life.

Summary

1. Because of the high mortality rate of bleeding varices in alcoholic cirrhosis, emergency therapy is of paramount importance.

2. Emergency diagnosis of bleeding varices can be made regularly within 4 to 5 hours of admission to the hospital by means of the history and physical examination, liver function tests (particularly ICG excretion, endoscopy, barium contrast upper gastrointestinal series roentgenograms, and wedged hepatic venous pressure measurements.

3. Six general measures of treatment should be employed in all patients. These are (a) prompt restoration of blood volume with fresh blood, (b) measures to prevent ammonia intoxication, (c) support of the liver with vitamins and glucose, (d) frequent monitoring of vital functions, (e) correction of metabolic alkalosis, and (f) treatment of the hyperdynamic state with digitalis and cardiotonic drugs.

4. Specific nonsurgical measures to control bleeding include esophageal balloon tamponade, systemic intravenous vasopressin, selective mesenteric intra-arterial vasopressin, percutaneous transhepatic embolization, and endoscopic sclerotherapy. None of these measures consistently achieves hemostasis. A prospective study of emergency and long-term EST involving 53 unselected patients at our institution showed rebleeding in 89% of patients, a mean requirement of 16.3 U of

blood transfusion, and a 2-year survival rate of only 17%.

5. Regarding emergency surgical procedures, currently three types of operations are being used: transesophageal varix ligation, esophagogastric devascularization procedures, and EPCS. Comparison of the results of medical treatment, varix ligation, and emergency shunt in a prospective study involving 342 unselected, consecutive patients showed that long-term survival is far better in patients treated by emergency shunt. Specifically, in an Early Group of 180 unselected, consecutive patients, emergency shunt resulted in an operative survival rate of 58% and a 5-year survival rate of 38%. In a Recent Group of 84 unselected, consecutive patients, the early survival rate has increased to 83%, and the 5-year survival rate to 72%, which is at least as good as the survival rate reported for elective shunt in highly selected patients.

6. Encephalopathy, the major complication of portacaval shunt, occurred in one-third of patients *before* the shunt, in 31% of the Early Group, and 16% of the Recent Group after the shunt, and was severe in only 7% of the total shunts.

7. Of 153 patients who were operated on 10 or more years ago, 45, or 29%, are alive 10 to 22 years after operation.

8. In a recent prospective randomized trial of EPCS and EMT followed by elective portacaval shunt, operation resulted in over a twofold greater survival rate, a markedly lower requirement for blood transfusions, and confirmed all of our earlier results. Similarly, comparison of our results of emergency shunt with our results of EST showed a survival rate following emergency shunt that was over fourfold greater than that of sclerotherapy.

9. The results of our studies show that EPCS, by preventing death from varix hemorrhage in alcoholic cirrhosis, makes it possible for a substantial number of patients to live a normal life span and enjoy an acceptable quality of life.

References

1. Ratnoff OD, Patek AJ Jr. Natural history of Laennec's cirrhosis of the liver. Analysis of 386 cases. *Medicine* 1942; 21:207–268.
2. Higgins WH Jr. The esophageal varix: A report of one hundred and fifteen cases. *Am J Med Sci* 1947; 214:436–441.
3. Atik M, Simeone F. Massive gastrointestinal bleeding: A study of 296 patients at City Hospital of Cleveland. *Arch Surg* 1954; 69:355–365.
4. Nachlas MM, O'Neil JE, Campbell AJ. The life history of patients with cirrhosis of the liver and bleeding esophageal varices. *Ann Surg* 1955; 141:10–23.
5. Cohn R, Blaisdell FW. The natural history of the patient with cirrhosis of the liver with esophageal varices following the first massive hemorrhage. *Surg Gynecol Obstet* 1958; 106:699–701.
6. Taylor FW, Jontz JG. Cirrhosis with hemorrhage. *Arch Surg* 1959; 78:786–790.
7. Merigan TC Jr, Hollister RM, Gryska PF, Starkey GWG, Davidson CS. Gastrointestinal bleeding with cirrhosis: Study of 172 episodes in 158 patients. *N Engl J Med* 1960; 263:579–585.
8. Orloff MJ. Emergency treatment of bleeding esophageal varices in cirrhosis. In: Longmire WP Jr, ed. Portal hypertension. *Current Problems in Surgery.* Chicago: Year Book Medical Publishers, 1966, pp. 13–28.
9. Orloff MJ, Thomas HS. Pathogenesis of esophageal varix rupture: A study based on gross and microscopic examination of the esophagus at the time of bleeding. *Arch Surg* 1963; 87:301–307.
10. Liebowitz HR. Pathogenesis of esophageal varix rupture. *JAMA* 1961; 175:874–879.
11. Garceau AJ, Chalmers TC, Boston Inter-Hospital Liver Group. The natural history of cirrhosis. I. Survival with esophageal varices. *N Engl J Med* 1963; 268:469–473.
12. Hoare AM. Comparative study between endoscopy and radiology in acute upper gastrointestinal hemorrhage. *Br Med J* 1975; 1:27–30.
13. Orloff MJ. Emergency portacaval shunt for bleeding esophageal varices. In: Fiddian-Green RG, Turcotte JG, eds. *Gastrointestinal Hemorrhage.* New York: Grune & Stratton, 1980:295–310.
14. Viamonte M Jr, Warren WD, Fomon JJ, Martinez LO. Angiographic investigations in portal hypertension. *Surg Gynecol Obstet* 1970; 130:37–56.
15. Sloop RD, Orloff MJ. An important syndrome of metabolic alkalosis in patients with cirrhosis, bleeding varices, and portacaval shunt. *Surg Forum* 1966; 17:37–38.
16. Del Guercio LRM, Commaraswamy RP, Feins NR, Woolman SB, State D. Pulmonary arteriovenous admixture and the hyperdynamic cardiovascular state in surgery for portal hypertension. *Surgery* 1964; 56:57–74.
17. Siegel JH, Greenspan M, Cohn JD, Del Guercio LRM. The prognostic implications of altered physiology in operations for portal hypertension. *Surg Gynecol Obstet* 1968; 126:249–262.
18. Siegel JH, Williams JB. A computer based index for the prediction of operative survival in patients with cirrhosis and portal hypertension. *Ann Surg* 1969; 169:191–201.
19. Ludington LG. A study of 158 cases of esophageal varices. *Surg Gynecol Obstet* 1958; 106:519–526.
20. Conn HO. Hazards attending the use of esophageal tamponade. *N Engl J Med* 1958; 259:701–707.
21. Read AE, Dawson AM, Kerr DNS, Turner MD, Sherlock S. Bleeding oesophageal varices treated by oesophageal compression tube. *Br Med J* 1960; 1:227–231.
22. Orloff MJ, Halasz NA, Lipman CA, Schwabe AD, Thompson JC, Weidner WA. The complications of cirrhosis of the liver. *Ann Intern Med* 1967; 66:165–198.
23. Villanueva A, Magnenat P. Resultats du traitement des hemorrhagies oesophagogastriques sur varices par la sonde de Sengstaken-Blakemore. *Gasttroenterologia* 1964; 102:242–246.
24. Hermann RE, Traul D. Experience with the Sengstaken-

Blakemore tube for bleeding esophageal varices. *Surg Gynecol Obstet* 1970; 130:879–885.

25. Pitcher JL. Safety and effectiveness of the modified Sengstaken-Blakemore tube: A prospective study. *Gastroenterology* 1971; 61:291–298.

26. Johansen TS, Baden H. Re-appraisal of the Sengstaken-Blakemore balloon tamponade for bleeding esophageal varices, results in 91 patients. *Scand J Gastroenterol* 1973; 18:181–183.

27. Novis BH, Duys P, Barbezat GO, Clain J, Bank S, Terblanche J. Fiberoptic endoscopy and the use of the Sengstaken tube in acute gastrointestinal hemorrhage in patients with portal hypertension and varices. *Gut* 1976; 17:258–268.

28. Terés J, Anastasio C, Bordas JM, Rimola A, Bru C, Rodés J. Esophageal tamponade for bleeding varices. Controlled trial between the Sengstaken-Blakemore tube and the Linton-Nachlas tube. *Gastroenterology* 1978; 75:566–569.

29. Orloff MJ, Bell RH Jr, Greenburg AG. Prospective randomized trial of emergency portacaval shunt and medical therapy in unselected cirrhotic patients with bleeding varices. *Gastroenterology* 1986; 90:1754.

30. Conn HO. Emergency portacaval anastomosis (EPCA): The long-awaited trial. *Hepatology* 1986; 6:1058–1060.

31. Conn HO, Simpson JA. Excessive mortality associated with balloon tamponade of bleeding varices. *JAMA* 1967; 202:587–591.

32. Schwartz SI, Bales HW, Emerson GL, Mahoney EB. The use of intravenous pituitrin in treatment of bleeding esophageal varices. *Surgery* 1959; 45:72–80.

33. Merigan TC Jr, Plotkin GR, Davidson CS. Effect of intravenously administered posterior pituitary extract on hemorrhage from bleeding varices. *N Engl J Med* 1962; 266:134–135.

34. Shaldon S, Sherlock S. The use of vasopressin ('pitressin') in the control of bleeding from oesophageal varices. *Lancet* 1960; 2:222–225.

35. Johnson WC, Widrich WC, Ansell JE, Robbins AH, Nabseth DC. Control of bleeding varices by vasopressin: A prospective randomized study. *Ann Surg* 1977; 186:369–376.

36. Chojkier M, Groszmann RJ, Atterbury CE, et al. A controlled comparison of continuous intra-arterial and intravenous infusions of vasopressin in hemorrhage from esophageal varices. *Gastroenterology* 1979; 77:540–546.

37. Orloff MJ. Emergency treatment of variceal haemorrhage. *Can J Surg* 1979; 22:550–553.

38. Orloff MJ, Bell RH Jr, Hyde PV, Skivolocki WP. Long-term results of emergency portacaval shunt for bleeding esophageal varices in unselected patients with alcohol cirrhosis. *Ann Surg* 1980; 192:325–340.

39. Orloff MJ, Bell RH Jr. Improved survival of unselected cirrhotic patients with bleeding esophageal varices treated by emergency portacaval shunt. *Gastroenterology* 1983; 84:1389.

40. Orloff MJ, Bell RH Jr, Greenburg AG. Prospective randomized trial of emergency portacaval shunt and medical therapy in unselected cirrhotic patients with bleeding varices. *Gastroenterology* 1986; 90:1754.

41. Conn HO. Emergency portacaval anastomosis (EPCA): The long-awaited trial. *Hepatology* 1986; 6:1058–1060.

42. Mols P, Hallemans R, Van Kuyk M, et al. Hemodynamic effects of vasopressin, alone and in combination with nitroprusside, in patients with liver cirrhosis and portal hypertension. *Ann Surg* 1984; 199:176–181.

43. Groszmann RJ, Kravetz D, Bosch J, et al. Nitroglycerin improves the hemodynamic response to vasopressin in portal hypertension. *Hepatology* 1982; 2:757–762.

44. Nusbaum M, Baum S, Sakiyalak P, Blakemore WS. Pharmacologic control of portal hypertension. *Surgery* 1967; 62:299–310.

45. Barr JW, Lakin RC, Rösch J. Similarity of arterial and intravenous vasopressin in portal and systemic hemodynamics. *Gastroenterology* 1975; 69:13–19.

46. Millette B, Huet P-M, Lavoie P, Viallet A. Portal and systemic effects of selective infusion of vasopressin into the superior mesenteric artery in cirrhotic patients. *Gastroenterology* 1975; 69:6–12.

47. Murray-Lyon IM, Pugh RNH, Nunnerley HB, Laws JW, Dawson JL, Williams R. Treatment of bleeding oesophageal varices by infusion of vasopressin into the superior mesenteric artery. *Gut* 1973; 14:59–63.

48. Nusbaum M, Younis MT, Baum S, Blakemore WS. Control of portal hypertension. Selective mesenteric arterial infusion of vasopressin. *Arch Surg* 1974; 108:342–347.

49. Conn HO, Ramsby GR, Storer EH, et al. Intra-arterial vasopressin in the treatment of upper gastrointestinal hemorrhage: A prospective, controlled clinical trial. *Gastroenterology* 1975; 68:211–221.

50. Johnson WC, Widrich WC. Efficacy of selective splanchnic arteriography and vasopressin perfusion in diagnosis and treatment of gastrointestinal hemorrhage. *Am J Surg* 1976; 131:481–489.

51. Kaufman SL, Harrington DP, Barth KH, Maddrey WC, White RI Jr. Control of variceal bleeding by superior mesenteric artery vasopressin infusion. *AJR* 1977; 126:567–569.

52. Getzen LC, Brink RR, Wolfman EF Jr. Survival following infusion of pitressin into the superior mesenteric artery to control bleeding esophageal varices in cirrhotic patients. *Ann Surg* 1978; 187:337–342.

53. Sherman LM, Shenoy SS, Cerra FB. Selective intra-arterial vasopressin: Clinical efficacy and complications. *Ann Surg* 1979; 189:298–302.

54. Lunderquist A, Vang J. Transhepatic catheterization and obliteration of the coronary vein in patients with portal hypertension and esophageal varices. *N Engl J Med* 1974; 291:646–649.

55. Passariello R, Rossi P, Simonetti G, Ciolina A, Rovighi L. Emergency transhepatic obliteration of bleeding varices. *Cardiovasc Radiol* 1979; 2:97–106.

56. Lunderquist A, Börjesson B, Owman T, Bengmark S. Isobutyl-2-cyanoacrylate (bucrylate) in obliteration of gastric coronary vein and esophageal varices. *AJR* 1978; 130:1–6.

57. Turner WW Jr, Ellman BA. Transhepatic embolization in patients with acute variceal hemorrhage. *Am J Surg* 1981; 142:731–734.

58. Bengmark S, Börjesson B, Hoevels J, Joelsson B, Lunderquist A, Owman T. Obliteration of esophageal varices by PTP. A follow-up of 43 patients. *Ann Surg* 1979; 190:549–554.

59. Smith-Laing G, Scott J, Long RG, Dick R, Sherlock S. Role of percutaneous transhepatic obliteration of varices in the management of hemorrhage from gastroesophageal varices. *Gastroenterology* 1981; 80:1031–1036.

60. Sos TA. Transhepatic portal venous embolization of varices: Pros and cons. *Radiology* 1983; 148:569–570.

61. Benner KG, Keefe EB, Keller FS, Rösch J. Clinical outcome after percutaneous transhepatic obliteration of esophageal varices. *Gastroenterology* 1983; 85:146–153.

62. Johnston GW, Rodgers HW. A review of 15 years experience in the use of sclerotherapy in the control of acute

hemorrhage from oesophageal varices. *Br J Surg* 1973; 60: 797–800.

63. Paquet KJ, Oberhammer E. Sclerotherapy of bleeding oesophageal varices by means of endoscopy. *Endoscopy* 1978; 10:7–12.

64. Terblanche J, Northover JMA, Bornman P, et al. A prospective evaluation of injection sclerotherapy in the treatment of acute bleeding from esophageal varices. *Surgery* 1979; 85:239–245.

65. DiMagno EP, George L, Gores A, Carlson GL. Does sclerotherapy alter the natural history of bleeding esophageal varices? *Gastroenterology* 1983; 84:1137.

66. Kjaergaard J, Fischer A, Miskowiak J, Lindahl F, Baden H. Sclerotherapy of bleeding esophageal varices. Long-term results. *Scand J Gastroenterol* 1982; 17:363–367.

67. Alwmark A, Bengmark S, Borjesson B, Gullstrand P, Joelsson B. Emergency and long-term transesophageal sclerotherapy of bleeding esophageal varices. A prospective study of 50 consecutive cases. *Scand J Gastroenterol* 1982; 17:409–412.

68. MacDougall BRD, Theodossi A, Westaby D, Dawson JL, Williams R. Increased long-term survival in variceal haemorrhage using injection sclerotherapy. Results of a controlled trial. *Lancet* 1982; 1:124–127.

69. Goodale RL, Silvis SE, O'Leary JF, et al. Early survival after sclerotherapy for bleeding esophageal varices. *Surg Gynecol Obstet* 1982; 155:523–528.

70. Barsoum MS, Bolous FI, El-Rooby AA, Rizk-Allah MA, Ibrahim AS. Tamponade and injection sclerotherapy in the management of bleeding oesophageal varices. *Br J Surg* 1982; 69:76–78.

71. Soehendra N, deHeer K, Kempeneers I, Runge M. Sclerotherapy of esophageal varices: Acute arrest of gastrointestinal hemorrhage or long-term therapy? *Endoscopy* 1983; (Suppl)15:136–140.

72. Terblanche J, Kahn D, Campbell JAH, et al. Failure of repeated injection sclerotherapy to improve long-term survival after oesophageal variceal bleeding. *Lancet* 1983; 2:1328–1332.

73. Westaby D, Williams R. The history of injection sclerotherapy for esophageal varices. *Gastrointest Endosc* 1983; 29:303 307.

74. Conn HO. Endoscopic sclerotherapy: An analysis of variants. *Hepatology* 1983; 3:769–771.

75. Health and Public Policy Committee, American College of Physicians: Position paper. Endoscopic sclerotherapy for esophageal varices. *Ann Intern Med* 1984; 100:608–610.

76. Orloff MJ, Krims P, UCSD Gastroenterology Division. Effect of endoscopic sclerotherapy on rebleeding and survival of cirrhotic patients with bleeding esophageal varices. *Gastroenterology* 1986; 90:1574.

77. Boerema I. Bleeding varices of oesophagus in cirrhosis of the liver and Banti's syndrome. *Arch Chir Neerl* 1949; 1: 253–260.

78. Ottinger LW, Moncure AC. Transthoracic ligation of bleeding esophageal varices in patients with intrahepatic portal obstruction. *Ann Surg* 1974; 179:35–38.

79. Rothwell-Jackson RL, Hunt AH. The results obtained with emergency surgery in the treatment of persistent haemorrhage from gastro-oesophageal varices in the cirrhotic patient. *Br J Surg* 1971; 58:205–215.

80. Wirthlin LS, Linton RR, Ellis DS. Transthoracoesophageal ligation of bleeding esophageal varices. A reappraisal. *Arch Surg* 1974; 109:688–692.

81. Orloff MJ. A comparative study of emergency transesophageal ligation and nonsurgical treatment of bleed-ing esophageal varices in unselected patients with cirrhosis. *Surgery* 1962; 52:103–116.

82. Futagawa S, Sugiura M, Hidai K, Shima F. Emergency esophageal transection with paraesophagogastric devascularization for variceal bleeding. *World J Surg* 1979; 3: 229–234.

83. Johnston GW. Treatment of bleeding varices by oesophageal transection with the SPTU gun. *Ann R Coll Surg Engl* 1977; 59:404–408.

84. Pugh RNH, Murray-Lyon IM, Dawson JL, Pietroni MC, Williams R. Transection of the oesophagus for bleeding oesophageal varices. *Br J Surg* 1973; 60:646–649.

85. Sugiura M, Futagawa S. Further evaluation of the Sugiura procedure in the treatment of esophageal varices. *Arch Surg* 1977; 112:1317–1321.

86. Yamamoto S, Hidemura R, Sawada M, Takeshige K, Iwatsuki S. The late results of terminal esophagoproximal gastrectomy (TEPG) with extensive devascularization and splenectomy for bleeding esophageal varices in cirrhosis. *Surgery* 1976; 80:106–114.

87. Johnston GW. Six years' experience of oesophageal transection for oesophageal varices using a circular stapling gun. *Gut* 1982; 23:770–773.

88. Osborne DR, Hobbs KEF. The acute treatment of haemorrhage from oesophageal varices: A comparison of oesophageal transection and staple gun anastomosis with mesocaval shunt. *Br J Surg* 1981; 68:734–737.

89. Wanamaker SR, Cooperman M, Carey LC. Use of the EEA stapling instrument for control of bleeding esophageal varices. *Surgery* 1983; 94:620–626.

90. Umeyama K, Yoshikawa K, Yamoshita T, Todo T, Satake K. Transabdominal oesophageal transection for oesophageal varices: Experience in 101 patients. *Br J Surg* 1983; 70:419–422.

91. Mir J, Ponce J, Morena E, et al. Esophageal transection and paraesophagogastric devascularization performed as an emergency measure for uncontrolled variceal bleeding. *Surg Gynecol Obstet* 1982; 155:868–872.

92. Van Beek DF, Gleysteen JJ, Malangoni MA, Klamer TW, Lewis JD. Mortality and rebleeding after hypertensive variceal disconnections. *Arch Surg* 1984; 119:446–449.

93. Orloff MJ. Emergency portacaval shunt. A comparative study of shunt, varix ligation, and nonsurgical treatment of bleeding esophageal varices in unselected patients with cirrhosis. *Ann Surg* 1967; 166:456–478.

94. Orloff MJ. Emergency treatment of bleeding esophageal varices. In: Markoff NG, ed. *The Therapy of Portal Hypertension.* Stuttgart: Georg Thieme Verlag, 1968:211–219.

95. Orloff MJ. Emergency treatment of bleeding esophageal varices in alcoholic cirrhosis. In: Sardesai VM, ed. *Biochemical and Clinical Aspects of Alcohol Metabolism.* Springfield, Illinois: Charles C Thomas, 1969:288–297.

96. Orloff MJ, Chandler JG, Charters AC, et al. Emergency portacaval shunt for bleeding esophageal varices. Prospective study in unselected patients with alcoholic cirrhosis. *Arch Surg* 1974; 108:293–299.

97. Orloff MJ, Chandler JG, Charters AC, et al. Portacaval shunt as emergency procedure in unselected patients with alcoholic cirrhosis. *Surg Gynecol Obstet* 1975; 141:59–68.

98. Bell RH Jr, Hyde PVB, Skivolocki WP, Brimm JE, Orloff MJ. Prospective study of portasystemic encephalopathy after emergency portacaval shunt for bleeding varices. *Am J Surg* 1981; 142:144–150.

99. Orloff MJ, Bell RH Jr. Long-term survival after emergency portacaval shunting for bleeding varices in patients with alcoholic cirrhosis. *Am J Surg* 1986; 151:176–183.

100. Isbell H, Fraser HF, Wikler A, Belleville RE, Eisenman AJ. An experimental study of the etiology of "rum fits" and delirium tremens. *Q J Stud Alcohol* 1955; 16:1–33.

101. Nielsen J. An intensive one-year study of delirium tremens in Copenhagen from August 1, 1961 to July 31, 1962. *Acta Psychiatr Scand* 1965; (Suppl 187)41:32–85.

102. Fischer JE. Hepatic coma in cirrhosis, portal hypertension, and following portacaval shunt. Its etiologies and the current status of its treatment. *Arch Surg* 1974; 108: 325–336.

103. Schenker S, Breen KJ, Hoyumpa AM Jr. Hepatic encephalopathy. Current status. *Gastroenterology* 1974; 66:121–151.

104. Zieve L, Nicoloff DM. Pathogenesis of hepatic coma. *Annu Rev Med* 1975; 26:143–157.

105. Clarke JS, Ozeran RS, Hart JC, Cruze K, Crevling V. Peptic ulcer following portacaval shunt. *Ann Surg* 1958; 148:551–563.

106. Phillips MM, Ramsby GA, Conn HO. Portacaval anastomosis and peptic ulcer: A nonassociation. *Gastroenterology* 1975; 68:121–131.

107. Papper S. Renal failure in cirrhosis (the hepatorenal syndrome). In: Epstein M, ed. *The Kidney in Liver Disease.* New York: Elsevier, 1976.

108. Wilkinson SP, Williams R. Renal failure in cirrhosis: Current views and speculations. *Adv Nephrol* 1977; 7:15–32.

109. Wong PY, McCoy GC, Spielberg A, Milora RV, Balint JA. The hepatorenal syndrome. *Gastroenterology* 1979; 77: 1326–1334.

110. Gabuzda GJ. Nutrition and liver disease. Practical considerations. *Med Clin North Am* 1970; 54:1455–1472.

Editorial Comment

Dr. Orloff's continuing, rather dramatic, approach to the management of bleeding esophageal varices with immediate emergency portacaval shunt is certainly impressive. To some, the mortality of emergency portacaval shunt may seem high and, in fact, when Dr. Orloff began his trials some years ago, the early mortality rate was in the 42% range. With increasing experience, the mortality has been recently reported at 17%, an impressive performance in what is described as an unselected series.

One can analyze Dr. Orloff's series and then try to initiate a comparison between his group of patients and those reported by Terblanche in Chapter 13B with endoscopic sclerotherapy employed as the treatment of choice.

Obviously, a valid comparison is not possible in two different series in different parts of the world with various types of inadvertent selection occurring but certainly, the information presented in this section does not permit one to easily discard emergency portacaval shunt as a valid choice and

possibly the treatment of choice, under these catastrophic circumstances.

There are a number of studies adjunctive measures that we have not found useful such as intra-arterial use of vasopressin and other relatively peripheral and unimportant adjuncts to diagnosis and treatment. We ourselves have not had a prospective randomized study on the emergency management of esophageal varices but the evaluation of our clinical efforts over the years have led to a fairly standardized approach, which consists of immediate diagnostic evaluation relying primarily on endoscopic visualization of the upper GI tract followed by ice water lavage, heavy doses of antacids, intravenous vasopressin and, when necessary, balloon tamponade. We have also felt that early shunt surgery provided the most effective immediate and long-term control but have termed our approach as "urgent shunt surgery" since we will often defer operation for 48 to 72 hours in order to achieve restoration of blood volume, reestablishment of urinary output, and support of cardiac and pulmonary function during the critical shock phase. Only after reasonable stabilization would we proceed to operation.

The enthusiasm for endoscopic sclerosis has led us to initiate in the Boston-New Haven Collaborative Group, a randomized study of the management of bleeding esophageal varices but the data from this study is too preliminary to warrant comment at this time.

One also would wonder of necessity if it is justified to operate on all cases since we inevitably encounter a significant percentage of individuals who are near terminal from their basic disease as well as from the hemorrhage, and for whom we feel operation would be intolerable.

In conclusion of this commentary, it is obvious to all who have provided management for this incredibly difficult problem of bleeding esophageal varices that there are enormous numbers of variables in any series and statistical comparisons become almost impossible across institutional boundaries. Nonetheless, we would continue to wonder if a certain selection process prior to urgent shunt surgery would not be the more rational approach. This does leave the surgeons and gastroenterologists somewhat more leisure to analyze the problems and to select the most appropriate shunt.

Chapter 14
Shunts

Chapter 14A
Elective Portasystemic Shunts

RONALD A. MALT

In the hemodynamic analysis of the splanchnic venous system, complex interplays among flow, resistance, shunting, and ignorance exceed the bounds of simple models (1–5) and heuristic arguments prevail over logic. But one overriding fact is that the principles of newtonian flow in rigid tubes do not hold when applied to the flexible, elastic veins. Moreover, the splanchnic venous system is not freely intercommunicating. Functional or anatomic blocks may isolate one part so that decompression of another part has no effect on it. For example, isolated splenic vein thrombosis causes left upper quandrant varices and is curable only by a splenectomy. To the contrary, the huge retroperitoneal collateral veins sometimes connecting the splenic vein to the renal vein in portal hypertension are ineffective decompression.

A "total" shunt in a normal person deprives the hepatocytes of all splanchnic venous blood and leads to portasystemic encephalopathy. Modern research into the problems actually began with just such a preparation in a patient whose portal vein was purposely resected in 1952 during a pancreatectomy for cancer, followed by an end-to-side anastomosis of the superior mesenteric vein to the inferior vena cava (6). By and large, however, total shunts are infrequent nowadays, as compared with 1977, a decade ago, and patients with a normal liver rarely undergo a total shunt except in cases of portal-vein injury.

In patients with long-standing portal hypertension inferences that some shunts are total shunts because of apparent flow patterns of radiographic contrast media are heavily influenced by artifacts and are thus inexact (2). Doppler duplex ultrasonography seems more valid; it shows that in a "total" side-to-side portacaval shunt total loss of splanchnic flow does not occur (7), an observation confirmed by other means (8). In almost every case, compensatory mechanisms increase hepatic arterial flow and collateral splanchnic venous flow so that perfusion of the hepatocytes continues— sometimes to a nearly normal level, sometimes very little; sometimes with considerable splanchnic venous blood, sometimes with almost none. Moreover, the relationship even between the classic Eck's fistula and "meat intoxication" in dogs (6) may have to be revised in light of studies showing that adequate nutrition prevents hepatic coma, but not hepatic atrophy (9).

By design, the end-to-side portacaval shunt removes residual direct splanchnic venous perfusion of the hepatocytes and should thus be "total." In addition, the side-to-side portacaval shunts, the proximal splenorenal shunts (with splenectomy), the mesocaval shunts, and the renoportal shunts also have the potentiality for being nominally total. Whether or not any one of them actually is depends on the balance among inflow pressures, intrahepatic and intravascular resistances, shunts between the hepatic arterial system and the portal venous system, and sites of decompression by collateral veins.

Only the selective distal splenorenal shunt is, indeed, selective in the sense of not depriving the liver of portal venous circulation in the early postoperative phase. But the choice of patients for a distal splenorenal shunt requires the preselection of those with "prograde" (centripetal) flow of portal-vein blood as candidates, thus coincidentally selecting the best-risk patients—those whose cirrhosis is not so bad as to create a high resistance to splanchnic venous perfusion or to cause hepatic arterial shunting into the portal circulation. The propensity of even selective shunts to become nonselective with time and to act as functional side-to-side shunts is addressed by Warren in Chapter 14B (10).

End-to-Side Portacaval Shunts

The end-to-side portacaval shunt is appropriate for both the emergency arrest of otherwise uncontrollable bleeding from esophageal varices and the elective control of varices in patients who have bled. Results following its use may be as good as those following use of any of the more complicated shunts. The trouble is predicting which patients will do so well that their lives are almost normal, except for the limits imposed by the primary disease, and which will do badly from hepatic failure and portasystemic encephalopathy.

Prophylactic shunts should not be done for patients whose varices have never bled because they only change the mode of death from bleeding to hepatic encephalopathy and failure (11). For the patient whose varices have bled, conventional wisdom derived from results of randomized trials also says there is no value to shunting in prolonging life. Yet, analysis of the statistics from the studies on which this conclusion was reached indicates to the surgeon potential flaws in the arguments (12–15). Most patients entered into the trials were good risks, stratification was imprecise, the populations examined were usually small, varying skills of different surgeons and hospitals could not be controlled, and the β-error and power of negative observations was never calculated; the issue of power was considered only in studies done in the early 1980s (15). Thus, studies describing a 20% increase in survival rate at 3 years after an end-to-side shunt may be more "significant" than they have been credited (12). An increase in the number of patients studied might have yielded generally accepted statistical significance.

Once it is granted that a shunt is appropriate treatment for a patient with varices that have bled—lesser measures having failed or being inappropriate—an end-to-side shunt is not only the easiest to do but the one most nearly certain to control variceal bleeding. An end-to-side shunt can even be done without preliminary imaging studies. It can be done with considerable confidence that the portal vein will be patent, otherwise suitable for use, and nearly certain to work. Doppler duplex ultrasonography promises to add certainty and reduce the need for preliminary angiography.

Although the techniques of end-to-side shunting are described elsewhere and will not be considered here, a few principles should be mentioned (16–19): (a) the focus of dissection should be limited to the relevant portion of the inferior vena cava and the nearby portal vein. (b) Initial exposure is facilitated by reflecting the duodenum with Kocher's maneuver, normally an easy dissection. (c) Other structures in the portal triad should be retracted from the portal vein, not dissected individually. (d) Only the exposure of the medial side of the portal vein entails a dangerous dissection. (e) Clamping the hepatic end of the vein does not require good visualization of it, if an appropriate method is used. (f) The vein must run in a good hemodynamic line to the medial aspect of the vena cava. The presence of a replaced hepatic artery running along the lateral aspect of the triad may require ingenious rerouting of portal vein; an impeding lip of pancreas or a wad of dense fat may require division. (g) Caution should be exercised in using the vena cava as a conduit for decompression if there is angiographic or hemodynamic evidence of its compression by an engorged liver (as in Budd-Chiari syndrome) or a nodular caudate "lobe"; nonetheless, most ostensible compression disappears when the patient is erect and any ascites present are drained. Actual anatomic obstructions in the vena cava (webs, for instance) are, of course, another story.

Failure of an end-to-side portacaval shunt to control esophageal varices usually means that two walls of the vessels have been stitched together or that a clot has been allowed to form in the portal vein. The presence of postoperative ascites does not mean the shunt is thrombosed, internists' views to the contrary.

Aside from its utility in relieving portal hypertension, the end-to-side portacaval shunt can be used to correct metabolic disease by eliminating hepatic transformation of substances in the splanchnic venous circulation. It (and its modifications) can ameliorate hypoglycemia and promote glycogenolysis in patients with some forms of glycogen storage disease, and can reduce synthesis of cholesterol and mobilize lipoprotein deposits in patients with homozygous familial hypercholesterolemia (2,3,20).

Side-to-Side Portacaval Shunt

Not only does the side-to-side portacaval shunt have the propensity for decompressing the distal portal vein and its tributaries, it can decompress the hepatic end of the portal vein, reducing intrahepatic portal venous pressure. While on the one hand this decompression may be desirable to remedy effects of a Budd-Chiari syndrome or to treat the now-rare case of intractable ascites, it has the potential liability of depriving the liver of even more portal circulation than an end-to-side shunt. That is, in cirrhotic patients the characteristic flow of hepatic arterial blood through arteriovenous shunts at the sinusoidal level could be diverted down the cephalic end of the side-to-side decompression, depriving the liver further of its vascular supply. As stated above, however, these arguments may not be valid. But because of this uncertainty and although it is widely used, the side-to-side shunt for emergency decompression of the splanchnic circulation is not considered appropriate by many authorities. It may, however, be useful in elective operations. Recent evidence suggests that controlled small-orifice side-to-side portacaval shunt has the potentiality for decompressing the portal circulation enough to prevent variceal bleeding, while permitting enough splanchnic hypertension to avoid the consequences of encephalopathy after total decompression (7,8).

The direct side-to-side shunt is more difficult to perform than the end-to-side portacaval shunt because the portal vein and the inferior vein may be too far apart to be joined easily or may have their potential route of connections blocked by an engorged caudate "lobe" of the liver. Generalized engorgement of the liver may compress the intrahepatic vena cava, raising its pressure considerably and vitiating use of the vena cava as a low-pressure avenue for decompression. Narrowing of a side-to-side shunt from tension on the anastomosis caused by pulling two distant veins together predisposes to thrombosis. Indeed, the very disease for which this operation is best (Budd-Chiari syndrome) is the one most likely to give rise to all these problems. Thus, if division of several lumbar veins and dissection of the portal vein do not produce enough mobility for easy approximation of the portal vein and the inferior vena cava, an interposition ("H") graft of a vascular prosthesis or of autogenous vein is required. A double-barrel end-to-side portacaval shunt is particularly efficacious when circumstances allow its construction (21).

Mesocaval Shunt (H-Graft)

The principle of a mesocaval shunt was originally proposed for decompression of portal hypertension in childhood, when the splenic vein and other peripheral splanchnic veins were considered too small for use.

Although one might anticipate this shunt would function like a mere side-arm tap off the portal vein—that is, like a side-to-side shunt—relationships of flow and resistance are such that it, too, can divert the much portal-vein blood into the systemic circulation. In terms of function, it has no advantage over a side-to-side portacaval shunt.

Nonetheless, the mesocaval shunt is undoubtedly valuable in decompressing the portal vein when the portal vein is occluded, but the superior mesenteric vein is open. It is an alternative to the side-to-side portacaval shunt for treatment of the Budd-Chiari syndrome. Extreme obesity and infrahepatic scarring may be relative indications for its use, as compared with a direct venovenous shunt. For glycogen storage disease and homozygous familial hypercholesterolemia, the mesocaval shunt should work like the end-to-side portacaval shunt.

In terms of ease of use, those well-versed say it is a simpler operation than the portacaval shunt (22,23). Even if this assertion is correct, the H-graft mesocaval shunt must be considered less desirable than a portacaval shunt because it introduces problems of kinking and occlusion of the superior mesenteric vein, of clotting in the prosthesis, of infection, and of erosion into the duodenum. The international incidence of thrombosis and other complications is certainly 20% (24) and may actually be over 30%. Use of autologous jugular vein as the H-graft offers no advantage in adult cirrhotics (25). In children with extrahepatic splanchnic venous occlusion or hypertension second to biliary atresia, cystic fibrosis, or congenital hepatic fibrosis, however, a high success rate may be possible, even if the vein has a diameter of only 5 millimeters (26).

For emergency shunting a small and imperfect randomized trial of the mesocaval shunt concluded it had no advantages over the end-to-side portacaval shunt for surgeons reared in the tradition of direct shunting (27). Instead, the facility of working with autogenous veins made the direct end-to-side portacaval shunt more appropriate.

Mesocaval Shunt (C-Graft)

Hemodynamics of this shunt are doubtless the same as those of the H-graft, and its range of applications is the same. Its overwhelming utility is that it is unlikely either to erode into the duodenum or another structure, or to kink the superior mesenteric vein, because lines of stress on the vein wall are better. Too few have been done for the likelihood of thrombosis overall to be accurately assessed. In expert hands, a prevalence of patency over 90% is possible (28).

Mesocaval Shunt (Side-to-End)

Obliteration of the portal vein and its intrahepatic branches from neonatal omphalitis and thrombophlebitis often spares the superior mesenteric vein. Until recently, the best shunt for children with portal hypertension from any extrahepatic block of this kind was a Marion-Clatworthy-Valdoni operation, which entails dividing the inferior vena cava, turning it up, and anastomosing it to the mesenteric vein for decompression (2). Nowadays the procedure is obsolescent because good results are possible by direct splenorenal anastomosis, even in small children, unless the splenic vein is also thrombosed (see below). The side-to-end shunt should never be used in adults because the frequent massive edema of the lower extremities is too great a price, as long as alternative forms of decompression exist.

Proximal Splenorenal Shunt with Splenectomy

Because it is harder to perform than any of the shunts previously discussed (29–31), twice as liable to clot than the end-to-side portacaval shunt (29% vs. 14%, worldwide), introduces the risk of overwhelming postsplenectomy sepsis in children, and is not suitable for emergency use because it decompresses the portal system too slowly, unique applications must be found if the proximal splenorenal shunt is to have a therapeutic role (29). The main acceptable indication is extrahepatic portal hypertension in children who have a patent splenic vein.

Figure 14A.1 shows that decompression with the expectation of long-term patency is possible in young children (32). Results such as these and the 94% patency rate in an earlier series (33) are

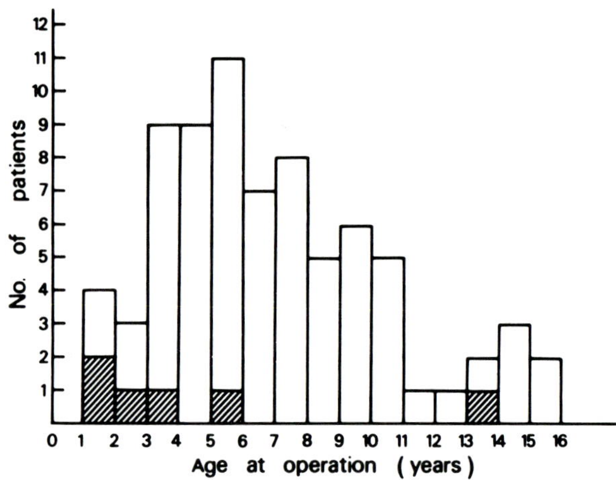

Figure 14A.1. Patency rates of splenorenal shunts in childhood. The hatched area represents the proportion of thrombosed shunts. (Reproduced by permission from Alvarez F, Bernard O, Brunelle F, Hadchouel P, Odievre M, Alagille D. Portal obstruction in children. II. Results of surgical portasystemic shunts. *J Pediatr* 1983; 5:703–707.)

putting to rest the old saw that bleeding varices in childhood should be treated nonoperatively, waiting until the child reaches his or her teens before attempting a shunt. While the traditional advice is true in the sense that children almost never die from variceal hemorrhage because their cardiovascular system is resilient, and some children stop bleeding as they age, the risks of hepatitis, cytomegalovirus infection, and acquired immune deficiency syndrome (AIDS) from blood transfusions may now be greater than those of surgery.

Relief of splanchnic venous hypertension and hypersplenism in patients with schistosomiasis and other forms of presinusoidal hypertension is also feasible with the proximal splenorenal shunt, but with the risk of a 31% incidence of encephalopathy over the short term (34). However, the alternative operation, a selective distal splenorenal shunt, gives results at least as good in terms of control of varices and preservation of the spleen, and is associated with only a 13% incidence of encephalopathy (34). (Esophagogastric disconnection may in fact, be superior to either.) The large splenic vein in these diseases facilitates either type of anastomosis.

Considering the number of cirrhotic American patients only, the great question is where the proximal splenorenal shunt with splenectomy stands in the priority list of operations for patients with bleeding varices. There is no question that some patients do superbly after this operation (35). Unfortunately, as with all portasystemic shunts, matching the type of shunt to the patient remains the dilemma. Some of the variables will be considered in Proximal Splenorenal and End-to-Side Portacaval Shunts: Results Compared, below, and the alternative of a selective distal splenorenal shunt will be analyzed in Chapter 14B.

As a result of an unpublished trial of 30 patients randomized between a proximal shunt and a distal shunt at our hospital, only two conclusions are justified: (a) It was impossible to predict from any preoperative study whether the proximal shunt or the distal shunt would be easier to do. Anatomic situations that looked difficult beforehand for one kind of operation turned out to be easy, and vice versa. (b) The patient with the worst encephalopathy had a selective distal splenorenal shunt.

Proximal Splenorenal and End-to-Side Portacaval Shunts: Results Compared

Analysis of the results of shunting 120 patients in the 8 years from 1966 through 1973 (portacaval shunt, 57% of total; proximal splenorenal shunt, 43%) showed no differences in survival rates or encephalopathy rates between patients who underwent a portacaval shunt or a splenorenal shunt. These data were compared with those of 141 patients in the 8 years from 1974 through 1981 (portacaval shunt, 23% of total; proximal splenorenal shunt, 58%; mesocaval shunt, 12%; distal splenorenal shunt, 6%; coronary-caval shunt, 1%) (36).

Although the Child-Turcotte criteria (Table

Table 14A.1. Child-Turcotte Classification of Cirrhotic Patients According to Functional Reserve

Variable	Class A	Class B	Class C
Serum bilirubin (mg/dl)	<2.0	2.0–3.0	>3.0
Serum albumin (g/dl)	>3.5	3.0–3.5	<3.0
Ascites	None	Minimal	Poorly controlled
Neurologic disorder	None	Minimal	Advanced, coma
Nutrition	Excellent	Good	Poor, "wasting"

Abbreviations: g/dl, grams per deciliter; mg/dl, milligrams per deciliter.
Adapted from Child GC III, Turcotte JG. Surgery and portal hypertension. In: Child CG III, ed. *The Liver and Portal Hypertension*, Vol. 1. Dunphy JE, ed. *Major Problems in Clinical Surgery*. Philadelphia, WB Saunders, 1964, pp.1–85.

Table 14A.2. Scale for Predicting Early Postoperative Mortality

	Points Assigned[a]		
Variable	0	1	2
Bilirubin (mg/dl)	≤0.99	1.00–1.99	≥2.0
Ascites	None	Stable	Uncontrollable
Operative urgency	Elective	Emergency	—

[a] Score is the sum of points established for all predictors: minimum = 0; maximum = 5.
Reproduced by permission from Lacame F, LaMuraglia GM, Malt RA. Prognostic factors in survival after portasystem shunts: Multivariate analysis. *Ann Surg* 1985; 202:729–734.

14A.1) (37) were useful in predicting the mortality rate of operations, the criterion of "encephalopathy" was not a specific one because it predicted the likelihood of future encephalopathy (83% accuracy) rather than the probability of survival. Nutritional status was rarely assessed accurately (38).

Considering the 1974–1981 patients, the validity of a simple six-point scale to predict the likelihood of a postoperative death was confirmed (Table 14A.2, Fig. 14A.2) using the last data collected before an operation (36). An equation derived by logistic regression identified independent prognostic significance for an emergency operation, serum albumin and bilirubin concentrations, age, and sex (men, worse). With these data the cutpoint

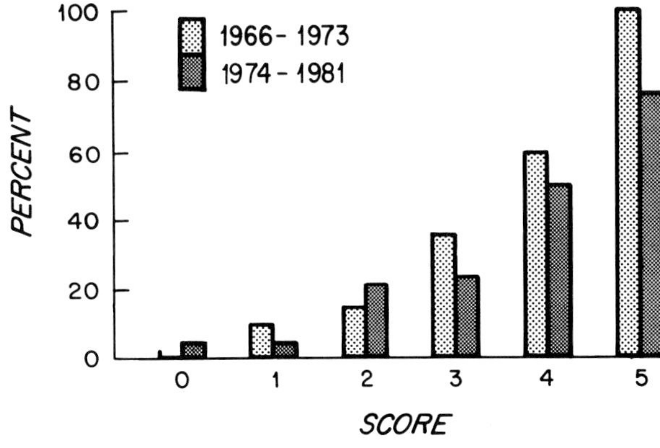

Figure 14A.2. Mortality rates of portacaval and splenorenal shunting by score (see Table 14A.2): comparison of two intervals. (Reprinted by permission from Lacaine F, LaMuraglia GM, Malt RA: Prognostic factors in survival after portasystemic shunts: Multivariate analysis. *Ann Surg* 1985; 202:729–734.)

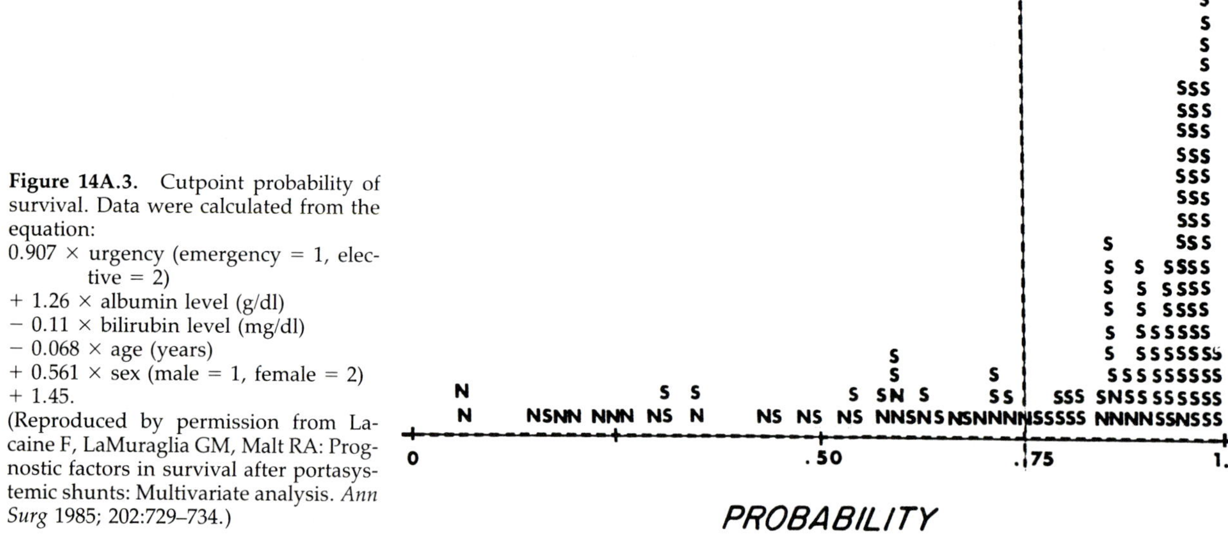

PROBABILITY

Figure 14A.3. Cutpoint probability of survival. Data were calculated from the equation:
0.907 × urgency (emergency = 1, elective = 2)
+ 1.26 × albumin level (g/dl)
− 0.11 × bilirubin level (mg/dl)
− 0.068 × age (years)
+ 0.561 × sex (male = 1, female = 2)
+ 1.45.
(Reproduced by permission from Lacaine F, LaMuraglia GM, Malt RA: Prognostic factors in survival after portasystemic shunts: Multivariate analysis. *Ann Surg* 1985; 202:729–734.)

probability of 0.75 separated patients who had an 84% chance of survival (above 0.75) from those below, who had at least a 77% chance of death (Fig. 14A.3).

A Cox regression model for long-term survival after an emergency operation defined male sex and a prolonged partial thromboplastin time as poor prognostic factors, while after an elective operation only the serum albumin level was prognostic. Once a patient had survived the emergency operation (46% mortality rate vs. 9% elective), his or her likelihood of 5-year survival (30%) was as good as that of survivors of elective operations (37%).

The rate of encephalopathy was 35% among all patients and over all time, if encephalopathy was defined by the most sensitive criterion (any report of encephalopathy by any physician); the severity of encephalopathy was not assessable. The frequency of encephalopathy after end-to-side portacaval shunts in a randomized trial has been examined in only one study (11). That study showed an incidence in of all encephalopathy control (nonshunted) patients rising from 18% to 38% during 4 years of observation, contrasted to 20%, rising to 53%, in shunted patients. The difference between 38% and 53% was not statistically significant. The rate of severe encephalopathy, however, was 3% in control subjects and 20% after portacaval shunts. Contemporary repetition of such a study with all modern controls and means of estimating

encephalopathy would be highly desirable, especially if extended to comparisons with proximal and the distal splenorenal shunts.

References

1. Donovan AJ. Surgical treatment of portal hypertension: A historical perspective. *World J Surg* 1984; 8:626–645.
2. Malt RA. Portasystemic venous shunts. *N Engl J Med* 1976; 295:24–29, 80–86.
3. Callow AD. Portacaval shunts. *World J Surg* 1984; 8:688–697.
4. Voorhees AB Jr, Price JB. An update of portal systemic shunting and its complications. *World J Surg* 1984; 8:698–701.
5. Inokuchi K. Present status of surgical treatment of esophageal varices in Japan: A nationwide survey of 3,588 patients. *World J Surg* 1985; 9:171–180.
6. McDermott WV Jr, Adams RD. Episodic stupor associated with an Eck fistula in the human with particular reference to the metabolism of ammonia. *J Clin Invest* 1954; 33:1–9.
7. Johansen K. The Harborview shunt: Initial experience with a small-caliber portacaval anastomosis. *Surg Gynecol Obstet* (in press).
8. Sarfeh IJ, Rypins EB, Mason GR. A systematic appraisal of portacaval H-graft diameters: Clinical and hemodynamic perspectives. *Ann Surg* 1986; 204:356–363.
9. Thompson JS, Schafer DF, Haun J, Schafer GJ. Adequate diet prevents hepatic coma in dogs with Eck fistulas. *Surg Gynecol Obstet* 1986; 162:126–130.
10. Warren WD, Millikan WJ Jr, Henderson JM, Abu-Elmagd KM, Galloway JR, Shires GT III, et al. Splenopancreatic disconnection: Improved selectivity of distal splenorenal shunt. *Ann Surg* 1986; 204:346–355.
11. Conn HO, Lindenmuth WW, May CJ, Ramsby GR. Prophylactic portacaval anastomosis. A tale of two studies. *Medicine* 1972; 51:27–40.
12. Jackson FC, Perrin EB, Felix WR, Smith AG. A clinical

investigation of the portacaval shunt: V. Survival analysis of the therapeutic operation. *Ann Surg* 1971; 174:672–701.

13. Resnick RH, Iber FL, Ishihara AM, Chalmers TC, Zimmerman H. A controlled study of the therapeutic portacaval shunt. *Gastroenterology* 1974; 67:843–857.

14. Rueff B, Degos F, Degos J-D, Maillard J-N, Prandi D, Sicot J, et al. A controlled study of therapeutic portacaval shunt in alcoholic cirrhosis. *Lancet* 1976; 1:655–658.

15. Reynolds TB, Donovan AJ, Mikkelsen WP, Redeker AG, Turrill FL, Weiner JM. Results of a 12-year randomized trial of portacaval shunt in patients with alcoholic liver disease and bleeding varices. *Gastroenterology* 1981; 80: 1005–1011.

16. McDermott WV Jr. *Surgery of the Liver and Portal Hypertension.* Philadelphia: Lea & Febiger, 1974, pp. 117–123.

17. Malt RA. Emergency and elective operations for bleeding esophageal varices. *Surg Clin North Am* 1974; 54:561–571.

18. Turcotte JG, Erlandson EE. Portacaval shunts. In: Rutherford RB, ed. *Vascular Surgery*, 2nd ed. Philadelphia: WB Saunders, 1984, 1013–1020.

19. Mikkelsen WP. End-to-side portacaval anastomosis. In: Malt RA, ed. *Surgical Techniques Illustrated.* Philadelphia: WB Saunders, 1985, pp. 436–441.

20. McNamara DJ, Ahrens EH Jr, Kolb R, Brown CD, Parker TS, Samuel P, et al. Treatment of familial hypercholesterolemia by portacaval anastomosis: Effect on cholesterol metabolism and pool sizes. *Proc Natl Acad Sci USA* 1983; 80:564–568.

21. McDermott WV Jr. The treatment of cirrhotic ascites by combined hepatic and portal decompression. *N Engl J Med* 1958; 259:897–901.

22. Gliedman ML. Mesocaval shunt. In: Malt RA, ed. *Surgical Techniques Illustrated.* Philadelphia: WB Saunders, 1985, pp. 442–448.

23. Sanfey H, Cameron JL. Mesocaval shunts. In: Rutherford RB, ed. *Vascular Surgery*, 2nd ed. Philadelphia: WB Saunders, 1984, pp. 1029–1051.

24. Cello JP, Deveney KE, Trunkey DD, Heilbron DC, Stoney RJ, Ehrenfeld WK, et al. Factors influencing survival after therapeutic shunts: Results of a discriminant function and linear logistic regressions analysis. *Am J Surg* 1981; 141: 257–265.

25. Stipa S, Ziparo V. Mesentericocaval shunt (MCS) with autologous jugular vein. *World J Surg* 1984; 8:702–705.

26. Valayer J, Hay J-M, Gauthier F, Broto J. Shunt surgery for treatment of portal hypertension in children. *World J Surg* 1985; 9:258–268.

27. Malt RA, Abbott WM, Warshaw AL, Vander Salm TJ, Smead WL. Randomized trial of emergency mesocaval and portacaval shunts for bleeding esophageal varices. *Am J Surg* 1978; 135:584–588.

28. Sarr MG, Herlong HF, Cameron JL. Long-term patency of the mesocaval C shunt. *Am J Surg* 1986; 151:98–103.

29. Bismuth H. End-to-side splenorenal anastomosis. In: Malt RA, ed. *Surgical Techniques Illustrated.* Philadelphia: WB Saunders, 1985, pp. 465–473.

30. Malt RA. Proximal splenorenal venous shunts. In: Rutherford RB, ed. *Vascular Surgery*, 2nd ed. Philadelphia: WB Saunders, 1984, pp. 1021–1028.

31. Barsoum MS, Rizk-Allah MA, El-Said Khedr M, Khattar NY. A new posterior exposure of the splenic vein for an H-graft splenorenal shunt. *Br J Surg* 1982; 69:376–379.

32. Alvarez F, Bernard O, Brunelle F, Hadchouel P, Odievre M, Alagille D. Portal obstruction in children. II. Results of surgical portasystemic shunts. *J Pediatr* 1983; 5:703–707.

33. Bismuth H, Franco D. Portal diversion for portal hypertension in early childhood. *Ann Surg* 1976; 183:439–446.

34. Raia S, Mies S, Macedo AL. Surgical treatment of portal hypertension in schistosomiasis. *World J Surg* 1984; 8:738–752.

35. Ottinger LW. The Linton splenorenal shunt in the management of the bleeding complications of portal hypertension. *Ann Surg* 1982; 196:664–668.

36. Lacaine F, LaMuraglia GM, Malt RA. Prognostic factors in survival after portasystemic shunts: Multivariate analysis. *Ann Surg* 1985; 202:729–734.

37. Child CG III, Turcotte JG. Surgery and portal hypertension. In: Child CG III, ed. *The Liver and Portal Hypertension*, Vol I. Dunphy JE, ed. *Major Problems in Clinical Surgery.* Philadelphia: WB Saunders, 1964, pp. 1–85.

38. Christensen E, Schlichting P, Fauerholdt L, Gluud C, Andersen PK, Juhl E, et al. Prognostic value of Child-Turcotte criteria in medically treated cirrhosis. *Hepatology* 1984; 4:430–435.

Editorial Comment

Dr. Malt has undertaken a review of elective total portal-systemic shunts and, in a remarkably succinct analysis, has presented us with a beautifully organized historical and current review of both the hemodynamics and the clinical aspects of shunt surgery. The logic of the presentation and the method of selection of patients for various operative procedures indicates the depth of the author's knowledge of the peculiar and fluctuating hemodynamics of portal hypertension, and ties in very well with Chapter 12B, in which Dr. Fischer presents an analysis of the hemodynamics of this physiologic abnormality.

There is something about portal hypertension that seems to preclude an entirely objective analysis, but somehow Malt has achieved this type of objectivity and provides the rational approach to the reader without any irritating dogma. Malt has purposely avoided the innovation of the selective shunt and has left this to Chapter 14B.

Chapter 14B
Selective Transsplenic Decompression Procedure: Current Status and Projected Role in the Treatment of Portal Hypertensive Bleeding

W. DEAN WARREN

Death from variceal bleeding has plagued humans for centuries (1). Therapy remains controversial (2–4). Historically, all therapy evolves in a cyclical pattern. A new treatment is discovered (or rediscovered) and stimulates a wave of excitement and uncontrolled testimony. Controlled trials follow, which either reinforce the superiority of the new treatment or define the need for other therapy.

Therapy for variceal bleeding exemplifies this cyclical pattern. Prior to 1945 there was no effective method to control variceal bleeding. Faced with this problem, A. O. Whipple reinstituted portacaval shunt (5). His initial success triggered a wave of enthusiasm (and acceptance) that lasted 25 years. However, experience reaffirmed observations first recorded by Pavlov (6). Diversion of portal flow caused hepatic encephalopathy and liver atrophy, and did not prolong survival from bleeding varices in cirrhotic subjects (7–12). These failings of portacaval shunt led to the use of therapy that preserved portal flow to the liver. Nonshunt procedures have a role in patients bleeding from varices but are plagued by high rebleeding rates (13–27). Selective shunt [distal splenorenal shunt (DSRS), transsplenic decompression] evolved with specific goals: prevention of rebleeding by transsplenic decompression of varices, and maintenance of postoperative portal perfusion and portal venous hypertension (28). Twenty years of experience has shown that selective shunt controls bleeding as well as portasystemic shunts and improves survival in nonalcoholics (29–32). During the period 1982–1988, endoscopic sclerosis has reemerged as the primary treatment for bleeding varices (33–43). Sclerotherapy can control acute bleeding and pro-

long survival when compared to standard medical treatment or shunt surgery. More controlled trials with longer follow-up are required to determine if the rebleeding rate with sclerosis (50%—1 year) represents a greater risk to patients than the morbidity of selective shunt surgery.

This report details the approach to portal hypertensive bleeding used at Emory University and defines the current status of distal splenorenal shunt relative to other therapeutic modalities. Our approach is to divide the spectrum of disorders that present with variceal bleeding into groups based on the anatomic point of obstruction to portal flow: prehepatic, intrahepatic, or posthepatic. This approach emphasizes the physiologic differences among these populations. Within each group, the patient is stratified by a series of clinical and quantitative studies that define the hepatic database (44–46) (Table 14B.1). Choice of therapy to control bleeding—further sclerosis, selective shunt, nonselective shunt—is based on a projected response to therapy plus our bias. We believe that no single therapy is the "best treatment" for all portal hypertensive bleeding patients, and that preservation of portal flow is better than loss of perfusion.

Prehepatic Block

Diseases producing prehepatic block include schistosomiasis, extrahepatic portal vein thrombosis, and ideopathic portal hypertension, and are frequently grouped as noncirrhotic portal hypertensive disorders. All are characterized by low intrahepatic pressure (low hepatic vein wedge pres-

Table 14B.1. Emory Hepatic Database

Child's score	Superior mesenteric angiovenography
Portal perfusion grade	Galactose clearance
Liver blood flow	First-pass nuclear cardiography
Cardiac output	Galactose elimination capacity
Quantitative liver function	NH$_3$-amino acid tolerance test
Liver size	CT scan

Abbreviations: CT, computed tomography.

sure), normal (or near-normal) liver morphology, and excellent liver function. Because pressure is high in the portal vein and low in the hepatic sinusoid, portal perfusion is maintained over time unless diverted by portasystemic shunt.

Schistosomiasis is the leading cause of portal hypertensive bleeding worldwide, but is infrequently seen in the United States (47). The true incidence of ideopathic portal hypertension is unknown but probably accounts for <5% of all cases of variceal bleeding in the United States and Europe (48). Extrahepatic portal vein thrombosis is also uncommon (<10%) but conceptually is important because experimental and clinical studies are available to show the crucial role of preserving portal flow (6,49,50). Pavlov showed that diversion of portal blood caused meat intoxication (hepatic encephalopathy) and hepatic atrophy (6). Pavlov also observed that occlusion of the Eck's fistula was followed by collateralization around the obstructed shunt and restitution of portal flow. When portal blood returned to the liver, meat intoxication resolved. This same experiment has been reported in a patient with extrahepatic portal vein thrombosis (51). This 43-year-old woman was referred to Emory with incapacitating hepatic encephalopathy. At age 21 she had been diagnosed as having portal vein thrombosis and underwent splenectomy with central splenorenal shunt to control bleeding varices. Eleven years later she developed alterations in mental status, which progressed over the next 10 years to severe portasystemic encephalopathy. When hospitalized at Emory University 21 years after shunt, the patient was encephalopathic and had been totally disabled for 8 years, requiring around-the-clock nursing care in the home. She had marked protein intolerance manifested by coma after a 10-gram protein meal. Fasting ammonia was in excess of 140 micro-

grams per deciliter and approached levels of 500 μg/dl after the 10-g protein meal. Her electroencephalogram (EEG) showed changes consistent with metabolic encephalopathy. Liver biopsy showed fatty change without fibrosis. Radiologic studies showed a patent central splenorenal shunt and reversal of portal venous flow on the wedge hepatic venogram. The central splenorenal shunt was ligated, which restored portal venous perfusion to the liver. Postoperatively, the patient developed a drug withdrawal response that corresponded temporally to a fall in plasma ammonia. Rapid improvement followed, and over the intervening 8 years there has been no further encephalopathy. The patient now consumes more than 100 g of protein per day and has a normal EEG. Fasting, postprandial ammonia, and standard liver tests are also within normal limits.

Other evidence documents the untoward effect of diverting portal venous blood in patients with schistosomiasis and ideopathic portal hypertension (52–54). In a clinical review of 71 publications, Raia and colleagues found a 72% incidence of encephalopathy after portasystemic shunt in patients with schistosomiasis (55,56). Similar rates of encephalopathy have also been reported by Machado et al. (57) and Habashi (58).

Michelson (48) published similar deleterious results after portacaval shunt in subjects with idiopathic portal hypertension. In a study of noncirrhotic portal hypertension published in 1965, Mikkelsen and colleagues found that 17 patients had patent portal veins and grossly normal livers. Ten patients (58%) rapidly developed encephalopathy and liver failure after portacaval shunt.

This clinical and experimental evidence shows that patients with extrahepatic portal vein thrombosis, idiopathic portal hypertension, and schistosomiasis suffer if portal blood is diverted from the liver. In patients with presinusoidal block presenting with esophageal variceal bleeding, sclerosis should be instituted. Because these patients have normal liver function, rebleeding is usually well tolerated. In fact, when Voorhees et al. documented the dire effects of portacaval shunt in patients with presinusoidal block, the recommendation was made that therapy should be limited to transfusions only (59).

However, patients with extrahepatic portal vein thrombosis and schistosomiasis have very large spleens, and in the Emory experience, frequently bleed from gastric varices that are not controlled by sclerotherapy. If patients with prehepatic block do not tolerate total diversion of portal flow, what is the response to selective shunt?

These patients with low sinusoidal pressure are the best candidates for selective shunt because portal perfusion is preserved in the long term after surgery. Two reports from our group have shown that patients with extrahepatic portal vein thrombosis maintain portal perfusion and quantitative function after selective shunt (51,60). Similarily, Raia and colleagues have reported excellent preservation of hepatic function and low rates of encephalopathy after selective shunt in patients with schistosomiasis (55,56). In 1984, Raia et al. reported the preliminary results of an important study in patients with schistosomiasis (55). In this controlled trial, selective shunt was randomized against central splenorenal shunt, and splenectomy with gastric devascularization. Nonselective shunt produced a higher incidence of hepatic encephalopathy than selective shunt (32% vs. 13%). Encephalopathy after selective shunt and splenectomy with gastric devascularization were similar. Further follow-up is required to determine if the anticipated rebleeding rate in the nonshunt group will evolve. Results to date reinforce the concept that therapy to control bleeding in patients with prehepatic block should preserve portal perfusion.

One additional aspect of noncirrhotic bleeding should be addressed—hypersplenism. Extrahepatic portal vein thrombosis usually develops during childhood. Splenomegaly, leukopenia, and thrombocytopenia are often detected before the onset of variceal bleeding, and splenectomy is recommended. We believe that splenectomy for hypersplenism is contraindicated in patients with extrahepatic block, for two reasons (61). First, the patient is usually asymptomatic. Splenomegaly and abnormal laboratory studies bother the physician, not the patient. Secondly, splenectomy may preclude DSRS. Although selective shunt has been performed in postsplenectomy patients, it is technically difficult to perform (62).

Intrahepatic Block

Intrahepatic block due to cirrhosis is the most common cause of portal hypertensive bleeding in the United States, Europe, and China (63–65). All cirrhotics are not the same. The natural history of alcoholic and nonalcoholic cirrhotics is different and the spectrum between and within these major subsets is wide. In 1971, Emory initiated a longitudinal follow-up program to monitor shunt patients with quantitative measures of hepatic function and hemodynamics. This hepatic database has recently been expanded to include subjects treated with chronic sclerotherapy. Results of these studies show that nonalcoholic cirrhotics have smaller livers, larger spleens, and lower intrahepatic resistance (wedge pressure) than alcoholics (66). These studies also demonstrate that hepatic function and hemodynamics vary widely in cirrhotics when they first present with variceal bleeding. Some patients have normal portal perfusion with excellent liver function and others have lost reversal of portal flow and have markedly decreased hepatic reserve.

These same studies have also shown that the response to shunt surgery is different in alcoholic and nonalcoholic cirrhotics. Unoperated cirrhotics whose bleeding is controlled by sclerotherapy preserve portal perfusion, total hepatic blood flow, and quantitative function for at least 2 years (67). When portal perfusion is maintained after selective shunt, as is the norm in nonalcoholic cirrhotics, function and liver blood flow are also preserved (31,66,67). However, when portal flow is lost after surgery, liver function is preserved only when liver blood flow also increases (66).

In nonalcoholic cirrhotics with gastric varices or in those not controlled by sclerosis, selective shunt is the surgical procedure of choice because (a) further bleeding is prevented, (b) postoperative portal perfusion is preserved, (c) postshunt encephalopathy is low, and (d) survival is improved. This superiority of selective shunt over nonselective shunt was first reported by Zeppa (68) and has also been shown by the 10-year Emory experience (44) and reinforced by the 11-year follow-up of Emory's prospective randomized trial (32).

In alcoholic cirrhotics, the problem of how to deal with sclerosis failures is more difficult because controlled trials do not show the superiority of selective shunt over nonselective shunt. Alcoholic cirrhotics respond differently to selective shunt than nonalcoholic cirrhotics because they frequently lose portal perfusion within 6 months of surgery. In 1984, Warren et al. advanced the physiologic concept of the "pancreatic siphon" to explain the mechanism by which portal perfusion

DSRS – The Pancreatic Siphon

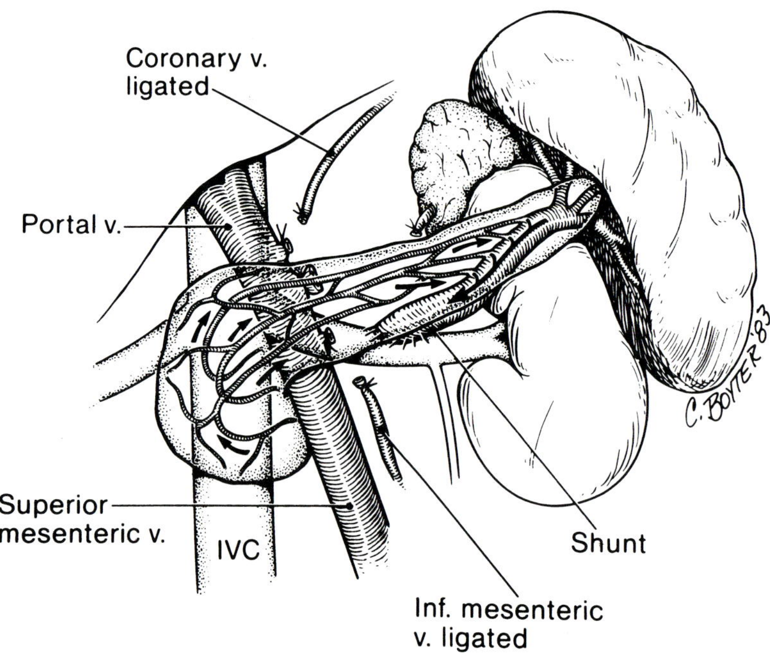

Figure 14B.1. Schematic of the "pancreatic siphon," which develops after DSRS resulting in the loss of hepatotrophic factors from the liver. *Arrows* denote route of blood flow from the high-pressure portal circulation to the low-pressure splenorenal anastomosis.

was lost after selective shunt in alcoholic cirrhotics (62) (Fig. 14B.1). The hypothesis was that portal perfusion was lost via transpancreatic collaterals (the pancreatic siphon), which developed after selective shunt between the high-pressure portal circulation and the low-pressure splenorenal anastomosis. Although similar collateral pathways develop in nonalcoholic cirrhotics, portal perfusion is preserved because intrahepatic resistance to portal flow is lower and peripheral resistance is higher in nonalcoholics. Similar observations documenting the hemodynamic importance of collateralization after selective shunt have been published by Inokuchi et al. (69). Warren et al. projected that complete separation of the splenic vein from the bed of the pancreas [splenopancreatic disconnection (SPD)] (Fig. 14B.2) during selective shunt would eliminate the pancreatic siphon and preserve portal perfusion in alcoholic cirrhotics. Data that support this projection are now available. More than 70 patients have now been operated on at Emory with this new variation of selective shunt, and 30 have been followed at least 1 year

after surgery and have been studied with serial angiogram to monitor portal perfusion. These studies show that selective shunt + SPD maintain portal perfusion better ($p < 0.05$; 88% vs. 25%) than selective shunt alone. Furthermore, the hyperdynamic state defined by an increase in cardiac output and liver blood flow that develops in alcoholics who lose portal perfusion after selective shunt does not evolve in alcoholics after selective shunt + SPD (70).

Further follow-up is required to determine if the hemodynamic and metabolic benefits of selective shunt + SPD persist over time. If they do, a significant advance in selective shunt will have been achieved and improved survival in alcoholics can be anticipated.

At the present time, the data from controlled trials do not show improved survival in alcoholics after selective shunt but support its use because of its lower risk of encephalopathy (31,71–75). We believe that selective shunt should be performed in alcoholic cirrhotics whose bleeding is not controlled by endoscopic sclerotherapy and that the

SPLENOPANCREATIC   DISCONNECTION

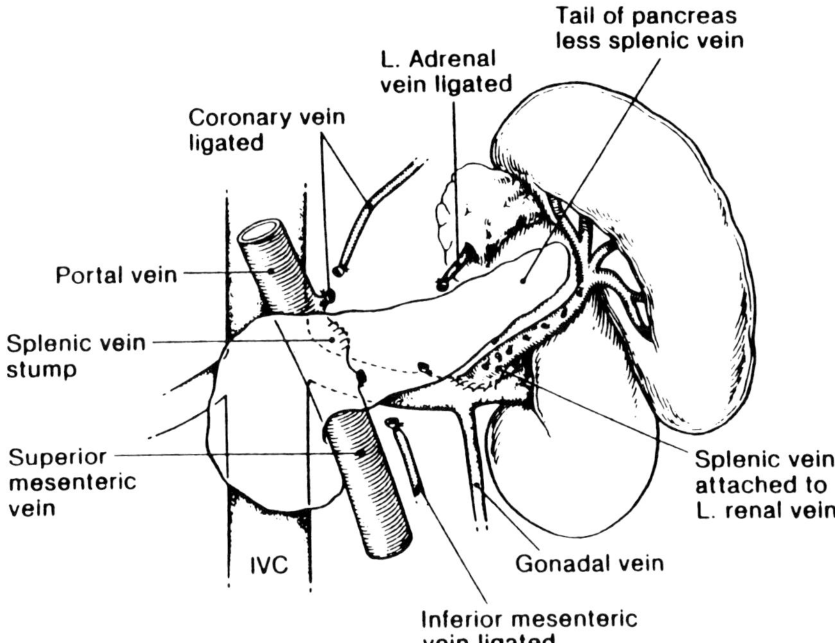

Figure 14B.2. DSRS + SPD. Note the complete separation of the splenic vein from the pancreas.

operation should include complete separation of the splenic vein from the bed of the pancreas (SPD).

In addition to data from controlled trials, there is now a large volume of uncontrolled experience that has recently been summarized by Henderson and Warren (76) to show that the original goals of DSRS have been achieved (77–93). More than 1000 patients operated with selective shunt have been reported in the literature. The majority of subjects reported in these series were good-risk patients (40% Child's class A, 40% Child's case B). Whereas 80% of the controlled trial patients were alcoholics, 60% were alcoholics in the uncontrolled experience. Rebleeding (8%) and operative mortality (9%) rates were low, which reinforce that selective shunt is effective in preventing rebleeding and is technically feasible. Encephalopathy rates were also low (12%–14%), which mimic the controlled trial data. Survival was improved in nonalcoholic cirrhotics.

What is the current status of selective shunt in cirrhotics with bleeding varices? Selective shunt is a safe and effective operative procedure that prevents rebleeding and prolongs survival in nonalcoholic cirrhotics. We propose that longer follow-up of controlled trials will show distal shunt is

better than sclerosis in nonalcoholic cirrhotics because of the high rebleeding rate associated with injection therapy. In good-risk alcoholic cirrhotics, selective shunt + SPD should be performed.

Posthepatic Block

Portal hypertensive bleeding from posthepatic block is rare in the United States and is almost always secondary to hepatic vein occlusion (Budd-Chiari syndrome) (94,95). This syndrome of ascites, hepatomegaly, and abdominal pain carries a very high mortality if the congested liver fails. In patients with liver failure and zone 3 necrosis on liver biopsy, the only hope for survival is either transplantation or to convert the portal vein to an outflow tract by side-to-side portasytemic shunt (96,97).

However, if the swollen liver obstructs the vena cava and elevates inferior vena caval pressures, side-to-side portacaval (mesocaval, mesorenal) shunt may not remain patent because the pressure gradient between the portal vein and vena cava is inadequate. As emphasized by Cameron, the cava can also occlude in Budd-Chiari syndrome (98). When the inferior cava is obstructed or occluded,

Table 14B.2. Approach for Patients with Budd-Chiari Syndrome.

Patient: Hepatomegaly, ascites, pain
   Diagnosis (24 hr)
      Step 1: Hepatic venogram: (infrahepatic cavagram,
         pressures)
      Step 2: Liver biopsy
   Treatment
      1. BCS + zone 3 necrosis → failing liver →
         shunt surgery to convert portal vein to outflow tract
        a. No intrahepatic caval obstruction →
          portacaval shunt
        b. Infrahepatic caval obstruction →
          mesoatrial shunt

Abbreviations: BCS, Budd-Chiari Syndrome.

mesoatrial shunt can convert the portal vein to an outflow tract and decompress the liver (99). Because of the propensity of long interposition grafts to occlude in the venous circulation (100), Warren et al. recommended that the mesoatrial shunt be converted to a short interposition portacaval shunt after the swollen liver decreases in size and inferior vena caval pressures return to normal (101). Cameron has recently advocated a modification of the ringed cortex mesoatrial graft (102). Combined with chronic anticoagulation therapy, this may lessen the risk of mesoatrial shunt occlusion.

The critical problem in patients with Budd-Chiari syndrome is deciding which patients require shunt surgery. In an attempt to address this question, the Emory group recently reviewed their experience with hepatic vein occlusion and found that the liver biopsy was different in patients who required shunt surgery and those who survived without surgery (103). Patients whose liver biopsy showed zone 3 necrosis responded well to shunt surgery. Patients whose biopsies showed no zone 3 necrosis have survived thus far without shunt. Because of these findings, the approach we recommend to patients presenting with Budd-Chiari syndrome is summarized in Table 14B.2. In patients where shunt surgery is withheld, hepatic database evaluations are performed every 3 to 6 months or immediately if there is clinical deterioration. More study is required to define the natural history of Budd-Chiari syndrome. Orthotopic liver transplantation offers a new dimension to patients with Budd-Chiari syndrome (104). If these patients do not require shunt surgery, transplantation is technically easier to perform.

Operative Protocol

Patient Population

The ideal patient for selective shunt has prehepatic block or is Child's class A-B cirrhotic with prograde portal flow. Details of the preoperative protocol have been published (105,106). Best results are obtained when patients are operated on an elective basis.

The reemergence of sclerotherapy has altered our patient population and affected acute and long-term survival. Over 80% of patients now undergoing selective shunt are sclerotherapy failures, and many are brought to surgery on an emergent or urgent basis. As a result, we are operating on sicker patients than before.

Operative Technique

The patient is positioned with the left side elevated 20 degrees and the left arm adducted across the chest. A left subcostal incision is extended across the right rectus muscle. After dividing the gastrocolic ligament from the pylorus to the short gastric vessels, the splenocolic ligament is taken down, which exposes the hilum of the spleen; provides access to the lesser sac, splenic artery, and tail of the pancreas; and interrupts the major collateral pathway between the splenic vein and mesentery of the splenic flexure.

SPD is complete dissection of the splenic vein from the pancreas to its bifurcation at the splenic hilum. Dissection of the splenic vein should proceed on the vein with the posterior, inferior surface isolated before approaching anterior and superior surfaces. The junction of the splenic and superior mesenteric vein should be controlled early in the dissection. Small splenopancreatic perforating veins are ligated and divided as they are encountered. Division of the splenic vein at its junction with the superior mesenteric vein facilitates dissection of the splenic vein from the pancreas, as does intermittent clamping of the splenic artery to decrease blood loss. Superiorly rotating the pancreas with the surgeon's left hand behind the gland aids exposure as the splenic vein passes through the upper border of the pancreas (the pancreatic groove). In most patients the splenic vein courses above the pancreas for several centimeters before entering the hilum of the spleen. Controlling the vein above the pancreas requires special care as injury to the vein at the hilum may cause irreversible harm. If dissection of the splenic vein from the pancreas is difficult, complete mobilization of the spleen from its bed with rotation of both spleen and pancreas medially allows dissection of the splenic vein from a posterior approach (Inokuchi's maneuver) (69,107,108).

Postoperative Care

Details of postoperative care have been published (105). Patients are maintained for 24 to 48 hours in the intensive care unit (ICU). Sodium and fat restriction are instituted prior to surgery in elective patients to minimize the risk of postoperative ascites. As our operative population had changed over the last 3 years, more patients with ascites have had surgery and the need for serial paracentesis and LeVeen's valve 4 to 6 weeks after operation have increased.

Future Goals for Selective Shunt

This review has attempted to define the role of selective shunt in the Emory approach to portal hypertensive bleeding. Because of the current enthusiasm for sclerosis, we project that at least for the next several years, selective shunt—and all surgery—will be relegated to a backup position for patients who fail or are not candidates for injection therapy. It is to be hoped that, as time passes, a better definition of sclerosis failure will evolve to decrease the volume of emergent shunt surgery. More controlled trials comparing chronic sclerosis and selective shunt are needed. Specifically, selective shunt with SPD and chronic sclerosis need to be compared in alcoholic cirrhotics. At present, the experience of the first 15 years with selective shunt can be summarized as follows:

1. DSRS is as effective as portasystemic shunt in preventing bleeding from varices.
2. Selective shunt should be performed in patients with noncirrhotic portal hypertension who fail sclerotherapy because portal perfusion is preserved for years after surgery.
3. Selective shunt also maintains postoperative portal perfusion, and improves survival in nonalcoholic cirrhotics.
4. Alcoholic and nonalcoholic cirrhotics respond differently after selective shunt. Portal perfu-

sion is frequently lost (50%) within 1 year in alcoholics.
5. Selective shunt with SPD preserves portal perfusion better in alcoholics than selective shunt without disconnection.

Cirrhosis is a killer disease in which therapy to control bleeding is improving. A major part of the improvement is due to the evolution of selective shunt coupled with the reemergence of endoscopic sclerosis therapy. We believe these two therapies are additive and together have the potential to markedly improve survival from variceal bleeding (1).

References

1. Warren WD. Control of variceal bleeding. Reassessment of rationale. *Am J Surg* 1983; 145:8–16.
2. Conn HO. Therapeutic portacaval anastomosis: To shunt or not to shunt. *Gastroenterology* 1974; 67:1065–1073.
3. Editorial. Bleeding oesophageal varices. *Lancet* 1984; 1:139–141.
4. Reynolds TB. What to do about esophageal varices? *N Engl J Med* 1983; 309:1575–1577.
5. Whipple AO. The problem of portal hypertension in relation to hepatosplenopathies. *Ann Surg* 1945; 122:449–475.
6. Hahn M, Massen O, Nencki M, Pavlov J. Die ecksche fistel zwischen der unteren hohlvene und der pfortaden und folgen fur den organismus. *Arch Exp Pathol Pharmakol* 1893; 32:162–210.
7. Resnick RH, Iber FL, Ishihara AM, et al. A controlled study of the therapeutic portacaval shunt. *Gastroenterology* 1974; 67:843–857.
8. Rueff B, Prandi D, Degos F, et al. A controlled study of the therapeutic portacaval shunt in alcoholic cirrhosis. *Lancet* 1976; 1:655–659.
9. Jackson FC, Perrin EB, Felix RW, et al. A clinical investigation of the portacaval shunt: V. Survival analysis of the therapeutic operation. *Ann Surg* 1974; 174:672–701.
10. Jackson FC, Perrin EB, Smith AG, et al. A clinical investigation of the portacaval shunt: II. Survival analysis of the prophylactic operation. *Am J Surg* 1968; 115:22–42.
11. Resnick RH, Chalmers TC, Ishihara AM, et al. The Boston Interhospital Liver Group: A controlled study of the prophylactic portacaval shunt. A final report. *Ann Intern Med* 1969; 70:675–688.
12. Reynolds TB, Donovan AJ, Mikkelsen WP, et al. Results of a 12-year randomized trial of portacaval shunt in patients with alcoholic liver disease and bleeding varices. *Gastroenterology* 1981; 80:1005–1011.
13. Wirthlin LS, Linton RR, Ellis DS. Transthoracoesophageal ligation of bleeding esophageal varices: A reappraisal. *Arch Surg* 1974; 109:688–692.
14. Linschoten H, Tytgat GN, The GT, Bakker DJ. Ligatuur transsecties van de oesophagus abdominaal zowel als thoracaal. *Acta Chir Belg* 1982; 4:423–427.
15. Wanamaker SR, Cooperman H, Carey LC. Use of the EEA stapling instrument for control of bleeding esophageal varices. *Surgery* 1983; 94:620–626.
16. Gouge TH, Ranson JHC. Esophageal transection with paraesophageal devascularization (the Sugiura proce-

dure) for bleeding esophageal varices. *Am J Surg* 1986; 151:47–53.

17. Hassab MA. Nonshunt operations in portal hypertension without cirrhosis. *Surg Gynecol Obstet* 1970; 131:648–654.

18. Skinner DB. Transthoracic, transgastric, interruption of bleeding esophageal varices. *Arch Surg* 1969; 99:447–453.

19. Estes NC, Pierce GE. Late results of extended devascularization procedure for patients with bleeding esophageal varices. *Am Surg* 1984; 50:381–385.

20. Ginsberg RJ, Waters PF, Zeldin RA, et al. A modified Sugiura procedure. *Ann Thorac Surg* 1982; 34:258–264.

21. Sugiura M, Futagawa S. Results of six hundred thirty-six esophageal transections with paraesophagogastric devascularization in the treatment of esophageal varices. *J Vasc Surg* 1984; 1:254–260.

22. Giordani M, Ravo B, Sacchi M, et al. Treatment of bleeding esophageal varices by portoazygos disconnection and esophageal transection with the button of Boerema and EEA stapler: A ten years' experience. *Surgery* 1985; 97:649–652.

23. Johnston GW. Six years experience of oesophageal transection for oesophageal varices using a circular stapling gun. *Gut* 1982; 23:770–773.

24. Weese JL, Starling JR, Yale CE. Control of bleeding esophageal varices by transabdominal esophageal transection, gastric devascularization and splenectomy. *Surg Gastroenterol* 1984; 3:31–36.

25. Johnson G, Womack NA, Gabriel OF, Peters RM. Control of the hyperdynamic circulation in patients with bleeding esophageal varices. *Ann Surg* 1969; 169:661–671.

26. Jaffe SW. Non-shunting procedures for control of variceal bleeding. *Semin Liver Dis* 1983; 3:235–250.

27. Keagy BA, Schwartz JA, Johnson G Jr. Should ablative operations be used for bleeding esophageal varices? *Ann Surg* 1986; 203:463–469.

28. Warren WD, Zeppa R, Foman JJ. Selective transplenic decompression of gastroesophageal varices by distal splenorenal shunt. *Ann Surg* 1967; 166:437–455.

29. Warren WD, Rudman D, Millikan WJ Jr, Galambos JT, Salam AA, Smith RB III. The metabolic basis of portasytemic encephalopathy and the effect of selective vs. nonselective shunts. *Ann Surg* 1974; 180:572–579.

30. Galambos JT, Warren WD, Rudman D, et al. Selective and total shunts in the treatment of bleeding varices. A randomized controlled trial. *N Engl J Med* 1976; 295:1089–1095.

31. Rikkers LF, Rudman D, Galambos JT, et al. A randomized, controlled trial of the distal splenorenal shunt. *Ann Surg* 1978; 188:271–282.

32. Millikan WJ Jr, Warren WD, Henderson JM, et al. The Emory prospective randomized trial: Selective vs. nonselective shunt to control variceal bleeding: Ten-year follow-up. *Ann Surg* 1985; 201:712–722.

33. Crafoord C, Frenckner P. New surgical treatment of varicose veins of the oesophagus. *Acta Otolaryngol* 1939; 27:422–429.

34. Moersch HJ. Esophageal varices: Further studies on the treatment of esophageal varices by injection of a sclerosing solution. *Ann Otol Rhinol Laryngol* 1941: 50:1233.

35. Johnston BW, Rogers HW. A review of 15 years' experience in the use of sclerotherapy in the control of acute hemorrhage from esophageal varices. *Br J Surg* 1973; 60: 797–800.

36. MacDougall BRD, Westaby D, Theodossi A, Dawson JL, Williams R. Increased long-term survival in variceal haemorrhage using injection sclerotherapy. Results of a controlled trial. *Lancet* 1982; 1:124–127.

37. Terblanche J, Northover JMA, Bornman P, et al. A prospective controlled trial of sclerotherapy in the long term management of patients after esophageal variceal bleeding. *Surg Gynecol Obstet* 1979; 148:323–323.

38. Paquet K-J. Prophylactic endoscopic sclerosing treatment of the esophageal wall in varices—a prospective controlled randomized trial. *Endoscopy* 1982; 14:4–5.

39. Mitchell KJ, MacDougall BRD, Silk DBA, Williams R. A prospective reappraisal of emergency endoscopy in patients with portal hypertension. *Scand J Gastroenterol* 1982; 17:965.

40. Novis BH, Duys P, Barbezat GO, Clain J, Bank S, Terblanche J. Fibreoptic endoscopy and use of the Sengstaken tube in acute gastrointestinal haemorrhage in patients with portal hypertension and varices. *Gut* 1976; 17:258.

41. Johnson AG, Simms JM, Stoddard CJ. Is there a role for injection sclerotherapy in the presence of active bleeding? In: Westaby D, MacDougall BRD, Williams, eds. *Variceal Bleeding*. London: Pitman, 1982. pp. 159–164.

42. Terblanche J, Yakoob HI, Bornman PC, et al. Acute bleeding varices. A five-year prospective evaluation of tamponade and sclerotherapy. *Ann Surg* 1981; 194:521–530.

43. Sclerotherapy after first variceal hemorrhage in cirrhosis. A randomized multicenter trial. The Copenhagen Esophageal Varices Sclerotherapy Project. *N Engl J Med* 1984; 311:1594–1600.

44. Warren WD, Millikan WJ Jr, Henderson JM, et al. Ten years portal hypertensive surgery at Emory: Results and new perspectives. *Ann Surg* 1982; 195:530–542.

45. Henderson JM, Millikan WJ, Wright L, et al. Quantitative estimation of metabolic and hemodynamic hepatic function: The effects of shunt surgery. *Surg Gastroenterol* 1982; 1:77–85.

46. Nordlinger BM, Nordlinger DF, Fulenwider JT, et al. Angiography in portal hypertension: Clinical significance in surgery. *Am J Surg* 1980; 139:132–141.

47. Ong GB. Helminthic diseases of the liver and biliary tract In: Wright R, Alberti KGMM, Karran S, Millward-Sadler GH, eds. *Liver and Biliary Disease*. London: Saunders, 1979, pp. 1267–1303.

48. Mikkelsen WP, Edmondson HA, Peters RL, et al. Extra- and intra-hepatic portal hypertension without cirrhosis (hepatoportal sclerosis). *Ann Surg* 1965; 162:602–608.

49. Warren WD, Muller WH. A clarification of some hemodynamic changes in cirrhosis and their surgical significance. *Ann Surg* 1959; 150:413–420.

50. Warren WD, Restrepo JE, Respess JC, et al. The importance of hemodynamic studies in management of portal hypertension. *Ann Surg* 1963; 158:387–394.

51. Warren WD, Millikan WJ, Smith RB, et al. Noncirrhotic portal vein thrombosis. Physiology before and after shunts. *Ann Surg* 1980; 192:341–349.

52. Carneiro, JLdeA. A circulacao colateral gastresofagica apos desconexao azigo-portal. Thesis, Centro Biom Univ Fed Esp Santo Vitoria, 1979.

53. Ramos OL, Saad F, Leser WP. Portal hemodynamics and liver cell function in hepatic schistosomiasis. *Gastroenterology* 1964; 47:241.

54. Warren KS, Reboucas G, Baptista AG. Ammonia metabolism and hepatic coma in hepatosplenic schistosomiasis. Patients studied before and after portacaval shunt. *Ann Intern Med* 1965; 62:1113.

55. Raia S, Mies S, Macedo AL. Surgical treatment of portal hypertension in schistosomiasis. *World J Surg* 1984; 8:738–752.

56. Raia S. *Descompressao Portal Selectiva: Na esquistossomose Mansonica*. Universidade de Sao Paulo, Brazil, 1978.

57. Machado AL, Filho JEB, Campos AB, et al. Selective distal splenorenal shunts: Technique and results. *Am J Surg* 1981; 142:281–284.

58. Habashi AHF. Transsplenic decompression of oesophageal varices by selective distal splenorenal shunt. *J Egypt Med Assoc* 1977; 60:23–28.

59. Voorhees AB, Chaitman E, Schneider S, Nicholson JF, Kornfield DS, Price JB. Portal systemic encephalopathy in the noncirrhotic patient. *Arch Surg* 1973; 107:659–663.

60. Henderson JM, Millikan WJ Jr, Galambos JT, Warren WD. Selective variceal decompression in portal vein thrombosis. *Br J Surg* 1984: 71:735–749.

61. El Kishen MA, Henderson JM, Millikan WJ Jr, Kutner MH, Warren WD. Splenectomy is contraindicated for thrombocytopenia secondary to portal hypertension. *Surg Gynecol Obstet* 1985; 160:233–238.

62. Warren WD, Millikan WJ, Henderson JM, Rasheed ME, Salam AA. Selective variceal decompression after splenectomy or splenic vein thrombosis—with a note on splenopancreatic disconnection. *Ann Surg* 1984; 199:694–702.

63. Reynolds TB. Portal hypertension. In: Diseases of the Liver. Philadelphia: JB Lippincott, 1975, p. 331.

64. Sherlock S. *Diseases of the Liver and Biliary System*, 6th ed. London: Blackwell Scientific Publications, 1981.

65. Galambos JT. Cirrhosis. In: *Major Problems in Internal Medicine*, Vol. 18. Philadelphia: WB Saunders, 1979, p. 253.

66. Henderson JM, Millikan WJ Jr, Wright-Bacon L, Kutner MH, Warren WD. Hemodynamic differences between alcoholic and nonalcoholic cirrhotics following distal splenorenal shunt—effect on survival? *Ann Surg* 1983; 198:325–334.

67. Warren WD, Henderson JM, Millikan WJ Jr, et al. Distal splenorenal shunt vs. endoscopic sclerosing in long-term management of variceal bleeding. Preliminary report of a prospective randomized trial. *Ann Surg* 1986; 203:454–462.

68. Zeppa R, Hansley GT, Levy JV, et al. The comparative survival of alcoholics versus nonalcoholics after distal splenorenal shunt. *Ann Surg* 1978; 187:510–514.

69. Inokuchi K, Bepu K, Koyanagi N, et al. Exclusion of nonisolated-isolated splenic vein in distal splenorenal shunt for prevention of portal malcirculation. *Ann Surg* 1984; 200:711–717.

70. Warren WD, Millikan WJ Jr, Henderson JM, et al. Splenopancreatic disconnection: Improved selectivity of distal splenorenal shunt. *Ann Surg* (in press).

71. Reichle FA, Fahmy WF, Golsorkhi M. Prospective comparative clinical trial with distal splenorenal and mesocaval shunts. *Am J Surg* 1979; 137:13–21.

72. Langer B, Rotstein LE, Stone RM, et al. A prospective randomized trial of the selective distal splenorenal shunt. *Surg Gynecol Obstet* 1980; 150:45–48.

73. Villamil F, Redeker A, Reynolds T, et al. A controlled trial of distal splenorenal and portacaval shunts (abstr). *Hepatology* 1981; 1:557.

74. Conn HO, Resnick RH, Grace ND, et al. Distal splenorenal shunt vs. portal-systemic shunt: Current status of a controlled trial. *Hepatology* 1981; 1:151–160.

75. Fischer JE, Bower RH, Atamian S, et al. Comparison of distal and proximal splenorenal shunts: A randomized prospective trial. *Ann Surg* 1981; 194:531–544.

76. Henderson JM, Warren WD. Selective variceal decompression: Current status and recent advances. In: *Advances in Surgery*. Chicago: Year Book Medical, 1984; 18: 81–115.

77. Saubier EC, Partansky C, Gouillat C. Early postoperative angiographic control of the Warren procedure in 40 patients. *World J Surg* 1982; 6:765–770.

78. Marqios C, Gertsch P, Mosimann R. Control angiographique, endoscopic et manometrique à long terme des anastomoses spleno-renales distales don Warren. *Helv Chir Acta* 1982; 49:633–636.

79. Prete F, Neri V, Montemurro S, et al. L'anastomosi splenorenale distale nel trattamento dell'ipertensione portale. *Minerva Chir* 1982; 37:405–408.

80. Kallio H, Lempiren M. Distal shunt for portal hypertension. *Ann Chir Gynaecol* 1981; 70:1–4.

81. Kieninger G. Der distal splenorenale shunt. *Chirurgie* 1981; 52:717–721.

82. Marni A, Trojst C, Belli L. Distal splenorenal shunt: Hemodynamic advantage over total shunt and influence on clinical status, hepatic function and hypersplenism. *Am J Surg* 1981; 142:281–284.

83. Vang J, Simert G, Hansson JA, et al. Results of a modified distal splenorenal shunt for portal hypersplenism. *Ann Surg* 1977; 185:224–228.

84. Mosimann R, Loup R. Efficacy and risks of the distal splenorenal shunt in the treatment of esophageal varices. *Am J Surg* 1977; 133:163–198.

85. Cuschieri A. Selective decompression for bleeding esophageal varices in patients with preparenchymal blocks. *J R Coll Surg Edinb* 1981; 26:229–231.

86. Funovics JM, Fritsch A, Appel WH, et al. Ergebnisse mit den distalen-splenorenalen shunt nach Warren. *Langenbecks Arch Chir* 1981; 354:81–88.

87. Maillare JN, Flamant Y, Hay JM. Operation de Warren et anastomose spleno-renale distale sans deconnexion. *Chirurgie* 1982; 108:523–525.

88. Soper NJ, Rikkers LF. Effects of operations for variceal hemorrhage on hypersplenism. *Am J Surg* 1982; 144:700–703.

89. Busutill RW, Brin B, Tompkins RK. Matched control study of distal splenorenal and portacaval shunts in the treatment of bleeding esophageal varices. *Am J Surg* 1979; 138:62–67.

90. Nabseth DC, Jonson WC, Widrich WC, et al. Splenorenal shunts in portal hypertension. *J Cardiovasc Surg* 1979; 20: 201–207.

91. Langer B, Patel SC, Stone RM, et al. Selection of operation in patients with bleeding esopahgeal varices. *Can Med Assoc J* 1978; 118:369–372.

92. Martin EW, Molnar J, Cooperman M, et al. Observations of fifty distal splenorenal shunts. *Surgery* 1978; 84:379–383.

93. Brittan RC. The clinical effectiveness of selective portal shunts. *Am J Surg* 1977; 13:506–511.

94. Budd G. *On Diseases of the Liver*. London: John Churchill, 1845, p. 146.

95. Chiari H. Ueber die seibstandige phlebitis obiliterans der hauptstamme der venae hepaticae ais todersursache. *Beitr Pathol Anat* 1899; 26:1–17.

96. Langer B, Stone RM, Colapinto RF, et al. Clinical spectrum of the Budd-Chiari syndrome and its surgical management. *Am J Surg* 1975; 129:137–145.

97. McDermott WV, Stone MD, Bothe A Jr, Trey C. Budd-Chiari syndrome: Historical and clinical review with an analysis of surgical corrective procedures. *Am J Surg* 1984; 147:643–647.

98. Powell-Jackson PR, Melia W, Canalese J, et al. Budd-

Chiari syndrome: Clinical patterns and therapy. *Q J Med* 1982; 201:79–88.

99. Rappaport AM. The microcirculatory acinar concept of normal and pathological hepatic structure. *Beitr Pathol* 1976; 157:215–243.

100. Smith RB, Warren WD, Salam AA, et al. Dacron interposition shunts for portal hypertension: An analysis of morbidity correlates. *Ann Surg* 1980; 192:9–17.

101. Warren WD, Potts JR, Fulenwider JT, et al. Two stage surgical management of the Budd-Chiari syndrome associated with obstruction of the inferior vena cava. *Surg Gynecol Obstet* 1984: 159:101–107.

102. Cameron JL, Herlong HF, Sanfey H, et al. The Budd-Chiari syndrome treatment by mesenteric-systemic venous shunts. *Ann Surg* 1983; 198:335–346.

103. Millikan WJ Jr, Henderson JM, Sewell CW, et al. An approach to the spectrum of Budd-Chiari syndrome— which patients require portal decompression? *Am J Surg* 1985; 149:167–176.

104. Starzl TE, Porter KA, Francavella JA, et al. A hundred years of the hepatotrophic controversy. In: *Hepatotrophic Factors*. Ciba Foundation Symposium. Elsevier/Excerpta Medica/North Holland, 1978, pp. 111–138.

105. Warren WD, Millikan WJ Jr. The liver and portal vein. In: Dudrick SJ, Baue AE, Eiseman B, et al., eds. *Manual of Preoperative and Postoperative Care*, 3rd ed. The American College of Surgeons. Philadelphia: WB Saunders, 1983, pp. 422–442.

106. Millikan WJ Jr, Warren WD. Recent advances in portal hypertensive bleeding. Syllabus for American College of Surgeons. October 21, 1986.

107. Warren WD, Millikan WJ. Selective transsplenic decompression procedure; Changes in technique after 300 cases. *Contemp Surg* 1981; 18:11–29.

108. Warren WD, Millikan WJ Jr, Henderson JM. Splenopancreatic disconnection: Improved selectivity of distal splenorenal shunt. *Ann Surg* (in press).

Editorial Comment

Probably the most stimulating clinical reports in the field of surgery of the liver and portal hypertension during the past two decades have been those emanating from the imaginative ideas and the extensive clinical applications provided by Dean Warren and associates and by Robert Zeppa, who was Dr. Warren's early collaborator in the first reports on the selective shunt.

The recognition that a total loss of portal perfusion resulted in a disastrous clinical syndrome, referred to as postshunt encephalopathy, cast a pall in 1954 (1) on the booming field of shunt surgery for bleeding esophageal varices. It became apparent that not only did a total shunt in the presence of a normal liver either in the clinic or the laboratory result in disastrous encephalopathy, but also that an unpredicatable but significant percentage of patients following shunt surgery for intrahepatic cirrhotic portal bed block also devel-

oped disabling neurologic syndromes. Thus, when Warren introduced the concept of selective shunting, enthusiasm was revived for the surgical management of bleeding esophageal varices. A number of prospective randomized studies were initiated to compare the total shunt with the selective shunt; these studies led to variable reported results, divided almost evenly between those showing a significant advantage in terms of decreased encephalopathy for the selective shunt and those indicating little or no statistically significant difference. Our own randomized study, stemming from the Boston Inter-Hospital Liver Group (BILG) (2), did not distinguish any difference between the two types of shunts but all the studies left a nagging feeling that the logic of Warren's efforts was almost incontrovertible, and perhaps it was the multifactorial nature of portal hypertension that made even randomized studies difficult to interpret.

Warren's studies have certainly made one point clear: there seems to be a difference in the results obtained from the selective shunt in the nonalcoholic cirrhotic compared to the chronic alcoholic. It has also become evident that selective shunting and continued pro grade perfusion of the liver tends to disappear gradually over the postoperative months and years so that ultimately many selective shunts are converted to total portal-systemic shunts. A third problem with the selective shunt is the fact that ascites are not controlled because of the lack of decompression of a postsinusoidal block, and that sometimes ascites appear to an incapacitating degree after the construction of a selective shunt. Thus, despite the superb contributions of Warren and colleagues, we still do not seem to have the answer that will permit us to select the exact and appropriate shunt for each individual case of portal hypertension. Certainly, the clinical and hemodynamic studies by Warren have led us further along this pathway to an ultimate goal.

References

1. McDermott WV Jr, Adams RD. Episodic stupor associated with an Eck fistula in the human with particular reference to the metabolism of ammonia. *J Clin Invest* 1954; 33:1–9. (Presented before the Society of Clinical Investigation, May 1953.)

2. Conn HO, Resnick RH, Grace ND, et al. Distal splenorenal shunt vs. portal-systemic shunt: Current status of a controlled trial. *Hepatology* 1981; 1:151–160.

Chapter 15
Nonshunting Procedures in Management of Bleeding Esophageal Varices

RICARDO L. ROSSI
CLAYTON L. WOOD

Bleeding from varices secondary to portal hypertension can be treated by decompression of the portal system or by nonshunting operations. The latter procedures attempt to obliterate, disconnect, or remove the varices or decrease the blood flow to the portal system. Many nonshunting techniques have been described (Table 15.1) (1), and several are now only of historical value as isolated procedures. Some, however, have been incorporated as part of more extensive and current operations.

Nonshunting procedures have the advantage of not interfering with portal flow and liver hemodynamics and therefore do not precipitate encephalopathy or lead to progressive liver failure. These operations preserve the portal vein so that liver transplantation can be performed in patients in whom this therapy may be indicated in the future. A long follow-up period is required to access the rate of rebleeding, a major complication of nonshunting procedures. The operative risk of nonshunting operations is related mainly to the condition of the patient as determined by Child's classification (Table 15.2) (2). The central hepatic clearance rate of amino acids as described by Clowes and associates (3) could become a useful technique to predict survival. Perhaps with the exception of sclerotherapy, most nonshunting procedures, compared with portasystemic shunting, do not decrease the operative mortality for patients with Child's class C alcoholic cirrhosis.

The lack of controlled trials, the heterogeneity of patient populations, and the frequently short-term follow-up data available in different studies make it difficult to define clearly advantages and disadvantages of different shunting and nonshunting procedures in patients with bleeding esophageal varices. Vasopressin (Pitressin) and balloon tamponade continue to be helpful in the early medical management of patients with bleeding varices. However, sclerotherapy, described in the 1930s (4), has become the preferred method to control the acute episode of variceal bleeding. Early limited devascularization techniques, such as Tanner's operation, have been replaced by more extensive devascularization operations, with a decrease in the rates of recurrent bleeding that has renewed interest in these techniques. Interest continues in identifying drugs that could decrease the portal pressure and be useful in the long-term management of patients with portal hypertension. Although early enthusiasm for percutaneous transhepatic portal techniques of embolization and obliteration of varices has decreased, improvements in technique now make it possible, in selected patients, to dilate shunts or to occlude collaterals that have transformed a selective shunt into a total shunt. Surgeons who deal with portal hypertension should be aware of these operations, as occasionally one of them might be necessary as a single procedure or as part of a more complex, extensive operation.

Nonshunting Procedures that Obliterate or Compress Varices

Balloon Tamponade

The use of balloon tamponade was suggested by Preble (5) in 1900 and was reported by Westphal (6) in 1930 and by Rowntree (7) in 1947. The technique was improved by Sengstaken and Blakemore (8) in 1950 and by Linton (9) in 1953. The

Table 15.1. Procedures for Bleeding Esophageal Varices

Nonshunting procedures
  Obliterate or compress varices
    Balloon tamponade
    Ligation of varices (transthoracic-transabdominal)
    Sclerotherapy
  Reduce portal blood volume
    Arterial ligation
    Infusion of vasopressin
    Beta-adrenergic blocking agents
    Percutaneous splenic arterial occlusion
  Promote new collaterals
    Omentopexy
    Splenic transposition
  Reduce varix bed
    Subtotal esophagectomy
    Esophagogastrectomy with interposition
  Interrupt flow to varices
    Transection (esophageal-gastric)
    Devascularization and transection—porta-azygos
      disconnection
    Tanner's operation
    Sugiura's procedure
    Modifications
    Percutaneous transhepatic coronary vein thrombosis

Reproduced by permission from Rossi RL, Jenkins RL, Nielsen-Whitcomb FF. Management of complications of portal hypertension. *Surg Clin North Am* 1985; 65(2):231–262.

Sengstaken-Blakemore tube has a gastric balloon, an esophageal balloon, and a port for suctioning the stomach. The Minnesota four-lumen esophagogastric tube (Davol, Providence, Rhode Island) adds a port for esophageal suction proximal to the gastric balloon.

Initial control of bleeding is achieved with the Sengstaken-Blakemore tube (Fig. 15.1) in approximately 80% of patients, but when the balloon is deflated or the tube is removed, approximately 40% to 50% of patients rebleed (Table 15.3) (10–12). Although Conn and Simpson (7) reported high morbidity and mortality rates using this tube (aspiration pneumonia, airway obstruction, esophageal tears), prospective studies (12,13) have demonstrated that, with attention to detail, these rates can be decreased appreciably (see Table 15.3).

Factors that decrease the morbidity and mortality are endoscopic proof of an accurate diagnosis of bleeding varices, placement of the tube after emptying the stomach, verification that the balloons and tubing are not leaking and that the tube has not become partially deflated to avoid migration to the mediastinum with resulting airway obstruction, radiologic confirmation of the position of the gastric balloon, suction of the proximal esophagus, use of pressure control of the esophageal balloon (25–30 millimeters of mercury), gentle traction on the tube using a nose pad or a helmet, and avoidance of traction devices with weights.

With the increasing popularity of sclerotherapy, balloon tamponade is used less frequently as a first therapeutic option. However, it should be considered when sclerotherapy is not available or when exsanguinating bleeding occurs and stabilization of the patient is required before sclerotherapy.

If bleeding continues after inflation of the gastric balloon, the esophageal balloon is inflated. The gastric balloon is left inflated for 24 hours while the esophageal balloon is deflated and reinflated several times during that 24-hour period to avoid injury to the distal esophagus. After 24 hours, the esophageal balloon is left deflated. If bleeding does not occur, the gastric balloon is deflated 12 to 24 hours later. With both balloons deflated, the tube is left in place for another 24 hours and is removed if no further bleeding has occurred.

Ligation of Varices (Transthoracic-Transabdominal Approach)

Direct surgical suture ligation to control variceal bleeding through a transthoracic approach was suggested by Boerema (14) in 1949 and is performed through the chest or the abdomen in both adults and children as reported by several authors (15–17) (Table 15.4). Bleeding was initially con-

Table 15.2. Child's Classification

Group	A	B	C
Serum bilirubin (mg/dL)	<2.0	2.0–3.0	>3.0
Serum albumin (g/dL)	>3.5	3.0–3.5	<3.0
Ascites	None	Easily controlled	Poorly controlled
Neurologic disorder	None	Minimal	Advanced
Nutrition	Excellent	Good	Poor (wasting)

Adapted by permission from Turcotte JG, Wallin VW Jr, Child CG III. End-to-side versus side-to-side portocaval shunts in patients with hepatic cirrhosis. *Am J Surgery* 1969; 117(1):108–116.

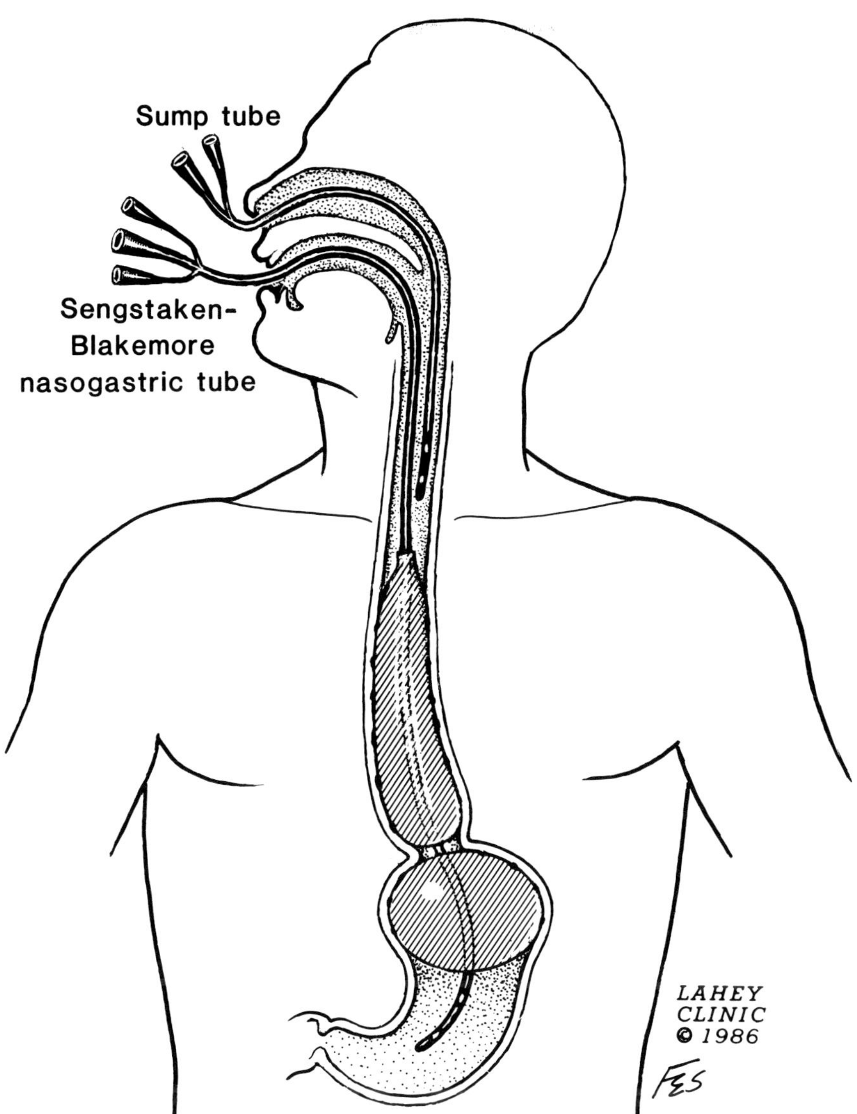

Figure 15.1. Proper placement of the double (Sengstaken-Blakemore) tube. (Reproduced by permission of Lahey Clinic.)

trolled in more than 80% of patients, but rebleeding was common and approached 100% in patients who had long-term survival, especially in children with extrahepatic portal hypertension. The operative mortality was high in patients with cirrhosis but low in patients with extrahepatic portal hypertension. Ottinger and Moncure (18) reported failure to control the initial episode of bleeding in 18% of their patients. The rebleeding rate at 2 months was 20%. The rate of esophageal leakage was 10% and was related to the patient's condition as categorized by Child's classification. Wirthlin et al. (19) reported on a staged approach in the management of the patient with bleeding varices that consisted of suture ligation of the varices followed by an

elective portasystemic shunt. This staged approach incurred the combined mortality of two operations with equivocal benefits in improving ultimate survival. Currently, direct ligation has been replaced by sclerotherapy or is included as part of more extensive devascularization operations.

Esophageal variceal ligation is performed by a left thoracotomy through the seventh intercostal space. The esophagus is isolated and dissected down to the gastroesophageal junction, transecting and ligating paraesophageal veins. The esophagus is opened longitudinally for about 6 centimeters in length down to the esophagogastric junction (Fig. 15.2). The column of varices is iden-

Table 15.3. Effectiveness and Safety of Sengstaken-Blakemore Tube

Author (No.)	No. Patients	Initial Control (%)	Ultimate Control (%)	Morbidity from Tube (%)	Mortality from Tube (%)	Overall Mortality (%)
Conn and Simpson (10)	90	56	—	40	20	—
Hermann and Traul (11)	75	81	50	10	4	28
Pitcher (12)[a]	50	92	76	16	2	36
Novis et al. (13)[a]	41	85	46	22	—	48

[a] Prospective studies.

tified and occluded with a running suture that is started superiorly. Cephalad traction on the suture permits an additional length of gastric varix to be pulled up into the esophagus and occluded. The esophageal defect is closed in two layers.

Sclerotherapy

Sclerotherapy is discussed in detail in Chapter 13B.

Methods that Reduce Portal Blood Flow

Reduction of the portal blood flow can be accomplished by surgical or radiologic interventional techniques of occlusion of arteries to the splanchnic circulation or by pharmacologic means.

Arterial Ligations and Splenectomy

Blain (20) in 1918 and Everson and Cole (21) in 1948 recommended ligation of the splenic artery, and Berman et al. (22) in 1951 presented experimental evidence in favor of ligating both the hepatic and splenic arteries. Mayo (23) in 1924 suggested the use of splenectomy. Rousselot (24) in 1940, Shumacker and King (25) in 1952, and Fonkalsrud et al. (26) in 1974 reported on splenectomy for bleeding esophageal varices. The latter two studies were performed on children, and all three studies included patients with extrahepatic portal hypertension and a normal liver. Rebleeding occurred in 60 to 95% of patients with a follow-up period of 1 to 25 years.

Although splenectomy was formerly used to control bleeding esophageal varices, splenectomy alone should only be performed in patients with simple splenic vein thrombosis and left-sided portal hypertension. It is otherwise a poor operation, rebleeding is the rule, and it eliminates the possibility of future shunts that use the splenic vein. Splenectomy is currently part of different extensive devascularization and disconnection operations.

Percutaneous splenic artery occlusion has been reported to be successful in treating patients with hypersplenism with improvement of peripheral cytopenia (27). Splenectomy should not be performed solely for pancytopenia or thrombocytopenia in portal hypertension. Thrombocytopenia by itself usually does not represent a problem. If the patient undergoes a shunting operation, pancytopenia usually improves (28). Complications of percutaneous splenic artery occlusion include infarcts and abscesses of the spleen. Del Guercio et al. (29)

Table 15.4. Suture Ligation for Bleeding Esophageal Varices

Author (No.)	No. Patients	Operative Mortality (%)	Rebleed (%)	Follow-up	Overall Survival (%)
Britton and Crile (15)					
Cirrhosis	14	43	29	3–14 yr	—
Normal liver	14	0	50	—	—
Cooperman and Hermann (16)					
Cirrhosis	13	25	100	1–10 yr	38
Normal liver	12	17	75	—	75
Fonkalsrud et al. (17)[a]	22	9.5[b]	100	1–25 yr	—

[a] Children.
[b] Includes reoperations.

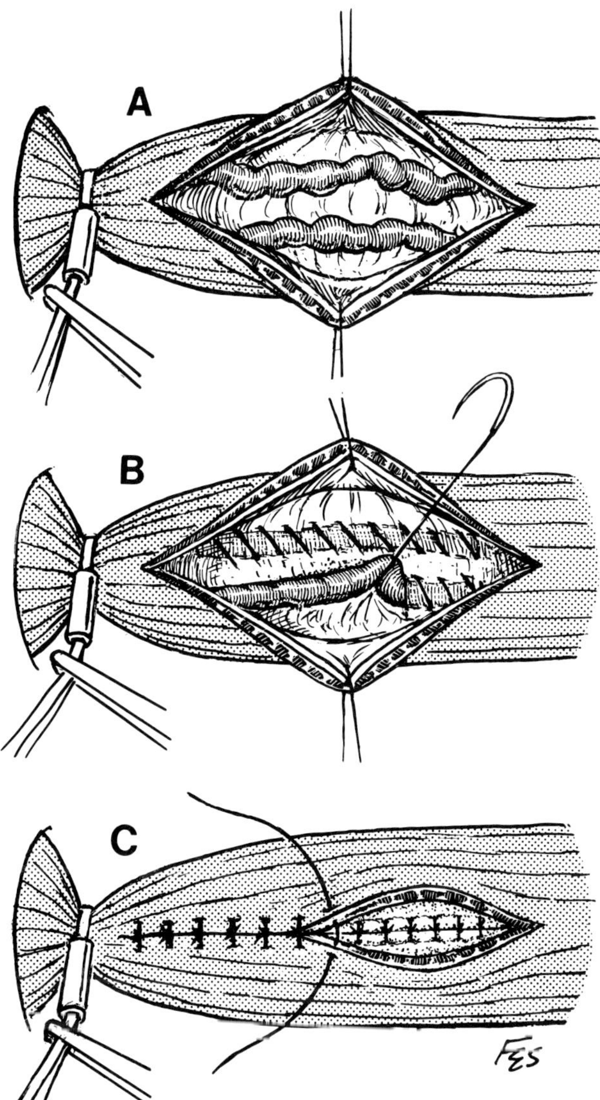

Figure 15.2. Transesophageal ligation of varices. (*A*) Esophagus opened longitudinally. (*B*) Varices occluded by running sutures. (*C*) Esophagus closed in two layers. (Reprinted by permission from Braasch JW, Rossi RL. Liver, gallbladder, biliary tract, pancreas, and spleen. In: Beahrs OH, Beart RW Jr, eds. *General Surgery: Therapy Update Service, Update 8.* Media, Pennsylvania: Harwal Publishing, 1982, p. 6-30.)

advocated the combination of percutaneous splenic artery occlusion and occlusion of the coronary vein and variceal collateral as a nonsurgical means in the emergency management of patients with bleeding esophageal varices. Their hospital mortality was 22%. The rate of recurrent bleeding was 46% and was believed to be less severe than the original episode of bleeding. The mean decrease in portal pressure was 8.5 cm. Their study suggested

that hepatic artery flow may increase after the procedure. The value of this technique requires further assessment.

Arteriovenous fistula between splanchnic arteries (hepatic, splenic artery) and branches of the portal system can be the result of trauma or rupture of arterial aneurysms. This can cause portal venous hypertension and bleeding varices. The treatment of choice is occlusion of the fistula by arterial ligation or radiologic catheter embolization techniques.

Pharmacologic Means to Decrease Portal Hypertension

Vasopressin decreases portal pressure by vasoconstriction of the splanchnic arterioles leading to a reduction in portal venous flow. In several studies (30–32), the mean reduction in portal pressure ranged from 17% to 29% and that of portal flow from 33% to 54%. Rebleeding occurs in about 62% of patients (33). Infusion through the superior mesenteric artery offers no advantage, and therefore the drug is given through a peripheral vein (34). A 20-unit bolus is given over 20 minutes, and thereafter a continuous infusion is started at 0.4 units per minute and is titrated to a lower dose. The patient should be on a cardiac monitor because vasopressin can cause decreased cardiac output, decreased heart rate, increased blood pressure, myocardial infarction, congestive heart failure, arrhythmias, and cardiac arrest. Skin necrosis ([scalp, nipples (35)]) has been reported. The use of nitroglycerin can reverse the cardiovascular side effects of vasopressin (36). In addition, small doses of intravenously administered nitroprusside have been reported to minimize the deleterious hemodynamic effects of vasopressin (37).

The beta-blocking agent, propranolol, has been used in an attempt to prevent recurrent bleeding. In a controlled trial, Lebrec et al. (38) demonstrated that propranolol decreased the rate of recurrent bleeding. In another controlled trial, however, Burroughs et al. (39) failed to demonstrate clear benefit. The effectiveness of propranolol in selected patients is being assessed. The drop in portal pressure appears to be secondary to the decrease in cardiac output and to the extracardiac effects of the beta-blocker.

Table 15.5. Resective Procedures for Bleeding Esophageal Varices

Author (No.)	Procedure	No. Patients	Status Liver	Operative Deaths[a]	Rebleed	Follow-up[b]
Habif (42)	Esophagogastrectomy with jejunal interposition	22	Normal, 17; cirrhosis, 4	3 (18%) 1 (25%)	2 (14%)	1–6 yr
Koop and Roddy (43)	Esophagogastrectomy with colon interposition	11	Normal, 11	0	3 (27%)	2–8 yr

[a] Three deaths were related to anastomotic leaks.
[b] All patients who survived were alive at the time of study, except for one accidental death.

Procedures that Promote New Collaterals

The Talma-Morrison omentopexy, splenopexy, and splenic transposition to the left chest in an attempt to provide collateral circulation through the pulmonary veins are only of historical interest as they do not provide any solution to the problem of bleeding varices.

Procedures that Reduce the Varix Bed

Phemister and Humphreys (40) reported in 1947 the use of total gastrectomy in one patient and esophagogastrectomy in another patient to control bleeding varices. Cooley and DeBakey (41) reported on the use of esophagogastrectomy. Habif (42), dealing mainly with patients with schistosomiasis, reported in 1959 on the use of esophagogastrectomy with jejunal interposition, and Koop and Roddy (43) employed esophagogastrectomy with colon interposition in the management of children with extrahepatic portal hypertension. Although these procedures can be carried out with a low operative mortality in patients with a normal liver and extrahepatic portal hypertension, they are a major undertaking in patients with cirrhosis and are therefore associated with substantial mortality. Rebleeding occurred in 14% of the patients followed up by Habif (42) and in 27% of the patients followed up by Koop and Roddy (43) (Table 15.5).

These procedures are now rarely performed as sclerotherapy, and extensive devascularization procedures are preferable to resective operations. Occasionally they may be justified in a patient with extrahepatic portal hypertension (normal liver) or in patients with presinusoidal block (schistosomiasis) when other shunting or nonshunting procedures have failed. The high rate of rebleeding and high mortality make these procedures unacceptable in patients with alcoholic cirrhosis.

Procedures that Interrupt Flow to the Varices

Esophageal Transection

Walker (44) in 1964 and George et al. (45) in 1973 reported on the circumferential transection of the distal esophagus (Table 15.6). The procedure is associated with a low operative mortality in patients with a normal liver (extrahepatic portal hypertension) but with a high mortality in cirrhotic patients. Bleeding recurred in about 50% of the patients and was believed to be the rule if the

Table 15.6. Esophageal Transection for Variceal Hemmorhage

Author (No.)	No. Patients	Operative Mortality (%)	Late Rebleed (%)	Follow-up
Walker (1964) (44)[a]				
Cirrhosis	28	25	43	1–12 yr
Normal liver	25	0	56	2–11 yr
George et al. (45)				
Cirrhosis	30	53	55	1–7 yr
Normal liver	5	0	20	2 mo–4 yr

[a] Esophageal dehiscence (rate of leakage), 10%.

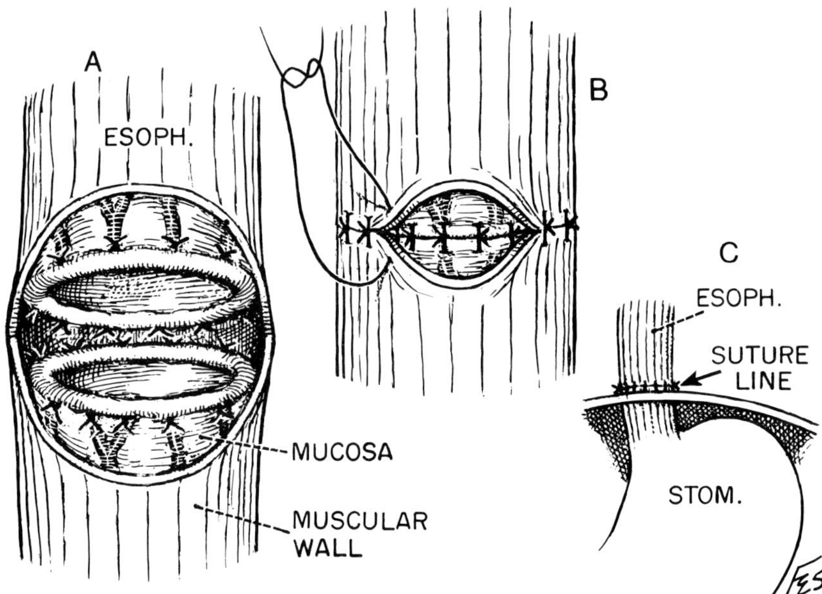

Figure 15.3. Esophageal transection. (*A*) Esophagus transected completely except for posterior muscular wall. Bleeding points secured with fine suture ligatures. (*B*) Mucosa of posterior wall is closed with interrupted absorbable sutures, and anterior wall is closed in two layers. (*C*) Esophagus resutured. (Reproduced by permission from Braasch JW, Rossi RL. Liver, gallbladder, biliary tract, pancreas, and spleen. In: Beahrs OH, Beart RW Jr, eds. *General Surgery: Therapy Update Service, Update 8.* Media, Pennsylvania: Harwal Publishing, 1982, p. 6-30.)

follow-up period was long. Hirashima et al. (46) reported on 63 patients with 55 survivors.

The esophagus is exposed through a left thoracotomy, and both the muscular layer and the mucosa of the anterior wall of the esophagus are divided in a transverse fashion about 2 cm above the gastroesophageal junction. Bleeding points are secured with suture ligatures. On the posterior wall, only the mucosa is transected, leaving the muscular layer intact (Fig. 15.3). The mucosa of the posterior wall is closed with absorbable interrupted sutures, and the anterior wall is closed in layers. The use of the Russian intraluminal stapling device to transect the esophagus was reported by Vankemmel (47) of France in 1974 and later by Johnston (48) in 1977 and Spence and Johnston (49), who later reported on an experience with 100 patients. Cooperman et al. (50,51) cited their experience with the use of the end-to-end anastomosis (EEA) stapler (United States Surgical Corp., Stamford, Connecticut).

Although these techniques control acute bleeding in more than 80% of patients, they result in high morbidity and mortality rates in high-risk patients. Therefore, if the alternative is sclerotherapy, there is probably a limited place for emergency esophageal transection. A prospective randomized trial comparing sclerotherapy and esophageal transection using the EEA stapler was

reported by Huizinga et al. (52). The perioperative mortality from sclerotherapy was 24% and that for transection was 33% ($p > 0.05$). The transected group had a lower rate of recurrent bleeding and required fewer reoperations, transfusions, and hospital readmissions.

Esophageal transection using the EEA stapler or a similar device (Fig. 15.4) is performed through a laparotomy, and the stapler is introduced through a gastrotomy on the anterior wall of the stomach into the distal abdominal esophagus and fired just above the cardia. The vagus nerves should be identified and preserved. If they are not identified, a gastric drainage procedure may be required.

Esophageal transection as a single procedure should be considered a temporizing operation. This procedure has been included in more extensive devascularization and disconnection operations in an attempt to improve long-term results and decrease the rate of recurrent bleeding. Esophageal transection by itself is not of benefit to the patient bleeding from gastric varices.

Devascularization and Transection: Porta-azygos Disconnection

Tanner (53) in 1950 reported a technique of devascularization of the greater and lesser curvature of the stomach for about 7 cm with division and

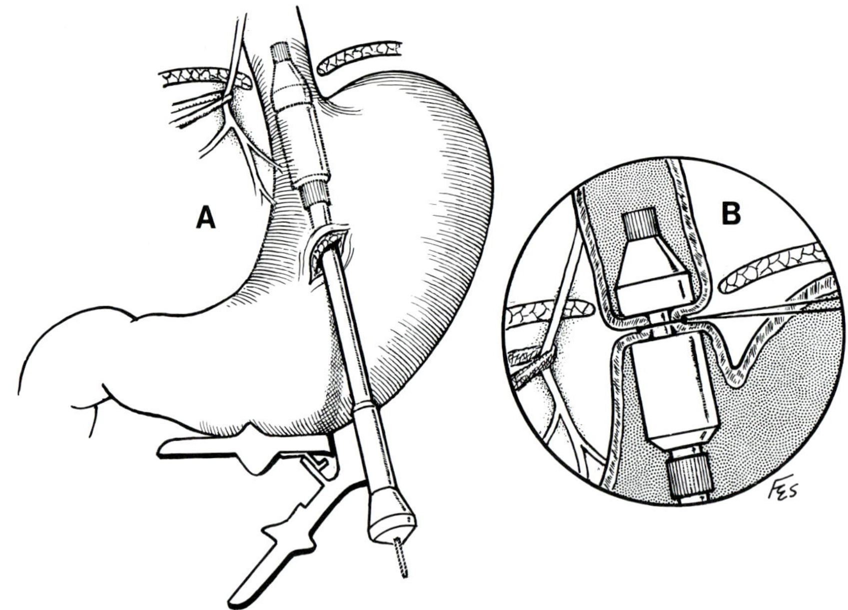

Figure 15.4. Esophageal transection using the EEA stapler. (*A*) Esophagus is isolated, and EEA stapler is placed through anterior gastrotomy. (*B*) EEA stapler is fired 1 to 2 cm above gastroesophageal junction. (Reprinted by permission from Braasch JW, Rossi RL. Liver, gallbladder, biliary tract, pancreas, and spleen. In: Beahrs OH, Beart RW Jr, eds. *General Surgery: Therapy Update Service, Update 8.* Media, Pennsylvania: Harwal Publishing, 1982, p. 6-31.)

resuturing of the stomach about 5 cm below the cardia (Fig. 15.5). Later Tanner added a limited external devascularization of the distal 5 cm of the esophagus. In 1961, Tanner (54) reported on 32 patients, 25 of whom had cirrhosis and 7 had a normal liver. The operative mortality was 24% and 0%, respectively, and the rate of recurrent bleeding was 44% and 70% during a follow-up period of 6 months to 10 years.

Womack and Peters (55) and Johnson et al. (56) described a more extensive procedure that included splenectomy, resection of the greater curvature of the stomach, ligation of arterial branches to the cardia, and transthoracic direct ligation of varices. Hassab (57) reported in 1972 on the use of extensive gastric devascularization in the treatment of bleeding varices from schistosomiasis. In 1973 Sugiura and Futagawa (58) described a new technique that differed from previous operations in the extent of the esophageal dissection and devascularization (Fig. 15.6). Through a left thoracotomy, the esophagus is mobilized and devascularized meticulously from the left pulmonary vein down to the cardia. The esophagus is transected above the cardia by dividing the anterior muscular wall and mucosa and preserving the posterior muscular wall. Fine vascular sutures are used to maintain hemostasis of the esophagus. The esophagus is closed with two layers of interrupted sutures. The first or thoracic stage of the operation is immediately followed in the same operation by the abdominal stage in the patient who is a good surgical risk. The second stage, performed through a midline laparotomy, consists of extensive devascularization of the lesser and greater curvature of the stomach, selective vagotomy, pyloroplasty, and splenectomy. However, this second stage can be deferred in the high-risk patient.

In 1977 Sugiura and Futagawa (59) published their results in 276 patients, with an operative mortality of 4.3%, a rate of recurrent bleeding of 2%, a 5-year survival of 83%, a rate of esophageal dihiscence of 7%, and a rate of stricture of 3%. Several factors in their experience favored these good results. Cirrhosis was the cause of portal hypertension in only two-thirds of the patients, while one-third of the patients had an extrahepatic cause. Of their patients, 73% were good or fair risks according to Child's classification. They also included 60 prophylactic operations in this series. It is, therefore, meaningful to consider their results in poor-risk patients (Child's class C) who had portal hypertension secondary to cirrhosis. In this group of patients, the operative mortality of 17% increased to 24% in emergency operations. The 5-year survival approached 60%, but the rate of recurrent bleeding remained below 5%, comparing favorably with that of portasystemic shunting. In a

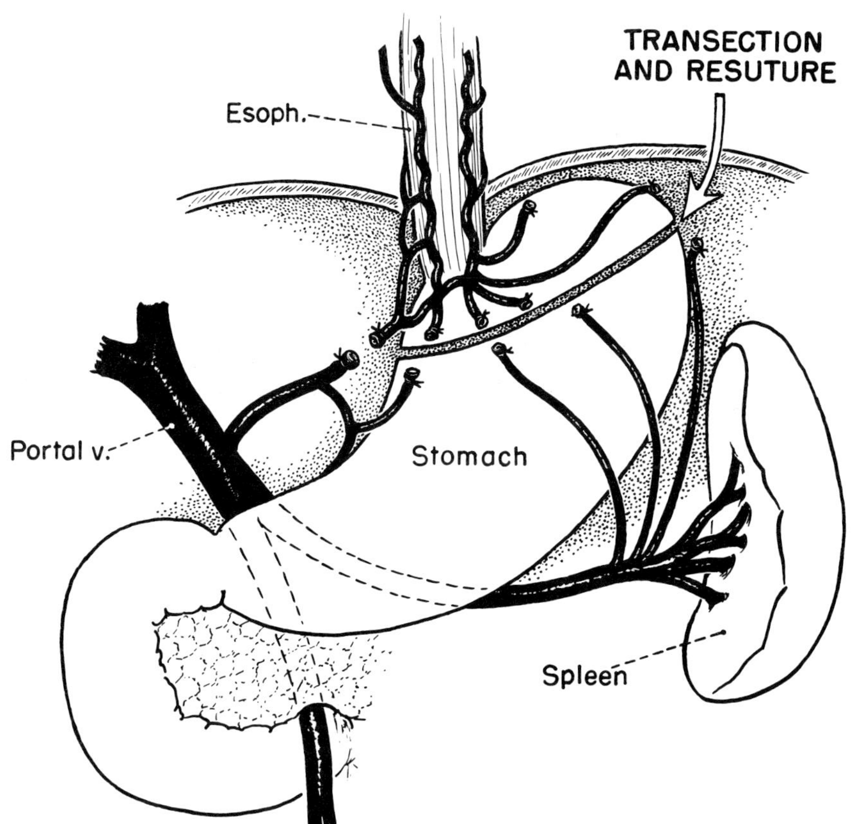

Figure 15.5. Tanner's method of porta-azygos disconnection is shown. (Reproduced by permission from Sedgwick CE, Poulantzas JR. Portal hypertension. Boston: Little, Brown, 1967, p. 243.)

review of their overall experience with 671 patients, Sugiura and Futagawa (60) reported that late rebleeding continued to be less than 5%. Koyama et al. (61) have reported similar results.

Sugiura's results with extensive devascularization have been difficult to reproduce in the Western world (62,63), where alcoholic cirrhosis is prevalent and where patients are frequently considered to be poor risks. Mortality is high in this group of patients, and rebleeding is frequent. It should be stated, however, that the procedures performed often are modifications of Sugiura's operation. Patient selection appears to be a critical factor. Sugiura and Futagawa (59) have not considered a patient for this procedure if ascites are present, encephalopathy does not improve with medical therapy, the bilirubin level is more than 3.0 milligrams per deciliter, or the albumin value is lower than 2.7 g/dL. These workers emphasized the importance of extensive paraesophageal devascularization and pointed out that in patients who had esophageal transection without periesophageal de-

vascularization, the rate of recurrent bleeding was 15%.

Extensive devascularization procedures appear to be indicated in patients who do not have vessels available for shunting, in patients with extrahepatic portal vein obstruction, in patients with preexistent encephalopathy, in some children (64) in whom sclerotherapy has failed or who are not suited for shunting, and in patients with schistosomiasis.

Modifications of extensive devascularization operations vary in the method preferred to open the stomach or esophagus, in the use of ligation of varices, and in the choice between stapling devices and manual suturing (65–68). Our modification consists of a first stage that includes a limited parietal cell (highly selective) vagotomy to devascularize the upper third of the lesser curvature of the stomach and the distal esophagus for about 5 to 7 cm (Fig. 15.7). This preserves the nerves of Latarjet and avoids pyloroplasty. Devascularization of the greater curvature of the stomach and

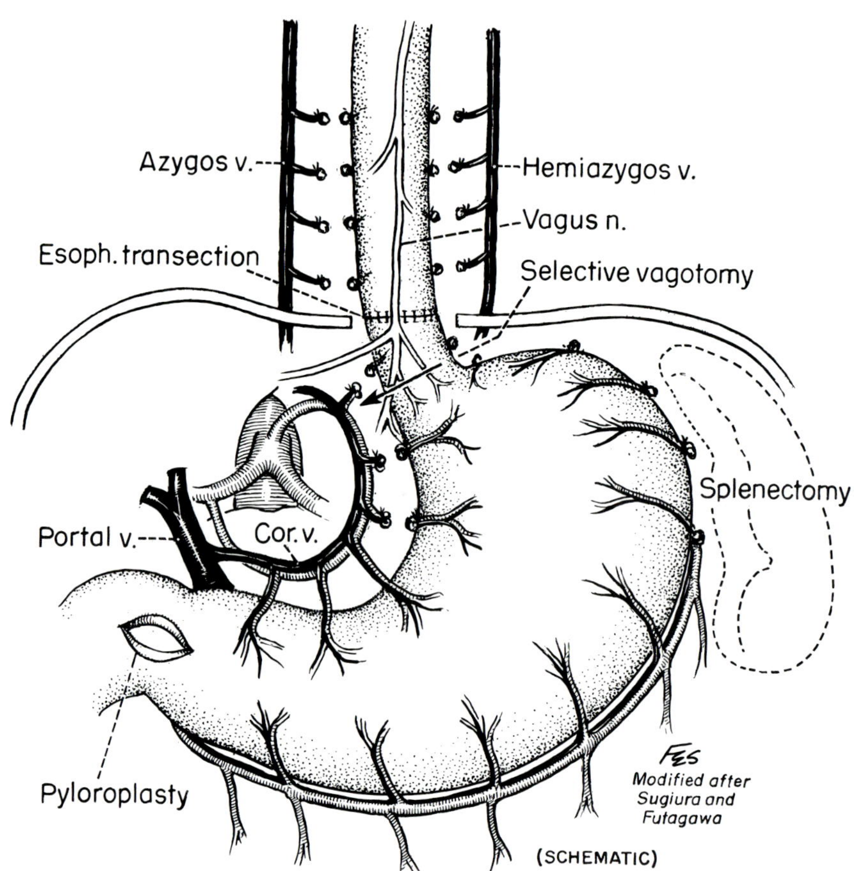

Figure 15.6. Esophageal transection with paraesophagogastric devascularization (Sugiura's procedure). (Reproduced by permission from Matory WE Jr, Sedgwick CE, Rossi RL. Nonshunting procedures for bleeding esophageal varices. *Surg Clin North Am* 1980; 60(2):289.)

splenectomy are performed next. Instead of esophageal transection, we employ a separate stapling technique, without transection of the anterior and posterior gastric wall, at the junction of the proximal third and middle third of the stomach using the TA-90 stapler or the gastrointestinal anastomosis stapler (GIA-S) (United States Surgical Corp., Stamford, Connecticut) without a knife blade. These staplers are positioned through small gastrotomies made in the lesser and greater curvature. Some of the recurrent episodes of bleeding after standard esophageal transection using the EEA stapler are the result of gastric varices. Bleeding from high gastric varices can be controlled better by stapling the stomach at the junction of the middle and upper thirds of the stomach at the time of the porta-azygos disconnection. The left gastric vein is identified over the pancreas and is ligated (Fig. 15.8). The second or thoracic stage, consisting of periesophageal devascularization up to the inferior pulmonary vein, is deferred for 6 to 8 weeks

or more, or is replaced by a plan of chronic sclerotherapy.

In patients who have undergone multiple previous abdominal procedures, including failed shunts, and in whom multiple vascular adhesions are anticipated, we prefer a single thoracic approach. A left thoracotomy is performed, the distal esophagus is devascularized from the inferior pulmonary vein down to the cardia, and the diaphragm is incised. Splenectomy is performed; the left gastric vein is ligated; and through two small gastrotomies, one in the lesser curvature and the other in the greater curvature, the anterior and posterior walls of the stomach are stapled separately (Fig. 15.9). Patients are followed up by serial endoscopy, and sclerotherapy is undertaken if varices are detected. These techniques are well tolerated in the patient with extrahepatic portal hypertension and in good-risk patients, but are associated with a high morbidity and mortality in patients with Child's class C alcoholic cirrhosis.

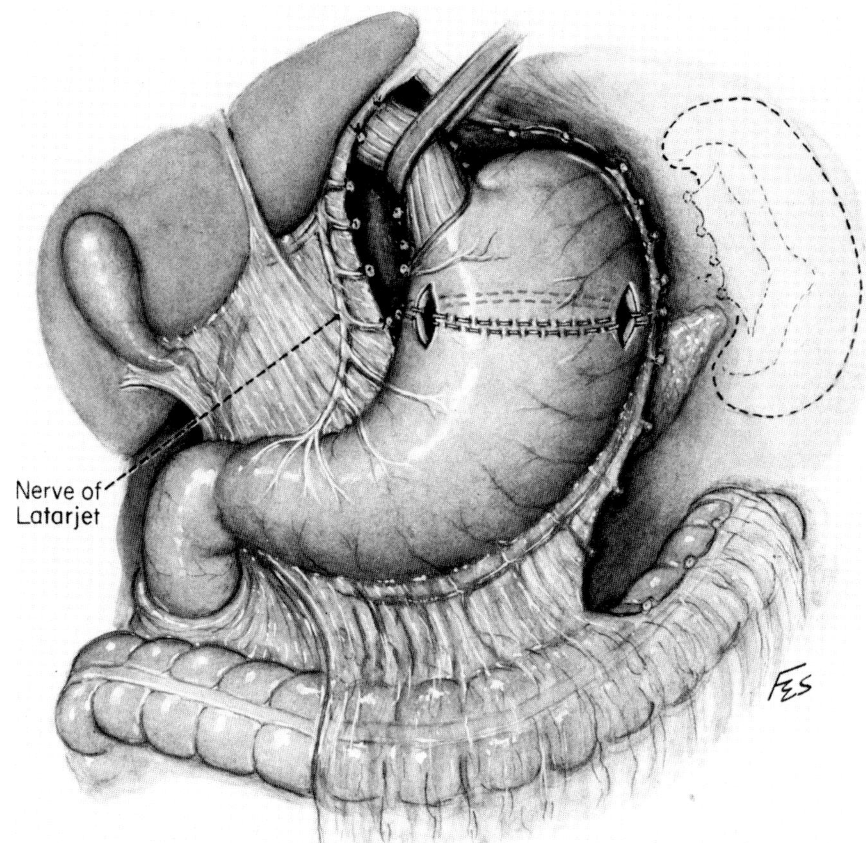

Figure 15.7. Devascularization technique. Parietal cell vagotomy, splenectomy, and gastrotomies for gastric stapling. (Reproduced by permission from Rossi RL, Jenkins RL, Nielsen-Whitcomb FF. Management of complications of portal hypertension. *Surg Clin North Am* 1985; 65(2):245.)

Sugiura and Futagawa (60) suggested that patients who have had recent sclerotherapy can have a higher incidence of esophageal dehiscence at the time of esophageal transection. In a prospective trial, Raia et al. (68) compared results using distal splenorenal shunt, a Linton central splenorenal shunt, and extensive esophagogastric devascularization in the management of bleeding esophageal varices caused by schistosomiasis. They used a technique of porta-azygos disconnection (Fig. 15.10) that consisted of splenectomy, devascularization of the proximal stomach, suture ligation of varices through a vertical esophagotomy and gastrotomy, and a 270-degree fundic wrap as an antireflux procedure and to protect the esophagotomy and gastrotomy used for suture ligation of the varices. The average follow-up period was 53 months. The incidence of recurrent bleeding was similar in patients who underwent a shunt and in those who had gastric devascularization (12%). Hepatic encephalopathy was present in more than 30% of patients in whom Linton's central splenorenal shunt was used, but occurred less frequently in patients who underwent a distal splenorenal shunt or had an extensive devascularization operation (13%). Some authors (64) have added a fundoplication to the devascularization procedures. Although the advantages of this modification are unclear, some data (69) suggest that an increase in the lower esophageal sphincter pressure decreases the flow through the varices.

Percutaneous Transhepatic Obliteration

In 1974 Lunderquist and Vang (70) introduced the method of catheterizing the portal vein transhepatically, embolizing the left gastric vein and other collaterals, and obliterating varices. Initially, it was thought that this procedure would have wide application in the management of patients with bleeding esophageal varices. However, appreciable expertise was required; intra-abdominal bleeding, portal vein thrombosis, and pulmonary emboli were not uncommon; and late rebleeding

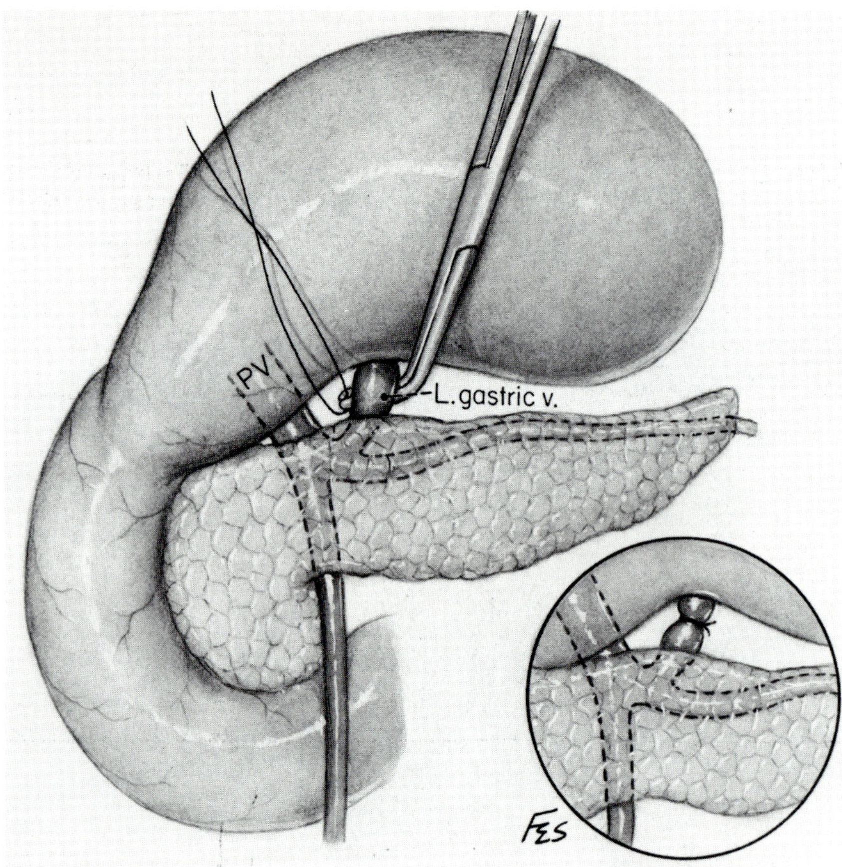

Figure 15.8. Modification of Sugiura's technique. Left gastric vein is tied above the pancreas. (Reproduced by permission from Rossi RL, Jenkins RL, Nielsen-Whitcomb FF. Management of complications of portal hypertension. *Surg Clin North Am* 1985; 65(2):246.)

frequently occurred, emphasizing that percutaneous transhepatic obliteration was also a temporizing procedure. Bengmark and associates (71) observed that a high rate of rebleeding and a high incidence of complications have considerably diminished earlier enthusiasm for this technique. In skilled hands and in well-selected patients, this procedure can be helpful as a temporizing maneuver. Different materials have been used to achieve thrombosis, such as thrombin, Gelfoam, collagen, autologous blood clot, sclerosing agents, and metal coils. Ohnishi et al. (72) have used stainless coils plus Gelfoam and hypertonic glucose with a 93% success rate in stopping the acute episode of bleeding. However, 29% of patients rebled within 2 months, and 56% rebled by 9 months.

Percutaneous techniques have been used to dilate stenotic shunts or to occlude collaterals in patients who have had selective shunts and in whom encephalopathy developed. Percutaneous transarterial occlusion can also be used to treat some arteriovenous fistulas.

Indications for Nonshunting Procedures

Selection of therapy for patients with portal hypertension and bleeding varices depends on multiple factors—the condition of the patient as defined by Child's classification, the urgent or elective nature of the operation, the cause and pathogenic mechanism of the portal hypertension, the patency and anatomic relationship of vessels in the portal system, the presence and degree of ascites and encephalopathy, the site of bleeding (esophageal or gastric), the age of the patient, the associated medical conditions, the previous surgical procedures, the expertise available in a given institution, and the likelihood of the patient becoming a candidate for liver transplantation.

The selection of therapy is controversial. Analysis of the literature demonstrates many variables and biases that make comparison of different surgical procedures and of the same surgical procedure in different series of patients difficult. Most studies are not controlled, and frequently the pe-

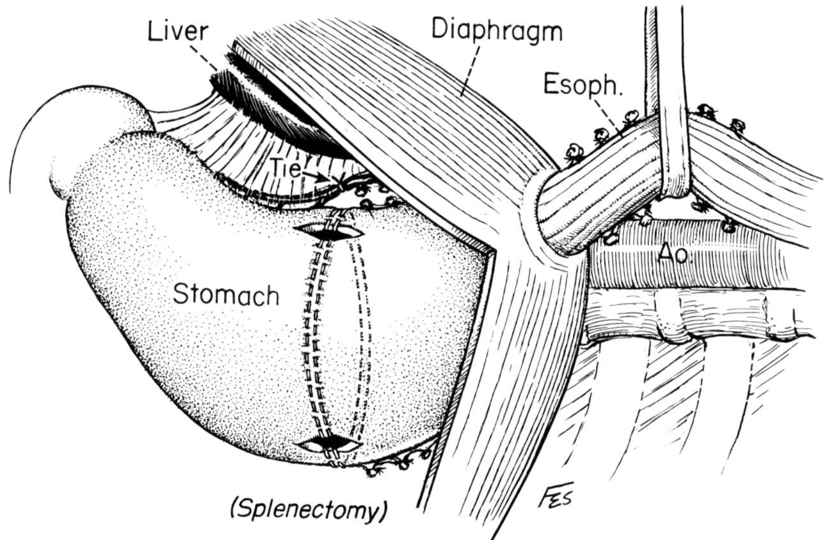

Figure 15.9. Devascularization of the stomach using the TA-90 stapler. (Reproduced by permission from Matory WE Jr, Sedgwick CE, Rossi RL. Nonshunting procedures in management of bleeding esophageal varices. *Surg Clin North Am* 1980; 60(2):293.)

riod of follow-up is limited. Reports of long-term results with such techniques as chronic sclerotherapy and extensive devascularization procedures and prospective studies comparing these techniques with medical therapy and with shunting operations are still too scarce to determine clearly the advantages and disadvantages of different therapeutic modalities.

We usually consider a nonshunting procedure (73) for patients with unsuitable veins for shunting in the portal system, for patients with severely impaired liver function (especially when emergency operations are required), for patients with encephalopathy, for patients who may become candidates for liver transplantation, when emergency surgical control of bleeding is required in patients who are hemodynamically unstable, when a selective shunt fails or is technically impossible at the time of operation, and with schistosomiasis where total shunts often result in a high rate of encephalopathy.

Sclerotherapy has become the procedure of

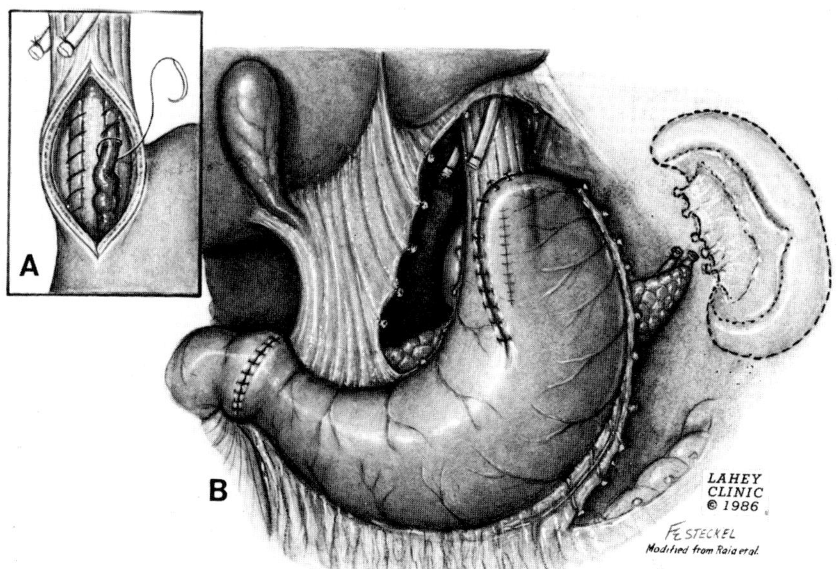

Figure 15.10. Devascularization procedure as described by Raia et al. (68). (Reproduced by permission of Lahey Clinic.)

choice in the management of patients with acute variceal bleeding. Although it is uncertain whether chronic sclerotherapy increases survival, prospective trials comparing it with medical therapy appear to demonstrate fewer episodes of bleeding in the group having sclerotherapy. In prospective trials, chronic sclerotherapy appears to have some advantages over distal splenorenal shunt as reported by Warren et al. (74) in a 2-year follow-up report and when compared with portacaval shunt in a study by Cello et al. (75) with a mean follow-up period of 263 days. However, longer follow-up is required to determine its usefulness.

Balloon tamponade and vasopressin continue to be good adjuncts in the treatment of an acute episode of bleeding, especially when sclerotherapy is not available or when bleeding is massive and must be controlled before sclerotherapy.

Although esophageal transection, variceal ligation, splenectomy, and limited devascularization procedures have, for the most part, been abandoned as isolated procedures, they have been included as part of more extensive devascularization operations. Splenectomy alone should be used only in the presence of isolated splenic vein thrombosis and left-sided portal hypertension. Extensive devascularization and disconnecting procedures, such as Sugiura's operation or variations of this technique, have become attractive because they have been able to decrease the rate of late rebleeding without inducing encephalopathy. As demonstrated by Sugiura and Futagawa (60), this procedure can be accomplished with a low operative mortality and with favorable long-term results in the good surgical risk patient (Child's class A and B) and in the patient with extrahepatic portal hypertension. In some children (64) in whom sclerotherapy fails or vessels are inadequate for shunting, devascularization techniques can be considered. In a prospective trial, Raia et al. (68) demonstrated that in patients with schistosomiasis, extensive devascularization can be performed with a low operative mortality and with long-term results similar to those of distal splenorenal shunts. The value of extensive devascularization in patients with alcoholic cirrhosis and in poor surgical risk patients remains controversial. Nonshunting operations offer an alternative to patients who are candidates for future liver transplantation as they preserve the portal vein—a structure that is necessary for the success of a liver transplant.

Further evaluation is required to assess the role of chronic sclerotherapy and extensive devascularization procedures in the management of patients with bleeding varices resulting from portal hypertension, and to determine whether these techniques have any effect on long-term survival compared with shunting operations and medical therapy exclusively, especially in alcoholic patients. We must also recognize that there is a group of terminally ill patients who are often alcoholic and have severe jaundice, ascites, malnutrition, and irreversible coagulopathy and for whom surgery has nothing to offer.

In patients with intestinal stomas and bleeding varices about the stoma, local procedures, such as suture ligation and sclerotherapy, have been used successfully. Occasionally, the stomas require reconstruction. Hemorrhoids associated with portal hypertension have also been treated successfully with surgical excision or sclerotherapy. Massive peristomal bleeding may require total portal decompression through a portasystemic shunt.

The patient who has the rare association of portal hypertension and bleeding varices from an arteriovenous fistula between a visceral artery and a branch of the portal system requires surgical or percutaneous catheter occlusion of the fistula.

Conclusion

The surgeon managing the patient with bleeding esophageal varices has a choice of many nonshunting procedures that attempt to stop the bleeding by obliterating or compressing varices, reducing the portal blood volume, or interrupting the flow to the varices. The selection of therapy is based on multiple factors and continues to be controversial. It includes the basic pathogenic mehanism of the portal hypertension, the status of the patient, the site of the block in the portal system, the caliber and anatomic relationship of the vessels available for anastomosis, the presence and severity of ascites or encephalopathy, the site of bleeding (esophageal or gastric), the techniques and expertise available at a given institution, previous procedures attempted on the patient, and the likelihood of the patient becoming a candidate for liver transplantation. Nonshunting procedures do not induce encephalopathy and, with the exception of extensive devascularization operations, are associated with a high rate of rebleeding. The new methods of extensive esophagogastric devascularization are attractive because of the low rate of recurrent bleeding. These extensive procedures can be accomplished with a low operative morbidity and mortality in the low-risk patient and in the patient with extrahepatic portal hypertension or schistosomiasis, but are associated with a high operative mortality in the patient with Child's class C alcoholic cirrhosis. Nonshunting procedures should be considered in patients with unsuitable veins for shunting, in patients with encephalopathy or poor liver function, in some children, and in patients with extrahepatic portal hypertension and schistosomiasis. Further evaluation is required to compare the benefits of nonshunting procedures with shunting operations, especially in alcoholic patients.

References

1. Rossi RL, Jenkins RL, Nielsen-Whitcomb FF. Management of complications of portal hypertension. *Surg Clin North Am* 1985; 65(2):231–262.
2. Turcotte JG, Wallin VW Jr, Child CG III. End-to-side versus side-to-side portacaval shunts in patients with hepatic cirrhosis. *Am J Surg* 1969; 117(1):108–116.
3. Clowes GH Jr, McDermott WV, Williams LF, Loda M, Menzoian JO, Pearl R. Amino acid clearance and prognosis in surgical patients with cirrhosis. *Surgery* 1984; 96(4): 675–685.
4. Crafoord C, Frenckner P. New surgical treatment of varicous veins of the oesophagus. *Acta Otolaryngol* 1939; 27(4): 422–429.
5. Preble RB. Conclusions based on sixty cases of fatal gastro-intestinal hemorrhage due to cirrhosis of the liver. *Am J Med Sci* 1900; 119(3): 263–280.
6. Westphal K. Uber eine Kompressionsbehandlung der Blutungen aus Ocsophagusvarizen. *Dtsch Med Wochenschr* 1930; 56(7):1135–1136.
7. Rowntree LG, Zimmerman EF, Todd MH, Ajac J. Intraesophageal venous tamponade: Its use in a case of variceal hemorrhage from the esophagus. *JAMA* 1947; 135(10):630–631.
8. Sengstaken RW, Blakemore AH. Balloon tamponade for the control of hemorrhage from esophageal varices. *Ann Surg* 1950; 131(5):781–789.
9. Linton RR. The emergency and definitive treatment of bleeding esophageal varices. *Gastroenterology* 1953; 24(1): 1–15.
10. Conn HO, Simpson JA. Excessive mortality associated with balloon tamponade of bleeding varices: A critical reappraisal. *JAMA* 1967; 202(7):587–591.
11. Hermann RE, Traul D. Experience with the Sengstaken-Blakemore tube for bleeding esophageal varices. *Surg Gynecol Obstet* 1970, 130(5):879–885.
12. Pitcher JL. Safety and effectiveness of the modified Sengstaken-Blakemore tube: A prospective study. *Gastroenterology* 1971; 61(3):291–298.
13. Novis BH, Duys P, Babezat GO, Clain J, Bank S, Terblanche J. Fibreoptic endoscopy and the use of the Sengstaken tube in acute gastrointestinal hemorrhage in patients with portal hypertension. *Gut* 1976; 17(4):258–263.
14. Boerema I. Chirurgische Hulp by bloedinger uit Varices van den Oesophagus by lever Cirrhose en by het Syndrom van Banti. *Nederl T Geneesk* 1949; 1:4174–4182.
15. Britton RC, Crile G Jr. Late results of transesophageal suture of bleeding esophageal varices. *Surg Gynecol Obstet* 1963; 117(1):10–14.
16. Cooperman AM, Hermann RE. Ligation procedures in the management of portal hypertension. *Surgery* 1977; 81(4): 382–385.
17. Fonkalsrud EW, Myers NA, Robinson MJ. Management of extrahepatic portal hypertension in children. *Ann Surg* 1974; 180(4):487–493.
18. Ottinger LW, Moncure AC. Transthoracic ligation of bleeding esophageal varices in patients with intrahepatic portal obstruction. *Ann Surg* 1974; 179(1):35–38.
19. Wirthlin LS, Linton RR, Ellis DS. Transthoracoesophageal ligation of bleeding esophageal varices: A reappraisal. *Arch Surg* 1974; 109(5):688–692.
20. Blain AW. Ligation of the splenic artery for Banti's disease. *Surg Gynecol Obstet* 1918; 26:660–662.
21. Everson TC, Cole WH. Ligation of the splenic artery in patients with portal hypertension. *Arch Surg* 1948; 56(2): 153–160.
22. Berman JK, Koenig H, Muller LP. Ligation of hepatic and splenic arteries in treatment of portal hypertension: Ligation in atrophic cirrhosis of the liver. *Arch Surg* 1951; 63(3):379–389.
23. Mayo WJ. The surgical treatment of hepatic cirrhosis. *Ann Surg* 1924; 80(3):419–424.
24. Rousselot LM. Late phase of congestive splenomegaly (Banti's syndrome) with hematemesis but without cirrhosis of liver; further observations on etiology of Banti's syndrome and effect on prognosis of certain variations in portal venous pattern. *Surgery* 1940; 8(1):34–42.
25. Shumacker HB Jr, King H. Splenic studies. II. Portal hypertension in children associated with gastroesophageal hemorrhage. *Arch Surg* 1952; 65(4):499–510.
26. Fonkalsrud EW, Myers NA, Robinson MJ. Management of extrahepatic portal hypertension in children. *Ann Surg* 1974; 180(4):487–493.
27. Zannini G, Masciariello S, Pagano G, Sangiuolo P, Zotti G, Iaccarino V. Percutaneous splenic artery occlusion for portal hypertension: A new mechanical technique for hypersplenism. *Arch Surg* 1983; 118(8):897–904.
28. el-Khisen MA, Henderson JM, Millikan WJ Jr, Kutner MH, Warren WD. Splenectomy is contraindicated for thrombocytopenia secondary to portal hypertension. *Surg Gynecol Obstet* 1985; 160(3):233–238.
29. Del Guercio LRM, Hodgson WJB, Morgan JC, Berman HL, Kinkhabwalla MN. Splenic artery and coronary vein occlusion for bleeding esophageal varices. *World J Surg* 1984; 8(5):680–687.
30. Bosch J, Kravetz D, Rodes J. Effects of somatostatin on hepatic and systemic hemodynamics in patients with cirrhosis of the liver: Comparison with vasopressin. *Gastroenterology* 1981; 80(3):518–525.
31. Tsakiris A, Haemmerli UP, Bühlmann A. Reduction of portal venous pressure in cirrhotic patients with bleeding from oesophageal varices, by administration of a vasopressin derivative, phenylalanine²-lysine⁸-vasopressin. *Am J Med* 1964; 36(6):825–839.
32. Sonnenberg GE, Keller U, Perruchoud A, Burckhardt D, Gyr K. Effect of somatostatin on splanchnic hemodynamics in patients with cirrhosis of the liver and in normal subjects. *Gastroenterology* 1981; 80(3):526–532.
33. Merigan TC Jr, Plotkin GR, Davidson CS. Effect of intravenously administered posterior pituitary extract on hem-

orrhage from bleeding esophageal varices. *N Engl J Med* 1962; 266(3):134–135.

34. Chojkier M, Groszmann RJ, Atterbury CE, et al. A controlled comparison of continuous intra-arterial and intravenous infusions of vasopressin in hemorrhage from esophageal varices. *Gastroenterology* 1979; 77(3):540–546.

35. Reddy KR, Iskandarani M, Jeffers L, Schiff ER. Bilateral nipple necrosis after intravenous vasopressin therapy. *Arch Intern Med* 1984; 144(4):835–836.

36. Groszmann RJ, Kravetz D, Bosch J, et al. Nitroglycerin improves the hemodynamic response to vasopressin in portal hypertension. *Hepatology* 1982; 2(6):757–762.

37. Mols P, Hallemans R, Van Kuyk M, et al. Hemodynamic effects of vasopressin, alone and in combination with nitroprusside, in patients with liver cirrhosis and portal hypertension. *Ann Surg* 1984; 199(2):176–181.

38. Lebrec D, Poynard T, Hillon P, Benhamou J-P. Propranolol for prevention of recurrent gastrointestinal bleeding in patients with cirrhosis: A controlled study. *N Engl J Med* 1981; 305(23):1371–1374.

39. Burroughs AK, Jenkins WJ, Sherlock S, et al. Controlled trial of propranolol for the prevention of recurrent variceal hemorrhage in patients with cirrhosis. *N Engl J Med* 1983; 309(25):1539–1542.

40. Phemister DB, Humphreys EM. Gastro-esophageal resection and total gastrectomy in the treatment of bleeding varicose veins in Banti's syndrome. *Ann Surg* 1947; 126(4):397–410.

41. Cooley DA, DeBakey ME. Subtotal esophagectomy for bleeding esophageal varices. *Arch Surg* 1954; 68(6):854–871.

42. Habif DV. Treatment of esophageal varices by partial esophagogastrectomy and interposed jejunal segment. *Surgery* 1959; 46(1):212–238.

43. Koop CE, Roddy SR. Colonic replacement of distal esophagus and proximal stomach in the management of bleeding varices in children. *Ann Surg* 1958; 147(1):17–25.

44. Walker RM. Esophageal transection for bleeding varices. *Surg Gynecol Obstet* 1964; 118(2):323–329.

45. George P, Brown C, Ridgway G, Crofts B, Sherlock S. Emergency oesophageal transection in uncontrolled variceal haemorrhage. *Br J Surg* 1973; 60(8):635–640.

46. Hirashima T, Hara T, Takeuchi H, et al. Transabdominal esophageal mucosal transection for the control of esophageal varices. *Surg Gynecol Obstet* 1980; 151(1):36–40.

47. Vankemmel M. Cited by Donovan AJ. Surgical treatment of portal hypertension: A historical perspective. *World J Surg* 1984; 8(5):626–645.

48. Johnston GW. Treatment of bleeding varices by oesophageal transection with the SPTU gun. *Ann R Coll Surg Engl* 1977; 59(5):404–408.

49. Spence RAJ, Johnston GW. Results in 100 consecutive patients with stapled esophageal transection for varices. *Surg Gynecol Obstet* 1985; 160(4):323–329.

50. Cooperman M, Fabri PJ, Martin EW Jr, Carey LC. EEA esophageal stapling for control of bleeding esophageal varices. *Am J Surg* 1980; 140(12):821–824.

51. Wanamaker SR, Cooperman M, Carey LC. Use of the EEA stapling instrument for control of bleeding esophageal varices. *Surgery* 1983; 94(4):620–626.

52. Huizinga WKJ, Angorn IB, Baker LW. Esophageal transection versus injection sclerotherapy in the management of bleeding esophageal varices in patients at high risk. *Surg Gynecol Obstet* 1985; 160(6):539–546.

53. Tanner NC. Gastroduodenal hemorrhage as a surgical emergency. *Proc R Soc Med* 1950; 43:147–152.

54. Tanner NC. The late results of porto-azygos disconnexion in the treatment of bleeding from oesophageal varices. *Ann R Coll Surg Engl* 1961; 28:153–174.

55. Womack NA, Peters RM. Ligation of gastric arterial supply and splenectomy in the treatment of acute hemorrhage from gastroesophageal varices. In: Ellison EH, Firesen SR, Mulholland JH, eds. *Current Surgical Management*, Vol. 3. Philadelphia: WB Saunders, 1965, 268–278.

56. Johnson G Jr, Dart CH Jr, Peters RM, Macfie JA. Hemodynamic changes with cirrhosis of the liver: Control of arteriovenous shunts during operation for esophageal varices. *Ann Surg* 1966; 163(5):692–703.

57. Hassab MA. Nonshunt operations in portal hypertension without cirrhosis. *Surg Gynecol Obstet* 1972; 131(4):648–654.

58. Sugiura M, Futagawa S. A new technique for treating esophageal varices. *J Thorac Cardiovasc Surg* 1973; 66(5):677–685.

59. Sugiura M, Futagawa S. Further evaluation of the Sugiura procedure in the treatment of bleeding esophageal varices. *Arch Surg* 1977; 112(11):1317–1321.

60. Sugiura M, Futagawa S. Esophageal transection with paraesophagogastric devascularizations (the Sugiura procedure) in the treatment of esophageal varices. *World J Surg* 1984; 8(5):673–682.

61. Koyama K, Takagi Y, Ouchi K, Sato T. Results of esophageal transection for esophageal varices: Experience in 100 cases. *Am J Surg* 1980; 139(2):204–209.

62. Bothe A Jr, Stone MD, McDermott WV Jr. Portoazygos disconnection for bleeding esophageal varices. *Am J Surg* 1985; 149(4):546–550.

63. Giordani M, Ravo B, Sacchi M, Smith N, Ger R. Treatment of bleeding esophageal varices by portoazygos transection with the button of Boerema and EEA stapler: Ten years' experience. *Surgery* 1985; 97(6):649–652.

64. Superina RA, Weber JL, Shandling B. A modified Sugiura operation for bleeding varices in children. *J Pediatr Surg* 1983; 18(6):794–799.

65. Delaney JP. A method for esophagogastric devascularization. *Surg Gynecol Obstet* 1980; 150(6):899–900.

66. Chaib SA, Souza Lessa B, Cecconello I, Felix WN, Chaib E. A new procedure for the treatment of bleeding esophageal varices by transgastric azygo-portal disconnection. *Int Surg* 1983; 68(4):353–356.

67. Romero-Torres R. Hemostatic suture of the stomach for the treatment of massive hemorrhage due to esophageal varices. *Surg Gynecol Obstet* 1981; 153(5):710–712.

68. Raia S, Mies S, Macedo AL. Surgical treatment of portal hypertension in schistosomiasis. *World J Surg* 1984; 8(5):738–752.

69. Lunderquist A, Alwmark A, Gullstrand, et al. Pharmacologic influence on esophageal varices: a preliminary report. *Cardiovasc Intervent Radiol* 1983; 6(2):65–71.

70. Lunderquist A, Vang J. Transhepatic catheterization and obliteration of the coronary vein in patients with portal hypertension and esophageal varices. *N Engl J Med* 1974; 291(13):646–649.

71. Bengmark S, Börjesson B, Hoevels J, Joelsson B, Lunderquist A, Owman T. Obliteration of esophageal varices by PTP. A follow-up of 43 patients. *Ann Surg* 1979; 190(4):549–554.

72. Ohnishi K, Takayasu K, Takashi M, et al. Transhepatic obliteration of esophageal varices using stainless coils combined with hypertonic glucose and gelfoam. *J Clin Gastroenterol* 1985; 7(3):200–207.

73. Jenkins RL, Benotti PN, Bothe AA, Rossi RL. Liver transplantation. *Surg Clin North Am* 1985; 65(1):103–122.

74. Warren WD, Henderson JM, Millikan WJ, Galambos JT, Brooks WS, Riepe SP, et al. Distal splenorenal shunt *versus*

endoscopic sclerotherapy for long-term management of variceal bleeding: Preliminary report of a prospective, randomized trial. *Ann Surg* 1986; 203(5):454–462.

75. Cello JP, Grendell JH, Crass RA, Trunkey DD, Cobb EE, Heilbron DC. Endoscopic sclerotherapy versus portacaval shunt in patients with severe cirrhosis and variceal hemorrhage. *N Engl J Med* 1984; 311(25):1589–1594.

Editorial Comment

At this point in time, either sclerotherapy or portal-systemic shunting, or a combination of the two, has been the most widely applied form of invasive therapy for bleeding esophageal varices. Understandable dissatisfaction with the results of either or both of these treatments has led to the emergence of a large number of other approaches to this difficult and highly lethal problem. Dr. Rossi has presented a scholarly review of the nonoperative programs that have included various pharmacologic and radiologic approaches. A number of ingenious operations have been devised over the years, such as multiple arterial ligations, various types of collateralization, ligations, and transections, and all have had transient periods of popularity. In reviewing this particular manuscript, the editor could not find a single procedure to which at least passing mention had not been given, and certainly this is one of the most complete historical reviews available.

Dr. Rossi focused on the only procedure classification that could be said to compete with sclerotherapy and/or shunting procedures—the forms of disconnection that have been introduced over the past decade and which in general terms could be referred to as porta-azygous disconnections. In general, these efforts have focused on dividing the collateralized channels between the high-pressure portal and the low-pressure azygous circulations. They involve multiple ligations of left gastric (coronary) gastroepliploic, splenic, and other venous channels with or without splenectomy, often combined with a form of gastric or esophageal transection, frequently using a stapling device. The so-called Sugiura's procedure is long and tedious and has not had as widespread acceptance in this country as in Japan, possibly because the categories of patients in these two geographically separate areas are significantly different. The disconnections most favored in the United States have extended the venous ligations described by Warren as adjunctive to the selective shunt with gastrotomies and anterior and posterior gastric wall stapling; we have described our own variant of this approach (1) and have applied it widely to a number of instances in which neither sclerotherapy nor portal-systemic shunting has been applicable or successful. This technique, which Dr. Rossi has described in some detail, is, we believe, useful in approaching the difficult and multifactorial problems that are often lumped under the main heading of bleeding esophageal varices. It is natural, however, for anyone who has spent years in this particular area of surgery to be skeptical about any "magical" solution to what has traditionally been one of the most difficult, discouraging, and frustrating disease entities.

References

1. Bothe A Jr, Stone MD, McDermott WV. Portal azygous disconnection for bleeding esophageal varices. *Am J Surg* 1985; 149:546–550.

Chapter 16

Hematologic Problems of Liver Disease: Coagulopathies and Hypersplenism

JAMES L. TULLIS

In normal individuals, clot formation and clot lysis are in a state of kinetic balance. The many proteins and accelerators that tend to convert blood from a liquid to a solid are in a precise equilibrium with a similarly complex set of enzymes and anticoagulants that inhibit this process and initiate lysis whenever clotting occurs. The clotting system is further reinforced by vascular hemostasis in which calcium, von Willebrand's factor, platelets, ADP, monoamines, intact endothelium, and nerve fibers interact in such a manner as to retain blood within the vascular space and simultaneously present a smooth semipermeable membrane for the egress of essential crystalloids and nutrients into the tissues.

Liver disease is frequently accompanied by gross derangements of these controls, as the bulk of the coagulation proteins and hemostatic factors are synthesized in this organ. Moreover, the phagocytic Kupffer's cells normally play the important role of removing from the blood any circulating fibrinogen/fibrin degradation products or activated clotting factors which might otherwise initiate diffuse intravascular coagulation (DIC). Either hypo- or hypercoagulable states can occur in liver disease, depending on whether synthesis or degradation is predominant at the moment. However, clinical bleeding disorders greatly outnumber thrombotic events in frequency and severity. In order to develop a rational approach to the management of such conditions, it is essential first to focus on the coagulant role of the liver under normal conditions.

The Liver in Normal Hemostasis

Of the 11 known coagulation proteins, at least 9 are made exclusively in the liver: factors I-II-V-VII-IX-X-XI-XII and XIII. One of the other two, factor VIII, is synthesized partly in the liver (Table 16.1). The remainder of the factor VIII is produced in the endothelial cells throughout the vascular bed. The relative contribution of hepatic synthesis to the circulating concentration of factor VIII recently has been demonstrated by the observation that a cirrhotic hemophiliac who underwent homologous liver transplantation from a nonhemophiliac showed spontaneous correction of his factor VIII deficiency (1). The other procoagulants, tissue thromboplastin and platelet factor III, are complex phospholipid, the precise origin of which are unknown. The circulatory concentrations of the coagulant proteins excepting only for fibrinogen are roughly an order of magnitude higher than is necessary for support of normal clotting. Moreover, the ability of the liver to synthesize the clotting factors apparently continues long after albumin synthesis is lost, and hence, underproduction rarely becomes clinically important except in preterminal liver disease.

There are three natural anticoagulants that also arise in the liver and serve highly important clinical roles: antithrombin III (AT_{III}), protein C, and protein S. Antithrombin$_{III}$ is a serine protease inhibitor that is the principal plasma antagonist of thrombin. It binds slowly to thrombin, otherwise normal clot formation could not begin. In the presence of heparin, AT_{III} converts to antithrombin II (AT_{II}) or heparin cofactor, and immediately blocks the action of thrombin on fibrinogen. Under normal circumstances there is a gross excess of AT_{III} in plasma. It has been estimated that 1 milliliter of normal plasma can inactivate the total thrombin that can be generated in the circulation. However, under conditions of chronic activation of

Table 16.1. Liver in Normal Hemostasis

> Synthetic
>   Prothrombin complex (II-VII-IX-X)
>   Fibrinogen (factor I)
>   Labile factor (factor V)
>   Surface factors (factors (XI + XII)
>   Inhibitors of activators of plasminogen
>   Factor VIII (25%–50%)
>   Proteins C and S
>   Antithrombin III
> Degradative
>   Removes FDP/fdp from circulation
>   Removes fibrin monomers from circulation
>   Removes activated factors VII_a-IX_a-X_a

Table 16.2. Abnormalities of Hemostasis in Liver Disease

> Portal congestion
>   Venous distention (varices and hemorrhoids)
>   Hypersplenism with thrombocytopenia
> Peripheral congestion
>   Vena caval constriction (hepatomegaly and ascites)
>   Reduced arterial Po_2 with endothelial anoxia
>   Hypoalbuminemia and edema
> Toxic
>   Hyperbilirubinemia with ↓ platelet function
>   Elevated bile salts with ↑ thrombin action on plasminogen
> Decreased R-E function
>   Delayed clearance of monomers
>   Delayed clearance of FDP/fdp
> Decreased hepatocyte function
>   Diminished synthesis of factors I, II, V, VII, IX, X, XII, XIII
>   Diminished synthesis of inhibitors of activators of
>   plasminogen
>   Diminished synthesis of AT_{III}

clotting, for example, stress, cigarette smoking, estrogens, or pregnancy, the AT_{III} in the circulation can be consumed more rapidly than it is replaced, thus leading to a potential hypercoagulable state and thrombotic disorders. In certain pathologic states, especially colon cancer with metastases to the liver (2), there is a deficiency of AT_{III} due both to overconsumption and underproduction (see Deficiencies of Vitamin K–Dependent Clotting Factors, and Diffuse Intravascular Coagulopathy, below).

Protein S and protein C are two recently identified natural anticoagulants of plasma. They function by inhibiting the activation of clotting factors V and VIII. Like the prothrombin complex, both are vitamin K–dependent. Approximately half of the protein S circulates in a free (active) state. The remainder is bound to C_4b, an inhibitor of the complement system (3). The free protein S interacts with a surface-active protein, thrombomodulin, on endothelium. It is then capable of converting protein C to an active form, which is a potent inhibitor of factors V and VIII in the intrinsic clotting system. Protein S has the further ability to potentiate fibrinolysis. Protein S is thus a key protein in determining the balance between bleeding and clotting and further represents a specific pathway by which the vascular bed interacts with the blood to help control liquidity.

Evidence suggests that the liver is the site of production of a potent inhibitor of plasminogen activation. This substance has been only partly defined chemically but appears to play a regulatory feedback role which limits the extent of fibrinogenolysis/fibrinolysis that normally occurs each time the intrinsic clotting system is activated (4). In liver disease (see Hypofibrinogenemia, below) its

diminished synthesis may have important physiologic implications.

Hemostasis in Liver Disease

The abnormalities of coagulation and hemostasis that may accompany liver disease are outlined in Table 16.2. Fortunately for the clinician, only a few of these disorders occur with sufficient frequency to complicate the pre- and postoperative management of patients with liver disease. The complexity of the coagulation disorders in liver disease has been well summarized in observations of the preoperative and intraoperative complications of liver transplantation (5).

In order to construct a rational approach to diagnosis and treatment, the coagulant disorders are grouped (see below) in terms of the principal proteins that are abnormal and then considered in descending order of occurrence.

Deficiencies of Vitamin K–Dependent Clotting Factors: Prothrombin Complex

Coagulation factors II, VII, IX, and X together comprise the prothrombin complex. All but factor IX are part of the so-called *extrinsic* clotting system and thus are measured by the prothrombin time (PT) test. If significant depression of factor IX synthesis is suspected, it is necessary to perform a partial thromboplastin time (PTT) test, a recalcification time test, a whole blood clotting time test, or some other assay of the intrinsic system. Classical prothrombin complex deficiency accompanies obstructive jaundice (6–8) due to a defective intake or absorption of vitamin K. It also can be seen after perioperative sterilization of the bowel with antibiotics or after biliary secretory failure, both of which may block normal vitamin K absorption. If hepatic function is reasonably normal and the prothrombin deficiency is from jaundice alone, a single dose of vitamin K may return the prolonged PT and/or PTT to normal. This may be used as a prognostic screening test (9). It has been shown that over 50% of the patients who do *not* correct by this maneuver will develop severe or often fatal hemorrhage during the same hospitalization. When prothrombin complex deficiency is due to icterus and malabsorption of vitamin K, protein synthesis of the basic prothrombin molecule still progresses normally. Vitamin K is essential only for the addition of the final carbohydrate moiety to the precursor protein present in the hepatic microsomes. This will occur in vitro even in tissue slices to which cyclohexamine has been added (10). Thus, the administration of vitamin K differentiates the patients who have only obstructive jaundice or malabsorption from those with impaired synthesis of prothrombin complex, factor V, or fibrinogen due to inflammatory or destructive parenchymal-cell disease (see below).

When prothrombin deficiency is not corrected by vitamin K therapy, temporary support can be given with fresh frozen plasma (FFP) or concentrates of prothrombin complex. Despite the ever-present hazards of transmissions of cytomegalovirus (CMV); Epstein-Barr (EB) virus; human T-cell lymphotropic virus-III (HTLV-III); hepatitis B; hepatitis A; and non-A, non-B hepatitis, the use of FFP can be justified on a cost risk basis in this type of liver disease if temporary control is important. In addition to prothrombin, FFP contains all of the coagulant and anticoagulant proteins such as factor V, fibrinogen, factor VIII, and antithrombin and thus can correct temporarily any deficiency that may be present. Because of the short half-life of factor VII, estimated between 3.7 and 6.1 hours, the transfusions must be repeated frequently. The use of concentrates of prothrombin complex for such circumstances was described as long ago as 1965 (11), but until the recent development of heat-treatment for the concentrate, it was rarely used due to the high risk of disease transmission that follows any product made from pooled human plasma. Although this hazard appears to

have been now encompassed, its use appears best confined to patients with single coagulant deficiencies or to patients on chronic coumarin therapy who need prompt correction of their deficiency of factors II, VII, IX, and X because of trauma or the need for emergent surgery. In liver disease patients, the concurrent presence of a deficiency of AT_{III} and/or proteins C and S can produce an underlying hypercoagulable state that could be grossly aggravated by the administration of prothrombin complex unless simultaneous heparinization is employed.

PROACCELERIN (FACTOR V) DEFICIENCY

This labile clotting factor is the next most common deficiency in liver disease. It usually follows concurrent or antecedent deficiency of prothrombin complex. As noted earlier, factor V deficiency indicates a poor prognosis. Its deficiency may be due either to decreased synthesis or to accelerated proteolysis from circulating plasmin, especially in acute, fulminant hepatitis (12). Since it is not vitamin K–dependent, its presence should be suspected whenever a prolonged PT fails to shorten after parenteral vitamin K therapy. This can be confirmed by the (prothrombin-proconvertin) P & P test in which normal absorbed plasma is added to the prothrombin test to supply an excess of fibrinogen and factor V. It also can be established by simple mixing studies with fresh plasma to supply labile factor V, which will correct the abnormality, whereas the addition of stored plasma to the test system will have no effect. No concentrates of factor V are available for clinical use. Therapy must be provided by transfusions of FFP.

HYPOFIBRINOGENEMIA

Striking deficiencies of fibrinogen can occur in liver disease, especially chronic cirrhosis, without any outward signs or symptoms of coagulant abnormality. It is highly important to diagnose this state while it is subclinical, as the subsequent interposition of an invasive procedure such as intubation or needle biopsy, or the development of an additional complication such as a ruptured varix or gastric hemorrhage, can result in an overwhelming exsanguination before the fundamental defect is identified and treated. Deficiencies of fibrinogen lead to prolonged clotting times in any assay, as fibrinogen is the final common pathway of all clotting reactions: PT, PTT, thrombin time (TT), and so forth. Thus, a prolonged PT on the chart of a patient with liver disease should not be assumed always to reflect prothrombin (complex) deficiency unless the prolonged PT is corrected by a subsequent in vivo dose of vitamin K or unless specific assays for factors II, VII, IX, or X show a deficiency. If the PT remains prolonged after vitamin K, an assay of factor V and/or fibrinogen should be obtained. Hypofibrinogenemia can be documented either by protein precipitation techniques or by immunologic assay. In an emergent situation the attending surgeon or house officer can perform a simple bedside physiologic assay for the adequacy of fibrinogen by adding 2 units of thrombin to 2 ml of (citrate or oxalate) anticoagulated venous blood (13) drawn from the patient. Failure to form a firm, well-defined clot within 30-45 seconds after adding thrombin can only occur if the amount of fibrinogen is inadequate or if it is in an abnormal form from prior proteolysis.

Contrary to many reports, asymptomatic hypofibrinogenemia in chronic cirrhosis is due as frequently to primary uncompensated fibrinogenolysis as to DIC with secondary fibrinolysis or to diminished fibrinogen synthesis. Whereas most of the clotting proteins are synthesized within the liver, the lytic system for fibrinogen/fibrin and its activators are chiefly extrahepatic in origin. Only the *inhibitors* of the plasminogen activators are synthesized in the liver. Plasminogen itself is produced chiefly in eosinophiles. The activators are kinases that are produced in different areas of the body such as urokinase in the kidney and bladder, tissue plasminogen activator (tPa) in endothelium, and streptokinase at sites of bacterial growth. The normal production of the inhibitor of these activators may be lost early in cirrhosis. Since the other components controlling lysis are extrahepatic in origin, their synthesis is not impaired in liver disease. Hence, the normal feedback mechanism to turn off plasmin activation before the excessive consumption of fibrinogen and other proteins of the intrinsic cascade is lost. It should be noted that this syndrome results primarily in fibrinogenolysis rather than fibrinolysis. Although the lytic end-products of both fibrinogenolysis (FDP) and fibrinolysis (fdp) are anticoagulant, and although neither a physical nor immunologic separation of

FDP/fdp has been achieved, the blocking effects of fibrinogenolytic breakdown products (FDP) on thrombin action are greater than the effect of fibrinolytic breakdown products (fdp). This is believed to explain the finding that TT is more prolonged in liver disease in proportion to the degree of hypofibrinogenemia than to comparable degrees of hypofibrinogenemia in other illnesses. Other anticoagulant effects of FDP/fdp include inhibition of polymerization of fibrin monomers and inhibition of platelet aggregation. Treatment can be effected by either replacement of the fibrinogen with cryoprecipitate or FFP, or by interruption of further plasmin activity through the administration of a proteolytic inhibitor like epsilon aminocaproic acid (EACA) (Amicar). This has a prompt beneficial effect and also has the advantage of avoiding plasma volume expansion. If the patient has evidence of encephalopathy, he should be watched carefully for aggravation of hepatic coma as EACA competes for essential amino acids and may further derange protein synthesis.

Confirmation of the presence of a fibrinogenolytic/fibrinolytic state should be established after demonstration of hypofibrinogenemia and before institution of therapy. This can be achieved by diverse immunologic, chemical, and physiologic assays, including whole blood clot lysis time, euglobulin lysis, fibrin plate lysis, serial TT, decreased plasminogen concentration, and by direct measurement of the concentration of fibrin split products (FDP/fdp) by tanned red cell hemagglutination inhibition or standard immunologic test kits.

Diffuse Intravascular Coagulation

The initiation of intravascular clotting (DIC) in liver disease has been attributed to the presence in the circulation of products of hepatic cell necrosis. However, it more commonly results from complications such as gram-negative septicemia or hemorrhagic shock. Hypofibrinogenemia is invariably present when the process is out of control due to excessive consumption of fibrinogen in clot formation as well as its destruction through secondary lysis. The presence of excessive thrombin in the circulation also leads to the consumption of the other factors of intrinsic clotting, including factors X, IX, VIII, V, II, and platelets. It also is usually accompanied by profound deficiency of AT_{III}, which is of course exhausted prior to the development of an uncontrolled consumptive state.

A Dutch study of the turnover rate of ^{125}I fibrinogen in cirrhotic patients showed a half-life of 76.7 hours ($\pm$15.2 hours), which compares with 109.4 hours ($+$8.8 hours) in normal subjects. Proof of the consumptive origin of this increased rate of fibrinogen utilization was obtained by infusing concentrates of AT_{III}. This caused a return of the fractional catabolic rate to normal and an elevation of the ^{125}I fibrinogen half-life to 108.4 hours ($\pm$ 17.6 hours). It should be noted that all of the cirrhotic patients in the study were in a clinically stable state at the time of evaluation, thus emphasizing the occult nature of DIC in its early preclinical phase (14). This lack of correlation between the presence or absence of compensated DIC and the degree of severity of cirrhosis has been noted by many investigators. Numerous clinical findings are helpful in making the diagnosis of DIC after the process gets out of control. These include not only a deficiency of clotting proteins but also the presence of fragmented red cells and a modest to severe thrombocytopenia. Hypofibrinogenemia and elevated FDP/fdp are of no use in diagnostic differentiation between DIC and primary fibrinogenolysis, as lysis occurs in both. It is a primary process in one and a secondary event in the other. The only definitive way to prove intravascular clotting is to show the presence of an end-product exclusively related to the action of thrombin on fibrinogen. These tests include: fibrinopeptide A (3% of the cleavage product of thrombin action on fibrinogen) (15); the D-cross-linked dimer of fibrin that occurs prior to the cleavage of later plasmin fragments; fibrin monomers that may be identified in the circulation prior to polymerization; and the presence of activated factor XIII. Through the development of monoclonal antibodies directed to specific protein fragments and by the use of enzyme-linked immunosorbent assay (ELISA) technology, highly sensitive and reproducible assays now exist to prove the presence of thrombin action on fibrinogen (16). However, for the most part these tests are suitable only for the research laboratory and are too complex to permit routine clinical availability for an occasional patient suspected of DIC. The ristocetin assay for fibrin monomers is an exception to this generalization (17,18). It can be performed without special treatment of the patient's plasma sample or the preparation of complex re-

agents. If monomers are present, a spontaneous precipitate will appear after mixing 1 ml of plasma and 1 milligram of ristocetin. Although the test is qualitative rather than quantitative in type, it permits prompt institution of therapy when positive.

Treatment of DIC should be directed first toward correction of the precipitating cause. If there is shock, it should be corrected with plasma volume expanders; if hemorrhage is present, it should be treated with blood replacement; if gram-negative sepsis is present, antibiotics should be given. In the vast majority of cases, restoration of the normal physiologic state will lead to spontaneous correction of the coagulopathy. Only rarely does heparin, FFP, or AT_{III} need to be infused to block further thrombin action.

PLATELET ALTERATION

Thrombocytopenia is not a common finding in liver disease. It is usually confined to those individuals with portal hypertension and hypersplenism (see Hypersplenism, below), wherein the grossly expanded vascular pool of the spleen and a simultaneously slowed blood transit time result in creased platelet sequestration (19). Acute alcoholic hepatitis may be accompanied by thrombocytopenia (20), but this appears to be due to toxic effects of alcohol itself more than to the associated hepatitis. Acquired thrombocytopathy, on the other hand, has been reported on a number of occasions. These changes have consisted of delayed platelet aggregation after exposure to ADP and a decrease in adhesiveness, resembling von Willebrand's disease (21). The cause of these qualitative changes is unknown. However, they may relate in part to antecedent icterus. High concentrations of unconjugated bilirubin are known to block ADP, adrenalin, and collagen-induced aggregation.

Hypersplenism

The term "hypersplenism" was coined many years ago to describe the thrombocytopenia and granulocytopenia that occur in patients with a large spleen but in whom there is a normoplastic or hyperplastic bone marrow. It was postulated that cellular production in such patients was adequate but that the storage and peripheral removal of cells was increased. Tests were established to prove the existence of an expanded splenic reservoir capable of contracting and liberating increased platelets and neutrophiles in response to epinephrine stimulation. Intraoperative observation of platelet counts drawn simultaneously from the afferent and efferent splenic vessels corroborated the striking ability of the spleen to filter and sequester cells in the red pulp and sinusoids and liberate them again in response to splenic contraction.

Portal blood passes through the liver at a rate of about 1100 ml/min in normal subjects. The blood volume in the hepatic veins and sinuses at any moment is about 650 ml. The splenic pool adds another 100 ml to this. Because of the marked distensibility of both organs, the amount of blood that can be trapped is at least a liter when there is an impediment to flow as in chronic cirrhosis. The most common single cause of hypersplenism is cirrhosis. It is uncommon, however, for the spleen to enlarge to more than double or triple its normal size in this condition. Hence, the pancytopenia is seldom sufficient to require therapeutic splenectomy. The same situation obtains for the hypersplenism that accompanies chronic connective tissue disorders such as lupus erythematosus or rheumatoid arthritis (Felty's syndrome).

An uncommon group of hypersplenism cases deserves special mention. These are the patients with malignant, myeloproliferative disease such as polycythemia vera or primary thrombocythemia who over a period of years gradually develop a massive splenomegaly secondary to repeated splenic infarction and extramedullary hematopoesis. Splenectomy can occasionally improve the morbidity even though it has no effect on the inexorable progression of the underlying disease. For many years it was believed that splenectomy in myeloid metaplasia patients would remove their major locus of blood formation. This has not proved to be true and indeed improvement in previously aplastic-appearing marrow has been noted after splenectomy. Another group of uncommon hypersplenism patients are those associated with primary lymphoma of the spleen. In this rare disorder, there may be no evidence of lymphoma in any other area of the body and the patient's only complaint may be that of a gradually increasing splenic size, accompanied by anemia, neutropenia, or thrombocytopenia either selectively or together. Splenectomy in such patients (22) has been followed by apparent clinical cure even when the spleen has reached a size as large as 2 kilograms.

Patients with autoimmune thrombocytopenic purpura, autoimmune hemolytic anemia, and the less common immune neutropenias should not be classified as having hypersplensim despite the existence of cytopenia in the presence of a hyperplastic anemia. The spleen is only minimally enlarged or not enlarged at all, and it is the basic process of blood cell destruction and removal in the red pulp that is abnormal. In idiopathic thrombocytopenic purpura (ITP), for example, the individual platelets have increased membrane-associated IgG leading to enhanced phagocytosis by the reticuloendothelial (RE) system. Splenectomy remains an important approach to therapy in all such patients who have failed a definitive course of steroids, antimetabolites, or cytotoxic drugs singly or together, even though the basic anomaly is not "hypersplenism" in the correct definition of the term. The removal of the spleen decreases the bed of RE phagocytic cells (red pulp) and a major locus of autoantibody production (white pulp).

Budd-Chiari Syndrome

This rare disorder is characterized by thrombosis of the postsinusoidal hepatic veins. It is usually seen as a late sequela of a primary hematologic disease that is accompanied by a hypercoagulable state or an intrinsic platelet defect. Among the most common of these antecedent causes are paroxysmal nocturnal hemoglobinuria, polycythemia vera, primary thrombocythemia, sickle cell disease, and chronic oral contraceptive use with the attendant depression of circulating AT_{III}. With the widespread use of low-estrogen-containing contraceptive pills in the 1980s and an awareness by smokers of the danger of two simultaneous thrombotic stimuli, the latter may diminish in the future. The clinical findings of right upper quadrant abdominal pain, hepatomegaly, and abrupt onset of ascites raises a suspicion of the disease. Splenomegaly may be present either as part of the primary (myeloproliferative) disease or because of an associated portal hypertension. Confirmation of hepatic vein thrombosis may be made by hepatic vein catheterization, percutaneous hepatic venography, or by comparison of computed tomography views pre- and postcontrast injection. Although numerous surgical approaches have been tried for treatment of this rare disorder, modern improvements in anticoagulant therapy and primary thrombolytic therapy make these approaches the appropriate first line of management, especially if the duration of the signs and symptoms is less than 1 week.

References

1. Lewis JH, Bontempo FA, Ragni MV, Starzl TE. Liver transplantation in a hemophiliac. *N Engl J Med* 1985; 312: 1189–1190.
2. Honegger H, Anderson N, Hewitt L, Tullis JL. Antithrombin III profiles in malignancy, relationship to primary tumors and metastatic sites. *Thromb Haemost* 1981; 46:500–503.
3. Comp PC, Miletich JP, Marlar RA. Thrombosis: The protein C pathway (abstract 17). New Orleans: American Society of Hematology, December 7–10, 1985, p. 8.
4. Tullis JL. CLOT. Springfield, Illinois: Charles C Thomas, 1976, p. 107.
5. Bontempo FA, Lewis JH, Van Thiel DH, Spero JA, et al. The relation of pre-operative coagulation findings to diagnosis, blood usage and survival in adult liver transplantation. *Transplantation* 1985; 39:532–536.
6. Ratnoff OD. In: Schiff LN, ed. *Diseases of the Liver*. Disordered Hemostasis in Hepatic Disease. Philadelphia: JB Lippincott, 1987, pp. 187–207.
7. Sherlock S. *Diseases of the Liver and Biliary Tract*. Oxford: Blackwell Scientific Publications, 1968.
8. Owen CA. *The Diagnosis of Bleeding Disorders*. Boston: Little, Brown, 1969.
9. Spector I, Corn M. Laboratory tests of hemostasis. The relation to hemorrhage in liver disease. *Arch Intern Med* 1967; 119:577–582.
10. Chandler AB, Nordöy A. Adenosine diphosphate induced thrombosis in hypothyroid rats. *Scand J Hematol* 1964; 1:89–93.
11. Tullis JL, Melin M, Jurigian P. Clinical use of human prothrombin complexes. *N Engl J Med* 1965; 273:667–674.
12. Tullis JL. *CLOT*. Springfield, Illinois: Charles C Thomas, 1976, p 359.
13. Tullis JL. *CLOT*. Springfield, Illinois: Charles C Thomas, 1976, p. 368.
14. Schipper HG, TenCate JW. Antithrombin III transfusions in patients with hepatic cirrhosis. *Br J Haematol* 1982; 52: 25–33.
15. Coccheri S, Mannucci PM, Palareti G, Gervasoni W, et al. Significance of plasma fibrinopeptide A and high molecular weight fibrinogen in patients with liver cirrhosis. *Br J Haematol* 1982; 52:503–509.
16. Kudryk B, Rohoza A, Ahadi M, Chin J, Wiebe ME. A monoclonal antibody with the ability to distinguish between NH$_2$-terminal fragments derived from fibrinogen and fibrin. *Mol Immunol* 1983; 20:1191–1200.
17. Watanabe K, Tullis JL. Precipitation of fibrin monomers and fibrin degradation products by ristocetin. *Am J Med Sci* 1978; 275:337–344.
18. Watanabe K, Tullis JL. Ristocetin precipitation test. A new simple test for detection of fibrin monomer and fibrin degradation products. *Am J Clin Pathol* 1978; 70:691–696.
19. Aster RH. Pooling of platelets in the spleen: Role in the pathogenesis of "hypersplenic" thrombocytopenia. *J Clin Invest* 1966; 45:645–657.
20. Ryback R, Desforges JF. Alcoholic thrombocytopenia in three inpatient drinking alcoholics. *Arch Intern Med* 1970; 125:475–487.
21. Thomas DP, Ream J, Stuart RK. Platelet aggregation in patients with Laennec's cirrhosis of the liver. *N Engl J Med* 1967; 276:1344–1348.
22. Wolf BC, Neiman RS. Malignant lymphoma presenting with permanent splenomegaly. A clinical pathologic study with special reference to intermediate cell lymphoma. *Cancer* 1985; 55:1948–1957.

Editorial Comment

The section on hematologic problems in liver disease by Dr. James Tullis, author of the text, *Clot*, and one of the world's leading experts in coagulopathies, has been beautifully geared to the needs of the practicing internist and surgeon. The esoteric and changing world of the "Coagulationists" is one in which many of us feel we face a "stern chase" when attempting to follow the intricacies of the problems presented by the experts. In this chapter, without minimizing the sophistication of the problems, the presentation is couched in a way that should be both understandable and useful to a student of liver disease and the practicing physician and surgeon who will perforce care for the great majority of patients with varying liver disorders.

Chapter 17
Hepatic Encephalopathy and the Hepatorenal Syndrome

WILLIAM V. McDERMOTT, JR.

The relationship between liver disorder and abnormalities in central nervous system function is not a new concept. It is always difficult to trace the thread of an idea but one cannot help but be intrigued by the verbal exchange in "Twelfth Night" between Sir Andrew Aguecheek (one of Shakespeare's most confirmed topers) and Sir Toby Belch. Significantly, the comment is made regarding Sir Andrew's liver that if he died and his liver were examined, "it would not contain enough blood to fill the foot of a flea"—a not inaccurate observation if one considers the extent of fibrosis in advanced alcoholic disease of the liver. Even more intriguing, however, is the remark by Aguecheek that, "I am a great eater of beef and I believe that does harm to my wit." Regardless of the absolute genesis of the concept, whether from Galen's nebulous description of "humors" relating the liver to abberations in disposition and temperament or from Shakespeare's astutely phrased observations, it is clear now that central nervous system disorders may accompany either fulminant hepatic disease in a chronic or progressive form or the effects of abnormal hemodynamics secondary to portal hypertension and portal-systemic shunting even when there is *minimal* disorder in measurable hepatic function.

Although references exist in the literature to the effects on the central nervous system of the ingestion of nitrogenous material and of abnormalities in ammonia metabolism, no general clinical recognition was given to these observations until about 1957 and, in fact, a high-protein diet was usually urged on patients until they finally slipped into an unresponsive state. Since a degree of hepatic coma effectively prevented protein intake in that era, miraculous, if temporary, recoveries occurred fre-

quently. It is only in the period 1947–1987 that increasing attention has been focused on the metabolic and hemodynamic disorders that in puzzling ways related to the development of variable central nervous system symptoms ranging from mild confusion and disorientation to deep and unresponsive coma.

Even after four decades of continuing clinical and biochemical studies, there has been no universally accepted pathogenesis or an organized pattern of biochemical changes that would be adaptable to all the variable clinical patterns that one encounters and that are lumped under the general heading of "hepatic encephalopathy." Although one could, and probably should, discuss two major entities that fall under this general heading and that could be referred to as *exogenous* (portal systemic encephalopathy) or *endogenous* (hepatocellular failure) hepatic coma, there are certain common denominators that can be identified.

The electroencephalographic tracings shown in Figure 17.1 range from normal to the pattern consistent with deep and unresponsive coma. Although similar tracings may be found occasionally in other metabolic disorders, they are so consistent in patients with varying degrees of hepatic encephalopathy as to be very helpful in diagnosis, prognosis, and in terms of response to treatment.

Postmortem examinations on patients who died in deep "hepatic coma" have quite consistently shown a characteristic pattern of microscopic changes in the central nervous system. This picture of proliferation of protoplasmic astrocytes is characteristic and, interestingly enough, may to some extent be correlated with the clinical neurologic syndrome. For instance, in a patient whose presenting signs and symptoms of postshunt en-

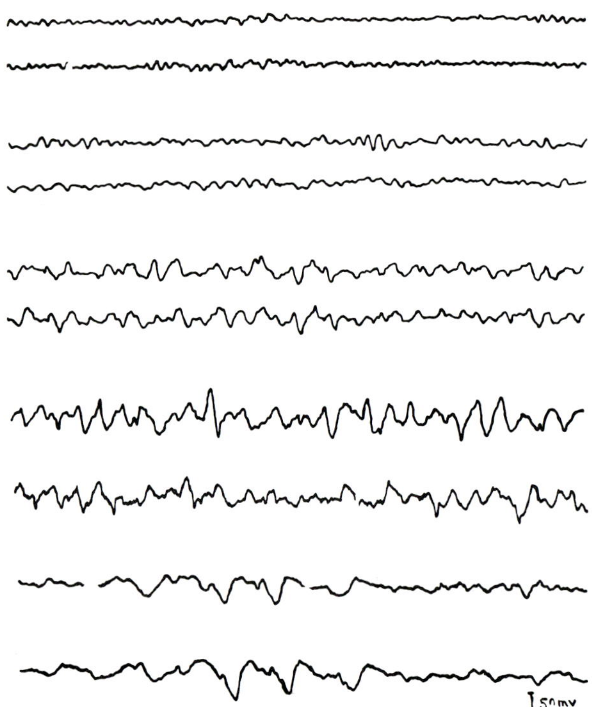

Figure 17.1. Electroencephalographic patterns ranging from normal to those seen in deep "hepatic coma."

cephalopathy were primarily those of choreoathetosis rather than cortical dysfunction, the heaviest concentration of protoplasmic astrocytes found at autopsy was in the basal of ganglia rather than in the cerebral cortex.

In addition to these two major clinical syndromes, disorders of the central nervous system may frequently be seen secondary to fluid and electrolyte disorders and renal dysfunction. These clinical patterns will be handled separately in the section Hepatorenal Syndrome, below, and also in Chapter 18, specifically directed toward the problems of ascites and liver disease. In Figure 17.2, a diagrammatic representation is given of the various factors that may cause or contribute to "hepatic coma."

Portal-Systemic Encephalopathy

The central nervous system disorders attendant on a development of an intrahepatic portal bed block and spontaneous portal-azygous collateral circulation have been grouped under the general heading of portal-systemic encephalopathy, or as it has

been also referred to in the literature, exogenous hepatic coma or episodic stupor. Initiation of work in this area began in 1877 when Eck demonstrated the feasibility of constructing an anastomosis between the portal vein and inferior vena cava; although seven of his animals died in the immediate postoperative period, one survived for 8 weeks before escaping from the laboratory and thus could be characterized under the heading of "lost to followup" (1). Nonetheless, this limited study did lead, as so many other physiologic questions have done, to a study 16 years later in Pavlov's laboratory. Hahn and colleagues (2), while working on this problem, observed that animals in whom Eck's fistula had been constructed manifested a pattern of central nervous symptoms that the authors related specifically to the ingestion of meat and to which the original investigators and subsequent observers referred to as "meat intoxication." This syndrome aroused considerable if intermittent interest over the subsequent decades but the variability and inconstancy of the symptoms and the inability to define a specific metabolic cause of the syndrome resulted in a confused and confusing picture. Many etiologic factors were suggested, including guanidine, amino acids, unknown toxins, and bacteriologic and viral infections of the central nervous system. Several observers over the years noted elevations in the peripheral blood ammonia in these dogs with Eck's fistula and Monguio and Krause (3) suggested as long ago as 1934 that this might be the cause of these peculiar symptoms. Our own review (4) in 1957 of the literature concerned with the metabolism and toxicity of ammonia and the recent medical progress survey on hepatic encephalopathy by Frazier and Arieff (5) would appear to indicate that the great weight of clinical and laboratory investigations concerned with this subject would emphasize the importance of portal systemic shunts in the genesis of the clinical syndrome.

The definition of the etiology in terms of a single biochemical disorder remains a subject of valid disputation. Although the syndrome of meat intoxication in the Eck fistula dog was described in 1892, it was not until 1927 that a disorder of ammonia metabolism was suspected by Burchi (6) of causing symptoms in humans. Five years later, Van Caulaert and associates presented a series of reports (7–10) that related the ingestion of ammonium chloride and other related substances by

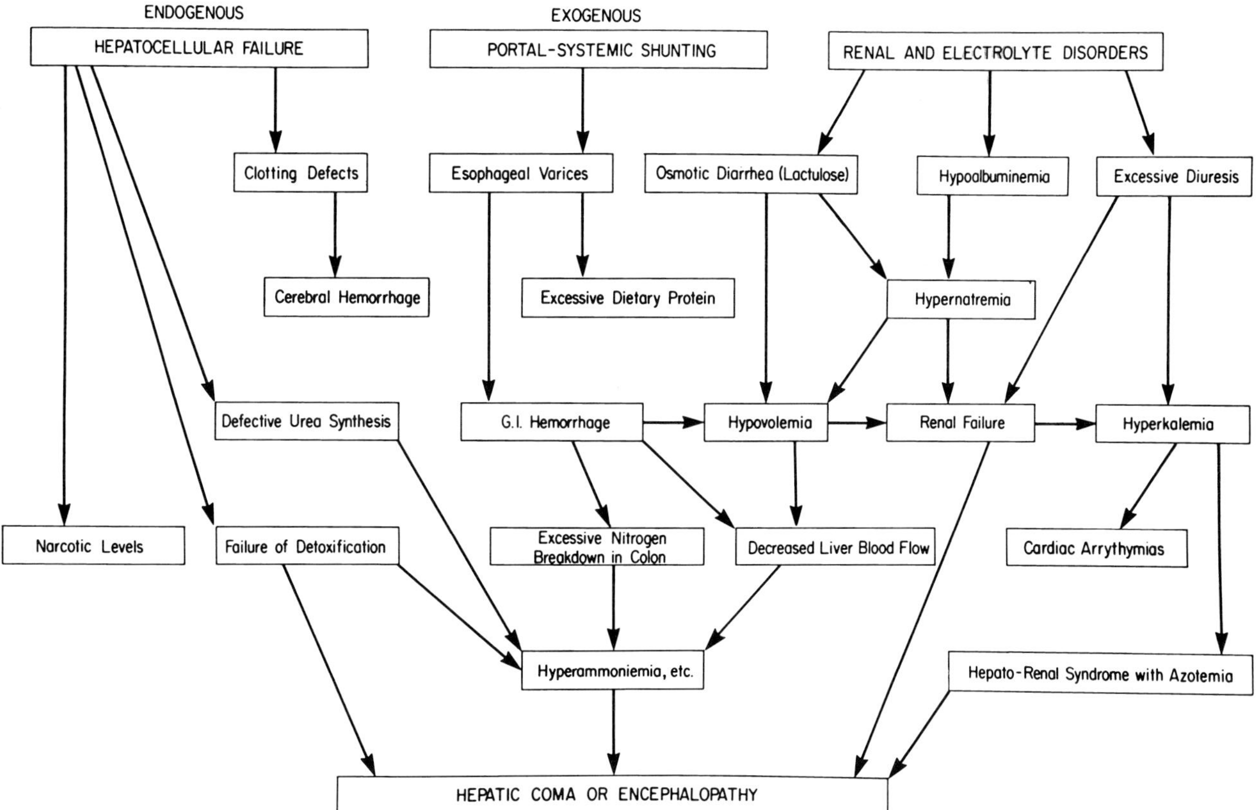

Figure 17.2. Microscopic changes in hepatic coma.

patients with cirrhosis of the liver to the subsequent symptoms of drowsiness, confusion, and coma.

In 1936 Kirk (11) found elevated levels of ammonia in blood drawn from collateral venous channels in the abdominal wall of a patient with cirrhosis, thus confirming indirectly in humans the observations of Folin and Denis (12) in animals that portal blood has a high ammonia concentration.

For over a decade, and during World War II, interest in this phase of liver disease lapsed and a high protein intake was still considered essential for adequate restoration of liver function until several significant reports appeared in the literature. In 1949 Gaustad (13) described a syndrome of "transient hepatargy" in which reversible coma was observed in patients with cirrhosis after either gastrointestinal hemorrhages or the ingestion of protein; based on these observations he attributed the disorder to absorption from the gastrointestinal tract of nitrogenous products of enzymatic

activity in the colon. In 1952 forceful attention to the dangers of ingestion of nitrogenous material by patients with liver disease was drawn by the reports of Gabuzda et al. (14) and of Phillips and colleagues (15) in the United States and by Stahl and associates in France (16). All of these reports emphasized that in certain patients with cirrhosis of the liver the ingestion of protein, ammonium salts, and iron exchange resins that liberated ammonia produces symptoms of varying severity that resemble the prodromal symptoms of hepatic coma. In the following year McDermott and Adams (17) reported on an extensively studied case that appeared to correlate the observations on the intoxication in the Eck's fistula dog with the effects of increased nitrogenous intake in a similar hemodynamic preparation in humans. Bizarre episodes of stupor and coma occurred at intervals in a patient in whom a superior mesenteric-caval shunt was constructed after resection of the portal vein for cancer of the pancreas, and in whom ordinary tests of liver function were within normal limits as was the liver biopsy taken at time of the operation. In observations over a number of months these episodes were seen to be associated with the ingestion of protein, urea, and ammonium salts and ion-exchange resins, all of which had the common denominator of liberation of ammonia in the gastrointestinal tract. These episodes were completely reversible but were correlated with increases in the blood ammonia and with electroencephalographic changes identical to those described by Foley and associates (18) in patients with chronic liver failure and "hepatic coma." Thus it appeared, as Kirk had suggested, that some of the disorders of consciousness in liver disease were caused not by hepatocellular dysfunction per se but by collateral channels between the portal and systemic circulation. The importance of portal blood bypassing the liver in the presence of an intrahepatic block was stressed again in 1954 by Sherlock and associates (19), who described several patients with this reversible neurologic disorder and referred to the syndrome as "portal-systemic encephalopathy."

At the time of writing, these and subsequent studies in the medical and surgical literature pointed to a common denominator relating to the formation of ammonia from any nitrogenous material reaching the colon as a major factor in the medical and clinical abnormalities seen in patients with bleeding esophageal varices, and ultimately led to alterations in therapy based on this assumption. Numerous and often conflicting observations began to appear relating to the old questions of ammonia metabolism as a major factor in the genesis of hepatic encephalopathy. The question was raised as to whether the elevation in blood ammonia levels seen so frequently in liver disease was similar to the azotemia one finds in renal failure, which is coincidental with but not a direct cause of this syndrome. This analogy is unsatisfactory because, unlike the situation in uremia, the precoma or coma of hepatic encephalopathy can be induced by a number of different nitrogenous substances or by certain exchange resins, the common denominator of which is a release of ammonia in the gastrointestinal tract. It is true that the actual level of ammonia in the blood does not correlate exactly with the clinical state, but in a number of reports in which levels have been carefully followed during the entire course of patients with episodes of portal-systemic encephalopathy in-

duced by bleeding or ingestion of other nitrogenous material, one finds that the elevation of blood ammonia occurs prior to the neurologic symptoms and that, as the source of ammonia production is controlled or eliminated, the ammonia level falls toward the normal range prior to the more gradual recovery of the patient from the episodes of precoma or coma. Bessman (20) stressed the importance of the arterial-venous differential in ammonia levels in blood taken from the carotid artery and jugular vein and was the first to suggest that a disorder in the tricarboxolic acid cycle initiated by high levels of ammonia binding to alphaketoglutarate was the direct biochemical cause of the coma.

Extensive studies over the past two decades have introduced a number of interesting theories relating to the biochemical genesis of the symptoms of hepatic encephalopathy but none have been generally accepted as a total and final explanation. A number of aromatic amino acids such as tryptophan, methionine, and the mercaptans have been implicated (21) as have short-chain fatty acids (22), but one of the more interesting series of observations has involved the alteration in concentration of various false neurotransmitter substances in the brain. Under this concept, it has been postulated that there is increased intestinal production of gamma-amino butyric acid, octopamine, and other amines by colonic bacteria as a cause of hepatic encephalopathy (23). It is intriguing to relate the aromatic amines to the genesis of hepatic encephalopathy because of the long-recognized clinical sign of "fetor hepaticus," which has been thought to be due to mercaptan (24). Again, an apparent association is variable and one does encounter frequently the odor of fetor hepaticus in patients who have no clinical or electroencephalographic changes relating to hepatic coma or precoma.

A simplified pathogenesis of the syndrome is shown in Figure 17.3. The *diagnosis* of the clinical syndrome of portal-systemic encephalopathy is thus based on a correlation of history, physical examination, and laboratory findings. Hyperammonemia may be found in the majority of patients but, as mentioned above, the level depends on the stage of syndrome at which one encounters the patient and thus is not an absolute criterion of diagnosis. Electroencephalography is much more useful and consistent, and of course laboratory studies indicating a disorder in liver functions is

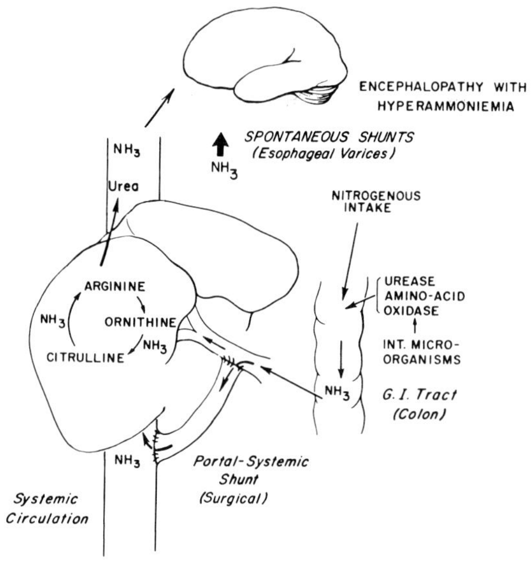

Figure 17.3. Factors in hepatic coma.

corroborative evidence. The most common triad consists therefore of the clinical observations (which should include the physical and neurologic findings consistant with basic liver disease and encephalopathy), characteristic electroencephalographic findings, and the history of either gastrointestinal bleeding (usually but not necessarily from esophageal varices) or the ingestion of an excessive amount of protein or other nitrogenous material.

The management of the patient with portal-systemic encephalopathy is based on the data relating to pathogenesis that have been reviewed, and consists in an orderly but vigorous approach to the problem, which can be summarized as follows:

1. control of gastrointestinal bleeding (which of course depends on accurate diagnosis of the source of the hemorrhage)
2. elimination of protein from the diet
3. vigorous efforts directed toward emptying the colon, through administration of cathartics and enemas
4. oral administration of antibiotics (Neomycin

has been a traditional therapy but has been somewhat supplanted by the safer and almost equally useful Ampicillin) in order to eliminate the coliform organisms that are the source of the enzymatic production of ammonia and other substances
5. the administration of lactulose which functions both as a cathartic but more importantly as a synthetic disaccharide, which is not absorbed and which will alter the acid base balance in the colon to the extent that ammonia production is decreased

Although many other methods of therapy have been suggested such as administration of soluble salts of glutamic acid (25), arginine (26), and innumerable other therapeutic agents, the simplistic outline described above forms a basis of controlling this particular form of hepatic encephalopathy. Of course, the number of associated disorders that may accompany this syndrome, including associated hepatocellular failure, immensely complicate the treatment and often result in extraordinarily high mortality not due so much to the coma itself as to the associated metabolic, hemodynamic and renal disorders.

In addition to the acute form of the syndrome, one encounters not infrequently the repetitive bouts of disordered mentation that are sometimes attendant on and presumably related to the construction of a portal-systemic shunt for the control of massive and life-threatening hemorrhage from esophageal varices. In fact, the development of this postshunt encephalopathy is one of the major reasons why one is reluctant to consider shunt surgery even with the recognition that fatal hemorrhage results if portal hypertension is not controlled. The recent introduction of endoscopic sclerosis of esophageal varices may provide an alternative solution that has, of course, been discussed in another section of this book. If one does, however, encounter the syndrome of chronic recurrent postshunt encephalopathy, which has been variably estimated to have an incidence ranging from 25% to 40% of all total shunts, one can embark on a series of corrective and prophylactic methods that include all forms of cathartics and bulk laxatives tending to ensure maintenance of as empty a colon as possible; this, of course, can be reinforced with appropriate use of enemas. This course of therapy will obviously involve some restriction of ingested protein, although, unfortunately, too rigid a proscription can further enhance deterioration in hepatocellular function. The judicious use of antibiotics and the well-established effectiveness of lactulose lends another addition to the therapeutic program that can be implemented. If all else fails and the syndrome is highly debilitating, it may be necessary to operatively eliminate the shunt and carry out some other procedure such as portal-azygous disconnection to prevent further hemorrhage or to carry out a subtotal colectomy (27) or perform colon-bypass procedure (28), all of which have been well documented to be major adjuncts in control of this distressing syndrome. In Chapter 14 on the use of portal-systemic shunts, the relative merits of total versus selective shunting have been extensively discussed and need not be repeated here, although it is clear that the genesis of this controversy is related to a decrease in liver blood flow, and that if shunting did not result in alteration of prograde flow to the liver, it would be an ideal solution to the problem of bleeding esophageal varices.

Hepatocellular Failure

This syndrome may be characterized as chronic, progressive, or fulminant and results either from sudden massive liver cell necrosis or from local or systemic stress on an already damaged liver with the apparently sudden onset of what may prove to be terminal liver failure. This series of events may, of course, result from a severe form of viral hepatitis, the culmination of extended continuous ingestion of alcohol (alcoholic hepatitis), from traumatic or surgical devascularization of the liver, or from the effects of a number of hepatotoxic agents, of which the otherwise effective anesthetic agent referred to as halothane has been recognized as an occasional idiosyncratic cause of fulminant liver failure. While controversy still continues about the actual incidence of toxicity from this agent, it would appear that it is rare to find serious disorders with the first administration, although subtle clinical and biochemical changes may occur. Subsequent administrations, however, may result in a massive disruption of functioning liver tissue.

Regardless of the cause, the syndrome of hepatic encephalopathy under these circumstances is caused by the sudden widespread dissolution of hepatic cells and is clinically manifested by rapidly developing jaundice, lethargy progressing to deep and unresponsive coma, fetor hepaticus, and evidence of widespread interference with the clotting mechanism as manifested by ecchymoses, nosebleeds, purpura, and bleeding from one or more organ systems. Laboratory tests relating to liver function show the expected bilirubinemia and a widespread and progressive alteration in so-called liver enzymes and evidences of gross disorder in the various synthetic mechanisms of the liver on which the body is so dependent. Although ammonia levels are frequently elevated in patients with this type of fulminant hepatocellular failure, it is clear that the extremely complex metabolic disorder that occurs under these circumstances is certainly not explicable on the basis of ammonia intoxication alone (as it may be in the syndrome of portal-systemic encephalopathy), and that the extraordinary reserve in urea synthesis permits clearance of a considerable portion of formed ammonia even when many other functions of hepatic cells have deteriorated to an extreme degree. Hypoglycemia may be one of the preterminal manifestations of fulminant liver failure even in the presence of continuous administration of concentrated glucose solutions. Until recently, a syndrome of fulminant hepatic failure from any one of the causes mentioned was attended by an extraordinarily high mortality.

Treatment of hepatic failure has involved a number of invasive therapies in addition to the measures described for portal-systemic encephalopathy. The introduction of orthotopic transplantation of the liver has, however, altered to some degree the prognosis of fulminant liver failure, albeit at the cost of tremendous expenditure of medical resources and with the requirement for available, highly trained personnel. Nonetheless, the occasional immediate recovery and long-term survival under these circumstances is one of immense gratification to the physicians and surgeons involved in this extraordinarily complex undertaking.

Exchange transfusions as originally suggested by Trey (28) were widely used at one point but are less and less applied to the management of this extremely complicated problem, similar to other efforts such as cross-transfusion, ex vivo pig liver, or other perfusion mechanisms. Thus, one provides every known form of metabolic support to the patient in fulminant hepatic failure and when it is clear that death is imminent or inevitable, then orthotopic liver transplantation is indicated.

Hepatorenal Syndrome

A combination of hepatic and renal failure has long been recognized as a clinical syndrome, although it has become increasingly clear that innumerable factors may come into play in the course of advanced liver disease that may effect renal function adversely. With increasing knowledge of hepatic and renal pathophysiology, groups of patients with both hepatic and renal failure have been identified separately and classified in terms of precipitating cause of the renal failure. In Table 17.1, an outline is given of the various subdivisions of the so-called hepatorenal syndrome that have been recognized and defined. In any individual case, one or more of these etiologic factors may be present but there has been increasing recognition that there are a significant number of cases in which oliguria and anuria accompany progressive liver failure without any of the recognized "precipitating" factors and without microscopically demonstrable disease in the kidneys. It is the patients in this group that are so puzzling. A number of efforts have been made over the years to establish experimental knowledge so that models of disease with possible humoral or neurohumoral factors could be studied. Although many have been implicated, there is still no generally accepted factor or factors that can be absolutely identified as major causes of the combined failure syndrome.

Table 17.1. Hepatorenal Syndrome

A. Hypovolemia and prerenal azotemia
  1. Gastrointestinal hemorrhage
  2. Massive and rapid accumulation of ascites
    a. Hepatic failure with postsinusoidal block and hypoalbuminemia
    b. Following paracentesis
    c. Subsequent to end-to-side portacaval shunt (in occasional cases with a high degree of postsinusoidal block)
    d. Gram-negative septicemia
B. Acute tubular necrosis (subsequent to any of the factors above causing renal ischemia)
C. Severe jaundice (usually causing renal failure when associated with depletion of blood or plasma volume)
D. Pre-existing renal disease
E. Other precipitating factors (congestive heart failure, severe pulmonary disease with hypoxia)
F. Dehydration (diuretics, primary water depletion)
G. Hepatic failure (without any of above and without microscopically demonstrable changes in kidneys)—idiopathic

Most of the categories in Table 17.1 are self-explanatory and need no extensive discussion. *Hypovolemia* from any cause results in decreased renal perfusion, and with or without liver disease causes decreased renal function. Unless a prolonged period of renal ischemia ensues, the syndrome is reversible, provided replacement with plasma is indicated and carried out vigorously. If, however, renal ischemia ensues as a result of the decreased renal perfusion, *acute tubular necrosis* may occur and follow a course similar to that seen in patients who develop this lesion without liver disease. Severe and progressive *jaundice* has been implicated both clinically and experimentally with renal failure. It is clear, however, that the presence of obstructive jaundice alone does not result in impaired renal function, but it would appear from clinical observations and from experimental studies that the presence of deep jaundice in some way sensitizes the kidneys to the effects of hypovolemic shock. These conclusions have resulted from studies in pure obstructive jaundice since the frequent presence of hypobilirubinemia in association with hepatocellular failure introduces the complexity of liver function as well as the effects of an elevated bilirubin alone. In the presence of *preexisting renal disease*, it is extremely difficult to evaluate the effects of liver failure and one must of necessity place these patients in separate categories.

In all the patients in whom coexisting hepatic and renal failure is analyzed and classified in a fashion similar to the outline in Table 17.1, there still remains a group of patients in whom the development of severe and progressive renal failure and association of liver failure occurs without any recognizable precipitating factor. It is this group that has particularly puzzled clinicians and stimulated a number of laboratory studies. Perhaps the most clearcut evidence that renal failure is reversible as liver failure is controlled comes from the report of transplantation of cadaveric patients who died with the so-called hepatorenal syndrome. In this report, a kidney from each of five patients and both kidneys from a sixth patient who died with terminal hepatic and renal failure were transplanted into seven patients with end-stage kidney disease whose liver function was normal. Diuresis and improvement of renal function occurred in all but one recipient; no disease was demonstrated microscopically in any of the transplanted kidneys. In our own experience, several patients with advanced and ultimately lethal hepatic failure had a diuresis and reversal of the biochemical abnormalities associated with oliguria and anuria, after ex vivo perfusion or exchange transfusion. Therefore, although the lethal nature of hepatorenal syndrome cannot be minimized, it is clear that patients with clinical cases of this dangerous combination may recover without any permanent renal damage and that the transplanted kidney functions immediately when transferred to a metabolic environment where normal hepatic function exists. Fischer's concept of the role of false neurotransmitters in the genesis of hepatic coma have also been applied by him in the hepatorenal syndrome (23), and Metarinol has had a preliminary and limited clinical trial; no practical clinical application has, however, stemmed from these interesting initial metabolic observations.

Treatment, therefore, of patients with combined hepatic and renal failure is directed toward the correction of any of the possible factors identified in Table 17.1 that might adversely affect renal function, and toward every possible support of the failing aspects of hepatic function.

Orthotopic liver transplantation, of course, reverses the renal failure as normal hepatic function is reconstituted.

References

1. Eck NVK. Cited in Child CG III. Eck's fistula. *Surg Gynecol Obstet* 1953; 96:375.
2. Hahn M, Massen O, Nencki M, Pawlow J. Die Eck'sche Fistel zwischen der unteren Hohlvene und der Pfortader und ihre Folgen fur den Organismus. I. *Arch Exp. Pathol. Pharmakol* 1893; 32:161–210
3. Monguio J, Krause F. Uber die Bedeutung des NH_3-Gehaltes des Blutes fur die Beurteilung der Leberfunktion: Studien am normalen, lebergeschadigten und Eckschen Fistelhund. *Klin* Wochenschr 1934; 13:1142–1147.
4. McDermott WV Jr. Metabolism and toxicity of ammonia. *N Engl J Med* 1957; 257:1076–1081.
5. Fraser CL, Arieff AI. Hepatic encephalopathy. *N Engl J Med* 1985; 313:865–871.
6. Burchi RI. I saggi della funzionalita epatica e le prova dell'ammoniemia spontanea e provocata: Studio dell'sufficenze funzionale del fegato. *Folia Clin Chim Microsc* 1927; 2:5–68.
7. Van Caulaert C, Deviller C. Ammoniemie experimentale après ingestion de chlorure d'ammonium chez l'homme à l'état normal et patholigique. *Comp Rend Soc Biol* 1932; 111:50–42.
8. Van Caulaert C, Deviller C, Halff M. Le taux de l'ammo-niemie dans certaines affections hepatiques. *Comp Rend Soc Biol* 1932; 111:735.
9. Van Caulaert C, Deviller C, Hofstein J. Epreuve de l'ammoniemie provoque: Repartition de l'ammoniaque dans le sang et les humeurs. *Comp Rend Soc Biol* 1932; 111:739.
10. Van Caulaert C, Deviller C, Halff M. Troubles provoqués par l'ingestion de sels ammoniacaux chez l'homme atteint de cirrhose de Laennec. *Comp Rend Soc Biol* 1932; 111:739.
11. Kirk E. Amino acid and ammonia metabolism in liver diseases. *Acta Med Scand* 1936; (Suppl 77):1–147.
12. Folin O, Denis W. Protein metabolism from standpoint of blood and tissue analysis: Origin and significance of ammonia in portal blood. *J Biol Chem* 1912; 11:161–167.
13. Gaustad V. Transient hepatargy. *Acta Med Scand* 1949; 135:354–363.
14. Gabuzda GJ Jr, Phillips GB, Davidson CS. Reversible toxic manifestations in patients with cirrhosis of liver given cation-exchange resins. *N Engl J Med* 1952; 246:124–130.
15. Phillips GB, Schwartz R, Gabuzda GJ Jr, and Davidson CS. Syndrome of impending hepatic coma in patients with cirrhosis of liver given certain nitrogenous compounds. *N Engl J Med* 1952; 247:239–246.
16. Stahl J, Roger S, Witz J. Essai d'interpretation du mecanisme de l'épreuve d'hyperammoniemie provoquée chez les cirrhotiques. *Comp Rend Soc Biol* 1952; 146:1787–1791.
17. McDermott WV Jr, Adams RD, Riddell AG. Ammonia metabolism in man. *Ann Surg* 1954; 140:539–556.
18. Foley JM, Watson CW, Adams RD. Significance of electroencephalographic changes in hepatic coma. *Trans Am Soc Neurol A* 1950; 75:161–165.
19. Sherlock S, Summerskill WHJ, White LP, Phear EA. Portal-systemic encephalopathy: Neurological complications of liver disease. *Lancet* 1954; 2:453–457.
20. Bessman SP, Bessman AN. Cerebral and peripheral uptake of ammonia in liver disease with hypotheses for mechanism of hepatic coma. *J Clin Invest* 1955; 34:622–628.
21. Ohihara K, Mozai T, Kirai S. Tryptophas as cause of hepatic coma. *N Engl J Med* 1966; 275:1255–1256.
22. Zieve L. Encephalopathy due to short and medium chain fatty acids. In: McCandless DW, ed. *Cerebral Energy Metabolism and Metabolic Encephalopathy.* New York: Plenum, 1985; pp. 163–178.
23. Fischer JE. Hepatic coma in cirrhosis, portal hypertension, and following portacaval shunt: Its etiologies and the current status of its treatment. *Arch Surg* 1974; 108:325–336.
24. McDermott WV Jr, Wareham J, Riddell AG. The treatment of "hepatic coma" with L-glutamic acid. *N Engl J Med* 1955; 253:1093–1102.
25. McDermott WV Jr, Henneman DH, Laumont C. The metabolic effects of glutamic acid and arginine in "hepatic coma" with hyperammoniaemiea. *J Clin Invest* 1957; 36:913.
26. Atkinson M, Goligher JC. Recurrent hepatic coma treated by colectomy and ileorectal anastomosis. *Lancet* 1960; 1:461–464.
27. McDermott WV Jr, Victor M, Point WW. Exclusion of the colon in the treatment of hepatic encephalopathy. *N Engl J Med* 1962; 267:850–854.
28. Trey C, Burns DG, Saunders SJ. Treatment of hepatic coma by exchange blood transfusion. *N Engl J Med* 1966; 274:473–481.

Chapter 18
Ascites

WILLIAM V. McDERMOTT, JR.

The term "ascites," which, from its Greek derivation, refers to a bag of fluid, is used in medical terminology to refer to any collection of free fluid within the peritoneal cavity. There are a number of different causes for the accumulation of ascites and one must establish some type of categorization in order to present a comprehensible discussion of the problem.

Classification

It has been customary to classify ascites under two major headings: *exudative* and *transudative*, terms that in a broad sense are self-explanatory. Since in this particular chapter we are primarily concerned with abnormalities associated with the liver, only a few introductory comments will be made relative to the disease processes classified under *exudative ascites*. This term refers, of course, to the accumulation of fluid in the peritoneal cavity that results from an excess outpouring of liquids of high specific gravity and high protein content from either an inflammatory or neoplastic process within the abdomen. Since there is free exchange between the peritoneal cavity and the vascular compartment, the exudation of fluid must be in excess of the resorptive capacity of the serous lining of the abdomen and the thoracic duct. In the process of equilibration under these circumstances, the ascitic fluid is more likely to draw water from the vascular compartment because of its high protein content than it is to be resorbed through lymphatic channels. In Figure 18.1, a simplified categorization of the various causes for the accumulation of ascites is given and the differential diagnosis between the two major categories of exudative and transudative ascites is made primarily on the specific gravity (with 1.020 as the dividing point) and the level of protein, which is ordinarily > 3.0 gram % in exudative ascites, and less than this when the fluid accumulation is a transudate. If these two simple measurements are made and the fluid is also analyzed in terms of cytology (in order to identify malignant cells) and with bacteriologic cultures, major steps will have been made toward identifying the cause of the disease presentation. As one can see from Figure 18.1, once the fluid obtained through paracentesis has been shown to have a specific gravity < 1.020, a protein content < 3.0 g%, and has no abnormal cells on cytologic examination and no growth from bacteriologic cultures, then the overwhelming likelihood is that this transudation is on the basis of intrahepatic disease.

Among the causes of exudative ascites, the one that is most likely to cause confusion in relation to cirrhotic ascites is a relatively rare syndrome referred to as *pancreatic ascites* (1). Occasionally, following trauma or inflammation, the rupture of the pancreatic ductile system may result in the establishment of a free communication with the peritoneal cavity rather than a localized inflammatory mass or a pseudocyst. Since many patients with pancreatitis are chronic alcoholics, accumulation of fluid under these circumstances and without overt signs of inflammation may easily lead to a confusion in a diagnosis based on features other than analysis of the fluid. If one, however, considers the possibility of pancreatic ascites, the syndrome is distinctive—the peritoneal fluid has a high specific gravity, a high protein content, a very high amylase level, and the serum amylase level is usually, although not invariably, elevated.

It is with the general phenomenon of *transudative ascites* and, more specifically, cirrhotic ascites that we will be primarily concerned in this chapter. Under these circumstances, accumulation of fluid within the abdomen is secondary to transudation

405

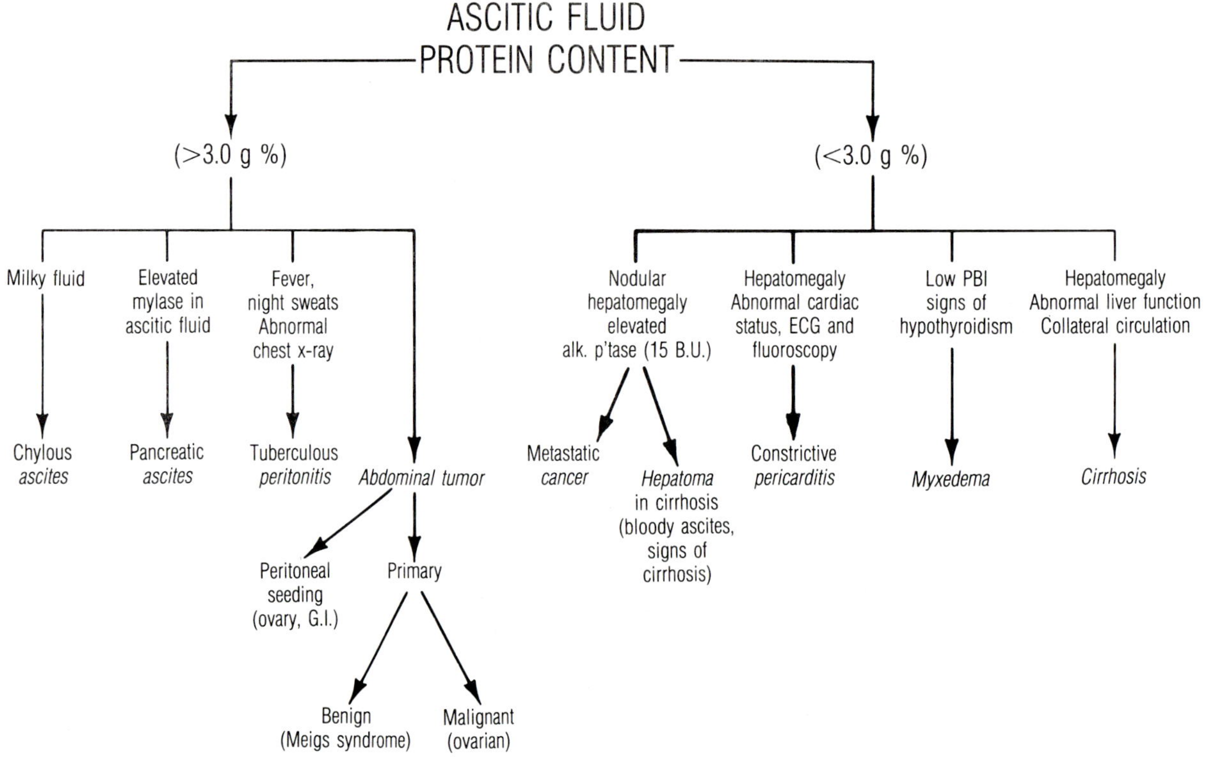

Figure 18.1.   BU, Bodansky units; ECG, electrocardiogram; GI, gastrointestinal; PBI, protein-bound iodine.

from capillary or sinusoidal beds and from the lymphatics of the splanchnic and hepatic circulations. This, in turn, may be caused by increased venous pressure secondary to a number of disorders of which the most common is some type of cirrhosis, usually macronodular in gross manifestations in which the destruction of the parenchyma has resulted in such a disorder of the hepatic architecture that an intrahepatic postsinusoidal obstruction is the ultimate result. On the other hand, it is important to realize that obstruction of the hepatic venous outflow, either from thrombosis or other abnormalities in the development of the inferior vena cava or hepatic venous circulation, from the retrohepatic extension of malignant disease, or from intrahepatic disease affecting the tributaries of the hepatic venous outflow, may also cause intractable ascites; this group of disorders is referred to in common parlance as the Budd-Chiari syndrome and will be discussed below in the section "Budd-Chiari Syndrome."

Pathogenesis of Cirrhotic Ascites

The mechanisms involved in the formation of cirrhotic ascites are still somewhat confusing because of the complex hemodynamic and metabolic changes that occur in varying degrees in different patients. Even with modern technology, it is difficult to define exactly the proportional impact of the various factors involved. At the risk of oversimplification, however, one can piece together sufficient experimental and clinical observations to provide a clearer picture of the disordered pathophysiology seen with cirrhotic ascites than was possible some years ago. A number of specific facts and observations are particularly significant:

1. Ascitic fluid has approximately the same composition as liver lymph.
2. Lymphatics in the liver hilus and gastrohepatic ligament are greatly increased in size and number (2) and, in experimental studies, transudation from these lymphatics and from the

liver itself accounts for a major portion of the accumulated intraperitoneal fluid.

3. The experimental production of ascites can be easily accomplished by any procedure that obstructs outflow from the liver but not by obstruction of the portal vein itself.

4. The increased intrahepatic portal pressure seen in cirrhosis with ascites does not fall within the normal range after occlusion of the portal venous inflow (3) and presumably this is on the basis of intrahepatic arterial-portal shunting.

5. In cirrhotic ascites, there is abnormal retention of water and sodium; restriction of salt alone may bring about an amelioration or dissipation of the accumulated fluid.

6. Increased aldosterone activity is a consistent pattern and it is probable that the increased aldosterone levels are related not to failure of detoxification by the damaged liver but rather to the effect on volume receptors of a decreased effective circulating arterial volume. Other mechanisms such as hypokalemia may also be related to the hyperaldosterone syndrome.

7. The serum albumin level and, therefore, the intravascular osmotic pressure are usually decreased and this, of course, increases the fluid lost by transudation from the capillary beds in the intrahepatic and splanchnic lymphatics.

While there are admittedly many factors in the formation of cirrhotic ascites, certainly an alteration of the normal hemodynamics of the liver plays a major role and an intrahepatic postsinusoidal outflow block is undoubtedly an important factor in the ascites seen with various forms of liver disease, particularly when the laboratory indices of liver function seem surprisingly good for the degree of accumulation of intraperitoneal fluid that exists. While the morphologic and hemodynamic changes found in association with cirrhosis vary widely, certain observations have been generally accepted. These tend to support the fact that postsinusoidal block of a varying degree does exist in most types of liver disease and that shunts between the arterial and portal circulations within the liver do exist as a part of the general pattern. It is difficult, however, on an individual basis to relate these changes specifically to the degree and

intractability of ascites because the postsinusoidal block is by no means the sole factor contributing to the retention of intraperitoneal fluid with liver disease. As mentioned above, the consistent depression of this serum albumin level that one sees in association with cirrhosis results in a fall in intravascular osmotic pressure, which is certainly an important factor in the transudation of fluid since the integrity of the vascular compartment is maintained primarily by circulating plasma proteins. Normally, the plasma proteins that leak from the proximal end of the capillary or sinusoidal bed are returned to the blood so that osmotic equilibrium remains undisturbed. With cirrhotic ascites, however, one frequently finds a combination of the depression in the serum albumin and a resulting drop in the osmotic pressure together with increased pressure at the distal end of the capillary or sinusoidal bed. Intravenous administration of human serum albumin may help in management, but a rapid equilibration occurs between the vascular and interstitial compartments and therapeutic value may be evanescent.

In addition to the hemodynamic and osmotic factors, it is important, as mentioned above, to recognize the role of endocrine factors and alterations in renal function that occur in the presence of ascites. The increased levels of aldosterone certainly play a major role in the abnormal retention of sodium and water as has been referred to above. An increased secretion of antidiuretic hormone that has been demonstrated under these circumstances may be an accessory endocrine factor in the syndrome, although it probably does not play a role comparable to that of aldosterone. The characteristic measurable change in renal function that occurs is a voracious retention of sodium by the kidney with an increased excretion of potassium in the urine. Thus, in most of the patients with relatively intractable ascites, one would find < 5 milliequivalents per liter of sodium in the urine and an incremental increase in the excretion of potassium by a factor of two or three times the normal amount.

In summary, therefore, one can say that the accumulation of ascitic fluid in connection with cirrhosis is caused in part by the development of a postsinusoidal block in association with the depression of serum albumin and resulting decrease in osmotic pressure. The endocrine changes are

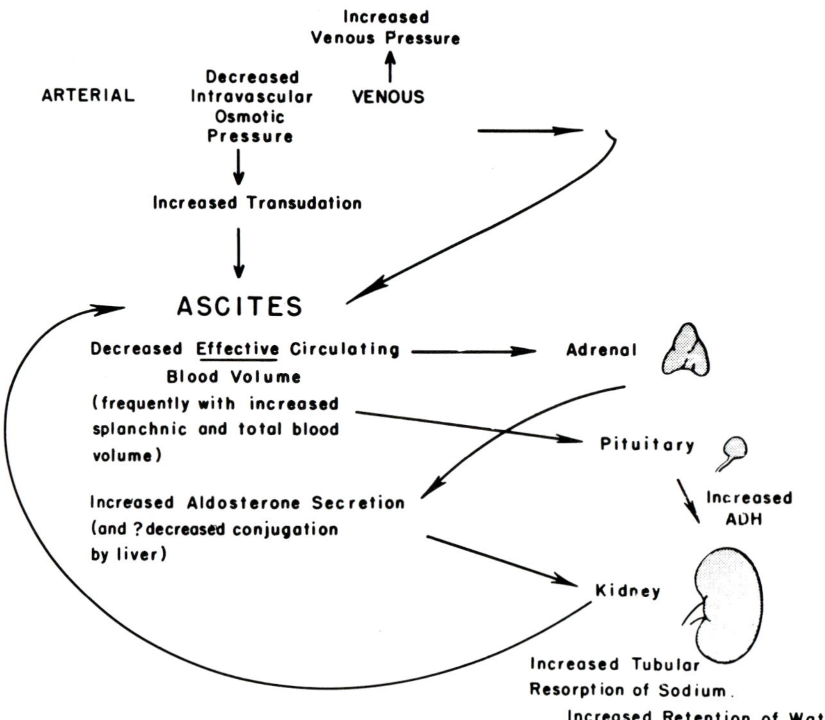

Figure 18.2. Pathogenesis of ascites. ADH, antidiuretic hormone.

probably secondary manifestations of changes in plasma volume, osmolarity, hypokalemia, and hepatic blood flow. A simplified diagram indicating the major factors involved in the pathogenesis of cirrhotic ascites is shown in Figure 18.2.

Treatment of Ascites

Medical

The patient with cirrhotic ascites is treated primarily as a problem in medical management, particularly since the introduction of effective diuretics and aldosterone antagonists over the past two decades. The surgeon, however, is not infrequently directly involved in the problem if there is associated bleeding from esophageal varices that require surgical intervention before a desirable period of a diuretic program can be completed, and in those instances in which refractory ascites can be shown to be due to one of the variants of the Budd-Chiari syndrome.

As described in the introduction above, the appearance of ascites is determined primarily by two factors, the serum albumin level and the increased intrahepatic postsinusoidal venous pressure. The rate at which ascitic fluid accumulates, however, is a reflection of the disparity between dietary sodium intake and sodium excretion; restriction of sodium intake is, therefore, a keystone of successful medical management, a factor that is commonly overlooked because of the high degree of effectiveness of modern diuretic drugs.

Under ordinary circumstances and in a normal external environment, an afebrile patient will rarely excrete more than 10 mEq of sodium in sweat. The major route of sodium excretion is the kidney and under normal circumstances, an individual with an intake of 5 to 8 g of salt daily will show a urinary excretion of 80 to 100 mEq/L of sodium in the urine, with concomitant potassium excretion in the range of 40 to 50 mEq/L. This amount and the ratio described is surprisingly consistent, although, of course, major variations in dietary intake will result in concomitant changes in the urinary concentration and total excretion.

With accumulating or refractory cirrhotic ascites, however, this situation is drastically altered and the sodium excretion in the urine may diminish to levels of 0 to 5 mEq/L because of voracious retention of sodium by the kidneys secondary to aldosterone activity. Therefore, in the patient who may be excreting only 15 to 20 mEq of sodium daily in combined urine and sweat, a dietary intake as low as 1 g daily will still result in a net daily increase in the total body sodium and concomitant retention of water, both of which are reflected primarily in a progressive increase in the ascites. Treatment must, therefore, focus on both rigid restriction of sodium intake (a diet of < 500 mg of salt daily can be prescribed by a good dietitian) and efforts made to increase the loss of sodium from the kidneys by effective use of diuretics and judiciously administered serum albumin.

The introduction of the chlorthiazide drugs (Diuril and Hydrodiuril), which effectively increase the excretion of sodium by the kidney, proved to be a major advance 30 years ago in the satisfactory medical management of ascites. Shortly after they were utilized widely, it became apparent that their use was occasionally attended by a form of hepatic encephalopathy or coma. Despite extensive studies of this phenomenon, it is still not clear as to whether the central nervous system disorder is caused by the recognized losses of potassium in the urine and the concomitant hypokalemia, by the increased production of ammonia by the kidney, or by some other as yet undefined metabolic disorder. At any rate, the use of a greatly increased intake of potassium in association with chlorthiazide administration appears to have limited the risks associated with the use of these drugs. Further improvement and medical management occurred when ethacrynic acid and furosemide (Lasix) were found to be significantly more effective than previously known diuretic agents including the chlorthiazide drugs. Of the two, ethacrynic acid appeared to be the more potent but furosemide exhibited an unusually broad dose-response curve and in large doses, its potency approached that of ethacrynic acid. The physiologic changes induced by these two agents were quite similar; they pointed to a dual site of action in the ascending limb of Henle's loop in the kidney and to a second site of action in the distal tubules where urinary dilution is accomplished. Because of a greater margin of safety and less toxicity, furosemide is commonly used at the time of writing in preference to ethacrynic acid. It should be noted, however, that the margin of safety of this drug is less than one finds with the thiazide agents and a patient receiving furosemide must be more carefully observed in order to prevent disastrous and rapid shifts in fluid and electrolyte balance with the concomitant development of encephalopathy and coma. Mercurial diuretics may be used cautiously in association with above agents but only when adequate renal perfusion and urinary output have been established.

When the importance of hyperaldosteronism in this syndrome was recognized, pharmacologic agents designed to counteract the effect of aldosterone were introduced. Treatment with spironolactones as aldosterone antagonists was followed by widespread acceptance and clinical usage but it was soon recognized that of themselves, the aldosterone antagonists were not as effective as a program in combination with the other diuretic agents described above. Certainly, they may be used as a solitary agent, but their effectiveness is synergistic and together with thiazide or furosemide will effect a more rapid diuresis than could be anticipated from the summation of the actions of the individual drugs alone.

The role of depressed intravascularized osmotic pressure, so commonly found with cirrhosis, has been emphasized in the pathogenesis of ascites. Therefore, the use of salt-free human serum albumin is extremely important in the depleted patient and should be administered cautiously to restore the serum albumin level to near normal; emphasis should be made, however, on the fact that injudicious use of human serum albumin may cause rapid rises in portal pressure and frequently precipitate bleeding from esophageal varices.

The malnutrition associated with cirrhotic ascites is usually impressive, and the patient commonly appears as a thin, wasted, almost cachectic individual with a huge, tense abdomen and clearly a negative nitrogen balance with a loss of lean body mass. A high carbohydrate intake is imperative, even if forced feeding through a soft tubing is necessary. A high protein intake is important from a nutritional standpoint and to restore positive nitrogen balance but, since portal-systemic shunting is so commonly found with cirrhosis, the induction of encephalopathy by high protein feedings is an ever-present threat and oral protein intake should be increased cautiously by small increments and reduced immediately if asterixis or neurologic symptoms appear. The efficiency and effectiveness of high caloric parenteral feeding has been an extremely valuable adjunct in the restoration of the nutritionally depleted patient with cirrhotic ascites to a normal state of health and an adequate lean body mass. The type of medical regimen outlined above has been extremely satisfactory in inducing diuresis in most patients with cirrhotic ascites unless they are in terminal phases of the disease or unless bleeding from esophageal varices does not permit a leisurely medical program. In such cases, surgical intervention may be required and will be discussed below.

Surgical

In order to clarify the selective group of individuals with whom we are dealing when we discuss surgical procedures for cirrhotic ascites, it should be understood that reference is made to three major classes of patients. First are those who are truly intractable to medical therapy but generally not in severe and progressive hepatic decompensation. The second group are those who are similarly intractable to a medical program but who are in an advanced state of depletion and for this and perhaps other concomitant medical disorders will present as prohibitive risk for any major surgical intervention. The third group would include those individuals in whom the onset of severe esophageal varices requires immediate consideration of surgical intervention despite the presence of ascites.

This last group is the one in which the existence of ascites presents an added complication to the primary problem of hemorrhage and which the type of shunt to be employed is a serious consideration.

The definition of intractability is a point that also requires considerable thought and analysis since this definition will obviously vary widely with each physician responsible for the management of a patient with ascites. As a generalization, it is not unreasonable to say that ascites might be considered intractable if they are not diminished or dissipated after several weeks of vigorous and consistent medical therapy designed along the guidelines referred to in the previous section. With these rough guidelines in mind, one might then

Table 18.1. Procedures for Ascites

I.	Establish collateral
	A. Talma-Morison omentopexy
	B. Spleen in abdominal wall, testicle in peritoneal cavity, excision of parietal peritoneum
II.	Reduce portal flow
	A. Arterial ligation
	B. Splenectomy
III.	Promote drainage or absorption
	A. Anastomosis of renal pelvis or bladder to peritoneum
	B. Button in subcutaneous tissue
	C. Saphenous vein to peritoneum
	D. "Rectus wick" (divided rectus to peritoneal cavity)
	E. Ileal entectropy
	F. Splenohepatic sinus
	G. Splenic transposition
IV.	Shunt surgery
V.	Venous infusion of ascitic fluid
VI.	Peritoneal-atrial shunt

proceed to consider what role the surgeon may play in the management of the patients with severe or intractable cirrhotic ascites, which either of itself is a factor for favoring surgical intervention or in which the gastrointestinal hemorrhage precipitates some kind of surgical intervention.

The long history of surgical efforts to dissipate ascites is summarized in Table 18.1. Many ingenious and sometimes bizarre procedures have been employed but the rather singular lack of success in most instances has made these procedures of historic interest rather than current significance. Nonetheless, there are occasions when one or a number of these procedures or devices might be utilized, and special circumstances for miscellaneous procedures will be referred to again at the end of the section.

Perhaps the most important surgical advance in the treatment of cirrhotic ascites occurred with the revival of shunt surgery in the treatment of this particular complication of cirrhosis (3). It is of historical interest to note that the first successful experimental shunt performed by Eck in 1877 (4) was carried out with the concept that it might be applicable to the problem of ascites in humans since the disasters of gastrointestinal hemorrhage in relationship to ascites had not been thoroughly categorized. With the introduction of shunting procedures into clinical usage some 60 years later by Whipple (5), it was hoped that variants of the shunt procedure might be effective in the dissipation of cirrhotic ascites. Initially, however, the high mortality and the lack of effectiveness of the end-to-side portacaval shunt in this group of patients led to the generally accepted concept that the existence of an appreciable amount of ascites was an actual contraindication to a shunting procedure. With the evolution and understanding of the pathophysiology associated with cirrhotic ascites, however, there was a revival of interest in shunt procedures specifically directed toward the alleviation of this problem (6–8). Surgeons involved in these clinical studies approached the problem with the concept that one of the major factors in intractable ascites was the existence of an intrahepatic outflow block producing what might be described as a physiologic analogue to experimental methods of obstructing hepatic outflow and to variants of the Budd-Chiari syndrome. Successful dissipation of cirrhotic ascites was achieved, utilizing either the side-to-side or double portacaval shunt, both of which procedures effected a combined decompression of the intrahepatic as well as the splanchnic bed and were effective in correcting the hemodynamic abnormalities. With the introduction of the modern diuretic and endocrine programs as described previously, the utilization of a shunt that accomplished combined hepatic and splanchnic decompression proved to be less widely applicable than in the previous era, but it should be kept in mind that the principle still applies whenever a shunting procedure is deemed applicable to a patient who also has severe ascites.

It should be emphasized strongly, however, that the clinical success and low mortality of combined portal and hepatic decompression in the treatment of cirrhotic ascites depend on careful selection of patients. In those with reasonably good liver function, one might anticipate that hemodynamic effects of an outflow block are prominent in the pathogenesis of the persistent ascites and that it is not purely a manifestation of progressive hepatocellular failure with inability to synthesize albumin and to maintain an intravascular osmotic pressure.

Postoperative management is obviously of extreme importance when the ascites have dissipated during the laparotomy with the construction of a combined decompressing shunt. The immediate postoperative period will be associated with rapid reaccumulation of at least some of the intraperitoneal fluid; why the reversal of the abnormal pathophysiology and abnormal hemodynamics does not result in immediate diuresis is not entirely clear, but it may be that the dissection required to construct the shunt leaves a large number of open

lymphatics. During this initial period of rapid although variable reaccumulation, urine output and the specific gravity should be followed at 2-hour intervals and maintained at adequate volume and moderate degree of concentration. This may require many units of plasma or salt-free albumin during the first 24 hours but eventually stabilization occurs as indicated by the maintenance of an adequate urine output and the cessation of rapid weight gain. If adequate volume replacement is not carried out, one encounters atypical azotemia and ultimately death. After stabilization, one can anticipate the increasing appearance of sodium in the urine and a progressive dissipation of the reaccumulated ascites; it is usually complete within 3 weeks and the patient may often leave the hospital without salt restriction or the necessity of any diuretic program.

It is well to emphasize, however, that only a combined shunt is hemodynamically effective in patients with severe ascites. Thus, a side-to-side double or interposition shunt will provide effective decompression of both the splanchnic bed (to control hemorrhage) and the sinusoidal bed (to control ascites). An end-to-side splenorenal shunt is basically a small side-to-side shunt and may have some degree of effectiveness in this particular situation, but a selective or distal splenorenal shunt or an end-to-side portacaval shunt precludes any retrograde decompression of the intrahepatic postsinusoidal block and thus is unlikely to be effective in the dissipation of ascites. This has been clearly shown in any number of clinical studies and should be kept in mind under the circumstances described in this section.

Before concluding, it should also be pointed out that there are many instances in which a shunting procedure may be considered of more magnitude than could possibly be tolerated by the individual in question. Under these circumstances, the insertion of a peritoneal-atrial shunt may provide effective palliation of the distressing and incapacitating ascites at much less risk than the more invasive construction of a portal systemic shunt.

Budd-Chiari Syndrome

The term "Budd-Chiari syndrome" is applied rather widely today to any clinical entity in which any one of a variety of pathologic processes causes an outflow block from the sinusoidal bed of the

Table 18.2. Budd-Chiari Syndrome (17 Cases)

Suprahepatic block (4)	
Inferior caval obstruction	2
Retrohepatic tumor	2
Intrahepatic block (12)	
Tumor	2
Veno-occlusive disease	2
Myeloproliferative disease	5
Hypercoagulable states	4

liver and results in progressive and usually refractory ascites.

Although many cases of cirrhosis, particularly those with a macronodular configuration, show the pathologic and hemodynamic features of the Budd-Chiari syndrome, these are usually excluded from that classification and have already been covered extensively in the preceding text.

From the historical point of view, it is interesting to read Chiari's original paper (9) in which he generously gave credit to Budd (10) for a rather vague case report and then proceeded to describe in great detail seven cases of his own. These apparently all had a very specific pathologic entity of "endophlebitis obliterans" of the small hepatic veins with ascites and all terminated in death. Chiari speculated on the etiology of this disease and raised the question of whether it might be due to either tuberculosis or to syphilis since both of those disorders were prevalent in the late nineteenth century. In fact, as one reads the details of the pathologic descriptions, the resemblance to

veno-occlusive disease as described by Bras et al. (11) is quite striking. Since veno-occlusive disease has been correctly ascribed to the injection of pyrollizidine alkaloids from Crotolaria or Senecio plants, it may well have been that Chiari's patients ingested bread made from grain that was contaminated by one of those two weeds.

In our own series (12) of 17 cases, one can view this from the anatomic location of the blood (Table 18.2) or by etiologic factors involved in the production of the postsinusoidal block (Table 18.3).

The criteria that have been generally accepted for the definition of Budd-Chiari syndrome consist of the rapid onset of ascites and the existence of a well-defined postsinusoidal block either in the retro- or superhepatic vena cava, the hepatic veins, or the intrahepatic venules with a microscopic pathologic picture of centrilobular congestion and necrosis and the clinical picture of a rapid onset of ascites.

The causative factors as noted in the tables included caval web or tumor, hepatic tumor, a hypercoagulable state with intravascular thrombosis, myoloproliferative disease with multiple venous occlusions, and the specific entity of veno-occlusive disease itself.

The hemodynamic analogy between the Budd-Chiari syndrome and patients with cirrhosis who demonstrate many of the features of the Budd-Chiari syndrome was reminiscent of the approach that we had used some years ago in utilizing surgical production of combined hepatic and

Table 18.3. Budd-Chiari Syndrome (17 Cases)[a]

Etiology (by Disease Process)	Treatment	Result
Vena caval obstruction (4)		
Congenital valve (1)	Transatrial fracture	Excellent
Primary tumor (leiomyosarcoma) (1)	Transatrial partial removal	Unsuccessful, died
Retrohepatic tumor (2)	None	Died
Myeloproliferative diseases (5) (polycythemia, lymphoma, idiopathic)	S-S portacaval shunts (2) Peritoneoatrial shunts (2)	Excellent result or palliation
Hypercoagulable states (4) (paroxysmal nocturnal hemoglobinuria, oral contraceptives)	S-S portacaval shunt (1) Expectant (3)	Excellent Died (1), resolution (2)
Veno-occlusive disease ("bush-tea poisoning")	S-S portacaval shunt (2)	Excellent
Liver tumor (hepatoma, cystadenoma) (2)	Peritoneoatrial shunt (1) Resection (1)	Palliation Excellent

Abbreviations: S-S, side-to-side.
[a] Numbers in parentheses represent number of cases.

splanchnic decompression in the treatment of otherwise intractable cirrhotic ascites (7). Based on this concept, we constructed side-to-side shunts in the treatment of five patients with Budd-Chiari syndrome, with excellent results. These were substantiated by the results of others (13–16) who applied the same type of analysis and the same surgical approach to the syndrome with equally satisfactory results.

This does not imply that every patient with the Budd-Chiari syndrome should be immediately brought to surgical treatment, but it is well to consider this type of operative procedure as a hemodynamic corrective for the disorder.

For those patients who represent too poor a risk for consideration of shunt surgery or whose primary disease has such a limited prognosis that one would not wish to consider major surgery, an alternative is the insertion of a peritoneal-atrial shunt, which, of course, is equally applicable to any form of intractable accumulation of ascites and which will be discussed below.

Peritoneal-Atrial Shunting

Over many years, efforts have been made to collect ascitic fluid that had been withdrawn from the peritoneal cavity under sterile conditions and re-infuse this into the circulation because of the full recognition that ultimate dissipation of the fluid required maintenance of circulating blood volume through the kidneys.

The development of equipment used to accomplish this goal stems from the introduction of a mechanism by LeVeen (17,18) for the closed and continuous routing of accumulating peritoneal fluid in patients with intractable ascites into venous circulation.

The relative success of this device led to the introduction of various improved systems, of which the most effective to date has been the so-called Denver shunt described in some detail by Lund and Newkirk (19).

The basic concept of these peritoneal-venous shunts depends on the implantation of a type of collecting system into the peritoneal cavity, which can be carried out under local anesthesia, and then the subcutaneous tunneling in a proximal direction towards the supraclavicular area, and the ultimate insertion of a tubing via the jugular vein into the superior vena cava. Within the system, there are one or two one-way valves so that the flow can be only in the direction of transmitting the fluid from the abdominal cavity to the venous circulation. In the later apparatus, a pump chamber is a part of the system so that rather than relying on changes in respiratory pressures, the patient or an attendant can exert external pressure on the pump chamber and increase the flow of the ascitic fluid through the system.

On the surface, this sounds very simple but in our own experience and in that of others (20–22), these or any of these devices may be associated with serious complications including sepsis, ascitic fluid leakage, disseminated intravascular coagulopathy, thrombosis of the major vessels in the chest (including the superior vena cava), pneumothorax, pneumonia, pulmonary edema, pulmonary emboli, shunt dislodgement or occlusion, and various other less serious problems. In our own continuing experience, there have been approximately three complications of moderate severity for every two insertions of this type of apparatus.

Thus, while this is a tool that can be used successfully and with considerable palliative effect in patients who have intractable ascites either from exudative fluid from intraperitoneal malignancy or from a type of outflow obstruction to the liver characteristic of the so-called Budd Chiari syndrome, nonetheless, it is important to recognize that the procedure, although carried out under local anesthesia, is attended by a significant percentage of complications and thus utilization of the procedure must be carried out advisedly.

References

1. Cameron JL, Kieffer RS, Anderson WJ, Zuidema GD. Internal pancreatic fistulas: Pancreatic ascites and pleural effusions. *Ann Surg* 1974; 184:587–593.
2. Baggenstoss AH, Cain JC. Hepatic hilar lymphatics of man: Their relation to ascites. *N Engl J Med* 1957; 256:531–535.
3. McDermott WV Jr. Evaluation of the hemodynamics of portal hypertension in the selection of patients for shunt surgery. *Ann Surg* 1972; 176(4):449–456.
4. Eck NV. Cited by Child CG III. Eck's fistula. *Surg Gynecol Obstet* 1953; 96:375.
5. Whipple AD. Problem of portal hypertension in relation to hepatosplenopathies. *Ann Surg* 1945; 122:449–473.
6. Welch CS, Attarian E, Welch HF. Treatment of ascites by side to side portacaval shunt. *Bull NY Acad Med* 1958; 34:249–255.
7. McDermott WV Jr. The treatment of cirrhotic ascites by combined hepatic and portal decompression. *N Engl J Med* 1958; 259:897–901.
8. McDermott WV Jr. The double portacaval shunt in the

treatment of cirrhotic ascites. *Surg Gynecol Obstet* 1960; 110: 457–469.

9. Chiari H. Ueber die selbstange phlebitis obliterans der hauptstamme der venae hepaticae als todesursache. *Beitr Pathol Anat* 1899; 26:1–17.

10. Budd G. *Diseases of the Liver*. Philadelphia: Blanchard and Lea, 1857, pp. 194–196.

11. Bras G, Jelliffe DD, Stuart KL. Veno-occlusive disease of the liver with nonportal type of cirrhosis, occurring in Jamaica. *Arch Pathol* 1954; 57:285–300.

12. McDermott WV, Stone MD, Bothe A Jr, Trey C. Budd-Chiari syndrome. *Am J Surg* 1984; 147:463–467.

13. Vons C, Bourstyn E, Bonnet P, Smadja C, Szekely AM, Franco D. Results of portal systemic shunts in Budd-Chiari syndrome. *Ann Surg* 1986; 203:366–370.

14. Franco D, Vons C, Lecompte Y, Nuzzo G, Smadja C. Portoatrial shunt in Budd-Chiari syndrome. *Surgery* 1986; 99:378–380.

15. Millikan WJ, Henderson JM, Sewell CW, Guyton RA, Potts JR, Cranford CA, et al. Approach to the spectrum of Budd-Chiari syndrome: Which patients require portal decompression? *Am J Surg* 1985; 149:167–176.

16. Malt RA, Dalton JC, Johnson RE, Gurewich V. Side-to-side portacaval shunt versus non-surgical treatment of the Budd-Chiari syndrome. *Am J Surg* 1978; 136:387–389.

17. LeVeen HH, Christoudias G, Ip M, et al. Peritoneal venous shunting for ascites. *Ann Surg* 1974; 180:580–590.

18. LeVeen HH, Wapnick S, Diaz C, et al. Further experience with peritoneal venous shunt for ascites. *Ann Surg* 1976; 184:574–580.

19. Lund LH, Newkirk JB. Peritoneal venous shunting system for surgical management of ascites. *Contemp Surg* 1979; 14: 31–38.

20. Lund LH, Moritz MW. Complications of denver peritoneal venous shunting. *Arch Surg* 1982; 117:924–928.

21. Echauser FE, Strodel WE, Knol JA, Turcotte JG, et al. Superior vena caval obstruction associated with long-term peritoneal venous shunting. *Ann Surg* 1981; 193:180–184.

22. Lerner RG, Nelson JC, Corines P, et al. Disseminated intravascular coagulation: A complication of LeVeen peritoneal venous shunts. *JAMA* 1978; 240:2064–2066.

PART V
Hepatic Trauma, Tumors, and Resection

Chapter 19
Surgical Management of Hepatic Trauma

ALEXANDER J. WALT

Interest in hepatic trauma goes back a long time and is shown graphically in Homer's *Iliad* where Achilles "stabbed with his sword at the liver, the liver was torn from its place, and from it the black blood drenched the fold of his tunic and his eyes were shrouded in darkness as the light went . . . ." For the next 2600 years liver wounds, with very few exceptions, were regarded as fatal. With the introduction of general anesthesia and antisepsis, however, many surgeons began to study hepatic wounds in animals and results improved. In 1872 Mayer (1) noted that the mortality of liver injury was 59% rather than the traditionally accepted 100%. By 1900 many fundamentals of hepatic injury were established and it was recognized that smaller wounds tended to stop bleeding spontaneously, that the liver regenerated rapidly, and that massive and significant hemorrhage could be controlled by a variety of suturing techniques. In 1906, in the second volume of *Surgery, Gynecology and Obstetrics*, Schroeder (2) of Cook County Hospital, in an article entitled "The Progress of Liver Hemostasis," succinctly reviewed the status of hepatic surgery, commented on the ease with which smaller wounds could be safely repaired, and described a practical method of balloon tamponade for missile tracks deep in the parenchyma. Two years later, Pringle (3), in a celebrated but grossly misinterpreted report, advanced the concept of temporary occlusion of the portal triad as a method of gaining control of hepatic hemorrhage, transection of the suspensory ligaments to provide access to posterior lacerations, and the use of gauze packing to achieve temporary hemostasis. Despite the logic of his advocacy, Pringle had no survivors with this technique. World War I brought few advances in hepatic surgery and little progress was made between the two world wars. If anything, unsubstantiated dogma was further entrenched, with ligation of the hepatic artery regarded as almost uniformly fatal, occlusion of the portal vein for more than 15 minutes as a virtual guarantee of hepatic necrosis, and the use of temporary guaze packing as tantamount to malpractice. Nevertheless, the trend toward earlier operation, adequate blood transfusion, and direct intrahepatic hemostasis was reflected in reduced mortality rates. Experience in the Vietnam War was discouraging due to the high velocity of the missiles used but later reflection influenced a new generation of surgeons who were well supplied with blood, antibiotics, and a healthy skepticism, which led them to reassess the problems posed by civilian injuries. Surgeons between 1970 and 1980 (4–6), recognizing the wide array of injuries encountered in the United States, ranging from the blunt trauma of motor vehicle accidents to the penetrating wounds of civilian weapons, and studying the outcome of different subsets, brought some order and a cautionary conservatism to the management of hepatic injuries.

Since 1980, with the development, refinement, and availability of technology such as ultrasonography and computed tomography (CT) scanning, a new conservative trend that espouses the avoidance of surgery in selected patients—especially children—is clearly discernible. In contrast, the need for an early, very aggressive approach to the salvage of patients with lacerations of large intra- and juxtahepatic veins (the major cause of death in hepatic injury) has gained many adherents (7,8). This chapter seeks to provide a perspective on the current management of liver injury and its complications.

Table 19.1. Mortality Rates of Patients with Hepatic Injury

Hospital	Country	Period	No. Cases	Mortality Rate (%)
Detroit Receiving	USA	1961–83	1592	12.4
Ben Taub	USA	1979–84	1000	10.5
San Francisco General	USA	1976–81	443	9.0
Kuala Lumpur	Malaysia	1961–80	379	15.8
Lincoln Memorial	USA	1977–85	345	19.4
Sunnybrook	Canada	1976–85	220	29.0[a]
Westmead	Australia	1979–84	97	22.0[a]

[a] Marked preponderance of blunt trauma.

Mortality of Liver Trauma

The liver is injured in approximately 30% of all abdominal injuries. Next to the spleen, the liver is the most commonly injured viscus in blunt trauma and it is the most frequently injured organ in penetrating wounds of the abdomen. Many institutions (9,10) have now reported series of hepatic injuries in excess of 1000 patients and the larger trauma centers expect to treat an average of one to three patients with liver injuries each week (11). The relative distribution of blunt and penetrating injuries varies greatly in different regions and cultures. In the Wayne State University series (9) of 1635 patients, blunt injury constituted about 12% and in the Ben Taub Hospital series (10), 13.6%. In contrast, the regional trauma center at Sunnybrook Hospital in metropolitan Toronto (12) and the Westmead Hospital in Australia (13) treated 143 and 97 cases of liver injury, respectively, of which 97% and 91% were due to blunt trauma. The relatively high mortality rates in blunt injury are due to the fact that major hepatic veins are injured in about 12% of these patients while about 20% to 25% have concomitant head injury.

The mortality rate in various series varies with the type of injury, length of elapsed time between injury and definitive treatment, and the organization and regionalization of the trauma services in the community. When stab wounds and low velocity missile gunshot wounds are frequent, the overall mortality rate is likely to be less than 6% in contrast to the 20% to 30% mortality rate when blunt injuries predominate. In the larger trauma centers that have a varying combination of the different types of injuries, the mortality rate has tended to plateau between 10% and 14% (4,11) (Table 19.1).

In an era when the phrase "quality control" has become an indispensable feature of administrative jargon and "outcome" the ultimate yardstick, it is essential before comparisons are made between institutions or regions that any series of liver injuries be carefully divided into subsets that take into account the nature of the wounding agent, the number of associated organs damaged, the degree of shock sustained by the patient when first seen, the age of the patient, and the volume of fluids required to resuscitate the patient. Ironically, the most sophisticated trauma centers to which a majority of moribund patients may be brought are likely to have a deceptively high mortality rate by virtue of the severity of injuries they treat.

Attempts have been made to categorize liver injuries much as has been done for the staging of malignancies. Most classifications are fundamentally anatomic in design and suffer the disadvantage of not being integrated with the physiologic changes in the more severely injured patients. Consequently, not all series necessarily show a linear increase in mortality, although the direction is always clear. One such limited but useful classification is illustrated in Table 19.2.

Table 19.2. A Classification of Civilian Hepatic Trauma

Class	Liver Injury	Frequency (%)
I	Capsular avulsion Parenchymal fracture < 1 cm deep	15
II	Parenchymal fracture 1–3 cm deep Subcapsular hematoma <10 cm diameter Peripheral penetrating wound	55
III	Parenchymal fracture > 3 cm deep Subcapsular hematoma > 10 cm diameter Central penetrating wound	25
IV	Lobar tissue destruction Massive central hematoma	3
V	Retrohepatic vena cava injury Extensive bilobar disruption	2

Reproduced by permission from Moore, EF. Critical decisions in the management of hepatic trauma. *Am J Surg* 1984; 148: 712–716.

Etiology

Most blunt injuries result from direct compression of the liver by external forces that, in approximately 80% of cases, injure other organs too, most often the diaphragm and organs in the upper abdomen and lower chest, but also more remote structures, such as the brain and skeletal system. In other patients, the main hepatic injury appears to be due to a deceleration injury with rotation of the liver and related lacerations in the area of one or other of the hepatic ligaments. In falls from heights, one may have a combination of these events with the production of an explosive type of parenchymal damage, and a constellation of fractures of the pelvis, os calcis, and spine.

Penetrating wounds are mostly caused by stabs, gunshot wounds, or shotgun wounds. What appears to be almost spontaneous bleeding may occur in patients with sickle cell disease, peliosis, coagulopathy, or pregnancy.

An increasing number of iatrogenic injuries are encountered today, mostly due to needle biopsy, percutaneous cholangiography, transhepatic stents, the inappropriately low insertion of chest tubes, or external cardiac compression in the course of resuscitation. The Wayne State University series (9) collected over 18 years is fairly typical of the patients encountered in the large trauma centers. The overall mortality rate was approximately 12%. Associated injuries were present in about 75% of patients. In order of descending frequency, the organs involved were thoracic (the lung, chest wall, diaphragm, and heart), stomach, colon, kidney, long bone fractures, small bone fractures, gallbladder, pancreas, duodenum, and spleen. If blunt trauma alone is considered, injury to the solid organs becomes relatively much more common. Due to the large number of organs that may be damaged, it is difficult to apportion with accuracy the precise cause of death in all patients with hepatic injury. When the liver alone is injured, the mortality is only 5% to 10%. As the number of concomitant injured viscera rises, the mortality rate increases in rough proportion. About half the deaths are due to the liver injury; a quarter to intra-abdominal extrahepatic causes; and a quarter to head, chest, or osseous injuries. Approximately 70% of patients die of hemorrhage (not necessarily from the liver), 20% of subsequent sepsis (most often in the abdomen or lungs), and about 10% of direct cerebral or cardiopulmonary injury.

With the causes of death now well recognized, attention has been directed to identifying these early and to instituting specific countermeasures. Restoration of blood volume and establishment of adequate ventilation take precedence. On infrequent but testing occasions, some exceptionally challenging decisions become necessary when a patient who has proven or suspected hepatic bleeding also has established or suggestive signs of a torn thoracic aorta, cardiac tamponade, massive hemothorax, or increased intracranial pressure. The priority of operation given to each lesion may be crucial to survival.

About one-third of patients who die do so in the emergency department or on the operating table, another third die within the first 24 hours (some due to continuing bleeding associated with a coagulopathy or a technical failure), and the remainder die after 24 hours, most often of sepsis or acute adult respiratory disease syndrome (ARDS). It is therefore imperative that attention be directed to ensuring adequate respiratory gas exchange first, combating the effects of hemorrhage, limiting the establishment of infection, and avoiding the physiologic side effects of hypothermia. The presence of established shock is a discouraging but by no means hopeless sign; similarly, the need for massive blood transfusion is ominous but does not preclude a successful outcome. Thirty-nine percent of our patients with a systolic blood pressure (SBP) below 90 millimeters of mercury on admission subsequently died, in contrast to only 1.5% of those whose SBP was above 90 mmHg. Fifty-six of 231 recent patients with liver injury required more than 10 units of blood; 27 lived. Paradoxically, 17 of 30 patients (56.6%) who required more than 20 U survived.

Pathology of Liver Injury and Relationship to Outcome

Blunt Injuries

The spectrum of hepatic damage is wide, ranging from a subcapsular hemorrhage to a linear crack that may be short and shallow or deep and long, an intraparenchymal hematoma that may be deceptively hidden beneath a relatively normal external surface, a soft parenchymal mush of shattered tissue, and a complex stellate series of cracks, classically found in the posterosuperior aspect of the right lobe under the diaphragm. The degree of damage may be difficult to assess initially, especially in blunt injury. Today, however, the CT scan may be very helpful preoperatively. At operation, palpation often gives a good indication of the degree of internal parenchymal damage but not necessarily so.

Stab wounds vary with the type of instrument used and may extend far deeper than surmised. The greatest dangers in managing stab wounds lie in the cirrhotic liver where vessels tend not to retract spontaneously, and in deep penetrating wounds where the continuation of bleeding may not be initially appreciated. Prediction of the degree of hepatic involvement by the site of entrance of a stab or bullet wound can be very misleading. All wounds below the fourth intercostal space on either side of the chest may be associated with liver injury, and in the case of missiles, no entry point is too distant from the liver to preclude involvement of that organ.

Patients with gunshot wounds have a mortality rate of about 15% to 25% depending on the weapon used. The muzzle velocity of the weapon varies from 970 feet per second in the .38 revolver to 2160 ft/sec in the .303 hunting rifle. While small-caliber missiles with low velocities may produce so small a track and so little adjacent necrosis that very limited débridement is necessary, a trajectory that causes the missile to enter or exit near the large vessels of the hilum or the large retrohepatic veins may obviously result in death or great morbidity. High-velocity wounds such as those encountered in the Vietnam War disrupt large segments of liver tissue with consequent extensive vascular and biliary injury. In these wounds, extensive débridement of the liver sequestra is mandatory and damage to other abdominal and thoracic viscera can be anticipated. Similarly, shotgun wounds are potentially very destructive, depending on the closeness of the patient to the point of discharge. These patients are also prone to sepsis, depending on the amount of foreign material introduced.

About 120 cases of apparently spontaneous hepatic subcapsular hemorrhage or rupture have been described in pregnancy (14). The mortality rate for these cases ranges between 60% and 75%. Early recognition is important and is aided by the association in most patients of eclampsia, right upper quadrant pain, and sudden hypotension due to bleeding. Concomitant hypercoagulability is usually present together with so-called hepatic necrosis and changes in the vessel walls. The subcapsular hematoma may be very extensive, spreading across the entire lobe of the liver, most often on the right, with or without rupture into the peritoneal cavity and into the parenchyma of the liver. Nonoperative treatment almost invariably leads to death. Operation is therefore essential and should be directed at the area of bleeding. About 50% of these patients and most of their babies may be saved. Ligation of the hepatic artery and, to a lesser extent, packing are far less likely to be successful.

Clinical Picture

The history of the injury is important but may not always be available. Similarly, physical examination may be invaluable but the physical signs and the reactions of the patient are often obscured by obtundation or inebriation. In assessing the likelihood of hepatic injury, certain clues are always sought, such as the presence of fractured ribs, signs of excoriation of the skin by a seat belt, the presence of subcutaneous ecchymoses or tire marks, distention of the abdomen, local tenderness, and shoulder tip pain. Surprisingly, a substantial percentage of patients who are subsequently proven to have blunt liver injury may be normotensive when admitted to the emergency department. Furthermore, some of these patients have few, if any, or only mild abdominal symptoms and signs. Patients may display remarkably little tenderness even though they have substantial damage visible on CT scan or are subsequently found to have a liter or more of blood in the peritoneal cavity. The presence of blood in the right pleural space in an injured patient with right upper quadrant abdominal pain suggests liver trauma and the possibility of a diaphragmatic laceration. While the subtleties of the clinical picture of hepatic injury are often stressed, the diagnosis is fairly obvious in most patients. Whenever a falling hemoglobin level cannot be accounted for by the presence of a scalp or other laceration, blood in the chest, or a major fracture, abdominal bleeding must be suspected and the high likelihood entertained that the liver is the responsible organ. Peritoneal aspiration and peritoneal lavage (of greater accuracy) is likely to reveal the presence of intraperitoneal blood but not the identity of the source (15). Specific involvement of the liver is best determined when necessary and feasible by a CT scan of good quality, which is very accurate in delineating the extent and type of parenchymal injury (16). Obviously, the patient must be stable and not restless at the time of the CT scan, which is also useful in detecting concomitant injuries to the spleen, kidneys, pancreas, and duodenum.

Use of hepatobiliary isotopic scanning has been advocated for liver injuries as a test to demonstrate the extent of parenchymal damage and the presence of bile leaks (17). As of 1985, the superior virtues of the HIDA scan in complex liver injuries have been advanced but the indications for this test do not extend beyond the uncommon circumstance when identification of a large and hazardous bile leak is sought (18). Bile leakage in itself is not an indication for operation and nonvisualization of the gallbladder on a HIDA scan in trauma does not indicate cholecystitis.

The need to assess, reassess, and treat the frequently concomitant injuries is an ever-present priority. The patient who does not respond to an accurately calculated fluid volume replacement may have a direct myocardial contusion or myocardial tamponade. The timing of aortography in the patient with a widened mediastinum and suspected hepatic injury is often debated. Again, this decision is a matter of clinical judgment determined by the physiologic status of the patient and the assessment of the amount of intraperitoneal blood present. When the abdominal injury is felt to be the cause of significant continuing hemorrhage, the abdominal exploration takes precedence and aortography and possible thoracotomy are delayed. Rarely, in the patient with an associated life-threatening head injury, it may be necessary to adopt a two-team approach so that the brain is decompressed while the abdominal bleeding is brought under temporary control at least. The sequencing of investigations and operative interventions is determined by judgments of which individual injury represents the most immediate threat to life.

Diagnosis and Preoperative Management

When a reasonable suspicion of hepatic injury is entertained, adequate intravenous lines are inserted for purposes of providing fluids to defend the intravascular volume. Errors of overenthusias-

tic commission are far safer than errors of omission. Ideally, a percutaneous polyethylene cannula is inserted percutaneously; in more serious cases, two or even three intravenous lines are needed. When the patient is in shock, series of rapid cutdowns on the antecubital veins with insertion of large-bore catheters should be performed. Some surgeons favor the insertion of a subclavian or internal jugular catheter in these circumstances but this technique is more hazardous in the shocked patient. When this approach is adopted, it is essential that immediate radiographs be taken to exclude the possibility of an iatrogenic pneumothorax, confirm the position of the catheter, and check that the catheter has not been placed through the wall of the vein with the consequent production of a hydrothorax. In selected emergency cases, the cutdown may be done on the saphenous vein at the ankle or even at the groin in desperate circumstances. While there is a theoretical objection to the use of veins in the lower limb on the grounds that the replacement fluid may leak from the hepatic or inferior vena cava (IVC) injury, this occurs very rarely. A Foley catheter is inserted to measure the urinary output, which serves as a valuable indicator of perfusion. Antibiotics are started prophylactically. No single regime has universal acceptance but cefoxitin or a combination of penicillin, gentamicin, and metronidazole (or clindamycin) are probably equally satisfactory in the initial stages.

Two to 3 liters of warmed Ringer's solution are administered over the first 10 to 20 minutes. If there is little response or if the patient deteriorates further, the possibilities of inadequate replacement, a tension pneumothorax, or a pericardial tamponade must be entertained. When possible, it is desirable to wait for fully cross-matched blood but this requires up to 40 minutes in most institutions. In severe injuries, the need for type-specific blood or type O blood is usually obvious within the first few minutes.

Ideally, before any definitive operation is embarked upon, the patient will be brought out of shock. In the severely injured patient with hepatic bleeding, however, this may never occur despite the most vigorous efforts. In such cases, surgical intervention is mandatory within minutes, even though the patient is in a poor physiologic state as evidenced by marked hypotension, tachycardia, obvious hypoxia, or an inability to increase the hemoglobin level. In all such cases, the operation becomes an integral part of the resuscitation process, which is best conducted from the start in the operating room. When deterioration is obvious and rapid, the surgeon is not permitted the luxury of further attempts at resuscitation and must of necessity operate close to the nadir of the patient's physiologic decline.

The operative approach will vary with the circumstances. If an associated chest injury is present, thoracotomy may take precedence, to achieve intrathoracic hemostasis and to permit clamping of the aorta above the diaphragm, which may serve to increase cardiac and cerebral perfusion and greatly decrease abdominal blood loss. The use of prelaparotomy thoracotomy, advocated initially for the patient with an abdominal tamponade and unrelenting shock that is little influenced by rapid infusion of fluids, remains controversial (19). Feliciano and colleagues report a 4.5% emergency center thoracotomy rate with 3.8% survival for abdominal injuries, although all 45 patients with liver injuries died (10). In the absence of a cardiac or thoracic injury, compression of the aorta below the diaphragm while resuscitative measures are continued probably achieves the same results, provided that aortic control is expeditiously obtained.

Nevertheless, the need for thoracotomy in patients with hepatic injury is not rare. In our recent series of 231 patients with hepatic injury, thoracotomy was performed in 40 patients (17.3%) at some time for a variety of reasons that included the need to deal with cardiac or pulmonary injuries, to obtain adequate exposure, and to treat subsequent fistulae or sepsis (9). Seventeen of the 40 patients (42.9%) survived.

Children

Most hepatic injury in children is blunt in origin and is caused by motor vehicle accidents, falls, and kicks. Some important features that differentiate these from injuries in adults also serve to influence treatment. The hepatic injury in the child is more likely to be isolated (about 30%) than in the adult, the degree of injury less extensive, and the association of intestinal injury much less likely. The hematoma is more often contained both extra- and intrahepatically, making conservative nonsurgical observation, well established now for splenic inju-

ries, more feasible. Series have been reported where operation was avoided in over 80% of cases (20). Nevertheless, while a nonoperative approach is more applicable to children than to adults, the overall mortality rate may be about the same—22% in a series from Toronto (21), or as low as 4%, depending on the composition of the series (22).

The use of CT provides knowledge of the extent of hepatic and extrahepatic injury and a rough estimate of the amount of blood in the peritoneal cavity. If the liver appears to be the only organ with significant injury and the patient remains hemodynamically stable, the child may be placed under close clinical surveillance and operation withheld unless bleeding continues to an unacceptable degree, for example, a requirement of more than 40 milliliters per kilogram to maintain vital signs. Operation is also mandatory if abdominal pain increases, and objective evidence is noted on sonography or CT of an enlarging subcapsular intrahepatic hematoma or if signs appear that are suggestive of injury to another abdominal organ.

Uncertainty remains about the best plan to obviate delayed rupture in these children when the bleeding has stabilized with nonoperative therapy. For safety, these children are confined to bed for about 2 weeks and restricted activity advised for 2 to 3 months after discharge. Meticulous recording of the detailed instructions to the mother should be placed in the hospital chart. As judged by serial CT scanning, most hepatic regeneration and disappearance of the parenchymal lesion requires about 3 months. It is important to stress that pursuit of a nonoperative approach requires the availability of a surgical intensive care unit and meticulous nursing and medical observation throughout. When these facilities and personnel are not available or if there is any doubt about the degree of liver injury, laparotomy should be performed as it is better to perform a relatively unnecessary operation than have an unquestionably avoidable death.

Operation

A midline incision is made from the xiphoid to below the umbilicus. This incision should be generous enough to ensure that good exposure is guaranteed from the start. Packs are thrust into the upper right and left quadrants to produce local pressure. Free blood is evacuated by sponges and suction. Note is taken of the general area from which hemorrhage appears to be coming and manual tamponade of any such region is instituted. If the patient is moderately hypotensive and bleeding is temporarily controlled, blood is given until the patient's vital signs have risen to a point where the intravascular volume appears to have been reasonably restored. During this time, any holes in the bowel may be temporarily closed with Allis's or Babcock's forceps or oversewn to prevent further spillage of intestinal contents. The abdomen may be irrigated with warm saline to reduce the bacterial contamination and to counteract from the start the possible occurrence of hypothermia. In selected patients, blood may be collected for autotransfusion.

A stable clot over the dome of the liver or a contained retrohepatic hematoma should be approached with considerable caution even in the stable patient. Detachment of clot by finger or sucker may be followed by a gush of venous blood difficult to control. This eventuality should be considered ahead of time and a plan of action established.

If bleeding cannot be adequately controlled and is noted to originate from the right upper quadrant, the subdiaphragmatic thoracic aorta is occluded digitally or by aortic compressor or by application of a vascular clamp through the lesser omentum, and the portal triad is occluded by a vascular clamp while the liver is manually compressed against packs. To obtain effective compression, it may be necessary to incise the suspensory ligaments of the liver so as to render the liver mobile and more easily tamponadable. Once more, if these temporizing maneuvers successfully bring the bleeding under temporary control but the patient remains in shock, attention is directed to vigorous resuscitation and repletion of the intravascular blood volume before the definitive operation begins again. This respite may be invaluable.

When, despite these maneuvers, bleeding continues, the source of the bleeding must be assumed to originate from the retrohepatic inferior vena cava or one or more major hepatic veins either within the parenchyma or in their short extrahepatic course. As the great majority of deaths from hepatic trauma occur in this group of patients, a decision on definitive treatment should be made rapidly at this point and is critical. The

options available vary with the topography of the lesion but are limited to (a) possible total or near-total lobectomy; (b) transhepatic parenchymal exposure and direct ligation or repair of the injured veins; (c) insertion of an intracaval shunt through the right atrium, the abdominal inferior vena cava, or the femoral vein; or (d) temporary packing of the area.

Fortunately, in 80% or more of patients, the injury to the liver poses few technical problems. In about 50% of patients, the liver laceration will have stopped bleeding by the time of laparotomy. The main decisions for the surgeon are whether to place sutures locally and whether to drain the area. If the patient is normotensive, there is probably no need to insert any sutures, although most surgeons choose to close the laceration with absorbable sutures when the lesion is superficial to produce a local tamponading effect. When good local control of bleeding and bile leakage is obtained, drainage of the area is superfluous and possibly predisposes to infection (23). Conversely, if there is any question about the quality of hemostasis, a Jackson-Pratt drain or similar soft sump drain should be brought out from the area through a separate incision and removed after 24 to 36 hours unless a significant amount of drainage continues.

In the other 20% of cases, the surgical approach is complicated by the presence of active bleeding from deep in a stab wound, parenchymal crack, or missile track. The principles accepted elsewhere in the body apply to the liver too. Good exposure and accurate ligation of any bleeding point is always desirable. In the liver, this objective may be achieved by deliberate extension of the parenchymal wound so that the floor and the walls of any track or cavity may be inspected. Use of the electrocautery and knife handle, together with finger-fracture, reduce the amount of bleeding caused by this iatrogenic extension of the wound, using the same principles that are applied to hepatic lobectomy. Individual vessels and bile ducts are suture-ligated or hemoclipped as they are encountered. At the end of the procedure, it is likely that the wound will be large; most such wounds are better drained. If the damaged area is fairly extensive, some surgeons favor the insertion of a pedicle of vascularized omentum—a so-called omental pack—to act as a tamponading and hemostatic agent (24). Care must be taken, however, to ensure that the omentum acts as a pack and not a plug that prevents the egress of active bleeding and leads to the collection of blood under high pressure.

Iatrogenic extension of the wound is easy when the laceration is situated in a readily accessible part of the liver or where the missile track is superficial. In contrast, when the missile track passes deeply through the liver parenchyma or when the hepatic fracture is situated under the dome of the diaphragm, control of bleeding and decisions associated with it become much more complex. In these circumstances, good mobilization of the liver is essential. With the falciform and round ligaments transected to act as a fulcrum of retraction helping to dislocate the liver, the coronary and triangular ligaments are incised round to the "bare area" posteriorly. Firm compression of the bleeding area by an assistant is essential while this is done. Once successful mobilization has been completed, the liver may be brought to the surface of the abdomen and the injured portion brought under direct vision. It is important not to preface the decision to mobilize the liver with repetitive frustrating attempts to visualize the area of bleeding by pulling on the unmobilized liver. When this is attempted, the cracks in the liver are often iatrogenically enlarged. It has been estimated that each such attempt may result in the loss of 200 to 300 ml of blood and expose the patient to the ever-present hazard of air embolism due to the differences in pressure between the open abdomen and the closed chest. Such substantial losses of blood cause further rapid deterioration in the general condition of the patient and may result in death on the operating table. This phase of the operation may be the most critical as opening of any hematoma posteriorly may result in torrential hemorrhage for which the surgical team should be prepared.

Once the liver has been delivered as a mobile, almost midline organ, care is taken not to rotate the liver excessively or to place packs or retractors in such a way as to limit the return of blood through the IVC to the right atrium. With the liver under direct vision, extensive resectional-débridement may now be undertaken and individual sources of bleeding ligated or clipped. In patients in whom a missile track has passed deeply through the liver, this track may be opened and a limited local resection performed. The middle hepatic vein is preserved whenever possible. At the end of the debridement, which may involve many different

segments of the liver, it is necessary to ensure hemostasis and bilostasis but it is not necessary to produce a cosmetically tidy liver. If oozing continues, some surgeons prefer to apply microcrystalline collagen or one of the newer antithrombin agents, with or without the application of omentum sewn over the area. When the latter is done, it is important to ensure that any blood and bile that may collect under the omentum has access to the drains that will need to be placed into position.

Certain caveats and alternatives warrant mention. The closure of deep stab wounds to the liver with suturing of the solitary entrance wound may be extremely dangerous. If bleeding continues within the parenchyma and the blood cannot decompress into the peritoneal cavity, excessive tension may build up within the liver over a matter of 12 to 24 hours, produce necrosis by pressure, and almost literally explode the lobe with consequent exsanguinating bleeding. A similar principle applies to the through-and-through missile wound that continues to bleed and that may be very difficult to manage if the track is not fully opened. It has been customary over the years to insert blindly a series of interrupted absorbable sutures with blunt-nosed liver needles at intervals of approximately 1 centimeter, with the sutures placed approximately 1 cm from the margins of the lesion. The intent has been to approximate the walls of the defect and by this maneuver, together with any incidental hemostatic effects of the ligatures, produce hemostasis. In practice, this maneuver is usually effective but it should be recognized that it cannot be totally relied upon. In recent years, this basic technique has been supplanted by direct visualization whenever possible. Some surgeons, reluctant to open tracks, have tried to compromise by placing some sutures blindly and then by insertion of a catheter placed on low suction into the track. This approach is even more uncertain and may, in fact, have the effect of removing essential clot. Variations on this theme are to be found. Bluett et al. (25) successfully produced hemostasis in nine penetrating wounds by placing a collection of 1-inch Penrose drains in the track to produce a tamponading effect. The drains were brought out through the abdominal wall and then slowly removed after about a week.

In 1987, use has been advocated of a special balloon catheter designed to exercise pressure on the walls of the track (26), much as was successfully reported by Schroeder in 1906 (2). While these nondefinitive attempts to produce hemostasis may be successful, none can be as certain as direct surgical visualization and occlusion of the bleeding points.

Enthusiasm for ligation of the hepatic artery blossomed rapidly in the early 1970s when it was realized that the common, right, or left hepatic arteries (but probably not the hepatic artery proper) can be ligated with few obvious clinical signs, thus contradicting a long-held belief that this action was usually lethal. Application of hepatic artery ligation was initially excessive and applied indiscriminately, as reflected in the 33.1% incidence in one series of 178 patients (27). As of 1987, the place of hepatic artery ligation had been clarified. Today, this technique is used in not more than 1% to 2% of patients with liver injury and is in essence a rival to subtotal or total lobectomy. Hepatic artery ligation may be tentatively tried when hepatic bleeding is arterial and incompletely responsive to local débridement or ligation of vessels in the injured parenchyma. Although the immediate reward may be rapid hemostasis, the delayed penalty may be local ischemia with subsequent sepsis, in which case exitus by infection may replace death by hemorrhage. In about 10% of patients in whom one or other hepatic artery is ligated, delayed rebleeding occurs anywhere from 24 hours after collaterals have opened to 10 to 14 days, usually a manifestation of secondary hemorrhage.

If the common hepatic or right hepatic artery is ligated, the gallbladder should be removed. In practice, the type of lesion that may lead to the use of hepatic ligation will not infrequently have damaged the gallbladder itself or the hilar area. Hepatic artery ligation, like packing, is not a substitute for assiduous attempts at local hemostasis.

In the United States, lobectomy for liver injury is done in only 2% to 4% of patients today. The mortality rate remains high and is estimated at 40% or more in most institutions. The use of the more conservative measures that are focused on local hemostasis produces better overall survival rates. This approach constrasts with that of Balasegaram (28), who reported 94 major hepatic resections in a series of 443 patients in Malaysia with a mortality rate of only 10.3% for the resections but an overall mortality rate of 15.3% for the entire series. The elapsed time from injury, the nature of the injuries, and the remarkably low incidence of concomitant injuries distinguishes this unique series from the type of hepatic injury encountered in the United States. Hepatic lobectomy is unavoidable in the patient with a shattered or completely devitalized lobe, or in whom parenchymal bleeding cannot be controlled by any other approach. Ideally the decision to perform a lobectomy should be made when the patient is not in deep or prolonged shock and every effort should be made to reduce hemorrhage by careful and sustained manual pressure while lobectomy is being performed. Hemostasis may be helped by a Penrose drain slung round the mobilized lobe or by the use of a special liver clamp. Although the principles associated with elective lobectomy pertain, lobectomy for trauma tends to be a less orderly procedure. A Pringle's maneuver is helpful; the appropriate hepatic vessels and bile ducts are ligated at the hilum; the line of ischemic demarcation is incised by the electrocautery; the parenchyma is separated by finger fracture with ligation or clipping of individual vessels; the posterior veins entering the IVC are occluded before they can be torn; and in right lobectomies, the large right hepatic vein is clamped within a fringe of parenchyma rather than neatly dissected and clamped as in elective procedures. Hemostasis of the residual liver surface is obtained, and may sometimes be supplemented by microcystalline collagen or omentum applied to the raw transected area.

As with any serious liver injury, drains are placed in the region of the resection and brought out laterally. Sump drains are usually employed, with or without a collection of Penrose drains. Some surgeons still favor removal of the 12th rib as the site of exit but most feel this to be unnecessary or even undesirable. Drains are left only as long as they are producing material, and can usually be removed within a week. During this time, the exit site must be kept meticulously clean to avoid the ingress of organisms. Drainage of the Penrose drains into a colostomy bag may be helpful.

Whereas T-tube drainage was a standard addition in major hepatic injuries until the early 1970s, the fact that the T-tube serves no purpose and may lead to infection, ductal damage, and erosive gastritis is now universally accepted (29). A T-tube should only be inserted when the extrahepatic biliary ducts are injured or when bile is to be diverted from the duodenum.

Hepatic Veins in Hepatic Trauma

Bleeding from the large hepatic veins, usually in the posterocentral area of the liver, is very difficult to control and is a potent cause of death. Access to the area and exposure of the lacerated veins is always associated with substantial or massive fresh bleeding and also the potential hazard of air embolism. Knowledge of the variable patterns of the hepatic venous drainage is important in planning the appropriate technique to obtain hemostasis, including the safe conduct of a lobectomy.

Many studies have been published on the anatomy of the hepatic veins (30,31). All studies agree on the wide variability of distribution of the hepatic veins, if not on the specific numerical distribution of these veins. Failure to recognize the unpredictability of venous drainage may lead to failure of the operation. Emergency surgery on the injured liver differs from elective surgery in certain important ways. The injured patient is often in profound hypovolemic shock, which greatly reduces the margin of physiologic reserve. In addition, hepatic parenchymal life-threatening bleeding has to be controlled at the same time as exposure is being obtained; a tidy and orderly operation may not be possible under these circumstances.

The anatomy of the hepatic veins is variable and individual differences abound but certain broad principles and caveats may be stated.

First, the right hepatic vein (RHV) is the most frequently injured of the large hepatic veins. In patients with this injury who survive to reach the hospital, the injury is much more likely to be in the intraparenchymal section of the vein than the free extrahepatic portion, which varies in length from 1 millimeter to 3 cm and has an average length of about 1.7 cm. The vein is often surrounded by a substantial fibrous sheath that extends into the parenchyma. Dissection of this portion of the vein may lead to an increased functional length of about 2 cm but this dissection is seldom feasible during emergency surgery. Tributaries joining the extrahepatic venous segment are not uncommon, thereby compounding the lethality of this lesion. Of those who survive RHV injury, almost all have penetrating rather than blunt injuries. Blunt injuries tend to shear the veins off the inferior vena cava, producing massive untamponaded hemorrhage, and these patients also have other hepatic and extrahepatic injuries. For anatomic reasons, it is therefore rare to be able to repair a major tear in the extrahepatic RHV. In lobectomy for trauma due to superoposterior injury with intraparenchymal RHV injury, the final transection of the liver is often more safely accomplished by placing hemostats through the parenchyma to include the hepatic vein rather than seeking to expose the RHV precisely for purposes of ligation.

In children, access to the RHV may be easier than in adults as the clinical picture tends to unfold more slowly and the injury is often less extensive when an isolated injury is present. Direct repair of the hepatic vein in the child is more likely to be feasible as direct surgical access through a median sternotomy and incision of the diaphragm to the IVC is easier.

Second, the right lobe of the liver is also drained by the middle hepatic vein (MHV); fairly constant posterolateral, posterior, and posteroinferior hepatic veins, a series of 5 to 20 small veins; and 2 caudate veins that pass directly from the posterior surface of the liver into the IVC.

When a right hepatic lobectomy is performed, attention should be directed to the RHV to the exclusion of the other veins draining the right lobe posteriorly. The need to preserve the MHV, which drains both the right and a portion of the left lobe, is widely recognized. The MHV usually begins deep in the liver and runs almost vertically to become superficial near its entry into the IVC. The MHV runs along a line roughly joining the gallbladder to the IVC diaphragmatic opening, and should be protected during resectional débridement and partial lobectomy to the extent possible.

The posterior and posteroinferior veins may be large. The posteroinferior vein in particular may be long (up to 1.5 cm) and on occasion may be almost as large as the RHV. The entry point of the posteroinferior vein into the IVC varies but is to be found anywhere between 3 and 7 cm below the point at which the right and left hepatic veins enter. These posterior veins may be the source of excessive intraoperative hemorrhage and therefore should be ligated or hemoclipped in continuity when the right lobe is mobilized during right hepatectomy. Loss of control of these sometimes neglected veins may easily lead to exsanguination.

Third, the left hepatic vein (LHV) is of variable length, ranging from a few millimeters to 3 cm.

While the LHV usually has a single entry point into the IVC, some patients may have one to three separate openings. Relationships of the LHV and the MHV vary widely and this confluence determines the local anatomy. In about 75% of patients, the MHV joins the LHV after a short extrahepatic course of about 1 cm to form a common vein of about 1 cm in length. In about 25% of patients, however, the MHV opens into the IVC separately from the LHV.

Fourth, theoretically, ligation of a large hepatic vein should be followed by resection of the parenchyma, which it drains so as to avoid congestion, hypoxemia, and necrosis. While in practice this is done almost invariably, there are reports of ligation of the left and middle hepatic veins (subsequently proven by venography) where the parenchyma has regained reasonable color and turgor intraoperatively and the patient has recovered well, despite the fact that the subtended parenchyma has not been resected (32). The degree of collateral venous drainage within the liver is probably greater than is conventionally accepted.

Approaches to Injuries of the Hepatic Veins and Inferior Vena Cava

As might be expected, most patients who survive long enough to reach the operating room have some natural containment of the perihepatic hemorrhage, which may be supplemented by temporary local pressure at laparotomy. Following the introduction of the atrial caval shunt (ACS) in 1968, uncertainty clouded its precise role in the salvage of patients with complex hepatic injuries. Only patients who have sustained really significant hepatic or extrahepatic venous injury, often with an element of massive parenchymal injury, qualify for the use of an intracaval shunt. Most of these patients have been in deep shock for a variable period. The mortality rate following the use of the ACS is predictably very high and is likely to be 100% if the technique has not been practiced in the morgue or laboratory preoperatively. As the reported results will also reflect the selection of cases, data on ACS should not be taken at their face value. In the mid-1970s a few relatively successful series were partly attributable to the use of the ACS in a number of highly favorable patients who could more easily have been managed by a direct approach to the bleeding

area through the hepatic parenchyma (4). With a greater readiness on the part of surgeons to mobilize the liver and to use adjunctive packing, ACS has become less commonly used in recent years. Above all, a rapid transhepatic finger-fracture approach down to the area of the injury with local ligation or venous repair under direct vision has an increasing number of adherents and may achieve superior results, such as those reported in the Bellevue series where both packing and shunting have been virtually abandoned (7). As part of the direct attack on complex vascular injuries, Pachter has employed adjunctive measures including the administration of intravenous methylprednisolone succinate (30 to 40 milligrams per kilogram) as a bolus, iced saline, hypothermia of the liver to reduce metabolism, and, where necessary, occlusion of the portal triad for periods in excess of the traditional 15 to 20 minutes. Few surgeons favor the use of steroids, which theoretically may predispose to the development of sepsis due to immunosupression, and the deliberate cooling of the liver in these emergency conditions is seldom practiced. Occlusion of the portal triad for an hour or more, however, is tolerated very satisfactorily by most patients although the period of hepatic hypoxia should still be kept to an unavoidable minimum, especially in the shocked patient.

ACS is of greatest value in the patient with a torn hepatic vein or lacerated retrohepatic IVC and bleeding so massive that the site of origin cannot be clearly exposed without the probability of exsanguination. Successful salvage of four of eight patients with very complex venous injuries of this variety has been reported in 1987 (33). If ACS is to be successful, certain principles of selection and management are essential: (a) the patient should be young; (b) the decision to shunt should be made early and, if possible, before large amounts of blood have been given and hypothermia and coagulopathy established; (c) the period of shock should be minimized—it is significant that 4 of the 18 survivors in the San Francisco General Hospital series never had a blood pressure below 80 mmHg at any time (8); (d) penetrating wounds lend themselves to shunting far more often than wounds due to blunt injury in which survival is very rare; (e) patients with a predominantly parenchymal source of bleeding are more likely to survive following shunting than those with central venous lacerations. (f) The team should have practiced the technique.

Of the intracaval shunts, the ACS is the most effective as the concomitant median sternotomy ensures excellent exposure to the supradiaphragmatic IVC and to the area of bleeding. Cardiac massage may be performed if necessary. A 38 or 40 French chest tube rapidly placed through a purse-string suture in the right atrium serves as the shunt. The tube should be carefully guided down the IVC to ensure that it does not pass into the venous laceration, tearing the vein further and virtually ensuring the demise of the patient. Holes must be cut in the atrial portion, the shunt sited with its lumen just below the renal veins, and tapes or tubing placed round the supra- and infra-hepatic vena cava to keep the shunt in position. A Pringle's maneuver is added and, on occasion, temporary clamping of the descending abdominal aorta may be necessary. With the field now relatively dry, direct exposure and repair of the injured veins may be carried out or a hepatic lobectomy performed.

Alternatively, a shunt may be placed through the abdominal IVC below the renal veins or inserted through the femoral vein. These approaches have also been successfully used but have not acquired the same acceptance as the ACS.

As many technical problems remain unresolved, new experimental approaches stimulated by experience with liver transplantation are being explored, such as the shunting of blood around the liver from the femoral vein to the subclavian vein with a rapid transfusion pump in the circuit. Use of heparin in the trauma patient, however, is not practical. Others are attempting to design new catheters with strategically placed balloons.

Finally, two new segments of dogma are being challenged. The first reflects the long-held view that occlusion of the venous return to the heart through the IVC results in shock, arrhythmia, and death. The second concerns the concept that ligation of a major intrahepatic vein inevitably results in necrosis of the subtended tissue and makes hepatic resection mandatory. There have been scattered reports in the past about successful ligation of the suprarenal IVC as a desperate measure. More recently, some surgeons have deliberately occluded the IVC below and above the liver to produce a dry field preparatory to a rapid direct attack on the intra- or retrohepatic site of hemorrhage while administering large volumes of compensatory fluid centrally. Successful use of this technique in prolonged elective hepatic surgery was reported by Huguet in 1978 (34) when he pointed out that humans, unlike dogs and pigs, have a natural venous collateral system and that during long operations, the reduction in core temperature provided by rapid transfusions of blood reduces hepatic metabolism. Results obtained with this approach are thought by some to be more favorable than results with the use of an intracaval shunt. In a few such cases, the injury in the dry field may even lend itself to application of a Satinsky's clamp or the insertion of a Foley catheter to produce temporary hemostasis preparatory to formal repair.

With regard to the ligation of large intrahepatic veins, the conventional view that complete or partial lobectomy is invariably necessitated when one or more of these veins is ligated, is also being questioned today.

Use of the Abdominal Pack

Use of abdominal packing to control hemorrhage fell into disfavor during and after World War II, mainly because of a high associated rate of infection but even more because of the regrettable tendency of surgeons to substitute this technique for proper mobilization of the liver, exposure of the area of the injury, and assiduous accomplishment of hemostasis by ligation of the bleeding points. This retreat from surgical principles well established for other areas of the body inevitably resulted in unacceptably high mortality rates. Unfortunately, these results also served to obscure the small but definite role for packing in selected patients.

The dogmatic rejection of packing under all circumstances was revisited and challenged in the mid-1970s (4), when it was recognized that in certain patients senseless prolongation of the operation in the shocked and oozing patient, instead of a planned and orderly retreat with the help of packs, was a certain recipe for death. Over the period 1977–1987, it has been shown that about 70% of patients survive in whom packing is inserted after attempts at acceptable hemostasis have failed and where the alternative is judged likely to be death. Most of these patients have additional adjunctive hemostatic techniques applied, such as débridement, ligation of a hepatic artery, or ligation of large veins.

Review of the incidence of packing provides us with some perspective. In the Ben Taub Hospital (35) and San Francisco General Hospital (36) experience, packing was used in 66 of 1348 patients (5.3%), and in 17 of 443 patients (4%) with good results. In contrast, the Lincoln Hospital experience was less satisfactory (37).

The decision to pack remains difficult and should not be abused. Packing is rarely justified for the active high-volume bleeder in the depths of the liver unless the patient is operated on as an emergency by a team with insufficient surgical expertise or in a hospital with inadequate facilities. Except under these latter circumstances, packing is not usually instituted until the liver has been widely mobilized as a preliminary to a full-scale attempt at hemostasis. The main indications for packing are (a) continuing oozing from the liver after maximal attempts at hemostasis have been made and when the oozing is an expression of a coagulopathy resulting from the administration of substantial or massive quantities of blood, (b) persistent bleeding from a relatively inaccessible area of the liver in a patient whose general condition is so poor that continued operation is adjudged to be too hazardous, (c) the presence of a deep crack that extends widely across both lobes of the liver, (d) an extensive nonenlarging subcapsular hematoma, (e) continued oozing from a large raw surface of the liver, and (f) as a temporizing measure in an inadequately equipped institution before transferring the patient to a trauma center.

Certain important principles must be respected when the surgeon resorts to packing. The large, dry gauze packs should be placed against the bleeding area to produce local compression, and this often necessitates packing both above and below the liver. Some continuing postoperative bleeding, albeit slow, may be anticipated. It is customary for the patient to lose 0.5 to 1.5 L blood over the ensuing 2 to 3 days, but blood and clots may collect in the peritoneal cavity producing distention and increased pressure and consequent oliguria. Care must also be taken not to compromise the venous return through the inferior vena cava by the packs as this may result in reduced cardiac output. Excessive intra-abdominal pressure (± about 25 mmHg) may be crudely assessed by indirect measurement of the intraperitoneal pressure through a Foley catheter (38).

Adequate ventilation must be ensured, as the diaphragm may be pushed cephalad and splinted by the presence of the packs, which interfere with ventilation; consequently, intratracheal intubation needs to be prolonged. Sepsis is an ever-present danger in the presence of packs with a varying reported incidence—40% in the Wayne State University series. While in the past some surgeons brought the packs out through an incision in the abdominal wall and subsequently removed these gradually, today the accepted technique is to close the abdomen over the packs, which are then removed later under general anesthesia. The timing of removal varies but ideally should be as early as possible, and removal can usually be accomplished within 48 to 72 hours. The packs should be removed when the patient is hemodynamically stable, normothermic, free of any clinical coagulopathy, and ready to be extubated. At the time of the laparotomy, further significant bleeding is seldom encountered after the pack has been gently removed. The opportunity should be taken, however, to débride obviously ischemic tissue and to check any other questionable areas in the abdomen. If an hepatic artery has been ligated as part of the original operation, the compressive effects of the pack enhance the development of local ischemic parenchyma and increase the potential need for débridement.

In the mid-1980s, mainly in Europe, attempts have been made to achieve hemostasis by the application of fibrin glue (39). Most reports on this biologic adhesive composed of concentrated human fibrinogen and thrombin recount animal experiments, but the mixture has been successfully used in a few humans with hepatic injuries. As yet, fibrin glue has not been released by the Food and Drug Administration. In time, fibrin glue may be of value in desperate cases but will not replace direct ligation of bleeding vessels.

Miscellaneous Complications

Nonoperative Management

Computed tomography scans have confirmed the clinical impression that subcapsular hematomas of the liver, parenchymal cracks, and central collections of blood and bile are far more common than has been previously recognized. As a significant number of such patients are stable and have no other overt intra-abdominal injuries warranting operation, the practice of close observation rather than laparotomy is increasing. Geis, in a series of

65 patients with hepatic injury in a larger group of 283 with severe blunt torso injury, chose to observe 16 (15.4%) (40). Six of the 16 patients required operation over the next month. Similarly, Olsen (41) found that 7 of 320 patients (2.2%) developed delayed parenchymal complications. Consequently, these patients must be closely observed both in hospital and following discharge. The most common complications of nonoperative treatment are continued enlargement of the hepatic hematoma with delayed severe hemorrhage, disruption of the liver if the bleeding is initially contained within the organ, sepsis, hemobilia, post-traumatic cyst formation, and arteriovenous fistulae. Consequently, a fall in hemoglobin, enlargement of an hepatic defect on sonography or CT scan, a developing hepatomegaly, fever, hematemesis, or melena are all indications for emergency measures.

Hemobilia

Hemobilia is an uncommon sequela of hepatic injury (42). Previously viewed almost exclusively in the context of blunt or penetrating major trauma, the majority of cases as of the time of writing are of an iatrogenic nature due to biopsy, percutaneous cholangiography, or the insertion of a stent. In classical external trauma, the incidence of hemobilia is about 0.002% as judged by only four cases of our last 1635 hepatic injuries.

Clinically, the hemobilia may appear early or be delayed for a year or more, may be small in quantity and intermittent or rapid and persistent, and may present as melena or hematemesis. Jaundice and fever may or may not be present. Occasionally, pigmented gallstones may be a subsequent complication.

Diagnosis is made by arteriography. With the advent of selective embolization through a catheter placed in the hepatic artery, the need for laparotomy and a direct attack on the parenchymal cavity is rarely necessary unless sepsis is present and catheter drainage is not feasible (43). Some small peripheral lesions have been observed to stop bleeding spontaneously and then regress, especially in children (44). Adoption of a plan that does not seek actively to occlude the vessel places the onus of failure directly on the physician and is a risky course to follow.

Biliary Fistulas

Bile ducts are almost inevitably damaged in any appreciable liver injury. Leakage of bile into the peritoneal cavity has been demonstrated angiographically, isotopically, and by direct vision. In most cases, symptoms are few and the bile leakage ceases spontaneously. On occasion, however, a bile leak may present as peritonitis or as a fistula through the abdominal wall, into the pleural cavity, or rarely into a bronchus (45). Most abdominal-biliary fistulae close within 1 to 6 weeks unless originating from an extrahepatic duct or a large intraparenchymal defect. The extent of the leak can often be delineated by a fistulogram and a direct surgical approach made to the area.

Bronchopleural leaks are drained through a thoracostomy tube in the first place (46). If draining persists, a thoracotomy is necessary with débridement of the source, ligation of the offending lesion, closure of the hole in the diaphragm, and rarely cortication of the lung.

Bronchobiliary fistulas are rare but may cause rapid death by flooding the bronchial tree with bile. The presence of bile in the sputum may be delayed but is always an ominous warning sign that demands immediate investigation. Excision of the fistula by means of a difficult lower lobectomy is usually necessary.

Arteriovenous fistula, not unexpectedly, are often demonstrable when arteriography is performed soon after hepatic injury. Most of these fistula heal spontaneously and rapidly. However, at least 15 cases have been reported where the arteriovenous fistula caused serious symptoms reflecting the chronicity and large size of the fistula. Clinical manifestations include an hepatic bruit, local hemorrhage, portal hypertension, esophageal varices, and upper gastrointestinal bleeding. Treatment by embolization with coils or other agents is usually effective, but operation may be necessary in the rare larger lesions. The varices disappear rapidly after successful occlusion of the fistula (47).

Conclusion

The great majority of liver injuries pose few technical problems to the surgeon; some blunt injuries, demonstrated on CT scan, may be followed nonoperatively. Fifteen percent of liver injuries, however, require a therapeutic selection from among a number of different approaches, and decisions may have to be made urgently regarding a patient who is in hypovolemic shock. Hemorrhage is always the immediate danger and is most threatening when originating from behind the liver or from deep within the parenchyma. In some cases, invaluable time may be bought by local compression while intensive fluid resuscitation is undertaken. In other patients, even this may not be feasible and a direct attack on the bleeding area through the parenchyma, with or without an intracaval shunt, may be unavoidable. In a few cases, this direct aggressive approach may be life-saving. In a small percentage of patients with a contained hemorrhage low-pressure bleed, or oozing due to the coagulopathy of shock and massive blood transfusions, temporizing packing may be optimal.

Over the decade 1977–1987, the importance of wide mobilization of the liver and adequate exposure has been universally accepted. Current research is concentrating on the development of occluding balloons, perihepatic shunts, and the local application of hemostatic substances such as fibrin sealant and coagulating lasers.

With the mortality of liver injury virtually plateaued in most institutions and an extensive experience with liver injuries, future advances will lie principally with the accurate objective demonstration by noninvasive means of how unneeded operations may be avoided and at the other extreme by very rapid control of hepatic injury before recalcitrant shock has supervened.

References

1. Mayer L. *Die Wunde der Leber and Gallerblase*. 1982.
2. Schroder WE. The progess of liver hemostasis—reports of cases. *Surg Gynecol Obstet* 1906; 2:52–61.
3. Pringle JH. Notes on the arrest of hepatic hemorrhage due to trauma. *Ann Surg* 1908; 48:541–549.
4. Walt AJ. The mythology of hepatic trauma or Babel revisited. *Am J Surg* 1978; 135:12–18.
5. DeFore WW, Mattox KL, Jordan GL, et al. Management of 1590 consecutive cases of liver trauma. *Arch Surg* 1976; 111:493–497.
6. Trunkey DD, Shires GT, McClelland R. Management of liver trauma in 811 consecutive patients. *Ann Surg* 1974; 179:722–728.
7. Pachter HL, Spencer FC, Hofstetter SR, et al. The management of juxtahepatic venous injuries without an atriocaval shunt: Preliminary clinical observations. *Surgery* 1986; 99:569–575.
8. Kudsk KA, Sheldon GF, Lim RC. Atrial-caval shunting (ACS) after trauma. *J Trauma* 1982; 22:81–85.
9. Walt AJ. Trauma to the liver. In: Moody FG, Carey LC, Jones RS, Kelly KA, Nahrwold DL, Skinner DB, eds. *Surgical Treatment of Digestive Disease*. Chicago: Year Book Medical, 1986, pp. 397–408.
10. Feliciano DV, Jordan GL, Bitondo CG, et al. Management of 1000 consecutive cases of hepatic trauma (1979–1984). *Ann Surg* 1986; 204:438–445.
11. Moore EF. Critical decisions in the management of hepatic trauma. *Am J Surg* 1984; 148:712–716.
12. Hanna SS, Maheshwari Y, Harrison AW, et al. Blunt liver trauma at the Sunnybrook Regional Trauma Unit. *Can J Surg* 1985; 28:220–223.
13. Little JM, Fernandes A, Tait N. Liver trauma. *Aust NZ J Surg* 1986; 56:613–619.
14. Stalter KD, Sterling WA. Hepatic subcapsular hemorrhage associated with pregnancy. *Surgery* 1985; 98:112–114.
15. Trunkey D, Federle MP. Editorial—Computed tomography in perspective. *J Trauma* 1986; 26:660–661.
16. Moon KL, Federle MP. Computed tomography in hepatic trauma. *AJR* 1983; 141:309–314.
17. Weissman HS, Byun KJ, Freeman LM. IDA scintigraphy in the evaluation of hepatobiliary trauma. *Semin Nucl Med* 1983; 13:199–212.
18. Gartman DM, Zeman RK, Cahow CE, et al. The value of hepatobiliary scanning in complex liver trauma. *J Trauma* 1985; 25:887–891.
19. Ledgerwood AM, Kazmers M, Lucas CE. The role of thoracic aortic occlusion for massive hemoperitoneum. *J Trauma* 1976; 16:610–615.
20. Cywes S, Rode R, Millar AJW. Blunt liver trauma in children: Nonoperative management. *J Pediatr Surg* 1985; 20:14–18.
21. Giacomantonio M, Filler RM, Rich RH. Blunt hepatic trauma in children: Experience with operative and nonoperative management. *J Pediatr Surg* 1984; 19:519–522.
22. Oldham KT, Guice KS, Ryckman F, et al. Blunt liver injury in childhood: Evolution of therapy and current perspective. *Surgery* 1986; 100:542–549.
23. Fischer RP, O'Farrell KA, Perry JF. The value of peritoneal drains in the treatment of liver injuries. *J Trauma* 1978; 18:393–398.
24. Stone HH, Lamb JM. Use of pedicled omentum as an autogenous pack for control of hemorrhage in major injuries of the liver. *Surg Gynecol Obstet* 1975; 141:92–94.
25. Bluett MK, Woltering E, Adkins RB. Management of penetrating hepatic trauma. *Am Surg* 1984; 50:132–142.
26. Morimoto RY, Birolini D, Junqueira AR, et al. Balloon tamponade for transfixing lesions of the liver. *Surg Gynecol Obstet* 1987; 164:87–88.
27. Flint LM, Mays ET, Aaron WS, et al. Selectivity in the management of hepatic trauma. *Ann Surg* 1977; 185:613–618.
28. Balasegaram MB, Joisny S. Hepatic resection in trauma. In: Shires GT, ed. *Advances in Surgery*. Chicago: Year Book Medical, 1984, pp. 129–170.
29. Lucas CE, Walt AJ. Analysis of randomized biliary drainage for liver trauma in 189 patients. *J Trauma* 1972; 12:925–930.
30. Nakamura S, Tsuzuki T. Surgical anatomy of the hepatic veins and the inferior vena cava. *Surg Gynecol Obstet* 1981; 152:43–50.
31. Hardy KJ. The hepatic veins. *Aust NZ J Surg* 1972; 42:11–14.
32. Depinto DJ, Mucha SJ, Powers PC. Major hepatic vein ligation necessitated by blunt abdominal trauma. *Ann Surg* 1975; 183:243–246.
33. Rovito PF. Atrial caval shunting in blunt hepatic vascular injury. *Ann Surg* 1987; 205:318–321.
34. Huguet C, Nordlinger B, Bloch P, et al. Tolerance of the

human liver to prolonged normothermic ischemia. *Arch Surg* 1978; 113:1448–1451.

35. Feliciano DV, Mattox KL, Burch JM, et al. Packing for control of hepatic hemorrhage. *J Trauma* 1986; 26:738–743.

36. Carmona RH, Peck DZ, Lim RC. The role of packing and planned reoperation in severe hepatic trauma. *J Trauma* 1984; 24:779–784.

37. Ivatury RR, Nallathambi M, Gunduz Y, et al. Liver packing for uncontrolled hemorrhage: A reappraisal. *J Trauma* 1986; 26:744–753.

38. Kron IL, Harman PK, Nolan SP. The measurement of intraabdominal pressure as a criterion for abdominal re-exploration. *Ann Surg* 1984; 199:28–30.

39. Giakoustidis E, Drosinopoulos P, Agouridakis K, et al. Surgical treatment of liver injuries by application of fibrinkleber. *World J Surg* 1985; 9:144–148.

40. Geis WP, Schulz KA, Giacchino JL. The fate of unruptured intrahepatic hematomas. *Surgery* 1981; 90:689–697.

41. Olsen WR. Late complications of central liver injuries. *Surgery* 1982; 92:733–743.

42. Goodnight JE, Blaisdell FW. Hemobilia. *Surg Clin North Am* 1981; 61:973–979.

43. Sclafani SJA, Shaftan GW, McAuley J, et al. Interventional radiology in the management of hepatic trauma. *J Trauma* 1984; 24:256–262.

44. Lockwood TE, Schorn L, Coln D. Nonoperative management of hemobilia. *Ann Surg* 1977; 185:335–340.

45. Boyd DP. Bronchobiliary fistulas. *Ann Thorac Surg* 1977; 24:481–487.

46. Franklin DC, Mathai J. Biliary pleural fistula; a complication of hepatic trauma. *J Trauma* 1980; 20:256–258.

47. Missavage AE, Jones AM, Walt AJ, et al. Traumatic hepatic arteriovenous fistula. *J Trauma* 1984; 24:355–358.

Editorial Comment

This excellent, complete, and well-organized review of the problems of liver trauma leaves little for the editor to accomplish in either additions or critique.

One problem that has been well-described on page 421 might benefit from further emphasis. It concerns the type of compression blunt trauma that results in massive hemorrhage but at laparotomy will show little except an innocuous stellate laceration on the posterior superior surface of the liver; it may not be bleeding actively and may not be easily visible. If the surgeon is lulled by the appearance and by the absence of visible hemorrhage into closing the abdomen, the extensive internal damage in which a large segment of the parenchyma of the right lobe is transformed into a clotted pulp, further lethal hemorrhage may occur or the cavity becomes infected and require extensive resection and drainage. A finger inserted into the laceration on the surface will reveal, by the feel of the mushy interior, the extent of the damage. Evacuation, débridement (or even resection), and hemostasis at that time will preclude the other life-threatening eventualities.

In terms of operative approach, the surgeon should always be prepared to extend the incision (either subcostal or mid-line) into the chest because of the frequent need to control the hepatic veins and the suprahepatic cava.

What is particularly impressive about this chapter is the meticulous description of operative approaches and maneuvers. This was not written by a theoretician with limited personal experience!

Chapter 20
Hepatic Tumors

BLAKE CADY

The surgery of liver tumors has become relatively standardized, with various procedures that are well recognized and performed by many surgeons with low operative mortality rates. In addition, the entire area of judgments about suitable candidates for liver tumor resection has been thoroughly investigated with a myriad of articles over the past fifteen years, so that now general criteria for liver tumor resection are fairly well recognized. This chapter deals with the natural history, presentation, and surgical therapy of a variety of liver tumors that constitute the most common neoplasms occurring in the liver.

Benign Liver Tumors

Benign liver tumors are not uncommon and in autopsy studies can be demonstrated as frequently as 1 or 2 cases out of every 100 (1). Although a variety of unusual and rare liver tumors occur that need not be mentioned here, the most common liver tumor in overall incidence and the most common benign liver tumor that the surgeon will need to address regarding decisions about management is hemangioma (1–6). The natural history of hemangiomas of the liver is not well worked out and is made confusing by the fact that occasional giant hemangiomas in the neonatal period undergo progressive growth to attain a huge size. Hemangiomas are considered hamartomatous and not neoplastic. In adults large hemangiomas rarely spontaneously rupture (5), occasionally seem to increase in size, sometimes have episodes of pain related to thrombosis of portions of the hemangioma, and sometimes produce massive bleeding when undergoing liver needle biopsy or even incisional biopsy in the operating room. Thus the potential for disaster with hemangiomas is well recognized and the incidence of such catastrophe

is unclear but probably extremely low. Hemangiomas can range in size from miniscule to giant hemangiomas, which occupy most of one lobe of the liver or even more. Angiographers frequently encounter hemangiomas as vascular structures in radiologic studies of the liver and can recognize them by the puddling and pooling of dye that occurs in the delayed phase in venous lakes that constitute the hemangioma (7). Thus the radiologic diagnosis of hemangioma is highly accurate and can be achieved by obtaining delayed pictures following hepatic angiography and by the use of computed tomography (CT) with vascular contrast material and repeated images (Fig. 20.1) (8).

Some authors recommend resecting the majority of hemangiomas encountered because of their concern about spontaneous rupture bleeding, pain, and progressive growth (9). However, a recent article from the Mayo Clinic, which followed 49 patients with hemangioma over a long period of time, noted that few required resection and that most resections were done either for complications of inappropriate needle biopsy or because of the unknown nature of the liver tumor (5). They noted as many patients with spontaneous shrinkage over time as with spontaneous progressive growth. Particularly in a group of children with hemangiomas of the liver, they did not show progressive growth in follow-up over several years. In their entire series not a single patient died from unexpected rupture of a hemangioma while being followed. Thus the need to resect a hemangioma of the liver should be seriously questioned, but would seem to be appropriate in patients who have repeated episodes of pain from spontaneous thrombosis or who had bleeding either inadvertently from a needle biopsy or surgical misadventure or from spontaneous rupture. In addition, in

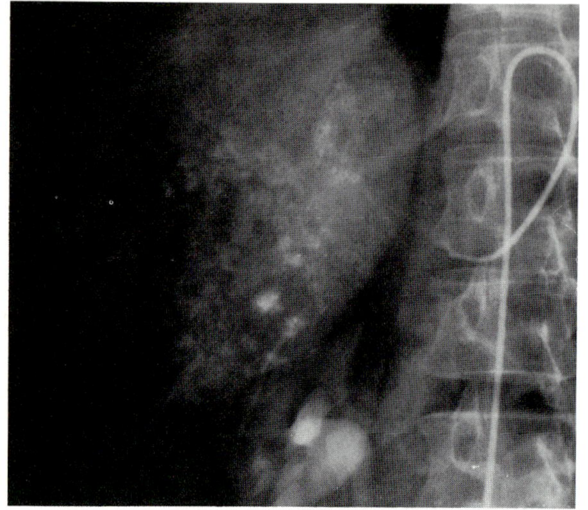

A

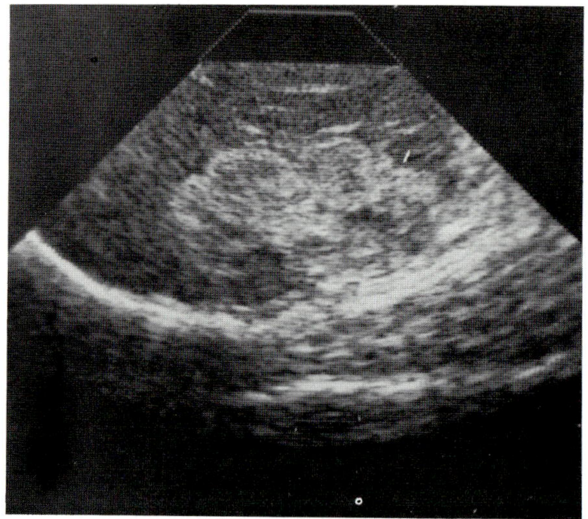

B

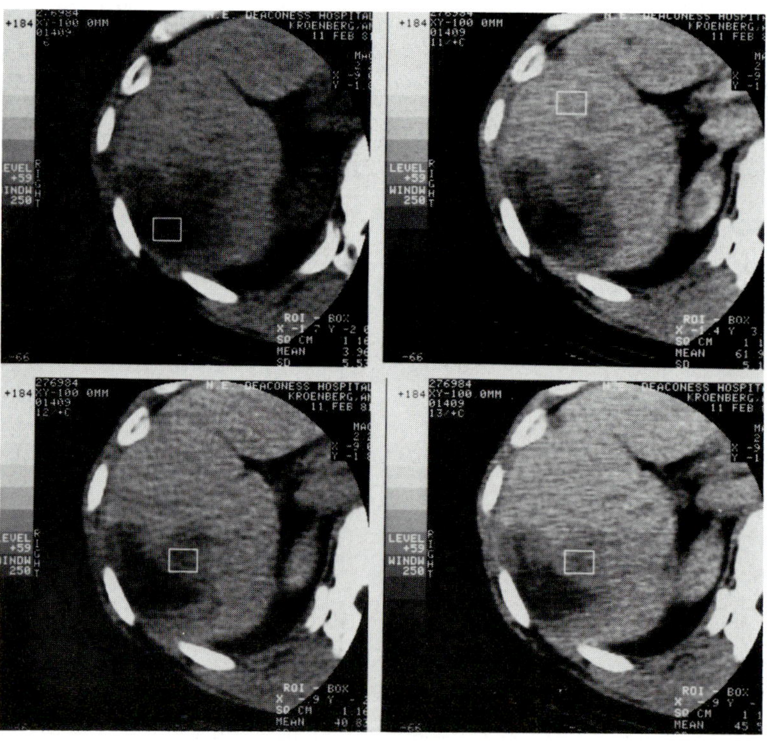

C

patients who had a large tumor that protruded below the costal margin and were in danger of traumatic injury, serious consideration should be given to resection. Similar attitudes are expressed in a 1985 article by Takagi (6). Rarely will lesions less than 4 cm in diameter require surgical resection (6,10,11).

When resection is contemplated, however, it is important to have a tumor that is lateralized enough to offer opportunities for anatomic resection. Surgery of a large hemangioma of the liver, indeed even biopsy, can be fraught with hazard from extraordinary bleeding that is difficult to control. Direct biopsy should be scrupulously avoided and no mass of the liver should be biopsied percutaneously without appreciating its probable nature by preliminary diagnostic workup. Hemangiomas frequently lie in the posterior portion of the posterior segment of the right lobe and this can be suspected by location alone. They rarely cause symptoms or cause any liver function abnormalities, unless very large. Ultrasonic study of the liver can produce the highly suggestive pattern of hemangioma that enables the clinician to undertake a cautious approach and avoid biopsy. Computed tomography with contrast or other diagnostic studies that are possible in hemangioma of the liver include administration of chromium-51-tagged red blood cells with a gamma camera survey of the liver to look for late localization and pooling of the blood in the vascular bed of the hemangioma. The combination of either CT with contrast or angiography with chromium-51-tagged red blood cells can provide an extremely accurate diagnosis of hemangioma. Angiography can provide a definitive diagnosis.

Therapeutic options with hemangiomas of the liver currently should include consideration of the arteriographic obliteration of feeding vessels angiographically before surgery is embarked on (6). The vascular obliteration can be performed by the use of angiographic metal coils, insertion of Ivalon particles, and other powders or material to provide the focus for thrombosis in the lesion. Radiation and the administration of steroids probably do not have any role in control of hemangiomas of the liver and should not be utilized (5,6).

In summary, hemangiomas of the liver are common, and provide frequent diagnostic dilemmas in patients undergoing studies for liver masses or other conditions, particularly cancers, because of the appearance of a mass on scans of the liver. They can be diagnosed with great accuracy nonoperatively. Biopsies should be avoided scrupulously because of the great potential for massive bleeding. Indications for surgery of hemangioma should be extremely limited and restricted to those patients who display multiple episodes of painful thrombosis, documented progression in size, spontaneous hemorrhage, huge size with exposure below the costal margin, hemorrhage after biopsy, or coagulopathy because of platelet consumption.

Focal Nodular Hyperplasia

Focal nodular hyperplasia (FNH) of the liver is a benign condition, sometimes considered localized cirrhosis, hamartomatous malformation, or localized vascular malformation (12) that is seen with some frequency. FNH offers confusion in diagnosis and in distinguishing it from a regenerating nodule in cirrhosis, a liver cell adenoma, or a low-grade hepatoma (Fig. 20.2). Nodules of focal nodular hyperplasia are usually small and asymptomatic and do not bleed spontaneously or with trauma (13). They infrequently exceed 5 centimeters in diameter and are usually less than 2 cm in diameter. Their etiology is unclear and their prime importance is in differentiation from more serious tumors since they seldom cause health problems and rarely are large enough to cause symptoms or undergo rapid enough progressive growth to be of concern. If the diagnosis is confusing they may be resected, and can be biopsied with a needle either intraoperatively or percutaneously under radiologic guidance because they are not highly vascular and do not cause bleeding when traumatized. If

---

Figure 20.1. An angiogram (*A*), ultrasound (*B*), and CT scan (*C*) of cavernous hemangioma. The contrast puddling in the vascular lakes seen on the angiogram is diagnostic. The ultrasound shows a hyperechoic lesion consistent with hemangioma. The CT scan is now frequently used to diagnose hemangiomas without arteriography. The CT scan shows four views of a study, first without contrast material, then after one bolus of contrast dye with filling-in of the periphery of the lesion, and then two views showing continued filling-in of the lesion with contrast material 15 and 20 minutes later, consistent with hemangioma.

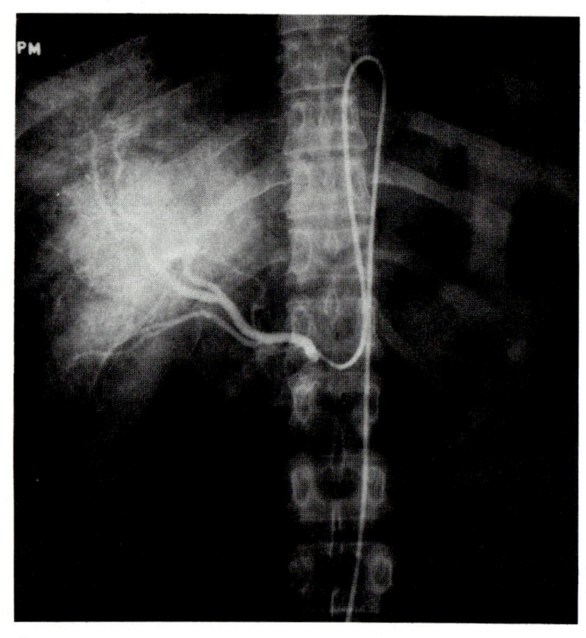

A

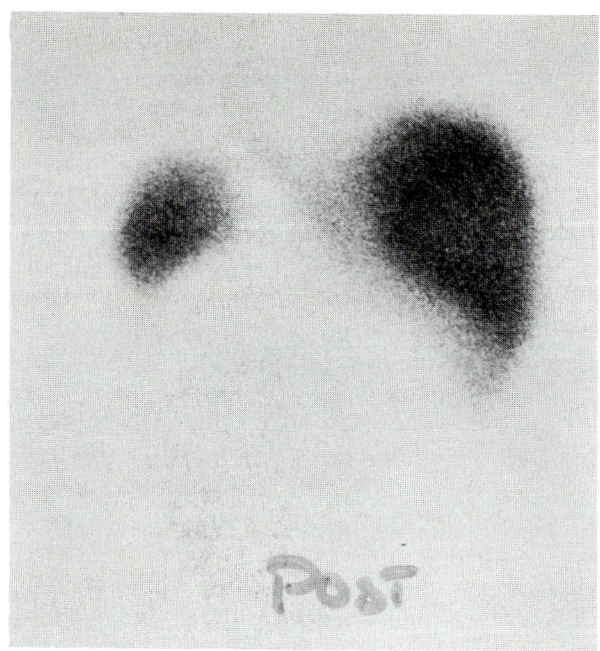

B

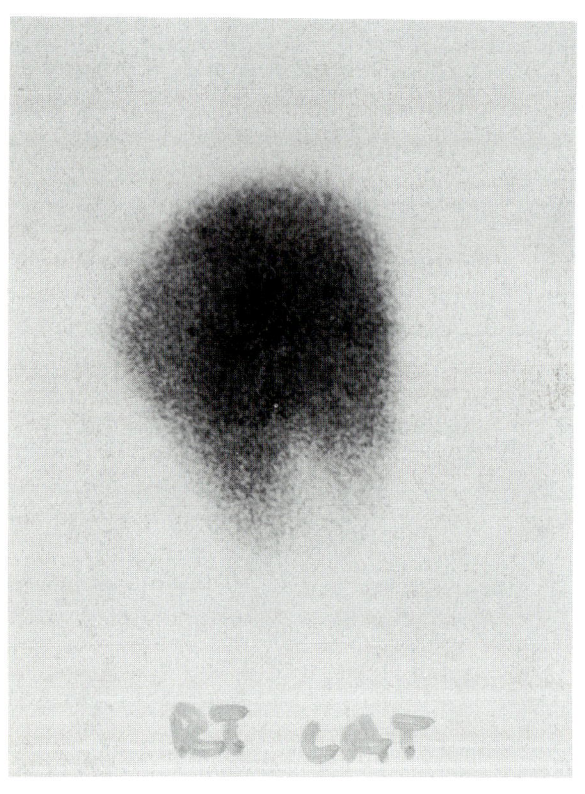

C

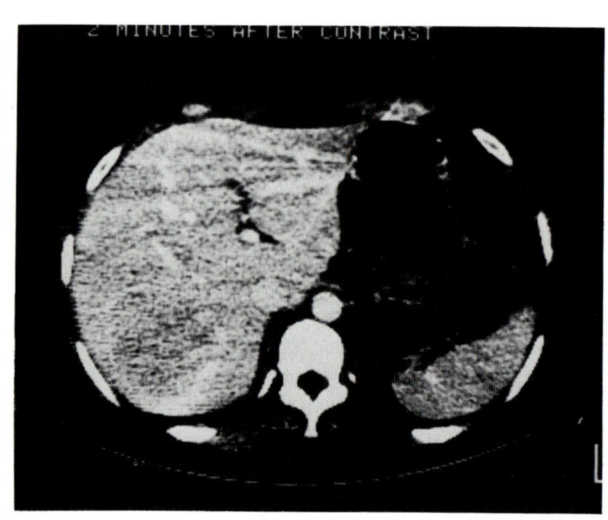

D

Table 20.1.

	Focal Nodular Hyperplasia (%)	Liver Cell Adenoma (%)
Age		
<20 yr	21	8
20–29 yr	21	49
30–39 yr	35	27
>40 yr	24	16
Presentation		
Mass	33	62
Incidental at surgery	52	3
Pain or symptoms	10	5
Rupture-hemorrhage	0	30
Size		
<5 cm	60	5
5–10 cm	16	38
>10 cm	24	52

Adapted by permission from Foster JH, Berman MM. *Solid Liver Tumors. Major Problems in Clinical Surgery*, Vol. 22. Philadelphia: WB Saunders, 1977, pp. 138–178.

after a needle biopsy there is still concern about the nature of the mass, resection may be warranted and should be done in as conservative a fashion as possible.

Table 20.1, adapted from Foster and Berman (13), displays the most useful division between liver cell adenoma and focal nodular hyperplasia. The separation of these two lesions histologically is highly controversial, however, and has not yet been fully resolved by pathologists. In particular, the epidemiology of the two lesions is unknown and there is enough overlap in their presentations so that diagnostic dilemmas arise with some regularity.

Liver Cell Adenoma

Liver cell adenoma (LCA), in contrast to FNH, is slightly less common but considerably more troublesome because of frequent spontaneous rupture, progressive growth, and large size (Fig. 20.3) (13). These lesions are frequently attributed to ingestion of steroid compounds and usually occur in women, but were recorded and well described long before steroids were available (14), and they do occur in men (13). A variety of steroids have been associated with their development including birth control pills, androgens, and cortisone substances. Massive hemorrhage with bleeding into shock and even death have been recorded repeatedly in LCA and therefore whenever LCAs are diagnosed, they should be resected. Generally they can be removed with a conservative margin of liver tissue and do not require an anatomic resection, but when extremely large may warrant even liver transplantation in order to technically remove the entire tumor (9). If patients have not bled from the LCA and have a lesion that is relatively small in size or is diagnosed while actually taking steriod medication, the cessation of steroid ingestion may sometimes cause spontaneous regression (15). Obviously this course of action should not be undertaken in an LCA that is demonstrating complications, particularly bleeding, but may be attempted in small lesions incidentally discovered. Cases have been reported of patients with more than one LCA, and Foster and Berman have described a family in which LCAs and hepatic cell carcinomas both occurred (13). Hepatocellular carcinoma has also been reported in patients who have ingested steroids, but it is not felt that a liver cell adenoma will progress to a hepatocellular carcinoma.

Primary Hepatic Malignancy

While a variety of primary tumors may arise in the liver, hepatocellular carcinoma is by far the most frequent. Cholangiocarcinomas arising from bile duct epithelium also occur in the liver but the ratio between the hepatocellular carcinoma and cholangiocarcinoma runs from 20:1 to 12:1 in various reports (17). Occasionally mixed forms of cancer occur in which features of both hepatocellular and cholangiocarcinoma can be recognized. These are also uncommon. Hepatocellular carcinoma is worldwide in distribution and, in many parts of the underdeveloped world, constitutes one of the

Figure 20.2. Angiograms (*A*) and radionuclide scans (*B, C*) of focal nodular hyperplasia. A catheter has been placed in the right hepatic artery from the superior mesenteric artery and outlines the posterior segment of the right lobe of the liver characterized by a diffuse hypervascular mass. The CT scan (*D*) shows that the mass is actually outlined by a slightly more hypervascular rim. The radionuclide study shows uptake in the lesion that would make it consistent with focal nodular hyperplasia since focal nodular hyperplasia contains Kuppfer's cells.

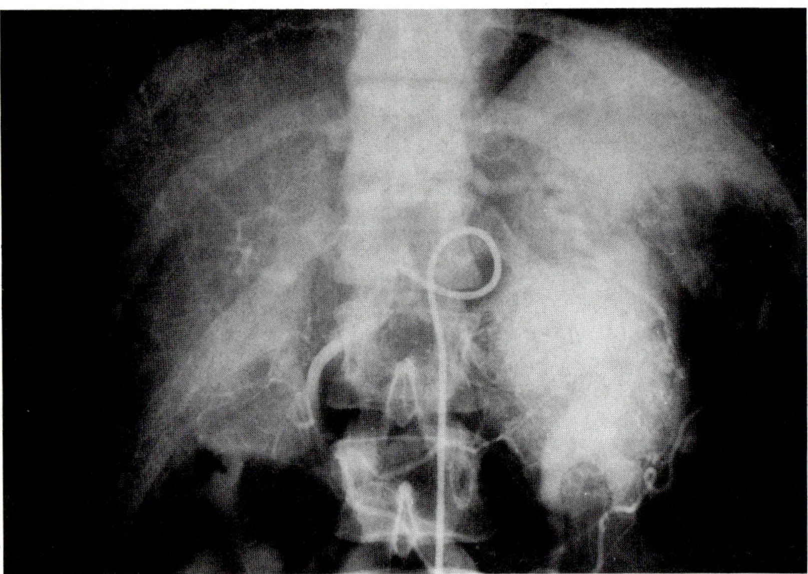

Figure 20.3. Arterial injection showing hypervascular blush in the left lobe of the liver consistent with a liver cell adenoma. Hepatic angiography alone cannot differentiate between benign and malignant tumors. However, a tagged red cell study will diagnose hemangioma, and a radionuclide scan will diagnose either a regenerating nodule or focal nodular hyperplasia by the lack of a "cold" area that would be seen in liver cell adenoma.

leading causes of death from cancer (19). The areas of particularly high risk include East Africa, the countries of Southeast Asia, and parts of the Orient. The epidemiology is undoubtably multifactorial and includes exposure to hepatitis virus; dietary factors, including malnutrition; ingestion of aflatoxins; and other as yet unknown factors. Cirrhosis is a common antecedent to a hepatocellular carcinoma and depending on the nature and etiology of the cirrhosis may demonstrate high incidences of a hepatocellular carcinoma complicating the cirrhosis (20,21). It has been reported that as many as 10% of patients with nutritional cirrhosis may eventually develop hepatoma, sometimes not discovered until autopsy, while the occurrence of cirrhosis secondary to viral hepatitis may produce an incidence of hepatocellular carcinoma of 20%. Untreated hemochromatosis with cirrhosis develops into hepatocellular carcinoma in an even higher percentage of cases (20) and roughtly 40% of patients with alpha$_1$ antitrypsin enzyme deficiency eventually develop hepatocellular carcinoma (22). A minority of hepatocellular carcinomas arise on the background of a noncirrhotic liver. This generally occurs in younger adults or even teenagers. Such patients have a higher frequency of hepatitis B exposure and this infection may play a role in its development (23).

In bottom-dwelling fish of the eastern United States seaboard areas, it has been shown that a high incidence of hepatocellular and cholangiocarcinomas occur in fish from the most contaminated harbors and polluted seawater, presumably with high levels of toxic wastes (24). Certain fish species and poultry and bird species are extraordinarily sensitive to minute amounts of aflatoxin, a toxin from fungal contamination in feed, which produces hepatocellular carcinoma (25). While these facts are well established, and seem to indicate a relationship between certain ingested carcinogenic agents and liver cancer, the incidence of hepatocellular carcinoma in Americans over the past five decades has declined significantly (26).

The possibility of vaccinating high-risk populations against hepatitis B offers the promise of wide-scale control of hepatocellular carcinoma in the Third World, where the high incidence makes it a true public health problem (27). Such a campaign would not be justified in this country because of the low incidence of the disease, and the high incidence of previous hepatitis B exposure in the small population at risk.

The pathologic varieties of hepatocellular carcinoma are quite distinct and involve at least three patterns (28). Hepatocellular carcinoma may grow as a diffuse process throughout the liver with diffuse, multiple nodules either as a result of a true multifocal origin or widespread early interhepatic dissemination from a small focus. The lesion may also arise as a single focus in one area with or without a background of cirrhosis. More recently, a particular variety labeled "fibrolamellar" has been described, which grows as a solitary nodule usually without a background of cirrhosis and displays prolonged survival and a highly suitable situation for surgical resection (29,30). This "fibrolamellar" pattern is quite distinctive microscopically as well as grossly. "Encapsulated" hepatocellular carcinomas are also reported that are not of the distinct "fibrolamellar" histology but of the more common histologic characteristics (31); encapsulated varieties seem to be more slowly progressive, metastasize later, and grow as a single focus. These two biologic varieties have a better prognosis and present much more suitable situations for resection; they represent as many as 10% or more of cases in some series reported (31–33).

A hepatoblastoma occurs in infants and children and has a more benign clinical course, with progressive local growth of a solitary focus, sometimes to a huge size before late dissemination with pulmonary metastases (34). Thus, hepatoblastomas also are highly suitable for surgical resection, sometimes after preliminary chemotherapy to reduce bulk and create a resectable situation (34).

Hepatocellular carcinoma has a propensity for growing into vascular structures, particularly the portal vein; marked exacerbation of portal hypertension may occur with complications of esophageal variceal bleeding and ascites (Fig. 20.4) (35). It may also grow into hepatic veins and may extend intravascularly centrally to the right heart. Occasionally hepatocellular carcinoma may grow intraluminally in the biliary system and produce jaundice, although this is less common (36). Paraneoplastic syndromes including fever, hypercalcemia, polycythemia, and hypoglycemia are not uncommon in hepatocellular carcinoma (37).

The clinical presentation of liver cancer is frequently masked by the underlying cirrhosis. Patients with underlying cirrhosis who are in a relatively steady state may clinically and biochemically deteriorate with the appearance of esophageal bleeding, liver failure, ascites, or pain. Such a sudden worsening of a stable clinical condition may be the result of the progressive growth of hepatocellular carcinoma with destruction of an already compromised hepatic mass or the sudden worsening of the already established portal hypertension. Esophageal bleeding occurs in liver cancer to a large degree in those patients with intraluminal portal venous extension (35). The

appearance of a Budd-Chiari syndrome may likewise herald hepatic venous intraluminal growth.

Some patients do not have previously diagnosed or obvious cirrhosis and present with the onset of pain, mass, liver decompensation, or ascites as their first manifestation of both tumor and cirrhosis. Patients without underlying cirrhosis may also present with a palpable mass, pain, symptoms from displacement of surrounding organs, ascites, bleeding, and evidence of portal hypertension. More subtle indications of hepatic dysfunction may appear such as weight loss, anorexia, etc. Hepatocellular carcinomas may occasionally first present with metastatic disease in bone or lung, but this is relatively uncommon. Spontaneous rupture of hepatic cell carcinoma occurs with some regularity and presents a dramatic picture of intraperitoneal hemorrhage and shock (38,39).

In parts of China where hepatocellular carcinoma is common, public health screening utilizing alpha-fetoprotein determination frequently detects hepatocellular carcinomas at an extraordinarily early stage and may lead to high cure rates by resection (40). Such screening, while not applicable to the population at large in this country because of the low risk of hepatoma, may be suitable for individual cirrhotic patients in follow-up examinations. Such early detection techniques have the possibility of improving survival if resection is possible. Patients with cirrhosis, who on biopsy have evidence of a hepatic cell dyscrasias or dysplasia, are at much higher risk for the development of hepatocellular carcinoma and should be evaluated appropriately or perhaps screened yearly with alpha-fetoprotein determinations (41).

Diagnostic studies in patients suspected of harboring hepatocellular cancer should be utilized to differentiate between progressive cirrhosis and the onset of cancer, by means of enzyme abnormalities, the presence of an elevated alpha-fetoprotein (42), and anatomic studies that display the presence of a mass. Many patients with hepatocellular carcinoma have a negative or normal alpha-fetoprotein; thus a negative test is no assurance that hepatocellular carcinoma does not exist. Anatomic studies of the liver include initial echograms as the least invasive and most cost-effective. Radionuclide scans are less useful in patients with cirrhosis since many underlying anatomic irregularities occur. Computed tomography scans of the liver are

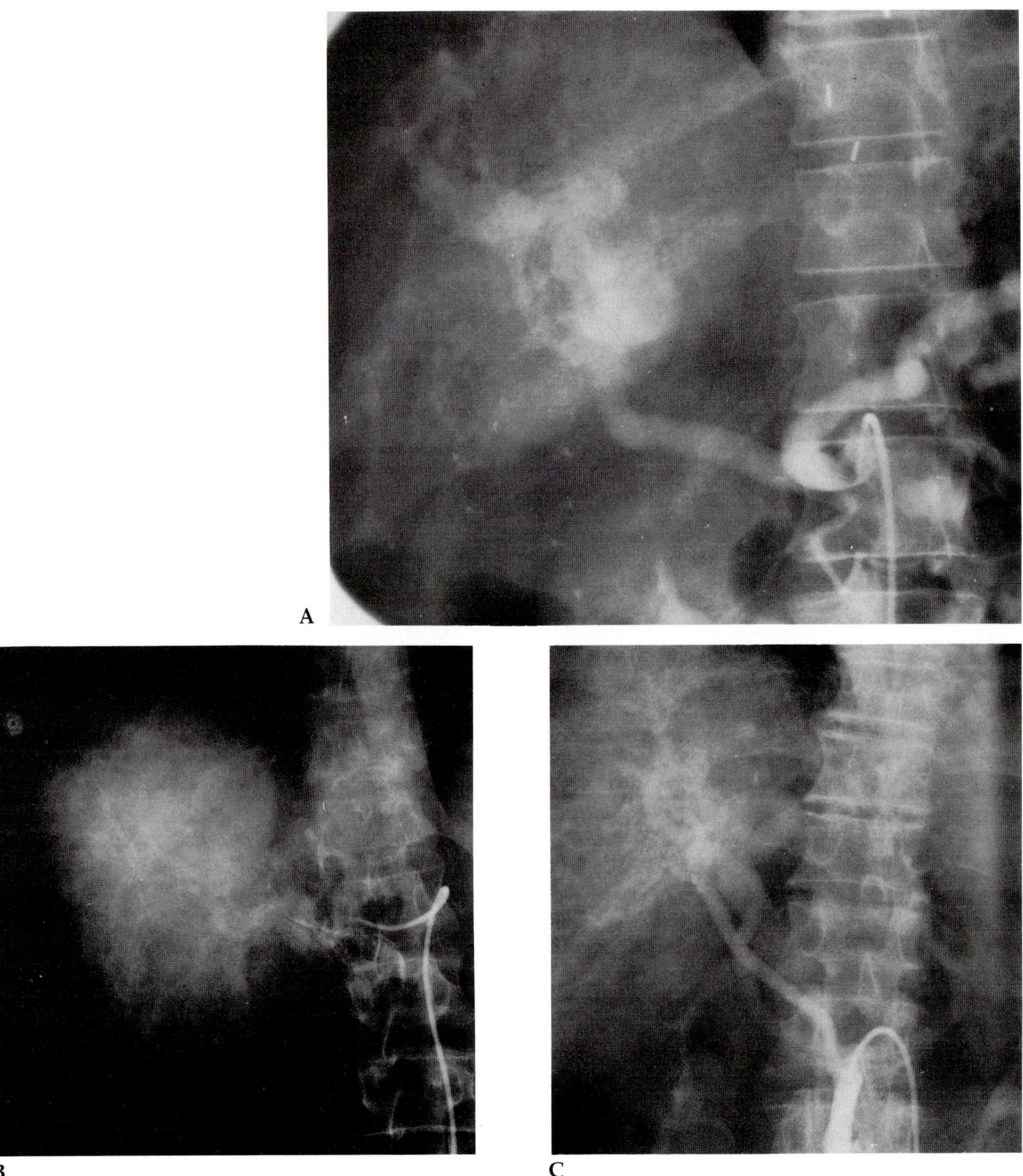

Figure 20.4. (*A*) A celiac arterial injection showing the splenic artery, the common hepatic artery, with rapid filling of the portal vein, which contains a large lucent defect consistent with hepatoma in the portal vein. (*B*) A selective injection into the proper hepatic artery. The film is in the later arterial and midcapillary phase, showing an excellent demonstration of a hypervascular blush throughout the liver consistent with hepatocellular carcinoma. There is a rapid portal vein filling with streaking of the left portal vein consistent with intravascular tumor thrombosis resulting from arterial to portal vein shunting. (*C*) A superior mesenteric artery injection with the right hepatic artery arising from it. Again there is a hypervascular blush in the midportion of the right lobe with rapid filling of the portal vein consistent with arteriovenous shunting and hepatofugal flow from a hepatocellular carcinoma.

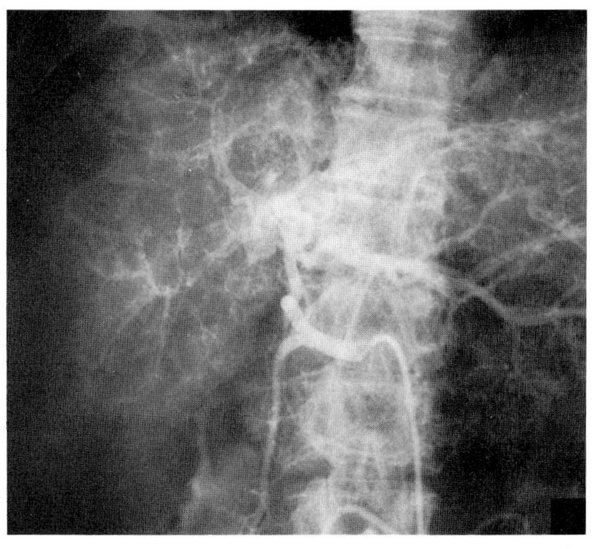

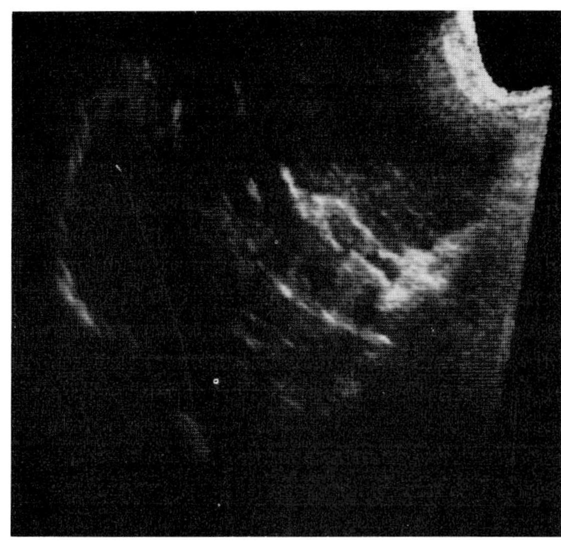

D   E

Figure 20.4 (continued).   (*D*) Hepatoma showing an injection into the common hepatic artery. There is a diffuse hypervascular blush throughout both lobes of the liver with rapid filling of the left as well as the right portal branches. (*E*) Sagittal ultrasound scan showing tumor thrombus in the portal vein.

moderately accurate but not invariably so. Even large hepatomas of the liver can be "blind" to CT scans, particularly in the presence of underlying cirrhosis, which distorts the configuration and normal pattern of the liver parenchyma. Fatty infiltration of the liver in cirrhosis and other situations such as hyperalimentation also render the CT scan less reliable. Computed tomography scans should always be done with contrast agents, which improves their accuracy. Hepatic angiography is highly reliable. Angiographically, only hepatocellular carcinomas, cancers of the pancreatic islet cells, and carcinoid tumors present as hypervascular relative to the surrounding liver (Fig. 20.5 A & B). Rarely will other cancers produce a liver metastasis that is similarly hypervascular. Thus an angiographic hypervascular mass in the liver is almost diagnostic of a hepatocellular carcinoma, if islet cell cancers and carcinoid are excluded. The combination of an alpha-fetoprotein determination that is over 400 milligrams per milliliter (42) and a typical angiogram is equivalent to a histologic diagnosis, eliminating the need for a biopsy in many cases.

Percutaneous transhepatic biopsies of suspected hepatocellular carcinomas should be avoided if the patient is a potential operative candidate because of the extremely vascular nature of these cancers, which can bleed massively and require emergency surgical control.

Once a diagnosis is suspected, surgical resection should be considered in all patients who are feasible resection candidates. Patients with multifocal hepatocellular carcinoma are not candidates for curative resection. Approximately 30% of patients with hepatoma require surgical exploration for complete confirmation of the diagnosis and evaluation of resectability. Large anatomic resections in cirrhotic livers lead to postoperative mortality and liver failure in a high percentage of cases. Peripheral wedge resections of small superficial hepatocellular carcinomas may be carried out on patients with cirrhosis with relative safety, but this is an uncommon clinical situation. In general, the presence of cirrhosis, even of relatively minor physiologic impact, precludes surgical resections of any significant size because of the incapability of hepatic regeneration or hypertrophy. Furthermore, most cancers arising on a background of cirrhosis are multifocal, advanced, and of extremely poor prognosis (18). Several surgeons with wide experience currently feel that no patient with underlying cirrhosis is a candidate for resection of hepatocellular carcinoma because of poor results, high

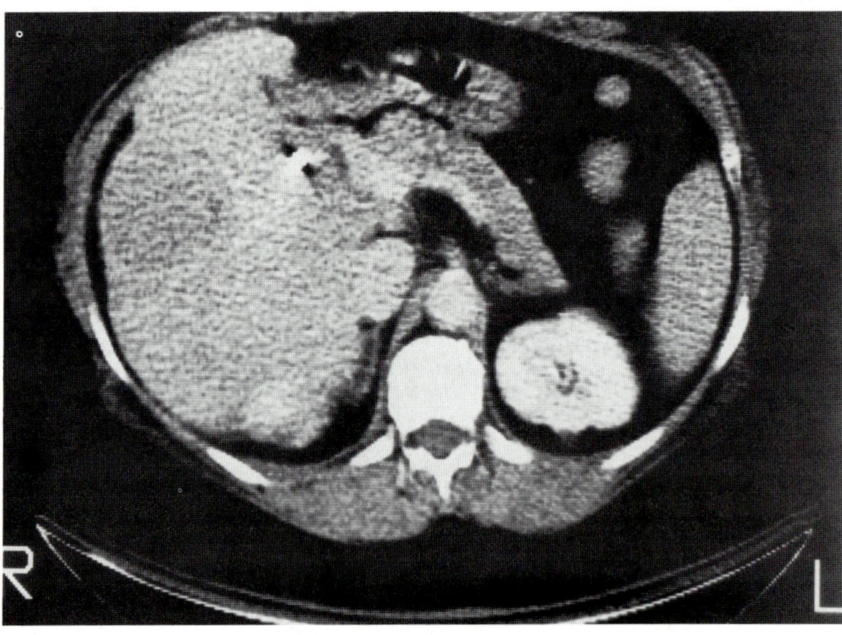

A

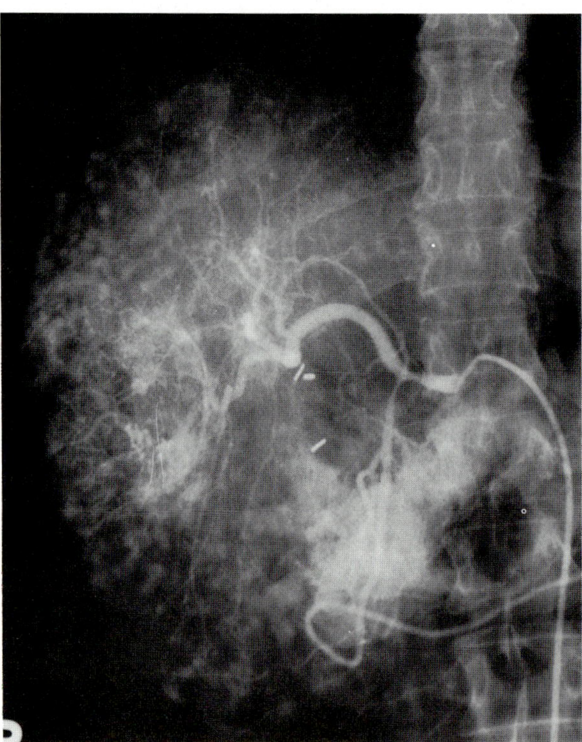

B

Figure 20.5. (*A*) Solitary hepatic cell carcinoma in the right lobe of the liver by CT, which is slightly less vascular than the rest of the liver. (*B*) Arteriogram showing the displacement of vessels around this hepatocellular carcinoma in the right liver with multiple hypervascular areas within it. In addition, there are diffuse hypervascular areas throughout the entire right and left lobes of the liver consistent with diffuse tumor, which would make the patient unresectable.

complication rate, increased blood loss, and high incidence of multifocal disease (43,44). The usual candidates for resection of hepatocellular carcinoma are those patients with solitary lesions arising on the background of a normal liver. In such candidates, resections of even large lesions can produce substantial cure rates since the biology of these "fibrolamellar," "encapsulated," or unifocal hepatomas is more favorable. Approximately 30% of patients who are explored will be able to undergo a curative resection. Of those patients resected, approximately 30% survive disease-free for long periods. Thus, of 100 patients with hepatoma, only 3% to 5% will be cured. Some reports from Japan indicate that in Oriental patients, resections despite underlying cirrhosis may still be associated with cure and moderate operative mortality, in contrast to the Western experience (45,46).

The particular surgical resection is less important if the criterion of a margin of normal liver of at least 1 cm is achieved. Preferably a 2-cm margin should be obtained. Large size is not a contraindication to surgical resection, since the most successful results occur in those biologic varieties that may grow to large size and metastasize late. Hepatocellular carcinomas that are small, focal, and lateral in the liver tissue can be easily removed with a wedge resection so long as the criterion of reasonable local margins is achieved. Anatomic resections of the right or left lobe are frequently required because of large size, and extended resections occasionally need to be performed, but almost never can be done safely in cirrhotic livers.

Recently, surgeons from China have reported a series of cases in which unifocal hepatocellular carcinomas arising on the background of cirrhosis were cured without resection by the use of intraoperative cryotherapy with liquid nitrogen delivered via specialized apparatus (47). This technique needs further exploration since it holds the promise of a safe and effective therapy in isolated cancers where surgical resection might be hazardous due to cirrhosis. Limitations of this technique include the inability to freeze large cancers because of rapid heat loss near the periphery of the frozen volume. At present, such a technique is probably not suitable for lesions larger than 3 to 4 cm in diameter. Other nonsurgical treatments of a hepatocellular carcinoma include the use of radioactive labeled ferritin antibody as reported by Order et al. (48). Order has described prolonged survivals and

possibly cures in otherwise untreatable patients. While it is difficult to know the exact usefulness of this technique because of its early development in small numbers of highly selected patients, such an approach offers unique and exciting therapeutic possibilities.

Other therapeutic techniques that can be utilized include radiotherapy for isolated areas of the liver to relieve pain and the use of angiographic or surgical dearterialization to produce palliation by the reduction in size or pain, and the control of bleeding in ruptured hepatocellular carcinoma. The use of a variety of nonoperative techniques probably does not extend survival over untreated control subjects, but may relieve symptoms (49,50).

Cholangiocarcinoma arising in the liver occurs with much less frequency than hepatocellular carcinoma, and may be associated with previous Thorotrast exposure (51). It is characterized by unifocal growth, hypovascular appearance angiographically, and absence of background cirrhosis, but unfortunately carries an even worse prognosis with few surgical resections and rare cures (17). A recent report is at some variance with this bleak background and may indicate that with earlier detection, successful resections are possible (52).

Other unusual primary malignant tumors arising in the liver include angiosarcoma, which is highly aggressive, rapidly growing, and an almost uniformly rapidly lethal tumor that has been associated with exposure to Thorotrast (53) and to various stages in the production of polyvinyl chloride (54). These and other sarcomas are rare and provide few opportunities for surgical resection (55,56).

Primary lymphoma of the liver occurs rarely, but can be cured by resection (57). The exact nature of such lesions may not be known until resection, and it appears that resection alone is adequate for treatment with a high cure rate.

Another category of liver cancer occurs by direct extension from an adjacent organ and thus invades the liver peripherally. These cancers most commonly arise in the gallbladder and extrahepatic bile ducts, but may also arise in the stomach, adrenal gland, duodenum, or colon. Appropriate in-continuity wedge resection of the involved liver may be performed in carcinomas of the gallbladder, stomach, adrenal gland, and colon (58). In general, liver resections for such adjacent tumors should be limited in extent. However, carcinomas of the gallbladder directly involving the liver do not warrant an extensive hepatic resection and are of such poor prognosis that extensive surgery seems inappropriate (59). While a cure has been reported in the literature of carcinoma of the gallbladder with direct invasion of a small portion of the adjacent liver (60), it would seem unnecessary to do a large anatomic resection in order to achieve whatever cure might be available in this unusual situation. A wedge excision of the gallbladder bed would seem to be the most appropriate solution in these highly selected cases where the gallbladder carcinoma arose on the hepatic surface without other demonstrated evidence of spread.

Anatomic resection of the right or left lobes of the liver may well be a logical extension of curative resection of cancers of the extrahepatic bile ducts that grow anteriorly into the liver substance and do not manifest metastases or unresectable local extension. Usually such cancers also involve the hepatic artery, portal vein, or opposite lobar hepatic duct to preclude cure, but a small proportion of cases may be candidates for an extended resection (61,62). Liver transplantation for primary liver cancer has been performed in a number of cases (63). While the results have been disappointing in clinical cancers, the fact that a number of hepatocellular cancers were cured when they were small in size and unsuspected, indicates that, at least theoretically, liver transplantation may be an acceptable treatment in the future. Almost 50% of patients with fibrolamellar hepatocellular carcinomas survived free of disease in a small number undergoing liver transplantation.

Hepatic Metastases

Metastatic carcinoma of the liver is a common cause of death from cancer. Unfortunately, liver metastases are usually but one manifestation of disseminated disease from cancers arising in the portal venous drainage area as well as in other parts of the body. Metastases to the liver are extremely common in carcinomas of the lung, breast, esophagus, stomach, pancreas, upper aerodigestive tract, and melanoma. Only in carcinomas of the colon, rectum, islet cell of the pancreas, sarcoma of the gastrointestinal tract, and carcinoid does the pattern of "hepatic only" metastases appear with any frequency (64). Of course, other cancers may develop solitary hepatic metastasis, but they rarely lend themselves to resection (65).

Of the cancers listed, only carcinoma of the colon and rectum presents frequently with solitary or few metastases only in the liver. Thus the vast majority of liver resections for metastatic cancer relate to carcinomas of the large bowel. In these cases, the "liver-only" pattern with only a few metastases may appear in between 3% and 6% of patients who fail their primary resection (64,65,66). While this is not a large proportion of the patients who fail, the high incidence of carcinomas of the large bowel indicates that with 6% of 40,000 annual deaths from the disease as many as 2400 cases may be suitable for hepatic resection each year. Studies indicate that patients suitable for resection of metastatic colorectal cancer with curative intent usually have only one, two, or three tumor nodules in the liver, and no other extrahepatic metastatic disease (67). Occasional patients with a larger number of separate nodules of metastatic cancer may also be salvaged. Rarely patients with metastasis to the liver from colon cancer may survive 5 years untreated (68), however, with resection, 5-year disease-free survival rates of 25% to 35% have been reported in many series (9,67–71). The particular biologic features that are associated with a higher long-term survival rate disease-free include a primary colon cancer that was staged as Dukes B rather than Dukes C, a disease-free interval longer than 1 year, hepatic metastases that were few in number and confined to one lobe, and a surgical resection margin of more than 1 cm (67). Patients with a normal or low serum carcinoembryonic antigen (CEA) level have a higher cure rate than those with a high value. In patients who display all these criteria, the survival rate disease-free at 5 years may approach 50%.

The ultimate surgical approach to "hepatic only" metastases with a large mass of disease is transplantation of the liver. Such patients frequently but not always die of other disseminated metastases following immunosuppression. Interestingly enough, these patients may display metastases in the transplanted liver at autopsy.

All studies so far indicate that the presence of extrahepatic metastases including portahepatis lymph nodes, peritoneal seeding, and pulmonary metastases almost precludes cure by hepatic resection (67,68). Thus, patients should be worked up before exploring for possible hepatic resection by means of a barium enema or colonoscopy, to search for local recurrence of a new primary cancer, and a bone scan and chest film to detect metastases. At surgical exploration, the remainder of the abdominal cavity should be inspected for evidence of peritoneal seeding, ovarian metastases, retroperitoneal lymph nodes, and portahepatis lymph nodes. Even though such extrahepatic spread is a bad prognostic sign, resection may be undertaken for palliation and prolongation of survival in appropriate situations.

The amount of hepatic tissue resected is of little prognostic consequence in the studies that have addressed that issue, if a minimum 1-cm margin of normal tissue surrounds the hepatic metastasis (67,69). If less than a 1-cm margin occurs, few patients are salvaged. Thus, wedge resection of the liver is perfectly suitable for small- to moderate-sized lesions, while anatomic resections are more suitable for larger lesions. Hughes has shown that for metastatic nodules larger than 4 cm in diameter, anatomic lobar resection provides a higher cure rate than wedge resection, indicating that margins might well be compromised when resecting large lesions with just a wedge resection (67).

It is important to keep in mind that the results by resection of liver metastases from large bowel carcinoma reflect a biologic rather than a temporal phenomena. Thus the resection of solitary metastases of the liver that are more than 8 cm in diameter and even 12 cm in median diameter are as successful as the resection of metastases that are less than 2 cm in diameter (67,68). In addition, the resection of asymptomatic patients detected by CEA screening of large bowel cancer patients following primary colon resection is no more successful than the detection and treatment of patients who present with symptoms and considerably larger hepatic metastases (72). Furthermore, the resection of small lesions by wedge-resection of the peripheral liver is no more successful than the resection of large anatomic regions for much larger metastases (67,68). Such facts point out that those patients who are cured after resection of a liver metastasis reflect a biologic peculiarity where the disease grows only in the liver and only in one or a few foci despite the inevitable showering of the body with tumor cells. That both large and small lesions are cured at the some rate indicates a unique biology, rather than early detection. Thus early resection of an unsuitable biologic situation

does not improve the cure rate, and delayed resection of a patient with appropriate biologic behavior of the metastatic disease does not impair curability by liver resection. How or why such a biologic phenomenon occurs in unknown, but this places our curative approach to liver metastases in a more logical light that enables us to focus on those patients who will benefit by an aggressive and vigorous surgical attack. Early detection by screening asymptomatic patients with CEA will therefore not lead to the increased cure rates as suggested by Minton, the leading proponent of second-look operations (72).

CEA is used as a screening technique for detecting patients with metastases from colorectal carcinoma in follow-up examinations so the earliest possible resection of metastatic disease may be carried out. Unfortunately, the vast majority of patients with metastases detected by CEA elevations have disease in multiple organs or in multiple nodules throughout the liver and are not suitable for hepatic resection of isolated metastasis or any curative treatment. It has been shown that the pattern of CEA rise also reflects the suitability for curative resection of liver metastases so that patients who have either a slow rise or a low absolute level of CEA do much better than those patients with a rapid rise or an extremely high CEA value. This phenomena again reflects the fact that the role of the surgeon is to select the suitable biologic situation rather than to select the earliest possible temporal framework in which to resect liver metastases.

Liver metastases from other primary cancer sites occasionally present with a solitary hepatic metastasis, but seldom result in cure when resected (13). Islet cell cancer of the pancreas and carcinoid tumors usually have multiple liver metastases throughout both lobes of the liver. Leiomyosarcomas of the gastrointestinal tract, while sometimes demonstrating only a few nodules in the liver, usually present with bilateral disease, which obviates the chance for curative resection. In Foster's collected series, only 7 patients without colorectal primary sites were cured after resection (13). These few cancers are known for unusual biologic behavior patterns (73).

In highly selected clinical situations, liver resections can be undertaken for strictly palliative intent and in the presence of metastases in other parts of the organ or in the presence of disease elsewhere in the body. These cases should be selected extremely carefully, since in only specialized situations will there be justification in terms of prolonged survival or decreased symptoms that outweigh the risks of the surgery itself. Such situations generally arise in those tumors that have a liver-only propensity for metastatic spread. Thus, carcinoid metastases that are unresponsive to chemotherapy and present with a bulky mass in one anatomic portion of the liver, that can be resected with significant reduction in the bulk of tumor, might well undergo amelioration of symptoms and be suitable for liver resection. Islet cell cancers of the pancreas that are secreting functional hormones and that fail to respond to chemotherapy should be pursued aggressively in terms of resecting symptomatic liver metastases since these patients frequently have a prolonged disease course, and the functional symptoms from the hormonal products elaborated by the tumor may cause severe disability and morbidity. Since the hormonal production is quantitatively related to the bulk of tumor, the resection of a large amount of hepatic metastases may achieve a dramatic clinical improvement and prolonged comfortable survival even though some disease remains. Hepatic metastases that are accompanied by hemorrhage or infarction with necrosis and symptoms from a large mass should also be resected to achieve significant palliation if operative mortality can be kept to a minimum, and survival expectation in these cases is prolonged, as in leiomyosarcomas of the gastrointestinal tract.

Technical Aspects of Surgical Resection

The technical aspects of hepatic resection are based on a thorough knowledge of hepatic anatomy, wide operative exposure of the liver and the right upper quadrant, adequate dissection of the porta hepatis for anatomic resections, a capacity for transfusing blood rapidly, and a system of dissecting through liver tissue that keeps the field clear enough to enable control of bleeding by cautery of small vessels and clamping and ligation of the larger vascular and biliary structures encountered. Numerous articles describe technical and judgmental aspects of hepatic resection (43,74–78). An ultrasonic dissector can also be used (79).

Wedge resections of the peripheral liver or a left lateral segment resection may not require portahepatis dissection or isolation and control of the central vascular structures since the periphery of the liver is devoid of large venous structures, and bleeding can be controlled readily with local clamps, coagulation, and ligature. It is vitally important, however, when performing wedge resections of the periphery of the liver, to orient the hepatic tissue dissection plane in such a way as to create a wide "saucer" removal of the liver substance rather than a deep narrow V-shaped resection. Resection in such a fashion produces wide exposure of the hepatic tissue and vascular structures and assurance of an adequate margin around the primary or metastatic cancer. The portion of liver to be resected must be grasped with one hand while the operating hand dissects through liver substance. The surgical assistants should control bleeding vessels and provide exposure. It is difficult, if not impossible, to re-resect a margin of liver substance after a primary inadequate removal of liver tissue because the flexibility, softness, friability, and vascularity prevents easy grasping and manipulation of fragments of thin sections of liver. Every attempt to achieve a 2-cm margin around the palpable hepatic mass should be made in order to ultimately achieve at least a 1-cm disease-free margin in the final specimen. While a wedge resection can achieve this with much less morbidity and mortality compared to a right hepatic lobectomy, wedge resection of posterior or superior portions of the right lobe demands extensive operative exposure. In tumor masses in these locations, it should be mandatory to open the right chest and diaphragm widely in addition to a large abdominal incision, so that complete visualization and mobilization of the liver can be achieved to perform the more limited wedge resection. Left hepatic wedge resections, left lateral segmental resections, and left lobectomies can almost always be performed without extending the abdominal incision into the chest.

If more exposure is necessary for left hepatic resections, the xiphoid can be resected and an inferior sternotomy performed to provide a wide view of the superior hepatic hilum and the inferior vena cava as it traverses the diaphragm (77). Supradiaphragmatic control of the inferior vena cava can also be achieved if required.

When anatomic resections of the right or left lobe or extended right or left trisegmental resections are considered, it is critical to completely and carefully dissect and isolate all the vascular and biliary structures of the porta hepatis before commencing the actual liver dissection. The biliary anatomy in the upper porta hepatis is just as variable as it is in other parts of the biliary tree. The anterior or posterior segmental duct on the right lobe may cross the apparent hepatic duct bifurcation and enter the left hepatic duct in up to 20% of patients (74). These ducts can be injured when performing a left hepatic resection; thus these anatomic variations must be kept in mind. With complete vascular and biliary isolation at the porta hepatis and suitable ligation of vascular structures to anatomic portions of the liver, blood loss can be minimized and extensive resections may be kept more rational. While the preferable technique for doing a right hepatic lobectomy should include opening the right chest widely to get excellent exposure of the vena cava and the right hepatic vein, some surgeons find that routine opening of the chest is not required. For safety's sake, I personally believe that the chest should usually be opened for a right hepatic resection to insure complete control of the hepatic veins, exposure of the vena cava above the liver, dissection of the superior hepatic hilum, and ligation of as many of the short hepatic veins draining directly into the anterior wall of the vena cava as can be achieved. Since the hepatic veins run within the anatomic intralobar and intrasegmental planes, actual division through liver substance should be kept slightly off the anatomic planes to avoid dissecting the hepatic vein or entering it in such a way as to interfere with its function of draining the portion of the retained liver adjacent to the resection line. Thus, for a right hepatic resection, the division through the liver substance should be 1 or 2 cm to the right of the intralobar fissure, while for a left hepatic resection, that division plane should be similarly placed to the left of the intralobar fissure. Variations on this technique have to be made to accommodate the location of the individual tumor. It is possible to do a central hepatic resection by removing the medial segment of the left lobe and the anterior segment of the right lobe for metastatic nodules centrally placed and bridging the intralobar fissure (76).

Currently an important adjunct to hepatic surgery is the use of intraoperative ultrasound. With this device, the extent, number, and nature of the hepatic nodules or metastases can be detected as well as their relationship to major venous structures and other aspects of the detailed anatomy of the liver. Routine liver resections do not warrant the use of intraoperative ultrasound; however, complicated or difficult resections or large tumors centrally placed may have surgery immeasurably aided by the careful intraoperative ultrasonic screening of the anatomy and the nature and outline of the tumor prior to actual commencement of the hepatic resection.

In 1985 we initiated a program of cryotherapy or freezing of hepatic metastases that enables us to freeze in situ, without resecting, critically placed nodules or second or third nodules, following an anatomic resection of one major portion of the liver that may lie in the opposite residual lobe (80).

Summary

Liver surgery has achieved a recognized role in the past 15 years such that the vast majority of cancers of the liver that present a suitable biologic situation for potential care can be resected for cure or substantial palliation with safety. Operative mortality after right hepatic resection in the United States as of 1987 should be less than 5%. The operative mortality for wedge resections and left hepatic resections of the liver should be no more than 1%, and in most reports is 0%. Postoperative management of these patients is such that they generally make a rapid recovery; the median hospital stay of patients undergoing major hepatic resections is less than 2 weeks in uncomplicated cases, even in elderly patients (62).

References

1. Henson SW Jr, Gray HK, Dockerty MB. Benign tumors of the liver. *Surg Gynecol Obstet* 1956; 103:23–30.
2. Ochsner JL, Halpert B. Cavernous hemangioma of the liver. *Surgery* 1958; 43:577–582.
3. Adami GJ. *Principles of Pathology.* Philadelphia: Lea & Febiger, 1910.
4. Edmondson HA. *Tumors of the Liver and Intrahepatic Bile Ducts.* Washington, DC: Armed Forces Institute of Pathology, 1958.
5. Trastek VF, van Heerden JA, Sheedy PF II, Adson MA. Cavernous hemangiomas of the liver: Resect or observe? *Am J Surg* 1983; 145:49–53.
6. Takagi H. Diagnosis and management of cavernous hemangioma of the liver. *Semin Surg Oncol* 1985; 1:12–22.
7. Moss AA. Computed tomography of the hepatobiliary system. In: Moss AA, Gamsu G, Genant HK, eds. *Computed Tomography of the Body.* Philadelphia: WB Saunders, 1983, pp. 599–698.
8. Bernett PH, Zerhouni EA, White RI, Siegelman SS. Computed tomography in the diagnosis of cavernous hemangioma of the liver. *AJR* 1980; 134:439–447.

9. Iwatsuki S, Shaw BW Jr, Starzl TE. Experience with 150 liver resections. *Ann Surg* 1983; 197:247–253.

10. Kawarada Y, Mizumoto R. Surgical treatment of giant hemangioma of the liver. *Am J Surg* 1984; 148:287–290.

11. Adam YG, Huvos AG, Fortner JG. Giant hemangiomas of the liver. *Ann Surg* 1970; 172:239–244.

12. Stocker JT, Ishak KG. Focal nodular hyperplasia of the liver: A study of 21 pediatric cases. *Cancer* 1981; 48:336–345.

13. Foster JH, Berman MM. *Solid Liver Tumors. Major Problems in Clinical Surgery*, Vol. 22. Philadelphia: WB Saunders, 1977, pp. 138–178.

14. Turner P. Case of excision of an adenoma of the liver which had ruptured spontaneously causing internal hemorrhage. *Proc R Soc Med* 1923; 16:60.

15. Ramseur WL, Cooper MR. Asymptomatic liver cell adenomas: Another case of resolution after discontinuation of oral contraceptive use. *JAMA* 1978; 239:1647–1648.

16. Pryor AC, Cohen RJ, Goldman RL. Hepatocellular carcinoma in a woman on long-term oral contraceptives. *Cancer* 1977; 40:884–888.

17. Okuda K, et al. Primary liver cancers in Japan. *Cancer* 1980; 45:2663–2669.

18. Foster JH, Berman MM. *Solid Liver Tumors. Major Problems in Clinical Surgery*, Vol. 22. Philadelphia: WB Saunders, 1977, pp. 62–104.

19. Sumithran E, Prathap K. Hepatocellular carcinoma in the Malaysian Orang Asli. *Cancer* 1976; 37:2263–2266.

20. Niederau C, Fischer R, Sonnenberg A, et al. Survival and causes of death in cirrhotic and in noncirrhotic patients with primary hemochromatosis. *N Engl J Med* 1985; 313: 1256–1262.

21. Purtilo DT, Gottlieb LS. Cirrhosis and hepatoma occurring at Boston City Hospital (1917–1968). *Cancer* 1973; 32:458–462.

22. Eriksson S, Carlson J, Velez R. Risk of cirrhosis and primary liver cancer in alpha$_1$-antitrypsin deficiency. *N Engl J Med* 1986; 314:736–739.

23. Blumberg BS, Larouze B, London WT, et al. The relation of infection with the hepatitis B agent to primary hepatic carcinoma. *Am J Pathol* 1975; 81:669–682.

24. Murchelano RA, Wolke RE. Epizootic carcinoma in the winter flounder, *Pseudopleuronectes americanus*. *Science* 1985; 228:587–589.

25. Alpert ME. Mycotoxins: A possible cause of primary carcinoma of the liver. *Am J Med* 1969; 46:325–327.

26. *CA: A cancer journal for clinicians*. 1986; 19–36.

27. Blumberg BS, London WT. Hepatitis B virus and the prevention of primary hepatocellular carcinoma. *N Engl J Med* 1981; 304:782–789.

28. Moertel CG. The liver. In: Holland JF, Frei E III, eds. *Cancer Medicine*. Philadelphia: Lea & Febiger, 1973, pp. 1541–1547.

29. Berman MM, Libbey NP, Foster JH. Hepatocellular carcinoma: Polygonal cell type with fibrous stroma: An atypical variant with a favorable prognosis. *Cancer* 1980; 46:1448–1455.

30. Craig JR, Peters RL, Edmondson HA, Omata M. Fibrolamellar carcinoma of the liver: A tumor of adolescents and young adults with distinctive clinico-pathologic features. *Cancer* 1980; 46:372–379.

31. Okuda K, Musch H, Nakajima Y, et al. Clinicopathologic features of encapsulated hepatocellular carcinoma: A study of 26 cases. *Cancer* 1977; 40:1240–1245.

32. Teitelbaum DH, Tuttle S, Carey LC, Clausen KP. Fibrolamellar carcinoma of the liver. *Ann Surg* 1985; 202:36–40.

33. Soreide O, Czerniak A, Bradpiece H, et al. Characteristics of fibrolamellar hepatocellular carcinoma. *Am J Surg* 1986; 151:518–523.

34. Exelby PR, Filler RM, Grosfield JL. Liver tumors in children in the particular reference to hepatoblastoma and hepatocellular carcinoma. *J Pediatr Surg* 1975; 10:329–337.

35. Nagasue N, Inokuchi K, Kobayashi M, Saku M. Hepatoportal arteriovenous fistula in primary carcinoma of the liver. *Surg Gynecol Obstet* 1977; 145:504–508.

36. Kojiro M, Kawabata K, Kawano Y, et al. Hepatocellular carcinoma presenting as intrabile duct tumor growth. *Cancer* 1982; 49:2144–2147.

37. Hall TC, ed. Proceedings: Paraneoplastic syndromes. *Ann NY Acad Sci* 1974; 230:1–377.

38. Okezi O, DeAngelis G. Spontaneous rupture of hepatoma: A misdiagnosed surgical emergency. *Ann Surg* 1974; 179:133–135.

39. Chearanai O, Plengvanit U, Asavanich C, et al. Spontaneous rupture of primary hepatoma: Report of 63 cases with particular reference to the pathogenesis and rationale treatment by hepatic artery ligation. *Cancer* 1983; 51:1532–1536.

40. Tang Z, Yu Y, Lin Z, et al. Small hepatocellular carcinoma. *China Med J* 1979;92:455.

41. Anthony PP, Vogel CL, Barker LF. Liver cell dysplasia: A premalignant condition. *J Clin Pathol* 1973; 26:217–223.

42. Chen DS, Jung JL. Serum alpha-feto protein in hepatocellular carcinoma. *Cancer* 1977; 40:779.

43. Balasegaram M, Joishy SK. Hepatic resection: Pillars of success built on the formulation of 15 years of experience. *Am J Surg* 1981; 141:360–365.

44. Foster JH. Commentary. *World J Surg* 1984; 8:365–366.

45. Okamoto E, Tanaka N, Yamanaka N, Toyosaka A. Results of surgical treatments of primary hepatocellular carcinoma: Some aspects to improve long-term survival. *World J Surg* 1984; 8:360–366.

46. Tsuzuki T, Ogata Y, Iida S, et al. Long-term survival of patients with hepatocellular carcinoma combined with liver cirrhosis: Report of two patients. *Cancer* 1985; 55: 2835–2838.

47. Zhou X, Tang Z, Yu Y. Cryosurgery for liver cancer: Experimental and clinical study. *Chinese J Surg* 1979; 17:480.

48. Order SE, Stillwagon GB, Klein JL, et al. Iodine 131 antiferritin, a new treatment modality in hepatoma: A Radiation Therapy Oncology Group study. *J Clin Oncol* 1985; 3:1573–1582.

49. Lai ECS, Choi TK, Tong SW, et al. Treatment of unresectable hepatocellular carcinoma: Results of a randomized controlled trial. *World J Surg* 1986; 10:501–509.

50. Falkson G, MacIntyre JM, Moertel CG, et al. Primary liver cancer: An Eastern Cooperative Oncology Group trial. *Cancer* 1984; 54:970–977.

51. Rubel LR, Ishak KG. Thorotrast-associated cholangiocarcinoma: An epidemiologic and clinicopathologic study. *Cancer* 1982; 50:1408–1415.

52. Kawarada Y, Mizumoto R. Cholangiocellular carcinoma of the liver. *Am J Surg* 1984; 147:354–359.

53. Underwood JCE, Huck P. Thorotrast associated hepatic angiosarcoma with 36 years latency. *Cancer* 1978; 42:2610–2612.

54. Makk L, Delmore F, Creech JL. Clinical and morphologic features of hepatic angiosarcoma in vinyl chloride workers. *Cancer* 1976; 37:149–163.

55. Wilson SE, Braitman H, Plested WG, Longmire WP Jr. Primary leiomyosarcoma of the liver. *Ann Surg* 1971; 174: 232–237.

56. Chang WWL, Agha FP, Morgan WS. Primary sarcoma of the liver in the adult. *Cancer* 1983; 51:1510–1517.

57. Osborne BM, Butler JJ, Guarda LA. Primary lymphoma of the liver: Ten cases and a review of the literature. *Cancer* 1985; 56:2902–2910.

58. Foster JH, Berman MM. *Solid Liver Tumors. Major Problems in Clinical Surgery*, Vol. 22. Philadelphia: WB Saunders, 1977, pp. 246–254.

59. Piehler JM, Critchlow RW. Primary carcinoma of the gallbladder (collective review). *Surg Gynecol Obstet* 1978; 147:929–938.
60. Brasfield RD. Right hepatic lobectomy for carcinoma of gallbladder: A five year cure. *Ann Surg* 1961; 153:563–566.
61. Cady B, Fortner JG. Surgical resection of intrahepatic bile duct cancer. *Am J Surg* 1969; 118:104–107.
62. Cady B, Bonneval M, Fender R. Elective hepatic resection. *Am J Surg* 1979; 137:514–521.
63. Iwatsuki S, Gordon RD, Shaw BW Jr, Starzl TE. Role of liver transplantation in cancer therapy. *Ann Surg* 1985; 202:401–407.
64. Pickren JW, Tsukada, Lane WW. Liver metastases: Analysis of autopsy data. In: Weiss L, Gilbert HA, eds. *Liver Metastases*. Boston: GK Hall, 1982.
65. Foster JH, Berman MM. *Solid Liver Tumors. Major Problems in Clinical Surgery*, Vol. 22. Philadelphia: WB Saunders, 1977, pp. 209–234.
66. Willett CG, Tepper JE, Cohen AM, et al. Failure patterns following curative resection of colonic carcinoma. *Ann Surg* 1984; 200:685–690.
67. Hughes KS, Simon R, Songhorabodi S. Resection of the Liver for Colo-Rectal Carcinoma Metastases: A Multi-Institutional Study of Indication for Resection (in press). *Surgery* (in press).
68. Adson MA, van Heerden JA, Adson MH, et al. Resection of hepatic metastases from colorectal cancer. *Arch Surg* 1984; 119: 647–651.
69. Cady B, McDermott WV. Major hepatic resection for metachronous metastases from colon cancer. *Ann Surg* 1985; 201:204–209.
70. Fortner JG, Silva JS, Golbey RB, et al. Multivariate analysis of a personal series of 247 consecutive patients with liver metastases from colorectal cancer. *Ann Surg* 1984; 199:306–316.
71. Petrelli NJ, Nambisan RN, Herrera L, Mittelman A. Hepatic resection for isolated metastases from colorectal carcinoma. *Am J Surg* 1985; 149:205–209.
72. Minton JP, Hoehn JL, Gerber DM, et al. Results of a 400-patient carcinoembryonic antigen second-look colorectal cancer study. *Cancer* 1985; 55:1284–1290.
73. Margolin KA, Pak HY, Esensten ML, Doroshow JH. Hepatic metastasis in granulosa cell tumor of the ovary. *Cancer* 1985; 56:691–695.
74. Linder RM, Cady B. Hepatic resection *Surg Clin North Am* 1980; 60:349–367.
75. Schwartz SI. Right hepatic lobectomy. *Am J Surg* 1984; 148: 668–673.
76. Starzl TE, Bell RH, Beart RW, Putnam CW. Hepatic trisegmentectomy and other liver resections. *Surg Gynecol Obstet* 1975; 141:429–437.
77. Miller DR. Median sternotomy extension of abdominal incision for hepatic lobectomy. *Ann Surg* 1972; 175:193–196.
78. Foster JH, Berman MM. *Solid Liver Tumors. Major Problems in Clinical Surgery*, Vol. 22. Philadelphia: WB Saunders, 1977, pp. 255–303.
79. Hodgson WJB. Initial experience in liver surgery using the CUSA system. *Surg Update* 1982. Vol. I 1. pp. 9–11.
80. Ravikumar TS, Kane R, Cady B, et al. Hepatic cryosurgery with intraoperative ultrasound monitoring for metastatic colon carcinoma. *Arch Surg* 1987; Vol. 122. pp. 403–409.

Editorial Comment

As in other areas of this surgical text, this chapter by Dr. Blake Cady contains areas where there is certainly duplication with other chapters and sections, particularly in the area of surgical technique and in radiologic diagnosis. No attempt has been made to avoid this since the editor feels that variations and even conflicts between the writings of various authors are stimulating and probably educational.

At any rate, there is very little one can disagree with in the conclusions drawn from the data presented.

Of particular importance is the section on hemangioma, which emphasizes the relatively few indications for surgical approach to these lesions and presents a healthy restraint regarding extensive resection even of large tumors. The indications for operation are clearly spelled out and are very useful guidelines for the general surgeon.

For some time the surgical literature was confusing in the area of "benign hepatomas," a poorly chosen name because of the equally unfortunate use of the term hepatoma for malignant hepatocellular carcinoma. At any rate, the distinction between the lesion and follicular nodular hyperplasia is useful, as is the information on natural history and relative risks of the two types of lesions.

In the areas concerned with malignant tumors of the liver, the subset of hepatocellular carcinoma referred to ordinarily as fibrolamellar variety is well described. No comment is made on the relatively rare type known as clear cell carcinoma, but this is a small proportion of the total number and important only because of its occasional very bizarre behavior and inexplicable long-term survival.

One of the burgeoning areas in surgical approaches to the liver is cryosurgery and Dr. Cady provides an excellent descriptive introduction to an area that many of us feel will be of increasing importance in the management of many benign and/or malignant tumors of the liver.

Experiences in western civilization with hepatocellular carcinomas is relatively rare compared to the frequency with which these tumors are encountered in the Third World. Reference is given below to a review of surgical disease in East Africa that emphasizes some of the etiologic and behavioral characteristics of these liver cancers.

Reference

1. McDermott WV. Surgical disease in East Africa. *Arch Surg* 1987; 122:397–402.

lacerations. (f) The team should have practiced the technique.

Of the intracaval shunts, the ACS is the most effective as the concomitant median sternotomy ensures excellent exposure to the supradiaphragmatic IVC and to the area of bleeding. Cardiac massage may be performed if necessary. A 38 or 40 French chest tube rapidly placed through a purse-string suture in the right atrium serves as the shunt. The tube should be carefully guided down the IVC to ensure that it does not pass into the venous laceration, tearing the vein further and virtually ensuring the demise of the patient. Holes must be cut in the atrial portion, the shunt sited with its lumen just below the renal veins, and tapes or tubing placed round the supra- and infrahepatic vena cava to keep the shunt in position. A Pringle's maneuver is added and, on occasion, temporary clamping of the descending abdominal aorta may be necessary. With the field now relatively dry, direct exposure and repair of the injured veins may be carried out or a hepatic lobectomy performed.

Alternatively, a shunt may be placed through the abdominal IVC below the renal veins or inserted through the femoral vein. These approaches have also been successfully used but have not acquired the same acceptance as the ACS.

As many technical problems remain unresolved, new experimental approaches stimulated by experience with liver transplantation are being explored, such as the shunting of blood around the liver from the femoral vein to the subclavian vein with a rapid transfusion pump in the circuit. Use of heparin in the trauma patient, however, is not practical. Others are attempting to design new catheters with strategically placed balloons.

Finally, two new segments of dogma are being challenged. The first reflects the long-held view that occlusion of the venous return to the heart through the IVC results in shock, arrhythmia, and death. The second concerns the concept that ligation of a major intrahepatic vein inevitably results in necrosis of the subtended tissue and makes hepatic resection mandatory. There have been scattered reports in the past about successful ligation of the suprarenal IVC as a desperate measure. More recently, some surgeons have deliberately occluded the IVC below and above the liver to produce a dry field preparatory to a rapid direct attack on the intra- or retrohepatic site of hemorrhage while administering large volumes of com-

pensatory fluid centrally. Successful use of this technique in prolonged elective hepatic surgery was reported by Huguet in 1978 (34) when he pointed out that humans, unlike dogs and pigs, have a natural venous collateral system and that during long operations, the reduction in core temperature provided by rapid transfusions of blood reduces hepatic metabolism. Results obtained with this approach are thought by some to be more favorable than results with the use of an intracaval shunt. In a few such cases, the injury in the dry field may even lend itself to application of a Satinsky's clamp or the insertion of a Foley catheter to produce temporary hemostasis preparatory to formal repair.

With regard to the ligation of large intrahepatic veins, the conventional view that complete or partial lobectomy is invariably necessitated when one or more of these veins is ligated, is also being questioned today.

Use of the Abdominal Pack

Use of abdominal packing to control hemorrhage fell into disfavor during and after World War II, mainly because of a high associated rate of infection but even more because of the regrettable tendency of surgeons to substitute this technique for proper mobilization of the liver, exposure of the area of the injury, and assiduous accomplishment of hemostasis by ligation of the bleeding points. This retreat from surgical principles well established for other areas of the body inevitably resulted in unacceptably high mortality rates. Unfortunately, these results also served to obscure the small but definite role for packing in selected patients.

The dogmatic rejection of packing under all circumstances was revisited and challenged in the mid-1970s (4), when it was recognized that in certain patients senseless prolongation of the operation in the shocked and oozing patient, instead of a planned and orderly retreat with the help of packs, was a certain recipe for death. Over the period 1977–1987, it has been shown that about 70% of patients survive in whom packing is inserted after attempts at acceptable hemostasis have failed and where the alternative is judged likely to be death. Most of these patients have additional adjunctive hemostatic techniques applied, such as débridement, ligation of a hepatic artery, or ligation of large veins.

While the LHV usually has a single entry point into the IVC, some patients may have one to three separate openings. Relationships of the LHV and the MHV vary widely and this confluence determines the local anatomy. In about 75% of patients, the MHV joins the LHV after a short extrahepatic course of about 1 cm to form a common vein of about 1 cm in length. In about 25% of patients, however, the MHV opens into the IVC separately from the LHV.

Fourth, theoretically, ligation of a large hepatic vein should be followed by resection of the parenchyma, which it drains so as to avoid congestion, hypoxemia, and necrosis. While in practice this is done almost invariably, there are reports of ligation of the left and middle hepatic veins (subsequently proven by venography) where the parenchyma has regained reasonable color and turgor intraoperatively and the patient has recovered well, despite the fact that the subtended parenchyma has not been resected (32). The degree of collateral venous drainage within the liver is probably greater than is conventionally accepted.

Approaches to Injuries of the Hepatic Veins and Inferior Vena Cava

As might be expected, most patients who survive long enough to reach the operating room have some natural containment of the perihepatic hemorrhage, which may be supplemented by temporary local pressure at laparotomy. Following the introduction of the atrial caval shunt (ACS) in 1968, uncertainty clouded its precise role in the salvage of patients with complex hepatic injuries. Only patients who have sustained really significant hepatic or extrahepatic venous injury, often with an element of massive parenchymal injury, qualify for the use of an intracaval shunt. Most of these patients have been in deep shock for a variable period. The mortality rate following the use of the ACS is predictably very high and is likely to be 100% if the technique has not been practiced in the morgue or laboratory preoperatively. As the reported results will also reflect the selection of cases, data on ACS should not be taken at their face value. In the mid-1970s a few relatively successful series were partly attributable to the use of the ACS in a number of highly favorable patients who could more easily have been managed by a direct approach to the bleeding area through the hepatic parenchyma (4). With a greater readiness on the part of surgeons to mobilize the liver and to use adjunctive packing, ACS has become less commonly used in recent years. Above all, a rapid transhepatic finger-fracture approach down to the area of the injury with local ligation or venous repair under direct vision has an increasing number of adherents and may achieve superior results, such as those reported in the Bellevue series where both packing and shunting have been virtually abandoned (7). As part of the direct attack on complex vascular injuries, Pachter has employed adjunctive measures including the administration of intravenous methylprednisolone succinate (30 to 40 milligrams per kilogram) as a bolus, iced saline, hypothermia of the liver to reduce metabolism, and, where necessary, occlusion of the portal triad for periods in excess of the traditional 15 to 20 minutes. Few surgeons favor the use of steroids, which theoretically may predispose to the development of sepsis due to immunosupression, and the deliberate cooling of the liver in these emergency conditions is seldom practiced. Occlusion of the portal triad for an hour or more, however, is tolerated very satisfactorily by most patients although the period of hepatic hypoxia should still be kept to an unavoidable minimum, especially in the shocked patient.

ACS is of greatest value in the patient with a torn hepatic vein or lacerated retrohepatic IVC and bleeding so massive that the site of origin cannot be clearly exposed without the probability of exsanguination. Successful salvage of four of eight patients with very complex venous injuries of this variety has been reported in 1987 (33). If ACS is to be successful, certain principles of selection and management are essential: (a) the patient should be young; (b) the decision to shunt should be made early and, if possible, before large amounts of blood have been given and hypothermia and coagulopathy established; (c) the period of shock should be minimized—it is significant that 4 of the 18 survivors in the San Francisco General Hospital series never had a blood pressure below 80 mmHg at any time (8); (d) penetrating wounds lend themselves to shunting far more often than wounds due to blunt injury in which survival is very rare; (e) patients with a predominantly parenchymal source of bleeding are more likely to survive following shunting than those with central venous

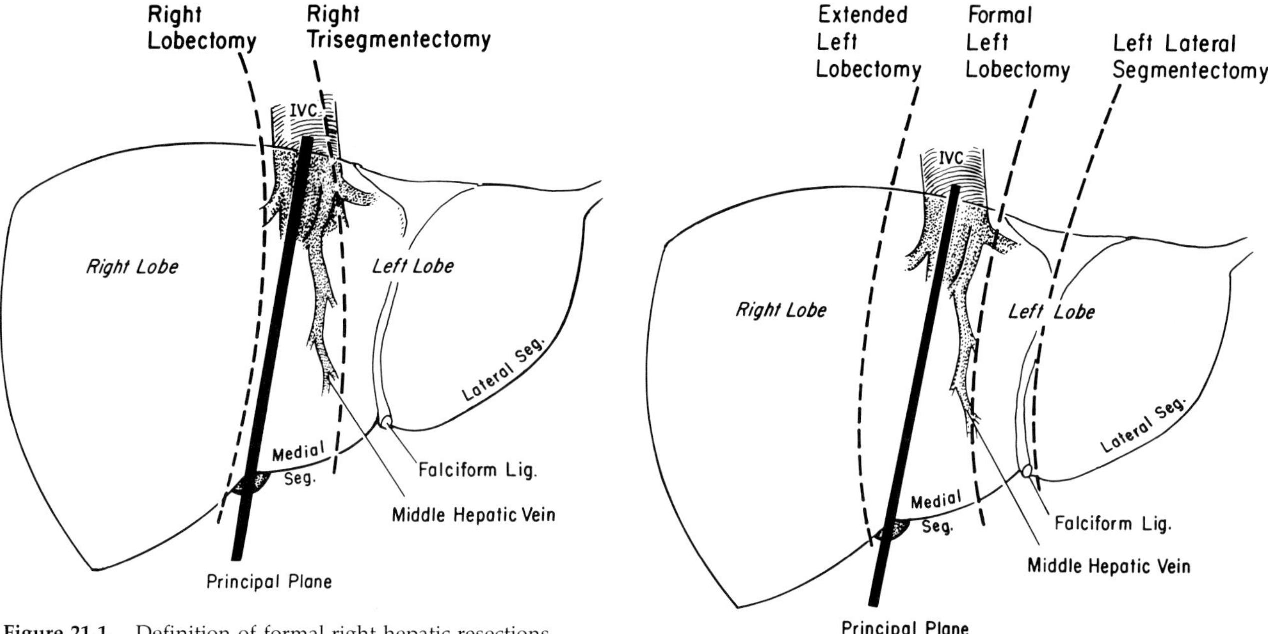

Figure 21.1. Definition of formal right hepatic resections.

Figure 21.2. Definition of formal left hepatic resections. One should note that the plan of dissection for the extended left is anterior to the right hepatic vein.

and postoperative mortality with this procedure. The surgeon who performs hepatic surgery only occasionally should not consider it. As a general rule, when contemplating extraordinary, nonanatomic hepatic operations, particularly in cases of metastatic disease, the surgeon should remember that the biology of the tumor often defeats the most adroit technique. Despite anecdotal exceptions, I believe that there is an inverse correlation between the extent of heroic measures applied in liver surgery for metastatic disease and the chance of curing a patient. There is no effective systemic therapy for any of the hepatic tumors we attempt to resect, and patients who are referred with primary or metastatic liver tumors should generally be approached only with curative intent. They should be operated on only if there is no evidence of extrahepatic disease spread and only if all of the liver tumor can be removed (11,12).

Preoperative Studies

The studies to be performed prior to hepatic resection for primary or metastatic cancer fall into two categories. First are studies done to rule out the presence of extrahepatic disease: chest roentgenograms and either pulmonary tomograms or computed tomography (CT) scans of the chest. In our experience, 15% of patients with normal findings

on chest posteroanterior (PA) and lateral roentgenograms have nonetheless been found to have colorectal pulmonary metastases (5). A prospective multiinstitutional study of hepatic resections for metastatic colorectal cancer now in progress should establish the frequency of insidious pulmonary metastases as documented by preoperative CT scans of the chest compared to conventional roentgenograms (13). When such extrahepatic metastases are found, one cannot easily justify a curative resection of the liver.

In patients with metastatic colorectal cancer, endoscopic screening of the large bowel should be performed as well as abdominal CT scan or, in its absence, abdominal ultrasound. Despite the increased resolution of the current generation of abdominal scanners, approximately one-third of patients predicted to have hepatic-only colorectal cancer metastases are found at surgery to have extrahepatic disease, intrahepatic metastases that are too numerous to resect, or intrahepatic disease that is anatomically unresectable (5,14).

The second mandatory preoperative study is obtained to define celiac arterial anatomy. I prefer standard hepatic arteriography, although the introduction of digital subtraction techniques may

Chapter 21
Technique of Hepatic Lobectomy, Trisegmentectomy, and a Variety of Hepatic Wedge Resections

GLENN STEELE, JR.

Present-day technique for hepatic resection of primary or metastatic disease is based on several foundations. First, an understanding of hepatic anatomy has resurfaced during the recent 10-year period in liver surgery. Second, new indications for performing primary tumor resection and hepatic metastectomy with curative intent have become acceptable. A more refined knowledge of the segmental distribution of hepatic arterial, portal venous, and biliary ductal architecture and thorough awareness of the "crossover" distribution of the hepatic venous architecture have meshed with the more aggressive treatment of diseases that until recently were considered uniformly lethal.

The historical establishment of priorities in hepatic surgery is difficult to sort out, but has been reviewed in the clinical expositions of Starzl, Adson, and Longmire (1–3). One of the best concise reviews of the history of advertent hepatic surgery is by H. Gans, who considers Wendel to be the forerunner of modern hepatic surgery (4). Dr. Gans defines modern hepatic surgery as that which is performed with some expectation of postoperative patient survival!

This chapter summarizes surgical technique for various kinds of liver resections. In it, the author's knowledge of the literature is filtered through his own hepatic resection experience (5,6).

The first precept in discussing hepatic surgery is to know what is meant when referring to a specific procedure. The best approach to the uniform anatomic definition of hepatic resections has been supplied by Balasegaram and co-workers (7). Figures 21.1 and 21.2 are modifications of Balasegaram's schematic drawings. Figure 21.1 shows the formal right hepatic lobectomy and the extended right hepatic lobectomy [referred to as right trisegmentectomy by Starzl et al. (1)], and Figure 21.2 shows the left hepatic lobectomy, the extended left hepatic lobectomy [referred to as left trisegmentectomy by Starzl et al. (8)], and the left lateral segmentectomy, which is the most frequently performed segmental resection for metastatic disease. Other anatomic segments can be removed individually from the periphery of the liver or in conjunction with major lobectomies.

This author's perspective on segmental hepatic anatomy has been simplified by his experience in the operating room. Although eight segmental divisions of the liver have been described anatomically (9,10), there are only four segments that can be easily surgically circumscribed: the right lobe (all of the liver to the right of a division extending from the gallbladder fossa down through the retrohepatic inferior vena cava), the medial segment of the left lobe (from the midplane of the liver to the falciform ligament), the left lateral segment (the part of the liver lateral to the falciform ligament), and the entire left lobe (both of the preceding segments).

If the surgeon defines other segments in planning the resection, he or she should be prepared for tedious dissection, encountering many vessels with significant blood loss. In particular, the left trisegmentectomy, a resection of the left hepatic lobe and an anterior segment of the right lobe, superficial to a coronal plane lying just above the right hepatic vein (8), is an anatomic fantasy. Even those who routinely perform "heroic" hepatic operations report significant intraoperative blood loss allow delineation of the celiac arterial road map after venous injection of contrast material on a more convenient outpatient basis. Some authors have denied the usefulness of arteriography (1), but I find that it is helpful to define particular variations of celiac arterial architecture preoperatively. For instance, if a patient is to undergo a segmental wedge resection of the lateral left lobe, the presence of an aberrant left hepatic artery arising from the left gastric artery would suggest that a formal left hepatic lobe resection should be performed instead. Transection of the aberrant artery in the course of the segmentectomy could produce a necrotic medial segment of the remaining left lobe, with resultant bleeding and infection. A second procedure might then be required in an unhappy attempt at nonanatomic completion lobectomy amid pus, blood, and bile. Knowing about a replaced left hepatic artery is also helpful when planning a right trisegmentectomy, since it becomes easier to dissect along the falciform ligament without inadvertently occluding the arterial blood supply to the remaining lateral segment of the left lobe.

A second important and common variation in the celiac anatomy is the replaced right hepatic artery, which usually arises from the superior mesenteric artery. The replaced right hepatic runs laterally and more posteriorly than usual as it courses out through the porta hepatis. Knowing this in advance helps the surgeon plan an efficient dissection of the porta.

Surgical Technique

The initial incision to be used for an hepatic lobectomy depends on the patient's physiognomy and the surgeon's preference. The author prefers a right subcostal incision, but has had several patients with right upper quadrant abdominal colostomies necessitating the use of other incisions. Regardless of the type of resection planned, a relatively limited abdominal incision is made to surgically stage the patient, ruling out extrahepatic disease or unresectable intrahepatic disease. If the surgical staging agrees with the preoperative staging, then the incision is extended. When a Kocher's incision is used, the abdominal extension is continued to the midline and brought up vertically to, and sometimes including, the xiphoid process.

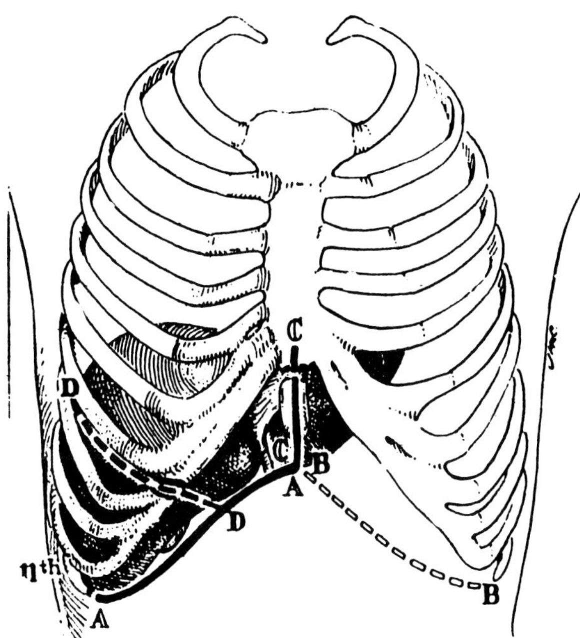

Figure 21.3. Incisions for hepatic resection. (Reproduced by permission from Starzl TE, Bell RH, Beart RW, Putnam CV. Hepatic trisegmentectomy and other liver resections. *Surg Gynecol Obstet* 1975; 141:429.)

Figure 21.3 summarizes the variety of incisions that can be used for hepatic resection.

In addition, the surgeon can use a median stenotomy extended up from a midline abdominal or Kocher's incision. This is often a standard approach for hepatic transplantation and can be used in patients who have large right lobe tumors with probable involvement of the right hepatic vein takeoff from the retrohepatic vena cava.

All patients with large right hepatic lobe tumors should be told that a thoracic extension is probable. The decision to make such an extension occurs at the time of surgery. The right thoracotomy can be carried up as a T from the middle of the right subcostal incision or can be brought up through the costachondral cartilage at the level of the sixth or the seventh rib from the midline at the xiphoid. In the author's experience, no more than 25% of right hepatic lobectomies have required extension into the right hemithorax. The major rationale for doing so is to visualize the right hepatic vein and to obtain vascular control prior to the hepatic finger fracture even when patients have large posterior, superior right lobe lesions. Although not always possible, when one can isolate and

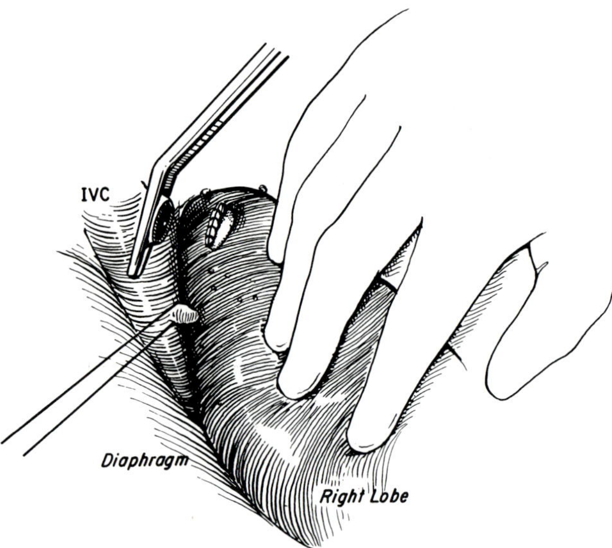

Figure 21.4. View of retrohepatic cava with medial retraction of right lobe after transection and suture of the right hepatic vein.

ligate the hepatic veins in an anatomic and surgically meticulous fashion, this obviates the less controlled approach of defining major venous structures at the base of the liver after finger fracture.

After ruling out extrahepatic disease and after examining and palpating the liver to define the anatomy of intrahepatic disease, attachments to the retroperitoneum and diaphragm should be freed up. Blunt and sharp dissection of triangular ligaments allow medial retraction of the right lobe and visualization of the entire right lateral border of the retrohepatic vena cava (Fig. 21.4).

If the tumor is lateral and posterior in the right lobe, there are often inflammatory extensions into the triangular ligaments, making the dissection to the vena cava more difficult. The surgeon should be careful to include as much of the inflammatory tissue in the resection as possible to avoid leaving tumor behind at the dissection margin. Extension of the tumor (whether primary or metastatic) from the surface of the superior aspect of the right lobe into the right hemidiaphragm has not dissuaded the author from curative resection. Free margins are obtained even if this entails considerable resection of the diaphragmatic musculature. The remaining hemidiaphragm can easily be repaired with prosthetic material or, more often than not, can be reopposed with interrupted zero-gauge silk horizontal mattress sutures.

Both the right and left lobes are routinely mobilized regardless of the position of the liver tumor. This necessitates blunt and sharp dissection of the triangular ligaments attaching the left lobe, even before performing a right hepatic lobectomy. Complete mobilization of the liver has enabled routine intraoperative ultrasound examination and provided the surgeon with better intrahepatic surgical staging (15). Numerous unsuspected metastases or multifocal primary tumors deep within the right or the left lobes have been discovered in this way. Intraoperative ultrasound has also helped to determine the extent of resection and obtain precise information about contiguity of the tumor to the right or middle hepatic veins or to the vena cava, eliminating the need for proceeding ahead with hepatic fracture and finding at the last minute that the tumor must be shaved off a right or middle hepatic vein or that the veins must be included in the resection to obtain a tumor-free margin.

After completing the ultrasound examination, the appropriate type of resection can be chosen. For a right hepatic lobectomy, a right trisegmentectomy, or a left hepatic lobectomy, the next surgical focus is the porta hepatis. For right-sided lesions necessitating formal lobectomy, the portal anatomy is defined by dissecting from anterior to posterior. The cystic artery and cystic duct are defined and transected. The right hepatic artery is next identified, but transected only after the left hepatic artery is visualized. The common duct bifurcation is usually within the substance of the liver at the uppermost margins of the porta. The right hepatic duct is transected only after the left hepatic duct has been visualized. The final structure defined and transected in the porta is the right portal vein. Placement of 6-0 Prolene vascular stitches rather than simple suture ligature or free ties prevents retraction and bleeding from either end. Retraction of an inadequately ligated portal vein stump on the liver side of the transected vein is particularly troublesome.

A somewhat different approach to the porta is helpful in performing a left lobectomy. The falciform ligament is dissected free down to the retrohepatic vena cava. The left portal venous branch can often be dissected more easily from the surrounding portal structures by proceeding from posterior to anterior. After complete dissection of the porta hepatis (Fig. 21.5), a color demarcation

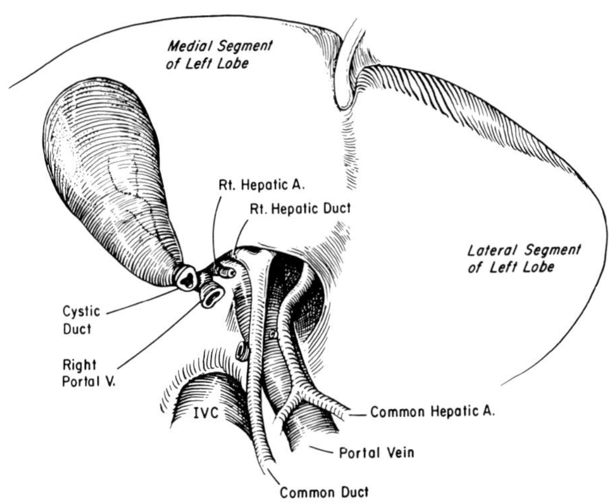

Figure 21.5. Dissecting the porta hepatis.

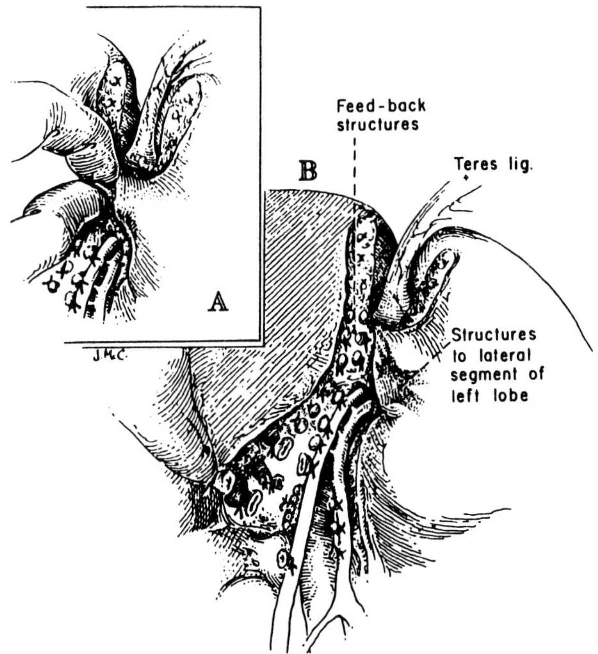

Figure 21.6. The right trisegmentectomy as described by Starzl et al. (Reproduced by permission from Starzl TE, Bell RH, Beart RW, Putnam CV. Hepatic trisegmentectomy and other liver resections. *Surg Gynecol Obstet* 1975; 141:429.)

anatomically defines the devascularized liver to be removed.

The anatomic extension of the porta hepatis dissection for a right trisegmentectomy or extended right hepatectomy has been well described by Starzl and colleagues (1). It consists of a dissection into the liver along the falciform ligament with definition and transection of the left hepatic arterial and left hepatic duct branches supplying the medial segment of the left lobe (Fig. 21.6). The so-called "crossover" anatomy of the hepatic venous structures and hepatic arterial and portal venous structures is important to understand before performing either a right hepatic trisegmentectomy or a left lateral lobe segmentectomy. Adherence to a line of transection contiguous to the falciform ligament rather than slightly to the right often devascularizes the remaining left lateral segment during right trisegmentectomy. During a lateral segmentectomy, performing the liver fracture directly through the falciform ligament rather than just to the left may devascularize a portion of the medial segment of the left lobe.

On completion of the porta hepatis dissection, the most appropriate approach to the hepatic venous anatomy must be chosen. In a patient undergoing a right hepatic lobectomy or an extended right hepatic lobectomy, the preferred technique is to visualize the right hepatic vein directly applying vascular clamps to its juncture with the retrohepatic vena cava, with placement of a running 6-0 Prolene stitch on the cava side and, if possible, on

the liver side after transection. As with the portal venous stump, slippage of the hepatic vein on the caval side can easily be repaired by applying sponges fore and aft of the caval venotomy. Slippage on the liver side is much more troublesome since the hepatic venous stump retracts up into the substance of the liver. This often marks a dramatic change in the operative rhythm, with a move to immediate hepatotomy when neither surgical assistants nor anesthesiologists are fully prepared.

Numerous small hepatic veins along the retrohepatic vena cava can easily be occluded with hemaclips and then transected. Forty-five-degree-angle hemaclip placers are perfect for applying medium- to large-sized clips. The undersurface of the liver, which is the caval resection plane, should be freed of all but the middle and/or left hepatic vein, which will be preserved.

Following hepatic venous dissection, the hepatic transection is performed in any of numerous ways. My own preference is to score the liver capsule at the point of vascular demarcation using a knife or cautery. By finger fracture, I proceed through the liver substance feeling veins, arteries, and bile ducts that will not easily yield to the fingers. These structures are clamped and tied with 3-0 or 4-0 silk sutures. Others prefer to use the Cavitron for the hepatotomy and it works quite nicely, in essence combining the blunt finger method with a suction device. As with finger fracture, major hepatic venous, portal venous, and arterial and biliary ductal structures still need to be clamped and tied. At completion of the dissection through the substance of the liver, all remaining bleeders are ligated. All devitalized tissue is removed even if this requires further formal resection of residual liver tissue. Tumor margins are checked by the surgical pathologist to assure clearance. Neither topical thrombin nor mattress sutures through the substance of the liver capsule should be necessary after formal lobectomy. The liver bed should be dry prior to closure. The large space that is left following a right hepatic lobectomy or a right trisegmentectomy is drained using multiple closed suction devices, such as Jackson-Pratt drains with 200 to 250-cc reservoirs. These are left in place until there is no biliary, blood, or seromatous drainage. Normally 5 to 6 days of such drainage is necessary following right and extended right lobectomy. Fewer days of drainage are needed following left or left lateral segmental resection since there is less dead space to drain.

The approach to hepatic venous anatomy during a left hepatic lobe resection is different than for right hepatic lobe resection. As is illustrated in Figure 21.7, one cannot define the major venous structures before doing the hepatotomy, and in general, major venous drainage from the left lobe is encountered only at the base of the hepatic fracture. The precise anatomic relationships between a large, medial left hepatic lobe tumor and the middle hepatic vein and its bifurcation into left and medial venous tributaries can be far more easily discerned with the aid of intraoperative ultrasound technique in advance of the transection. At the base of the finger fracture hepatotomy, the left hepatic vein is defined at its junction from the middle hepatic vein. Right-angled clamps are placed, the vein is transected, and the left liver lobe is removed. The decision to place free suture ties or to apply a 6-0 running Prolene stitch at the base of the hepatic vein can be made following removal of the lobe, and depends on the particular hepatic venous anatomy found.

The major technical challenge in hepatic resection involves the hepatic venous anatomy. The

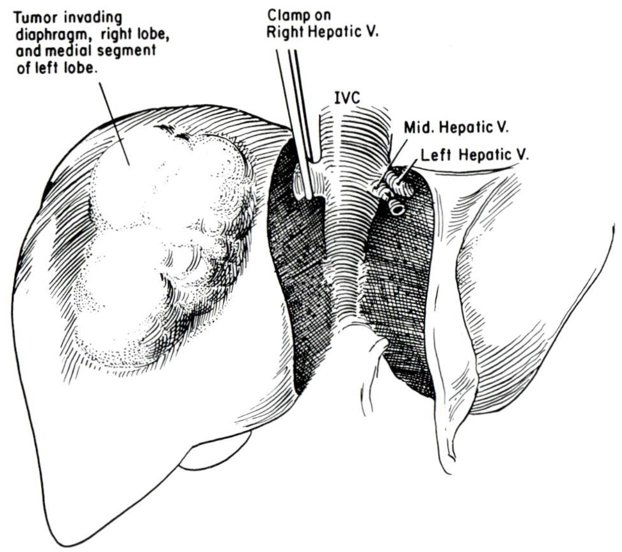

Figure 21.7.   View of major hepatic veins at the base of the hepatotomy.

only potentially lethal technical error that a competent hepatic surgeon can make is the inadvertent vertical transection of the middle hepatic vein in the midst of a right hepatic or extended right hepatic lobectomy. If this laceration extends downward into the branching points of the vessel as it retracts back into the medial segment of the left lobe, a completion trisegmentectomy for vascular control might have to be performed. If manual compression of the residual left lobe cannot be released without substantial bleeding, several technical salvage maneuvers can be tried. The liver can be completely isolated by applying a vascular clamp across the remaining structures in the porta hepatis (known as Pringle's maneuver), and the retrohepatic vena cava can be clamped above and below the liver. Warm ischemia will be tolerable for up to 1 hour. The cardiac index will decrease but not unacceptably, particularly if the anesthesiologist is forewarned of the development and can increase the patient's intravascular volume before the placement of caval clamps. Such complete vascular isolation of the liver can give the surgeon time to define the extent of the technical problem with the middle hepatic vein, and to decide in a calm environment whether to perform a completion trisegmentectomy or to attempt direct repair of the retracted, lacerated branches of the middle hepatic vein. Although techniques such as isolation/perfusion, popularized a number of years ago by Fortner et al. (16), are no longer necessary for routine hepatic resection, modifications like those of Huguet and the hepatic transplanters (17,18) have demonstrated the feasibility of complete vascular isolation as a temporary fallback in case of trouble.

Hepatic wedge resections can be performed in a number of ways. Before choosing to do a wedge resection, the surgeon must remember that a large wedge resection may be more difficult to perform than a formal hepatic lobectomy simply because vascular control cannot be accomplished with anatomic precision. Wedge resections of tumor on the lateral aspects of the right or the left lobe are preceded by placement of O-Chromic mattress sutures using a large blunt-tipped needle. The liver capsule is scored just lateral to this stitch with cautery or a knife, and the liver substance is resected by finger fracture or Cavitron. Visual and proprioceptive tumor margins should be confirmed by the pathologist. Major venous, arterial, and biliary duct structures are clamped and ligated with 3-0 or 4-0 silk. The previously placed chromic mattress sutures are tied tightly enough to compress but not cut through the liver capsule. All bleeding must be meticulously controlled. The use of various natural and non-natural substances (e.g., omentum and topical thrombin) to abut the bare area of residual liver should be avoided. Cautery (at the highest setting) can occasionally be used to stop minor bleeding. After a major wedge resection, as after formal hepatic lobectomy, the patient should be left with closed tube drainage of the right upper quadrant until there is no further drainage.

Numerous authors have described the use of various liver clamps in performing hepatic resection. Figure 21.8 illustrates the typical placement of such a clamp (19). This figure also illustrates why the author does not use such clamps. The shape of the human liver in the author's patient population simply does not allow such clamp placement as depicted in the figure. Laser techniques for scoring the liver capsule and performing hepatotomy have also been described, but probably offer no advantage over the surgeon's blade, at least for present indications for liver resection.

Conclusion

The median hospital stay for patients who have had major liver surgery in the author's series is 12 days (5). Patients recover quickly with surprisingly little serious morbidity. The development of ade-

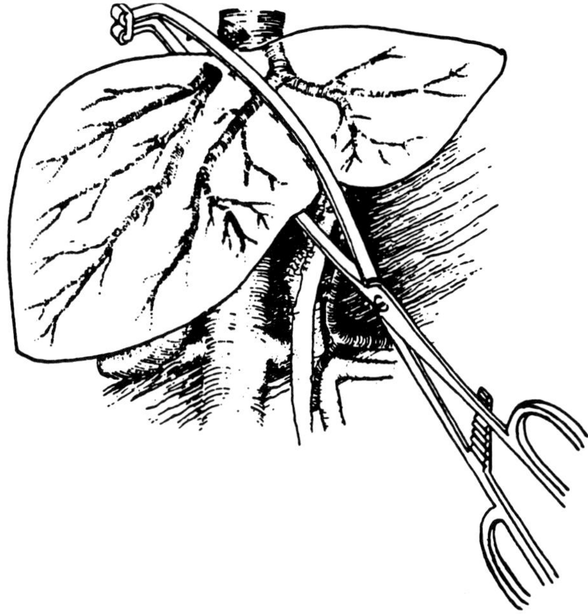

Figure 21.8. Conceptual view of hepatic clamp placement. (Reproduced by permission from Nagasue N, Hirose S. Hepatic trisegmentectomy using the Lin liver clamp. *Surg Gynecol Obstet* 1983; 156:302.)

quate closed drainage systems is a distinct improvement over the earlier use of multiple Penrose or polyethylene drains placed through the lateral aspect of the subcostal incision, which probably allowed as much contamination from the outside in as drainage from the inside out. Occasionally, clinically significant collections of bile and serum occur after removal of Jackson-Pratt drains, often causing temperature spikes a week or two after the patient has been discharged from the hospital. These collections can easily be defined by ultrasound examination and drained by percutaneous ultrasound or CT-guided pigtail catheter placement necessitating only a short rehospitalization.

The published mortality in studies of major liver resection varies from 3% to 20%. Major liver surgery should not be done in centers where there is a 10% or greater mortality. The key to success in these cases is the combination of excellent anatomic understanding with surgical expertise and, above all, good surgical judgment in choosing patients. The usual deficit is not in technique. The adept and aggressive surgeon must remember that regardless of his or her heroism and brilliance, a primary or metastatic tumor too large or multifocal often reflects an intrinsically bad biology that will determine an unhappy outcome despite the surgeon's will.

References

1. Starzl TE, Bell RH, Beart RW, Putnum CV. Hepatic trisegmentectomy and other liver resections. *Surg Gynecol Obstet* 1975; 141:429–437.
2. Adson MA, Van Heerden JA. Major hepatic resections for metastatic colorectal cancer. *Ann Surg* 1980; 191:576–583.
3. Thompson HH, Tompkins RK, Longmire WP. Major hepatic resection. *Ann Surg* 1983; 197:375–388.
4. Gans H. Tradition and innovation: Reflections on selected historical highlights in the field of hepatic surgery. *Surgery* 1975; 77:593–601.
5. Steele G Jr, Osteen RT, Wilson RE, Brooks DC, et al. Patterns of failure after surgical "cure" of large liver tumors—a change in the proximate cause of death and a need for effective systemic adjuvant therapy. *Am J Surg* 1984; 147:554–559.
6. McDermott WV, Cady B, Steele G Jr. Major hepatic resection: A 20 year experience (abstr 335). Presented at the Hepato-Pancreatico-Biliary Surgery First World Congress, Lund, Sweden, 1986. June 12.
7. Joishy SK, Balasegaram M. Hepatic resection for malignant tumors of the liver: Essentials for a unified surgical approach. *Am J Surg* 1980; 139:360–369.
8. Starzl TE, Iwatsuki S, Shaw BW Jr, Waterman PM, et al. Left hepatic trisegmentectomy. *Surg Gynecol Obstet* 1982; 155:21–27.
9. Cournaud C. Lobes et segments hepatiques. *Presse Med* 1954; 62:709.
10. Ellis H, Petly D. Gross anatomy of the blood vessels and ducts within the human liver. *Am J Anat* 1952; 90:59.
11. Hughes KS, Simon R, Songhorabodi S, Adson MA, et al. Resection of the liver for colorectal carcinoma metastases: A multi-institutional study of patterns of recurrence. *Surgery* 1986; 100:278–284.
12. Ekburg H, Tranberg KG, Andersson R, et al. Pattern of recurrence in liver resection for colorectal secondaries. *World J Surg* (in press).
13. Gastrointestinal Tumor Study Group Trial GITSG 6584.
14. Hughes K, Simon R, Songhorabodi S, et al. Patterns of failure following hepatic resection for colorectal metastases: A multi-institutional study. *Cancer* (in press).
15. Ravikumar TS, Onik G, Kane R, et al. Hepatic cryosurgery with intraoperative ultrasound monitoring for metastatic colon carcinoma. *Arch Surg* (in press).
16. Howland WS, Schweizer O, Fortner JG, Shiu MH, et al. Intraoperative physiologic monitoring and management during hepatic lobectomy using the liver isolation-perfusion technic. *Am J Surg* 1975; 129:608–615.
17. Delva E, Barberousse JP, Nordlinger B, Ollivier JM, et al. Hemodynamic and biochemical monitoring during major liver resection with use of hepatic vascular exclusion. *Surgery* 1984; 95:309–318.
18. Shaw BW, Martin DJ, Marquez JM, Kang YG, et al. Venous bypass in clinical liver transplantation. *Ann Surg* 1984; 200:524–534.
19. Nagasue N, Hirose S. Hepatic trisegmentectomy using the Lin liver clamp. *Surg Gynecol Obstet* 1983; 156:302–304.

Editorial Comment

Three points relative to this excellent chapter on the techniques concerned with hepatic resection perhaps deserve further comment or amplification.

First, in regard to the ultrasonic scalpel (or Cavitron), the utilization of this particular technologic advance has had a mixed reception. To some surgeons, it is tedious and seems to offer no specific advantages. To others (the editors of this book included), there is a considerable advantage to the appropriate use of this tool in terms of blood loss, minimization of necrotic tissue, and identification and preservation of ducts and vessels prior to transection and ligation. While utilization of the instrument throughout the total transection of the liver may seem tedious to some, it is certainly of considerable advantage. It offers protection against inadvertent blood loss, when one is dissecting deeper in the hepatic parenchyma where one begins to encounter major afferent and efferent blood vessels. Its use in identification of medium to small biliary radicals does protect the patient, to an added degree, against a biliary leak in the postoperative period. Thus, if used judiciously, the instrument may prove of considerable value to the surgeon who has the patience to become accustomed to this particular and somewhat peculiar method of traversing the parenchyma of the liver itself.

Reference has been made to the intraoperative use of ultrasonography in identification of otherwise unrecognizable liver tumors. Not only is this useful in the diagnostic sense but also it can be applied as a guide to the introduction of a freezing probe for cryosurgical destruction of a limited number of tumors in the contralateral lobe.

Among the excellent and experienced hepatic surgeons in the world, there is tremendous variation in the technologies described in the literature and it would be hard to select one. Foster (1) has used an automatic applicator and has outlined its advantages in hepatic surgery, while others feel that the use of nonabsorbable foreign material in hepatic surgery is precluded by the risk of fistulas or a gradual invasion of the foreign material into the biliary tract. The very diversity of the minor variations in technology indicate that, as so often is true in surgical technique, there is more than one way of performing a given surgical task.

References

1. Foster JH. Automatic clip applier as an aid to liver resection. *Am J Surg* 151:289–290, February, 1986.

Chapter 22
Liver Abscess

LOUIS B. RICE
ADOLF W. KARCHMER

Despite remarkable advances in the past three decades, the diagnosis and management of hepatic abscesses continues to pose difficult problems for the practicing clinician. Ever-improving imaging techniques, a constantly expanding armamentarium of antibiotics, and rapidly evolving perspectives on modes of treatment provide the physician with a powerful array of tools to identify and combat these lesions. Nevertheless, because the presentation of hepatic abscesses may be subtle, the clinician must maintain a high index of suspicion to recognize the often obscure and nonspecific clues offered by the patient and to take advantage of these tools. The two main types of liver abscess, pyogenic (or bacterial) and amebic, share many features. However, their diagnosis and treatment are quite different. Therefore, this chapter addresses these entities separately. It attempts to provide an overview of the incidence, clinical and laboratory presentation, diagnostic evaluation, and therapeutic options for both pyogenic and amebic abscesses of the liver, acknowledging their similarities but, more importantly, emphasizing their differences.

Pyogenic Liver Abscess

Incidence

The incidence of pyogenic hepatic abscess has not changed significantly over the past five decades, ranging from 5 to 16 per 100,000 hospital admissions (1–7). Autopsy studies have shown a higher incidence, ranging from 29 to 59 per 100,000 autopsies (6,8,9). The majority of studies published about this illness have shown a slight male predominance with the male–female ratio ranging from 1:1 to 3:1 (10,11). The introduction of antibi-

otics and the aggressive surgical treatment of appendicitis in the 1940s coincided with an increase in the average age of those suffering from hepatic abscess, from the fourth to the sixth and seventh decades of life. The major part of this change took place between publication of the classic study by Ochsner, DeBakey, and Murray in 1938 (7) and the subsequent major autopsy study by Sherman and Robbins in 1960 (9). There has been little change in the average age of patients with this disorder since 1960. Although some studies have suggested a racial predilection for liver abscesses (12), this distinction is not supported by recent studies of racially mixed populations (13). There is little variation in the incidence of pyogenic hepatic abscesses between geographic regions, although the frequency of amebic abscesses relative to pyogenic abscesses is strongly affected by geography as a function of the endemicity of amebiasis (13,14).

The majority of pyogenic liver abscesses are solitary and occur in the right lobe of the liver. The reason for the right-lobe predominance is not known, though it has been suggested by numerous authors that this may result either from the larger size of the right lobe or from the preferential portal venous flow to this region. In 20% to 40% of cases abscesses involve both lobes, a distribution seen more commonly in the presence of obstructive biliary tract disease.

Pathogenesis

Predisposing conditions can often be identified in patients who develop pyogenic liver abscesses. Among these conditions are biliary tract disease (either intrahepatic or extrahepatic), infection in a region drained by the portal venous system (diverticulitis, appendicitis, perforated colon), arterial hematogenous seeding during bacteremic episodes, direct trauma to the liver (either penetrating or nonpenetrating), suppurative infection in a contiguous site, or necrotic malignant lesions within the liver itself. No predisposing condition can be identified for a significant number of abscesses; these are termed cryptogenic (15–17).

Prior to the antibiotic era, appendicitis was the most commonly identified predisposing condition for pyogenic liver abscess (7). As a result of aggressive surgical treatment of appendicitis and the use of antibiotics, liver abscess is now rarely associated with appendicitis. The most common predisposing factor at present is biliary tract disease (1,5,18). The frequency of the major predisposing conditions among patients with liver abscess is presented in Table 22.1. Finally, depression of immune defenses may allow the development of liver abscess, as evidenced by the occurrence of the lesions in patients with compromised immunity, such as those with childhood leukemia with granulocytopenia and chronic granulomatous disease.

It is generally accepted that some pre-existing liver damage is necessary for the development of a pyogenic liver abscess. The normal liver efficiently clears bacteria from both the portal and the systemic circulations, making it unlikely that portal bacteremia by itself (unless the inoculum is overwhelming) is sufficient to cause liver abscess. The infrequency of liver abscess as a complication of inflammatory bowel disease, a condition that predisposes to portal bacteremia, supports this concept (19). Hepatic injury (e.g., obstructed bile ducts, ischemia from hypotension, direct trauma, space-occupying lesions) may alter the liver's normal antibacterial defense and makes abscess formation more likely. Early liver transplant experience suggested that an infarcted area in the liver is especially susceptible to abscess formation (20). The damaged hepatic parenchyma can be seeded by bacteria that are delivered by the bile ducts, the portal vein, or the systemic circulation. Organisms then multiply in an area sequestered from normal tissue defenses, leading to abscess formation.

In cases of cryptogenic abscess the nature of the pre-existing liver damage, if in fact such damage is present, is less obvious. Lee and Block speculate that these abscesses occur in the setting of "idiopathic intrahepatic thromboembolism" (21), with subsequent infarction and bacterial invasion. They use as supportive evidence for this theory the frequent isolation of anaerobic bacteria from the cryptogenic abscesses. The anaerobic nature of the abscesses suggests, in their view, that the infection must have started in an area sequestered from the normal circulation.

Clinical Features

The clinical presentation of pyogenic liver abscess is varied and often nonspecific. Symptoms and physical findings from representative studies are given in Table 22.2. The duration of illness varies from days to months. Presentation can be insidious, with vague complaints of anorexia and malaise, or fulminant, with septic shock (22). The most common presenting complaints are fever, anorexia, malaise, weight loss, abdominal pain, nausea, and vomiting. The physical examination is equally nonspecific, the most common findings being an abnormal right lower lung field examination (29% to 62%) (13,23), abdominal tenderness (which may not be localized to the right upper quadrant)(28% to 76%)(21,24), and hepatomegaly or a right upper quadrant mass (23% to 92%)(21,24). Jaundice is rare but has been reported to be a poor prognostic sign.

Laboratory findings are also nonspecific. Most patients present with an elevated leukocyte count with an increase in the percentage of band forms.

Table 22.1. Frequency of Predisposing Factors for Pyogenic Liver Abscess

Source (Ref. No.)	Biliary Tract Infection (%)	Infections in Areas Drained by Portal Vein (%)	No Predisposing Factor (%)
Pitt and Zuidema, 1975 (5)	51	14	20
Balasegaram, 1981 (10)	35	12	5
Greenstein et al., 1984 (1)	44	16	21
Land et al., 1985 (24)	20	12	44
Conter and Tompkins, 1987 (22)	37	22	12
Gyorffy et al., 1987 (18)	35	19	15

Table 22.2. Frequency of Presenting Symptoms and Abnormalities on Physical Examination in Patients with Pyogenic Hepatic Abscess

		Presenting Symptoms			Physical Findings		
Source (Ref. No.)	No. of Patients	Fever (%)	Abdominal Pain (%)	Nausea/ Vomiting (%)	Pulmonary (%)	Abdominal Tenderness (%)	Hepatomegaly (%)
Lazarchick et al., 1973 (36)	80	87	77	53	21	41	69
Rubin et al., 1974 (6)	53	87		28	11	47	51
Balasegaram, 1981 (10)	125	98	97	68	36	95	87
Miedema and Dineen, 1984 (2)	106	93		24	35	71	52
Neoptolemos et al., 1982 (4)	44	91	73			52	50
Greenstein et al., 1984 (1)	38	95	84	47	37	42	39
Land et al., 1985 (24)	25	80	48			24	28	24

The erythrocyte sedimentation rate is usually elevated and the hematocrit depressed. Liver function abnormalities vary. Alkaline phosphatase elevations, reported in 12% to 100% of cases, will vary with the degree of coexisting biliary obstruction. Transaminase elevations, which are generally mild, have been reported in 30% to 90% of cases. Hypoalbuminemia has been frequently noted and is felt to be a poor prognostic sign. Bilirubin elevations, if present, are usually mild. In sum, the clinical and laboratory presentation of pyogenic liver abscess is often nonspecifc, requiring that the clinician have a high index of suspicion to pursue the diagnosis.

Diagnostic Imaging

No technologic advances in the past two decades have had a more profound effect on the diagnosis and treatment of liver abscesses than the improvements in hepatic imaging capabilities. Prior to the 1960s, the only noninvasive radiologic modalities used in the diagnosis of liver abscesses were routine chest and abdominal radiographs. Although chest x-ray findings are abnormal 35% to 85% of the time (1,17), the abnormalities are nonspecific (pleural effusion, right lower lobe atelectasis, raised right hemidiaphragm). Abdominal x-ray films are abnormal less often, although they may be of value if they reveal an abnormal gas or fluid collection in the right upper quadrant.

The first major advance in the diagnosis and localization of liver abscesses came in the 1960s with the introduction of the technetium colloid liver/spleen scintiscan. Initial reports were extremely encouraging, with some publications claiming 100% accuracy (15,21,25). More recent

reports suggest an accuracy ranging from 70% to 100% (2,22,23). Despite these impressive results, the liver/spleen scan has limitations. Although it is able to identify space-occupying lesions within the liver, it offers no information about the nature of these lesions. Smaller abscesses are below the resolution of the scintiscan. Finally, interpretation of these scans may be difficult in the presence of infiltrative or inflammatory disease in the liver.

Ultrasonography, introduced in the 1970s, has a diagnostic accuracy of 70% to 100% (2,10,22). More importantly, it allows the distinction of solid masses from those that contain liquid, thus aiding in the distinction between tumor and abscess. Finally, ultrasound provides a means by which the path of a percutaneously introduced needle can be monitored, making percutaneous aspiration of abscess contents a precise, safe diagnostic procedure. The major limitation of ultrasonography in the diagnosis of liver abscess is its inability to image the entire liver simultaneously, thereby increasing the likelihood that a smaller abscess in an area that is difficult to visualize will be missed.

The introduction of computed tomography (CT) has further improved diagnostic capabilities by allowing visualization of the entire liver, distinction between solid and liquid on the basis of measured density, and visualization of multiple small abscesses. CT can also be used to guide percutaneous abscess drainage and monitor response to therapy. Although studies using this modality are limited, some series suggest that the diagnostic accuracy approaches 100% (10,13,18, 22,26).

Excluding considerations of cost and radiation exposure, ultrasonography and CT are comparable technologies for the initial step in diagnosing a liver abscess. Although there are some situations in which a liver/spleen scintiscan may be helpful, this modality has to a large extent been supplanted by ultrasonography and CT. Magnetic resonance imaging may prove to be a useful tool in the future, but additional information is required in order to evaluate this modality.

Bacteriology

Cultures of the contents of a pyogenic liver abscess will yield bacteria in 70% to 100% of cases. The ability to recover bacteria from pyogenic liver abscess is influenced by prior treatment of patients with antibiotics, the actual microbiologic culture techniques used, and the care with which the specimens are collected and processed. These considerations are particularly important when attempting to recover organisms that are highly susceptible to antibiotics, are fastidious and difficult to culture, or are obligate anaerobes. Gram stains of abscess contents not only provide immediate information about the organisms present but also may reveal organisms that are not subsequently recovered in cultures. Blood cultures will be positive in almost 50% of patients with a pyogenic hepatic abscess. However, the positive blood cultures frequently fail to reflect the polybacterial nature of some abscesses.

Microbiologic culture techniques, particularly for anaerobic bacteria, have improved significantly. Although the frequency with which anaerobic bacteria are recovered from pyogenic liver abscesses has increased, the spectrum of bacteria causing these lesions has changed little over the past five decades. Enteric Gram-negative bacilli, most commonly *Escherichia coli* and *Klebsiella* species, are the organisms most often found in these abscesses. Streptococcal species, including enterococci and other group D streptococci, microaerophilic streptococci, and anaerobic streptococci (peptostreptococci), are also commonly found. Other anaerobic bacteria, including *Bacteroides fragilis*, other *Bacteroides* species, and *Fusobacterium* species are found in up to 45% of abscesses when the contents are properly handled (not exposed to air) and cultured (27). Organisms found less commonly, and often in association with underlying immune abnormalities or specific settings, are *Staphylococcus aureus* (chronic granulomatous disease, intravenous drug abuse, penetrating trau-

ma), *Candida albicans*, and *Pseudomonas aeruginosa* (immunosuppressive and cytotoxic chemotherapy).

Many liver abscesses contain more than one organism, with anaerobic bacteria often recovered in association with other organisms. The incidence of polybacterial abscesses is reported to be between 20% and 50% (6,10,13), reinforcing the importance not only of broad-spectrum antibiotic coverage but also of assiduous attention to both aerobic and anaerobic culturing techniques.

The bacteriologic profile of any given abscess is in part related to the underlying conditions that have predisposed the patient to abscess formation. Abscesses resulting from obstructive biliary tract disease commonly contain Gram-negative bacilli. Portal and cryptogenic abscesses are likely to harbor anaerobic bacteria. External penetrating trauma will predispose to staphylococcal abscesses, as will chronic granulomatous disease of childhood. Such associations only serve as general guidelines, as there is considerable variation within any given group and overlap between groups.

A particularly noteworthy cause of pyogenic liver abscess is *Streptococcus milleri*. This microaerophilic streptococcus is known to produce cryptogenic abscesses in many organs. In one study of 16 liver abscesses, *S. milleri* was recovered as the sole pathogen from 10 patients and in conjunction with other organisms in three others (28). Although this series is atypical, particularly in terms of the underlying conditions that predisposed to the formation of the reported abscesses, it emphasizes the importance of this organism. *S. milleri*, unlike the anaerobic streptococci, is resistant to metronidazole, an antibiotic frequently relied upon for the treatment of anaerobic bacteria causing these infections.

Complications

The complications associated with pyogenic liver abscesses are usually the result of either the hematogenous dissemination of organisms or the direct rupture of the abscess into an adjacent anatomic space. The most common complication noted by Ochsner, DeBakey, and Murray (7) was rupture of the abscess superiorly through the diaphragm into either the pleural space or the right lung itself. Less frequent complications included direct rupture of the abscess into the peritoneal space, with subsequent peritonitis, and rupture into the pericardium, the subphrenic space, the abdominal wall, the vena cava, or the thoracic duct (7). Complications are generally associated with a higher mortality rate. Septicemia is listed as the most common complication in more recent studies (2,4), suggesting that improved diagnostic techniques have allowed intervention prior to abscess rupture.

Treatment

The cornerstone of treatment of pyogenic liver abscess has always been drainage of the abscess. This procedure offers three distinct advantages. First, it markedly decreases the organism load and it enhances antibiotic efficacy by altering the conditions of the infection. Second, it decreases the tension on the abscess wall, thereby decreasing the potential for septic complications. Third, it provides the material from which a microbiologic diagnosis is established and thus allows for specific, rather than broad-spectrum, empiric antibiotic therapy. Some authors suggest that in many cases antibiotics alone will provide effective therapy (13,29). However, other bacteria, in addition to those recovered in blood cultures, have frequently been isolated when the contents of the abscesses have been cultured; furthermore, these additional isolates have often required a change in antibiotic therapy (13). Hence, it is generally accepted that all nonamebic liver abscesses should undergo at least simple aspiration, if not some form of continuous drainage.

Open surgical drainage has been the rule in the vast majority of studies published on liver abscesses over the past 50 years. Early studies suggested a high mortality despite surgical drainage. For example, Ochsner, DeBakey, and Murray reported a mortality of more than 60% in their surgically treated patients (7). This high mortality was due in part to the difficulty in establishing the diagnosis and in part to the lack of intraoperative antibiotic use. With current diagnostic techniques and vigorous perioperative antibiotic therapy, the number and location of liver abscesses can be accurately identified before an operation and the complications that result from intraoperative spillage of abscess contents can be avoided. As a result, more recent reports suggest a mortality rate with open surgical drainage ranging from 8% to 22% (18,22,24).

In the past decade, considerable interest has been focused on the drainage of liver abscess through catheters that are placed percutaneously using ultrasound or CT guidance. Although encouraging results with percutaneous drainage were actually first reported in 1953 (30), this form of drainage did not gain wide acceptance until reliable radiologic techniques for guiding catheter placement were available. Numerous recent studies suggest a high rate of successful drainage through percutaneously placed catheters, with few reported complications (27,31,32). In general, Silastic catheters are introduced into each identifiable fluid collection and left in place to allow for continuous egress of fluid until drainage ceases, at which time the catheters are removed. Empiric broad-spectrum antimicrobial therapy, based on the organisms commonly isolated from pyogenic abscesses and the predisposing circumstances in a given patient, should be started immediately before the procedure. This concomitant antibiotic therapy will provide protection against septicemia and local infection due to abscess leakage but is not likely to invalidate the cultures of the abscess. Although infrequent, complications of the percutaneous catheter drainage include invasion of the pleural space, perforation of the gall bladder, leakage of abscess fluid into the peritoneum, and bacteremia (33). Proper patient selection and experience using percutaneous drainage techniques are important if complications are to be avoided and therapy successful (31–34). Retrospective studies comparing surgical drainage and drainage through percutaneously placed catheters in the treatment of pyogenic liver abscess suggest that these techniques, in properly selected patients, are associated with comparable cure rates, average duration of hospitalization, and procedure-related morbidity (31,32).

Who should undergo open surgical drainage and who percutaneous catheter drainage, and when will antibiotics alone be effective? For patients with abscesses that are accessible to percutaneous drainage and for whom surgery is not required to correct a predisposing illness (obstructed bile duct, diverticular abscess), percutaneous drainage should be attempted initially. If the number or location of the abscesses precludes adequate drainage, or if, after percutaneous drainage, antibiotic therapy does not result in amelioration of the patient's fever in one week or abatement after two weeks, surgical exploration should be considered. If, despite percutaneous drainage and antibiotic therapy, there is evidence of clinical worsening (e.g., persistent bacteremia, hypotension, or depressed mental status), surgical drainage should be undertaken more promptly. Percutaneous drainage should not be utilized in patients who have predisposing illnesses that will subsequently require laparotomy. In most settings these patients should be treated surgically to effect drainage of the liver abscesses and to correct the predisposing abnormalities.

The efficacy of antibiotic therapy in the absence of aspiration or drainage remains to be defined. One recent study suggests a high rate of success without continuous percutaneous catheter drainage (13). In patients who have positive blood cultures and who are stable clinically, antibiotic therapy alone can be considered. However, it is prudent to recall that in patients with pyogenic liver abscesses the blood culture isolates often fail to indicate the full complement of infecting organisms in the abscess and that antibiotic therapy based solely on the blood culture isolates often does not provide effective therapy for all of the organisms in the abscess. To be certain that antibiotic therapy is both effective against all of the infecting organisms and not unnecessarily broad or potentially toxic, the precise bacteriology of pyogenic hepatic abscess should be determined. Consequently, aspiration of an abscess is a minimum requirement before embarking upon a prolonged course of antibiotic therapy in the absence of drainage. Antibiotic therapy of multiple small abscesses resulting from arterial seeding of the liver by bacteria from a distant infected focus (e.g., liver abscesses associated with acute *S. aureus* endocarditis) is an exception to this caveat. Further studies are required to define the patients who are likely to be cured by antibiotic therapy without drainage.

Antibiotic Therapy

Empiric antibiotic treatment for pyogenic abscesses should be effective against enteric Gram-negative bacilli, streptococci, and anaerobic bacteria, including *B. fragilis*. There are currently available a wide range of antimicrobial agents that can be used alone or in combination to achieve this goal. Table 22.3 lists some of these agents and their relative in vitro activity against organisms commonly isolated from hepatic abscesses. An exhaustive detailing of the possible antibiotic combinations for empiric therapy is beyond the scope of this discussion, but a few points can be made. (a) There are several agents whose spectrum of activity is sufficiently broad that in non-life-threatening settings they may be considered as single-agent empiric therapy (amoxicillin-sulbactam, mezlocillin, piperacillin, cefoxitin, cefotetan, imipenem-cilastatin). (b) There are many alternatives to the use of aminoglycosides for the empiric coverage of Gram-negative bacilli. The toxicity of the aminoglycosides and their questionable activity within abscess cavities (poor activity in acidic pH) suggest that use of these agents should be restricted to situations where infection with resistant Gram-negative bacilli is suspected or in patients with history of allergy to other available agents. (c) If metronidazole is chosen as therapy for anaerobic bacteria, it must be used in conjunction with an agent active against streptococci, including *S. milleri*, and Gram-negative bacilli (e.g., piperacillin, mezlocillin, or a third-generation cephalosporin). The antibacterial action of metronidazole is limited to anaerobic Gram-negative and Gram-positive bacteria. (d) If a patient has been treated with cephalosporins prior to development of a liver abscess, empiric coverage should include an agent active against the enterococcus. This organism, which is resistant to the cephalosporins, has been known to cause abscesses in patients who have been treated with cephalosporins (35).

Once abscess fluid has been obtained, a Gram stain should be performed. The preliminary information from the Gram stain may suggest revision of empiric therapy. Once the antibiotic susceptibility of the organisms recovered from aerobic and anaerobic cultures is known, the empiric antibiotic regimen should be revised to provide effective therapy for the responsible pathogens.

There are limited data on the optimal duration of antibiotic therapy in the treatment of pyogenic liver abscess. Most authors suggest at least 3 to 4 weeks of treatment for solitary abscesses that have been well drained and 6 to 8 weeks of therapy for multiple abscesses or those that have been aspirated but not fully drained. Parenteral antimicrobial therapy is recommended until abscesses are

Table 22.3. Antibiotics Effective in Vitro Against Bacteria Commonly Found in Pyogenic Liver Abscesses

Antimicrobial Agent	Antibiotic Efficacy for Selected Organisms				
	Enteric Gram-Negative Bacilli (E. coli, Klebsiella)	Streptococci (nonenterococcal)	Enterococci	S. aureus	Anaerobic Gram-Negative Bacilli B. fragilis, Bacteroides sp.
Penicillins					
Ampicillin/Amoxicillin	2	3	3	0+	0
Amoxicillin-Sulbactam	3	3	3	3	3
Piperacillin	3	3	3	0+	2-3
Mezlocillin	3	3	3	0+	2
Azlocillin	3	3	3	0+	2
Cephalosporins					
Cefazolin	2	3	0	3	0
Cefamandole	2	3	0	3	0
Cefuroxime	3	3	0	3	1
Cefoxitin	3	3	0	2	3-2
Cefotetan	3	3	0	2	2-3
Ceftriaxone	3	3	0	2	1
Ceftizoxime	3	3	0	2	1
Cefoperazone	2-3	3	0	1	1
Cefotaxime	3	3	0	2	1
Ceftazidime	3	3	0	1	1
Aminoglycosides					
Gentamicin	3	0	3*	—	8
Netilmicin	3	0	2*	—	0
Tobramycin	3	0	2*	—	0
Amikacin	3	0	2*	—	0
Others					
Imipenem-Cilastatin	3	3	3	3	3
Ciprofloxacin	3	2	2	3	0
Chloramphenicol	3	2	2	2	3
Clindamycin	0	3	0	3	3
Metronidazole	0	0	0	0	3
Vancomycin	0	3	3	3	0

+ = not active against beta-lactamase-producing strains.
* = must be used in combination with penicillin, ampicillin, or vancomycin to achieve effect.
3 = >90% inhibited by clinically achievable concentration; high potency.
2 = 70% to 85% inhibited by clinically achievable concentration; moderate potency.
1 = 25% to 75% inhibited by clinically achievable concentration; low potency.
0 = <25% inhibited by clinically achievable concentration; little or no antibacterial activity.

decompressed and fever has abated for at least a week. If an effective oral regimen can be devised, it might be considered thereafter. Sonography and CT provide convenient noninvasive techniques with which to follow the resolution of abscesses and to guide decisions regarding duration of antimicrobial therapy.

Prognosis

The prognosis for a patient with pyogenic liver abscess has improved dramatically over the past five decades. Whereas mortality rates in earlier studies commonly exceeded 50%, recent surgical series have claimed mortality rates of 8% to 22%. Among clinically comparable patients, the outcome of those treated with percutaneous drainage is at least as good as that of patients treated surgically. Certain factors such as Gram-negative bacteremia, multiple abscesses, underlying malignancy, biliary obstruction, age above 50 years, jaundice, hypoalbuminemia, and the presence of complications are associated with increased fatality rates. However, with improved diagnostic and therapeutic techniques, the mortality associated with liver abscesses continues to approach that associated with the concurrent underlying disease. Further improvements in outcome will depend on a heightened awareness of this diagnosis, prompt use of diagnostic imaging techniques, and aggressive drainage and antimicrobial therapy.

Amebic Liver Abscess

Liver abscess is the most common complication of *Entamoeba histolytica* intestinal infection. In contrast to pyogenic abscesses, amebic liver abscesses occur much more commonly in men and tend to occur in younger patients (13,37). In the United States, amebic liver abscess occurs primarily in patients who have emigrated from or traveled to areas with a high rate of endemic amebic disease such as Mexico and Southeast Asia. Although a prior intestinal amebic infection is presumed, a significant number of patients report no prior history of amebic dysentery, and those that do often report only a remote history (38). In 85% of patients with amebic abscess, it occurs as a solitary lesion, with 65% to 70% of these abscesses confined to the right lobe of the liver. Unlike pyogenic abscesses, amebic liver abscesses are not associated with any specific predisposing conditions.

Microbiology

The protozoa *Entamoeba histolytica* exists in two forms, a cyst and a motile trophozoite. The trophozoite is the invasive form. This form lives in the wall or lumen of the colon. Trophozoites, which are excreted in diarrhea but not in normal stool, are unable to survive outside the body. When bowel movements are normal, the trophozoites encyst prior to excretion. The cysts, which are the infectious form of the organism, resist drying and freezing and can withstand the acid pH of the stomach. Once ingested, the walls of the cyst break down in the small intestine and trophozoites are released. The trophozoites are carried to the colon, where they remain. They may become invasive, the severity of invasion ranging from small, punctate lesions to large ulcerations reminiscent of ulcerative colitis. Occasionally, trophozoites enter the portal circulation and move to the liver, where they produce areas of hepatic necrosis surrounded by hemorrhage that ultimately progress to a debris-filled abscess cavity.

Clinical Features

The presentations of amebic and pyogenic liver abscesses are similar (10,13,37,39). Patients commonly report having fever, often with rigors. Right upper quadrant pain, which is frequently pleuritic in nature, is more common with amebic than with pyogenic abscess, perhaps because of the larger size generally attained by amebic abscesses. Diarrhea is an infrequent presenting symptom, occurring in as few as 11% of cases (12). The duration of symptoms ranged from days to months. In rare cases, patients will present with complaints referable to those areas into which the abscess has ruptured: the peritoneal cavity, pleural space, lung parenchyma, or pericardial space. Thus, patients may present with signs of an acute abdomen, shortness of breath and chest pain, hemoptysis, cough with purulent phlegm, or signs of pericardial tamponade. The direction of rupture is determined to some extent by the location of the abscess. Rupture into the pericardial space, for example, occurs exclusively as a complication of amebic abscesses in the left lobe of the liver.

Findings on physical examination that are related to amebic liver abscess are often localized to the upper right abdomen (10,13,37,39). Right upper quadrant tenderness, mass, or hepatomegaly are commonly noted. Findings on lung examination consistent with consolidation, effusion, or atelectasis are noted in a majority of cases. Clinical jaundice is uncommon. In some cases, the physical examination is unrevealing.

Laboratory tests characteristically reveal a leukocytosis with an increase in the percentage of band forms, which in most cases is not as marked as that seen with pyogenic abscess. Anemia is also common, and appears to be related to the duration of symptoms. Although elevations of alkaline phosphatase are frequently noted, this is not a universal finding (11). Katzenstein et al. reported a direct correlation between the magnitude of alkaline phosphatase elevation and the duration of symptoms (37). As with pyogenic liver abscess, hyperbilirubinemia is uncommon, and when found it is associated with a poor prognosis. Eosinophilia is not associated with amebic liver abscesses.

Complications

Three important complications have been associated with amebic liver abscess: rupture into an adjacent body cavity or organ, superinfection by bacteria, and multiple abscess formation in other organs. Most common among these complications is rupture of the abscess into the thoracic cavity. Depending upon the location of the abscess and the degree of tissue inflammation, rupture may occur into the pleural space, the lung parenchyma, or the pericardium. Rupture into the lung parenchyma carries the best prognosis, probably because the connection with the bronchial tree provides a means of egress for the infected material. Fortunately, pericardial rupture, the most morbid of these complications, occurs in only 1% to 2% of cases (39,40). Abscesses may also rupture into the peritoneum, producing a diffuse peritonitis with physical findings consistent with an acute abdomen or multiple abdominal abscesses. Rupture of amebic abscesses carries a higher mortality rate than is seen in uncomplicated cases (1%): rupture into pulmonary parenchyma (6%), rupture into the pleural cavity (14%), intraperitoneal rupture (18%), pericardial rupture (30% to 60%) (39,40). Amebic abscesses also rarely rupture into the bowel, producing an intrahepatic gas collection and passage of necrotic debris and pus per rectum, or into the biliary tree, producing hemobilia and hematemesis.

Other complications are rare and include bacterial superinfection and distant amebic abscesses, most commonly in the lung or brain. The most common cause of bacterial infection is a prior invasive procedure, although contamination may also occur when an amebic abscess ruptures into a nonsterile area, or by hematogenous seeding. Occasionally the mechanism of secondary infection cannot be established (13,37).

Radiologic Imaging

Abnormal chest radiographs have been found in 50% to 85% of patients with amebic liver abscess (13,38). As with pyogenic abscess, the most common findings are right lower lobe atelectasis, right pleural effusion, and a raised or bulging right hemidiaphragm. Abdominal radiographs are rarely helpful. Currently the most useful imaging technique for the diagnosis of amebic liver abscess is ultrasonography. Recent studies have consistently shown that ultrasonography is able to identify amebic abscesses in more than 90% to 95% of cases (13,41). Although a number of different imaging criteria have been proposed as diagnostic of hepatic amebic abscess, a recent large-scale blinded study comparing pyogenic and amebic abscesses found only a "round or oval shape" or "a hypoechoic appearance with fine low level echoes

at high gain" to be predictive of amebic etiology (13,42). Although liver/spleen scan is able to reveal the majority of lesions, the limited value of this modality in defining structure has led to a decline in its use. Finally, although good results have been obtained with computed tomography, its superiority over ultrasonography has not been demonstrated. Given the cost and radiation exposure associated with CT, ultrasonography is the technique of choice for imaging amebic hepatic abscesses.

Diagnosis

Although freshly collected or appropriately preserved specimens of stool from patients with suspected amebic abscess should be examined for amebae, the vast majority of patients will not have parasites detectable in stool. Thus, this is a highly unreliable test with which to establish amebic infection. In contrast, serologic tests that detect antibody to *E. histolytica* have become central in the diagnosis of amebic abscess (43,44). Although many test methods have been developed to detect an antibody response to *E. histolytica*, including latex agglutination, immunoelectrophoresis, complement fixation, indirect immunofluorescence, counter immunoelectrophoresis and enzyme-linked immunosorbent assay, the indirect hemagglutination (IHA) and agar gel diffusion (AGD) tests have gained wide acceptance. Recent studies with these two tests have shown them to be very sensitive and specific (they identify individuals with disease as infected and uninfected individuals as disease-free) (42) and very useful in the identification of patients with amebic liver abscess (13,37). These tests detect antibody in patients with invasive intestinal amebiasis as well as those with extraintestinal amebic infection. The IHA and AGD tests may be negative if performed early in the acute phase of illness, but both will usually turn positive if repeated two weeks later. The IHA test remains positive for many years after infection (often for 10 or more years). In regions where amebic colitis is endemic, a positive IHA test in a patient with possible liver abscess is difficult to interpret because it may reflect old but eradicated infection rather than active amebic disease. In contrast, AGD titers usually become negative within 6 to 12 months after eradication of infection, and thus when positive the AGD test reflects active amebic disease. Among patients with clinical and imaging studies suggestive of a hepatic abscess, a positive serologic test (particularly with the AGD system) in persons who have not previously resided in an area where amebiasis is endemic is highly suggestive of an amebic etiology for the abscess. Among those with a similar clinical picture who have resided in an endemic area, a positive serologic test is still likely to reflect the nature of the abscess, but it must be interpreted with more caution. This is particularly true if conditions are present that would predispose the patient to pyogenic hepatic abscess. In any event, negative serologic studies, except in very acute illness (whereupon the tests should be repeated several weeks later), provide strong evidence against amebae as the cause of a hepatic abscess.

Amebic liver abscess can be diagnosed with relative certainty when a probable abscess of the liver is imaged and the results of serologic tests for ameba are positive. Although diagnostic aspiration was performed routinely in the past, there is little reason to perform this procedure at present. Even when a percutaneous biopsy of the abscess wall (the site where amebic trophozoites are most likely to be found) is performed in conjunction with aspiration of the abscess contents, microbiologic examination of the specimens only establishes the diagnosis of an amebic abscess in 25% to 40% of cases. Thus, from a diagnostic perspective, the major role of aspiration is to evaluate possible bacterial infection, particularly in those patients who have not responded as anticipated to amebicidal therapy. Aspiration might also be justified in patients when clinical considerations suggest bacterial superinfection or when, despite clinical and epidemiologic evidence of amebic abscess, the serologic tests are negative and the diagnosis remains uncertain. Lastly, therapeutic aspiration has been recommended when abscesses are larger than 10 centimeters in diameter and rupture appears imminent, particularly if the lesion is in the left lobe, threatening rupture into the pericardial space (45).

The characteristic fluid obtained from an amebic liver abscess has been described as having the appearance of "anchovy paste," although in fact many different appearances have been described. Amebae are seen on wet mount examinations in less than 50% of aspirates. The diagnostic yield may be improved by performing a wet mount examination on the last few drops aspirated and on tissue obtained by biopsy of the abscess wall and by examination of the abscess wall using periodic acid-Schiff staining of histologic specimens.

Treatment

Metronidazole, in a dosage of 750 milligrams every 8 hours for 10 days, is currently the treatment of choice for amebic liver abscess. In recent studies metronidazole has been effective in 85% to 100% of treated patients (13,37,40,46). Occasional failures of metronidazole therapy have been noted, however (47,48). One recent study showed that 94% of metronidazole responders demonstrated dramatic improvement within 72 hours of initiating therapy (49). In another study the median time to defervescence during metronidazole therapy was 3 days, with 90% of patients free of fever after a week of treatment (13). Alternative medical therapy or drainage of the abscess has been suggested for patients who do not respond after a week of treatment with metronidazole. For alternative medical therapy use dehydroemetine at a dose of 1.0 to 1.5 milligrams per kilogram of body weight per day (maximum 90 mg per day) intramuscularly for up to 5 days, followed by oral chloroquine phosphate 600 mg base per day for 2 days and 300 mg base per day for 3 weeks (each 500 mg chloroquine phosphate tablet contains 300 mg chloroquine base). Dehydroemetine is probably as effective as emetime (1 mg per kg of body weight per day, maximum dose 60 mg per day), which has also been used in the alternative regimen. Although dehydroemetine is thought to be less toxic, both dehydroemetine and emetine are associated with neuromuscular and cardiac toxicity. When receiving these drugs, patients should remain sedentary and be monitored electrocardiographically. Patients treated for amebic hepatic abscess with metronidazole or an alternative regimen should be treated subsequently to eradicate nondysenteric intestinal infection (cyst passage) since the tissue amebicidal therapy is not fully effective for infection in the intestinal lumen. To accomplish this, administer orally three times daily either iodoquinol (Yodoxin), 650 mg for 21 days, or diloxanide furoate (Furamide), 500 mg for 10 days. Diloxanide furoate and dehydroemetine are available in the

United States from the Centers for Disease Control, Atlanta, Georgia.

The role of surgery in the treatment of amebic liver abscess is to prevent or treat abscess rupture. Routine, ultrasonographically guided percutaneous aspiration is still advocated by some authors, with reports of high success rates and no complications in experienced hands (39). Despite these results, the success of amebicidal medical therapy alone suggests that there is little justification for aspirating amebic abscesses on a routine basis. Although aspiration is a safe procedure, there is always the attendant risk of introducing bacterial infection into the cavity. Aspiration should be reserved for nonresponders, especially those in whom rupture is feared, and for those settings in which bacterial infection must be excluded. Surgical treatment for amebic hepatic abscess should be avoided unless abscesses requiring drainage are inaccessible to needle aspiration or rupture requires surgical intervention.

Prognosis

The prognosis for uncomplicated amebic liver abscess is excellent, with most series reporting nearly 100% survival. As noted above, however, mortality increases significantly in the presence of complications, serving to emphasize the importance of making the diagnosis and instituting appropriate treatment as soon as possible. With prompt diagnosis, thorough evaluation, and appropriate treatment, overall mortality associated with amebic liver abscesses should be very low.

References

1. Greenstein AJ, Lowenthal D, Hammer GS, Schaffner F, Aufses AH. Continuing changing patterns of disease in pyogenic liver abscess: A study of 38 patients. *Am J Gastroenterol* 1984; 79:217–226.
2. Miedema BW, Dineen P. The diagnosis and treatment of pyogenic liver abscess. *Ann Surg* 1984; 200:328–335.
3. Fischer MG, Beaton HL. Unsuspected hepatic abscess associated with biliary tract disease. *Am J Surg* 1983; 146:658–662
4. Neoptolemos JP, Macpherson DS, Holm J, Fossard DP. Pyogenic liver abscess: A study of 44 cases in two centuries. *Acta Chir Scand* 1982; 148:415–421.
5. Pitt HA, Zuidema GD. Factors influencing mortality in the treatment of pyogenic hepatic abscess. *Surg Gynecol Obstet* 1975; 140:228–234.
6. Rubin RH, Swartz MN, Malt R. Hepatic abscess: Changes in clinical, bacteriologic and therapeutic aspects. *Am J Med* 1974; 57:601–610.
7. Ochsner A, DeBakey M, Murray S. Pyogenic abscess of the liver. *Am J Surg* 1938; 40:292–319.
8. de la Maza LM, Naeim F, Berman LD. The changing etiology of liver abscess: Further observations. *JAMA* 1974; 227:161–163.
9. Sherman JD, Robbins SL. Changing trends in the casuistics of hepatic abscess. *Am J Med* 1960; June:943–950.
10. Balasegaram M. Management of hepatic abscess. *Curr Probl Surg* 1981; 18:282–340.
11. Dietrick RB. Experience with liver abscess. *Am J Surg* 1984; 147:288–291.
12. Barbour GL, Juniper K. A clinical comparison of amebic and pyogenic abscess of the liver in 66 patients. *Am J Med* 1972; 53:323–334.
13. Barnes PF, DeCock KM, Reynolds TN, Rallis PW. A comparison of amebic and pyogenic abscess of the liver. *Medicine* 1987; 66:472–483.
14. Wintch RW, Reines HD, Rambo WM. Liver abscess: A changing entity. *Am Surgeon* 1982; 48:11–15.
15. Ribaudo JM, Ochsner A. Intrahepatic abscesses: Amebic and pyogenic. *Am J Surg* 1973; 125:570–574.
16. Young AE. The clinical presentation of pyogenic liver abscess. *Br J Surg* 1976; 63:216–219.
17. Ranson JHC, Madayag MA, Localio SA, Spencer FC. New diagnostic and therapeutic techniques in the management of pyogenic liver abscesses. *Ann Surg* 1975; 131:508–518.
18. Gyorffy EJ, Frey CF, Silva J, McGahan J. Pyogenic liver abscess: Diagnostic and therapeutic strategies. *Ann Surg* 1987; 206:699–705.
19. Valero V, Senior J, Watanakunakorn C. Liver abscess complicating Crohn's disease presenting as thoracic empyema. *Am J Med* 1985; 79:659–663.
20. Starzl TE, Putman CW. *Experience in Hepatic Transplantation.* Philadelphia: WB Saunders, 1969, pp. 309–327.
21. Lee JF, Block GE. The changing clinical pattern of hepatic abscesses. *Arch Surg* 1972; 104:465–470.
22. Conter RL, Tompkins RK. The changing face of hepatic abscess. *Surgical Rounds* 1987; January:31–40.
23. Hill FS Jr, Laws HL. Pyogenic hepatic abscesses. *Am Surgeon* 1982; 48:49–53.
24. Land MA, Moinuddin M, Bisno AL. Pyogenic liver abscess: Changing epidemiology and prognosis. *South Med J* 1985; 78:1426–1430.
25. Abbruzzese AA, Khaja NU. Pyogenic abscess of the liver. *Am J Gastroenterol* 1972; 58:288–298.
26. Sheinfeld AM, Steiner AE, Rivkin LB, Dermer RH, Shemesh ON, Dolberg MS. Transcutaneous drainage of abscesses of the liver guided by computed tomography scan. *Surg Gynecol Obstet* 1982; 155:662–666.
27. Sabbaj J, Sutter VL, Finegold SM. Anaerobic pyogenic liver abscess. *Ann Intern Med* 1972; 77:629–638.
28. Moore-Gillon JC, Eykyn SJ, Phillips I. Microbiology of pyogenic liver abscess. *Br Med J* 1981; 283:819–821.
29. Maher JA, Reynolds TB, Yellin AE. Successful medical treatment of pyogenic liver abscess. *Gastroenterology* 1979; 77:618–622.
30. McFadzean AJS, Chang KDS, Wong CC. Solitary pyogenic abscess of the liver treated by closed aspiration and antibiotics: A report of 14 consecutive cases of recovery. *Br J Surg* 1953; 41:141–152.
31. Bertel CK, van Heerden JA, Sheedy PF. Treatment of pyogenic hepatic abscesses: Surgical vs. percutaneous drainage. *Arch Surg* 1986; 121:554–558.
32. Gerzof SG, Johnson WC, Robbins AH, Nabseth DC. Intrahepatic pyogenic abscesses: Treatment by percutaneous drainage. *Am J Surg* 1985; 149:487–493.

33. Crass JR. High incidence of sepsis in percutaneous liver abscess drainage. *Minn Medicine* 1985; January:13–15.

34. McCorkell SJ, Niles NL. Pyogenic liver abscesses: Another look at medical management. *Lancet* 1985; 1:803–804.

35. Thomas CT, Berk SL, Thomas E. Enterococcal liver abscess associated with moxalactam therapy: Review of literature on enterococcal superinfections in association with moxalactam. *Arch Intern Med* 1983; 143:1780–1781.

36. Lazarchick J, de Souza e Silva M, Nichols DR, Washington JA. Pyogenic liver abscess. *Mayo Clin Proc* 1973; 48:349–355.

37. Katzenstein D, Rickerson V, Braude A. New concepts of amebic liver abscess derived from hepatic imaging, serodiagnosis, and hepatic enzymes in 67 consecutive cases in San Diego. *Medicine* 1982; 61:237–246.

38. Ochsner A, DeBakey M. Diagnosis and treatment of amebic abscess of the liver: A study based on 4484 collected and personal cases. *Am J Digest Dis* 1935; 2:47–51.

39. Adams EB, MacLeod IN. Invasive amebiasis: II. Amebic liver abscess and its complications. *Medicine* 1977; 56:325–334.

40. Ibarra-Perez C. Thoracic complications of amebic abscess of the liver: Report of 501 cases. *Chest* 1981; 79:672–675.

41. Abul-Khair MH, Kenawi MM, Korashy EEDA, Arafa NM. Ultrasonography and amoebic liver abscesses. *Ann Surg* 1981; 193:221–226.

42. Ralls PW, Colletti PM, Quinn MF, Halls J. Sonographic findings in hepatic amebic abscess. *Radiology* 1982; 145:123–126.

43. Patterson M, Healy GR, Shabot JM. Serologic testing for amoebiasis. *Gastroenterology* 1980; 76:136–141.

44. Milgram EA, Healy GR, Kagan IG. Studies on the use of the indirect hemagglutination test in the diagnosis of amebiasis. *Gastroenterology* 1966; 50:645–649.

45. Van Sonnenberg E, Mueller PR, Schiffman HR, Ferrucci JT, Casola G, Simeone JF, et al. Intrahepatic amebic abscesses: Indications for and results of percutaneous catheter drainage. *Radiology* 1985; 156:631–635.

46. Powell SJ, Wilmot AJ, MacLeod I, Elsdon-Drew R. Metronidazole in amoebic dysentery and amoebic liver abscess. *Lancet* 1966; 2:1329–1331.

47. Henn RM, Collin DB. Amebic abscess of the liver: Treatment failure with metronidazole. *JAMA* 1973; 224:1394–1395.

48. Griffin FM Jr. Failure of metronidazole to cure hepatic amebic abscess. *N Engl J Med* 1973; 288:1397.

49. Thompson JE Jr, Forlenza S, Verma R. Amebic liver abscess: A therapeutic approach. *Rev Infect Dis* 1985; 7:171–179.

Editorial Comment

In this chapter Rice and Karchmer follow the evolution of diagnosis and treatment of liver abscess and demonstrate that the striking improvement in mortality over the years is certainly a triumph of the modern era. A number of points would be worth further comment. In our own experience, occult diverticulitis has proved to be a not uncommon source for the development of liver abscess, and sometimes the local findings are so minimal that the source of the hepatic infection is obscure; recognition of the source is of vital importance because recurrence after drainage may be directly attributable to failure to eliminate the original infection.

Another unsettled problem is the duration of antibiotic therapy necessary after drainage. There is no reason in this era to allow inadequate drainage to occur, so the prolonged antibiotic therapy is probably unnecessary. Certainly, if guided catheter evacuation of the one or more abscessed cavities within the liver has not provided demonstrably satisfactory drainage, one should not hesitate to revert to open evacuation of residual cavity, thus negating the necessity for, and the possible complications of, long-term antibiotic therapy.

Technically, one might refer to the echinococcal cyst as an abscess since it is caused by an invading infectious organism and establishes itself within the liver in a surrounding fibrous capsule similar to a low-grade infectious process. The relative rarity of this problem in the continental United States is reflected in the lack of material within this text addressing itself to the problem. Probably, a few simple words would suffice. One should always be suspicious of this diagnosis in any person with a liver mass demonstrably cystic by ultrasonography, and confirmation can be achieved with serologic testing. The cyst may be sterilized prior to drainage by the injection of 3% saline at operation. Once the surgeon is satisfied by repeated aspirations and injections that the small daughter cysts are dead, the cyst can then be evacuated and the inner lining stripped from the outer fibrotic encasement, which is in direct contact with the liver itself.

PART VI
Special Problems in Liver Surgery

Chapter 23
Liver Transplantation

ROGER L. JENKINS
C. WRIGHT PINSON
MICHAEL D. STONE

Fueled by the development of new immunosuppressive agents and improved surgical technique, liver transplantation has evolved into a viable treatment option for a growing number of patients suffering from liver failure. Considered the most technologically complex of existing organ transplant procedures, liver transplantation has become a relatively common therapeutic procedure performed in the later stages of otherwise terminal liver disease.

Although the technical details essential to eventual human application of liver replacement were enthusiastically developed in animal models in the 1950s, it was not until 1963 that the first human liver transplant was carried out by Starzl in Denver (1). Although this important milestone was followed by similar attempts in scattered transplant centers, failure was universal with death invariably related to technical complications or uncontrollable graft rejection. Chiefly through the pioneering spirit and untiring efforts of Starzl and colleagues, solutions to the technical and immunologic problems were evolved leading to the first long-term survival following liver transplantation in 1967 (2). Stimulated by the growing success of kidney transplantation and the promise of liver replacement, Calne in Cambridge, England, initiated a clinical and investigative program in liver transplantation achieving effective patient survival in 1968 (3). Although sporadic attempts at liver replacement ensued in a number of centers throughout the world, marginal results and prohibitive costs restricted the implementation of this therapy for almost two decades. The introduction of cyclosporine as an effective immunosuppressive agent in 1980 considerably simplified the immunosuppression management of solid organ recipients and was associated with a near doubling of patient survival (4,5). In the period to follow, interest was rekindled in many medical centers so that by 1986 more than 40 centers were routinely performing liver transplants in the United States joined by a similarly growing number of medical centers in other countries (6). Despite the improved survival following liver replacement, the process of liver transplantation remained a formidable undertaking requiring significant institutional resources and an intense dedication of the medical support personnel. Rapid spread of this complex technology was limited by rising concerns at the state and federal level about the introduction of costly new medical treatments and its effect on total health care expenditure. Even as third-party payers recognized their responsibility to reimburse for such procedures, transplant personnel were cautiously restricted by local and regional health care planning agencies (7). In Boston, this led to the development of a consortium effort now known as the Boston Center for Liver Transplantation (BCLT). This organization serves to coordinate the activities of four major medical institutions in the provision of optimal liver transplant availability and quality while simultaneously supporting the state's efforts to control its impact on hospital resources (8). The material outlined here reflects the experience of the transplant team at the New England Deaconess Hospital, which has functioned as the most active member of the BCLT (9).

Although cyclosporine has been given credit for much of the improvement and survival with the transplantation of major solid organs, it is likely that improvements in patient selection and surgical technique have played equally important roles in the burgeoning success of the liver replacement process. With potentially more effective organ preservation techniques and immunosuppressive agents on the horizon, further improvements in survival will lead to more widespread applicability. As the technical impediments to successful liver replacement find solutions, however, the chief limitation to the widespread application of this treatment process, namely, the availability of adequate numbers of donor organs, will become the dominating concern for the future.

Candidate Selection

The indications for liver transplantation span virtually the entire range of advanced liver disease states managed by hepatologists. Open-minded approaches by clinicians treating patients with liver disease have gradually expanded the list of disorders treated by liver replacement while simultaneously identifying those patient characteristics that optimize the potential for survival. Categories of liver failure amenable to treatment by liver transplantation may be divided into acute and chronic disease states. The natural history and predictable complications of each disease usually allow careful patient evaluation for appropriately timed transplant intervention. Acute hepatic failure may present, however, in such fulminant form that rapid transplantation is crucial to survival. Similarly, if observation of the patient with chronic liver disease is unnecessarily prolonged, infection, malnutrition, bone disease, neurologic dysfunction, or bleeding may intercede to complicate an otherwise easily manageable situation. Improper planning of procedures performed for portal hypertension or biliary obstruction complicates eventual recipient hepatectomy contributing to higher perioperative mortality in otherwise favorable disease states. The primary or referring physician managing the patient's underlying disease therefore plays a major role in the ultimate success of any transplant venture.

Much of the uncertainty relating to proper transplant timing relates to our inability to accurately assess the severity of liver damage until standard biochemical parameters are markedly deranged. Prothrombin time, serum albumin, and fibrinogen are considered standard functional assays of hepatic mass but may also become altered in states of malnutrition or sepsis. In situations where the amount of hepatic reserve is unclear, more com-

plex assays like measurement of the central plasma clearance rate of amino acids (CPCR-AA) that reflect the liver's ability to clear an amino acid load may arbitrate the need for transplant versus management by more traditional operative interventions (biliary reconstruction, portosystemic decompression, hepatic resection) (10).

Despite the importance of monitoring biochemical parameters as indicators of declining hepatic junction, it is more common for a major disease related complication to precipitate urgent hospitalization and consideration for transplantation. Sclerotherapy, portasystemic shunting, peritoneovenous shunts, and other operative or radiologic interventions have taken on new importance with the growth of liver transplantation as an effective treatment modality. Used cautiously with an eye toward the eventual need for liver replacement, they serve as important therapeutic bridges to transplant. Used indiscriminately without regard for the logistic concerns of the transplant process, they can diminish the possibilities of success by creating excessive delay and prohibitive operative risk. Prior right upper quadrant surgery seriously complicates the hepatectomy because of the densely vascularized adhesions that result.

If portasystemic shunting is necessary to manage episodes of variceal hemorrhage that recur despite aggressive sclerotherapy, we prefer that the portal vein not be used because of the technical difficulties encountered in reconstructing portal inflow at the time of graft implantation. Proximal or distal splenorenal shunting may just as effectively control variceal hemorrhage without introducing complex anatomic difficulties in patients with marginal hepatic reserve.

Although categories for appropriate patient selection have been established (Tables 23.1 and 23.2), few predictors for survival have been specific enough to be applicable within the widely varying disease entities facing an already active liver referral service. As we initiated our own liver transplant program in 1983, our approach to patient selection allowed broad inclusion of potential candidates presenting with disease processes previously demonstrated to be curable by transplant. Although there was concern that this approach might open floodgates to the transplantation of marginal candidates, this broad experience permitted us to identify unfavorable characteristics in several disease categories, contributing to a more

Table 23.1. Indications for Liver Transplantation

Primary biliary cirrhosis
Chronic active hepatitis
Sclerosing cholangitis
Secondary biliary cirrhosis
Fulminant/subfulminant hepatic failure
  Toxic
  Viral
Primary hepatic tumors
Budd-Chiari syndrome
Polycystic liver disease
Alcoholic cirrhosis (inactive)
Metabolic disorders
  Wilson's disease
  Alpha$_1$-antitrypsin deficiency
  Glycogen storage disease
  Hemochromatosis
  Tyrosinemia
Biliary atresia
Failed prior transplant

precise focus on those patients with greatest chance for the longest and qualitatively best survival in a situation of scarce organ resources.

Specific Indications

Primary biliary cirrhosis (PBC) represents one of the major indications for transplantation in the adult (11). The majority of patients are women in their third or fourth decade of life when their disease becomes manifest with pruritus and jaundice. Variceal hemorrhage, encephalopathy, ascites, and malnutrition are complications that develop progressively over one to two decades with death resulting from complications of liver failure. Despite the prospects for prolonged survival with this chronic liver disorder, a debilitating consequence of the disease can be hepatic osteodystrophy sec-

Table 23.2. Contraindications to Liver Transplantation

Absolute
  Advanced systemic sepsis
  Extrahepatic malignancy
  Active drug or alcohol abuse
  Advanced cardiopulmonary disease
  Multiple, uncorrectable, congenital anomalies

Relative
  Age > 60 years
  Irreversible renal failure
  Extensive prior biliary surgery
  Portal vein thrombosis
  HTLV-III–positive state
  HB$_s$AG-positive state

Abbreviations: HTLV-III, human T-cell lymphotropic virus III; other abbreviations as in text.

ondary to altered vitamin D metabolism (12,13). Numerous spontaneous fractures may occur leading to major orthopedic deformity, further complicating the prospect for return to a reasonable quality of life following successful liver engraftment. Although few technical problems are posed during the operation replacement of the liver in this disease, the more advanced age of these candidates makes them less tolerant of operative stress and postoperative complications, highlighting the importance of transplant intervention before the patient becomes too fragile.

Chronic active hepatitis (CAH) includes a constellation of diseases that may be of autoimmune, toxic, or viral origin. Much attention has been focused upon the group of candidates known to be hepatitis B surface antigen (HB$_s$Ag)-positive because of the existence of blood markers that allow tracking of the B-virus activity following liver replacement. Re-emergence of the surface antigen universally occurs within several weeks of liver replacement despite the administration of large doses of hepatitis B immune globulin at the time of hepatectomy (14). Recurrent clinical disease is not universal, however, and when it does recur may not lead to major hepatic dysfunction. Four of our recipients with Hb$_s$AG-positive cirrhosis remain antigen positive up to 2 years following liver replacement without biochemical or histologic evidence of recurrent disease. Transplantation for this disease process does expose participating medical personnel to potential viral inoculation, emphasizing the importance of active immunization of individuals lacking detectable antibody titers. Technical aspects of transplantation for this form of cirrhosis are more problematic because of the intense portal hypertension and contraction of diaphragmatic attachments, which make dissection in the bare area of the liver during recipient hepatectomy particularly treacherous. These problems are further magnified in the presence of prior right upper quadrant surgery. Relative preservation of hepatic synthetic capacity is an important aid at the time of hepatectomy to minimize blood loss and hemodynamic instability. In our experience, patients with prior right upper quadrant surgery who present with chronic active hepatitis and prothrombin times greater than 18 to 20 seconds and serum albumin less than 2.0 gms% make poor candidates and are no longer offered transplantation.

Sclerosing cholangitis is an ideal disease process managed by liver replacement since most candidates are patients in the middle decades of life with excellent prospects for long-term survival. The greatest concern in these patients relates to the extensive prior operative history experienced before referral for transplant. When a patient is newly diagnosed with sclerosing cholangitis, it is crucial to outline an operative strategy that avoids multiple operative procedures upon the biliary strictures that are the hallmark of this disease. Although dominant strictures within larger biliary radicals may be best managed initially by aggressive operative resection or bypass in states of excellent hepatic reserve, percutaneous radiologic dilatation of peripheral or recurrent biliary strictures affords relief of symptoms and preserves the potential for future transplant. Our approach to the management of dominant strictures of the extrahepatic and proximal intrahepatic biliary system currently entails resection of the involved bile duct with reconstruction of the biliary tree through use of a Roux-en-Y jejunal limb. This method allows endoscopy and dilatation of recurrent strictures through the externalized jejunal limb, which later serves as a suitable conduit for biliary reconstruction of the hepatic allograft. Most importantly, deterioration in hepatic synthetic activity should be an indication for transplant intervention rather than attempts at biliary stricture dilatation. Survival rates of greater than 70% may be achieved with carefully selected recipients, illustrating the importance of thoughtful patient management prior to transplant referral (15).

A variety of toxic drugs and viral agents may precipitate *fulminant hepatic failure* with progression to death from liver failure, generally over 3 to 4 weeks. Subacute forms of hepatic necrosis follow a less catastrophic course with clinical deterioration over 8 to 12 weeks (16). Because even the more fulminant forms of hepatic necrosis are compatible with recovery and return of function by the native liver, delay in patient referral is common, diminishing the chances of finding a suitable donor organ in time to salvage the patient. Intervention ideally should precede the development of hypoglycemia, sepsis, gastrointestinal bleeding, renal failure, or hemodynamic instability for best chance of survival. Waiting until the development of stage 3 or 4 encephalopathy may allow successful transplantation but may not allow neurological recovery (17,18). Removal of an acutely insulted liver is considerably less complex than removal of one deformed by chronic scarring and portal hypertension. The most important variable determining eventual patient outcome is the immediate adequate function of the liver allograft. One rarely gets a chance to implant a second graft successfully because of the high incidence of sepsis and neurologic deterioration following initial graft failure. With careful attention to these concerns, 50% or better survival rates can be achieved in this disease category.

Neoplasms of the liver considered for transplant management have historically included both primary and metastatic lesions with high recurrence rates in both categories. Although transplantation for hepatocellular tumors is carried out commonly in many centers, Scharschmidt reported only 20%, 3-year survival in the combined experience of four major transplant centers as of 1983 (19). In an update on the Pittsburgh experience, Iwatsuki and colleagues identified favorable characteristics in a series of 54 patients undergoing transplant for a variety of liver tumors (20). Survival was uniformly excellent in patients harboring incidental hepatomas in their cirrhotic native livers. Of the 41 patients undergoing transplant because of the otherwise unresectable nature of their malignancy, only 30% remained alive at the end of a year with death almost invariably related to disease recurrence. The observation that incidental tumors fare so well following resection by transplant proves the potential utility of liver replacement as an effective tool for the cure of hepatomas. Operative staging of nodal status and carefully conceived preresectional chemotherapy regimens may offer improved survival possibilities for patients otherwise doomed by hepatoma. The limiting factor is the lack of a biologically active chemotherapeutic agent effective against this class of tumors. The fibrolamellar variant of hepatoma deserves special attention because of the relatively lengthy prolongation of survival achieved even in the presence of disease recurrence. The favorable biology of this malignancy warrants aggressive attempts at radical resection or removal by transplantation (21).

Results of liver replacement for intrahepatic cholangiocarcinoma or Klatskin tumors have been far more discouraging. Eighteen-month survival of less than 20% was reported at the Consensus Development Conference in 1983 with four centers pooling their results since 1967 (8). Encouraged by our experience with intraoperative radiotherapy and resection of proximal bile duct cancers, we have recently embarked on a protocol including operative exploration for staging of otherwise unresectable Klatskin tumors in the absence of extrahepatic disease. Despite a 3- to 4-week course of 5-fluorouracil (5-FU) infusion and radiation delivered to the hepatic hilum and celiac nodal tissue, our first three patients were found to have disseminated intra-abdominal metastases at the time of re-exploration for transplant, illustrating the aggressive nature of the tumor. Transplantation is unlikely to improve patient survival without the development of effective adjuvant therapy.

With the possible exception of occasional slow-growing neuroendocrine tumors manifesting persistent liver involvement in the absence of gross extrahepatic disease, it is unlikely that the biology of most metastatic tumors will allow meaningful survival following liver transplantation without a major breakthrough in chemotherapy. The critical scarcity of donor organs and the lengthy process of recovery from liver replacement make transplantation for palliation alone an unacceptable goal.

A number of less common hepatic disorders occasionally progress to the development of liver failure. Budd-Chiari syndrome may be managed with side-to-side portocaval shunting but is best treated by liver replacement if disease has progressed to the point of declining synthetic activity. Polycystic disease is far more commonly associated with renal failure but occasionally demonstrates need for liver replacement to relieve the debilitating abdominal mass effect when resectional techniques either have failed or are not suitable. Alcoholic liver disease represents a common disorder in modern society and remains a common disease referred for transplant consideration. The vast majority of potential candidates, however, are either too ill with associated dysfunction of other organ systems from long-term substance abuse or have obviously failed attempts to abstain from the use of alcohol for a reasonable length of time. Rarely, a patient presents with progressive chronic liver failure despite abstinence for a significant interval and demonstrates a stable psychosocial makeup allowing transplant consideration. Although we initially approached this disease category with trepidation, the few individuals who have successfully undergone liver replacement have remained free of alcohol use and have returned to productive existence.

Biliary atresia is the major indication for liver transplantation in the pediatric population. Most candidates with this disease category have previously undergone portoenterostomy (Kasai) procedures in an attempt to establish adequate biliary drainage. Although the presence of prior biliary surgery complicates eventual recipient hepatectomy, even a partially successful Kasai procedure may effectively slow the development of cirrhosis to buy valuable time for the growth of an afflicted child to a size more suitable for donor organ identification and implantation. Liver replacement clearly represents the most effective treatment for any liver disorder secondary to destruction of intrahepatic bile ducts. However, the experience within the BCLT as reported by Vacanti suggests that infants weighing less than 12 kg have diminished survival, chiefly as a result of a higher incidence of both hepatic artery thrombosis and primary graft nonfunction (22). The serious scarcity of donor organs in this age and weight category make successful transplantation a rare event. It is hoped that developing techniques of segmental liver engraftment will offer a more successful solution to the small liver donor scarcity (23).

A host of metabolic disorders may present in childhood or early adulthood with opportunities for cure by liver replacement. Wilson's disease is an autosomal-recessive disorder with organ damage resulting from excessive copper deposition within the liver, central nervous system, and kidneys. Copper chelation with D-penicillamine may effectively forestall the development of chronic liver disease but occasional patients may present with fulminant hepatic failure and hemolytic crisis. Liver replacement following stability of the patient is curative, although patients presenting in stage 4 coma have a poor prognosis (24). Hereditary tyrosinemia commonly leads to death within the first 6 months of life from acute hepatic failure but may also result in cirrhosis and liver failure at a later age. The chronic form of this disease is associated with a very high incidence of hepatocellular carcinoma developing in the native liver. Liver replacement has been most commonly carried out in the chronic form with cure of the metabolic defect and an acceptable recurrence rate for patients with associated malignancies (25). Alpha$_1$-antitrypsin deficiency is not strictly confined to the pediatric age group but typically presents in the child with progressive macronodular cirrhosis with or without advancing obstructive pulmonary disease. Transplantation of the liver provides the deficient protease inhibitor, normalizes the electrophoretic phenotype, and establishes normal levels of antitryptic activity in the serum (26). A similar cirrhotic state may develop in the adult in association with mild to moderate obstructive pulmonary symptoms. It is unclear whether the progressive destruction of lung tissue that leads to an emphysematous state is entirely halted.

Other unusual liver-based metabolic disorders have merited consideration for treatment by transplantation. Crigler-Najjar syndrome, protoporphyria, glycogen storage diseases, and lipid storage diseases present unusual circumstances where hepatic replacement may be considered in the absence of chronic liver disease. A particularly dramatic example of the potential for organ replacement in the management of life-threatening metabolic disorders was described in a young child with homozygous familial hypercholesterolemia complicated by end-stage atheromatous heart disease. Combined heart and liver transplant was carried out to replace the terminally scarred heart and to correct the liver-based metabolic defect responsible for the metabolic deficiency (27).

Retransplantation

Considering the potential for early allograft loss from primary graft nonfunction, hepatic artery thrombosis or acute rejection and late allograft loss from biliary complications, disease recurrence, or chronic rejection, hepatic retransplantation remains an important concept in the strategy for maximizing patient survival. Retransplant rates as high as 25% have been reported by Shaw, with 40% to 50% of such recipients surviving an otherwise hopeless situation (28). Hepatic artery thrombosis is the most frequent technical complication leading to graft failure with the majority of such situations arising in the small pediatric recipient. Hepatic arterial thrombosis is not synonymous with graft failure since occasional patients remain minimally symptomatic or develop drainable intrahepatic abscesses. Early arterial thrombosis, however, frequently presents with fulminant graft failure or bile duct necrosis with fistularization or

subhepatic abscess formation (29). Retransplant then offers the only chance for survival.

Primary graft nonfunction is a potentially devastating cause of immediate graft failure associated with high perioperative mortality. Unrecognized donor disease, improper preservation techniques, and technical problems during organ retrieval and implantation are but several of the possible factors to be considered in the genesis of this devastating problem. Persistent hepatocellular enzyme and prothrombin time elevation beyond 48 hours following transplant are ominous signs indicating the need to consider retransplant to avoid patient death from bleeding, sepsis, or neurologic deterioration.

Retransplantation within 3 months of primary graft implantation is generally technically uncomplicated because of the paucity of vascularized adhesions. Later retransplantation may be somewhat more difficult because of the development of dense adhesions and impairment of hepatic synthetic activity. It is therefore important to consider the possible need for retransplantation earlier in situations of remote graft failure to ensure the assistance of remaining hepatic reserve.

Contraindications

Experience has contributed to the identification of a number of absolute and relative complications to liver transplantation. Both extrahepatic malignancy and systemic sepsis present obvious prohibitive risk factors to patient survival. Although the stress of the transplant procedure mandates sufficient cardiopulmonary reserve, the potential for multiorgan replacement has demonstrated the need to maintain an open-minded attitude in the management of patients with associated multisystem failure. Wallwork and associates have reported simultaneous heart-lung and liver replacement in a young woman suffering from primary biliary cirrhosis and progressive pulmonary insufficiency leading to congestive heart failure (30). Properly orchestrated, multiple sequential organ implantation within a single recipient is likely to become more common as the limits of graft acceptance, technical expertise, and immunology are tested.

Advanced age is generally considered a relative contraindication to the transplantation of any organ. A more subjective "physiologic age" is probably more important in estimating risks and benefits of transplant intervention. We have offered transplantation to patients well into the sixth decade of life when prospects for long-term survival otherwise appeared favorable.

With the potential for disease recurrence, many transplant centers consider the Hb_sAG-positive disease states to be relative contraindications to liver replacement. Similarly, considering the devastating neoplastic and infectious implications of human immunodeficiency virus (HIV)-positive disease, all potential recipients are carefully screened for the presence of antibody and excluded from transplantation if positive. Retrospective review of survival in a series of seven liver recipients exposed to HIV-infected blood during management of pre- and post-transplant complications demonstrated only two long-term survivors, with both of these patients suffering an abundance of infectious complications (31).

Operative Procedure

Although numerous technical developments have simplified the hepatectomy and implantation phases of liver transplantation, a number of logistic impediments prevents the process from achieving routine operative status (32). Chief among the problems faced by transplant surgeons is the difficulty in identifying suitable numbers of compatible organs for the long list of deserving recipients with liver disease. Legislation newly introduced in several states attempts to encourage the identification and reporting of potential organ donors so that families can be offered the lifesaving option of organ donation. The organ supply situation is even more critical when the number of potential pediatric recipients below 12 kg in weight are considered. Historically almost half of such recipients in the Boston area have died before a size-matched organ became available, and prospects for retransplantation in situations of early graft failure have been even more discouraging (22). The scarcity of organ supply is further compounded by the limited techniques of organ preservation that until recently have restricted the period of reversible cold organ ischemia to 8 to 10 hours. Clinical introduction of the University of Wisconsin (UW) preservation solution for liver and pancreas grafting has dramatically extended preservation periods to 24 to 30 hours, optimizing the

practical radius of organ retrieval and the potential for efficient organ sharing arrangements with both neighboring and distant organ procurement agencies (33). Currently, a national network organization exists for the central registration of all potential organ recipients, stratifying patient need by severity of illness, time waiting for an organ, and regional proximity to an organ donor. The goal of this point award system is to maximize the equality of access to both regional and distant donor organ resources.

Potential organ donors are generally victims of head trauma or asphyxiation meeting the criteria for brain death but maintained in an otherwise stable hemodynamic state on conventional life support systems. Maintenance of circulatory perfusion of the solid organs until the period of organ dissection and in vivo cold perfusion with a fluid preservate virtually eliminates the normothermic destructive injury that rapidly accompanies the onset of circulatory arrest. The short viability periods historically afforded by preservation with Collin's solution limited matching of recipient and donor pairs on the basis of identical blood type and suitable size range alone. The urgencies of the transplant process have not allowed precise histocompatibility typing for the potentially more favorable immunologic matching of donor organs with recipients. Indeed, transplantation in the presence of preformed cytotoxic antibodies has generally been carried out without significant decline in survival (34). More desperate recipient situations occasionally force implantation of blood group– or size-incompatible organs but not without a discernible reduction in patient survival (35). It is unclear whether the extended preservation periods allowed by the new UW solution will affect graft success rates through histocompatibility matching.

The disparity between the number of potential organ donors and waiting recipients has effectively broadened the acceptable physiologic limits acceptable in the donor for most transplant centers. Functioning hepatic allografts have been obtained from newborn donors as well as donors well into their 50s and 60s. Hepatocellular enzyme elevations three or four times normal do not necessarily predict poor early graft function following implantation. Initial fears over the influence of moderate doses of pressor agents (dopamine, etc.) have not been borne out in our own experience. Key elements for final acceptance of a potential liver donor include adequate oxygenation and maintenance of adequate perfusion pressure.

Operative Techniques

Donor Hepatectomy

Since virtually all organ donors are now considered for multiple organ donation, relative standardization of the organ retrieval techniques is important to smooth interaction among the various teams required for the removal for satisfactorily functioning grafts (36). The standardization, however, does allow technical variations ranging from rapid in situ flushing with later organ dissection to meticulous vascular and ligamentous dissection before final cooling. Although most programs currently favor procuring their own organs, it is becoming more common for a single team to remove several or all the organs for distribution to the transplant teams as experience with the technical details becomes more widely disseminated.

A midline incision extending from the suprasternal notch to the symphasis pubis provides maximal exposure for both the thoracic and abdominal organs (Fig. 23.1). Because of the short preservation times allowed for cardiac and pulmonary grafts, initial immobilization of the mediastinal structures is carried out to ascertain the suitability of the heart and lungs for transplantation. Hepatic mobilization then begins by division of the left triangular and coronary ligaments with exposure of the supraceliac aorta for eventual clamp placement. The hepatic artery is identified in the porta hepatis and dissected proximally toward the celiac origin, ligating the gastroduodenal, splenic, and left gastric arteries as they are encountered. A replaced hepatic artery originating from the left gastric artery should be carefully preserved in continuity with the common hepatic artery. Care must also be taken to avoid injury to any right hepatic arteries that originate more proximally on the common hepatic artery and proceed posterior to the portal vein to the right lobe of the liver. A replaced hepatic artery may also originate from the superior mesenteric artery and should be recognized early in the course of the hilar dissection (Fig. 23.2). Kocherization of the duodenum and head of the pancreas allows proximal dissection of a replaced hepatic artery back to the superior

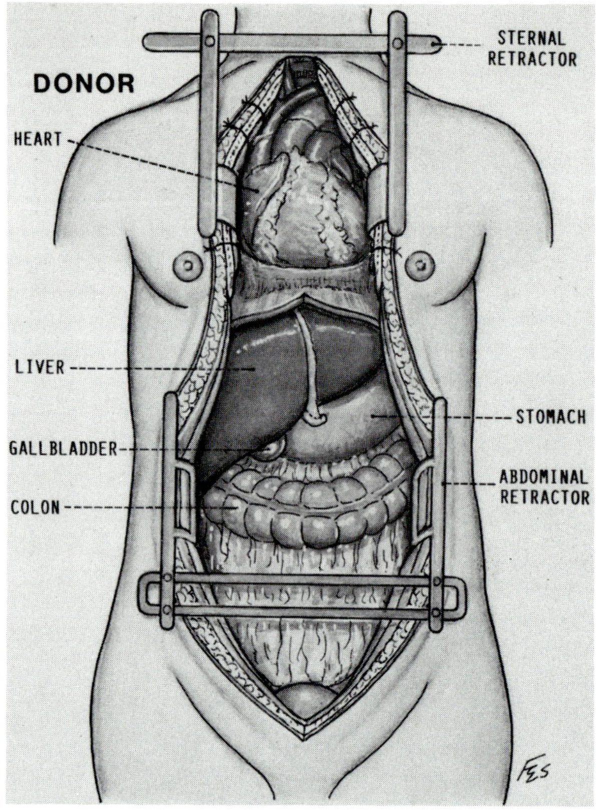

Figure 23.1. Sternal laparotomy incision for thoracic and abdominal organ exposure.

mesenteric artery and its origin at the aorta. The goal in such instances is to eventually excise a button of aorta around the continuous origins of the celiac and superior mesenteric artery for eventual bench reconstruction as described by Gordon (37) (Fig. 23.3). The common bile duct is transected just superior to the duodenum to maximize length. A cholecystostomy is made to allow irrigation of the biliary tree with saline solution to remove bile that may cause slugging in the biliary tree following implantation. If the pancreas is not being removed for implantation, it may be transected overlying the portal vein to allow cannulation of the splenic vein for final cooling of the liver. If the entire pancreas is to be retrieved, there are a number of modifications to the technique that preserve arterial supply to both liver and pancreas. To date, in six such instances we have simply transected the hepatic artery distal to the splenic artery takeoff, preserving the celiac axis and superior mesenteric artery origin with the pancreatico-

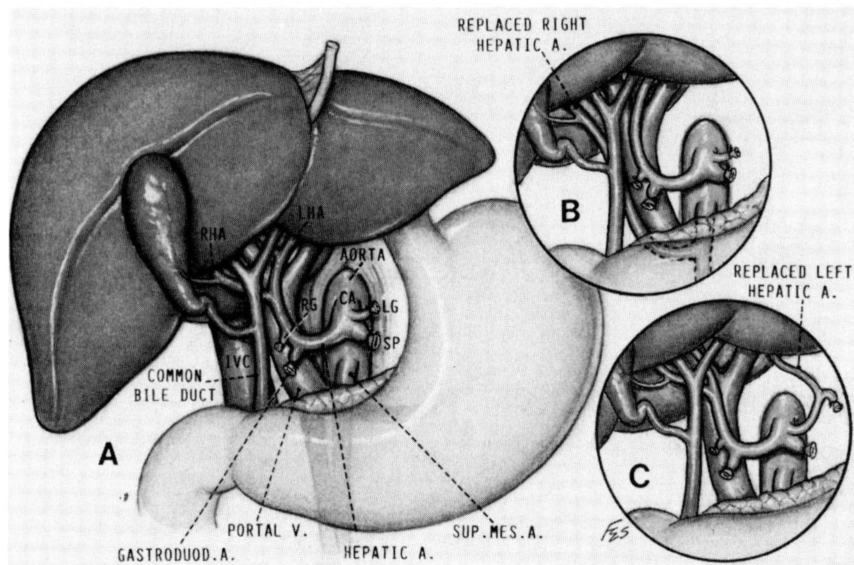

Figure 23.2. Dissection of hepatic arterial blood supply to the level of the aorta.

duodenal allograft. The gastroduodenal artery is sacrificed and a somewhat shortened hepatic artery is accepted for implantation in the liver recipient. Replaced left or right hepatic arteries may be managed by implantation into the gastroduodenal stump or anastomosed to a bifurcated segment of donor iliac artery graft. In situations where both the liver and pancreaticoduodenal allografts are

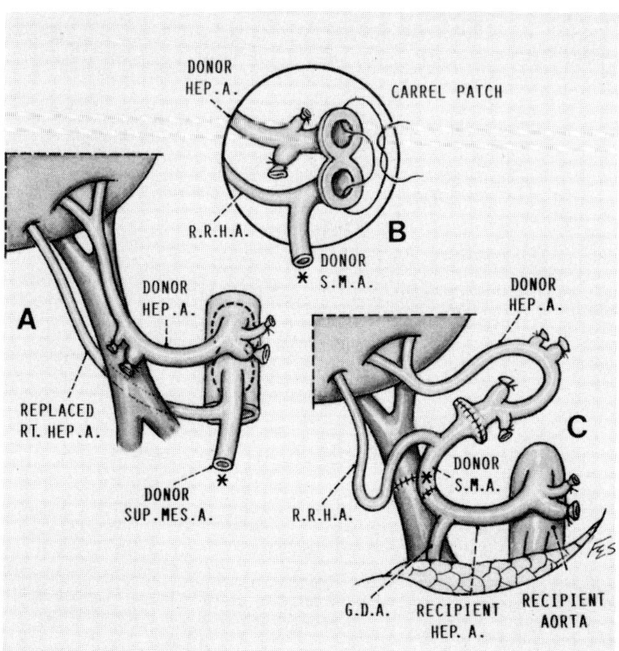

Figure 23.3. Technique of managing a replaced right hepatic artery.

being procured, the portal cannula is placed in the inferior mesenteric vein for final flushing of the liver. Once the aorta and hilar structures have been adequately visualized, mobilization of the right lobe of the liver with division of the right adrenal vein may be carried out if desired. Leftward rotation of the right colon and the base of the mesentery then allows full visualization of the abdominal aorta and inferior vena cava to the level of the iliac bifurcation. The superior mesenteric artery is ligated at its base in situations of normal arterial anatomy but must be encircled distal to any replaced right hepatic artery. Mobilization of the kidneys and ureters is then carried out with identification of the renal artery origins. Mobilization of the spleen and distal portion of the pancreas may also be carried out at this time. Cannulas are then placed in the aorta and the inferior vena cava. Prior to ascending aortic cross clamping for cardiectomy, cold lactated Ringer's solution is infused through the portal venous cannula. Cold UW solution is infused through the aortic cannula for renal, hepatic, and pancreatic flushing while overdistention of the organs is prevented by venting through the inferior vena caval cannula (Fig. 23.4). As cooling proceeds, removal of the heart or heart-lung grafts is accomplished followed by removal of the liver graft. A button of aorta is excised with the origins of the hepatic arterial supply and the suprahepatic vena cava is left with a surrounding cuff of diaphragm after its division from the right

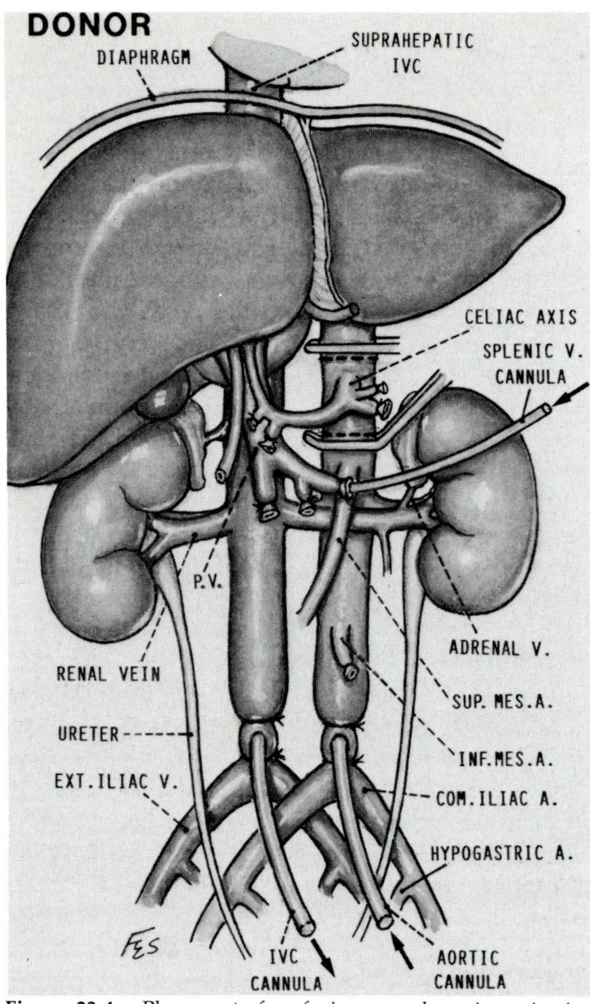

Figure 23.4.   Placement of perfusion cannulas prior to in situ flushing.

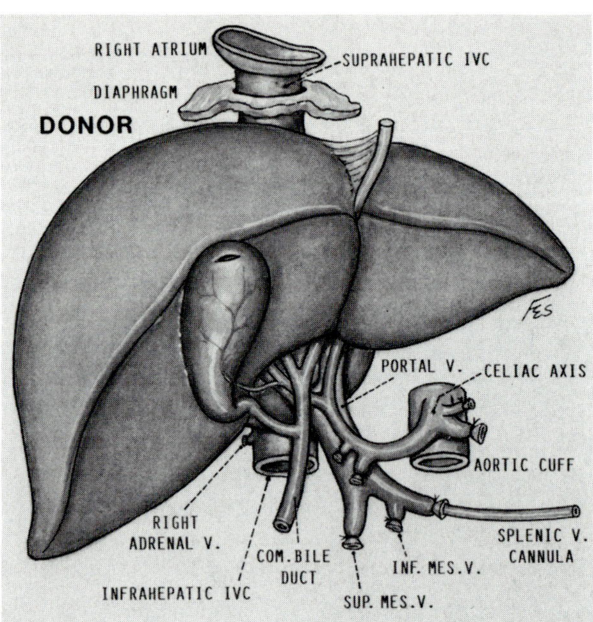

Figure 23.5.   Hepatectomy specimen demonstrating residual diaphragmatic attachments, retained portal cannula, and segment of aorta in continuity with celiac axis.

atrium (Fig. 23.5). The infrahepatic vena cava is transsected cephalad to the renal veins and, with division of the superior mesenteric vein, the liver graft is removed to the back table for further flushing with UW solution and subsequent packaging in crushed ice. Removal of the kidneys and ureters is accomplished en-bloc with the aorta and inferior vena cava for later separation and cold storage. Both iliac arteries and segments of the iliac veins are salvaged to serve as vascular grafts if more complicated arterial reconstructions are necessary.

Recipient Operation

With the extended preservation times currently permitted through use of the UW solution, the recipient operations can generally be scheduled as semielective operative procedures awaiting return of the donor organ. Patients suffering from fulminant hepatic failure, however, are considered more urgent candidates, requiring closer coordination of the donor and recipient operations for more expeditious transplantation before neurological deterioration ensues. In preparation for possible significant blood loss during the recipient operation, multiple large-bore peripheral and central lines are inserted along with a pulmonary artery catheter for cardiovascular monitoring. In patients with chronic liver disease and extensive portal hypertension, a continuous infusion of pitressin is begun early in the operative procedure and discontinued just prior to reperfusion of the implanted graft. This may help to minimize blood loss during the tedious recipient hepatectomy phase of the operative procedure. Use of an intraoperative red blood cell salvaging system (Haemonetics, Inc., Braintree, MA) routinely allows reinfusion of shed blood suctioned from the operative field, significantly reducing the need for blood bank component infusions (38). Clotting factors and platelets are aggressively replaced since they are deficient in the reprocessed blood.

Exposure of the operative field is facilitated by a

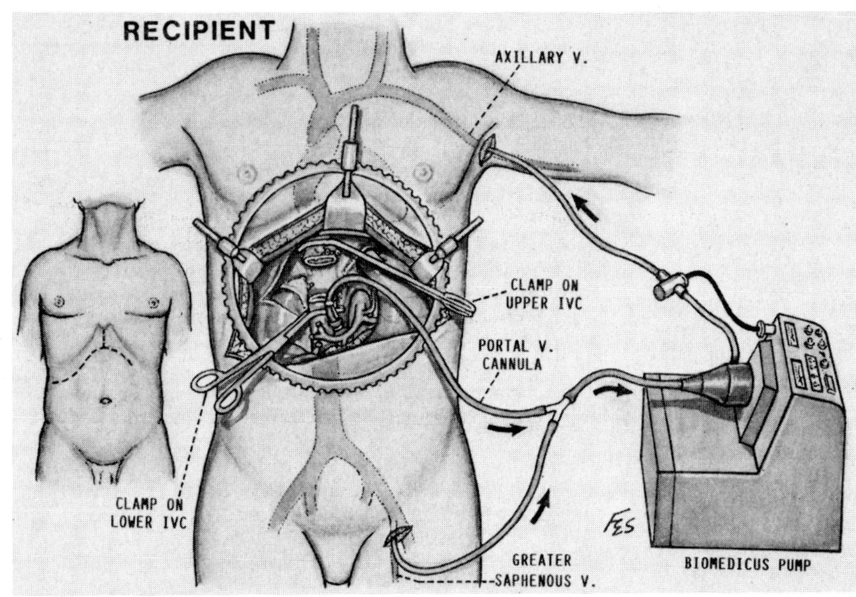

Figure 23.6 Venovenous bypass system during the anhepatic phase of orthotopic liver transplant.

generous bilateral subcostal incision with upper midline incision extension and excision of the xiphoid process. Cautery is used extensively with generous use of silk ligatures to control variceal collaterals in the hepatic ligaments and adhesive bands. Ligation of the round ligament is followed by division of the falciform ligament to the level of the suprahepatic vena cava. The left triangular and coronary ligaments are divided between ligatures, followed by division of the gastrohepatic ligament. Dissection of the portahepatis is carried out high in the hilum of the liver to maximize lengths of the vascular and biliary structures in the recipient. After division of the cystic duct and cystic artery, the common hepatic duct is transsected just below the level of the bifurcation of the left and right hepatic ducts. The left and right hepatic arteries are identified and traced proximally to the level of the gastroduodenal artery to expose all potential sites for eventual arterial anastomosis. Care must be taken to avoid traction on these vessels as intimal disruption easily results, leading to dissection and obliteration of the entire celiac axis. Further division of remaining lymphatic and variceal structures allows identification of the portal vein. Occasionally the portal vein is found to be thrombosed or recannalized, requiring dissection back under the superior aspect of the pancreas to achieve an adequate lumenal size.

Subsequent to hilar dissection, the infrahepatic vena cava is encircled below the caudate lobe and the suprahepatic vena cava as it leaves the liver and traverses the diaphragm. Although mobilization of the right lobe of the liver and division of the right adrenal vein may be carried out at this time, it is advisable in situations of extreme portal hypertension to perform this maneuver after venovenous bypass has been established. Although venovenous bypass is not essential in all circumstances, particularly in the pediatric population, it facilitates the implantation of the liver allograft by preserving cardiac output and hemodynamic stability during the anhepatic phase of the operative procedure (39,40). Heparin-bonded cannulas are inserted in the left femoral vein and portal vein for systemic and splanchnic decompression with blood return accomplished through the left axillary vein (Fig. 23.6). Once the hepatic artery has been ligated and venovenous bypass initiated, clamps are placed across the suprahepatic and infrahepatic vena cavae. Any remaining ligamentous attachments to the right lobe of the liver are severed and the substance of the liver is divided axially over the suprahepatic vena cava. This is carried into the parenchyma of the liver by blunt finger fracture technique until it is possible to identify hepatic venous structures 2 to 3 cm inferior to their junction with the vena cava where they are divided (Fig. 23.7). At this same level, further posteriorly, the vena cava is divided to maximize caval length below the level of the cross clamp. Inferiorly, the infrahepatic cava is divided at its junction with the

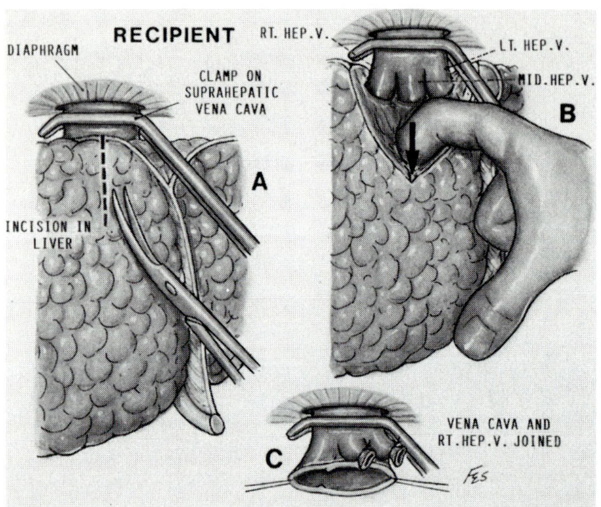

Figure 23.7. Completion of recipient hepatectomy with fracture of liver substance over hepatic veins to maximize length of suprahepatic caval cuff.

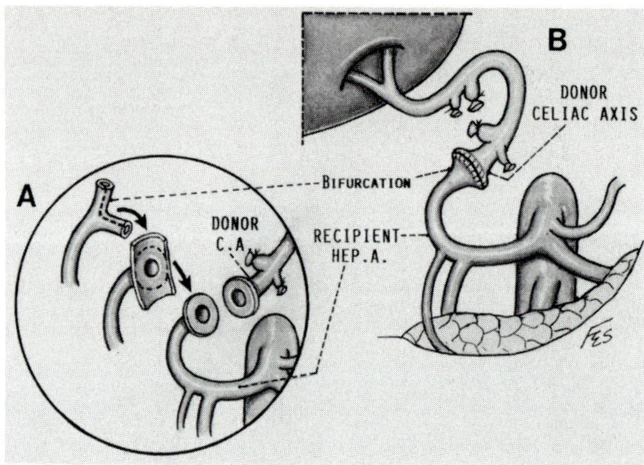

Figure 23.9. Branch patch technique for hepatic arterial anastomosis.

caudate lobe of the liver, allowing removal of the diseased organ. Hemostasis in the retroperitoneal region is obtained using a running heavy polypropylene suture to approximate the divided triangular and coronary ligaments over bare retroperitoneal surface areas (Fig. 23.8). The suprahepatic vena cava cuff is tailored to an appropriate size match to the donor suprahepatic cava by either ligating the hepatic vein stumps or dividing septations to incorporate them into the common lumen

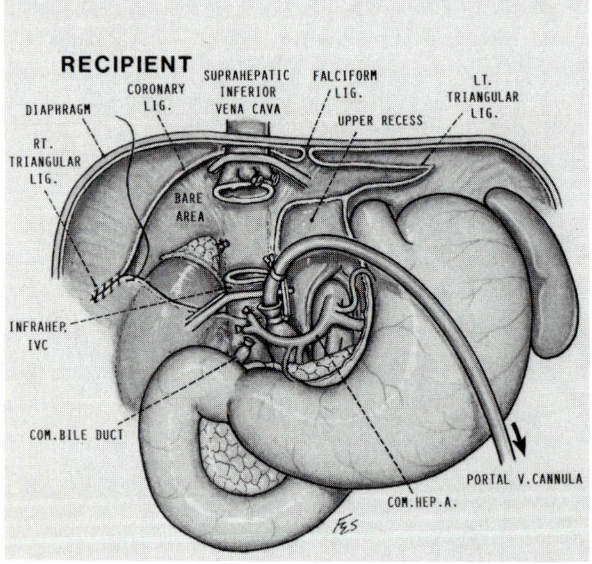

Figure 23.8. Anhepatic phase with portal cannula in place and hemostasis of retroperitoneum with continuous running suture technique.

of the vena cava. The donor organ is then placed in the right upper quadrant for implantation. The suprahepatic caval anastomosis is initiated with a running continuous 3-0 polypropylene suture using an everting technique as previously described (41). The intrahepatic vena caval anastomosis is performed in an identical fashion using 4-0 polypropylene suture, taking the precaution of flushing the liver graft through the retained portal cannula with cold lactated Ringer's solution to remove trapped air and residual potassium from the preservation solution. Following completion of the caval anastomoses, the portal cannula for the bypass system is clamped and removed to allow portal anastomosis. Donor and recipient portal vein lengths are trimmed to an appropriate length and anastomosed in a running continuous fashion with 5-0 polypropylene suture. The portal vein is flushed to remove any clot prior to completion of this anastomosis. Clamps are removed from the portal vein and both vena cavae to allow reperfusion of the hepatic graft with splanchnic blood. All anastomotic sites are checked for bleeding and cannulas are removed from the axillary and femoral veins to terminate venous bypass. For arterial reconstruction, a Carel patch of donor aorta around the celiac axis is anastomosed to a trumpet-shaped segment of recipient hepatic artery created by opening the bifurcation of the left and right branches of the recipient hepatic arteries (Fig. 23.9). A similar anastomosis can be constructed at the level of the gastroduodenal artery if desired. Anastomosis is performed using running continuous 6-0 or 7-0 polypropylene. If the recipient

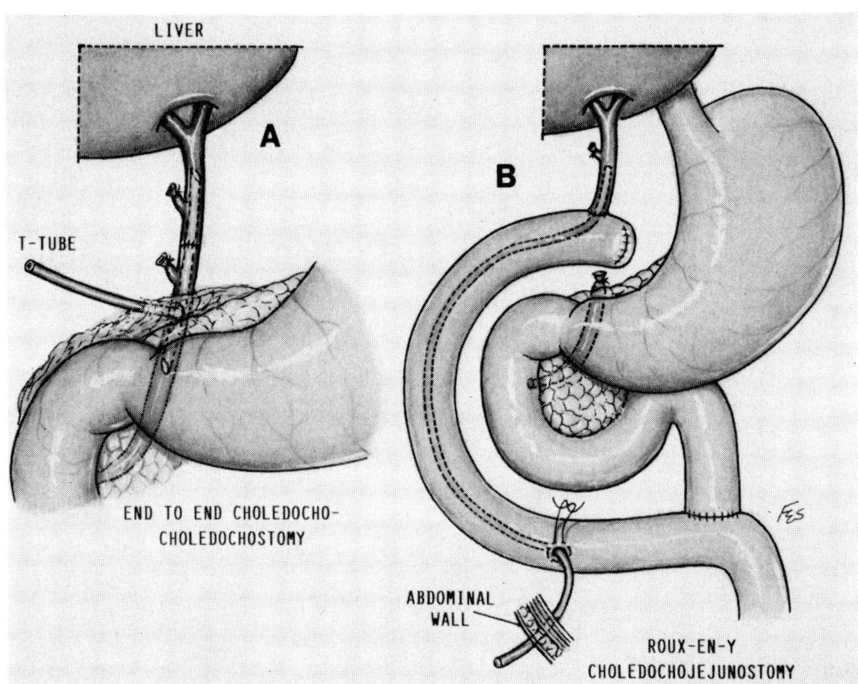

Figure 23.10. Techniques of duct-to-duct and duct-to-jejunal biliary anastomosis.

hepatic artery is unsuitable as an inflow conduit, an iliac artery graft obtained from the donor may be used in the supraceliac or infrarenal position to provide inflow for the graft arterial structures. Adequacy of arterial inflow is assessed intraoperatively using Doppler flow probes to be sure that no technical errors exist that may contribute to later hepatic artery thrombosis.

Following revascularization of the liver allograft, satisfactory function is heralded by rapidly improving prothrombin time and diminished blood loss from all raw surface areas. The donor gallbladder is then removed and the cystic duct and artery ligated. A choledocho-choledochostomy is constructed between donor and recipient common bile ducts using 5-0 PDS (Ethicon, Inc., Somerville, NJ) suture, stenting the anastomosis with a T-tube. When the recipient bile duct is unsuitable for biliary drainage as in situations of sclerosing cholangitis, biliary atresia, or retransplantation, a Roux-en-Y limb of jejunum is created for end-to-side choledochojejunostomy (Fig. 23.10). At the completion of implantation (Fig. 23.11), suction drains are placed above and below the liver, and the abdominal wall is closed with interrupted buried nylon sutures and skin staples. A portion of the midline fascia at the level of the xiphoid process is left unclosed to allow easy access to the left lateral segment of the liver in the postoperative

period. Removal of the overlying skin staples in that location allows needle biopsy of the liver in a safe manner with perfect hemostasis (42,43).

Duration of the recipient operation may range from 6 to 12 hours depending on the complexity of prior surgical interventions and clotting abnormalities. In our adult population, packed red blood cell use averages 18 U with a range from 0 to well over 100 U in more difficult cases.

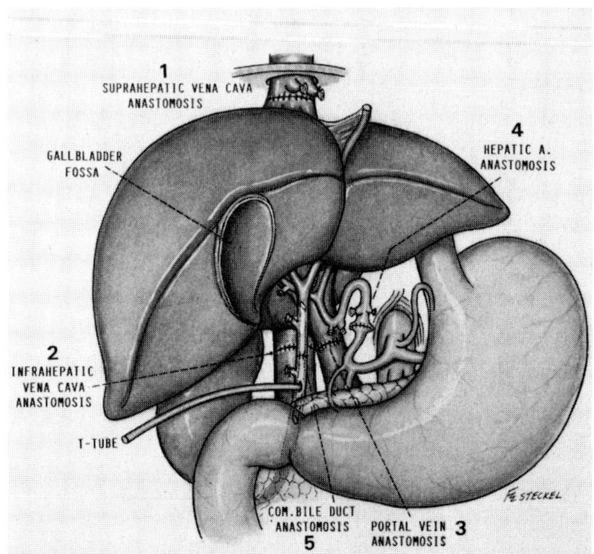

Figure 23.11. Completed anastomotic suture lines prior to drain placement and abdominal closure.

Postoperative Care

Conventional Supportive Care

The complexity of supportive care required in the initial postoperative period depends largely upon the severity of the preoperative illness and the quality of function of the newly implanted hepatic allograft. The extent of the injury incurred during the retrieval/implantation process is reflected in the early biochemical values obtained within the first 12 to 24 hours following completion of the transplant procedure. Transaminase values [aspartate aminotransferase (AST), alanine aminotransferase (ALT)] below a level of approximately 1000 μg/dl are usually accompanied by prothrombin times below 18 to 20 seconds, indicating mild insult to the hepatic parenchyma. Levels above 2000 μg/dl that do not decline rapidly within the first 48 hours may be associated with more protracted prolongation of the prothrombin time, often accompanied by altered mental status, intraabdominal hemorrhage, and oliguria signaling the potential for a considerably more complicated clinical course and even the need for hepatic retransplantation. Blood volume is judiciously maintained with infusions of packed cells and platelets as needed, although fresh frozen plasma is generally not administered unless prothrombin times are elevated above 20 seconds or there are clinical signs of ongoing blood loss. In the absence of fresh frozen plasma infusions, the time course for the return to a normal prothrombin time is a helpful indicator of the normalization of graft synthetic capacity. Excellent initial graft function is usually associated with a benign initial course allowing early extubation and the resumption of oral intake within 3 to 4 days. Closed suction drains left above and below the liver to monitor the character of perihepatic fluid accumulation are generally removed within the first 48 hours following surgery, irrespective of the volumes of ascites that they evacuate. The one exception is the drain in proximity to the biliary anastomosis, which is left in place until the seventh or eighth day after cholangiography has confirmed absence of leak or stenosis.

Varying degrees of metabolic alkalosis, related to the infusion of citrate with stored blood products, requires correction with hydrochloric acid infusions to minimize the compensatory respiratory (ventilatory) suppression that ensues (44). Potassium chloride is given sparingly because of the frequent presence of postoperative oliguria and the risk of sudden hyperkalemia in situations of acute graft necrosis from rejection or hepatic artery thrombosis. Patients are begun on an aggressive parenteral nutrition regimen within 24 hours of surgery to begin restoration of the protein-calorie deficits generated by steady progression of the pretransplant disease state (45). As gastrointestinal function improves, parenteral nutrition infusions are weaned in an overlapping manner with oral diet supplemented with nasoenteric feedings.

Hypertension is seen in most recipients beginning in the early postoperative period and may be refractory to simple management by diuresis and afterload reduction. A combination of agents is generally required to obtain initial blood pressure control with eventual long-term management based on administration of a diuretic and a beta-blocking agent. Locally acting antacids are administered in preference to H-2-blocking agents because of the unclear drug interaction potential with cyclosporine. Antibiotics are administered prophylactically for the first 72 hours to cover for exposure to enteric pathogens from enteric or biliary sources and gram-positive organisms introduced by way of invasive monitoring catheters. Patients undergoing liver replacement in the presence of pre-existing local or systemic infection are treated with selective antibiotic agents for a full therapeutic course. Although bacterial infections appear to be more easily controlled under immunosuppression with cyclosporine, mortality rates are, not unexpectedly, much higher in patients exhibiting infection early in their postoperative course (46). Frequent surveillance cultures and the expertise of an aggressive infectious disease team allow more rational management of the various bacterial, fungal, parasitic, and viral organisms encountered in these complex patients (47).

Immunosuppression and Rejection

Immunosuppression has continued to evolve rapidly since the initial introduction of cyclosporine for clinical liver grafting, as reported by Starzl in 1981 (4,48). Concern for the toxicity of existing agents, the introduction of new immunosuppressive agents, and the more aggressive histologic study of liver allografts have all compelled a more flexible approach to immunosuppression. Initial concerns about diminished metabolism of intravenously infused cyclosporine in the presence of poor initial graft function and the almost universal early renal dysfunction that accompanies its immediate use have obliged us to avoid the use of cyclosporine until satisfactory urine output is established. Intravenous cyclosporine is generally begun as a continuous infusion in a dose of 2 to 4 mg/kg/day and overlapped with an oral dose of 10 to 12 mg/kg/day as gut function returns. Attempts are made to maintain whole blood trough cyclosporine levels in the range of 250 to 500 μg/ml, depending on clinical events and biopsy results. Intercurrent events such as the clamping of the biliary tube may cause sudden elevation of previously stable cyclosporine levels, while the administration of several drugs that are potent hepatic enzyme inducers (phenytoin, rifampin) may cause abrupt lowering of previously effective cyclosporine levels by increasing drug elimination. The kinetics of cyclosporine dosing may be even more unpredictable in the pediatric recipient, with doses as high as 30 mg/kg/day having been recorded in several patients within the BCLT experience. In conjunction with steroids and low dose azathioprine, however, many of our patients are maintained chronically on only 2 to 5 mg/kg/day of oral cyclosporine as long as blood levels are monitored serially. Although recognized as a potent and effective immunosuppressive agent, use of cyclosporine following liver grafting requires constant vigilance.

Corticosteroids still represent an important component of the immunosuppression regimen, although at doses considerably reduced from those required when used in conjunction with azathioprine alone. A 500-mg bolus of methylprednisolone is administered in the operating room just prior to reperfusion of the implanted organ. Postoperatively, methylprednisolone is delivered in a decremental fashion, beginning at 200 mg/day and declining by 40 mg each day until a maintenance dose of 20 mg/day is reached by the sixth postoperative day. Children are generally begun at a daily dose of 100 mg of methylprednisolone the first day with reduction by 20 mg/day until a maintenance dose of 10 to 20 mg/day is established. If renal dysfunction is compromised enough to force significant reduction in cyclosporine dosing, mainte-

nance levels of steroids may be higher to provide effective immunosuppression. Reduction of steroid dosage is generally accomplished within the first postoperative year to a level of 10 to 15 mg/day in the average adult, as permitted by biochemical and histologic parameters. Several of our survivors beyond 2 years are maintained on less than 5 mg of methylprednisolone per day, while one patient requires cyclosporine alone to maintain normal liver function.

Azathioprine historically represented an important advance in the management of immunosuppression, which was combined with corticosteroids to allow significant prolongation of renal allograft survival. The development of cyclosporine as a more potent immunosuppression agent more effectively improved survival of extrarenal allografts, displacing azathioprine from many immunosuppression regimens. Concern for the nephrotoxic side effects of cyclosporine has led to a resurgence in use of azathioprine as part of a three-pronged approach to immunosuppression for liver grafting. Use of azathioprine in doses as low as 1 to 2 mg/kg/day allows more rapid reduction in both cyclosporine and corticosteroid dosages without compromising graft function. Azathioprine is begun intravenously in the immediate postoperative period and continued indefinitely in oral form unless signs of bone marrow suppression become evident. The immediate drop in white blood count and platelet count that occurs in the first 3 to 4 days following liver replacement probably represents a washout phenomenon and does not contraindicate the use of azathioprine.

While the three-drug regimen described represents the cornerstone of our immunosuppression induction and maintenance, the development of monoclonal antibody directed against specific lymphocyte receptors has given rise to a class of immunosuppressive agents that are particularly effective in the treatment of acute rejection refractory to the basic core of pharmacologic immunosuppression, including the addition of high-dose corticosteroids. Although polyclonal antilymphocyte or antithymocyte preparations [antilymphocyte serum (ALS), antithrombocyte globulin (ATG)] have been shown to be effective in the management of refractory renal allograft rejection and are tolerated extremely well despite the heterologous nature of the antibody preparation, monoclonal antibodies are conceptually more desirable because of their homogenous nature and their more strictly defined specificity (49). OKT3 (Orthoclone, Ortho Pharmaceuticals, Raritan, NJ) is a murine-derived monoclonal agent produced by hybridoma techniques with a specificity for the T3 (CD3) receptors present on all mature human T-lymphocytes.

Following reported trials on the use of OKT3 monoclonal antibody and the management of renal allograft rejection, the BCLT hospitals instituted the controlled clinical trial to study the use of OKT3 in the treatment of established liver allograft rejection (50,51). From November 1984 through May 1986, 57 consecutive recipients undergoing liver transplantation became eligible for inclusion in the trial. At that time, cyclosporine and low-dose steroids were used for maintaining immunosuppression, with azathioprine reserved for more refractory cases. When rejection was clinically suspected and confirmed by liver biopsy, ruling out anatomic factors with cholangiography and arteriography as indicated, patients were randomized to receive up to three 1-g boluses of intravenous methylprednisolone over a 48-hour period or a 10-day course of OKT3. Twenty-eight of the recipients had rejection severe enough to require randomization in the trial, 15 receiving OKT3 and 13 receiving steroids as the primary acute rejection therapy. Twenty-three of these recipients (82%) survived with their original allograft. Only 3 of the 13 patients assigned to the steroid group responded with good return of liver function, while OKT3 was required for rescue in 10 patients. Eleven of the 15 OKT3 recipients demonstrated improved allograft function, while two of these required additional steroids before clinical improvement ensued. One patient underwent retransplantation for the vanishing bile duct syndrome and one patient died of sepsis from a biliary leak. Subsequent to this trial, interest in the use of OKT3 as a prophylactic immunosuppressive agent spurred the initiation of a multi-institutional randomized trial in the use of OKT3 with imuran and prednisone versus conventional azathioprine-cyclosporine-prednisone therapy in the early postoperative period. This study is currently underway with almost 100 patients so far randomized among the six institutions. Cyclosporine was not administered for the first 10 days in patients receiving OKT3 therapy because of the concern for a higher incidence of cytomegalovirus or other infectious

complications. To date, however, we have noted several severe rejections in patients on OKT3 prophylaxis in the absence of cyclosporine, which could be managed only by the administration of high-dose corticosteroid. We are currently, therefore, monitoring peripheral circulating T cells to better define the need for earlier institution of cyclosporine therapy while on prophylactic OKT3.

Management of Graft Dysfunction

The causes of hyperbilirubinemia in the postoperative period following liver transplantation are extremely diverse, as outlined in Table 23.3 (52).

The height of the rise in transaminase levels (AST, ALT) reflects the degree of ischemic injury to the liver graft during the procurement preservation process. Later elevations within the first week may herald hepatic artery thrombosis with extensive hepatic necrosis and the onset of acute cellular rejection, which can occur as early as the fifth or sixth day following graft implantation. The onset of fevers, rising white blood count, diarrhea, a change in the bile quality, graft tenderness, and rising liver enzymes should prompt rapid diagnostic and therapeutic intervention. Blood cultures and cultures of other body fluids are drawn for bacterial, fungal, and viral agents and a 48-hour course of antibiotics is instituted while the evaluation process continues. Cholangiography through the bile tube is obtained to rule out biliary leak or obstruction, and a Doppler ultrasound examination is performed to ascertain the patency of the hepatic arterial and portal venous structures. Ultrasonography will also indicate the presence of any perihepatic collections that may require further percutaneous sampling. A liver biopsy is invariably obtained to better delineate the need for changes in the immunosuppression regimen during periods of changing biochemical pa-

Table 23.3. Causes of Hyperbilirubinemia in the Postoperative Period

Preservation procurement injury
Rejection
Hepatic artery thrombosis
Drug toxicity
Hemolysis
Systemic sepsis
Hepatitis
Cholangitis
Biliary obstruction or leak

rameters. We currently perform liver biopsies one to three times per week during the first month following transplantation. Supplementing standard laboratory and clinical observations, liver biopsy assists in the management of immunosuppression in both the late and early postoperative periods.

The histologic pattern most diagnostic of acute rejection is described elsewhere in this book but can be summarized as portraying a mixed lymphocytic polymorphonuclear portal infiltrate with associated lymphocytic damage to the bile duct epithelial cells and varying degrees of central vein endothelialitis (53,54). Cholestasis and ballooning of centrilobular hepatocytes may accompany the infiltrates. More severe patterns of rejection usually associated with more marked elevations of the hepatocellular enzymes may demonstrate confluent areas of necrosis. Successful treatment of the acute rejection process will lead to disappearance of the infiltrates but there may be a delay before the cholestasis and hepatocyte ballooning improves. Chronic patterns of rejection are associated with portal fibrosis in expanded tracts with gradual destruction or disappearance of bile ducts. Foamy macrophages accumulate in the subintimal areas of large- or medium-sized hepatic arteries, leading to their obliteration. A striking absence of bile ducts without dense portal infiltrate is occasionally seen as a chronic rejection process (vanishing bile duct syndrome). Most importantly, many of the biopsy specimens demonstrate mixed histologic patterns consistent with partial treatment or concurrent disorders, and it is the trend in the histologic pattern as well as clinical response that dictates the direction of clinical management. Lymphocytic infiltrates in portal triads are common even in patients with normal biochemical patterns, highlighting the need for an integrated clinical approach to the biopsy specimens.

Drug toxicity may be inferred in the presence of biochemical jaundice and in the absence of significant portal infiltrates. Cholangiography and evaluation of hepatic arterial inflow are important considerations before attributing the jaundice to a drug-related cholestasis. Occasionally patients are found in the early postoperative period to have dislodged T-tubes or leaks from around the sidearm of the T-tube, prompting the need for mechanical drainage. Hepatic arterial thrombosis may be dramatic in its presentation with a massive rise in hepatocellular enzymes well into the thousands, but occasionally presents surreptitiously with a progressive rise in the bilirubin and the development of an abscess within the hepatic parenchyma. Most acute cases of hepatic arterial thrombosis lead to graft failure requiring retransplantation, although later cases of hepatic arterial thrombosis may be managed conservatively with drainage of infection and the institution of antibiotics (29). Biliary leakage from a disrupted ischemic donor bile duct may indeed be the first sign of hepatic arterial thrombosis. Although repair is occasionally successful, retransplantation may provide the only option for recovery.

Hemolytic anemia may attend the implantation of ABO mismatch grafts, related to the passenger lymphocytes from the donor that continue to make antibody to recipient red blood cells (55). This condition typically manifests within the first 2 weeks following transplantation as a drop in hematocrit and a precipitous rise in the serum bilirubin level. Expectant management will allow most patients to recover uneventfully, although occasional patients have such severe hemolytic reactions that a variety of therapeutic approaches are required. In situations of known mismatch, the recipient can be transfused with donor-compatible red blood cells at the conclusion of the transplantation process to minimize the severity of postoperative hemolysis. When severe hemolysis has become clinically evident, the recipient is transfused again with donor-compatible red blood cells to minimize the number of red blood cells available for coating by donor-cell-produced antigen. Although patient and graft survival in ABO mismatching has been reported by Gordon to be reduced, it may well be that that reflects the late diagnosis of hemolysis and inappropriate management with heightened levels of immunosuppression (35,56).

Systemic sepsis is occasionally associated with elevations of the serum bilirubin level even when the infection is in sites removed from the liver. The mechanism for this is not understood. Systemic cytomegalovirus infection with liver involvement can lead to a dramatic elevation of the transaminase and alkaline phosphatase levels along with a progressive jaundice. Differentiation of this entity from rejection is crucial because the treatment is reduction in immunosuppression. Diagnosis is most rapidly made by identification of microabscesses and intracellular viral inclusions on liver biopsy specimens long before the virus can be cultured from blood.

The development of jaundice and other abnormalities of liver biochemical tests in the later postoperative period often reflects a different set of circumstances than those found in the early postoperative period. Chronic rejection that is refractory to all immunosuppressive intervention may be seen as a persistent mononuclear cellular infiltrate in the portal triads associated with dense fibrosis. Manipulation of cyclosporine levels or the administration of higher doses of steroids does not appear to affect this type of rejection and only contributes to more patient disability from bone disease and infection. Retransplantation becomes the only option in these recipients. Late abnormalities of graft function may also reflect recurrent disease, particularly in the case of hepatic neoplasms with metastatic disease often found within the graft itself as well as in other organ systems. Viral hepatitis may recur in the graft anywhere from several weeks to several years following transplantation and has been described most commonly in the case of B-antigen–positive CAH (34). The absence of markers for non-A, non-B CAH makes recurrence of this entity difficult to differentiate from a chronic rejection process. Although recurrence of primary biliary cirrhosis has been described, there has been some doubt that this does occur since the histologic pattern highly resembles a chronic rejection process (57–59). Key to the differentiation of these graft dysfunction syndromes is an organized approach highlighting the use of liver biopsy, invasive radiologic techniques, biochemical evaluations, and patient examination.

Complications and Results

From July 1983 through February 1988, over 200 transplants were performed within the BCLT. Ninety-two recipients received a total of 107 transplants at the New England Deaconess Hospital; ages of these patients ranged from 17 to 65 years. Table 23.4 lists the diagnostic categories for each of the recipients.

From our own experience, the most important early determinants of survival following liver replacement have been the preoperative condition of the patient and the quality of immediate graft function. The majority of deaths occur within the

Table 23.4. Diagnoses of Liver Recipients

Primary biliary cirrhosis	24
Chronic active hepatitis, HB$_s$AG negative	20
Chronic active hepatitis, HB$_s$AG positive	5
Sclerosing cholangitis	12
Acute HB$_s$AG-negative hepatitis	10
Acute HB$_s$AG-positive hepatitis	2
Acute toxic hepatitis	2
Alcoholic cirrhosis	6
Alpha$_1$-antitrypsin deficiency	3
Hepatoma	2
Polycystic disease	2
Autoimmune chronic active hepatitis	1
Cryptogenic cirrhosis	1
Hemochromatosis	1
Drug-induced cirrhosis	1
Total	92

first 30 days following liver replacement from a variety of factors related to technical problems, poor or marginal graft function, and ongoing infection. Indeed, five of the patients presented insurmountable technical challenges related to prior portacaval or biliary tract surgery leading to hemodynamic instability and death from hemorrhage before the new liver could even be sewn in place. Two additional patients continued to manifest severe coagulopathy following implantation of the new graft, culminating in death from hemorrhage. Six patients died within the first week following liver replacement from primary graft nonfunction, although in many of these situations the patients were morbidly ill at the time of transplantation, presenting with marked hemodynamic instability and pressor requirements throughout the entire operative procedure. Three patients died from sepsis, usually in the face of marginal graft function and preoperative antibiotic use. Only two patients died from acute rejection episodes, unable to be salvaged by retransplantation because of the lack of available donor organs. Death following the initial 3-month post-transplant period chiefly relates to the development of infection, which often established itself during periods of acute or chronic graft rejection when immunosuppressive regimens were augmented. From a technical perspective, only two of the adult recipients suffered graft failure from hepatic arterial thrombosis. Interestingly, in both cases, clot was not found at the anastomotic suture line but in more destal branches of the hepatic artery in association with acute rejection and graft swelling. One patient who underwent portal vein reconstruction for a

Table 23.5. Reasons for Retransplantation

Primary graft nonfunction	8
Vanishing bile ducts	3
Chronic rejection	1
Acute rejection	1
Hepatic artery thrombosis	2
Total	15

completely thrombosed portal vein rethrombosed her vein at the level of the confluence of the splenic vein and superior mesenteric vein. This was felt to be related to residual calcified thrombotic material, within the venous lumen that extended well out into the superior mesenteric vein. Death resulted when a second graft could not be identified in time. An additional patient thrombosed her portal vein within the first week following liver transplantation, again in association with an episode of acute rejection, but underwent successful thrombectomy and heparinization with documented patency 2 years following engraftment. Retransplantation was carried out in 15 instances (Table 23.5) and might have served to salvage additional patients had there been suitable numbers of available grafts. Eight patients received second grafts because of initial poor function of the liver allograft. Although initial failure of the liver allograft was usually associated with implantation into a patient with unstable hemodynamics, three of the grafts were implanted in stable patients and failed to function without definable cause. One patient underwent retransplantation for acute rejection, while four patients underwent retransplantation for chronic rejection. The two patients with hepatic arterial thrombosis were successfully retransplanted.

Our philosophy is that an aggressive reoperative stance must be maintained to minimize the morbidity and mortality of the transplantation process. Our current survival data demonstrate an actuarial survival of 62% at 1 year and 50% at 3 years. Of interest is that the younger patients who died in the postoperative period were more often transplanted in the face of extensive prior abdominal surgery for biliary reconstruction or portal hypertension. Excessive blood loss and associated high pressor requirements intraoperatively frequently contributed to poor initial graft function and early death. On the other hand, the advanced age and chronic debilitation of the older recipients made them less tolerant of the physiologic insults of the perioperative period, even in the absence of extensive prior abdominal surgery. Frequently transplanted late in their disease course, these patients remained at continued risk of infection and late death in the postoperative period. Although the older patients appear to have reduced survival characteristics, earlier consideration for transplantation generally allows a more successful result by capitalizing on remaining hepatic and nutritional reserves.

Although biliary complications such as leaks or stricture formation were common in the early reported experiences with liver transplantation, reliable reconstructive techniques have reduced their occurrence to reasonably low levels (60). Four of our recipients developed early biliary leaks and one patient developed biliary obstruction from hilar lymphadenopathy in the early postoperative period. An additional three patients experienced dislodgement of their T-tubes, which were managed conservatively by applying suction to the T-tubes and continuing antibiotic administration. One patient died from sepsis following an attempted repair of a late biliary stricture at the site of the original choledochojejunostomy. Ultrasound imaging had failed to reveal any biliary ductal distention, making the diagnosis elusive until a percutaneous cholangiogram demonstrated obstruction. In the meantime, excessive administration of immunosuppressive agents during evaluation contributed to death from overwhelming sepsis following biliary reconstruction. Both early and late abnormalities of liver function require aggressive study of the biliary tree to rule out atypical presentations of biliary obstruction.

Analysis of factors associated with excessive risk of death following liver replacement has allowed us to further refine our indications and contraindications to liver replacement for better utilization of scarce donor resources by maximizing patient survival. Although we initially approached liver transplantation with a broadly persuasive attitude embracing patients with virtually any liver disease state that was reportedly curable with liver transplantation, we have since modified certain disease categories to restrict the use of liver transplantation to patients that we feel have the best chance for survival. Clearly, those individuals that have had extensive prior right upper quadrant surgery can be successfully transplanted with anticipated good results following a higher perioperative risk period. However, patients with multiple operations who have prothrombin times above 17 or 18 seconds, or who have markedly depressed albumin levels below the level of 2.2 to 2.5 gm%, are generally the patients who experience profound hemodynamic instability and hemorrhagic complications during the operative procedure later, with excessive risk of death from hemorrhage or poor intral graft function. Likewise, older patients who have debilitating orthopedic deformities from progressive bone disease and associated malnutrition with extensive muscle wasting may have suitable initial early graft function, but are less able to tolerate the immunosuppressive regimens necessary to prevent graft rejection and often experience infectious complications or anguish from persistent handicaps leading to recurrent hospitalization. Earlier intervention is unquestionably the most effective approach to the management of these patients. As in the adult situation, however, intervention should be planned before invasive infection and profound malnutrition result. It is clear that a much more selective approach to liver transplantation can effectively improve survival, as has been reported by Krom (61) and Busittil (62). Such an approach, however, will certainly require the informed cooperation of referring physicians to achieve the goal of maximal survival. Further improvements in patient survival will relate to the improved methods of graft preservation and more selective methods of immunosuppression that are currently undergoing development. The most serious problem that will then face transplantation teams will be the relative scarcity of donor organs.

References

1. Starzl TE, Marchioro TL, von Kaulla K, Hermann G, Brittain RS, Waddel WR. Homotransplantation of the liver in humans. *Surg Gynecol Obstet* 1963; 117:659.
2. Starzl TE, Groth CG, Brettschneider L, Moon JV, Fulginiti VA, Cotton EK, et al. Extended survival in 3 cases of orthotopic homotransplantation of the human liver. *Surgery* 1968; 63:549.
3. Calne RY, Williams R. Liver transplantation in man. I. Observations on technique and organization in five cases. *Brit Med J* 1968; 4:535.
4. Starzl TE, Klintmalm GB, Porter KA, et al. Liver transplantation with use of cyclosporin-A and prednisone. *N Engl J Med* 1981; 305:266–269.
5. Starzl TE, Iwatsuki S, Van-Thiel DH, et al. Evolution of liver transplantation. *Hepatology* 1982; 2:614–636.
6. Bismuth H, Castaing D, Ericzon BG, Otte JB, Rolles K, Ringe B, et al. Hepatic transplantation in Europe. First report of the European Liver Transplant Registry. *Lancet* 1987; 2:674–676.
7. Annasa GJ. Regulating the introduction of heart and liver transplantation. *Am J Pub Health* 1985; 75:93–95.
8. Jenkins RL. The Boston Center for Liver Transplantation (BCLT). Initial experience of a new surgical consortium. *Arch Surg* 1986; 121:424–430.
9. Jenkins RL, Benotti PN, Bothe AA, et al. Liver transplantation. *Surg Clin North Am* 1985; 65:103–122.
10. Pearl RH, Bosari S, Clowes G Jr, et al. Amino acid clearance in cirrhosis: A predictor of postoperative morbidity and mortality. *Arch Surg* 1987; 122:468–473.
11. Kaplan MM. Primary biliary cirrhosis. *N Engl J Med* 1987; 316:521–528.
12. Cuthbert JA, Pak CY, Zerwekh JE, et al. Bone disease in primary biliary cirrhosis: Increased bone resorption and turnover in the absence of osteoporosis or osteomalacia. *Hepatology* 1984; 4:1–8.
13. Stellon AJ, Webb A, Compston J, et al. Low bone turnover state in primary biliary cirrhosis. *Hepatology* 1987; 7:137–142.
14. Demetris AJ, Jaffe R, Sheahan DG, et al. Recurrent hepatitis B in liver allograft recipients. Differentiation between viral hepatitis B and rejection. *Am J Pathol* 1986; 125:161–172.
15. Marsh JW, Iwatsuki S, Makowka L, et al. Orthotopic liver transplantation for primary sclerosing cholangitis. *Ann Surg* 1988; 207:21–25.
16. Bernau J, Reuff B, Benhamou JP. Fulminant and subfulminant liver failure: Definitions and causes. *Semin Liver Dis* 1986; 6:97–106.
17. Iwatsuki S, Esquivel CO, Gordon RD, et al. Liver transplantation for fulminant hepatic failure. *Semin Liver Dis* 1985; 5:325–328.
18. Bismuth H, Samuel D, Gugenheim J, Castaing D, Bernvau J, Reuff B, et al. Emergency liver transplantation for fulminant hepatitis. *Ann Intern Med* 1987; 107:337–341.
19. Scharschmidt BF. Human liver transplantation; analysis of data on 540 patients from four centers. *Hepatology* 1984; 4(Suppl):95S–101S.
20. Iwatsuki S, Gordon RD, Shaw BW, et al. Role of liver transplantation in cancer therapy. *Ann Surg* 1985; 202:401–407.
21. Starzl TE, Iwatsuki S, Shaw BW Jr, et al. Treatment of fibrolamellar hepatoma with partial or total hepatectomy and transplantation of the liver. *Surg Gynecol Obstet* 1986; 162:145–148.
22. Vacanti JP, Lillehei CW, Jenkins RL, Donahoe PK, Cosimi AB, Kleinman R, et al. Liver transplantation in children: The Boston Center experience in the first 30 months. *Transplant Proc* 1987; 19:3261–3266.
23. Bismuth H, Houssin D. Reduced-sized orthotopic liver graft in hepatic transplantation in children. *Surgery* 1984; 95:367.
24. Rakela J, Kurtz SB, McCarthy JT, et al. Fulminant Wilson's disease treated with post dilution hemofiltration and orthotopic liver transplantation. *Gastroenterology* 1986; 90:2004.
25. Starzl TE, Zitelli BJ, Shaw BW Jr, et al. Changing concepts: Liver replacement for hereditary tyrosinemia and hepatoma. *J Pediatr* 1985; 106:604–606.
26. Esquivel C, Vincente E, Van Thiel D, et al. Orthotopic liver transplantation for Alpha$_1$-antitrypsin deficiency: An experience in 29 children and 10 adults. *Transplant Proc* (in press).
27. Starzl TE, Bilheimer DW, Bahnson HT, et al. Heart-liver transplantation in a patient with familial hypercholesterolemia. *Lancet* 1984; 1:1382–1383.

28. Shaw BW, Gordon RD, Iwatsuki S, et al. Retransplantation of the liver. *Semin Liv Dis* 1985; 5:394–401.

29. Tzakis AG, Gordon RD, Shaw BW Jr, et al. Clinical presentation of hepatic artery thrombosis after liver transplantation in the cyclosporine era. *Transplantation* 1985; 40:667–671.

30. Wallwork J, Williams R, Calne RY. Transplantation of liver, heart, and lungs for primary biliary cirrhosis and primary pulmonary hypertension. *Lancet* 1987; 2:182–185.

31. Shaffer D, Pearl RH, Jenkins RL, Hammer SM, Dzik WJ, Groopman JE, et al. HTLV-III/LAV infection in kidney and liver transplantation. *Transplant Proc* 1987; 19:2176–2178.

32. Starzl TE, Iwatsuki S, Esquivel CO, et al. Refinements in the surgical technique of liver transplantation. *Semin Liver Dis* 1985; 5:349–356.

33. Kalayoglu M, Sollinger HW, Stratto RJ, D'Alassandro AM, et al. Extended preservation of the liver for clinical transplantation. *Lancet* 1988; 1:617–619.

34. Gordon RD, Fung JJ, Markus B, et al. The antibody crossmatch in liver transplantation. *Surgery* 1986; 100:705–715.

35. Gordon RD, Iwatsuki S, Esquivel CO, et al. Liver transplantation across ABO blood groups. *Surgery* 1986; 100:342–348.

36. Starzl TE, Hakala TR, Shaw BW Jr, et al. A flexible procedure for multiple cadaveric organ procurement. *Surg Gynecol Obstet* 1984; 158:223–230.

37. Gordon RD, Shaw BW Jr, Iwatsuki S, et al. A simplified technique for revascularization of homografts of the liver with a variant right hepatic artery from the superior mesenteric artery. *Surg Gynecol Obstet* 1985; 160:474–476.

38. Dzik WH, Jenkins RL. Use of intraoperative blood salvage during orthotopic liver transplantation. *Arch Surg* 1985; 120:946–948.

39. Wall WJ, Grant DR, Duff JH, et al. Liver transplantation without venous bypass. *Transplantation* 1987; 43:56–61.

40. Shaw BW Jr, Martin DJ, Marquez JM, et al. Venous bypass in clinical liver transplantation. *Ann Surg* 1984; 200:524–534.

41. Starzl TE, Iwatsuki S, Shaw BW Jr. A growth factor in fine vascular anastomosis. *Surg Gynecol Obstet* 1984; 159:164–165.

42. Williams JW, Vera SR, Peters TG. A technique for safe, frequent biopsy of the liver after hepatic transplantation. *Surg Gynecol Obstet* 1986; 162:592–594.

43. Jenkins RL, Gallik-Karlson CA, Georgi BA, et al. Safety and utility of a simple technique of liver biopsy following liver transplantation. *Transplant Proc* 1987; 19:2480–2482.

44. Driscoll DF, Bistrian BR, Jenkins RL, Randall S, Dzik WH, Gerson B, et al. Development of metabolic alkalosis after massive transfusion during orthotopic liver transplantation. *Crit Care Med* 1987; 15:905–908.

45. Hehir DJ, Jenkins RL, Bistrian BR, Blackburn GL. Nutrition in patients undergoing orthotopic liver transplant. *J Parental Enteral Nutr* 1985; 9:695–770.

46. Cuervas-Mons V, Millan I, Gavaler JS, et al. Prognostic value of preoperatively obtained clinical and laboratory data predicting survival following orthotopic liver transplantation. *Hepatology* 1986; 6:922–927.

47. Dummer JS, Hardy A, Poorsattar A, et al. Early infections in kidney, heart, and liver transplant recipients on cyclosporine. *Transplantation* 1983; 36:259–267.

48. Calne RY, Rolles K, White DJD, et al. Cyclosporine-A in clinical organ grafting. *Transplant Proc* 1981;13:349–358.

49. Delmonico FL, Cosim AB. Monoclonal antibody treatment of human allograft recipients. *Surg Gynecol Obstet* 1988; 166:89–98.

50. Cosimi AB, Burton RC, Colvin RB, et al. Treatment of acute renal allograft rejection with OKT3 monoclonal antibody. *Transplantation* 1981; 36:535–539.

51. Cosi AB, Cho SI, Delmonico FL, et al. A randomized clinical trial comparing OKT3 and steroids for treatment of hepatic allograft rejection. *Transplantation* 1987; 43:91–95.

52. Esquivel CO, Jaffe R, Gordon RD, et al. Liver rejection and its differentiation from other causes of graft dysfunction. *Semin Liver Dis* 1985; 5:369–374.

53. Porter KA. Pathology of liver transplantation. *Transplant Rev* 1969; 2:129–170.

54. Snover DC, Sibley RK, Freese DK, et al. Orthotopic liver transplantation: A pathological study of 63 serial liver biopsies from 17 patients with special reference to the diagnostic features and natural history of rejection. *Hepatology* 1984; 4:1212–1222.

55. Ramsey G, Nusbacher J, Starzl TE, et al. Isohemagglutinins of graft origin after ABO-unmatched liver transplantation. *N Engl J Med* 1984; 311:1167–1170.

56. Jenkins RL, Georgi B, Dzik W, Karlson C, Rohrer RJ. ABO mismatch and liver transplantation. *Transplant Proc* 19:4580–4585.

57. Neuberger J, Portmann B, Macdougall BR, et al. Recurrence of primary biliary cirrhosis after liver transplantation. *N Engl J Med* 1982; 306:1–4.

58. Fennell RH Jr. Ductular damage in liver transplant rejection: Its similarity to that of primary biliary cirrhosis and graft-versus-host disease. *Pathol Annu* 1981; 16(Pt 2):289–294.

59. Portmann B, O'Grady J, Williams R. Disease recurrence following orthotopic liver transplantation. *Transplant Proc* 1986; 18:136–143.

60. Lerut J, Gordon RD, Iwatsuki S, et al. Biliary tract complications in human orthotopic liver transplantation. *Transplantation* 1987; 43:47–51.

61. Krom R. Liver transplantation at the Mayo Clinic. *Mayo Clin Proc* 1986; 61:278–282.

62. Busuttil RW, Colonna JO II, Hiatt Jr, et al. The first 100 liver transplants at UCLA. *Ann Surg* 1987; 206:387–401.

Addendum
G.H.A. Clowes

Hepatic Transplantation

CPCR-AA and Patient Selection

Clinical transplantation of the liver, based on technical developments and improved methods for control of rejection, has become a practical method for treatment of end-stage liver disease. Nevertheless, an appreciable risk is associated with this procedure. Therefore, in addition to clinical signs, such as jaundice, ascites, bleeding, protein depletion, and histologic evidence from liver biopsies, specific measurements of important liver metabolic functions are needed to confirm the selection of certain patients for the irreversible procedure of liver transplantation. Such measurements also can assist in guiding postoperative management. CPCR-AA serves admirably for these purposes.

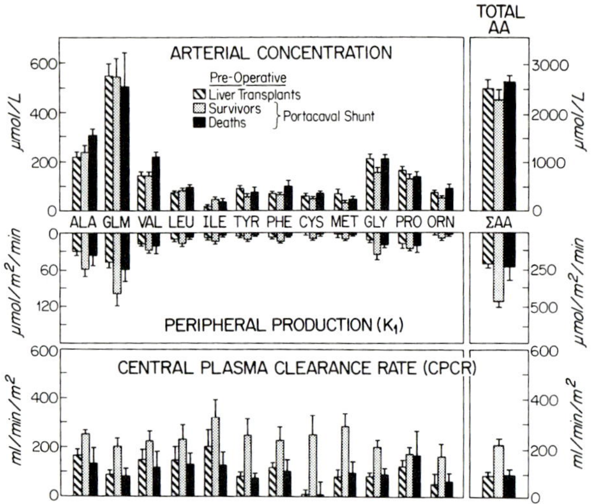

Figure A.1. Arterial plasma concentrations, peripheral release rates, and CPCR-AA comparing fasted preoperative liver transplant candidates with fasted preoperative patients who survived or died following other operations. Note the similarity of values between the transplant candidates and the group who died following other procedures.

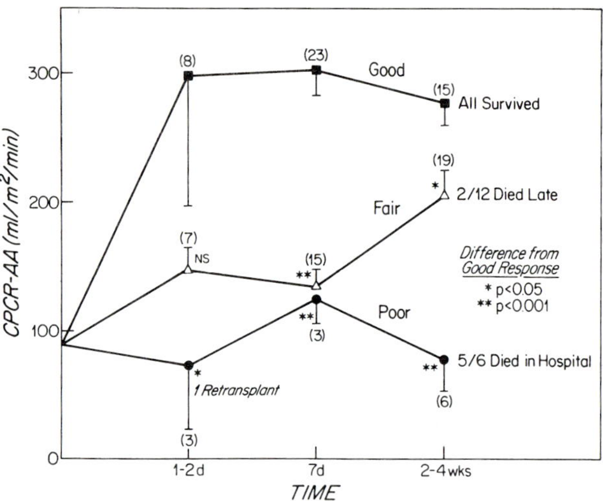

Figure A.2. Serial CPCR-AA values in 36 patients during the post-transplant period. Note the correlation of the clinical courses with the metabolic responses of these groups, as measured by CPCR-AA (see text).

Whereas the mean CPCR-AA of all patients who died following nontransplant surgical operations was 89 ± 8 ml/m^2/min, with a mortality of 38% (see Table 3A.5), the preoperative CPCR-AA value in the 46 patients in this series (1,2), who were studied and subsequently selected for transplantation, was 91 ± 9 ml/m^2/min. The hospital mortality in this group of patients was 31%. The diagnoses made by preoperative needle biopsies included, principally, primary biliary cirrhosis, CAH, submassive hepatic necrosis, and sclerosing cholangitis. Only two alcoholic cirrhosis and two miscellaneous types were accepted for transplantation. Culture evidence of some degree of infection, bacterial or viral, was present in 37% of the entire group.

Data presented in Figure A.1 reveal that the preoperative concentrations, peripheral production rates, and CPCR-AA values of individual amino acids (AAs) as well as total AAs of transplantation candidates are almost identical to those of patients who died following portacaval shunts. For individual AAs, the clearance of the aromatic AA, sulfur-containing AA, glycine, and ornithine are the most depressed. Thus, in end-stage liver disease, as represented by these patients, metabolic function of the hepatocytes is markedly impaired. However, it is noteworthy that the clearances of all AAs are significantly less than those of patients who survived portacaval shunts. This finding indicates that the utilization of AAs by all tissues is reduced.

Post-transplantation

CPCR-AA values obtained 104 times in this series during the postoperative period were found to correlate with the histologic pattern observed in simultaneous needle biopsies of the transplanted liver. Grade I, "normal transplanted liver," had a mean CPCR-AA of 263 ± 22 ml/m^2/min within 2 days after transplantation. Their recovery rate was 89%. In grade II, which showed the "presence of viral inclusion bodies," the CPCR-AA was 195 ± 13 ml/m^2/min, with a recovery rate of 67%. Of the patients with grade III, "viral hepatitis," 50% survived and CPCR-AA was 186 ± 37 ml/m^2/min. Finally, only 17% of patients with grade IV, "severe injury" (ischemia or rejection) survived. They had a mean CPCR-AA of 93 ± 19 ml/m^2/min.

The post-transplant clinical course also was closely related to the CPCR-AA values, as shown in Figure A.2. Eighteen patients with an "early response" had a rapid rise of CPCR-AA of 296 ± 92 ml/m^2/min, which was sustained during recovery. The average time for this group in the intensive care unit (ICU) was 10 ± 4 days and discharge from the hospital was 1.5 ± 0.4 months. The CPCR-AA of a second group of 12 patients with "delayed response" remained below 150 ml/m^2/min for several days to weeks. Subsequently, the CPCR-AA rose to 210 ± 15 ml/m^2/min. The average ICU stay for these patients was 30 days; two patients required retransplantation, and there were two deaths. In the third group, CPCR-AA failed to rise above 112 ± 12 ml/m^2/min; five patients died, despite retransplantation in three. Since death and prolonged convalescence after hepatic transplantation are usually associated with progressive viral and bacterial infection, it is evident from these data that patients with high post-operative CPCR-AA values are those who are capable of synthesizing the proteins essential to immunocompetence and cellular function. They are the patients who adequately counter the stresses of surgery and recover promptly.

References

1. Jenkins RL, Clowes GHA Jr, Bosari S, Pearl RH, Knettry U, Trey C. Survival from hepatic transplantation: Relationship of protein synthesis to histological abnormalities in patient selection and postoperative management. *Ann Surg* 1986; 204:364–374.
2. Pearl RH, Clowes GHA Jr, Bosari S, et al. Amino acid clearance in cirrhosis: A predictor of postoperative morbidity and mortality. *Arch Surg* 1987; 122:468–473.

Chapter 24
Nutritional Support in Surgery of the Liver

RAGU L. K. SHANBHOGUE
DOMINIC NOMPLEGGI
STACEY J. BELL
GEORGE L. BLACKBURN

The liver conducts the metabolic orchestra involving carbohydrates, lipids, proteins, hormones, and vitamins, and it is the principal organ that incorporates nutrients into the body cell mass. Therefore, metabolic disorders that accompany the end-stage liver disease can be considerable. The liver does have tremendous functional reserve and considerable ability to regenerate, and the metabolic disorders observed and appropriate modifications in the nutritional support vary depending on the functional ability of the liver and the nutritional status of the patient. Severe protein-calorie malnutrition, which is unfortunately very common in this group of patients, can seriously undermine the capacity for visceral protein synthesis and thus hepatic regeneration (1). At one end of the spectrum there is a healthy young adult having a segmental resection of the liver for a benign lesion who may not need any nutritional support at all, while at the other end of the spectrum one finds a malnourished, critically ill patient in the intensive care unit who has had two liver transplants in 1 week, needing aggressive and specialized nutritional support. It can be visualized that the remaining patients are within this spectrum needing varying degrees of nutritional support.

Once surgery is performed on the liver, apart from the technical aspects, the outcome is very much influenced by the control of infection, and by metabolic and nutritional management. Of all the various factors that are known to influence regenerative powers of the liver, such as insulin, glucagon, ileal factor, growth hormone, and nutrition, only nutrition could easily be manipulated by the physician. Therefore, it is not surprising that

many researchers have been actively involved for more than a decade in evolving effective nutritional therapy for patients with severe liver disease and hepatic encephalopathy. Although nutritional support in liver disease is discussed in general in this chapter, emphasis is on the end-stage liver disease (ELD) where specialized nutritional support appears to be particularly indicated.

Metabolic Derangements in Liver Disease

Fischer and Bower have reviewed the myriad of metabolic disturbances that occur when this master metabolic organ is severely diseased (2). Those particularly relevant to nutritional support are discussed here.

Carbohydrate Metabolism

The liver is the site of glycogen synthesis, glycogenolysis (along with muscle), gluconeogenesis (the kidney also plays a minor role), and the metabolism of glucose substitutes such as fructose, galactose, and xylitol (3).

The liver is unique in possessing the glucose-6 phosphatase enzyme; as a result, it is the only organ that can release free glucose into the circulation, meeting the demands of glucose-dependent organs (3,4) [such as brain, renal medulla, red blood cells (RBCs)]. In patients with loss of more than 80% of normal liver parenchyma, glycogen stores and gluconeogenesis are affected to such a degree that episodes of hypoglycemia may occur, particularly during surgical stress (5). The uptake and conversion of glucose substitutes reduces the energy-rich substances in the liver such as ATP, thus impairing energy-dependent metabolic activities of the liver such as protein synthesis. Therefore use of glucose substitutes such as fructose and xylitol in large amounts is not recommended when hepatic function is compromised (5).

Lipid Metabolism

The liver, along with peripheral tissues, plays an active role in lipid metabolism via B-oxidation of fatty acids, triglyceride synthesis, and formation of large quantities of phospholipids and cholesterol. Liver is the site of synthesis of fatty acids, lipoproteins (along with intestine), and ketone bodies (3,4). Plasma triglyceride, ketone body, and lipoprotein levels are variable in liver disease and no definite pattern has been established. Furthermore, lipolysis and ability to utilize ketone bodies and fatty acids by the peripheral tissues is often increased in liver disease (5).

Recent studies of patients with end-stage liver disease (ESLD) have focused on the effects of severe liver disease and subsequent liver transplantation on cholesterol and essential fatty acid metabolism (6). In comparison with healthy adults, these patients had significantly decreased concentrations of plasma lecithin:cholesterol acyl transferase (LCAT), apolipoprotein A-1, total phospholipids, and both total and esterified cholesterol. The increased concentration of saturated fatty acids coupled with reduced concentrations of polyunsaturated fatty acids was indicative of impaired essential fatty acid metabolism in ESLD. Following transplantation, plasma concentrations of total cholesterol, phospholipids, LCAT, and apolipoprotein A-1 were normalized. Essential fatty acid patterns of the plasma phospholipid and cholesterol ester fractions were also normal within 6 months following hepatic replacement. Thus, liver transplantation effectively restores both cholesterol and essential fatty acid metabolism in patients with prior ESLD.

Protein Metabolism

The body cannot dispense with the services of the liver in protein metabolism (4). The principal functions of liver in protein metabolism are deamination of amino acids, synthesis of urea, formation of plasma proteins, and transamination reactions that are involved in synthesis of all nonessential amino acids (4). Phenylalanine, tyrosine, and tryptophan are the aromatic amino acids (AA) that are metabolized in the liver while leucine, isoleucine, and valine are branched-chain amino acids (BCAA), which are preferentially used by the peripheral tissues (5). In ELD, synthesis of urea is impaired, clearance of AA is decreased, and the ratio between plasma BCAA and AA is decreased. Hyperinsulinemia is probably responsible for decrease in BCAA while hyperglucagonemia increases gluconeogenesis in the liver leading to accelerated muscle protein catabolism and increased flux of AA into plasma (Fig. 24.1).

Miscellaneous Disturbances

There is hyperinsulinemia, hyperglucagonemia, and a decreased insulin/glucagon ratio. This is due to impaired catabolism of these hormones by the liver and increased stimulus for glucagon secretion as a result of impaired gluconeogeneic functions of the liver. Hyperglucagonemia and other stress hormones seem to be mainly responsible for the glucose intolerance observed in these patients (5).

In addition, in ELD, storage and activation of vitamins such as A, D, E, vitamin B12, folic acid, thiamine, and storage of minerals such as iron, zinc, and magnesium are impaired (7,8). Rudman and associates have demonstrated that there is also impaired phenylalanine hydroxylation to tyrosine (9) and disturbances in transsulfuration pathway leading to impaired cysteine (10) and carnitine synthesis (11). Therefore, tyrosine, cysteine, and carnitine, which are normally dispensable, may become essential in the face of failing liver function.

Decreased synthesis of coagulation factors I, II, VII, IX, and X increases the risk of coagulopathy (4), while decreased levels of antithrombin III (a naturally occurring anticoagulant in blood, synthesized in liver) increases the risk of thrombotic episodes (12). Metabolic derangements in ELD are summarized in Figure 24.1.

Nutritional Assessment

The first step in the treatment of malnutrition is nutritional assessment. The purpose of the nutritional assessment is to identify and categorize patients with different types and degrees of mal-

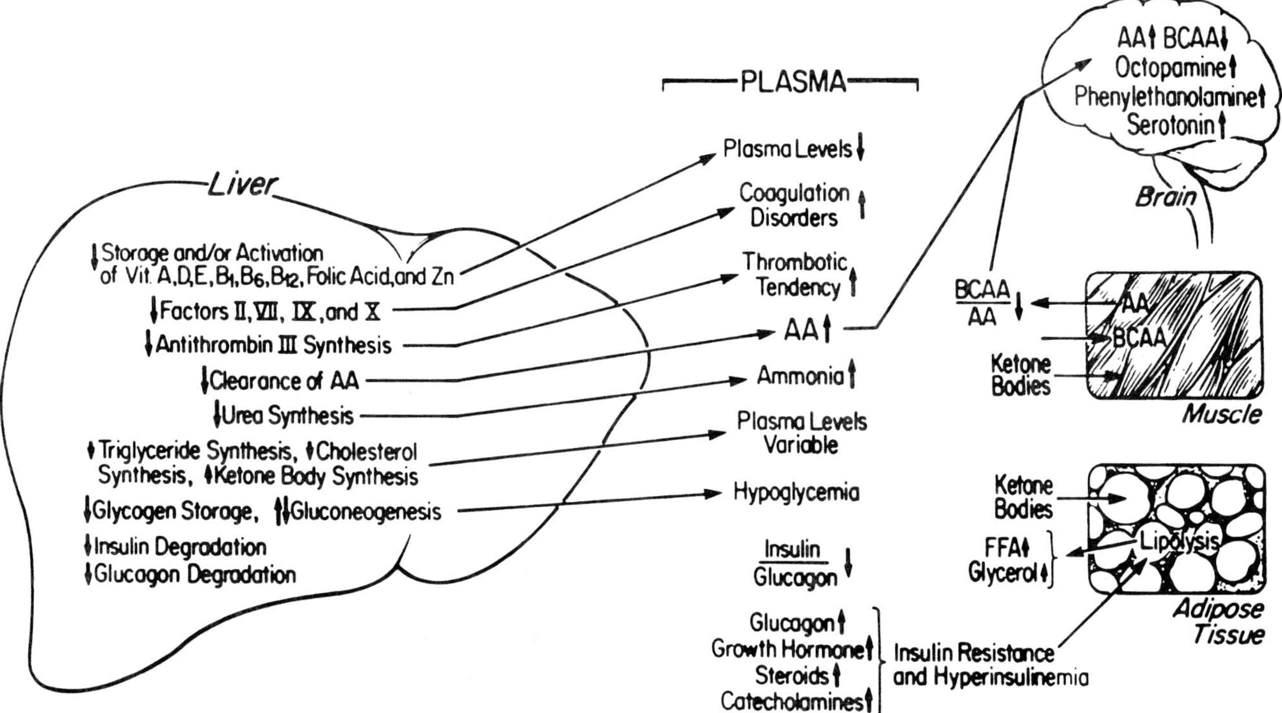

Figure 24.1. Diagram depicting different metabolic derangements relevant to nutritional support in liver disease. Actual metabolic disturbances observed depend on the severity of the liver disease.
AA, aromatic amino acids; BCAA, branched-chain amino acids; FFA, free fatty acids.

nutrition and relate these to morbidity and mortality attending a major stress such as surgery (13).

Clinical Evaluation

A detailed history of the patient's appetite, nausea, epigastric discomfort, steatorrhea, previous health, and operative procedures performed is obtained. Details regarding socioeconomic status, dietary habits, and alcoholic consumption often gives useful information. A clinical impression of the fluid status is provided by the presence of dependent edema, ascites, and fluid balance charts. It is important to look for signs of vitamin deficiency such as glossitis, cheilitis, anemia, and easy bruisability, which are often overlooked. The availability of the gastrointestinal tract is assessed by the absence of active bleeding, abdominal distension, and presence of active bowel sounds. When intravenous feeding is considered, evaluation of the coagulation status and possible approach for the central venous access is necessary. If there is any existing central catheter, this can be

changed over a guidewire by Seldinger's technique onto a new catheter and used for nutritional purposes. Presence of sepsis or other metabolic stress that would confound nutritional support should be documented.

Percentage weight loss in the last 6 months, serum albumin level, and total lymphocyte count are probably the most practical and most commonly used parameters for nutritional assessment (13,14). Anthropometry, creatinine height index (CHI), serum transferrin, and delayed hypersensitivity skin tests are also frequently used (15,16). Some of these are further discussed below and the nutritional assessment in liver disease is summarized in Table 24.1.

Body Weight

Body weight as a percentage of ideal body weight is generally used. Current weight of 70% to 80% of ideal body weight is suggestive of moderate caloric malnutrition and less than 70% of severe caloric malnutrition. Although there are ideal body

Table 24.1. Nutritional Assessment in Liver Disease

Body Compartment	Measurement	Mild	Moderate	Severe	Comments
Total body mass (lean, fat, water)	Percentage of actual weight lost in last 6 months	5%	5%–10%	>10%	Altered by edema, ascites, and tumor
Fat	Triceps skinfold thickness (TSF)	—	—	<5th percentile	Anthropometry is observer-dependent, but still these are more sensitive even when there are ascites, as fluid doesn't tend to accumulate in the arm
Skeletal muscle	Mid arm muscle Circumference = mid arm circumference minus π TSF	—	—	<5th percentile	
	Creatinine height index = $\dfrac{\text{Actual 24-hr urinary creatinine}}{\text{Ideal urinary creatinine for height}} \times 100$	80%–90%	60%–80%	<60%	Accurate 24-hr urine collections are difficult
Visceral proteins	Serum albumin	28–35 g/l	21–28 g/L	<21 g/L	Serum levels altered in severe liver disease, enteropathy, nephrotic syndrome, and metabolic stress
Immune competence	Total lymphocyte count = $\dfrac{\text{\% lymphocytes} \times \text{WBC count}}{100}$	1200–1500/mm^3	800–1200/mm^3	<800/mm^3	Immune competence may be affected by steroids, chemotherapy, or general anesthesia
	Delayed hypersensitivity to common skin antigens	Reactive	Partially reactive	Anergic	
	Induration at the site of antigen injection >5 mm		<1–5 mm	No response	
Vitamins[a]	Thiamine (vitamin B$_1$)		<40 ng/ml		Water-soluble vitamins are the principal vitamins deficient in alcoholic cirrhosis
	Pyridoxene (vitamin B$_6$)		<25 ng/ml		
	Folic acid		<3 ng/ml		
	Cyanacobalamine (vitamin B$_{12}$)		<200 pg/ml		
	Vitamin A		<20–40 mg/dl		Fat-soluble vitamins are the principal vitamins deficient in nonalcoholic cirrhosis
	Vitamin D		<15 ng/ml		
	Vitamin K		Prothrombin time more than 2 sec prolonged		
Trace minerals[a]	Zinc		<112 g/dl		Serum levels of zinc may not reflect body stores
Electrolyte	Magnesium		<1.3 mEq/L		Magnesium deficiency is one of the common electrolyte disorders in hospitalized patients
Others	Carnitine		<400 nmol/dl		Carnitine deficiency can manifest as muscular weakness

[a] Normal serum vitamins and trace mineral values depend on individual laboratory standards.
Adapted from Bistrian BR. In: Hill GL, ed. *Nutrition and the Surgical Patient*. Edinburgh: Churchill Livingstone, 1981, pp. 39–54; Grant JP, Custom PB, Thurlow J. Current techniques of nutritional assessment. *Surg Clin North Am* 1981; 61:437–463; Reilly JJ, Gerhardt AL. (Ravitch M, ser. ed.) Modern surgical nutrition. *Curr Prob Surg* 1985; 22:1–75; Hehir DJ, Jenkins RL, Bistrian BR, et al. Nutrition in patients undergoing orthotopic liver transplantation. JPEN 1985; 9:695–700.
Abbreviations: WBC, white blood cells.

weight tables for men and women, they have little clinical basis, and interpretation of these by the physicians for clinical use varies (15). Recent weight loss is determined by relating the percentage of weight change derived from the following formula:

$$\frac{\text{usual weight} - \text{current weight}}{\text{usual weight}} \times 100$$

Loss of 10% of body weight or more over any brief period of time is clinically significant (15). However, in the setting of ELD, weight becomes an insensitive parameter due to excessive total body water (17).

Arm Anthropometry

Triceps skinfold thickness and arm muscle circumference provide an estimate of body fat reserves and muscle mass, respectively. These are probably more sensitive measures even in the presence of excess body water, as fluid does not accumulate to the same degree in the arm (17,18). These also serve as useful baseline values, should the patient need long-term nutritional support (15). There are age- and sex-specific reference values developed for American men and women and these are expressed in percentiles. Values of less than fifth percentile for the age range and sex indicate severe protein-calorie malnutrition (15).

Creatinine Height Index

Several investigators have demonstrated creatinine excretion in the human to be a good predictor of lean body mass using ^{42}K dilution, ^{40}K total body counting, or total body water as a measurement of lean body mass (13). This is true even when protein malnutrition exists. CHI is a ratio of the 24-hour creatinine excretion of a patient to the expected 24-hour creatinine excretion of a normal adult of the same sex and height expressed as a percentage (19). CHI is a sensitive indicator of lean body mass but it is important to consider factors that alter creatinine excretion such as a creatine-free diet, trauma, sepsis, and end-stage renal failure.

Visceral Proteins

Serum albumin has been classically used in population as an indicator of kwashiorkor.

Hypoalbuminemic malnutrition is characterized by depletion of visceral protein mass, and signs and symptoms of depletion of visceral mass are quite elusive. The measurement of visceral proteins such as serum albumin and transferrin is an attempt to define that a decrease in the serum concentrations of these proteins is a consequence of decreased liver biosynthesis, which in turn is due to limited supply of the substrate due to malnutrition and an actual decrease in organ mass (15).

Since albumin synthesis occurs in liver, it is worthy of further comment as to the prognostic value of albumin levels. Studies in our laboratory have shown albumin synthetic rates to be at lower range of normal in end-stage liver disease (Shanbhogue LKR, Lakshman K, Bistrian BR, et al., unpublished observations). It is also observed that these patients have an increased protein turnover due to accelerated protein catabolism. Thus the more likely cause for the low serum albumin in these patients with liver disease is an increased catabolic rate, uncompensated for by increases in albumin synthetic rates, which could reflect inadequate synthetic reserve and/or inadequate protein intake (17).

Measurement of Immune Competence

Hypoalbuminemic malnutrition or a combination type of malnutrition may often be associated with depression of host's immune responsiveness. Decrease in total lymphocyte count, depressed neutrophil chemotaxis, and depression of skin test reactivity to standard antigens have all been observed as malnutrition progresses. Total lymphocyte count and skin test reactivity are most commonly used and the most practical parameters for assessing immune function. There is a strong correlation between lymphopenia and anergy (15). There is also a strong correlation between cutaneous anergy and mortality in general surgical and in cirrhotic patients. One study showed total anergy in 60% of cirrhotic patients with an incidence of 93% in fulminant hepatic failure and found that 50% of anergic cirrhotic patients died while in the hospital and 91% had documented bacterial sepsis in the week before death (18).

Vitamins A, D, and K and trace minerals such as zinc and magnesium may be deficient due to malabsorption, inadequate storage or activation, or increased urinary excretion. The cause generally tends to be multifactorial. It is a part of the nutritional assessment to look for and detect any specific nutrient deficiency.

Whenever moderate or severe malnutrition is diagnosed in a patient, the patient should be provided with nutritional support for at least 7 to 10 days preoperatively if the surgery is elective. Mullen and associates have documented reduction in postoperative complications and mortality when a malnourished patient receives adequate nutritional support preoperatively (20).

Energy Requirements

It is generally stated that the resting energy expenditure (REE) of the patients with liver disease is not different from that of patients without hepatic disorders (21). This result could be anticipated when the Harris-Benedict equation (22) is employed to estimate the energy expenditure. The validity of the Harris-Benedict equation depends on the theory that there is a close relationship between REE and the body cell mass and therefore can be predicted from the variables such as height and weight suitably corrected for age and sex. The hypercatabolism associated with ELD would be offset by the overestimate of body cell mass by body weight due to excess of total body water (23). In a recent study carried out in our laboratory, REE of 10 patients with relatively stable ELD and 10 normal control subjects was measured by indirect calorimetry and expressed as kilocalories per gram of urinary creatinine so that REE is related to lean body mass. Patients with ELD were found to have the mean REE of 1900 kcal/g creatinine versus 1370 kcal/g in normal control subjects ($p < 0.05$). When correlated to lean body mass, patients with ELD had increased REE (23,24). Therefore, it is advisable to measure the REE by using a mobile metabolic cart (Sensor Medics, Anaheim, California), which has oxygen and carbon dioxide sensors and employs the principle of indirect calorimetry (25).

If the facility to actually measure the REE is not available, it is advisable to predict the basal energy requirements by using the Harris-Benedict equation and making appropriate adjustments for the degree of stress, such as infection or surgery, rather than ignoring the problem (26). These data are summarized in Table 24.2.

Administering adequate calories is critical for adequate use of the protein sources, which attains greater importance in patients who are protein restricted. However, the enthusiasm to provide excess calories should be tempered and reassessed, since excess calories, particularly in the form of glucose, can foster hepatic lipogenesis and hepatic dysfunction, and can lead to increased production of carbon dioxide and thus respiratory work (26,28).

Fuels in Liver Disease

The concept of mixed fuel system, using both fat and carbohydrate for nonprotein calories, evolved to minimize the complications accompanying the excessive administration of glucose calories alone, as well as to offer the benefits of fat emulsions.

Glucose

This carbohydrate is an essential substrate for brain, RBCs, and renal medulla, and it is a source of energy even in the absence of oxygen through anaerobic glycolysis.

As a caloric source, glucose provides 3.4 kcal/g hydrous glucose. Utilization of glucose is optimal when administered at a rate of 4 to 5 milligrams per kilogram per minute. Administration in excess of 7 mg/kg/min, even with insulin, may only enhance the glucose clearance rate but does not affect the oxidation rate (29). Considering these

Table 24.2. Determination of Energy Requirements

1. Basal energy expenditure (BEE)
   BEE in men = $66.47 + 13.75W + 5H - 6.76A$
   BEE in women = $655.1 + 9.56W + 1.85H - 4.68A$
   [A = age (yr); H = height (cm); W = weight (kg)]
2. Stress factor: the correction factor for the degree of stress

	Stress factor
Mild starvation	0.85–1.00
Postoperative (no complication)	1.00–1.05
Peritonitis	1.05–1.25
Severe infection	1.30–1.55
Cancer	1.10–1.45

3. Activity factor = 1.25 for ambulatory patients
4. Total energy expenditure = BEE × stress factor × activity factor

Adapted from Harris JA, Benedict FG. *A Biometric Study of Basal Metabolism in Man.* Carnegie Institute of Washington, DC, Pub. no. 279, 1919; Elwyn DH, Kinney JM, Askanazi J. Energy expenditure in surgical patients. *Surg Clin N Am* 1981; 61:545–555; Wilmore DW. *The Metabolic Management of Critically Ill*, 1st ed. New York: Plenum, 1977.

factors, insulin resistance, and possible impairment of gluconeogenesis in ELD, it is advisable to supply 200 to 250 g of glucose in a day, which approximates the amount of glucose produced by the normal liver via gluconeogenesis.

Protein

The usual source of protein is a standard synthetic amino acid solution containing a mixture of essential and nonessential amino acids providing 4 kcal/g.

It has been established by whole-body protein turnover studies that patients with ELD have substantial elevations of up to three times normal rates for protein catabolism (30). Therefore, protein requirements of these patients is at least the same as that of the patients without liver disease. A nonstressed patient needs 250 mg nitrogen/kg/day (1 g nitrogen = 6.25 g protein), while a stressed patient may need up to 400 mg/kg/day (31). Requirements of the protein-intolerant patients and role of BCAA in encephalopathy will be discussed in Hepatic Encephalopathy and BCAA, below.

Serum albumin, as mentioned above, is a marker of the malnutrition and metabolic stress. Administration of exogenous albumin is unlikely to improve the prognosis. Nevertheless, if serum albumin is less than 2 grams per deciliter, 25 to 50 g of albumin may be infused to maintain the oncotic pressure.

Lipid Emulsions

Lipid emulsions are mainly polyunsaturated long-chain triglycerides (LCT). They are isotonic, can be administered peripherally, have a caloric value of 9 kcal/g, and provide essential fatty acids. There is evidence that emulsions of LCT in excess of 50% of calories under certain conditions can cause impaired bacterial clearance, and may compromise neutrophil and reticuloendothelial system (RES) function (32). Therefore, it is our practice to administer a maximum of 1.5 g/kg body weight or 100 g/day for a 70 kg adult.

Medium-Chain Triglycerides

Medium-chain triglycerides (MCT) are esters of saturated fatty acids. These are commercially available only in some parts of Europe. They supply 8.1 kcal/g and do not need carnitine for metabolism (B-oxidation). MCT emulsions do not seem to block RES and show a great promise as caloric source in septic patients. However, it is to be emphasized that MCT do not contain significant amounts of essential fatty acids and therefore a mixture of MCT and LCT is commonly used.

While investigators are busy in establishing the role of BCAA in hepatic encephalopathy, the exact role of fat emulsions in liver disease has not been completely defined. There is some evidence that fatty acids can displace the bound tryptophan in the plasma and thus theoretically increase the risk of encephalopathy (33), but it has also been demonstrated by means of indirect calorimetry that fat degradation in patients with liver disease is increased from 50% to 84% of the normal value (21). However, at present, fat seems to be an important source of calories in patients with ELD who are often intolerant to glucose and protein restricted, particularly in the face of increased lipolysis, fatty acid oxidation, and ketone body utilization (21) (see Fig. 24.1).

If the serum triglyceride levels are significantly elevated (i.e., more than 800 mg/dl), it is probably inadvisable to administer lipid emulsions.

Micronutrients

Vitamins act as coenzymes in various metabolic processes. Divalent cations like calcium, magnesium, copper, and zinc are important for enzyme function, while phosphate plays a major role in the contractility of muscles. Therefore, it is important that recommended dietary allowance of vitamins, electrolytes, and trace minerals is provided to patients via enteral or total parenteral nutrition (TPN) formulae. Furthermore, any specific nutrient deficiency should be appropriately treated.

Enteral Nutrition

It should be emphasized that the preferred route for satisfying the nutritional needs is via the gastrointestinal tract, and parenteral alimentation becomes necessary only when the gut is unavailable for long periods. The reason for this is physiologic in that the maximal effects of the first pass of the nutrients through the liver are operative and the hormonal interplay, particularly that of insulin and glucagon, is optimal. The presence of intraluminal

Table 24.3. Enteral Formulae

Product	Pro	Fat	CHO	Na$^+$	K$^+$	Cal/cc	Osmolality
		(g/L)			(mEq/L)		(mOsm/kg)
Sustacal[a]	61	23	140	40	53	1	625
Osmolite[b]	37	39	145	24	26	1	300
Magnacal[c]	70	80	250	44	32	2	590
Vital HN[d]	42	11	188	17	30	1	460
Travasorb MCT[e]	49	29	108	15	45	0.78	312
Hepatic Aid II[f]	45	37	172	5	—	1.2	560
Traumaid HBC[g]	56	12	166	23	30	1	675
		(g/20 g)			(mEq/100 g)		
Propac[h]	15	—		10	13	—	—
Polycose[i]	—	—	20	5	1	—	—

Abbreviations: CHO, cholesterol.

[a] Sustacal: a 1 cal/cc, protein-rich formula that is the formula of choice unless volume or electrolyte restriction is necessary (note high K$^+$ content).

[b] Osmolite: a 1 cal/cc iso-osmotic, moderate protein formula useful when osmolality is a concern.

[c] Magnacal: a 2 cal/cc moderate protein formula useful when volume or electrolyte restriction is necessary (note low K content).

[d] Vital HN: a predigested formula useful when decreased digestive/absorptive function is present.

[e] Travasorb MCT: a low-sodium, high-protein formula, which has MCT as the main fat source.

[f] Hepatic Aid II: a high-branched-chain (46%), low-aromatic-amino-acid formula with minimal electrolytes, useful in hepatic failure and other protein and/or electrolyte restricted situations. Note that it contains no vitamins or minerals.

[g] Traumaid HBC: a high-branched-chain (50%) amino acid formula that contains all necessary vitamins and minerals. It contains significant levels of sodium and potassium.

[h] Propac: a protein module used to increase a formula's protein content.

[i] Polycose: a carbohydrate module used to increase a formula's caloric density.

contents is essential for maintenance of immunity of the GI tract, possibly mediated by IgA production (34), and for improving barrier to bacterial toxins, particularly endotoxins.

Anorexia and encephalopathy are the primary factors in the reduced oral intake (35). Daily calculation of protein and calories consumed is required to demonstrate the adequacy of oral intake. Nursing and dietetic staff play a significant role in encouraging the oral intake and providing palatable supplements. If malabsorption and steatorrhea are significant factors, diets high in protein and low in fats (except medium-chain fatty acids), pancreatic exocrine replacement, and abstinence from ethanol constitute the important aspects of management (35).

If the oral intake is not adequate in spite of encouragement, nasogastric tube feeding is essential. If there is any doubt as to the mental status of the patient, the feeding tube should be manipulated beyond the pylorus, if necessary with the help of an endoscope, thus reducing the risk of aspiration. Introduction of the feeding tube should not be withheld even if there is a history of esophageal varices. *If an endoscopist can introduce an endoscope, one could definitely introduce a fine feeding tube without inducing bleeding.* A surgeon undertaking laparotomy should give careful thought to the present and future nutritional problems and consider a tube jejunostomy or a needle catheter jejunostomy, thus avoiding long-term TPN postoperatively due to oral intake limited by anorexia or encephalopathy.

Standard enteral nutritional formulas are available for dietary supplementation or administration via feeding tube (Table 24.3). They vary in caloric density, osmolality, electrolytes composition, and palatability. Elemental diets or chemically defined diets are low in fat content and contain peptides or amino acids. As a result, they tend to be hypertonic and do not carry any advantage over standard formulas unless absorptive functions of the small bowel are severely impaired. As a general rule, patients on fluid restriction need high-density formulas (e.g., Magnacal) and patients with marked metabolic abnormalities needing multiple modifications in caloric sources, protein, and electrolytes can be managed by modular diets. By using the nutrient modules, the nutritionist can prepare enteral solutions that are tailored to specific patient requirements such as low Na$^+$, K$^+$, or protein. Enteral nutrition may be employed as an adjunct to TPN or as a transition phase while TPN is being tapered. Meanwhile, the patient should be encouraged per oral intake. If it is felt that the tube feedings are interfering with the oral intake, feeds could be cycled at nighttime, thus reducing the fullness of stomach that some patients complain of and allowing the patient mobility.

Gastrointestinal obstruction, active GI infection, and active GI bleeding are common contraindications for enteral feeding (36). Misplacement of feeding tubes, aspiration of enteral feeds, diarrhea, dehydration, and hypophosphatemia are important complications of enteral nutrition to be borne in mind (36). The role of the BCAA in hepatic encephalopathy is discussed in Hepatic Encephalopathy and BCAA, below.

Parenteral Nutrition

Peripheral Intravenous Nutrition

By using fat emulsions to provide 30% to 60% of caloric input, full energy and protein needs can be met through a peripheral vein. Solutions with an osmolarity of greater than 600 mosmoles or with potassium concentrations greater than 60 millimoles per liter are more likely to cause phlebitis (37). Therefore, a larger fluid volume than with central venous feeding will be needed for TPN.

Protein-sparing therapy is the provision of standard amino acid solutions through a peripheral intravenous line providing 1.0 to 1.5 g protein/kg body weight without supplemental fat or dextrose (38). In a moderately stressed, well-nourished patient, if adequate oral intake is anticipated in 5 to 7 days, protein-sparing therapy is recommended. This will improve protein synthesis and minimize skeletal muscle catabolism.

However, protein-sparing therapy is not indicated in patients who are severely stressed, and peripheral nutrition is less applicable in patients who need complete nutritional replacement, are fluid restricted, or have inadequate peripheral venous access.

Central TPN

If the patient is a candidate for complete nutritional replacement, and GI function is uncertain, it would be in the patient's best interest to insert a central catheter and start TPN early. Hypertonicity of the TPN solutions necessitates its delivery to the superior vena cava (SVC), thus ensuring distribution of the nutrients at isotonic concentrations.

The SVC may be cannulated by a percutaneous

Table 24.4. Management of Catheter Infection and Sepsis

PBC	CBC	CTC	Diagnosis	Treatment
+	+	−	Sepsis probably	Change catheter over
+	−	−	not related to	guidewire once a week
			catheter	
−	−	+	Catheter infection	Change catheter over a
−	+	−	or contamination	guidewire employing
−	+	+		Seldinger's technique
+	+	+	Catheter sepsis	Remove catheter and
+	−	+		change to a new site

Additional rules
1. All catheter sites should be inspected at least twice a week and dressings changed aseptically.
2. If patient is septicemic and catheter is not the source, change catheter over guidewire once a week to prevent seeding of the catheter tip.
3. In case of *Staphyloccocus aureus* sepsis or fungal septicemia due to any source, change catheter to a new site.
4. Change catheter to a new site if there is catheter exit site infection.

Abbreviations: CBC, blood culture drawn through the central line; CTC, catheter tip culture; PBC, peripheral blood culture. Adapted from Bozzetti F. Central venous catheter sepsis—collective review. *Surg Gynecol Obstet* 1985; 61:293–301; Hopkins SB. Clinical Consultations in nutritional support. In: Blackburn GL, ed. 1st ed. Chicago: Medical Directions, 1982, pp. 14–16; Pettigrew RA, Lang SDR, Haydock DA, Parry BR, Bremmer DA, Hill GL. Catheter related sepsis in patients on intravenous nutrition; a prospective study of quantitative catheter cultures and guidewire changes for suspected sepsis. *Br J Surg* 1985; 72:52–55.

puncture of subclavian, internal jugular, or external jugular vein. An infraclavicular puncture of the subclavian vein is the most commonly used approach. It is acceptably safe and the catheter exit site is easier to manage. An internal jugular vein puncture may be preferred in severely wasted, emphysematous patients on ventilators as they run a greater risk of pneumothorax. Although a formidable number of mechanical complications of central line insertions is listed, these could be reduced to nearly zero with increasing experience and appropriate supervision during line placement (39).

A major complication during maintenance of central access is catheter sepsis. The key to the whole issue of prevention of catheter sepsis is a rigid protocol for catheter maintenance and dressings and keeping the line violation for the purpose of administration of drugs, blood, and blood products to a minimum (40). Management of catheter infection or sepsis is outlined in Table 24.4. It is essential to thoroughly investigate other possible sources of septic focus before the catheter sepsis is diagnosed (41,42).

Electrolyte imbalances, hyperglycemia, rebound hypoglycemia, and acid-base imbalance are some of the common metabolic complications that occur during TPN and warrant close monitoring of the patient. It is very important to recognize that glucose administered parenterally stimulates release of less insulin than the enterally administered glucose. Therefore, blood glucose levels should be carefully monitored during early days of TPN and the exogenous insulin administered if necessary. Protein synthesis and anabolism that occur with TPN can lead to hypophosphatemia. Therefore, serum phosphate levels should be closely monitored and at least 30 mmol of phosphate administered each day with TPN unless the patient has acute renal failure.

Hepatic Encephalopathy and BCAA

The most controversial area in the hepatology is probably the pathogenesis of hepatic encephalopathy (HE). A number of metabolic alterations observed in patients with hepatic encephalopathy have given room for various hypotheses. Currently there are two predominant hypotheses that have generated a lot of experimental data and interest.

Synergism Hypothesis

In the presence of hepatic failure, encephalopathy and ultimately coma result from synergistic effects of accumulating toxins with coma. Ammonia, mercaptans, and fatty acids are the commonly identified toxins. The toxins interact synergistically to produce neurologic alterations that are out of proportion to the resulting abnormality when administered singly. Accumulation of ammonia and its effects on the central nervous system are central in the synergism hypothesis. The metabolic abnormalities such as hypoxia, acid-base disturbances, electrolyte disturbances, and hypoglycemia augment the effects of accumulating toxins. Thus, this hypothesis recognizes that the etiology of HE is multifactorial; there is a large body of experimental data supporting it, and it correlates with the clinical observations. The principal criticism of this hypothesis is poor correlation between blood ammonia levels and HE. This discrepancy is explained by the fact that only a small portion of ammonia that passes through the circulation gets into the brain (43).

False Neurotransmitter Hypothesis

The plasma amino acid ratio of the BCAA to AA in liver disease, shown below,

$$\frac{\text{leucine} + \text{isoleucine} + \text{valine (BCAA)}}{\text{phenylalanine} + \text{tyrosine} + \text{tryptophan (AA)}},$$

is decreased and leads to increased entry of AA into the brain and synthesis of false neurotransmitters such as octopamine and decreased synthesis of dopamine and norepinephrine. Fischer and associates formulated this hypothesis in 1971 and ammonia was not considered to be a primary factor in the pathogenesis of HE (43). The same group developed a unified hypothesis in 1979, noting that patients with HE have elevated levels of glutamine in the cerebrospinal fluid. According to them, ammonia entering the brain is rapidly combined with glutamate to form glutamine, and the brain, in its efforts to normalize neutral amino acid levels, rapidly exports glutamine by the same mechanism responsible for the influx of neutral amino acids. Thus, ammonia indirectly contributes to the HE by increasing amino acid imbalance in the brain (45,46). Animal experiments do indicate a relationship between octopamine and coma (46), but changes in brain dopamine and norepinephrine have never been shown to cause coma (43). However, there is plasma amino acid imbalance in HE and this may have some causal relationship with HE.

The nutritional support in HE has evolved to a great extent from the pseudoneurotransmitter hypothesis. Fischer demonstrated initially that administration of BCAA-enriched solution to patients with HE corrects the amino acid pattern with improvement in the encephalopathy (47). Since then, there have been many BCAA trials and the results have been conflicting. Some of the important controlled trials are summarized in Table 24.5. It is very important to realize the difficulty in organizing a BCAA trial, which ideally demands selecting patients without secondary stress factors such as infection or GI hemorrhage, ensuring randomization, supplying the solution of amino acid for an adequate length of time, supplying nutritionally complete formulae, and providing adequate caloric sources for patients on both arms of the trial. Therefore, it becomes difficult to interpret the results of these trials since they are de-

Table 24.5. Controlled Trials of BCAA

Author/Ref. No.	No. Patients	Route	Treatment Groups	Results
Rossi-Fanelli (46)	34	IV	Lactulose Pure BCAA	Decreased level of HE in 47% lactulose and in 70% BCAA group
Wahren (47)	50	IV	Placebo D5W Pure BCAA, high leucine	No difference in HE or survival in BCAA group
Cerra (48)	22	IV	Neomycin F080 (Hepatamine)	HE improved in 25% and 25% mortality in control group, HE improved in 56% and no mortality in F080 group
Cerra (49)	59	IV	Neomycin + 25% dextrose Placebo + dextrose + F080	Slow improvement in encephalopathy and 35% mortality in control group Striking improvement in encephalopathy and 20% mortality in F080 group
Horst (50)	36	PO	Dietary protein A662 (Hepaticaid) supplement	HE developed in 58% diet group, 7% of BCAA group Nitrogen balance improved in both groups
Ericksson (51)	7	PO	Placebo Pure BCAA solution	No difference in HE, amino acid pattern returned to baseline within 12 hr with BCAA solution
McGhee (52)	4	PO	Casein Casein + Hepaticaid	No difference in HE Nitrogen balance improved in both groups
Christie (53)	8	PO	Casein supplement BCAA supplement	No significant change in encephalopathy or nitrogen balance between two groups

Abbreviations: D5W, 5% dextrose in water; F080, experimental enteral tube feeding diet.

signed differently. However, some conclusions can be drawn regarding protein supply in HE.

1. BCAA are safe orally (52) and parenterally (50).
2. Orally, BCAA (52), casein modular diet (55), and vegetable protein (56) seem to be better tolerated than the dietary meat protein.
3. BCAA can induce positive nitrogen balance, but it is essential to supply at least 75 g of protein for an adequate length of time (5).
4. It should be emphasized that BCAA are to be administered as a usual mixture of essential and nonessential amino acids enriched up to 50% with BCAA.
5. There have been no trials comparing BCAA and standard amino acid solutions in HE.

BCAA have also been shown to improve hepatic protein synthesis (57), reduce postinjury catabolism (58,59), and reverse the catabolic state characteristic of cirrhosis (60). Although more confirmation is needed regarding the anticatabolic properties of BCAA, at present it seems wise to administer BCAA when the protein intake is restricted, at least for metabolic reasons if not for neurologic reasons.

Nutritional Support in Liver Transplantation

Consequences of massive blood transfusions; frequent acute renal failure in the early postoperative period; interactions of immunosuppressive drugs, particularly cyclosporine; and manifestations of rejection necessitate specialized nutritional support in the posttransplant period. Probably *the most important factor in the nutritional management of these patients is close rapport with the transplant team.* Anywhere from 40 to 250 units of blood products may be transfused during liver transplantation in a significant load of citrate (61). One report has estimated the average load of citrate from blood products to be 750 milliequivalents (62). Metabolism of the delivered citrate load by the liver is believed to initiate the metabolic alkalosis, which may be potentiated by the use of the diuretics and corticosteroids (61). Infusion of hydrocholoric acid (HCl) (HCl is not compatible with lipid emulsions) in calculated amounts along with TPN can correct the acid-base abnormality and prevent compensatory hypoventilation, thus facilitating early weaning from the ventilator. However, if there is acute renal failure and hyperkalemia, enthusiasm for acid therapy should be tempered until the hyperkalemia resolves, to avoid life-threatening increases in serum potassium levels.

Cyclosporine, which forms an important component of the immunosuppressive regimen, can cause a disproportionate rise in blood urea nitrogen (BUN), in relation to the level of serum creatinine, and tubular defects leading to hyponatremia and hyperkalemia (63). Whenever BUN is more than 100 mg/dl, it is important to discuss with the transplant team possible adjustments in the immunosuppressive regimen so that there is reduction in cyclosporine dosage or dialysis, rather than reducing protein supply in TPN.

Methylprednisolone, which is often used supplementary to cyclosporine, can cause hyperglycemia and phosphaturia. Therefore, close monitoring of the blood glucose and phosphate levels is indicated.

Immunosuppressed patients are more prone to sepsis, therefore close monitoring of the catheter exit site and periodic blood cultures are indicated. Meanwhile, it is wise to remember that these patients can often have episodes of pyrexia related to organ rejection, unrelated to catheter sepsis, and thus avoid unnecessary interference with the catheter.

These patients can often have nonspecific disturbances in liver function tests unrelated to the rejection phenomenon and biopsy of the liver may indicate cholestasis. As many of these patients are on TPN, it would be essential to consider the possibility of TPN-induced cholestasis. TPN-induced liver damage can occur as early as the second week of TPN. It is more common in patients receiving large quantities of glucose in excess of the energy requirements with no supple-

mentation of fat emulsions; it is also common in patients after abdominal surgery, sepsis, and in patients who are only on TPN with no enteral diet (64). Considering these factors, liver transplant patients are at a high risk of developing TPN-induced liver damage. On the other hand, it is also possible that the cholestasis observed in the early posttransplant period may be due to the ischemic insult suffered by the liver during organ retrieval and transport (65). Therefore, a balanced judgment is called for as to the cause of cholestasis and appropriate action. Whatever may be the cause of cholestasis, commencement of enteral feedings as soon as the GI tract permits should reduce the risk of TPN-induced liver damage and improve the hepatic perfusion. Furthermore, Starzl and associates have found portal vein insulin to be one of the important factors in liver regeneration (66).

Nevertheless, it should be emphasized that all liver transplant patients do not need TPN. At the time of writing, some of our patients have attained excellent oral intake by the fifth postoperative day and they have been managed on close dietary supervision and oral supplements alone.

Monitoring of Nutritional Support

Accurate daily weight recordings are useful in assessing the patient's fluid status. Serum electrolytes may be needed twice a week or more often, depending on the degree of electrolyte disturbance. Actual bicarbonate and arterial blood gas values are needed for assessing the acid-base status and planning appropriate therapy, particularly in critically ill patients.

Urinary electrolytes assist in planning electrolyte replacement. Nitrogen balance studies carried out at least once a week with 24-hour urine collections will help in dynamic assessment and reflect nitrogen retention by the patient. The relationship among these factors is shown by the following equation.

$$\text{nitrogen balance (g)} = \frac{\text{protein intake (g)}}{6.25} - \text{24-hour urinary urea nitrogen (g)} + 4$$

Delayed hypersensitivity skin testing can be an early parameter indicating the patient's return to normal following adequate nutritional repletion. However, if the patient is immunosuppressed, this measurement may not return to normal as long as immunosuppression continues. Serum transferrin (half-life of 10 days) and serum albumin (half-life of 20 days) respond more slowly. If significant metabolic stress persists, the serum albumin level may not respond in spite of adequate nutritional support (13).

References

1. Blackburn GL, Bistrian BR, Maini B, Schlamm HT, Smith MF. Nutritional and metabolic assessment of the hospitalized patient. *JPEN* 1977; 1:11–22.
2. Fischer JF, Bower RH. Nutritional support in liver disease. *Surg Clin North Am* 1981; 61:653–660.
3. Martin DW, Mayes PA, Rodwell VW, Granner DK, eds. *Harper's Review of Biochemistry*, 20th ed. Los Altos, California: Lange Medical Publications, 1985; pp. 230–239.
4. Guyton AC. The liver and biliary system. In: Guyton AC, ed. *Textbook of Medical Physiology*, 6th ed. Philadelphia: WB Saunders, 1981; pp. 861–869.
5. Holm E, Kasper H, eds. *Metabolism and Nutrition in Liver Disease*. Boston: MTP Press, 1985.
6. Palombo JD, Lopes SM, Zeisel SH, Jenkins RL, et al. Effectiveness of orthotopic liver transplantation on the restoration of cholesterol metabolism in patients with end-stage liver disease. *Gastroenterology* 1987; 93:1170–77.
7. Russell RM. Vitamin and mineral supplements in the management of liver disease. *Med Clin North Am* 1979; 63: 537–544.
8. Lindeman RD. Assessment of trace element depletion. In: Wright RA, et al., eds. *Nutritional Assessment*. Boston: Blackwell Scientific Publications, 1984.
9. Rudman D, Kutner M, Ansley J, Jansen R, Chipponi J, Bain RP. Hypotyrosinemia, hypocystinemia and failure to retain nitrogen during total parenteral nutrition of cirrhotic patients. *Gastroenterology* 1981; 81:1025–1035.
10. Chawla RK, Berry CJ, Kutner MH, Rudman D. Plasma concentrations of transsulfuration pathway products during nasoenteral and intravenous hyperalimentation of malnourished patients. *Am J Clin Nutr* 1985; 42:577–584.
11. Rudman D, Sewell CW, Ansley JD. Deficiency of carnitine in cachectic cirrhotic patients. *J Clin Invest* 1977; 60:716–723.
12. Imperial JA, Bistrian BR, Bothe A, Bern M, et al. Limitation of central vein thrombosis in total parenteral nutrition by continuous infusion of low dose heparin. *J Am Coll Nutr* 1983; 2:63–73.
13. Bistrian BR. Assessment of protein energy malnutrition in surgical patients. In: Hill GL, ed. *Nutrition and the Surgical Patient*, 1st ed. Edinburgh: Churchill Livingstone, 1981, pp. 39–54.
14. Reinhardt GF, Myscofski JW, Wilkens DB, Dobrin PB, Mangan JE, Stannard RT. Incidence and mortality of hypoalbuminemic patients in hospitalized veterans. *JPEN* 1980; 4:357–359.
15. Grant JP, Custer PB, Thurlow J. Current techniques of nutritional assessment. *Surg Clin North Am* 1981; 61:437–463.
16. Reilly JJ, Gerhardt AL. (Ravitch M, ser. ed.) Modern surgical nutrition. *Curr Prob Surg* 1985; 22:1–75.
17. Hehir DJ, Jenkins RL, Bistrian BR, Wagner D, et al. Nutrition in patients undergoing orthotopic liver transplantation. *JPEN* 1985; 9:695–700.
18. O'Keefe SJD, Carraher TE, El-Zayadi AR, Davis M, Williams R. Malnutrition and immuno-incompetence in patients with liver disease. *Lancet* 1980; 615–617.
19. Bistrian BR, Blackburn GL, Sherman M, Scrimshaw NS. Therapeutic index of nutritional depletion in hospitalized patient. *Surg Gynecol Obstet* 1975; 141:512–516.
20. Mullen JL, Buzby GP, Matthews DL, Smale BF, Rosato EF. Reduction of operative morbidity and mortality by combined preoperative and postoperative nutritional support. *Ann Surg* 1980; 33:2119–2127.
21. Kleinberger G. Energy supply during parenteral nutrition in liver insufficiency. In: Holm E, Kasper H, eds. *Metabolism and Nutrition in Liver Disease,* 1st ed. Boston: MTP Press, 1985, pp. 303–312.
22. Harris JA, Benedict FG. *A Biometric Study of Basal Metabolism in Man.* Carnegie Institute of Washington, DC, Pub. no. 279, 1919.
23. Vitale GC, Neill GD, Fenwick MK, Wilson WS, Cuschieri A. Body composition in the cirrhotic patient with ascites: Assessment of total exchangeable sodium and potassium with simultaneous serum electrolyte determination. *Am Surg* 1985; 51:675–681.
24. Shanbhogue RL, Bistrian BR, Jenkins RL, Randall S, Blackburn GL. Increased protein catabolism without hypermetabolism after human orthotopic liver transplantation. *Surgery* 1987; 101:146–149.
25. Beckman Instruments, Inc., Schiller Park, Illinois. Using the Beckman metabolic cart for indirect calorimetry, Bulletin no. 5125. Presented at the ASPEN Fifth Clinical Congress, New Orleans, LA, Jan. 1981.
26. Elwyn DH, Kinney JM, Askanazi J. Energy expenditure in surgical patients. *Surg Clin North Am* 1981; 61:545–555.
27. Wilmore DW. *The Metabolic Management of Critically Ill*, 1st ed. New York: Plenum, 1977.
28. Elwyn DH. Nutritional requirements of adult surgical patients. *Crit Care Med* 1980; 8:9–20.
29. Wolfe RR, Allsop JR, Burke JF. Glucose metabolism in man: Response to IV glucose infusion. *Metabolism* 1979; 28: 210–220.
30. O'Keefe SJD, Abraham R, El-Zayadi A, Marshall W, et al. Increased plasma tyrosine concentrations in patients with cirrhosis and fulminant hepatic failure associated with increased plasma tyrosine flux and reduced hepatic oxidation capacity. *Gastroenterology* 1981; 81:1017–1024.
31. Hill GL, Church J. Energy and protein requirements of general surgical patients requiring intravenous nutrition. *Br J Surg* 1984; 71:1–9.
32. Hamawy KJ, Moldawer LL, Georgieff M, Valicenti AJ, et al. Effect of lipid emulsions on the reticuloendothelial system function in the injured animal. *JPEN* 1985; 9:559–565.
33. Muscaritoli M, Cangiano C, Casuino A, Ceci F, Rossi-Fanelli F. Effect of lipid infusion on plasma amino acid pattern in liver cirrhosis (abstr). European Society of Pareteral and Enteral Nutrition Clinical Congress, 1985.
34. Alverdy J, Sang H, Sheldon GF. The effect of parenteral nutrition on gastrointestinal immunity. The importance of enteral stimulation. *Ann Surg* 1985; 202:681–684.
35. Wade JE, Echenique M, Blackburn GL. Enteral feeding in liver failure. In: Johnston IDA, ed. *Advances in Clinical Nutrition*. Boston: MTP Press, 1982; pp. 149–162.
36. Bothe A, Wade JE, Blackburn GL. Enteral nutrition; an overview. In: Hill GL, ed. *Nutrition and the Surgical Patient*. Edinburgh: Churchill Livingstone, 1981; pp. 76–103.
37. Gazitua R, Wilson K, Bistrian BR. Factors determining peripheral vein tolerance to amino acid solutions. *Arch Surg* 1979; 114:897–900.
38. Blackburn GL, Flatt JP, Clowes GHA, O'Donnell TF,

Hensle TE. Protein sparing therapy during periods of starvation with sepsis and trauma. *Ann Surg* 1973; 177: 588–594.

39. Nehme AE. Nutritional support of the hospitalized patient. The team concept. *JAMA* 1980; 243:1906–1908.

40. Bozzetti F. Central venous catheter sepsis—collective review. *Surg Gynecol Obstet* 1985; 61:293–301.

41. Hopkins SB. *Clinical consultations in nutritional support*. In: Blackburn GL, ed. 1st ed. Chicago: Medical Directions, 1982; pp. 14–16.

42. Pettigrew RA, Lang SDR, Haydock DA, Parry BR, Bremmer DA, Hill GL. Catheter related sepsis in patients on intravenous nutrition; a prospective study of quantitative catheter cultures and guidewire changes for suspected sepsis. *Br J Surg* 1985; 72:52–55.

43. Zieve L. The mechanism of hepatic coma. *Hepatology* 1981; 1:360–365.

44. Fischer JE, Baldessarini RJ. Hypothesis; false neurotransmitters and hepatic failure. *Lancet* 1971; 2:75–79.

45. James JH, Jepsson B, Ziparo V, Fischer JE. Hyperammonemia, plasma amino acid imbalance and blood-brain amino acid transport: A unified theory of portal-systemic encephalopathy. *Lancet* 1979; 2:772–775.

46. Fischer JE. Amino acids in hepatic coma: Editorial. *Dig Dis Sci* 1982; 27:97–102.

47. Fischer JE, Rosen HM, Ebeid AM, James JH, Keane JM, Soeters PB. The effect of normalization of plasma amino acids on hepatic encephalopathy in man. *Surgery* 1976; 80: 77–79.

48. Rossi F, Riggio O, Cangiano C, Cascino A, et al. Branched-chain amino acids vs. lactulose in the treatment of hepatic coma, a controlled study. *Dig Dis Sci* 1982; 27:929–935.

49. Wahren J, Denis J, Desurmont P, Eriksson LS, et al. Is intravenous administration of branched-chain amino acids effective in the treatment of hepatic encephalopathy? A multicentric study. *Hepatology* 1983; 4:475–480.

50. Cerra FB, Cheung NK, Fischer JE, Kaplowitz N, et al. A multicenter trial of branched chain enriched amino acid infusion (F080) in hepatic encephalopathy (HE). *Hepatology* 1982; 2:699.

51. Cerra FB, Cheung NK, Fischer JE, Kaplowitz N, et al. Disease specific amino acid infusion (F080) in hepatic encephalopathy: A prospective randomized double blind controlled trial. *JPEN* 1985; 9:288–295.

52. Horst D, Grace ND, Conn HO, Schiff E, et al. Comparison of dietary protein with an oral branched chain enriched amino acid supplement in chronic portal-systemic encephalopathy: A randomized controlled trial. *Hepatology* 1984; 4:279–287.

53. Eriksson S, Persson A, Wahren J. Branched chain amino acids in the treatment of chronic hepatic encephalopathy. *Gut* 1982; 23:801–806.

54. McGhee A, Henderson M, Millikan JW, Bleier JC, et al. Comparison of the effects of hepatic aid and a casein modular diet on encephalopathy, plasma amino acids and nitrogen balance in cirrhotic patients. *Ann Surg* 1983; 197: 288–293.

55. Christie ML, Sack DM, Pomposelli J, Horst D. Enriched branched chain amino acid formula versus a casein-based supplement in the treatment of cirrhosis. *JPEN* 1985; 9: 671–678.

56. Greenberger NJ, Carley J, Schenker S, Bettinger I, et al. Effect of vegetable and animal protein diets in chronic hepatic encephalopathy. *Dig Dis Sci* 1977; 22:845–855.

57. Sobrado JS, Pomposelli JJ, Yamazaki K, Maiz A, et al. BCAA enriched elemental diets support hepatic protein synthesis in injured rats. *Nutr Res* 1985; 5:737–748.

58. Blackburn GL, Moldawer LL, Usui S, Bothe A, et al. Branched chain amino acid administration and metabolism during starvation, injury and infection. *Surgery* 1979; 86:307–315.

59. Cerra FB, Upson D, Angelico R, Wiles C, et al. Branch chains support postoperative protein synthesis. *Surgery* 1982; 92:192–199.

60. Marchesini G, Zoli M, Dondi C, Bianchi G, Cirulli M, Pisi E. Anticatabolic effect of branched chain amino acid-enriched solutions in patients with liver cirrhosis. *Hepatology* 1982; 2:420–425.

61. Jenkins RL, Benotti PN, Bothe AL, Rossi RL. Liver transplantation. *Surg Clin North Am* 1985; 65:103–122.

62. Priscoll DF, Bistrian BR, Jenkins RL, Randall S, et al. Development of metabolic alkalosis after massive transfusion during orthotopic liver transplantation. *Cut Care Med* 1987; 15:905–908.

63. Bennett WM, Pulliam JP. Cyclosporine nephrotoxicity; editorial. *Ann Intern Med* 1983; 99:851–854.

64. Roy CC, Belli DC. Hepatobiliary complications associated with TPN: An enigma. *J Am Coll Nutr* 1985; 4:655–660.

65. Williams JW, Vera S, Peters TG, Van Voorst S, et al. Cholestatic jaundice after hepatic transplantation. *Am J Surg* 1986; 151:65–70.

66. Starzl TE, Francavilla A, Halgrimson CG, Francavilla FR, et al. The origin, hormonal nature and action of hepatotrophic substances in portal venous blood. *Surg Gynecol Obstet* 1973; 137:179–199.

Editorial Comment

Malnutrition is such an integral part of the clinical picture presented by so many patients with progressive liver disease, and the corrections of the resulting defects so important to the operating surgeon, that this chapter is an invaluable adjunct to the overall text on surgery of the liver.

There is a section within the chapter on hepatic encephalopathy that provides an additional view of the neurologic problems associated with the construction of a surgical shunt or the progressive and rapid deterioration of hepatocellular function. As mentioned in the previous chapters specifically directed towards this metabolic abnormality, there are still gaps in our understanding of the exact biochemical sequence that certainly involves the metabolism of ammonia and probably is a result of subsequent defect in the tricarboxylic acid cycle of the brain. The entire metabolic picture has not as yet been completely clarified and there are still gaps existing which must be filled before complete understanding of the biochemical process is available.

Chapter 25
Anesthesia and the Liver

ISTRATI A. KUPELI
JAMES S. GESSNER
ELLISON C. PIERCE

The challenging surgical approaches utilized in the treatment of liver disease, especially in the most advanced stages, demand equally innovative anesthetic techniques. The medical and technical problems can appear to be overwhelming and the patient's optimal physical state is frequently compromised. Issues of management are made even more complex by the lack of clearcut studies addressing administration of anesthesia to patients with liver disease. Many suggestions and recommendations found in literature are based purely on experimentation or controversial speculation. Nevertheless, careful assessment and utilization of available resources will allow one to anesthetize safely such patients with an outcome appropriate to the clinical picture.

As Sherlock has stated, the liver is a mystery, its functions "only exceeded by the number of biochemical methods designed to test them" (1). It is unfortunate that a small degree of impairment may be significant but hard to detect and, once detected, just as hard to interpret (2).

Preoperative Assessment

The preoperative patient can be placed into one of the following classifications:

Class 1: Hepatobiliary disease without systemic or other organ involvement

Class 2: Severe hepatobiliary disease with systemic and other organ involvement

Class 3: Terminal hepatic disease with either impending or florid hepatic failure

This simple clinical classification allows the anesthesiologist to correlate disease entity, pathophysiologic alterations, and surgical procedure.

Furthermore, the technical aspects of the anesthetic—methodology; equipment; monitoring; laboratory workup; correction of abnormal metabolic, hematologic and respiratory parameters—can be accomplished by establishing priorities within the framework provided above.

The assessment of these patients follows the usual principles applied for any preoperative patient, emphasizing problems associated with liver disease and others unrelated to the existing primary process. Obviously, as the patient's physical status moves to a higher risk level, or the complexity of the surgical treatment increases, objective preoperative assessment by invasive means, particularly in older patients and in patients with important physiologic deficits, becomes necessary (3).

Simple clinical evaluation may fail to reveal hidden deficits and may introduce subjective bias in setting priorities for preoperative attention. Of particular interest is the changing approach to patients with recent history (3 to 6 months) of myocardial infarction. The high risk of infarction and mortality associated with surgery and anesthesia during this period has been documented by many (4–6). However, recent studies were able to demonstrate a substantial decrease in risk by the judicious application of invasive monitoring and appropriate therapy (7).

Routine use of nonspecific tests with low sensitivity and specificity, like the electrocardiogram (EKG) and chest films in the absence of past history, contribute little to the overall evaluation (8–10). These tests are obtained primarily as baseline data for future comparison, for example, in patients under the age of 50 with class 1 hepatobiliary disease.

Nonspecific tests of high specificity and sensitivity (hemoglobin, hematocrit, and urinalysis) may contribute as much as tests for the primary hepatic disease. Anemias must be investigated fully. Preoperative transfusion should be reserved for those patients with critically diminished oxygen-carrying capacity and for those who are at risk for cardiovascular instability with surgical bleeding. In any event, the potential complications of blood transfusion must not outweigh the potential benefits.

Liver function tests have been discussed elsewhere (see Chapter 3 and 3A of this book). Many of these tests have both a monitoring function as well as a screening-profile one. An elevated alkaline phosphatase or bilirubin level may have little value at surgery but great importance in screening for disease and in biochemical follow-up after surgery. On the other hand, altered albumin and simple coagulation tests can indicate severe hepatocellular dysfunction and require proper attention preoperatively (11). The anesthesiologist must review tests that pertain to function at the time of surgery.

Screening-profile tests with normal values serve as a baseline should hepatic dysfunction complicate surgery. Tests that have been abnormal in the past may be entirely normal at the time of surgery, important historical data for the anesthesiologist who may contemplate using potentially hepatotoxic drugs. Liver function tests are useful in diagnosing liver disease but may remain only marginally helpful when used as monitors to quantify the extent of disease or hepatic damage preoperatively. The physiologic basis of many tests is not fully understood and it is not surprising that certain ones correlate poorly with others when used as indices of hepatocellular function (11).

The Concept of Hepatic Clearance

The liver is an important organ for drug disposition. Anesthesia and surgery can affect hepatic function in rather unpredictable ways (12,13). Similarly, hepatic dysfunction disrupts pharmacokinetic and pharmacodynamic events, thus altering anesthetic management. The difficulty in making predictions of drug metabolism in the presence of liver disease lies in the fact that the functional abnormality associated with any particular disease

Table 25.1. Classification of Drugs Based on Pharmacokinetic Parameters Obtained in Normal Subjects

	Hepatic Extraction	Protein Binding	Effect of Shunting on Systemic Availability	Examples
Enzyme limited, binding insensitive	<0.25	<90	—	Antipyrine Amobarbital Caffeine Theophylline Aminopyrine
Enzyme limited, binding sensitive	<0.25	>90	—	Chlordiazepoxide Diazepam Diphenylhydantoin Indomethacin Phenylbutazone Rifampicin Tolbutamide Warfarin
Flow and enzyme sensitive	0.25–0.60	0–100	+	Acetaminophen Chlorpromazine Isoniazid Meperidine Metoprolol Nortriptyline Quinidine
Flow limited	>0.60	0–100	+++	Galactose Indocyanine green Labetalol Lidocaine Morphine Pentazocine Propoxyphene Propranolol Verapamil

Reproduced by permission from Larrey D, Branch RA. Clearance by the liver: Current concepts in understanding the hepatic disposition of drugs. *Semin Liver Dis* 1983;3(4):285–297.

varies widely within the clinical and laboratory criteria for rating the severity.

At this moment, the most useful assessment of the overall functional efficiency of the liver utilizes the concept of hepatic clearance (14). Clearance profiles for any given drug are developed through measurements of drug extraction ratios in perfused preparations and allow hepatocellular function to be characterized mathematically, independent of both descriptive components and elimination by other organs. Drugs are found to have high, intermediate, or low hepatic clearance (Table 25.1).

Clearance Formula

Hepatic clearance (Cl_h) can be expressed as a function of hepatic blood flow and hepatic extraction (15).

$$Cl_h = \frac{QC_i - QC_o}{C_i}$$

$$Cl_h = \left[Q \frac{C_i - C_o}{C_i} \right]$$

where

Cl_h = hepatic extraction
Q = blood flow
C_i = concentration of drug in the inflowing blood
C_o = concentration of drug in the outflowing blood

If C_o tends toward 0 (maximum hepatic extraction), then Cl_h approaches Q. Maximally extracted drugs have a Cl_h greater than $.6Q$. Drugs with low extraction have Cl_h less than $.25Q$, and intermediate extraction lies between the two extremes. The formula demonstrates a strong relationship between hepatic clearance and blood flow. Again, other factors modifying clearance but not represented in the formula are the efficiency of the drug's cellular disposition and the amount of plasma protein binding.

Functional Hepatic Microunit

The functional hepatic microunit is the hepatic lobule, classically described as a central vein and a peripheral portal triad (portal vein, hepatic artery, and bile duct) with the intervening sinusoids lined by hepatocytes. Hepatic blood flow and its correlation with metabolic function can best be appreciated, however, by considering an alternative model for the hepatic subunit as described by Rappaport (16).

In this model, arterial and portal inflow, rather than venous outflow, assume primary importance. Hepatocytes residing in the lobule are defined as being in areas of luxuriant, adequate, or scant perfusion.

The subunit (acinus) consists of a three-dimensional aggregate of hepatocytes and sinusoids whose origin is a terminal branch of the portal vein and hepatic artery. Blood flowing from the hepatic arteriole and portal venule bathes the hepatocytes and drains into branches of the central vein. There are gradients of oxygen, substrate, and hormones between the inflow and outflow regions of this Rappaport hepatic subunit. Hepatocytes can be grouped into different zones of metabolic activity

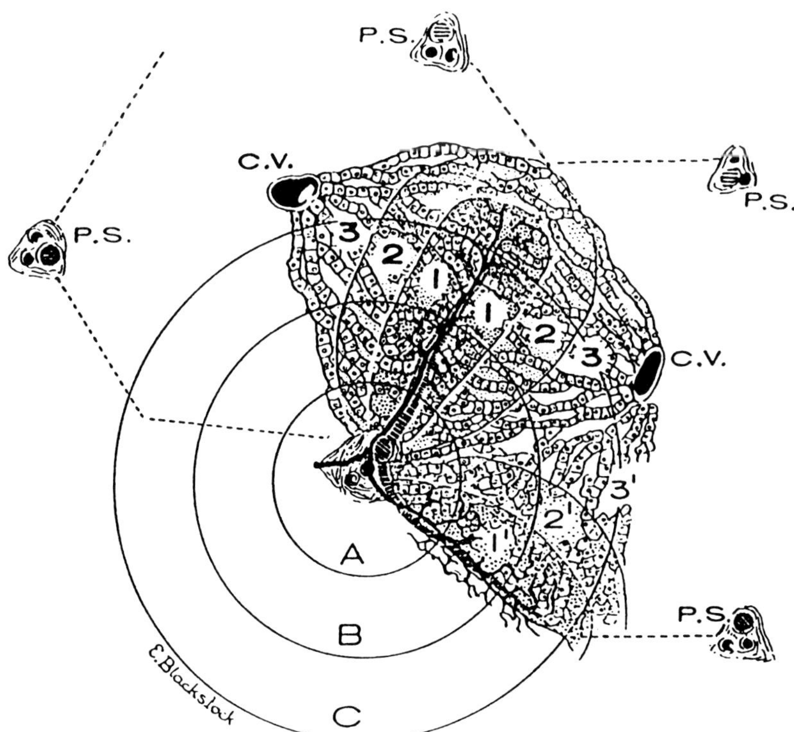

Figure 25.1. Blood supply of the hepatic structural unit. The structural unit occupies adjacent sectors of neighboring hexagonal fields. Zones 1, 2, and 3, respectively, represent areas supplied with blood of first, second, and third quality with regard to oxygen and nutrients. These zones center about the terminal afferent vascular twigs and extend into the periportal field from which these twigs originate. Zones 1', 2', and 3' designate corresponding areas in a portion of an adjacent structural unit. In zones 1 and 1', the afferent vascular twigs empty into the sinusoids. The circles A, B, and C delimit concentric bands of hepatic parenchyma arranged around a small portal field. (Reproduced by permission from Rappaport AM, et al. Subdivision of hexagonal liver lobules into a structural and functional unit: Role in hepatic physiology and pathology. *Anat Rec* 1954; 119:11–27.)

based upon their perfusion. Those in zone 1 are very close to vessels receiving blood rich in substrates and hormones. They have the highest metabolic activity and have been shown to perform protein catabolism, energy production, and gluconeogenesis. Hepatocytes in zone 3 are near the central vein or in areas not well overlapped by other vascular twigs. These hepatocytes receive less substrate and are more susceptible to anoxic damage. Their metabolic functions include lipid synthesis, biotransformation, and glycolysis (17, 18). Zone 2 hepatocytes are intermediate between zones 1 and 3.

Hepatocellular Function and Clearance

The zonal architecture may explain the histologic patterns observed after sustained hepatic ischemia where physiologically the perivenous hepatocytes are most vulnerable. In the Rappaport model, the perivenous cells are in zone 3 and might be expected to demonstrate the necrosis observed following hypoperfusion.

The majority of drugs used during the perianesthetic period undergo biotransformation in the hepatocytes of zone 3. There are two distinct phases of this process. During phase I the target compound or drug is prepared for subsequent conjugation by the addition of polar groups (hydroxy, carboxy, amino, and sulfhydryl) with which the conjugating molecule can later react. It is a complex reaction taking place in the smooth endoplasmic reticulum and involves a number of reactions, including oxidation, reduction, and hydrolysis. Phase II reactions include glucuronidation, acetylation, methylation, dihydrodiol formation, and conjugation with glycine taurine, sulfate, and glutathione (17).

In contrast to phase I, conjugation reactions remain relatively intact in acute viral hepatitis and established cirrhosis (19). Considering these, one can choose drugs such as oxazepam or lorazepam, which require only phase II glucuronidation, over related compounds such as diazepam and chlordiazepoxide, which require both phase I and phase II for their elimination.

An interesting aspect of biotransformation is the production of certain intermediate metabolites that are capable of combining with certain subcellular structures ultimately causing cellular injury and death. Free radical formation from carbon tetra-

chloride by zone 3 hepatocytes and the characteristic pattern of necrosis that follows is a classic example of liver injury being generated through normally functioning cellular processes (17).

The efficiency of cellular extraction may seem to be of paramount importance, yet hepatic clearance is also very sensitive to both hepatic blood flow and serum protein binding.

Hepatic Blood Flow and Clearance

In chronic liver disease, functional hepatic blood flow must be differentiated from total hepatic blood flow, which includes blood entering the hepatic bed but shunted through the liver without contact with hepatocytes. An opportunity for a "metabolism-perfusion" mismatch is created, much the same as the "ventilation-perfusion" mismatch of the lung in equivalent pathologic states (17). Hemodynamic changes induced by anesthesia further alter hepatic perfusion in both normal and abnormal patients with obvious effects on hepatic drug disposition.

Plasma Protein Binding and Clearance

Plasma protein binding of drugs in the blood can change significantly in the presence of liver disease. The ratio of unbound to bound drug may be altered because of protein binding deficiency, displacement of drug from binding sites, or decreased hepatic biotransformation of drug. Each of these distinct causes for changes in plasma protein binding leads to an increased, unbound fraction of drug and, thus, to increased pharmacodynamic action of that drug at the target site.

In many clinical studies authors have mistakenly confused changing serum drug levels, plasma protein drug binding, and hepatic extraction in the strict pharmacologic sense. For example, if changes in plasma levels are used to measure systemic drug clearance, the systemic plasma clearance of tolbutamide will be found to be increased by 50% in patients with acute viral hepatitis. This paradox is explained when plasma drug clearance is corrected for the significant decrease in drug-protein binding, which allows much more rapid extravascular distribution and brisk declines in serum levels. Hepatic clearance under these circumstances shows no difference when measured in ill or well patients. Again, pharmacokinetics of diazepam were studied in patients with cirrhosis and investigators noted an altered protein binding of the drug with an increased unbound fraction (14). They might have assumed that the extra unbound drug available to the systemic circulation accounted for the prolonged effects but further analysis revealed substantially reduced hepatocellular metabolism, initially masked by the increased amount of drug available.

Altered binding characteristics are not always due to or reflected by changes in serum albumin. For example, the elevated circulating levels of unconjugated bilirubin seen in patients with acute viral hepatitis have been suggested to account for change in binding of some drugs through a mechanism involving competitive displacement of drug from albumin by bilirubin (14).

Extrahepatic Tissues and Clearance

Hepatic clearance, strictly defined, ignores the affinity of the drug to extrahepatic tissues. In a clinical setting, this effect may be important and dramatic. For example, the narcotic anesthetic, fentanyl, shows a high degree of hepatic extraction and pharmacologically has rapid hepatic clearance. When studied in patients, this drug exhibits a long metabolic elimination, primarily due to its affinity for and slow release from extrahepatic tissues. Its highly lipophilic nature accounts for its rapid hepatic extraction yet slow release from extrahepatic tissues.

Extraction and Systemic Clearance

In general, drugs with low extraction have systemic clearances that are independent of flow. Clearance depends more on cellular performance than blood flow. Metabolism is enzyme-limited and intrinsic cellular function is most important. Protein binding can limit drug availability if the drug is highly bound (19), but changes in blood flow, intrahepatic shunting, or extrahepatic shunting have a lesser effect on clearance.

Drugs with high hepatic extraction have clearances that are blood flow limited. Metabolism is more sensitive to hepatic blood flow than protein binding. For example, in studies on cirrhotic patients, drugs with high clearance like propranolol and lidocaine demonstrate reduced clearance proportional to decreased blood flow and decreased

intrinsic clearance (20,21). When given orally, many drugs with high clearance are rapidly absorbed through the gastrointestinal tract and presented to the liver before reaching the systemic circulation. The "first-pass effect" describes the attenuated pharmacodynamic effects attributed to the large amounts of drug extraction by the liver prior to systemic delivery. As portal-systemic shunting develops, the first-pass effect of these drugs is significantly and further reduced, leading to enhanced bioavailability and adverse consequences. It is for this reason that highly extracted drugs with good oral absorption, such as propranolol or Demerol, must be reduced by at least 50% in patients with chronic liver disease.

Drugs and the Liver

Inhalational Anesthetic Agents

While it is not known whether administration of anesthesia to a patient with chronic liver disease exacerbates liver dysfunction, it is well accepted that some anesthetic agents have the potential to be toxic to the liver.

Halothane

Epidemologic, toxicologic, and immunologic studies have demonstrated several possible mechanisms for toxicity from halothane.

Early examinations provided epidemiologic evidence for a population at risk for damage after exposure to halothane. Analysis, exposure-rechallenge, and population studies led to the definition of a specific clinical syndrome (22). Genetic factors were implicated when kindreds with susceptibility to halothane were identified (23). At the time of writing, most authorities agree that halothane causes a mild form of hepatotoxicity at a low frequency, and a severe form that is relatively rare (24). Epidemiologic studies have refined the characteristics of susceptible patients, suggesting that toxicity may be increased by exposure in middle age, obesity, the female sex, and following multiple administrations within a short time (25).

Simple mechanisms for toxicity were proposed initially. Administration of halothane to patients with undisguised viral hepatitis, reactivation of latent hepatitis by anesthesia or surgery, and hypersensitivity to halothane proved as illusive to study as the more involved theories. Sophisticated toxicologic and immunologic analyses have provided helpful insights into other possible mechanisms.

Halothane can be metabolized by reductive and oxidative pathways. Under conditions of hypoxia and enzyme induction, a reductive pathway using the cytochrome P_{450} complex predominates. Free radicals are produced within the hepatocyte. These highly reactive, short-lived intermediaries are available to bind to microsomal proteins and lipids with the potential to destroy organelle and enzyme function (26–28). Under aerobic conditions, the cytochrome P_{450} system metabolizes halothane to oxidative metabolites, which react with water to form nontoxic substances. Experiments done in the mid-1980s, however, have suggested that these oxidative metabolites can acetylate tissues. Enzyme-linked immunoassay and direct immunofluorescent staining have located products of oxidative metabolism within the membrane of the hepatocyte, raising the possibility of altered cellular function under relatively normal clinical conditions (24).

Patients with the fulminant form of halothane-associated hepatotoxicity have antibody to hepatocytes obtained from animals exposed to halothane (29,30). Antibodies found by several investigators appear to be specific for hepatocytes affected with the syndrome. Other specific membrane-directed antibodies have been discovered in cases of hepatotoxicity from alpha-methyldopa and ethanol (31). It is postulated that these antibodies are directed against an antigen on the surface of the hepatocyte. The antigen may be produced by a reactive metabolite or other metabolic products. Variability in the immune response of an individual may account for the incidence and severity of the reaction. Thus, the presence of disease may not depend on the activity of an enzyme that can form a biologically active compound but on the immunogenicity of the altered membrane and the variability of an individual's immune response. Studies attempting to locate the genes responsible are now being reported (32).

Halothane remains a primary anesthetic choice for pediatric patients, who appear to be affected minimally by this toxicity, and is also widely used throughout the world in adults (33).

Enflurane and Isoflurane

There has been no uniform agreement concerning the existence of the newer inhalational anesthetics, enflurane and isoflurane. Scattered case reports of liver damage in association with these agents have not been supported by epidemiologic or experimental evidence of a syndrome or mechanism (34,35). Enflurane is metabolized to a very limited extent in oxygen, and isoflurane to an even lesser degree, if at all. Neither appears to be metabolized under conditions of hypoxia. Damage to hepatocytes during enflurane and isoflurane anesthesia has been demonstrated experimentally under conditions of hypoxia, but a mechanism other than interaction of toxic metabolites may be involved. Hypoxia alone may be responsible for the damage documented (36).

Since inhalation anesthetics alter hepatic perfusion, some may be better choices for patients undergoing hepatic surgery. In unanesthetized patients the splanchnic bed receives blood in proportion to cardiac output. Mild decreases in portal flow to the liver are compensated by increases in hepatic arterial blood flow. Within small ranges, total hepatic blood flow is preserved (37). Under anesthesia both cardiac output and systemic blood pressure may be reduced. Portal flow is similarly reduced.

Isoflurane has been demonstrated to allow an increase in hepatic arterial flow by either vasodilation or preservation of limited autoregulation. Halothane has been associated with depressed portal and hepatic artery blood flow. While neither agent has been shown to cause a decrease in metabolic demand, isoflurane may allow a greater supply of oxygen and substrate to the liver (38).

At this time, there is no reliable evidence to contraindicate the administration of isoflurane or enflurane to a patient with documented halothane hepatotoxicity. However, it may be clinically prudent to abstain from the use of other halogenated agents unless a compelling indication exists.

Intravenous Agents

BARBITURATES

The most widely used drugs, thiopental and methohexital, have a smooth, pleasant induction with rapid onset and recovery. They have different pharmacokinetic properties, a factor important in the presence of liver disease (39–41).

For both drugs, the plasma level rises very rapidly after intravenous administration, inducing sleep within a few seconds. As the plasma level falls precipitously, patients regain consciousness (usually within 10 to 15 minutes). After this distribution phase, the plasma level still continues to fall but at a much slower rate attributed to elimination and metabolism.

The percentage of protein binding of thiopental varies with the amount injected. As the plasma concentration increases, the percentage of bound thiopental decreases, making more drug available to the tissues (42). The changes in binding due to liver disease may further increase plasma concentration of unbound drug.

The increased delivery of drug to peripheral tissues other than the central nervous system may reduce the risk of a markedly prolonged effect of thiopental, for example, in patients with cirrhosis. Thiopental is a low-extraction drug and its metabolism is not dependent on blood flow to the liver. Clearance ultimately depends on intrinsic hepatic metabolism and protein binding. Redistribution to peripheral tissues helps limit the amount of drug available for metabolism at any given moment. It is also conceivable that an apparent prolonged effect in severe hepatic disease may be due to a sensitizing of the brain to depressants by nitrogenous byproducts of bacterial action in the bowel (43).

Thiopental and methohexital have similar initial distribution phases but different terminal elimination half-lives, methohexital having the shorter half-life (97 minutes) and thiopental the longer (403 minutes). This dramatic difference is attributed to the greater lipid solubility of thiopental (44).

Methohexital has high hepatic extraction and is dependent on blood flow to the liver for rapid clearance. It is much less dependent on effects of protein binding than thiopental because of its rapid extraction.

It has been recommended that doses of thiopental be decreased by as much as 50% in patients with liver disease. Similar empiric and clinical reasoning might support reduced doses of methohexital.

OPIATES

Morphine, a highly extracted drug, is inactivated by glucuronidation and subsequent renal excretion. Like other high-clearance drugs (lidocaine, propranolol) it undergoes extensive "first-pass" clearance and might be considered a poor choice for patients with advanced liver disease. It can be safely used, however, at reduced dose.

Studies of inpatients undergoing liver transplantation have shown a normal distribution phase and prolonged elimination half-life consistent with severely reduced hepatic function. However, during the anhepatic phase of the procedure and 2 hours after the administration of morphine, conjugated metabolites appear in the urine, increasing with time. This observation strongly suggests extrahepatic biotransformation in humans (45). Animal experimentation has demonstrated wide variability in the metabolism of morphine at extrahepatic sites (46).

Moderate to advanced stable cirrhosis does not appear to impair the disposition of morphine (47). When administered to cirrhotic patients in a dose of .15 milligrams per kilogram to a maximum of 15 mg IV, no differences were seen in any dispositional characteristics when compared to controlled patients. In both groups, 60% of injected morphine was recovered in 24 hours and 80% in 72 hours. Terminal elimination was similar (150 to 200 minutes) and no encephalopathy was noted. Pharmacodynamic correlates have not been fully investigated, and caution in the use of morphine must be emphasized.

Fentanyl, a very potent synthetic narcotic, differs from morphine by having rapid onset and short clinical duration of action. It is a highly lipophilic drug and, like thiopental, its effects are attributed to rapid penetration through membranes of the central nervous system (CNS). The lipophilic nature minimizes excretion of unmetabolized drug in normal and hepatectomized patients and accounts for a terminal half-life much longer than that of morphine (in healthy volunteers 219 ± 10 minutes). Primary clearance of this highly extracted drug is accomplished through hepatic metabolism. Extrahepatic sites of biotransformation are postulated because hepatectomy reduces but does not eliminate excretion of metabolites (48,49).

The biphasic respiratory depression observed by Becker et al. may be due to enterohepatic circulation (50). After intravenous administration, unmetabolized fentanyl appears almost instantly in the gastric juice. It has been calculated that the stomach can secrete and store about 16% of an injected dose. Later, reabsorption from the gut may cause respiratory depression.

When Kang et al. recorded fentanyl pharmacokinetics in patients with end-stage hepatic disease, they noted some patients had decreased biotransformation while others had entirely normal pharmacokinetics (51). The functional state of the liver in their patients was not reported and it is possible that preservation of enough hepatic function may have accounted for this variability.

The unpredictability of fentanyl pharmacokinetics in patients with significant hepatic disease is underscored by these and other studies (48). Patients may exhibit delayed metabolism of this highly extracted drug. In addition, the depressed "first-pass" effect of drug sequestered in the gut may lead to significant changes in bioavailability.

Meperidine is also highly extracted by the liver and has highly distinctive properties. Like morphine, it can produce hypotension after intravenous administration, which is attributed to a decrease of systemic vascular resistance from histamine release (52). However, unlike morphine and fentanyl, meperidine has been shown to have a direct myocardial depressant effect in both isolated cardiac tissue and whole animals (53). In equipotent doses, the negative inotropic action is 200 times that of morphine.

Meperidine is eliminated primarily by metabolism in the liver. The major metabolite, normeperidine, is a product of N-demethylation and is excreted unchanged in the urine (54). It is the only metabolite with significant pharmacologic activity. Meperidine in doses of 5 mg/kg (equivalent to 0.5 to 0.7 mg/kg of morphine) may induce CNS stimulation and seizures in humans (52). Normeperidine is twice as potent as a convulsant but only half as potent as the parent compound as an analgesic. Elimination is much slower than meperidine, and normeperidine can accumulate in patients receiving repeated doses. While plasma levels of normeperidine may not be detectable in normal volunteers or patients with cirrhosis or acute hepatitis following a single dose, measurable

levels can easily be found in patients with cancer and terminal renal failure (55).

Meperidine given orally undergoes substantial metabolism in the liver before reaching systemic circulation—the "first-pass effect." Approximately 50% of orally given meperidine is eliminated by this presystemic metabolism (56). The established oral-intravenous dose ratio of 2/1 reflects this fact as well.

In cirrhotic patients, reduced hepatic extraction and portocaval shunting markedly lower the presystemic metabolism of meperidine. Under these circumstances, the bioavailability of orally given meperidine increases substantially when compared with the parenteral route. Therefore, reduction of meperidine dosage in patients with cirrhosis or hepatitis should be greater for oral than the intravenous route (57–59).

KETAMINE

The popularity of ketamine in advanced liver disease derives from its effects on the cardiovascular system, producing a dose-related rise in the rate-pressure product, a transient rise in cardiac index, but no significant alteration of stroke index. The sympathomimetic actions of ketamine appear to be caused by the direct stimulation of the CNS, and in the absence of autonomic control it has direct myocardial depressant properties (60). In experimental hemorrhagic and septic shock, a significant increase in both systolic and diastolic pressure is noted, but maintenance of such cardiovascular parameters is associated with greater base deficit and increase in arterial lactate concentration (61,62).

Critically ill patients occasionally respond to ketamine with an unexpected drop in blood pressure, which may result from the inability of the sympathomimetic actions of ketamine to counterbalance its direct myocardial depressant and vasodilatory effect.

Ketamine demonstrates a rapid onset, relatively short duration, and high lipid solubility, like thiopental. Moreover, it is extensively metabolized by the liver. Experimentally, the duration of anesthesia is not affected by either the induction or inhibition of drug-metabolizing enzymes or decreases in renal clearance of the drug. Redistribution of ketamine from the brain to other tissues is responsible for the termination of its anesthetic effect.

Pharmacokinetically, the distribution phase of ketamine has a 7- to 11-minute half-life, while the elimination phase, reflecting both metabolic and excretory processes, has a half-life ranging between 120 and 180 minutes. Halothane, in addition to inhibiting hepatic metabolism, has been shown to slow the distribution and redistribution of ketamine. Both contribute to the prolonged effects of the drug on the CNS.

Anesthetic Management

The preoperative evaluation of a patient undergoing hepatobiliary surgery follows the usual standards given any surgical patient. Pertinent historical information includes prior experience with anesthetics, familial occurrence of anesthetic problems, current medications and medication allergies, substance abuse, prior blood transfusions, and hepatitis. Laboratory assessment should include evaluation of cardiopulmonary, liver, and renal function with documentation of coagulation parameters. Using both the classification of hepatobiliary disease described earlier and the American Society of Anesthesiologists (ASA) physical status, the anesthesiologist can define requirements for invasive monitoring. Additional predictive criteria for survival of patients with advanced hepatic disease have been discussed (63).

The likelihood of excessive bleeding dictates care in placing monitoring devices such as esophageal stethoscopes and temperature probes. Additional care must be exercised during endotracheal intubation and insertion of gastric tubes as well. Patients whose coagulation profiles deteriorate during surgery may show dramatic bleeding following apparently benign positioning of these devices. Monitoring may be simple and routine or invasive as the patient's status dictates. End-tidal carbon dioxide analysis can provide useful information regarding the changes in respiratory status and the occurrence of air embolism, most likely in hepatic surgery where major venous channels are transected.

The possibility of massive transfusion can be predicted with reasonable accuracy. In such cases, both the laboratory and blood bank should be notified in advance. Additional preparation should include adequate cannulation for large-volume infusions (the internal jugular, subclavian, axillary, and antecubital veins can accommodate large catheters) and methods for rapid warming of fluids. At the New England Deaconess Hospital, a rapid infusion device (Fig. 25.2) is frequently used during major hepatic surgery and transplantation. Its usefulness in vascular reconstruction, trauma, and other procedures with rapid excessive loss has been proven.

The major problems facing the anesthesiologist are listed in Table 25.2.

For patients assessed as class 3 in the hepatobiliary profile, and for all patients with massive transfusion, maintenance of coagulation becomes extremely important. Table 25.3 reviews the laboratory determinations and blood products used to maintain normal clotting profiles. Each test is uncomplicated and easily reproducible in a stat lab by relatively inexperienced personnel. These tests are ordered whenever transfusions equivalent to the patient's blood volume have been administered, or more frequently if indicated.

A white count is obtained as a crude indication of hemodilution, and thrombin time is obtained as a measure of heparin contamination in the samples used for other hematologic studies. Thrombin time is exquisitely sensitive to physiologic amounts of heparin. It becomes significantly elevated with any heparin contamination in the blood sample. Thus, normal thrombin time in the face of an elevated prothrombin time (PT) indicates need for further component therapy, whereas an abnormal thrombin time might suggest that repeat sampling be done before therapeutic decisions are based on the simultaneously elevated PT. The PT is used as the primary determination for administration of fresh frozen plasma. It is maintained at values of 15 seconds or less, and the platelet count is maintained in the 100,000 range by infusions of platelets. Whenever the fibrinogen level falls below 100 mg%, cryoprecipitate is administered.

Blood component therapy can begin preoperatively if abnormal coagulation is present. Casual crystalloid administration may lead to dilutional coagulopathy and should be avoided. In the case of hepatic transplantation, venous access may be restricted. Transection of the vena cava during surgery diminishes venous return from the lower extremities causing substantial declines in cardiac output. A passive pumping device is frequently placed from the femoral and portal circulations to the axillary vein. Thus, intravenous lines cannot be

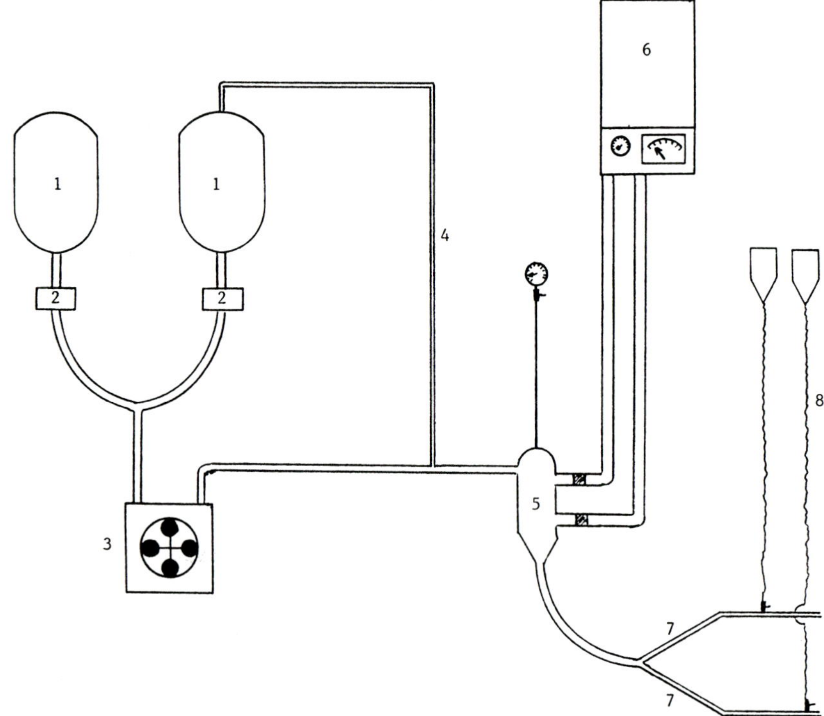

Figure 25.2. 1 = reservoir (blood and fluids), 2 = filters, 3 = pump, 4 = recirculation line, 5 = air trap and blood warming system, 6 = water circulation for blood.

placed in the left arm or lower extremities for this procedure.

Heat loss and hypothermia during surgery are related to the duration of surgery, degree of abdominal exposure, infusion of chilled parenteral solutions, low ambient room temperature, and inhalation of cold gases during mechanical ventilation (64). In hepatic transplantation, reperfusion of a large organ preserved in ice for several hours leads to further heat loss. One liter of inspired cold dry gas requires 15 calories to be warmed to 37°C and saturated with water vapor. This loss of about 12 kilocalories per hour can be substantially decreased by using a heater-humidifier in the anesthesia circuit.

Heating parenteral solutions to body temperature probably contributes little to uncomplicated surgery in a healthy patient but provides substantial caloric savings to patients needing large volumes intraoperatively. Blood transfusions should be warmed near body temperature. During hepatic transplantation where the possibility of massive blood transfusion is real, special provisions to heat the transfused blood must be made.

These measures for the prevention of heat loss are of little value if initiated in the presence of cold ambient operating room air temperature (65,66).

Table 25.2. Problems of Anesthetic Management During Liver Surgery

Coagulation
Hypothermia
Massive transfusion
Citrate intoxication[a]
Hyperkalemia[a]
Air embolism[a]
Acid-base disturbance[a]

[a]Generally during liver transplantation.

Table 25.3. Basic Coagulation Testing and Suggested Treatment

Test	Use/Normal Value	Product Used
WBC	Index of dilution	
Thrombin time	Index of heparin contamination in samples	
Prothrombin time	15 sec	Fresh frozen plasma
Platelet count	90,000	Platelet infusion
Fibrinogen	100 mg%	Cryoprecipitate
Hct	25%	Pooled red blood cells
Ca^{2+}	2.5 mg%	$CaCl_2$

Abbreviations: Hct, hematocrit; WBC, white blood cells.

Temperatures between 21 and 24°C appear to be optimal in limiting patient heat loss during major surgery. Heating blankets have no practical value and may cause nerve palsies and burns. Only 30% of the body surface area is in contact with the device and those portions are insulated by fat, bone, and muscles. Blankets are cumbersome and expensive as well.

Citrate Intoxication

The work of many investigators from Bunker, a generation ago, to more recent studies has documented that blood transfusions in excess of 1 to 2 cubic centimeters per kilogram per minute can be associated with hypocalcemia (67–69). The citrate anticoagulant, which is found in excess in blood and fresh frozen plasma infusions, binds the patient's own calcium, causing a transient decrease in serum ionized calcium. Myocardial function is disturbed when ionized calcium falls below 2 milliequivalents per liter. Poor blood pressure response to transfusion and depressed cardiac output with increased filling pressures can be seen during these periods. A prolonged Q-T interval on the EKG can also be documented but is not invariably present. Calcium chloride is administered sparingly when these circumstances are suspected or documented clinically. With injudicious administration of calcium chloride it is possible to give much more calcium chloride than is needed to temporize cardiovascular function during these periods. In the presence of diminished hepatic function, much of the administered calcium chloride may be temporarily bound to unmetabolized citrate. With return of hepatic function, for example, during a transplant, the exogenous citrate becomes metabolized. Previously bound calcium is released to the circulation and significant hypercalcemia can result.

Cardiovascular Support

Judicious use of both alpha- and beta-vasopressors is made during long periods of massive transfusion to minimize administration of calcium, control changes in systemic vascular resistance (SVR), and augment myocardial function. In any patient suspected of having the hepatorenal syndrome and in situations where the likelihood of acute renal failure from acute tubular necrosis is real, certain preventive measures may help protect renal function. Dopamine in dosages of 2 to 3 micrograms per kilogram per minute and mannitol infusions are useful in these circumstances. On rare occasions, when cardiovascular function seems poorly responsive to all therapeutic maneuvers, glucose/potassium/insulin infusions have been employed in an attempt to augment intracellular function (70).

Hyperkalemia

Hyperkalemia is seen during hepatic transplantation when the donor liver, preserved by prior flushing with iced crystalloid and transported in packed ice, is placed into the recipient. Although the organ is vigorously flushed before implantation, the anoxic liver can continue to release considerable amounts of potassium. Hyperkalemic arrests have been noted, particularly in children and occasionally in adults. Hyperventilation, glucose insulin infusions, and administration of calcium chloride are therapeutic maneuvers proven to be useful in control of hyperkalemia. Hypokalemia may be documented as organ function returns.

Air Embolism

Patients with significant portal systemic shunting and patients having major dissections of hepatic vasculature are at risk for inadvertent air embolism, which may be documented by capnography. Therapeutic maneuvers in this situation depend on the magnitude of air entrained. Surgeons must be alerted to limit their dissections, attempt positional changes, and flood the field with fluid. Positive end-expiratory pressure added to the breathing circuits is helpful. Vigorous chest compression may be required for brief periods as well.

Acid-Base Disturbances

Acid-base disturbances must be treated with caution. Liberal use of sodium bicarbonate may increase intracellular acidosis, causing functional disturbances in important tissues such as myocardium (71).

References

1. Sherlock S. *Diseases of the Liver and Biliary System,* 6th ed. Oxford: Blackwell Scientific Publications, 1981, p. 14.

2. Riding JE. Anaesthesia and the liver. *Br J Anaesth* 1972; 44: 123.

3. Del Guercio LRM, Cohn JD. Monitoring operative risk in the elderly. *JAMA* 1980; 243:1350–1355.

4. Tompkins MJ, Artusio JF. Myocardial infarction and surgery, a five year study. *Anesth Analg* 1964; 43:716–720.

5. Tarhan S, Moffitt EA, Taylor WF, Giuliani ER. Myocardial infarction after general anesthesia. *JAMA* 1972; 220:1451–1454.

6. Steen PA, Tinker JH, Tarhan S. Myocardial reinfarction after anesthesia and surgery. *JAMA* 1978; 239(24):2566–2570.

7. Rao TLK, Jacobs KH, El-Etr AA. Reinfarction following anesthesia in patients with myocardial infarction. *Anesthesiology* 1983; 59:499–505.

8. Kaplan EB, Sheiner LB, Boeckmann AJ. Usefulness of preoperative laboratory screening. *JAMA* 1985; 253:3576–3581.

9. Lundberg GD. Is there a need for routine preoperative laboratory tests? *JAMA* 1985; 253:3589.

10. Robbins JA, Mushlin AI. Preoperative evaluation of the healthy patient. *Med Clin North Am* 1979; 63:1145–1156.

11. McIntyre N. The limitations of conventional liver function tests. *Semin Liver Dis* 1983; 3:265–274.

12. Gelman SI. Disturbances in hepatic blood flow during anesthesia and surgery. *Arch Surg* 1976; 111:881–883.

13. Harper MH, Collins P, Johnson BH, Eager E II, Diara CG. Post anesthetic hepatic injury in rats: Influence of hepatic blood flow, surgery, and anesthetic time. *Anesth Analg* 1982; 61:79–82.

14. Wilkinson GR, Schenker S. Effects of liver disease on drug disposition in man. *Biochem Pharmacol* 1976; 25:2675–2681.

15. Williams RL. Drug administration in hepatic disease. *N Engl J Med* 1983; 309:1616–1622.

16. Rappaport AM, Boruwy ZJ, Lougheed WM, Lotto WN. Subdivision of hexagonal liver lobules into a structural and functional unit. Role of hepatic physiology and pathology. *Anat Rec* 1954; 119:11–27.

17. Corless JK, Middleton HM. Normal liver function. A basis for understanding hepatic disease. *Arch Intern Med* 1983; 143:2291–2294.

18. Larrey D, Branch RA. Clearance by the liver: Current concepts in understanding the hepatic disposition of drugs. *Semin Liver Dis* 1983; 3:285–297.

19. Shull HJ, Wilkinson GR, Johnson R, Schenker S. Normal disposition of oxazepam in acute viral hepatitis and cirrhosis. *Ann Intern Med* 1976; 84:420–425.

20. Huet PM, Villeneuve JP. Determinates of drug disposition in patients with cirrhosis. *Hepatology* 1983; 3:913–918.

21. Pessayre D, Lebrec D, Descatoire V, Peignoux M, Benhamou JP. Mechanism of reduced drug clearance in patients with cirrhosis. *Gastroenterology* 1978; 74:566–571.

22. Babion P, Tracy C. Drug hepatitis. In: Dykes MHM, ed. *Anesthesia and the Liver*. Boston: Little, Brown, 1970.

23. Hoft RH, Bunker JP, Goodman HF, Gregory PB. Halothane hepatitis in three pairs of closely related women. *N Engl J Med* 1981; 304(17):1023–1024.

24. Satoh H, Fukuda Y, Anderson DK, Ferrans VJ, Gillette JR, Pohl LR. Immunological studies on the mechanism of halothane-induced hepatology: Immunohistochemical evidence of trifluoroacetylated hepatocytes. *J Pharmacol Exp Ther* 1985; 233:857–862.

25. Cousins MJ, Plummer JL, Hall PD. Toxicity of volatile anesthetic agents. *Can Anaesth Soc J* 1985; 32:S52–S55.

26. de Groot H, Noll T. Halothane-induced lipid peroxidation and glucose-6-phosphatase inactivation in microsomes under hypoxic conditions. *Anesthesiology* 1985; 62:44–47.

27. Plummer JL, Beckwith ALJ, Bastin FN, Adams JF, Cousins MJ, Hall P. Free radical formation in vivo and hepatotoxicity due to anesthesia with halothane. *Anesthesiology* 1982; 57:160–166.

28. Hatano H, Nomura F, Ohnishi K, et al. Respective roles of hypoxia and halothane metabolism in halothane-induced liver injury in rats. *Hepatology* 1985; 5(2):241–244.

29. Vergani D, Mieli-Vergani G, Alberti A, et al. Antibodies to the surface of halothane-altered rabbit hepatocytes in patients with severe halothane-associated hepatitis. *N Engl J Med* 1980; 303:66–71.

30. Neuberger J, Gimson AES, Davis M, Williams R. Specific serological markers in the diagnosis of fulminant hepatic failure associated with halothane anesthesia. *Br J Anaesth* 1983; 55:15–19.

31. Kenna JG, Neuberger J, Williams R. An enzyme-linked immunosorbent assay for detection of antibodies against halothane-altered hepatocyte antigens. *J Immunol Methods* 1984; 75:3–14.

32. Otsuka S, Yamamoto M, Kasuya S, et al. HLA antigens in patients with unexplained hepatitis following halothane anesthesia. *Acta Anaesthiol Scand* 1985; 29(5):497–501.

33. Brown BR. Halothane hepatitis revisited. *N Engl J Med* 1985; 313(21):1347–1348.

34. Dykes M. Is enflurane hepatotoxic? *Anesthesiology* 1984; 61: 235–237.

35. Lewis JH, Zimmerman HJ, Ishak KG, Mulleck FG. Enflurane hepatotoxicity: A clinicopathologic study of 24 cases. *Ann Intern Med* 1983; 98:984–992.

36. Berman ML, Kuhnert L, Phythyon JM, Holaday DA. Isoflurane and enflurane-induced hepatic necrosis in triiodothyronine-pretreated rats. *Anesthesiology* 1983; 58:1–5.

37. Richardson PDI, Withrington PG. Liver blood flow. I. Intrinsic and nervous control of liver blood flow. *Gastroenterology* 1981; 81:159–173.

38. Gelmans S, Fowler KC, Smith LR. Liver circulation and function during isoflurane and halothane anesthesia. *Anesthesiology* 1984; 61:726–730.

39. Ghoneim M, Van Harnme M. Pharmacokinetics of thiopentone: Effect of enflurane and nitrous oxide anesthesia and surgery. *Br J Anaesth* 1978; 50:1237–1241.

40. Breimer D. Pharmacokinetics of methohexitone following intravenous infusions in humans. *Br J Anaesth* 1976; 48: 643–649.

41. Morgan DJ, Blackman GL, Paull JD, Wolf LJ. Pharmacokinetics and plasma binding of thiopental, I: Studies in surgical patients. *Anesthesiology* 1981; 54:468–473.

42. Pendele G, Chaux F, Salvadori C, Farivotti M, Duvaldestin P. Thiopental pharmacokinetics in patients with cirrhosis. *Anesthesiology* 1983; 59:123–126.

43. Ghoneim MM, Pandya H. Plasma protein binding of thiopental in patients with unpaired renal or hepatic function. *Anesthesiology* 1975; 42:545–549.

44. Hudson RJ, Stanski DR. Barbiturates—pharmacokinetics and pharmacodynamics. *Clin Anaesthesiol* 1984; 2(1):27–41.

45. Hug Jr CC. Pharmacokinetics of Drugs Administered Intravenously. *Anesthesiology* 1978; 57:704–723.

46. Patwardham RV, Johnson R, Hoyumpa AM, et al. Normal metabolism of morphine in cirrhosis. *Gastroenterology* 1981; 81:1006–1011.

47. Hug Jr CC, Murphy MR, Sampson JF, Terblanche J, Aldrete JA. Biotransformation of morphine and fentanyl. in anhepatic dogs. *Anesthesiology* 1981; 55:A261.

48. Hug Jr CC, Murphy MR. Tissue redistribution of fentanyl and termination of its effects in rats. *Anesthesiology* 1981; 55:369–375.

49. Duvaldestin P, Habere JP, Coudere E, Shoeffler P. Fen-

tanyl pharmacokinetics in surgical patients with cirrhosis. *Anesthesiology* 1982; 57:A237.

50. Becker LD, Paulson BA, Miller RD. Biphasic respiratory depression after fentanyl-droperidol or fentanyl alone used to supplement nitrous oxide anesthesia. *Anesthesiology* 1976; 44:291–296.

51. Kang YG, Uram M, Shin GK, Bleyaert A, Martin DJ, Nemoto E, et al. Pharmacokinetics of fentanyl in end-stage liver disease. *Anesthesiology* 1984; 61:A380.

52. Moldenhauer CC, Hug Jr CC. Use of narcotics analgesics as anaesthetics. *Clin Anaesthesiol* 1984; 2:107–138.

53. Freye E. Cardiovascular effects of high doses of fentanyl, meperidine and naloxone in dogs. *Anesth Analg* 1974; 53:40–47.

54. Inturrisi EC, Umans JG. Pethidine and its active metabolite, norpethidine. *Clin Anaesthesiol* 1983; 1:123–138.

55. Szeto HH, Inturrisi CE, Houde R, Saal S, Cheigh J, Reidenberg, MM. Accumulation of normeperidine, an active metabolite of meperidine, in patients with renal failure of cancer. *Ann Intern Med* 1977; 86:738–741.

56. Pond SM, Tong T, Benowitz NL, Jacob P, Rogod J. Presystemic metabolism of meperidine to normeperidine in normal and cirrhotic patients. *Clin Pharmacol Ther* 1981; 30:183–188.

57. Neal AE, Meffin PJ, Gregory PB, Blaschke TF. Enhanced bioavailability and decreased clearance of analgesics in patients with cirrhosis. *Gastroenterology* 1979; 77:96–102.

58. Klotz U, McHorse TS, Wilkinson GR, Schenker S. The effect of cirrhosis on the disposition and elimination of meperidine in man. *Clin Pharmacol Ther* 1974; 16:667–675.

59. McHorse TS, Wilkinson GR, Johnson RF, Schenker S. Effect of acute viral hepatitis in man on the disposition and elimination of meperidine. *Gastroenterology* 1975; 68:775–780.

60. White PF, Way WL, Trevor AJ. Ketamine—its pharmacology and therapeutic uses. *Anesthesiology* 1982; 156:119–136.

61. Wong DHW, Jenkins LC. An experimental study of the mechanism of action of ketamine on the central nervous system. *Can Anaesth Soc J* 1974; 21:57–67.

62. Waxman K, Shoemaker WC, Lippmann M. Cardiovascular effects of anesthetic induction with ketamine. *Anesth Analg* 1980; 59:355–358.

63. Garrison RN, Cryer HM, Howard DA, Polk HC. Clarification of risk factors for abdominal operations in patients with hepatic cirrhosis. *Ann Surg* 1984; 199(6):648–655.

64. Vale RJ. Normothermia: Its place in operative and postoperative care. *Anaesthesia* 1973; 28:241–245.

65. Holdcroft A, Hall GM. Heat loss during anaesthesia. *Br J Anaesth* 1978; 50:157–164.

66. Morris RH. Operating room temperature and the anesthetized, paralyzed patient. *Arch Surg* 1971; 102:95–97.

67. Bunker JP, Bendixen HH, Murphy AS. Hemodynamic effects of intravenously administered sodium citrate. *N Engl J Med* 1962; 266:372–377.

68. Olinger GN, Huttenrott C, Mulder DG, et al. Acute clinical hypocalcemic myocardial depression during rapid blood transfusion and postoperative hemodialysis. *J Thorac Cardiovasc Surg* 1976; 72:503–511.

69. Kahn RC, Jascott D, Graziano CC, Schweizer O, Howland WS, Goldiner PL. Massive blood replacement: Correlation of ionized calcium, citrate, and hydrogen ion concentration. *Anesth Analg* 1979; 58:274–278.

70. Whitlow PL, Rogers WJ, Smith LR, et al. Enhancement of left ventricular function by glucose-insulin-potassium infusion in acute myocardial infarction. *Am J Cardiol* 1982; 49:811–820.

71. Park R, Arieff AI. Lactic acidosis: Current concept. *Clin Endocrinol and Metab* 1983; 12:339–358.

Editorial Comment

There are few if any chapters or sections in this book that do not, in some way or another and in varying degrees of detail, refer to hepatocellular function, and this chapter is certainly no exception.

In fact the excellent description of the mechanisms involved in cellular extraction of drugs are almost specific to this chapter and add a great deal to the overall understanding of liver function under the combined stress of anesthesia and complex surgical procedures.

The concept of a "metabolism-perfusion" mismatch similar to the "ventilation-perfusion" mismatch that may occur in the lung is a fascinating idea, and in the view of the authors of this chapter can occur secondary to the hemodynamic changes induced by anesthesia with obvious effects on hepatic drug disposition.

It is obvious that the pharmacokinetics of the large number of drugs is of primary concern of the anesthetist, who is so often faced with an unstable patient with primary liver disease and with the superimposed major hemodynamic and metabolic disorders related to the combined effects of anesthesia and surgical intervention.

The section on halothane as an anesthetic agent is a rather abbreviated summary of a complex problem, but this is probably relevant to the combined attitude of the departments of anesthesia and surgery in this particular academic unit. Because of our interests years ago in extracorporeal pig liver perfusion as a support for patients in severe and presumably terminal liver failure, a surprising number of patients with massive liver injury secondary to halothane administration were referred to this department of surgery. A natural result of this has been an almost automatic resistance to the concept of using this particular drug as an anesthetic agent, although we all admit that there are innumerable other advantages, which in the eyes of many anesthesiologists, outweigh the actual but rare hazard of toxicity. Despite the number of cases seen in this unit, the rarity of the problem is emphasized by the fact that initial studies almost negated the concept of halothane toxicity to the liver, but further studies in depth on a national level defined that there was, in fact, a specific and disastrous syndrome. These studies all emphasize, however, the fact that there was no specific case of severe reaction to the initial administration of halothane and that it was a second or third exposure which could be documented as associated with massive liver necrosis. Whether or not this agent should be used in anesthesia is a decision that can only be made by individual units, and it may well be that the major advantages of halothane could well outweigh the extremely rare incidence of massive hepatic toxicity during one or subsequent administrations.

The pharmacology of barbiturates, the opiates, and other analgesics and narcotic agents have been given excellent coverage and provide a concise review for the education of the general surgeon interested in this particular segment of operative procedures.

It may be of specific interest to surgeons and anesthetists reading this text to see the details of a rapid infusion device used at the New England Deaconess Hospital, which was introduced because of the volume of hepatic surgery, particularly orthotopic transplantation of the liver, and the rapid massive blood loss occasionally associated with these procedures. This ingenious but simple mechanism has, in the view of all of us associated with these problems, been an extraor-

dinarily helpful and frequently life saving piece of technology.

Any discussion of cardiovascular support and volume replacement secondary to massive blood loss would be incomplete without reference to the "cell saver," which has been in widespread use by surgeons of this department for a number of years. The technical name for this device, manufactured by the Haemonetics Co., is the Red Cell Harvester. An additional virtue to the recirculation of blood lost during surgical procedures has been added by the increasing fear among patients of contracting AIDS from ordinary bank blood. Reassurances about the safety of the blood in our particular unit, where clinical and laboratory investigations in depth are carried out prior to administration of any banked unit, have not overcome patient fears as much as the assurance that whenever possible their own blood will be restored. It is rare in many of these instances that there is any opportunity for preadmission storage of self-donated blood, but this mechanism is also utilized whenever possible.

In summary, it would be difficult, I think, for any person involved to any degree in the various problems related to the liver to carry out any of these procedures without the background knowledge contained in this excellent chapter.

Chapter 26
Pediatric Liver Disease

W. HARDY HENDREN
JOSEPH P. VACANTI

Although some surgical pathology of the liver in infants and children is similar to that seen in adults, such as trauma, most of the conditions seen by the pediatric surgeon differ from those needing surgery in adults. This chapter will emphasize those entities unique to infancy and childhood. Operative management of children with liver disease has other differences as well. For example, sudden uncontrolled loss of just a few ounces of blood can be fatal in a newborn whose entire blood volume is less than one adult 500-milliliter blood transfusion unit. A 6-pound neonate's blood volume, calculated at 100 milliliters per kilogram of body weight, is only 300 ml. Skillful anesthetic management is mandatory, for the ranges of safety are much more narrow in infants and children with respect to blood volume, acid-base balance, oxygen saturation, depth of anesthesia, and temperature regulation. In our opinion the single greatest advance in pediatric surgery in the past decade has been the refinement in pediatric anesthesia that has occurred as more individuals have taken special interest in this field. Also of great importance has been the development of pediatric intensive care units for continued monitoring, ventilation, and overall management of the young patient after major surgery.

Biliary Atresia

Biliary atresia is the most common hepatic surgical disorder in the newborn. It presents as jaundice with clay-colored stools, usually within the first 3 to 4 weeks of life. It should be emphasized, however, that jaundice in the newborn includes differential diagnostic consideration of a different spectrum of entities from what might be considered in adults. For example, jaundice occurs in a high percentage of healthy newborn infants, due to a temporary inability of the hepatocyte to excrete bilirubin. This has been termed "physiologic jaundice of the newborn." However, jaundice may be also the first indication of surgically treatable disease. When a neonate presents with jaundice we first rule out those medical problems that can cause icterus. They include toxoplasmosis, cytomegalic virus inclusion disease, nenonatal sepsis, hematologic disorders, and rare metabolic disorders such as the Crigler-Najjar syndrome, the Dubin-Johnson syndrome, and alpha$_1$-trypsin deficiency. When these conditions have been excluded there remains a large group of jaundiced neonates whose problem will be either biliary atresia or neonatal hepatitis. In adults there is little diagnostic confusion between obstructive jaundice and jaundice from hepatitis. In neonates, however, this is a very difficult differential diagnosis, which usually cannot be solved by laboratory tests (1). Levels of serum bilirubin can be identical in infants with neonatal hepatitis and bile duct atresia. The differential diagnosis cannot be made with certainty by levels of liver enzymes or liver function tests. Radioisotope imaging with a technetium 99m immunodiacetic acid (IDA) derivative can exclude obstruction if it appears in the bowel. However, no excretion can be seen in some cases of hepatitis just as will be observed in complete obstruction. Ultrasound evaluation is not diagnostic. Even the histologic picture of a needle biopsy specimen from the liver in hepatitis and biliary atresia can overlap in appearance, making it impossible to differentiate between biliary atresia and giant cell hepatitis. Thus, surgical exploration is necessary in the majority of these jaundiced neonates to resolve the dilemma. About one-third of

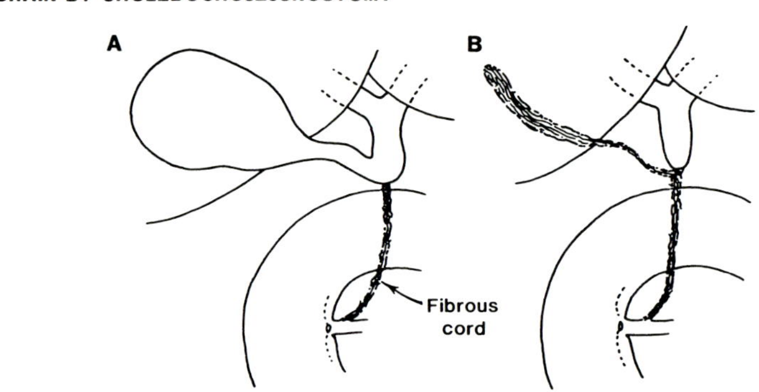

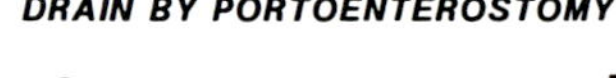

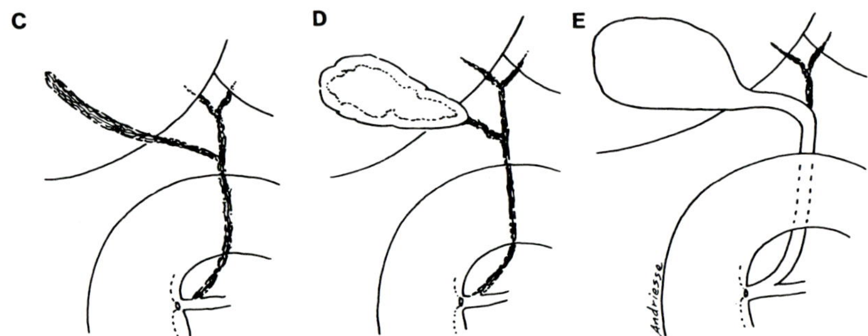

Figure 26.1. Most common types of biliary atresia and method for drainage.

such infants will prove to have hepatitis; two-thirds will have biliary atresia.

In Figure 26.1 are shown the principal types of biliary atresia. In Figure 26.1A and B are shown the relatively rare types where only the extrahepatic ducts are missing, but proximal ducts are present and allow choledochojejunostomy to be performed, with relief of jaundice. This was formerly called "the correctable form of biliary atresia." It is seen in about 5% to 10% of cases. Successful outcome depends on prompt recognition with early drainage before onset of severe biliary cirrhosis and also on whether there is a progressive obliterative process present. In Figure 26.1C, D, and E are shown what is present in the majority of infants with biliary atresia, which requires vastly different operative management. Surgical therapy for biliary therapy is relatively recent. In 1928 William E. Ladd (2), father of pediatric surgery in America, showed biliary obstruction could be relieved in those few cases with a dilated extrahepa-

tic duct by joining it directly to the duodenum. Sterling later demonstrated that inserting multiple silver rods into the liver hilum could result in drainage of bile in some cases (3). In 1959 Kasai reported in Japan success in establishing bile drainage in biliary atresia by what is essentially the method used by most surgeons today (4).

As shown in Figure 26.2 a minilaparotomy is performed, just enough to expose the gallbladder and perform an operative cholangiogram. Shown in Figure 26.3 is a cholangiogram from an infant with hepatitis. Main bile ducts are clearly seen, and there is free flow of contrast medium into the duodenum. With these findings, a liver biopsy would be taken, and the procedure terminated.

However, when there is nonfilling of the ductile system, even with gentle compression of the portahepatis with a small bulldog clamp, formal exploration of the liver hilum is performed. The technique for biliary exploration is shown in Figure 26.4. The superior attachments of the liver are

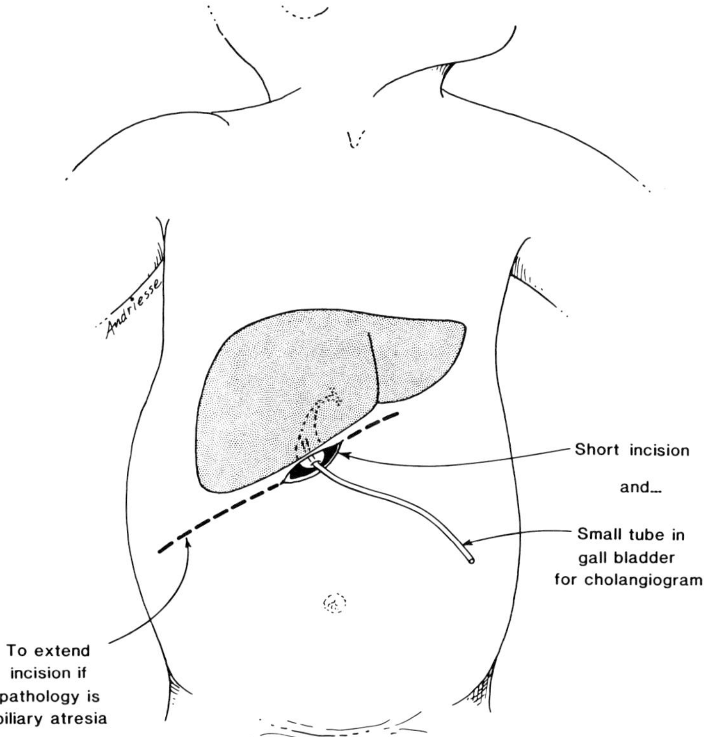

Figure 26.2. Minilaparotomy for cholangiography, which can be extended for biliary exploration.

incised. This allows rotating the liver to have a better view of the hilum. It is important to be aware that dislocating and retracting the liver can compress the inferior vena cava, causing circulatory collapse of an infant. Thus, cardiovascular monitoring and close communication between anesthesiologist and surgeons is important. The extrahepatic obliterated fibrous cords representing the biliary ducts, and often the gallbladder, are dissected up into the hilum of the liver. This requires brilliant illumination with an operative head lamp and magnification of the hilar structures by an operating microscope or high-power operating loupes. The naked eye is simply not able to accurately delineate the small structures and tiny ducts that may be encountered in this dissection. The dissection is carried into the liver hilum, posterior to the bifurcation of the portal vein, shaving the scar from the surface of the liver to identify microscopic ductules that can drain bile. This leaves a bare area when surface scar has been removed, to which can be sutured a Roux-en-Y loop of bowel by end-to-end or end-to-side technique. The dissection is not carried deep in the substance of the liver, for ductules that may be

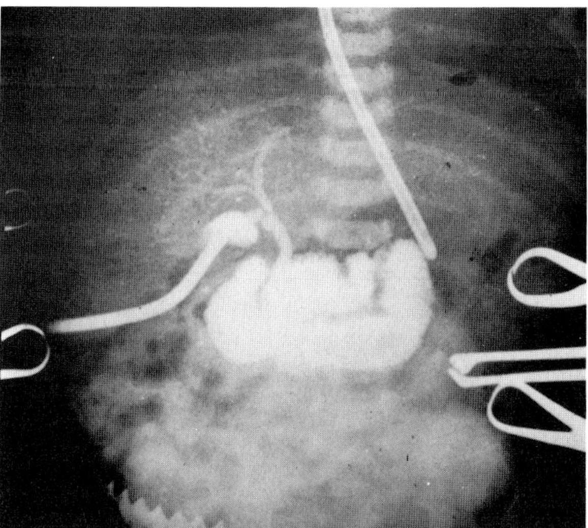

Figure 26.3. Cholangiogram in jaundiced infant with differential diagnosis of biliary atresia versus hepatitis. Note filling of hepatic ducts and duodenum, ruling out biliary atresia. Infant had hepatitis.

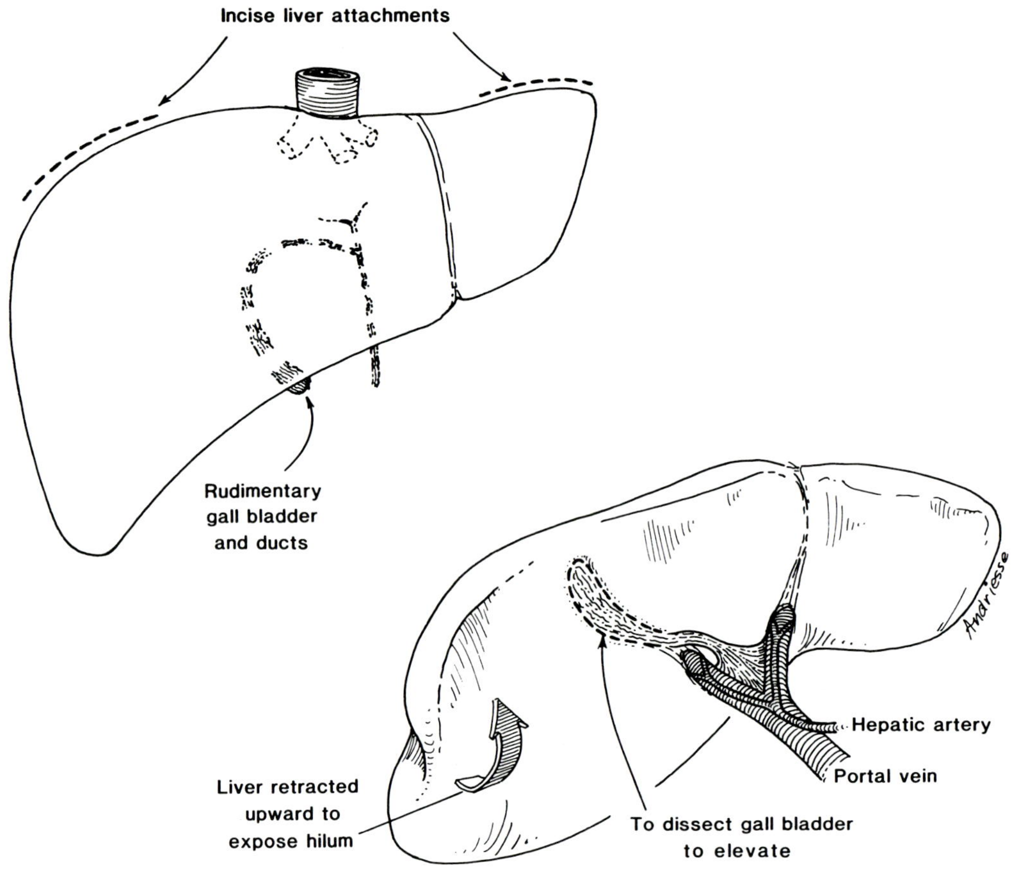

A

Figure 26.4. Portoenterostomy operation. (*A*) Liver attachments are incised, and the liver is retracted to expose the hilum.

present tend to later scar and obliterate after deep dissection is performed.

There are several variations in the type of Roux-en-Y loop that can be performed in hope of preventing ascending cholangitis (Fig. 26.5), which is the major complication seen in these patients. Some surgeons temporarily exteriorize the Roux-en-Y loop. Others perform a nipple valve to prevent reflux of intestinal contents to the biliary tree. In a recent conference about biliary atresia the subject remained controversial regarding which method of drainage provides the most effective relief of jaundice and the smallest incidence of cholangitis (1).

In Kasai's most recent experience jaundice was relieved by portoenterostomy in 66% of 53 patients (1). If corrective surgery is performed within 60 days after birth, serum bilirubin level was nor-malized in 80% of patients. In some infants bile flow ceases after an initial apparently successful result. In some this may result from a continuing obliteration of bile ducts by the process that causes biliary atresia initially. That process is not well understood, but in some it is thought to be related to a prenatal infection with reovirus type 3 (5). Reexploration should be performed in cases where there was satisfactory bile flow initially after a first operation. Ohi and associates reported their experience with reoperation in 23 patients (6). Excellent bile drainage after reoperation was obtained in 13 of 15 patients where good bile flow had been noted after the original operation. Reoperation does not meet with success in the majority of cases if active bile flow was not obtained at the first operation.

When portoenterostomy fails to provide satisfac-

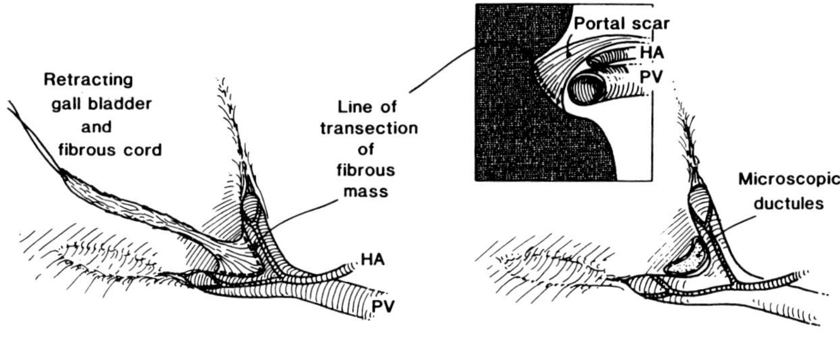

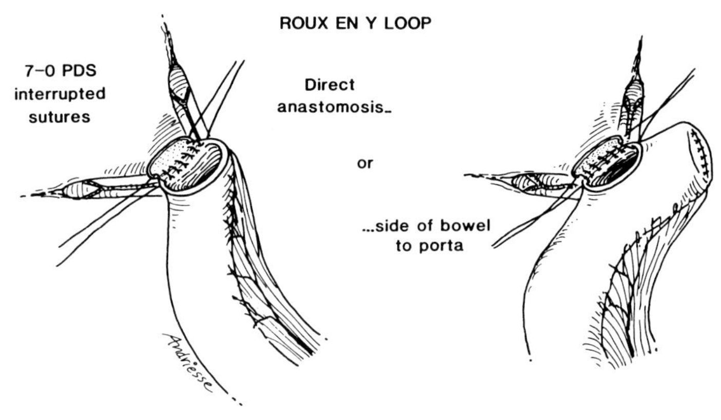

B

Figure 26.4 (continued).   Portoenterostomy operation. (*B*) Dissecting into hilum to expose microscopic ductules and drainage by Roux-en-Y loop.

tory bile flow, progressive liver failure and portal hypertension occur, with ultimate death of the child unless liver transplantation is performed. This method for treatment of end-stage liver disease in childhood, pioneered by Starzl, is now being performed in many medical centers in America and Europe (7). This is discussed in Chapter 6.

There are two rare conditions, biliary hypoplasia and Alagille's syndrome, that are in the spectrum of biliary atresia. In the former, ducts are present but they are very small. In the latter there is a paucity of intrahepatic bile ducts.

Choledochal Cyst

The term "choledochal cyst" denotes congenital cystic dilatation of the common bile duct. The principal types are shown in Figure 26.6. Addition-

ally, there is a rare variant in which there are multiple areas of cystic dilatation of the intrahepatic or extrahepatic biliary tree, or both. Choledochal cyst is reported in greater numbers in Orientals than whites (8), and it occurs about three times more often in females than males.

A young infant with a choledochal cyst may present with jaundice, just as in biliary atresia. An older child often presents with a clinical triad of jaundice, intermittent abdominal pain, and a palpable right upper abdominal mass. Fever may be present if there is cholangitis.

The diagnosis of choledochal cyst can be made by several means. Formerly, as shown in Figure 26.7, upper gastrointestinal (GI) series was performed, demonstrating compression and displacement of the duodenum. Today abdominal ultrasound is a very useful screening study to

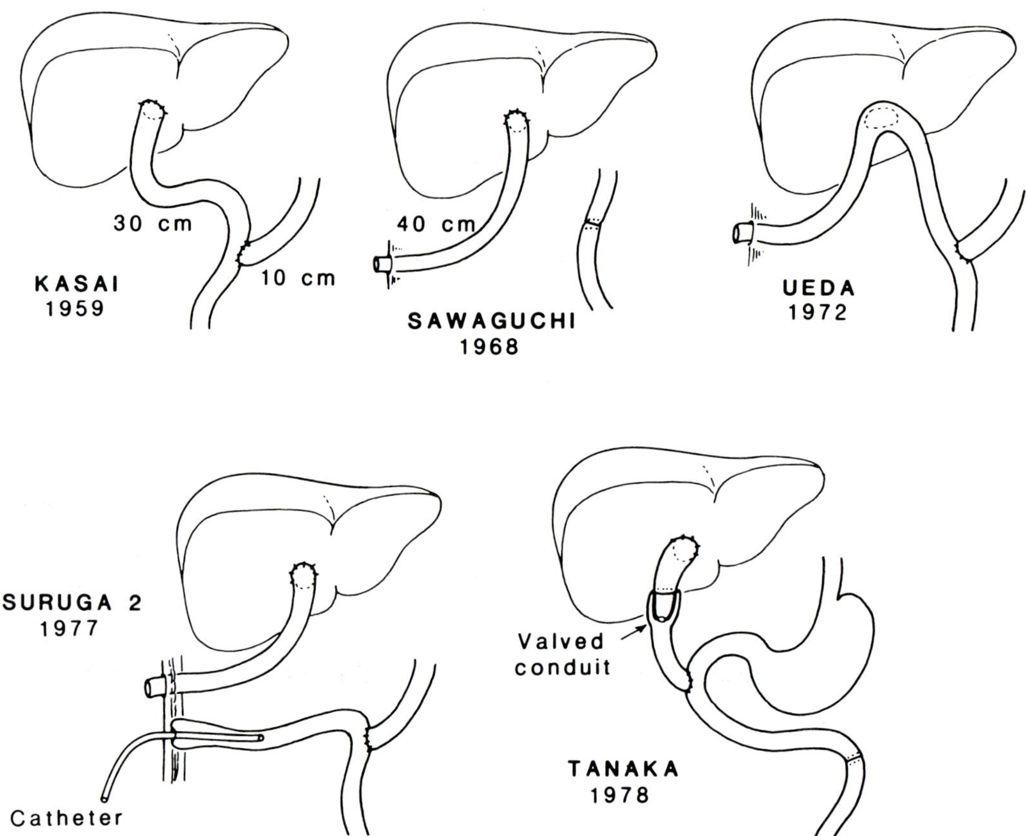

Figure 26.5.   Various methods for portoenterostomy with aim of draining bile and averting ascending cholangitis.

demonstrate the abnormally dilated biliary system. Other helpful imaging studies include radionucleide imaging with an IDA derivative, computed tomography (CT), and percutaneous transhepatic cholangiography. More recently endoscopic retrograde cholangiopancreatography has been used to demonstrate choledochal cysts, and in particular the anatomy of the ampulla of Vater, lower common bile duct, and main pancreatic duct. It has been recognized that in about one-third of cases the lower common bile duct empties directly into the main pancreatic duct (9,10). It has been proposed that reflux of pancreatic juice into the lower common bile duct may be an etiologic factor in choledochal cyst.

The treatment of choledochal cyst has changed over the past three decades (11). Originally they were often drained by a simple side-to-side cyst-duodenostomy (12). Later Roux-en-Y cyst jejunostomy became the procedure of choice because of a smaller incidence of ascending cholangitis from reflux of intestinal contents into the biliary tract (13–16). Roux-en-Y drainage may make the patient more susceptible to peptic ulcer by diverting the bile downstream distal to the duodenum. After the Japanese surgeons described excision of choledochal cysts (17,18), it has become the preferred method of treatment by most pediatric surgeons throughout the world (19). In most common forms of choledochal cyst, where there is fusiform dilatation of the common bile duct, most of the cyst is excised, draining the common hepatic duct into a Roux-en-Y loop of jejunum, shown in Figure 26.8. An intussuscepted nipple can be created as an additional safeguard against reflux into the biliary ducts. Excision of the lower end of the cyst can risk injury to adjacent structures. Therefore the outer wall is preserved, stripping the mucosa from the cyst, down to the point where it narrows, where it is transected and oversewn. It is important not to carry this dissection too low lest the main pancreatic duct be compromised in those cases where the

CHOLEDOCHAL "CYST"

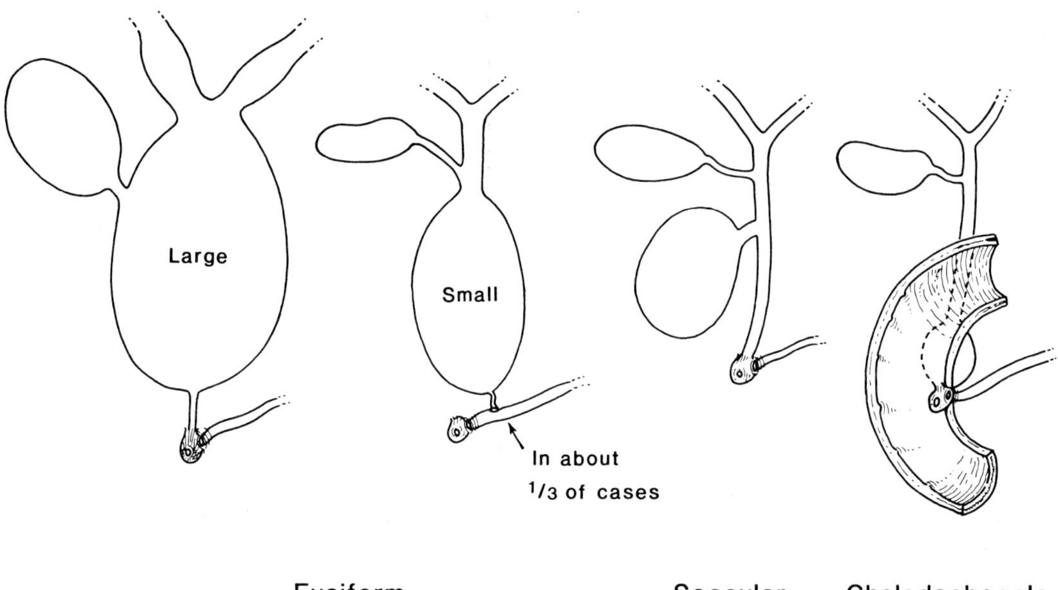

Figure 26.6. Types of choledochal cyst.

common duct joins the pancreatic duct. In the so-called choledochocele, where there is localized dilatation of the distal end of the common bile duct, it can be drained internally into the adjacent duodenum. The adjacent main pancreatic duct should be identified and protected, and enlarged if necessary. Cholecystectomy should be performed simultaneously with surgery for choledochal cysts because stasis in the gallbladder, and subsequent formation of gallstones, will result if it is not removed. Long-term follow-up of patients with choledochal cyst showed complications associated with cholangitis in 58% after cyst-duodenostomy, 34% after Roux-en-Y cyst jejunostomy, and only 8% following complete cyst excision (16). Other series have shown similar findings. It is not surprising, therefore, that cyst excision has become the procedure of choice. Bile duct carcinoma has been reported in patients with choledochal cyst, which is another reason to favor excision of the cyst.

A 1985 report described use of an isolated bowel conduit between the common hepatic duct and the duodenum, incorporating a nipple to prevent reflux (20), shown in Figure 26.9. Although follow-up is short, this would appear to have several advantages. The nipple prevents reflux from the bowel into the biliary tree. It drains the bile into the normal level of the GI tract, and the bacterial flora is less in the duodenum than further downstream in the jejunum. This is the method we currently employ. Long-term follow-up will be necessary to prove its superiority over the more conventional Roux-en-Y choledochoenterostomy.

Gallbladder Disease

Although uncommon as compared to adults, several diseases of the gallbladder occur in infants and children.

Hydrops of the Gallbladder

Since the advent of abdominal ultrasonography, acute hydrops of the gallbladder has been more commonly recognized in sick infants and children. It has been seen in association with long-term vomiting, prolonged total parenteral alimentation, sepsis, metabolic disorders, Kawasaki's disease, and in infants with diarrhea (21). The common denominator appears to be gallbladder stasis with resorption of bile and filling of the gallbladder with

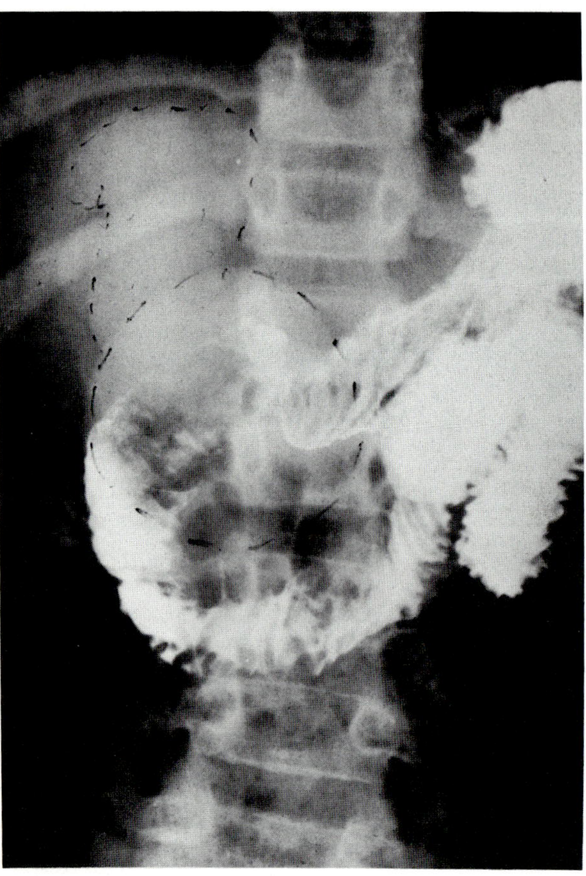

Figure 26.7. Upper GI series showing marked displacement of duodenum by large choledochal cyst. There is faint opacification of large cyst and hepatic ducts by contrast medium given previously.

a clear, serous transudate. By ultrasound the gallbladder loses its teardrop shape, becomes more oval, and can approach the size of the adjacent kidney. It does not contract well when stimulated with cholecystokinin. Serial ultrasonography provides a useful means for continuing assessment. If there is tenderness, laparotomy may be indicated, with the choices of performing either cholecystectomy or cholecystostomy.

Acalculous Cholecystitis

Acute cholecystitis without stones has been observed in various clinical states including generalized sepsis, dehydration, prolonged parenteral alimentation, prolonged gastrointestinal ileus, and after surgery requiring multiple transfusions. This entity should be suspected in a child with right upper quadrant tenderness, sometimes with a subcostal mass, with ultrasonic evidence of distention of the gallbladder. Cholecystectomy is usually indicated.

Cholelithiasis

Gallstones are rare in infants, but are seen with increasing frequency with increasing age. In about 20% of cases there is a hemolytic disorder that produces excessive bile pigment excretion, resulting in pigment stones (22–24). In about 80% of pediatric cholelithiasis, however, the etiology of gallstones is not so clear.

The most common hemolytic disorders associated with gallstones are congenital hereditary spherocytosis, sickle cell anemia, and thalassemia (25). Right upper quadrant symptoms in a patient with hemolytic disease should always prompt evaluation of the gallbladder. Ultrasonography and radionucleide scanning have largely replaced oral cholecystography in diagnosis of gallstones in pediatric patients. When splenectomy is to be performed in children for spherocytosis, gallbladder evaluation should be performed even when there are no symptoms suggesting stones, to determine whether simultaneous cholecystectomy should be performed. Acute pancreatitis has been reported secondary to previously asymptomatic pigment stones when a stone became impacted in the ampulla of Vater (26).

Sickle cell disease affects about 50,000 children in the United States (27). Gallstones secondary to hemolysis are seen in about 10% of those children less than 10 years of age, and the incidence rises to about 50% during the next several years. Cholecystectomy should be performed, particularly when the gallstones are symptomatic. It should not be done during a hemolytic crisis. Risk of perioperative complications in these children can be reduced by partial exchange transfusion preoperatively to reduce the level of hemoglobin S and avoiding dehydration and acidosis, which can precipitate sickling.

About 80% of gallstones in pediatric patients occur in the absence of a hemolytic disorder. Whereas the female/male ratio is 4:1 in adults with gallstones, it is much higher in adolescent girls.

Prolonged total parenteral nutrition has been noted to cause cholestasis and increased risk of gallstones in infants and children (28,29). Exten-

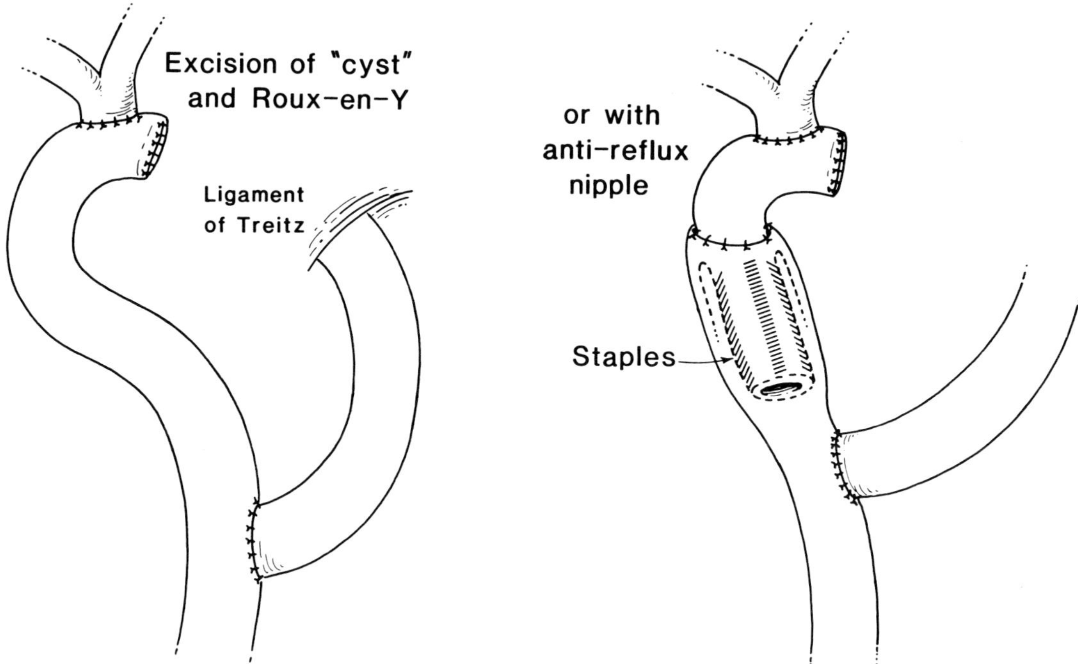

Figure 26.8. Roux-en-Y drainage of biliary tract after excision of choledochal cyst.

sive bowel resection in children with necrotizing enterocolitis, midgut volvulus, and irreducible intussusception may include distal small intestine. This upsets the enterohepatic transport of bile salts, which can contribute to gallstone formation. Rare congenital anomalies of the gallbladder described many years ago by Gross (30) can have stasis with stone formation. In a recent review of teenage girls with gallstones, two-thirds had been or were pregnant (22).

Some children with gallstones are asymptomatic. Others may have intolerance to certain foods. The most common symptom, however, is abdominal pain. The difficulty of diagnosing gallbladder disease in children is reflected by the considerable incidence of prior appendectomy because gallbladder disease had been overlooked (31). Physical findings in pediatric cholecystitis may be similar to those in adults, only more difficult to evaluate because a child in distress is often not very cooperative. Ultrasonography and radionucleide imaging have given a high degree of accuracy in diagnosis. As in adults, cholecystectomy is the procedure of choice (32). Decision to explore the common bile duct is based on the same general surgical principles as in adults.

Liver Tumors

Several types of benign and malignant masses in the liver are seen in infants and children. In a review by the Surgical Section of the American Academy of Pediatrics, 67% of primary liver tumors were found to be malignant (33). Weinberg and Feingold reported a 72% incidence of malignancy in primary liver tumors in children (34). Most often a child with a liver tumor is noted to have an upper abdominal mass or generalized abdominal enlargement. This may be accompanied by anorexia, weight loss, pain, and vomiting. Jaundice and ascites are uncommon. Laboratory analysis of liver function may be normal, although abnormal liver function tests may be seen if there is widespread involvement of liver parenchyma with cancer. Anemia may be present. Alphafetoprotein (AFP) is a serum protein that is produced in utero by immature hepatocytes. Its level normally decreases rapidly in the first few weeks of postnatal life and is not usually detected in the serum of children and adults. It has been found to be one of the most helpful markers for primary hepatic malignancy, being elevated in 90% of patients with hepatoblastoma (35). Levels of AFP

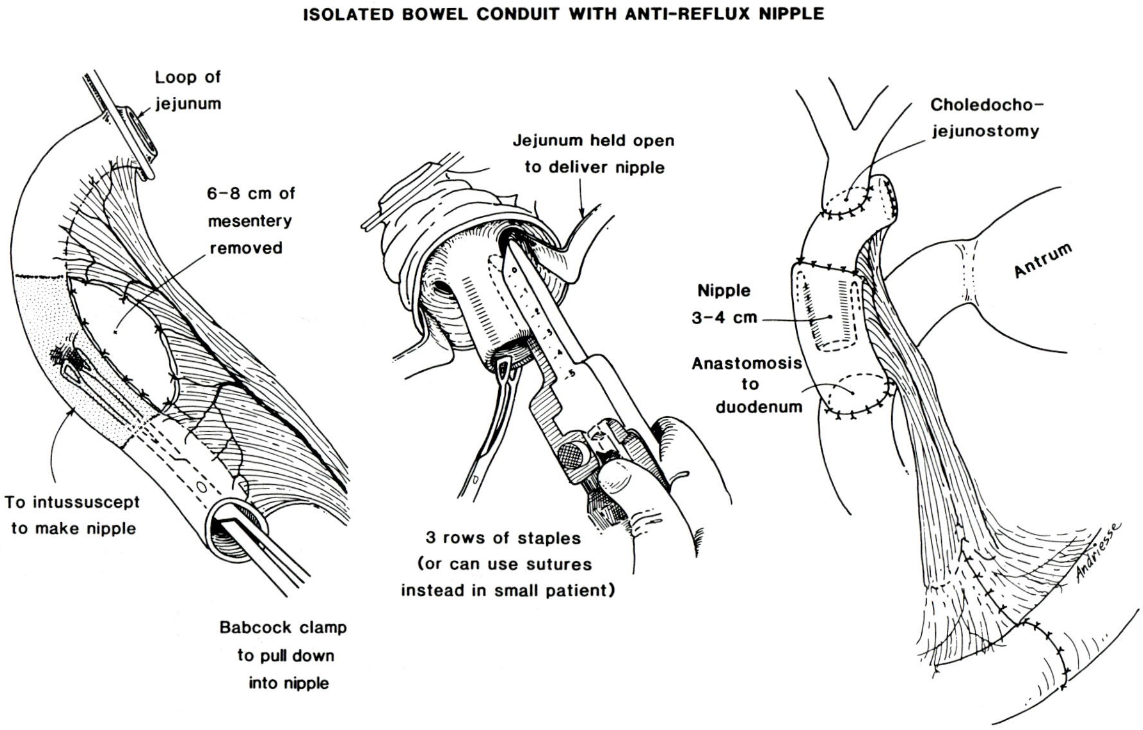

Figure 26.9. Use of nippled isolated bowel conduit to join biliary tract to duodenum.

have been shown to decrease after surgical removal of a tumor or after effective chemotherapy, and can rise if there is recurrence of tumor (36).

Because of the remarkable advances in radiology in the past decade the extent and type of an hepatic mass can usually be accurately determined preoperatively. Ultrasound can differentiate the solid mass from a cystic mass. Contrast-enhanced abdominal CT scanning is quite accurate to show tumor extent and location. Technetium-99m sulfur colloid liver-spleen scan is useful preoperatively because hepatocellular carcinoma does not take up the radionuclear material. However, some benign lesions of the liver likewise do not take up technetium. Radionuclear imaging is also useful postoperatively to assess the rate of regeneration in patients who have had hepatic resection (Fig. 26.10). Arteriography is useful to delineate intrahepatic neoplasm, their extent, and whether they are surgically resectable. Figure 26.11 shows the angiographic appearance of a large hepatoblastoma in the right lobe of the liver. Arteriography can demonstrate the abnormal neovascularization of the tumor as well as normal vessels displaced from their usual location.

Malignant Tumors

All types of cancers in children are relatively rare, as compared to adults. About 1 child in 600 develops a malignant tumor before age 15 years. Nonetheless, cancer remains second only to trauma as a cause for death in childhood. Also in contrast to adults, cancers of the epithelial origin are rare in children, who instead develop malignancy of the reticuloendothelial system, the central nervous system, and the mesenchymal tissues. Pediatric cancer is most prevalent in children less than 4 years of age (37). Primary tumors of the liver are very uncommon in children (38). In the majority of pediatric patients with malignancies of the liver it is metastatic neuroblastoma or Wilms's tumor (Fig. 26.12). Neuroblastoma often presents as a mass in the liver as the first sign of malignancy. Primary malignant tumors of the liver occur in only 1.9 per million population of children under 15 years of age in the United States. The majority are carcinomas of hepatic cell origin. Hepatomas, or liver cell carcinomas, are divided into two major histologic types, hepatoblastoma and hepatocellular carcinoma. Hepatomas occur more frequently in Asia

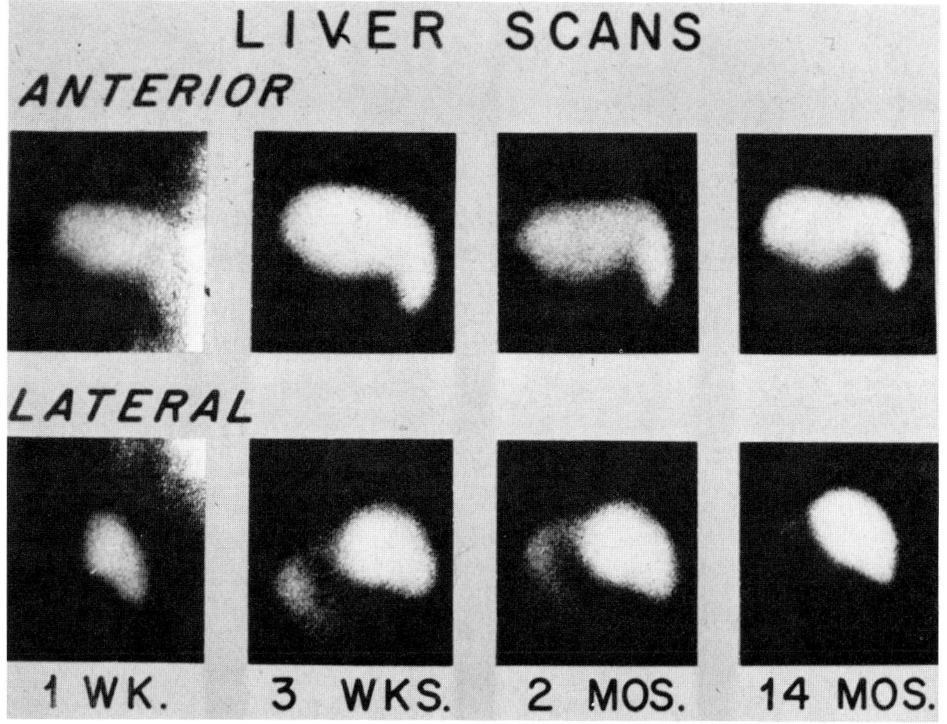

Figure 26.10. Liver scans after right hepatic lobectomy for large liver tumor. Note rapid regeneration by 3 weeks.

and Africa. In Japanese children carcinoma of the liver is the third most common form of abdominal cancer, and it has a much higher incidence in Japan than in other countries (39). Environmental factors may play a role in hepatomas, since hepatitis B virus (HBV)-associated antigens and antibodies are more common in patients with hepatoma than in the general population (40).

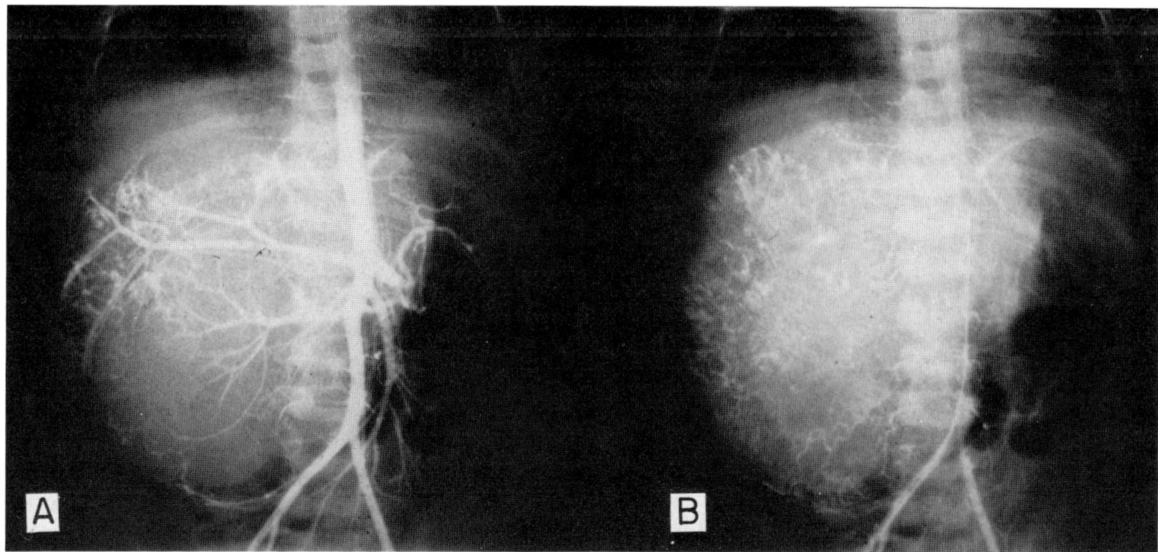

Figure 26.11. Aortogram, (*A*) early and (*B*) late phase in baby with large malignant tumor of right lobe of liver. Note "tumor blush" in late phase of study. Tumor was removed via thoracoabdominal exposure, with long-term survival.

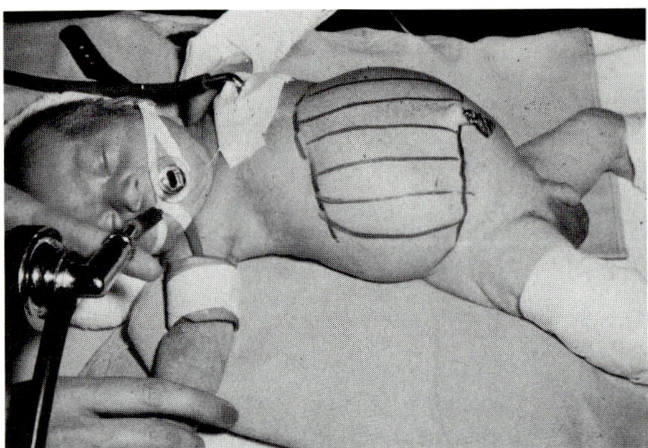

Figure 26.12. Newborn with diffuse involvement of liver with metastatic neuroblastoma from small primary in right adrenal. This unusual tumor, termed stage IV-S (special), has an 80% long-term survival despite what would seem an initially hopeless outlook.

ation therapy. Knowledge of the functional anatomy of the liver allows segmentectomy to be performed in resecting liver tumors to achieve curative resection without functional disturbance of remaining liver tissue (45). As much as 85% of the hepatic parenchyma can be resected with subsequent regeneration and recovery (46). The surgical techniques for resections are described in other chapter(s) in this book. As reported in a 1982 work, unresectable hepatoblastoma has been treated initially with multiple chemotherapeutic agents, which reduced tumor size and allowed subsequent resection (47). In general, however, chemotherapy has not been curative for children with residual disease in liver cancer (48), as it has been so often in Wilms's tumor and rhabdomyosarcoma.

Hepatoblastoma is seen mostly in infancy and seldom after 3 years of age. Histologically the tumor cells are smaller than normal hepatocytes and often contain osteoid and immature fibrous tissue. Hepatoblastoma has been classified into two epithelial types, a fetal and embryonal form. Patients with the fetal form appear to have the best prognosis (41). The prognosis for hepatoblastoma is better than for hepatocellular carcinoma.

Hepatocellular carcinoma occurs rarely before the age of 5 years. It has a peak incidence between 10 and 15 years of age. It has a male predominance of 2:1. Pre-existing cirrhosis is present in only 5% of children with hepatocellular carcinoma, whereas 79% of adults with this tumor have cirrhosis (42,43). Patients with a certain type of hepatocellular carcinoma, known as fibrolamellar carcinoma, have a high likelihood of localized disease with improved survival. Other diseases associated with the development of hepatocellular carcinoma include hepatitis B virus infection, biliary atresia, type 1 glycogen storage disease, Fanconi's syndrome, and the Beckwith-Wiedemann syndrome with hemihypertrophy.

Surgical excision is the only treatment that is potentially curative in hepatoblastoma and hepatocellular carcinoma (44). Since only one-half of patients with hepatoblastoma can be completely resected, and about two-thirds of patients with hepatocellular carcinoma have multicentric or unresectable disease, surgical resection in some should be combined with chemotherapy and radi-

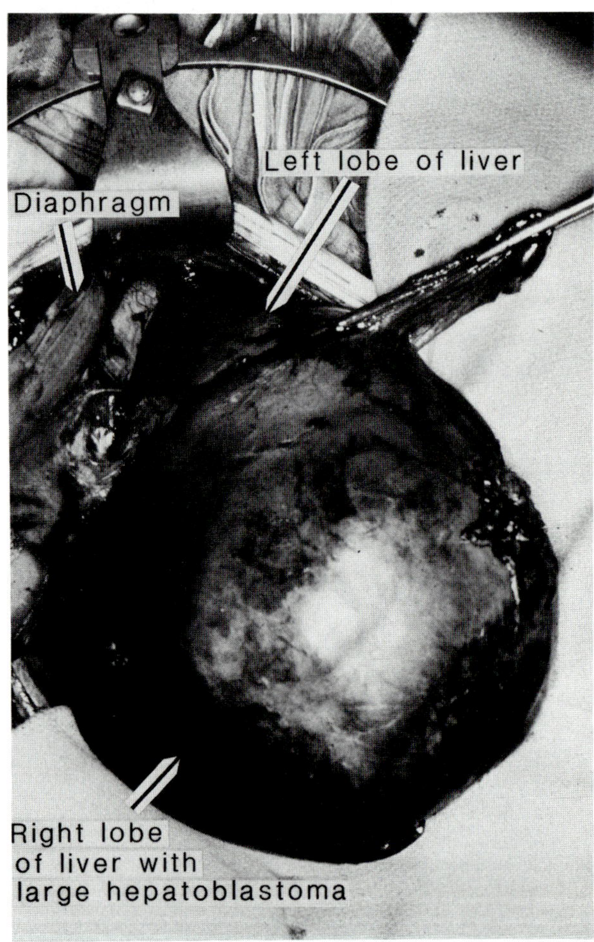

Figure 26.13. Operative exposure of large right hepatoblastoma through thoracoabdominal approach.

We prefer to use a thoracoabdominal incision in resecting large liver tumors (Fig. 26.13). This affords ideal operative exposure of not only the liver hilum, but also the suprahepatic vena cava and hepatic veins, which can be technically difficult to manage otherwise. Others have described the use of cardiopulmonary bypass with profound hypothermia in liver resection (49) and resection using hemodilution (50).

In addition to hepatomas there are several other types of rare malignant tumors in children. Most are of mesenchymal cell origin. Malignant mesenchymoma occurs in about 5% of all primary liver tumors. Undifferentiated sarcoma of the liver is usually found in patients less than 15 years of age. Childhood hepatic angiosarcoma is thought to be a malignant form of infantile hemangioendothelioma (51). Primary teratoma of the liver has been reported in childhood and roughly half were malignant (52).

Benign Tumors

Sometimes it is difficult to determine preoperatively whether a lesion in the liver is malignant or benign. Angiography is useful, together with abdominal CT scanning and ultrasound. However, occasionally the differential diagnosis cannot be made even in the operating room, and, therefore, histology must be obtained.

Vascular Tumors

Hemangiomas and hemangioendotheliomas are the most common benign tumors of the liver. Hemangiomas are composed of very large vascular lakes lined by fattened cells. Hemangioendotheliomas have both dilated and compressed vascular spaces and are lined by layers of endothelial cells. In some specimens both types occur in the same patient (Figs. 26.14, 26.15). It has been postulated that hemangiomas may be one of the regressive pathways for infantile hemangioendothelioma (53). Hemangioma, also called cavernous hemangioma, or a vascular malformation of the liver, is usually not associated with hemangiomas elswhere in the body. Management of this tumor does not require operation unless there are significant complications. It is unusual for this lesion to cause congestive heart failure from arteriovenous shunting, thrombocytopenia from sequestering of

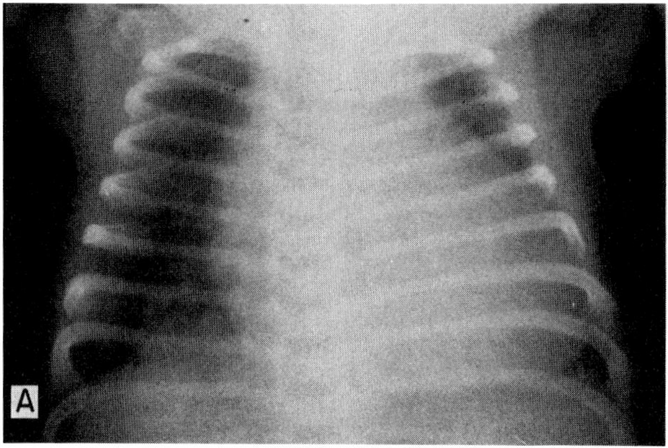
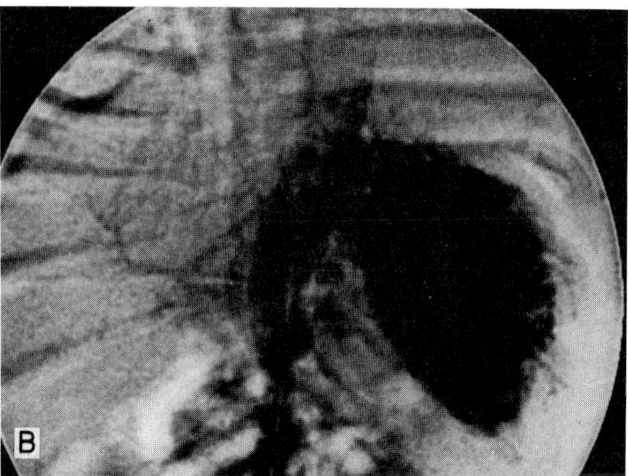

Figure 26.14. Infant with large, benign hemangioma in left lobe of liver. (*A*) Chest roentgenogram, showing cardiomegaly. There was congestive heart failure secondary to the large shunt in this tumor. (*B*) Hepatic angiogram showing marked vascularity of lesion.

platelets, or massive bleeding due to rupture. In contrast, hemangioendothelioma is more often associated with the above significant complications. More than 90% of these lesions are discovered before age 6 months. These children can present with massive hepatomegaly and congestive heart failure from shunting. Coagulopathy due to platelet sequestration occurs in about one-half of these children. Intraperitoneal hemorrhage from rupture has been reported (54). About 40% of these children have cutaneous manifestations of hemangioma. No treatment is required if the child is asymptomatic. Unfortunately this is unusual. Nonsurgical management includes diuretic therapy and digitalis if there is congestive heart failure (55). Corticosteroids have been shown to be useful in promoting involution. If medical management

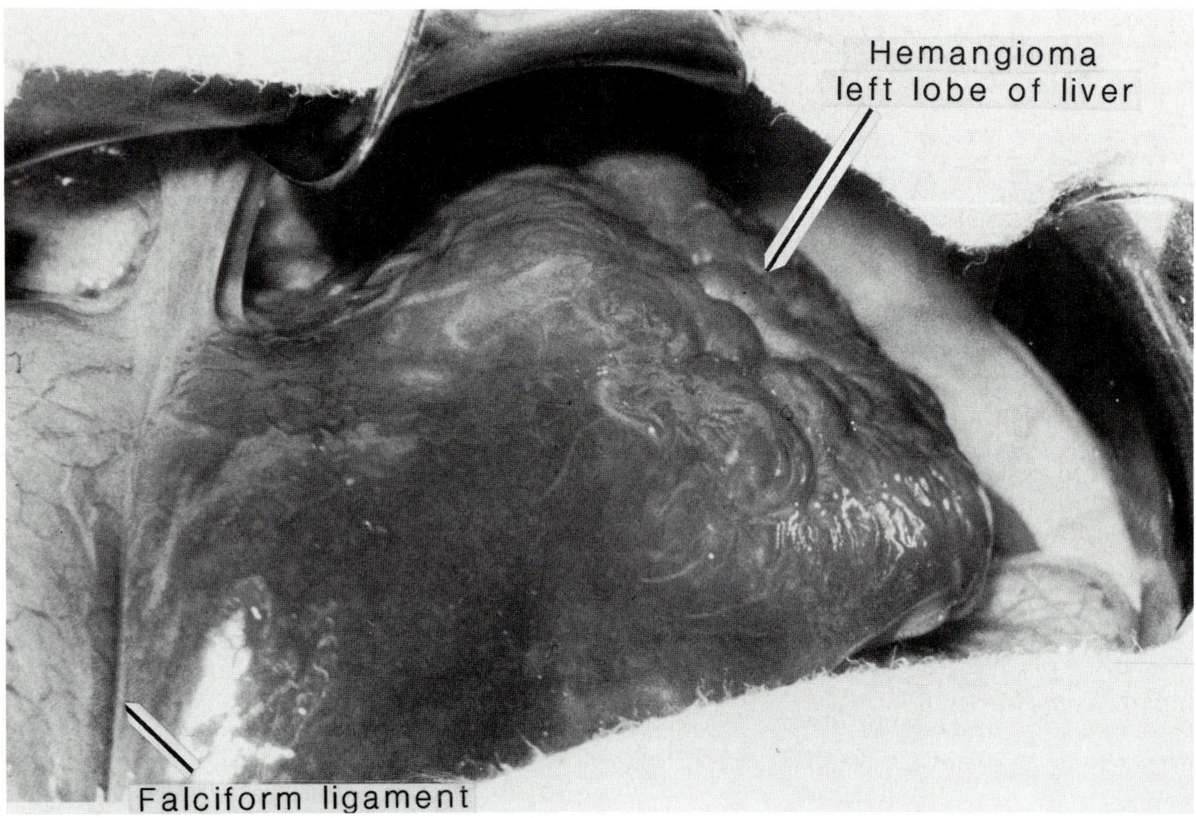

Figure 26.15.   Operative photograph showing lesion in left lobe of liver, which was removed, thereby curing the problem.

fails there should be consideration of ligating the hepatic artery (56), radiation therapy, or surgical excision if the tumor is localized. We have recently employed embolization of the feeding arteries in an attempt to control congestive failure. If a child can be treated without surgery, spontaneous resolution of the lesion may occur.

There are also other benign solid and cystic masses seen in the liver. The solid ones include liver cell or bile duct adenomas, hamartomas with both epithelial and mesenchymal elements, and "pseudo" tumor, such as focal nodular hyperplasia (57). There are congenital cysts (Fig. 26.16) and those secondary to infection such as chronic granulomatous disease and hydatid cysts. The origin of simple congenital cysts is not known. Treatment of a solitary one depends on its size and location. If resectable without damage to adjacent structures, this is the treatment of choice. For large cysts involving both lobes of the liver, internal drainage to a Roux-en-Y loop of jejunum should be considered. Alternatively the cyst can be unroofed

and the edges oversewn, making certain there is no bile leak. Hepatic adenoma is a rare benign lesion usually located in the right lobe of the liver. It can present with an acute abdominal emergency from hemorrhage. Wedge resection or lobectomy is the preferred treatment. Focal nodular hyperplasia can present as a circumscribed nodular mass.

Mesenchymal hamartoma is a rare lesion that occurs most often in the first year of life. It is a solitary tumor that usually involves the right lobe. It can be cystic or solid. When possible, removal of enucleation of the encapsulated lesion is recommended, but formal lobectomy may be necessary (58).

Portal Hypertension

Portal hypertension occurs in infants and children, but the causes are different from those in adults, which are mainly cirrhosis from alcoholism and hepatitis. Further, portal hypertension in childhood can be secondary not only to diseases that

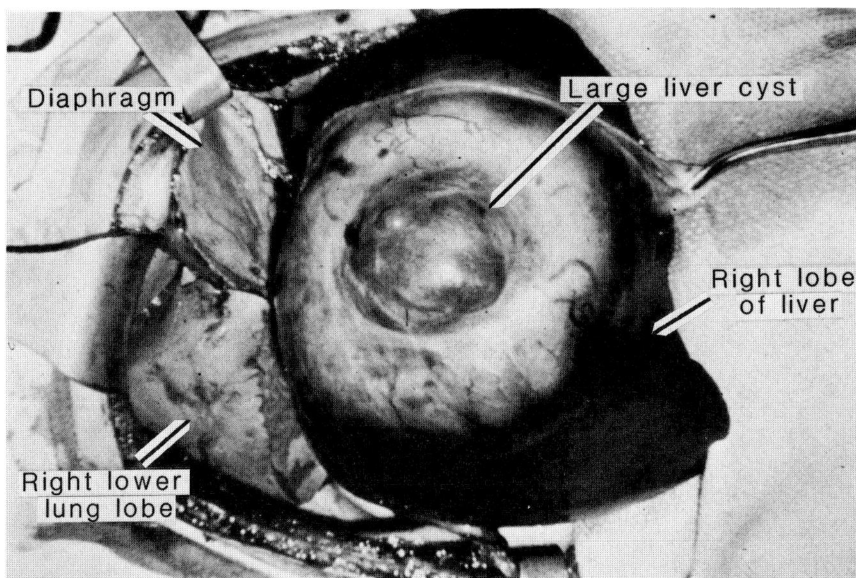

Figure 26.16. Large cyst of liver in 6-month-old infant, viewed through thoracoabdominal exposure. Cyst was enucleated, saving all of liver parenchyma.

cause scarring of the liver, but also from thrombosis of the extrahepatic portal venous system. Blockage of flow from the portal vein into the liver can cause tremendous dilatation of the entire portal system and secondary esophageal varices (Figs. 26.17, 26.18).

Causes for intrahepatic portal hypertension, that is, diseases that cause hepatic fibrosis, include

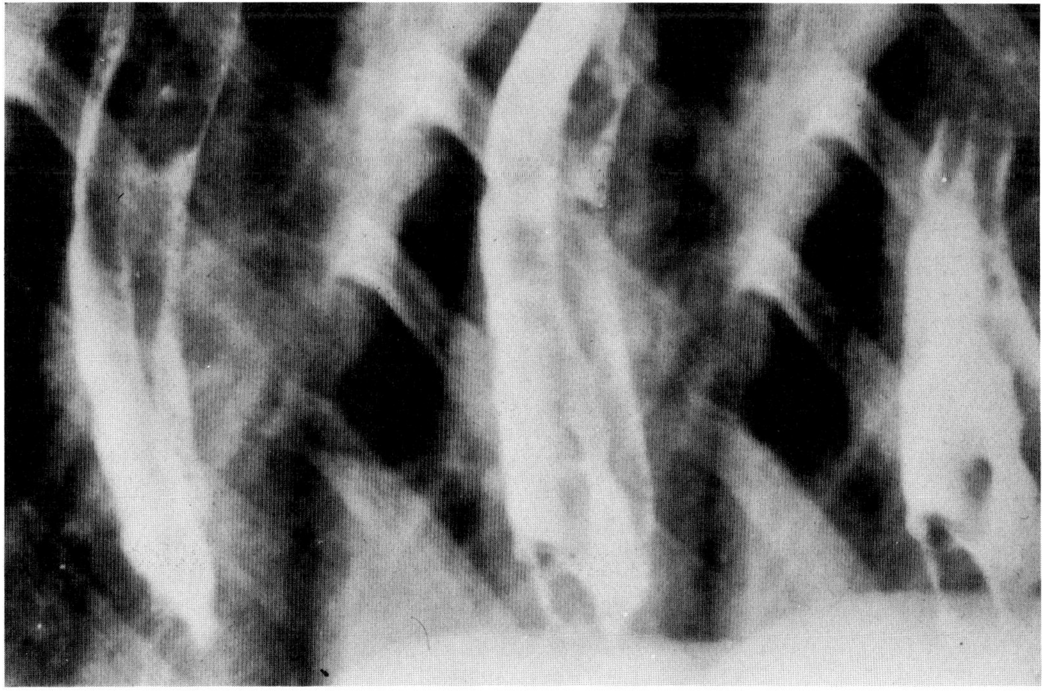

Figure 26.17. Esophageal varices in 10-year-old boy with portal hypertension. Note that they are large and extensive.

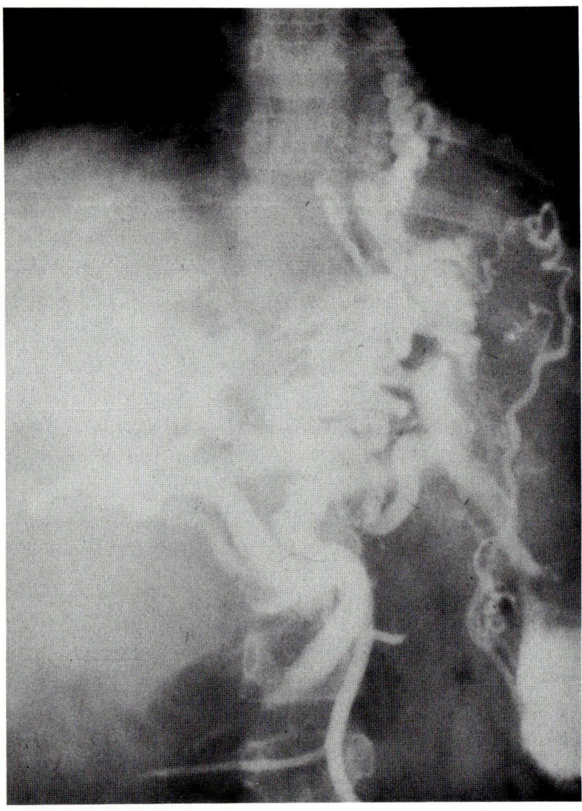

Figure 26.18. Splenoportogram in patient with extrahepatic portal hypertension, or Banti's disease. Note large, convoluted venous collaterals in abdomen, which extend up along esophagus.

biliary atresia, neonatal hepatitis, congenital hepatic fibrosis, Wilson's disease, cystic fibrosis, glycogen storage disease, and alpha$_1$-trypsin deficiency. All of these pathologic states can result in scarring of the liver and portal hypertension with varices, ascites, malnutrition, and liver failure. Extrahepatic portal hypertension, rarely seen in adults, is common in childhood, accounting for about one-half of all cases (59). In some there is a history of perinatal omphalitis or use of the umbilical vein for exchange transfusion as a neonate. In others there may have been a neonatal illness with profound dehydration and sepsis (60). In some children there is no history of an event that might have caused portal vein thrombosis. An important difference in this group of patients is that they have a normal liver and normal liver function tests, in contrast to those patients with intrahepatic portal hypertension who usually have profound liver disease and all of the usual secondary prob-

lems. These children are basically a healthier group who are better able to withstand intermittent GI hemorrhage secondary to portal hypertension with esophageal varices.

A rare and distinct type of portal hypertension seen occasionally in childhood is that caused by acquired obstruction of the hepatic venous drainage into the vena cava (Budd-Chiari syndrome) (61–63). This condition can be caused by certain senechio alkaloids found in imperfectly processed wheat in Africa and bush tea in the West Indies. This disease is known to the veterinarian when cattle ingest certain plants and develop ascites. Tumors that extend into the intrahepatic vena cava (Wilms's tumor in children and renal carcinoma in adults) can produce a similar pathologic picture. The patient is usually an older child with congestive splenomegaly and ascites. The outlook is generally poor, although we have treated one with success using a portosystemic shunt and another by removing intracaval tumor with long-term survival. Recently liver transplantation has been reported as a treatment of Budd-Chiari syndrome (64).

The diagnosis of portal hypertension in childhood should be suspected in acute GI bleeding in an infant or older child. Barium swallow usually discloses esophageal varices. However, with massive acute hematemesis in a child, immediate endoscopy should be considered. This can quickly differentiate between bleeding from varices of the esophagus versus peptic ulceration, or gastritis. Superior mesenteric arteriogram can disclose portal venous collateral enlargement. Equally effective is injection of contrast medium into the spleen (65) (Fig. 26.18), which can allow simultaneous measurement of portal venous pressure. Percutaneous needle splenoportogram has the slight risk of continued bleeding from the spleen. However, we have performed many such studies without encountering this complication.

Treatment of a child with acute gastrointestinal hemorrhage secondary to portal hypertension is usually supportive, and includes adequate blood replacement. When bleeding is massive, or persists, temporary balloon tamponade can be utilized. The Linton gastric balloon can be inflated and pulled up against the cardia to compress the gastroesophageal varices. We do not favor use of the classic Sengstaken tube which also has an intraesophageal balloon, having witnessed one

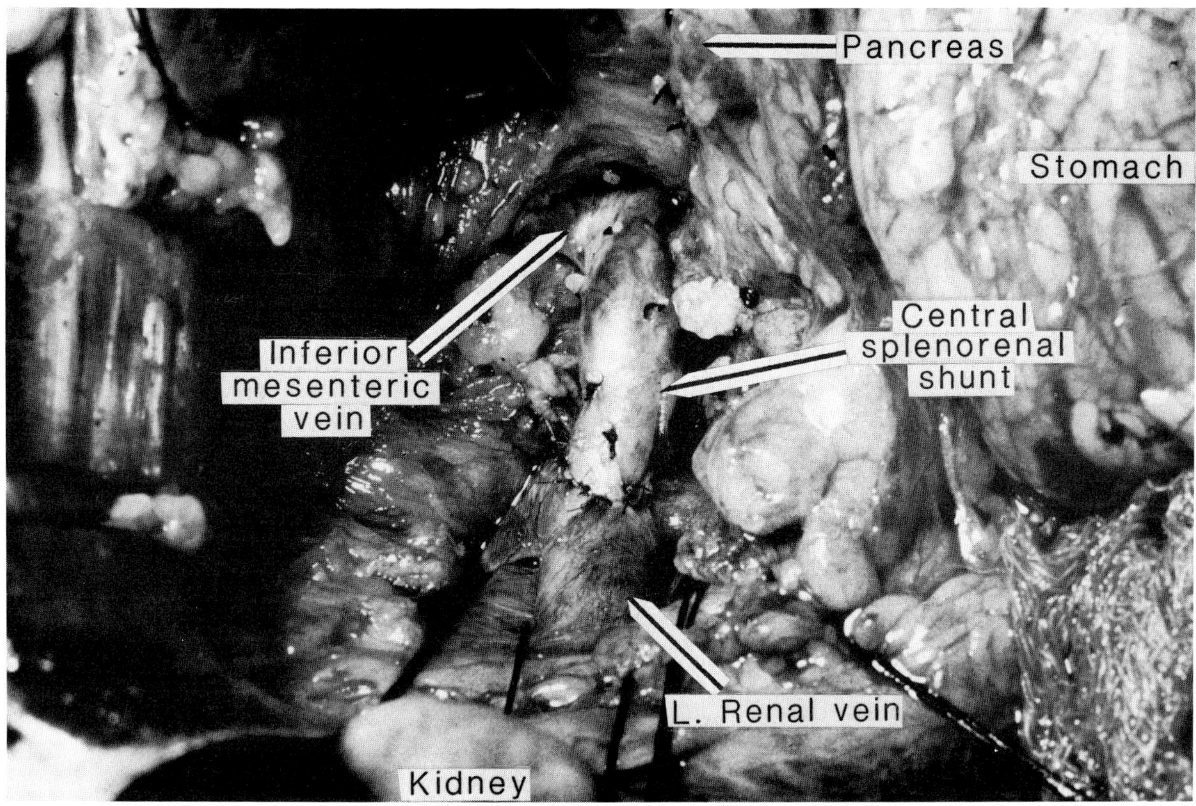

Figure 26.19. Central splenorenal shunt. Note that kidney has not been mobilized. Splenic vein has been dissected meticulously back to inferior mesenteric vein, leaving a short segment of proximal splenic vein to be joined without angulation to anterior aspect of left renal vein.

slip up into the pharynx and asphyxiate the patient. Intravenous pitressin has been effective in controlling gastrointestinal bleeding in some of these patients (66,67). As reported in 1980, endoscopic sclerotherapy has found its place in control of variceal bleeding (68). We have seen, however, one pediatric patient whose entire portal venous system was occluded following sclerotherapy. Other possible hazards from this method of treatment include intramural injection of the sclerosing solution with tissue necrosis and stricture formation.

Portosystemic venous shunts can be used in childhood, just as in adults, for decompression of the portal venous system (69,70). Experience has shown that technical success in constructing a shunt that remains open in childhood is less than in adults, principally because of the size of the veins available for shunting. Follow-up has shown in general that the vein to be decompressed should be 1 centimeter in diameter for a shunt to remain

open. Nevertheless, improved suture materials and optical magnification have made shunt construction more successful today than in 1968. We favor the use of the central splenorenal shunt (Fig. 26.19) described in 1947 by Linton (71) and applied to children by Clatworthy and Boles (72). If the splenic vein is mobilized all the way to its junction with the inferior mesenteric vein, it comes to lie very close to the adjacent renal vein. At that point it can be turned down and anastomosed end-to-side to the renal vein with maximum diameter of the anastomosis and minimal chance for angulation of the shunt. A splenorenal shunt in childhood was depicted many years ago by bringing the kidney into the operative field, performing a shunt between the renal vein, and replacing the kidney into its fossa (73). This technique has a high likelihood of angulation of the shunt, as compared to the central splenorenal shunt in which the kidney remains in situ. In one of our patients a splenorenal shunt was done at age 18 months and

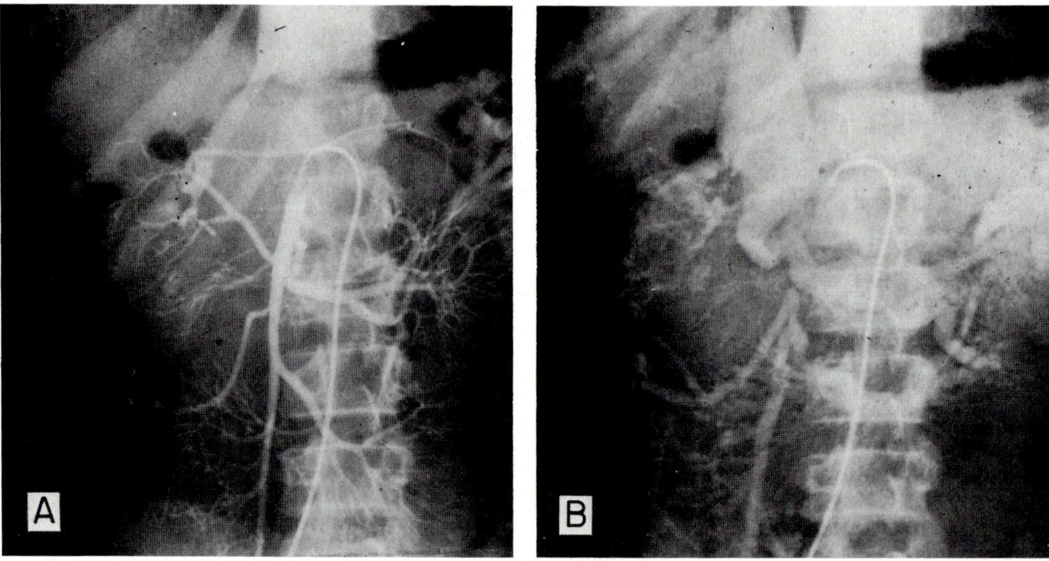

Figure 26.20.   Postoperative superior mesenteric arteriogram 1 year after mesocaval shunt in 16-year-old boy with recurrent massive bleeding from esophageal varices. The patient had extrahepatic block. He bled massively at age 10 years, and underwent splenorenal shunt, which remained open on long-term by angiography, but subsequently obliterated. An interposition H-shunt with prosthetic graft was performed at age 15. It was functional by angiography postoperatively, but later thrombosed. Because there was recurrent massive bleeding from varices, side-to-end mesocaval shunt was performed at age 16. The patient, now age 30 years, has had no further bleeding. (*A*) Early phase of study. (*B*) Blood filling vena cava via superior mesenteric vein.

was shown to be patent angiographically on long-term follow-up. The patient is now an adult. Since splenectomy is performed with the classic splenorenal shunt, certain precautions are necessary to avoid the well-recognized complication of late overwhelming sepsis secondary to splenectomy (74,75). Pneumococcus vaccine is given preoperatively when possible. The patient is maintained postoperatively on long-term prophylactic penicillin therapy. The classic side-to-side portacaval shunt can be used in certain children with portal hypertension, but it will be contraindicated in virtually all of those with extrahepatic block where dissection in the portahepatis is made extremely difficult by the presence of many large thin-walled venous collaterals. In patients with portal hypertension who may be liver transplant patients in the future, a shunt in the portahepatis in particular greatly decreases the likelihood of technical success in liver transplantation. Martin described end-to-side anastomosis of the portal vein into either the vena cava or left renal vein (76). Warren described division of the splenic vein, with anastomosis of the distal end into the renal vein (77). After dividing the coronary vein, gastroesophageal varices decompress via the short gastric and gastroepiploic vessels into the splenic hilum and from there into the renal vein. We have no experience with use of this shunt in children. The mesocaval shunt has been useful in selected children not suitable for other types of shunts, such as the child with extrahepatic portal hypertension who has had a previous failed splenorenal shunt, or splenectomy for splenomegaly with hypersplenism. The vena cava is divided just above its bifurcation, and rotated to be joined end-to-side with the superior mesenteric vein. Although there have been long-term successes with this shunt (Fig. 26.20), dividing the vena cava has the possible long-term complications of edema of the lower extremities. Drapanas described an interposition shunt of prosthetic material between the portal vein and vena cava (78), but that has the obvious disadvantage of thrombosis in a prosthetic graft in the venous system where pressures and flows do not result in the same degree of success as in the arterial system. We used one such shunt in a teenage boy but it thrombosed and was replaced by an autologous shunt (Fig. 26.21).

Distal esophagectomy and proximal gastrectomy

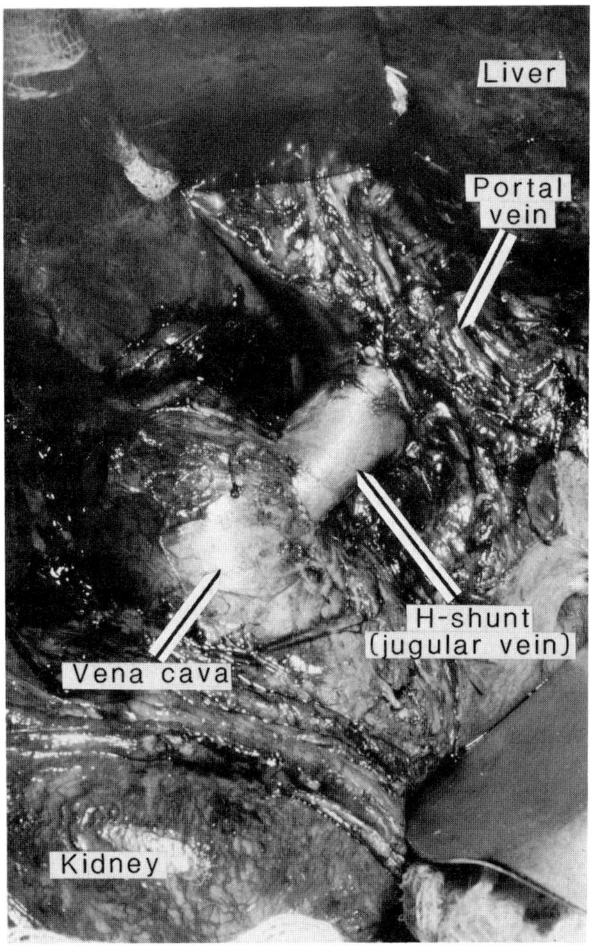

Figure 26.21. H-shunt using jugular vein in patient with extrahepatic portal hypertension. There was cavernous transformation of the portal venous system. Previous surgery had included splenorenal shunt, which closed, and mesocaval shunt, which did not function well and large varices persisted. Varices decompressed after this shunt, which has remained open for 6 years as shown by angiography and disappearance of varices.

is another option that should be considered in selected patients with portal hypertension and recurrent bleeding who are not good candidates for a shunt because of previous splenectomy or failed shunts. We have two such patients, both treated as children more than 25 years ago. On long-term follow-up they remain well without further GI bleeding (79).

Portosystemic shunt has been used in type I glycogen storage disease (Von Gierke's disease) where there is deficiency of the enzyme glucose-6-phosphatase. These children store ingested glucose in the liver as glycogen but cannot mobilize it back into glucose when the blood sugar falls several hours postpradially. This leads to severe hypoglycemia, which causes brain damage. Further, as a compensatory mechanism, lipids are mobilized and broken down, causing acidosis and coating of platelets, which results in prolonged bleeding time.

Starzl et al. (80) showed that portacaval shunt helped these children maintain normal glucose levels by bypassing the liver. Folkman et al. (81) showed that continuous infusion of 20% glucose into the vena cava prevents intraoperative and postoperative bleeding in these patients by maintaining blood glucose and preventing compensatory mobilization of the lipids secondary to severe hypoglycemia. In a 1978 report, Crigler and Folkman (82) showed that a more effective approach to management of these unfortunate children is continuous feeding with glucose, which is absorbed in the duodenum. Through a gastrostomy tube glucose is delivered during the night at a rate of .5 grams per kilogram per hour, which maintains blood glucose levels, thereby preventing the need for a portosystemic shunt, which was used formerly. During the daytime these children eat normally, but take supplementary amounts of glucose periodically throughout the day. At night glucose is administered continually through the tube. Some of these patients are now young adults, without brain damage. A further step in management of these patients has been to prescribe oral ingestion of cornstarch, which is a slow-to-release polymer that assures a more steady postprandial level of glucose than seen after ingestion of regular food (83).

Liver Trauma

Trauma is the leading cause for death in children. Intra-abdominal injury to the liver accounts for a significant percentage of this mortality. At the Children's Hospital National Medical Center in Washington, D.C., trauma accounted for 12% of all admissions and 13% of all intensive care unit admissions (84). Although head injury was most common, 14% of the children had major abdominal injuries. In large series of adult liver trauma, penetrating gunshot and knife wounds predominated (85–87). Rupture of the liver in childhood, however, is usually the result of blunt trauma (88,89).

In a monograph on liver trauma published in 1965 definitive treatment of all liver wounds was considered to be surgical (90). The authors commented that abdominal exploration was the only reliable index of intra-abdominal injury and they believed it was presumptuous to maintain that there are liver lacerations and ruptures that pass undetected. However, recent advances in diagnostic imaging of the traumatized child, especially CT (91), have increased our ability to detect and define the extent of many intra-abdominal injuries, particularly rupture of the liver, spleen, and kidney. Improvement in diagnosis has made it possible to be more selective regarding which children should be explored and which can be treated nonoperatively. When a child enters the emergency room following trauma, immediate resuscitation and systematic evaluation for extent of injuries are performed. The extent of diagnostic evaluation and urgency of decision making will depend on the amount of blood that has been lost and the child's response to initial resuscitative measures, including blood transfusion. In an extreme case immediate operation may be required for a child who enters with severe liver trauma, often in association with contusion over the liver and palpably broken ribs, and profound shock that does not improve with immediate transfusion. When major hepatic veins are sheared from the vena cava there may be profound shock that does not improve with blood transfusion, and immediate laparotomy may be required, foregoing the benefit of any diagnostic measures. We recall one 12-year-old boy with that injury, who had been struck by a bus, for whom more than 50 units of blood were given between entry to the emergency room and transfer to the intensive care unit after operation. He survived.

Fortunately in the majority of children with abdominal trauma, initial resuscitation will give more time for diagnosis and evaluation. If there is a head injury as well, peritoneal lavage can be helpful in determining whether there is blood in the abdominal cavity. Intraperitoneal blood by itself is not a criterion for exploratory laparotomy. However, it alerts physicians to the possibility that there is also an intra-abdominal injury. It is vital that the injured child be examined repeatedly by the same individual(s) who examined the child from the outset. In the awake patient this will be most important in determining whether abdominal findings are becoming more or less evident. Computed tomography scanning has become invaluable in assessing injury to the liver, spleen, kidneys, and pancreas. Observation includes also vital signs, serial hematocrit determination, central venous pressure monitoring, hourly urinary output, and repeated physical examination. If the patient's clinical course is stable, and there is no other indication for abdominal exploration, such as free air in the abdomen, it is feasible to watch closely a child with hepatic injury identified by CT scan. At the Children's Hospital of Buffalo (92) a recent series of 17 children with liver injuries were reported. In 32 there were other associated injuries. One required immediate exploration for an avulsed kidney. A second child had increased transfusion requirement on the fourth post-injury day and was explored. The other 15 children were managed nonoperatively in the intensive care unit for a mean stay of 6 days. The mean time required for resolution of the hepatic injury as judged by CT scan was 4 months.

Sandblom described the entity of traumatic hemobilia (93) in which a patient with recent liver trauma develops biliary colic and GI bleeding. Typically delayed bleeding in the liver fills the biliary tree with blood, which causes pain and which is relieved by decompression of the biliary tree into the GI tract via the common bile duct, with accompanying hematemesis. We treated two children, aged 5 and 6 years, in whom the bleeding point in the liver was defined by angiography (94). Although both had further bleeding during close observation in the hospital, it eventually stopped. Healing was demonstrated by later angiography in both children. Embolization therapy has been used for nonoperative management of intrahepatic hemorrhage after blunt trauma (95).

When operation is required in a child with liver trauma we prefer use of a midline incision for initial evaluation, with the patient draped and positioned so as to be able to extend into a thoracoabdominal exposure or sternal split, which is especially useful to approach major rupture through the dome of the right lobe of the liver where major hepatic vein injury may exist. Temporary occlusion of the structures at the portahe-

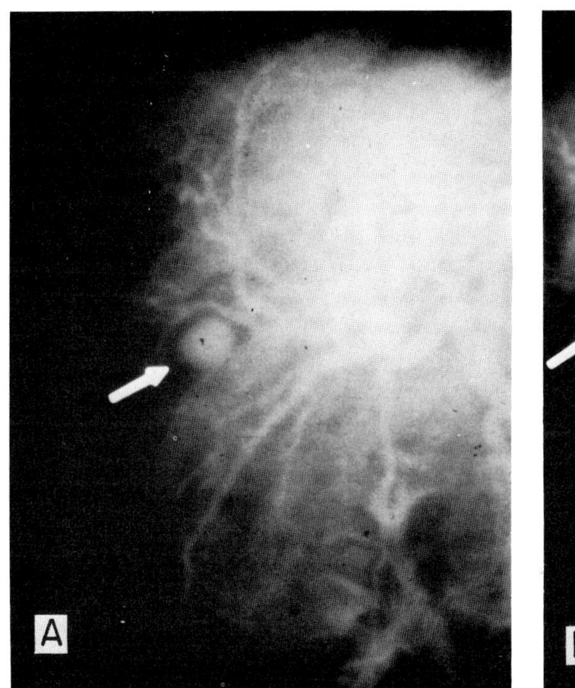
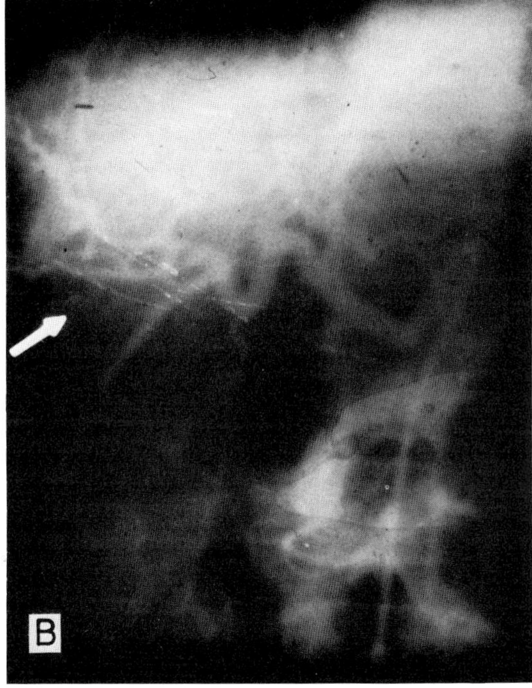

Figure 26.22. Hepatic arteriogram of 5-year-old boy with traumatic hemobilia. Ten days after repair of a laceration of the right lobe of the liver, hematemesis occurred. Five days later he developed back pain, epigastric pain, hematemesis, and jaundice. (*A*) Arteriogram 15 days after initial injury. Extravasation of contrast medium in intermediate segment of right lobe of liver (*arrow*). (*B*) Hepatic arteriogram 12 weeks after liver injury with healing of defect.

patis by applying a soft noncrushing clamp, the Pringle maneuver, will help control parenchymal bleeding in lacerations of liver parenchyma. When there is a major venous disruption, however, an intracaval shunt (85) may prove vital in repair of vena cava–hepatic vein disruption.

We have encountered subcapsular hematoma of the liver in the newborn, both from vigorous resuscitative measures at birth and from iatrogenic trauma during laparotomy for another problem. This can be managed successfully by covering the area with a piece of Teflon felt and suturing that to the liver with gently placed atraumatic sutures.

References

1. *Biliary Atresia: Proceedings of the Fourth International Symposium on Biliary Atresia Sendai, Japan.* Ohi R, ed. Professional Postgraduate Services, United States, United Kingdom, Mexico, Switzerland, Singapore, Japan, 1987.
2. Ladd WE. Congenital atresia and stenosis of the bile ducts. *JAMA* 1982; 91:1082–1087.
3. Sterling JA. Artificial bile ducts in the management of congenital biliary atresia. *J Int Coll Surg* 1961; 36:293–298.
4. Kasai M, Kimura S, Asakura Y, et al. Surgical treatment of biliary atresia. *J Pediatr Surg* 1968; 3:665–675.
5. Morecki R, Glaser J, Cho S, et al. Biliary atresia and neovirus type 3 infection. *N Engl J Med* 1982; 307:481–485.
6. Ohi R, Hanamatsu M, Mochizuki I, Ohkohchi N, Kasai M. Reoperation in patients with biliary atresia. *J Pediatr Surg* 1985; 20:256–259.
7. Vacanti JP, Lillehei CW, Jenkins RL, et al. Liver transplantation in children: The Boston Center Experience in the first 30 months. *Transplant Proc* 1987; 29(4):3231–3266.
8. Yamaguchi M. Congenital choledochal cyst: Analysis of 1433 patients in the Japanese literature. *Am J Surg* 1980; 140:653–657.
9. Okada A, Oguchi Y, Kamata S, et al. Common channel syndrome—diagnosis with endoscopic retrograde cholangiopancreatography and surgical management. *Surgery* 1983; 93:634–639.
10. Todani T, Watanabe Y, Fujii T, et al. Anomalous arrangement of pancreaticobiliary ductile system in patients with choledochal cyst. *Am J Surg* 1984; 147:672–676.
11. Cheney M, Rustad DG, Lilley JR. Choledochal cyst. *World J Surg* 1985; 9:244–248.
12. Gross RE. *The Surgery of Infancy and Childhood.* Philadelphia: WB Saunders, 1953.
13. Hays DM, Goodman GN, Snyder WH, et al. Congenital cystic dilatation of the common bile duct. *Arch Surg* 1969; 98:457–461.
14. Flanigan DP. Biliary cysts. *Ann Surg* 1975; 182:635–643.

15. Spitz L. Choledochal cyst. *Surg Gynecol Obstet* 1978; 147:444–452.

16. Kim SH. Choledochal cyst: Surgery by the Surgical Section of the American Academy of Pediatrics. *J Pediatr Surg* 1981; 16:402–407.

17. Kasai M, Asakura Y, Taira Y. Surgical treatment of choledochal cyst. *Ann Surg* 1970; 172:844–851.

18. Ishida M, Tsuchida Y, Saito S, et al. Primary excision of choledochal cysts. *Surgery* 1970; 68:884–889.

19. Lilly JR. Total excision of choledochal cyst. *Surg Obstet Gynecol* 1978; 146:254–256.

20. Reynolds M, Luck SR, Raffensperger JG. The valve conduit prevents ascending cholangitis: A follow-up. *J Pediatr Surg* 1985; 20:696–702.

21. Todd DW, Rosen WC, Miller RH. Hydrops of the gallbladder in infants and children—diagnosis and management. *Minn Med* 1983; 66:81–86.

22. Holcomb GW Jr, O'Neill JA Jr, Holcomb GW III. Cholecystitis, cholelithiasis, and common duct stenosis in children and adolescents. *Ann Surg* 1980; 191:626–635.

23. Law GE, Andrassy RJ, Mahour GH. A thirty year review of the management of gallbladder disease at a children's hospital. *Am Surg* 1983; 49:411–418.

24. Holcomb GW Jr. Gallbladder disease. In: Welch KJ, Randolph JG, Ravitch MM, O'Neill JA, Rowe MI, eds. *Pediatric Surgery*. Chicago, London: Year Book Medical Publishers, 1986, pp. 1060–1067.

25. Borgna-Pignotti C, deStefano P, Pajno D, et al. Cholelithiasis in children with thalassemia major: An ultrasonic study. *J Pediatr Surg* 1981; 99:243–248.

26. Hendren WH, Greep JM, Patton AS. Pancreatitis in childhood: Experience with 15 cases. *Br Arch Dis Child* 1965; 40:132–145.

27. Burrington JD, Smith MD. Elective and emergency surgery in children with sickle cell disease. *Surg Clin North Am* 1976; 56:55–66.

28. Roslyn JJ, Berquist WE, Pitt NA, et al. Increased risk of gallstones in children receiving total parenteral nutrition. *Pediatrics* 1983; 71:784–789.

29. Bell RL, Ferry GD, Smith EO, et al. Total parenteral nutrition-related cholestasis in infants. *J Parenteral Enteral Nutr* 1986; 10:356–360.

30. Gross RE. Congenital anomalies of the gallbladder. *Arch Surg* 1936; 32:131–162.

31. Kiesewetter WB. Cholecystitis and cholelithiasis. In: Benson CD, Mustard WT, Ravitch MM, et al., eds. *Pediatric Surgery*. Chicago: Year Book Medical Publishers, 1969, pp. 925–932.

32. Pieretti R, Auldist AW, Stephens CA. Acute cholecystitis in children. *Surg Gynecol Obstet* 1975; 140:16–18.

33. Exelby PR, Filler RM, Grosfield JL. Liver tumors in children in particular reference to hepatoblastoma and hepatocellular carcinoma: American Academy of Pediatrics-Surgical Section Survey—1974. *J Pediatr Surg* 1975; 10:329–337.

34. Weinberg AG, Finegold MJ. Primary hepatic tumors of childhood. *Hum Pathol* 1983; 14:512–537.

35. Lack EE, Neave C, Vawter GF. Hepatoblastoma: A clinical and pathologic study of 54 cases. *Am J Surg Pathol* 1982; 6:693–705.

36. McIntire KR, Vogel CL, Primack A. Effect of surgical and chemotherapeutic treatment on alpha-fetoprotein levels in patients with hepatocellular carcinoma. *Cancer* 1976; 37:677–682.

37. Altman AJ, Schwartz AD. The cancer problem in pediatrics: Epidemiologic aspects. In: Altman AJ, Schwartz AD, eds. *Malignant Diseases of Infancy, Childhood, and Adolescence*. Philadelphia: WB Saunders, 1983, pp. 1–21.

38. Altman AJ, Schwartz AD. Tumors of the liver and pancreas. In: Altman AJ, Schwartz AD, eds. *Malignant Diseases of Infancy, Childhood and Adolescence*. Philadelphia: WB Saunders, 1983, pp. 524–537.

39. Kasai M, Kimura S, Watanabe I. Primary carcinoma of the liver in infancy and childhood. *Z Kinderchirung* 1967; 4:347–351.

40. Lutwick LI. Relationship between aflatoxin, hepatitis B virus, and hepatocellular carcinoma. *Lancet* 1979; 1:755–762.

41. Ishak KG, Glunz PR. Hepatoblastoma and hepatocarcinoma in infancy and childhood: Report of 47 cases. *Cancer* 1967; 20:396–401.

42. Purtilo DT, Gottlieb LS. Cirrhosis and hepatoma occurring at Boston City Hospital (1917–1968). *Cancer* 1973; 32:458–462.

43. Jones E. Primary carcinoma at the liver with associated cirrhosis in infants and children: Report of a case. *Arch Pathol* 1960; 70:5–9.

44. Randolph JG, Guzzetta PC. Tumors of the liver. In: Welch KJ, Randolph JG, Ravitch MM, O'Neill JA, Rowe MI, eds. *Pediatric Surgery*. Chicago, London: Year Book Medical Publishers, 1986, pp. 302–311.

45. Bismuth H. Surgical anatomy and anatomical surgery of the liver. *World J Surg* 1982; 6:3–9.

46. Starzl TE, Bell RH, Beart RW, Putnam CW. Hepatic trisegmentectomy and other liver resections. *Surg Obstet Gynecol* 1975; 141:429–437.

47. Weinblatt ME, Siegel SE, Siegel MM, Stanley P, Weitzman JJ. Preoperative chemotherapy for unresectable primary hepatic malignancies in children. *Cancer* 1982; 50:1061–1064.

48. Evans AE, Land VJ, Newton WA, Randolph JG, Sather HN, Teft M. Combination chemotherapy (Vincristine, Adriamycin, Cyclorphasphamide, and 5-Fluorouacil) in the treatment of children with malignant hepatoma. *Cancer* 1982; 50:821–826.

49. Ein SH, Shandling C, Williams WG, et al. Major hepatic tumor resection using profound hypothermia and circulatory arrest. *J Pediatr Surg* 1981; 16:339–342.

50. Schaller RT, Schaller J, Morgan A, et al. Hemodilution anesthesia: A valuable aid to major cancer surgery in children. *Am J Surg* 1983; 146:79–84.

51. Falk H, Herbert JT, Edmonds L, et al. Review of 4 cases of childhood hepatic angiosarcoma—elevated environmental arsenic exposure in one case. *Cancer* 1981; 47:382–391.

52. Todani T, Tabuchi K, Watanabe Y, et al. True hepatic teratoma with high alpha fetoprotein in serum. *J Pediatr Surg* 1977; 12:591–595.

53. Braun P, Ducharme JC, Riopelle JL, et al. Hemangiomatosis of the liver in infants. *J Pediatr Surg* 1975; 10:121–126.

54. Pereyra R, Andrassy RJ, Mahour GH. Management of massive hepatic hemangiomas in infants and children: A review of 13 cases. *Pediatrics* 1982; 70:254–258.

55. Nguyen L, Shandling B, Ein S, et al. Hepatic hemangioma in childhood: Medical management or surgical management? *J Pediatr Surg* 1982; 17:576–579.

56. deLorimier AA, Simpson EB, Baum RS, et al. Hepatic artery ligation for hepatic hemangiomatosis. *N Engl J Med* 1967; 277:333–337.

57. Christopherson WM, May SET. Liver tumors and contraceptive steroids: Experience with the first one hundred registry patients. *J Natl Cancer Inst* 1977; 58:167–171.

58. Sroujc MN, Chatten J, Schulman WM, et al. Mesenchymal

hamartoma of the liver in infants. *Cancer* 1978; 42:2483–2489.

59. Altman RP, Krug J. Portal hypertension: American Academy of Pediatrics, Surgical Section Survey. *J Pediatr Surg* 1982; 17:567–570.
60. Shaldon S, Sherlock S. Obstruction to the extrahepatic portal system in children. *Lancet* 1962; 1:63–67.
61. Case Records of the Massachusetts General Hospital. *N Engl J Med* 1965; 273:156–163.
62. Nakamura T, et al. Inferior vena cava and hepatic vein thrombosis (Budd-Chiari syndrome): Characteristics of Japanese cases, including 18 authors' cases and 165 literature cases. *Jpn J Clin Med* 1967; 25:705–802.
63. Mitchell MC, Bortnott JK, Kaufman S, et al. Budd-Chiari syndrome: Etiology, diagnosis and management. *Medicine* 1982; 61:199–204.
64. Putnam CW, Porter KA, Weill R, et al. Liver transplantation for Budd-Chiari syndrome. *JAMA* 1976; 236:1142–1146.
65. Foster JH, et al. Splenoportography: An assessment of its value and risk. *Ann Surg* 1974; 179:773–781.
66. Baum S, et al. Gastrointestinal hemorrhage. II. Angiographic diagnosis and control. *Adv Surg* 1973; 7:149–153.
67. Chojkier M, Groszmann RJ, Atterbury CE, et al. A controlled comparison of continuous intra-arterial and intravenous infusions of vasopressin in hemorrhage from esophageal varices. *Gastroenterology* 1979; 77:540–547.
68. Clark AW, MacDougal BRD, Westaby D, et al. Prospective controlled trial of injection sclerotherapy in patients with cirrhosis and repeat variceal hemorrhage. *Lancet* 1980; 2:552–557.
69. Bismuth H, Franco D, Alagille D. Portal diversion for portal hypertension in children, the first ninety patients. *Ann Surg* 1980; 192:18–23.
70. Alvarez F, Bernhard O, Brunelle F, et al. Portal obstruction in children. II. Results at surgical portosystemic shunts. *J Pediatr* 1983; 103:703–708.
71. Linton RR, Jones CM, Volwyler W. Portal hypertension: Treatment by splenectomy and splenorenal anastomosis with preservation of the kidney. *Surg Clin North Am* 1947; 27:1162–1170.
72. Clatworthy HW Jr, Boles ET Jr. Extrahepatic portal bed block in children: Pathogenesis and treatment. *Ann Surg* 1959; 150:371 383.
73. Gross RE. *Surgery of Infancy and Childhood.* Philadelphia: WB Saunders, 1953.
74. King H, Shumacker HB. Splenic studies: Susceptibility to infection after splenectomy performed in infancy. *Ann Surg* 1952; 136:239–242.
75. Eraklis AJ, Kevy S, Diamond LK, Gross RE. Hazard of overwhelming infection in a child following splenectomy. *N Engl J Med* 1976; 276:22–27.
76. Martin LW. Changing concepts of management of portal hypertension in children. *J Pediatr Surg* 1972; 7:559–564.
77. Warren WD, Zeppa R, Foman JJ. Selective transplenic decompression of gastroesophageal varicies by distal splenorenal shunt. *Ann Surg* 1967; 166:437–455.
78. Drapanas JT. Interposition mesocaval shunt for the treatment of portal hypertension. *Ann Surg* 1972; 176:435–456.
79. Hendren WH, Hendren WG. Colon interposition for esophagus in children. *J Pediatr Surg* 1985; 20:829–839.
80. Starzl TE, Marchioro TL, Sexton AW, Hessmann TJ. The effect of portocaval transposition on carbohydrate metabolism: Experimental and clinical observations. *Surgery* 1965; 57:687–692.
81. Folkman J, Philippart A, Tze W, Crigler J. Portacaval shunt for glycogen storage disease: Value of prolonged intravenous hyperalimentation before surgery. *Surgery* 1972; 72:306–314.
82. Crigler JF, Folkman J. *Glycogen Storage Disease: New Approaches to Therapy. Hepatotrophic Factors, Ciba Foundation Symposium 55.* Elsevier/Excerpta Medica/North-Holland and Elsevier/North-Holland, 1978.
83. Chen YT, Cornblath M, Sidbury JB. Cornstarch therapy in type 1 glycogen storage disease. *N Engl J Med* 1984; 310:171–175.
84. Eichelberger MR, Randolph JG. Abdominal trauma. In: Welch KJ, Randolph JG, Ravitch MM, et al., eds. *Pediatric Surgery,* 4th ed. Chicago: Year Book Medical Publishers, 1986, pp. 154–174.
85. Trunkey DD, Shires GT, McClelland R. Management of liver trauma in 811 consecutive patients. *Ann Surg* 1974; 179:722–728.
86. Walt AJ. The mythology of hepatic trauma—or babel revisited. *Am J Surg* 1978; 135:12–18.
87. Patcher HL, Spencer FC. Recent concepts in the treatment of hepatic trauma—facts and fallacies. *Ann Surg* 1979; 190:423–429.
88. Kaufman JM, Burrington JD. Liver trauma in children. *J Pediatr Surg* 1971; 6:585–594.
89. Susan EM, Klotz D Jr, Kottmeier PK. Liver trauma in children. *J Pediatr Surg* 1975; 10:411–417.
90. Madding GF, Kennedy PA. *Trauma to the Liver,* Vol. 3. Philadelphia: WB Saunders, 1965.
91. Federle MP, Crass RA, Jeffrey RB, et al. Computed tomography in blunt abdominal trauma. *Arch Surg* 1982; 117:645–650.
92. Karp MP, Cooney DR, Pros GA, Newman BM, Jewett TC. The nonoperative management of pediatric hepatic trauma. *J Pediatr Surg* 1983; 18:512–518.
93. Sandblom P. Hemorrhage into the biliary tract following trauma, "Traumatic Hemobilia." *Surgery* 1948; 24:571–578.
94. Hendren WH, Warshaw AL, Fleischli DJ, Bartlett MK. Traumatic hemobilia: Non-operative management with healing documented by serial angiography. *Ann Surg* 1971; 174:991–993.
95. Lambeth W, Ruin BE. Nonoperative management of intrahepatic hemorrhage and hematoma following blunt trauma. *Surg Gynecol Obstet* 1979; 148:507–511.

Editorial Comment

This superb chapter on the special problems of surgical diseases of the liver that appear in infants and children is almost an abbreviated textbook in itself. Certainly this chapter by Drs. Hendren and Vacanti represents an excellent addition to the overall view of surgery of the liver, which has naturally focused, in the main, on adult problems.

Dr. Starzl has already presented an intriguing and challenging chapter on portal-systemic shunting as a method of correcting certain congenital metabolic disorders (Chapter 6). Drs. Hendren and Vacanti have referred to the experience of the Children's Hospital in Boston, in which Crigler and Folkman showed a more effective approach to the management of these unfortunate children by utilizing continuous night feeding of glucose and utilizing oral ingestion of cornstarch, a slow-to-release polymer that assures a more steady postprandial level of glucose than seen after ingestion of regular food. At least both points of view and results of surgical versus medical management have been well presented to the reader.

In the section of Chapter 21 on biliary atresia, it is obvious that pediatric surgeons have a problem in distinguishing between giant cell hepatitis and biliary atresia. As an editor who has little or no experience with these problems of infants, I could appreciate that the differential diagnosis certainly is of great importance and I could not help but wonder if a technique of percutaneous transhepatic cholangiography could be adopted for this purpose. It would provide discrimination and might prevent some unnecessary surgical explorations. Dr. Hendren feels, however, that in the absence of significant dilatation of the intrahepatic ducts, transhepatic cholangiogram would not help in differential diagnosis.

At any rate, the present chapter and the accompanying figures have been meticulously constructed, and this section provides an added dimension to our understanding of surgery of the liver.

Index